# CARE
# OF THE
# ADULT
# PATIENT

**Dorothy W. Smith,**
R.N., Ed.D.

*Professor of Nursing,*
*College of Nursing, Rutgers,*
*The State University of New Jersey*

**Carol P. Hanley Germain,**
R.N., M.S.

*Nurse Clinician and Consultant;*
*Coadjutant Assistant Professor, Continuing Education*
*Program for Nurses, Rutgers, The State University*
*of New Jersey*

# CARE OF THE ADULT PATIENT

## MEDICAL · SURGICAL NURSING

### Fourth Edition

**J. B. Lippincott Company**
PHILADELPHIA · NEW YORK · TORONTO

Copyright © 1975, 1971, 1966, 1963 by J. B. Lippincott Company

Distributed in Great Britain by Blackwell Scientific Publications Oxford, London and Edinburgh

CLOTHBOUND: ISBN 0-397-54165-1

PAPERBOUND: ISBN 0-397-54171-6

Library of Congress Catalog Card Number 75-9532

**Printed in the United States of America**

5 7 9 8 6

**Library of Congress Cataloging in Publication Data**

Smith, Dorothy W.
   Care of the adult patient.

   Includes bibliographies.
   1. Nurses and nursing.   2. Surgical nursing.
I. Germain, Carol P. Hanley, joint author.
II. Title.   [DNLM: 1. Nursing care. WY156 S645c]

RT41.S578   1975                610.73                75-9532

CLOTHBOUND: ISBN 0-397-54165-1

PAPERBOUND: ISBN 0-397-54171-6

# Consultants and Contributors to the Fourth Edition

Robert R. Abel, M.D., Assistant Clinical Professor of Dermatology, Cornell University Medical College, and Assistant Attending Physician, The New York Hospital, New York, N.Y., contributed to the material concerning dermatologic conditions.

Connie L. Addicks, M.A., C.C.C., Department of Speech and Audiology, Overlook Hospital, Summit, N.J., contributed to the chapter concerning diseases of the nasopharynx or larynx.

Ronald Altman, M.D., Director, Epidemiologic Services, New Jersey State Department of Health, Trenton, N.J., contributed to the chapter on venereal disease.

Mary Jo Aspinall, R.N., M.N., Nursing Care Specialist, Cardiac Surgery, Long Beach Veterans Administration Hospital, Long Beach, Calif., assisted in the preparation of the chapter on heart surgery.

Gail Ballweg, M.D., Attending Neurologist, St. Vincent's Hospital Medical Center, New York, N.Y., contributed to the material concerning neurologic disorders, spinal cord impairment, and cerebrovascular disease.

W. Hayman Behringer, M.D., Chief of Otolaryngology, Veterans Administration Hospital, Wilmington, Del., and Clinical Instructor of Otolaryngology, Thomas Jefferson University, Philadelphia, Pa., assisted in the preparation of the material on diseases of the nasopharynx or larynx.

Lowanna Schlotter Binkley, R.N., M.A., Nephrology Nursing Coordinator, Veterans Administration Hospital, and Instructor in Medical-Surgical Nursing, Vanderbilt University School of Nursing, Nashville, Tenn., contributed to the chapter concerning renal failure.

John Buckley, M.A., C.C.C., Director, Department of Speech and Audiology, Overlook Hospital, Summit, N.J., contributed to the material concerning diseases of the nasopharynx or larynx.

Arlan Cohen, M.D., N.I.H. Fellow in Gastroenterology, University of California Medical Center, San Francisco, Calif., contributed to the chapter on disorders of the liver, gallbladder, or pancreas.

Armand F. Cortese, M.D., Assistant Professor of Surgery, The New York Hospital, New York, N.Y., assisted in the preparation of the material on disorders of the liver, gallbladder, or pancreas.

## CONSULTANTS TO THE FOURTH EDITION

Joyce Crane, R.N., M.S.N., Associate Professor of Nursing, School of Nursing, The University of Michigan, Ann Arbor, Mich., contributed the material titled "Assessment and the nursing process."

Troy E. Daniels, D.D.S., Division of Oral Biology, School of Dentistry, University of California Medical Center, San Francisco, Calif., contributed to the chapter on disorders of the mouth.

Mary W. Denk, M.D., formerly director, Department of Radiation Oncology and Nuclear Medicine, The Cooper Hospital, Camden, N.J., contributed to the material concerning the oncologic patient and radiotherapy.

George E. Ehrlich, M.D., Professor of Medicine and Rehabilitation Medicine, Temple University School of Medicine, and Director, Arthritis Center and Section of Rheumatology, Albert Einstein Medical Center and Moss Rehabilitation Hospital, Philadelphia, Pa., contributed to the chapter on diseases of the bones and joints.

Solomon Garb, M.D., F.A.C.P., Scientific Director, American Medical Center at Denver, Colo., contributed to the chapter on accident and disaster.

Eileen DeGarmo, R.N., Maternal-Newborn Department, Yale University School of Nursing, New Haven, Conn., contributed to the material concerning the female reproductive pattern and disorders of the female reproductive system.

Timothy Gee, M.D., Assistant Professor, Cornell University Medical College; Director, Bone Marrow Laboratory, Memorial Hospital for Cancer and Allied Diseases; and Assistant Attending Physician, Memorial Sloan-Kettering Cancer Center, New York, N.Y., contributed to the chapter on blood or lymph disorders.

Mario P. Grasso, M.D., Medical Director, State of New Jersey Hospital for Chest Diseases, Glen Gardner, N.J., contributed to the chapter on pulmonary tuberculosis.

Raymond Haming, M.D., New Haven, Conn., contributed to the material on the female reproductive pattern and disorders of the female reproductive system.

Harold T. Hansen, M.D., F.A.C.S., A.A.O.S., Attending Orthopedist, New Jersey Orthopoedic Hospital, Orange, New Jersey, assisted with the preparation of the chapter on care of orthopoedic patients.

Raymond Harrison, M.D., F.A.C.S., Attending Surgeon, Manhattan Eye, Ear, and Throat Hospital, and Attending Ophthalmologist, The New York Hospital, New York, N.Y., contributed to the chapter concerning the patient with a visual problem.

Robert F. Hickey, Ph.D., Director, Division of Drug Abuse, and Assistant Professor of Preventive Medicine and Community Health, New Jersey Medical School, Newark, N.J., contributed to the material on the abuse of tobacco, alcohol, and drugs.

Sister Mary Louise Hoeller, R.N., B.S., N.Ed., Coordinator, Surgical Technology Program, Division of Continuing Education, Frost Park Community College, St. Louis, Mo., assisted in the preparation of the chapters on the surgical patient.

Carmen Diaz Janosov, Associate Professor of Nursing, University of Puerto Rico, Mayaguez, P.R., assisted in the preparation of the material concerning visual problems and hearing disturbances.

Elizabeth Katona, R.N., M.A., Community-General Hospital of Greater Syracuse, Syracuse, N.Y., contributed to the chapter on colostomy and ileostomy.

Eugene R. Kelly, M.D., Attending Physician in Internal Medicine and Cardiology, Overlook Hospital, Summit, N.J., assisted in the preparation of the chapter on shock.

John G. Keuhnelian, M.D., Clinical Associate Professor of Surgery (Urology), Cornell University Medical College; Associate Attending Surgeon (Urology), The New York Hospital, Cornell Medical Center; and Attending Urologist, Lenox Hill Hospital, N.Y., contributed to the material on the urologic patient and disorders of the genitourinary system.

# CONSULTANTS TO THE FOURTH EDITION

Martha L. Kiff, R.N., M.A., Instructor, Overbrook Hospital, arranged for and contributed illustrative materials to this edition.

Robert L. Kozam, M.D., Clinical Assistant, Professor of Medicine, State University of New York, Downstate Medical Center, Brooklyn, N.Y., and Assistant Attending Physician, St. Vincent's Hospital Medical Center, New York, N.Y., contributed to the chapters concerning acute and chronic respiratory disease.

Arthur Krosnick, M.D., F.A.C.P., Coordinator, Endocrine and Metabolic Disease Program, New Jersey State Department of Health, Trenton, N.J., contributed to the chapter concerning diabetes mellitus.

Georgie Labadie, R.N., Ed.D., Assistant Professor, Nursing Education, Teachers College, Columbia University, New York, N.Y., assisted in the preparation of the material on abuse of tobacco, alcohol, and drugs, venereal disease, and plastic surgery.

Joanne Lagerson, R.N., M.A., A.R.I.T., Clinical Specialist in Respiratory Care Nursing and Director, The Better Breathing Bureau, New York, N.Y., contributed to the material on acute and chronic respiratory disease and ventilatory insufficiency and failure.

Irving M. Levitas, M.D., Medical Director, Bergen County Heart Association, Cardiac Work Evaluation Unit, Hackensack Hospital, Hackensack, N.J., assisted in the preparation of the chapter on rehabilitation of the patient with heart disease.

H. Mildred McIntyre, R.N., M.A., formerly Associate Professor of Nursing, School of Nursing, University of California, San Francisco, Calif., contributed to the material concerning heart disease and congestive heart failure.

Kathleen Mahoney, M.Ed., Associate Director, Nursing Education, Mt. Sinai Hospital, New York, N.Y., contributed to the material on neurologic disturbance, spinal cord impairment, and cerebrovascular disease.

Alvin Mancusi-Ungaro, M.D., Diplomate American Board of Plastic and Reconstructive Surgery, and Attending Plastic Surgeon, St. Barnabas Hospital, Livingston, N.J., Clara Maas Hospital, Belleville, N.J., and Presbyterian Hospital, Newark, N.J., contributed to the material on plastic surgery.

Stanley R. Mandel, M.D., Associate Professor, Division of General Surgery (Vascular, Trauma, Transplantation), University of North Carolina School of Medicine, Chapel Hill, N.C., contributed to the chapter concerning peripheral vascular disease.

Henry Mannix, Jr., Director of Surgery, St. Francis Hospital, Hartford, Conn., assisted in the preparation of the chapter concerning endocrine disorders.

David A. Mathison, M.D., Associate, Division of Allergy and Immunology, Scripps Clinic and Research Foundation, La Jolla, Calif., contributed to the chapter on allergy.

William F. Minogue, M.D., F.A.C.P., Director of Medical Education, Overlook Hospital, Summit, N.J., and Associate Clinical Professor of Medicine, College of Medicine and Dentistry of New Jersey, Rutgers Medical School, New Brunswick, N.J., contributed to the material concerning coronary heart disease, cardiac arrhythmias, and acute myocardial infarction.

Virginia Nehring, R.N., Medical-Surgical Department, Yale University School of Nursing, New Haven, Conn., assisted in the preparation of the material on the female reproductive pattern and disorders of the female reproductive system.

Hugh D. Palmer, M.D., Director, Tuberculosis Service, New Jersey State Department of Health, Trenton, N.J., contributed to the chapter concerning pulmonary tuberculosis.

Guy F. Robbins, M.D., Acting Chief, Breast Service, Department of Surgery, Memorial Hospital for Cancer and Allied Diseases, New York, N.Y., contributed to the chapter on breast cancer.

Kay T. Roberts, R.N., M.A., Assistant Professor of Nursing, University of Evansville, Evansville, Ind., contributed to the material concerning water and electrolytes.

# Acknowledgments

The present edition of CARE OF THE ADULT PATIENT has, of course, evolved from previous editions. The contributions of consultants and of others who helped us with previous editions are acknowledged with thanks. The names of consultants to the third edition are listed below. The names of consultants and contributors to this edition are listed at the front of the book. It would be impossible to specify the many ways in which they contributed, as our working relationships with them were highly individual and varied.

The senior author expresses her deep gratitude to Claudia D. Gips, friend, and co-author of the first two editions, who died in 1966. We began the project together, and it has now grown, with the contributions of many others and with changes in nursing education. Claudia's enthusiasm and interest in the work were significant in the development of the original material.

David T. Miller, of the J. B. Lippincott Company, has been involved with the book from its beginning, and his participation in the project has provided a sense of continuity over time. We thank Dave for his support of the book's development according to the values and beliefs of the authors and contributors. This freedom to develop the material has meant a great deal to us.

Mary Dennesaites Morgan, of the J. B. Lippincott Company, through her understanding of the authors' values and goals and her belief in the project, played a crucial role in the development of this edition, as well as the previous one. Her outstanding integrity and ability to deal with others constructively steered the project through many difficult phases. We are deeply grateful to Mary and glad for the privilege of working with her.

We extend our thanks also to Diana Intenzo, who helped us with this edition.

Dr. Donald B. Louria, of the New Jersey College of Medicine and Dentistry, provided help with the material on drug abuse. Beverly Whipple, R.N., M.A., assisted with library research.

Our students and colleagues share with us their concern for patients and their enthusiasm. Their enlivening interest in the issues of patient care continues to stimulate our own.

## CONSULTANTS TO THE THIRD EDITION

The following consultants graciously contributed their time, thought and background to the preparation of the manuscript. The true value of their help is inestimable. They were chosen because of their special preparation, interest and experience in a particular field. Represented are physicians, nurses, a nutritionist, a physical therapist, and other specialists.

## ACKNOWLEDGMENTS

The authors used the material and the suggestions in their own way, and any errors which may have occurred are their responsibility alone.

Robert R. Abel, M.D.
Stephen M. Ayres, M.D.
Charles W. Clarke, Jr., M.D.
Armand F. Cortese, M.D.
Eugene Covington, M.D.
Maximilian Fabrykant, M.D.
Agnes Fahey
Kathleen S. Felix, R.N.
Donald J. Fishman, M.D.
Solomon Garb, M.D., F.A.C.P.
Timothy S. Gee, M.D.
Mario P. Grasso, M.D.
Frances Gutowski, R.N.
Harold I. Hansen, M.D., F.A.C.S., A.A.O.S.
Raymond Harrison, M.D., F.A.C.S.
Sister Mary Louise Hoeller, R.N., B.S.N.
John S. Johnson, M.D.
Elizabeth A. Katona, R.N., M.A.
Eugene R. Kelly, M.D.
John G. Keuhnelian, M.D.
Robert L. Kozam, M.D.

Ronald W. Lamont-Havers, M.D.
Irving M. Levitas, M.D.
C. Walton Lillehei, M.D., Ph.D.
Alvin Mancusi-Ugaro, M.D.
Henry Mannix, Jr., M.D.
Irwin R. Merkatz, M.D.
Gerald Mundy
Warren B. Nestler, M.D.
Sanford M. Reiss, M.D.
Guy F. Robbins, M.D.
Morton J. Rodman, Ph.D.
Barbara Rogoz, R.N., B.S.N., M.S.N.
Allen S. Russek, M.D.
Jules Saltman
Alan C. Scheer, M.D.
John N. Sheagren, M.D.
Owen A. Shteir, M.D.
Gertrud B. Ujhely, R.N., Ph.D.
Ferdinand LaVenuta, M.D.
Dabney R. Yarbrough III, M.D., F.A.C.S.

# Preface

The present edition has been extensively revised, and reflects not only changes in the care of patients, but changes in the role of the professional nurse in giving care. We have added considerable material on the nursing process including a chapter containing an overview, with emphasis on assessment of the patient. Discussion of the nurse's role in physical and psychosocial assessment and in carrying out the other phases of the nursing process are included in the various chapters where the material is applicable.

As in previous editions, the first section of the book deals with human development and change during the period of adulthood, and with concepts basic to the care of adults with medical-surgical conditions. It is our belief that medical-surgical nursing is not confined to the acutely ill hospitalized adult, although we have included material on this topic, but includes care of patients with acute and long-term conditions in the community as well as in hospitals and extended care facilities.

Prevention of illness, maintenance of health, and education of the patient for his role as a member of the health team are emphasized.

We have tried to bring to our readers' attention not only the physical aspects of care, but also the many ways in which illness is related to biopsychosocial and cultural factors. The chapters on drug abuse and tuberculosis are examples.

The care of seriously ill hospitalized patients (typically, those in intensive care units) is a field of growing importance, and we have continued therefore to devote a section of the book to the needs of this group of patients, with consideration of the complex physiological, emotional, and social problems facing them and their families.

Because of the growing complexity of the field, we have again sought consultation with and contributions from nurse and physician specialists. It has been our task to utilize these diverse and specialized contributions in ways which further the goals of the book—a task of rather formidable proportions. We believe that in the long run our readers are best served by opportunities to learn from various specialists as well as from us.

Amid such rapid growth and change as has occurred recently in the practice of nursing, it has become especially important to take, and to state, one's stand concerning values and beliefs about nursing. Our stand is that nursing, through its particular emphasis on humanistic values, has much to share with physicians and other health professionals, and has much to learn from them, also, in the interests of patients. Therefore we see physical assessment and data collection as important aspects of nursing, but not as its entirety. We view the process of obtaining data as more than medical history taking (although some aspects of a medical history may be included) and the process of assessment as more than physical assessment. In view of recent data indicating the striking relationship between the onset of physical illness and the occurrence of stress and change, such as loss of a spouse or a child, we continue to be convinced of the necessity to care for the medical-surgical patient in relation to patho-physiological and psycho-social-cultural factors, and to consider the therapeutic aspects of human relationships, as well as of drugs and surgery. Thus, while we draw upon the "medical model" for knowledge about disease and its treatment, we view nursing as distinct from that model.

Dorothy W. Smith
Carol P. Hanley Germain

# Contents

# UNIT ONE

## Concepts Basic to the Care of Patients

# Assessment and the Developmental Process

## CHAPTER 1

## ASSESSMENT OF THE PATIENT

Patient assessment, which provides the basis for planning nursing care, involves more than just an evaluation of a patient's physical condition. Of equal importance are his age and his stage of development. While these factors are sometimes viewed as being of primary importance during childhood and old age, they play an equally vital role in the years from young adulthood to old age—the longest and usually the most socially productive period of life. During these vital years, many important physiologic and psychological changes occur, affecting such aspects of an individual's living as his work, his relationships with others, his satisfactions and frustrations, and his response to illness, injury, and death.

It is interesting to note that emotional, social, and developmental factors affect not only a patient's response to illness, but also the likelihood of his becoming ill. At a conference held at the City University of New York in 1973, Dr. Thomas H. Holmes and his colleagues reported on a study of stress and its relation to physical illness. Their findings revealed that the death rate for widows and widowers is ten times higher during the first year of bereavement than for others of a comparable age; that following divorce, divorced persons have an illness rate twelve times higher than married persons of the same age; and that as many as 80 per cent of serious physical illnesses seem to develop at times when the individual feels helpless and hopeless (*Nurs. '73*). Dr. Holmes constructed a scale of major sources of stress, based on information from hundreds of individuals of varying social and economic groups. He found that such diseases as myocardial infarction,

3

peptic ulcer, and so on tend to occur after one or several stressful events.

The manner in which an individual responds to stress is influenced by numerous factors, including age. For example, adolescents typically display a greater resilience in recovering from loss, illness, and other setbacks than many people in older age groups. Social factors and the degree to which developmental tasks have been achieved also affect an individual's response to stress. The person who requires constant bolstering of his self-esteem is likely to have a more adverse response to the loss of a job than an individual who has an inner feeling of confidence in his abilities. A person who has close family ties and a stable income is usually better able to cope with the emotional or financial problems involved in illness or bereavement than a person who does not have these supports.

The material in Chapters 1 through 5 concerns the psychosocial and developmental aspects of assessment rather than the immediately presenting symptoms such as pain and nausea. The purpose of this material is to indicate the role of the following factors in assessment:

- **Expected physiologic response in relation to the patient's age.**
- **Social and economic factors and their influence on the patient's response to illness.**
- **The patient's achievement of some of the developmental tasks expected of adults in our culture.**
- **The relationship between nurse and patient.**

However, before entering into a detailed discussion of these factors, it might be well to discuss briefly the general approach to assessment and an overall view of human development.

## ACQUIRING ASSESSMENT DATA

Some of the data needed to make a patient assessment may be obtained quickly by simply asking the patient for the information, i.e., age, marital status, occupation, and name of the nearest relative or friend. If the patient is hospitalized, such information is usually obtained in the admission office, from either the patient or a relative or friend who has accompanied him to the hospital. However, if a patient is highly anxious or very ill, even simple brief questions may be burdensome or impossible for him to answer.

The patient is usually most willing to answer questions about his symptoms: where the pain is,

how long he has had it, what brought it on, and so on. Such questions convey to the patient a concern about his illness and imply an effort to help him in his distress.

It is extremely important to consider the patient's immediate concerns in anticipating how he is likely to respond to various types of questions. For patients who are under severe stress (and this includes most patients entering a hospital) it is important that the nurse's initial interaction with him focus on his concerns—his symptoms and his worries about what is happening to him—rather than on seemingly unrelated topics such as whether he gets along well with his children, whether his marital relationship is happy, what breakfast foods he most enjoys, and how he likes to spend his leisure time. While such information *is* useful and appropriately becomes part of the assessment of the patient, the timing and the context of the questions are the important considerations. Take, for example, the case of a newly admitted surgical patient who is plunged into activity upon admission—the anesthesiologist arrives to discuss the anesthetic to be used; the surgeon comes in to perform an examination; there is a flurry of getting into hospital clothing—itself a stark reminder that patienthood is a reality. Under such circumstances, what questions would be appropriate and useful to ask during the first nurse-patient meeting—questions which by their nature not only yield essential information, but also convey to the patient a concern for him? The following are a few suggestions:

- "Have you ever been in the hospital before?" (If so, ask him about that experience.)
- "Have you ever had surgery before?" (If the answer is "yes" ask the patient to describe that experience.)
- "What has your surgeon explained to you about the operation you will be having tomorrow?"
- What person(s) do you turn to now to help you? (The patient may give names of relatives or close friends.)

It is important for the nurse to have in mind the types of questions she wishes to ask, so that she can gather data in a disciplined fashion. For example, the nurse may have decided she needs information about the patient's family in order to plan for his home care. She may ask, "Are you expecting some of your family to come this evening?" The patient's response may be, "My wife died a year ago, but my son and daughter-in-law will be here." The patient may then continue to talk about his son and daughter-in-law—that they live nearby and will help him when he first goes home from the hospital. Thus the nurse gathers the data she needs to help her plan nursing care.

The disciplined thinking so essential to effective assessment requires that the nurse consider carefully the types of information needed and that she adapt the way she asks the questions, as well as their timing and context, to the patient's situation. Such a process is not static. It undergoes constant change and adaptation because it responds to what the patient says. Thus, once the nurse (or a team of health workers) has defined those categories of information which she needs for planning care, it is important that she be flexible in her approach to the patient about the way she asks the questions, what further questions should be raised, and what topics may best be left for discussion at another time. It is also important for her to remember that asking questions as a basis of assessment is not an isolated, mechanical task; it is part of her relationship with the patient and thus requires tact and thought about the effect the process will have upon the patient and upon his relationship with her.

It is also important that the nurse ask questions in a way which recognizes varied life styles and circumstances. For example, a brief question about the patient's marital status, especially if this is the only question asked about relationships with others, can give the unmarried patient a feeling of being ignored. In addition, such a question will not yield the information the nurse may really be seeking, such as, "To whom do you turn for help when you are sick?" The greater the nurse's sensitivity and flexibility, the more able she will be to phrase questions in a way which shows respect for the patient's life style and his immediate experience.

## SOME DEVELOPMENTAL TASKS OF ADULTS IN OUR CULTURE: AN OVERVIEW

Every stage of development has its own tasks—hurdles to be climbed over, things to be learned, changes to be accomplished. The baby under two must learn to walk. The six-year-old is taught to read. The adolescent is expected to establish a relationship with the opposite sex that is different from his childhood associations. The young adult in our society is expected to establish his own home and career. The person in middle life is asked to assume increasing community responsibilities, while

the elderly share with others the wisdom gathered through a lifetime.

Developmental tasks are achieved most readily at certain ages; failure to accomplish these at one time may make their later realization difficult or impossible. The best time is the stage of life at which they normally occur.

It is important and appropriate for a 16-year-old to invest time and effort in the techniques of dating. If he pays no attention to this social task at 16 and at 35 he is still socially unskilled, his dignity suffers both in his own eyes and in others'. What he should have learned earlier is harder to learn later. Similarly a woman who has remained dependent on her parents and has never left home or married may find adjustments in middle life to the death of her parents very difficult.

There is a progressive increase in the scope of developmental tasks as the individual grows from childhood to adulthood. For example, in the area of adjusting to one's own body, the following progression may be noted. It is the young child's task to learn what is part of his physical self and what is not (his toy is not, but his back and toes are). He must also develop skill in using his body for walking, holding a spoon, dressing, running, and so on. It is the adolescent's task to make a socially satisfactory adjustment to the maturing changes that his body undergoes, and to accept and utilize well his appearance. It is the adult's task to maintain a healthful physical regimen in spite of the pressures of his life and to learn what new motor skills are needed in his work, home, or recreation; and it is the task of the older adult to adapt his living to diminished strength and agility.

Development of satisfying sexual experience is another of life's tasks. It often looms large for the young adult whose sexual drives are especially strong. With maturity comes the task of establishing a mutually satisfying relationship with a partner. However, sexual adjustment is by no means a static thing; its achievement over a lifetime requires adaptability. For example, sexual desires of women are often affected by pregnancy. Lessening of sexual vigor with aging may affect one partner earlier in life than the other. An illness like heart disease may make it necessary to curtail marital relationships for a time. In some conditions, such as impotence due to paraplegia, sexual relationships may be permanently disrupted. Patients who develop long-term illnesses, such as tuberculosis, may be separated from their families for months, or even for years. Such lengthy separation can create problems for both husband and wife.

It is important to note that there is a wide variation in the extent to which adults achieve various tasks. Thus an individual should be considered in light of his particular achievements rather than in terms of a stereotyped view of what an adult of his age should be. One man may be a loving husband and father but a poor provider. Another may earn a large salary but spend little time with his family.

Thus, it is essential to guard against oversimplifying the concept of developmental tasks. Adjustments must be made over and over as each period of life or each change in the environment makes new demands. Rather than viewing developmental tasks as achieved or not achieved, it is more accurate to recognize that people of all ages are in the process of achieving them, and that the degree of success with each task may vary markedly at different periods of life.

**Some Intangibles**

While the more tangible accomplishments of establishing a home and earning a living are easier to observe, the search for meaning, for identity, and for lasting values involves tasks which determine the quality of a person's life and relationships. The effort to accomplish these tasks has different emphases at different stages of adulthood. For the youth the search for his own identity, for meaning, and for lasting values can be a new and compelling challenge. For the person in middle life it can involve re-examining his values and ideals in light of changed circumstances, such as responsibility for the care of others and to his work, and continuing his search for meaning with an understanding and humility deepened by these experiences. For the elderly person it can mean finding worthwhileness in the life he has lived, the efforts he has made, and the achievements he has earned.

Whether the individual is successfully dealing with these psychological tasks is especially likely to become evident in times of stress such as occur during illness or bereavement. Some people are aided in these tasks by a strong religious faith. Illness, aging, and the loss of loved ones bring fundamental questions to the fore, such as, "What is the purpose of my life?" or "Now that I am old and cannot work, what use am I?" Patients sometimes voice these thoughts to the nurse when given an opportunity; however, many patients do not ask these questions directly, but may imply them by their attitudes and reactions.

The nurse sees people under circumstances which tax inner strength. Understanding the concept of developmental tasks can help the nurse accept the patient where he is, in terms of his achievement of various life tasks and his response to the stress of illness. Some patients mobilize themselves after illness and misfortune; others, seemingly no worse off, do not. The inner strength which an individual has may not be known, even to him, until it is tested by an ordeal. This inner strength is often related to how able and willing a person is to stand the pain and anxiety of facing some of the fundamental issues of his life and accepting help from others when it is needed.

Inherent in this last point is the ability and willingness to develop a sense of trust in others. The seriously ill patient or the surgical patient is at least temporarily helpless and dependent upon the skill and goodwill of others. While such a situation can arouse much anxiety in a person who has difficulty trusting others, it can also provide opportunity to develop trusting relationships—opportunities which may not occur with the same intensity when the individual is feeling self-sufficient and is immersed in his usual daily activities.

Yet if the patient is primarily concerned with surface events and continues to focus on them during illness, the nurse should respect this and not try to change it. On the other hand, if the patient shows that he wishes to discuss some of his concerns about the meaning of life or his illness, the nurse can help by listening and showing concern. At the same time she cannot presume to know all the answers. What can the nurse say to a question such as, "Why must I suffer so much pain?" or "Why did my husband have to die so young?" She is not in a position to provide the answers—and especially not for another person whose values and experiences may be quite different from her own. She can, however, listen to the patient and convey concern for him as he explores these questions and seeks his own answers to them.

## REFERENCES AND BIBLIOGRAPHY

FRANKL, V. E.: *From Death Camp to Existentialism,* Boston, Beacon Press, 1959.
_____: *Man's Search for Meaning,* Boston, Beacon Press, 1963.

HAVIGHURST, R. J.: *Human Development and Education,* New York, Longmans, 1953.

JENNINGS, M., et al.: Physiologic functioning in the elderly, *Nurs. Clin. N. Am.,* 7:237, June 1972.

JOEL, LUCILLE A., and DAVIS, SHIRLEY M.: A proposal for base line data collection, *Perspec. in Psych. Care* II, 2:48, 1973.

LIDZ, T.: *The Person: His Development Throughout the Life Cycle,* New York, Basic Books, 1968.

LITTLE, DELORES, and CARNEVALI, DORIS: *Nursing Care Planning,* Philadelphia, Lippincott, 1969.

MOSES, D. V.: Assessing behavior in the elderly, *Nurs. Clin. N. Am.,* 7:225, June 1972.

MURPHY, G., and KUHLEN, R. G.: *Psychological Needs of Adults,* Chicago, Center for Study of Liberal Education for Adults, 1955.

Nurse's Notebook, *Nurs. '73,* 3:51, May 1973.

PRESSEY, S. L., and KUHLEN, R. G.: *Psychological Development Through the Life Span,* New York, Harper and Row, 1957.

SUTTERLEY, D. C., and DONNELLY, G. F.: *Perspectives in Human Development—Nursing Throughout the Life Cycle,* Philadelphia, Lippincott, 1973.

TILLICH, P.: *The Courage to Be,* New Haven, Yale University Press, 1952.

_____: *The Eternal Now,* New York, Scribner, 1963.

THORNDIKE, E. L.: *Adult Interests,* New York, Macmillan, 1935.

WILLIAMS, F.: Intervention in maturational crises, *Perspec. in Psych. Care,* 9:240, November-December 1971.

WOODY, MARY, and MALLISON, MARY: The problem oriented system for patient centered care, *Am. J. Nurs.,* 73:1168, July 1973.

# Assessment and the Nursing Process

## CHAPTER 2

## INTRODUCTION

The nursing process encompasses a deliberative, problem-solving approach to the practice of nursing. It reflects in its implementation the dynamic nature of the nurse's interactions with others and highlights the interdependence of process and content in nursing practice. It emphasizes rational, careful planning. Through application, it interrelates the cognitive or intellectual, technical, and interpersonal skills of the nurse. The process itself is a series of progressive, interdependent steps, or subprocesses, which unite judgment making with nursing action. Throughout the process these subprocesses may be used concurrently as well as recurrently, depending upon the demands of a particular patient care situation.

It is hardly possible to read nursing literature today without finding numerous references to nursing process. In many, the components of the process are cited and frequently described. While these descriptions vary somewhat, and in that sense may seem dissimilar and confusing to the reader, it should be noted that they all identify these major components: assessment, planning, implementation (intervention), and evaluation. Figure 2-1 is a model of the nursing process which depicts the relationship among its several components.

The American Nurses' Association has stated its standards for practice according to a systematic approach to nursing practice—the nursing process: assessment of the patient's status, planning nursing actions, implementation of the plan, and evaluation (ANA *Standards for Nursing Practice,* 1973). The emphasis on the process of nursing is apparent throughout these standards.

The nursing process is both dynamic and flexible. It is dynamic, in that it allows for and facilitates adjustment to the ever-changing nature of the nurse's interactions with others. Its flexibility is evident in the fact that its subprocesses may be employed sequentially and/or concurrently. For example, if during the planning step it becomes obvious that there are inadequate data to define a particular problem, the nurse may return to the assessment phase to collect these data while proceeding to the implementation phase for those problems which have had adequate definition and planning.

Another dimension of the flexibility of the nursing process is reflected in its applicability to nursing practice in any setting, whether its focus is episodic or distributive. Episodic nursing, as defined by the National Commission for the Study of Nursing and Nursing Education (1973), stresses practice that is curative and restorative, usually acute or chronic in nature, and usually provided in an inpatient facility. Through the nursing process, the nurse giving episodic care directs her efforts toward assessing, planning, and implementing activities which deal primarily with health maintenance and restoration, and with helping the patient and his family to adapt during crisis. Less emphasis is placed on promotion of health and prevention of illness.

In distributive nursing, emphasis is placed on nursing practice directed primarily toward health maintenance and disease prevention, usually continuous in nature, seldom acute, and often given in the community or in newly developing institutions. Nursing process is the basic framework for giving distributive care; emphasis is placed on anticipatory guidance to prevent crises.

## ASSESSMENT

The prominence given to nursing assessment is evident throughout the *Standards of Nursing Practice* recently adopted by the American Nurses' Association (1973). The first standard advocates systematic and continuous data collection about the health-illness status of the patient and specifies that these data should be accessible to all members of the health care team. Determination of nursing care needs and subsequent comprehensive care are dependent upon complete and ongoing data collection and nursing assessment. The relationship of the assessment process to nursing practice is inherent in each of the seven additional statements relating to professional practice.

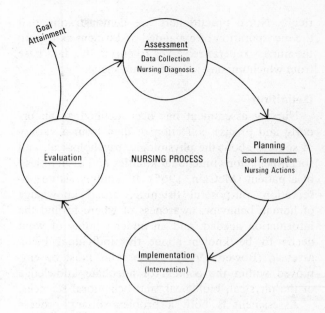

**Figure 2-1.** Model of the nursing process.

It is becoming increasingly evident to nurses that nursing care regimens must stem from precise nursing assessments which culminate in nursing diagnoses, just as medical regimens of care are based on systematically derived medical diagnoses. Reasoned judgments about health care needs cannot be made without an adequate data base, regardless of the professional background of the decision maker.

In addition to providing the base for nursing practice, systematic assessment promotes the individualization of nursing care, maximizes the amount and quality of data that can be collected in a limited time span, and facilitates the establishment of a relationship with the patient and his family. It provides baseline data about the patient's functional abilities and disabilities for later determination of changes in status and evaluation of outcomes of care.

As nursing practice has expanded to encompass greater accountability for nursing-related judgments and actions as well as the incorporation of previously defined medical tasks, there has been considerable debate about the depth and scope of the assessment process appropriate to professional nursing practice. While today many nurses are still asking if expanding nursing practice dictates the need for expanded assessment skills, educational programs in nursing are adding the teaching of these skills—including physical appraisal—to their curricula. Nurse practitioners are demonstrating that the incorporation of expanded assessment skills into the nurse's repertoire serves to enrich the data base from which nursing judgments are made.

## Definition

Nursing assessment has been defined as an orderly and precise collection of data from a variety of sources about the physiologic, psychological, and social behavior (functional abilities and disabilities) of a patient (McCain, 1965). It requires astute observation, purposeful listening, broad knowledge of human behavior, awareness of where to find the information needed, and an understanding of what needs to be known about the individual being assessed (Bower, 1972). These skills must be employed within the context of adequate knowledge of the physical, biological, and behavioral sciences.

Assessment is both a problem-solving process and a communicative, interactive process. Its implementation clearly reflects the practitioner's philosophy of nursing, as well as that of the agency in which she is employed. A philosophy of nursing is a system of beliefs and values about what nursing should encompass, and includes beliefs about the patient, the nurse, and the nature of nursing itself (Little and Carnevali, 1969). For example, if the nurse believes that the patient is a unique individual, she will include in her data-collecting activities information about his uniqueness and its influence on his nursing care needs. Similarly, if she believes that patient care should be family-centered, she will seek information about the family, its needs, and its coping patterns. If the nurse values her own uniqueness as a professional practitioner, this too will influence her approach to nursing assessment. Thus, a nurse who values critical thinking and is willing to be held accountable for her own nursing decisions and actions will demonstrate her ability to participate in independent and interdependent decision making.

Nursing assessment consists of two basic subprocesses: data collection and nursing diagnosis. Data collection entails seeking relevant information to provide a better understanding of (1) the needs of the patient and his family (or other significant persons), (2) factors in the environment which affect these needs, and (3) resources available to the patient for meeting them. Physical appraisal data are included, but the scope and depth of such data depend upon the skills of the practitioner, her role, and the requirements of the patient. To a limited extent, physical appraisal skills, such as assessment of blood pressure, pulse, and body temperature, have been a component of nursing assessment since its inception. As nurses become adept in physical appraisal skills, this will be clearly reflected in the data base from which decisions are made about *nursing* care needs, and provide a further basis for collaboration with other professionals.

Once an adequate data base has been established, the process of formulating nursing diagnoses assumes prominence. Nursing diagnoses are statements of (1) functional disabilities which, in the best judgment of the nurse, require specifically defined nursing actions, and (2) identified functional abilities that should be maintained and supported by nursing actions. When assessment decisions have been made and nursing diagnoses established, the second phase of the nursing process—nursing care planning—can be initiated. Specific information about the latter three phases of the nursing process —planning, implementation, and evaluation—will be found throughout this text as it applies to adult patients with specific health-illness problems.

## The Process of Data Collection

The data-collecting process should be systematic and ongoing, focusing on both subjective and objective data. Objective data are those which can be observed and measured by another individual, such as the size and appearance of a surgical incision. Subjective data relate to phenomena that can be felt or experienced only by the affected individual (e.g., nausea) (Byers, 1973).

Major areas in which data about the patient should be sought include:

1. Patient reactions, including those pertaining to previous health-illness experiences and current problems.
2. Expectations and goals of patient and his family and close associates.
3. Functional abilities, including developmental tasks, and emotional resources.
4. Functional disabilities.
5. Significant relationships and interaction patterns.
6. Environmental factors.
7. Resources available to the patient, both human and material.
8. Level of knowledge and understanding about current situation, including health-illness status.
9. Coping behaviors.
10. Cultural and religious patterns.

11. Life style.
12. Biopsychosocial behaviors.

In reporting on the first phase of a three-phase study designed to discover the criteria used by community health nurses in assessing a patient's status at a given time, Mayers lists nine such assessment items (Mayers, 1972). These include: ability to act independently, physical condition, congruent feelings or affect, interpersonal ability, verbal ability, ability to meet role expectations, congruent life style, appropriateness of future plans, and intellectual ability. The nurses' studies found these categories most useful in making assessment decisions. According to Mayers, these criteria tend to reflect a holistic view of patient assessment and appear to be generally applicable to any patient setting or to any diagnostic category.

## Sources of Data

Data are collected from a variety of sources, both primary and secondary. The primary source is the patient. Secondary sources are used to validate and supplement the data collected from the patient. These include: family, other significant persons, members of the nursing team, members of the health care team, individuals within the immediate environment (i.e., other patients) or the community (i.e., neighbors), and the patient's health care records. Secondary sources are particularly useful when the patient is unable to respond or communicate, or is unable to do so accurately. Validation, by either primary or secondary sources, is useful when there are discrepancies apparent in the data collected from the patient.

Whenever the patient is capable of providing data, his participation in this process should be emphasized. Thus an elderly person who is capable of responding and participating in planning his care should be approached directly, rather than having questions directed to his children, thus leaving him out of the process or conveying doubt about his competence to give information concerning himself. Exceptions are made when the patient is temporarily or permanently incapable of participating.

Data may be collected in a variety of settings, including the hospital, nursing homes, clinics, physicians' offices, community health agencies, industrial health offices, and the patient's home.

**Confidentiality.** Consideration for confidentiality and for the patient's right to privacy must be care-fully considered when seeking information from secondary sources. Judgment is required concerning the type of data sought and its relevance to the patient's health care status, and its urgency. For example, seeking data about a patient's venereal disease is essential for his welfare and for that of others who may have had sexual contact with him. However, such data must be sought and dealt with in a way which carefully considers the patient's privacy, and the effect such tracing may have upon his employment status and his relationship with other significant persons.

In general, it is essential that the patient be informed, and consent to, the seeking of information concerning his health status from secondary sources. To provide opportunities for the patient's participation and to obviate any questions and doubts he may have about confidentiality, it is desirable to include him in discussions about his welfare—for example, to talk with him and with members of his immediate family together. This approach can also yield valuable data about interactions and relationships among family members.

## Techniques Used in Data Collection

Techniques for collecting data include interview; history taking by other means, such as computers or written questionnaires; observation; physical appraisal, including inspection, palpation, percussion, and auscultation; and reading records and reports. The assessor must become skillful at utilizing all of these techniques for accurate and complete data collecting. In addition to the use of these techniques, Judge refers to two irrevocably interdependent elements which are essential in this stage of the assessment process: the sensory or perceptual act and the conceptual process. The sensory act involves perceiving, while the conceptual process relates the sensory stimuli to relevant knowledge or past experience (Judge and Zuidema, 1968).

**Interview.** The interview provides the means by which the nurse systematically gathers the patient data that she is seeking. The initial assessment interview should be conducted within a short time of the patient's admission to the unit or agency, preferably within the first 24 hours. This is crucial if the nurse believes that professional nursing care can be justified only if it is based on a thorough assessment of the patient's situation and the problems with which he is confronted. At the same time, the realities of the patient care setting or the acuteness of the patient's situation may necessitate nursing intervention prior to a thorough assessment. When this occurs, the nurse must establish priorities which best meet the patient's immediate needs.

It is extremely difficult, perhaps impossible, for the nurse to interview the patient and collect the necessary assessment data while attempting to carry out other nursing activities. Her undivided attention is demanded during the interview as she must actively listen at the same time that she is perceiving both verbal and nonverbal behavior—hers and that of the patient—responding to the patient as he offers information, and structuring the interview as it proceeds. The interview is usually semistructured in that the nurse enters the situation having thought through and identified some specific areas in which data are needed. Additional areas may become evident during the interview. The patient should be encouraged to tell his story; however, the success of the interview will depend on the nurse's ability to guide the patient through the process, keeping communication open and relevant to the health problem. The interview is often most usefully started by dealing with a functional area that is of concern to the patient. For example, if he comments on his inability to sleep even before the nurse initiates the interview, this might well be an appropriate topic to discuss.

The time required for the initial interview varies, depending upon the needs of the patient, the skills of the nurse, and the complexity of the problems. It is important for the nurse to allow time for the patient to bring up whatever concerns him, giving him the opportunity to decide what he will discuss. Participation by the patient can be initiated by such a comment as, "What else would you like to bring up?" or "What other things do you want to tell me?" Relevant information is often obtained in this way—such as that the spouse just lost his job, that a close friend has just died, or that the patient fears cancer and is afraid to ask his physician about the possibility of having a malignancy. This approach is also important in conveying to the patient that what is important to *him* will be considered. Although assessment is begun upon first contact with the patient, the process is continued, as the patient's condition changes, as new data become available, and as the relationship with the nurse develops.

**History Taking.** The optimal time and place for the history-taking interview are determined by the nurse and will be influenced by the particular patient care situation at hand. It is preferable to conduct the interview without interruption, and plans for this should be made in advance. This can often be accomplished by carefully selecting the time to coincide with a time when competing activities are not anticipated—for example a physician's visit, a scheduled diagnostic test, or a meal hour. Privacy and a nondistracting environment are important for both the interviewer and the interviewee. The patient may be reluctant to offer information when he knows that other patients can overhear.

In addition to data collection, there are many beneficial effects of the assessment interview. Mayers has cited five such benefits (Mayers, 1972). First, he points out that the interview initiates the nurse-patient relationship by providing the patient with an opportunity for dialogue with the nurse who will be assuming responsibility for his care. It also provides an early opportunity for the patient to become involved in planning his own care, and enhances the nurse's understanding of the patient and increases her commitment to him. (Nurses frequently claim that they feel closer to those patients with whom they have participated in assessment interviews.) In the long run the interview saves time, since patient needs and problems can often be anticipated and prevented. Last, it provides a medium for establishing a nurse-patient contract, an agreement between the two regarding the purposes and mutual expectations of their association.

**Observation.** Skilled observation may well be the most difficult technique used in assessing the patient and his situation. Observation is the act of perceiving through directed and careful analytical attention; it involves both a perceptual act and a conceptual process. It is a descriptive act, not one of interpretation or evaluation. Observation requires practiced discipline and employs all five senses: hearing, seeing, smelling, touching, and, infrequently, tasting. Bower (1972) describes observation as being readily influenced by the observer's past experiences, as well as by her ability to pick up subtle clues, to be thorough, and to remain objective.

The problems inherent in making reliable observations can be demonstrated by having a number of individuals observe the same phenomenon.

Observations are readily influenced and biased by an individual's previous experiences. They can often be assigned meaning in light of a person's own frame of reference and therefore are subject to error. For this reason, the skilled observer must be deliberate in making reliable observations, and in using the validation process to minimize bias. Observations may be validated with the patient, his family, and other health care professionals.

The nurse's subjective responses to the patient, when recognized as such, also provide useful data. She may feel shy in talking with an older and very successful professional person; she may feel inadequate when a patient says he believes he is going to die, or angry when she realizes that a patient is ill because he did not follow his diet. It is important that she register these responses, and take account of them, since they influence her interaction with the patient. By developing increasing awareness of her subjective responses, the nurse will be less likely to confuse them with objective data, thereby sharpening the accuracy of her observations.

In spite of the difficulties inherent in achieving skilled observation, it is an extremely valuable assessment tool when combined with other sources of data. Observation of an individual's body language indicates the behavioral patterns that he uses to communicate nonverbal messages: gestures, facial expressions, body position and posture, and body movements. Body language often depicts an individual's mood. For example, a person who is frightened may verbally deny this, although an observer notes that his hands are trembling and that his body is very tense.

The nurse can collect significant data about a patient's health-illness status by observing his general appearance. Gross abnormalities are often apparent. Body build, nutritional state, appearance of the skin, the patient's gait and general mobility, use of eye contact are all among the observations that provide useful assessment data. Significant data can also be obtained through observation of the patient's interpersonal behavior.

**Physical Assessment.** Physical appraisal encompasses the use of four specific techniques: inspection, palpation, percussion, and auscultation.

There are a variety of ways in which the acquisition of physical appraisal skills enhances nursing practice. Nurses working in intensive care areas rely on such methods to assess changes in their patients' conditions and to determine the need for further nursing intervention. Command of these skills enables the nurse to manage a greater range of patient care problems—some independently and others interdependently. In addition, they can be used to confirm hypotheses arising from the assessment interview and initial observation of the patient. There is little doubt that physical appraisal skills enrich the data base from which nursing judgments are made, and therefore increase the nurse's capacity for decision making (Lynaugh and Bates, 1974). Some nurses may employ these skills without direct opportunity for collaboration, for example, the family nurse practitioner who is the sole provider of health care in a remote rural community.

Nurses are increasingly using physical appraisal skills in providing primary health care (i.e., being the first health worker to have contact with the patient, and referring the patient as necessary.) The nurse's role of primary health care giver is being developed chiefly among deprived populations who otherwise lack health care, but is not limited to these settings.

In the following sections, the basic characteristics of the physical appraisal techniques of inspection, palpation, percussion and auscultation will be discussed.* For detailed descriptions of the procedures inherent in these techniques and their specific application in the practice setting, the reader should refer to one of several texts which have recently been written specifically for nurses who are interested in incorporating these skills into their nursing practice. Several of these texts are cited in the bibliography following this chapter.

INSPECTION. Inspection is the visual examination of the patient for detection of significant physical features. It combines detailed and focused observations with comparisons with established norms. Inspection differs from observation in that it focuses primarily on specific physical phenomena. It entails the ability to see relationships between that which is seen and that which is known, and to discern (1) what it normal and expected according to established standards or norms, (2) what is unusual but still "normal" for a given individual, and (3) what is abnormal. Lewis (1970) points out that the nurse's own senses are the most im-

*The material included in this section on physical appraisal has been adapted with permission of the author and publisher, from Crane, Joyce, "Physical Appraisal: An Aspect of the Nursing Assessment" in Sana, Josephine, and Judge, Richard, *Physical Appraisal Methods: Nurse Evaluation of Patients.* Boston: Little, Brown Company, 1975.

portant tools that are employed in clinical inspection: "eyes that see, ears that hear, hands that feel, a nose which detects odors, and a mind that understands."

It is important that inspection be conducted systematically to avoid overlooking significant findings, and in a manner which enables the nurse to give full concentration and scrutiny to the observations being made. Whatever approach is used, it must be both efficient and comfortable for the nurse using it, and sufficiently flexible to account for variations in particular patient situations. In one approach, the nurse might focus on identified assessment areas, such as the 13 categories identified by McCain: social, mental, special senses, motor ability, body temperature, circulatory, respiratory, nutritional, elimination, reproductive, skin and appendages, physical rest and comfort, and emotional (McCain, 1965). In this approach, she would carry out inspection activities as they relate to each category successively. In another approach, the nurse might proceed according to the systems of the body, for example: cardiovascular, respiratory, integumentary, and so on, completing the appraisal of one system before proceeding to the next. In a third approach, she might proceed with inspection from the patient's head to feet, symmetrically inspecting both sides of the body in the process. This is the approach most frequently used by physicians. A combination of several of these approaches may be the most productive.

Regardless of the format used, critical inspection should note both the general appearance of the area being inspected and its specific characteristics. Characteristics to be noted include: size, position, anatomical location, color, texture, appearance, temperature, presence or absence of unusual landmarks, type and degree of movement (and potential movement), symmetry, and comparison with the opposite side of the body. In addition, information should be sought about the nature, extent, history, duration, and precipitating factors relating to any findings that are considered significant on inspection. While inspection may be performed alone, it is a technique which is frequently used in combination with auscultation, palpation, or percussion.

PALPATION. Palpation is the process of examining the body by using the sense of touch to assess the characteristics of the body structures underlying the skin. It is usually employed in combination with inspection. In addition to utiliz-ing the sense of touch and feeling, palpation requires perception of position, vibration, motion, temperature, consistency, and form. With this technique, all accessible parts of the body including skin, hair, muscles, bones, organs, glands, and blood vessels, are examined. Palpation enables the examiner to appraise the presence, absence, and characteristics of the following phenomena: tenderness or pain, organ enlargement, swelling, muscular spasm or rigidity, elasticity, pulsatility, moisture, differences in texture, vibrations of voice sounds, and crepitus. The nurse has traditionally used this technique in taking the patient's pulse; palpation provides a means for assessing the character and quality of the heartbeat by allowing the nurse to feel changes in blood movement occurring in arteries located just below the skin.

To use palpation effectively as an assessment technique, the nurse must have a clear understanding of anatomical relationships. It is important that she be able to concentrate her senses on what is being felt, and to perceive, discriminate, and interpret the significance of what is being sensed.

The tools used for palpation are the hands of the appraiser. Since it is imperative that fine discriminations be made, the hands must be sensitive to subtle differences relating to the phenomenon being assessed. Different parts of the hand are utilized for detecting the various sensations for which they have particular affinity. The dorsa and the fingers are utilized for temperature perception because the skin is thinner and enables more finite detection of temperature differences. Fine tactile discriminations, such as the texture of the skin and hair and the size of lesions present under the skin, are most readily made by the fingertips. The grasping action of the fingers is used to detect position and consistency; because the palmar aspects of the metacarpophalangeal joints are particularly sensitive to vibration, they are used to distinguish vibratory sense.

The placement of the hands in relation to the structure to be palpated is also significant, as is the amount of pressure applied. The technique used to detect rebound tenderness, for example, involves exerting pressure on the organ being examined and then rapidly releasing the pressure to assess the impact on rebound. When deep palpation of the abdomen is indicated, a bimanual technique is employed. Both hands are used in such a manner that one, a passive or "sensing" hand, is placed against the abdomen while the other serves in an active capacity by applying pressure to the sensing hand. In this situation, the cushions and palmar surface of the sensing hand are used to perceive differences in sensations in deep structures. Both light and deep palpation are utilized in physical examination.

In preparing the patient for the palpatory portion of the examination, the nurse should explain what he can expect. This necessitates an initial general explanation and specific directions as the examination proceeds. It is especially important that the patient be relaxed. Muscular tension can interfere with the detection of significant problems by preventing adequate palpation or by distorting findings. Several techniques may be used to facilitate the patient's relaxation: providing him with an adequate explanation of what will happen and what will be expected of him; instructing him to take deep breaths through his mouth, particularly during deep palpation; palpating those areas which are tender last; avoiding unnecessary touching of the skin except when it is purposeful for the examination; and warming the hands before touching the patient's skin. It is often useful to note the patient's facial expression and body movements in response to palpation; this will give feedback about the degree of pain or discomfort experienced, as well as the individual's response to the examination itself.

Use of palpation in nursing assessment may be seen in breast examination performed to detect the presence of abnormal growths. The nurse incorporates this procedure into the assessment examination and also teaches it to the patient as a measure for early case finding.

PERCUSSION. Percussion is a physical appraisal technique which involves striking the body surface to produce sounds which enable the appraiser to determine the size, position, and density of underlying structures. Interpreting the effects of percussion requires the use of two senses, hearing and feeling. The character of the sounds elicited vary according to the density of the underlying tissue.

Percussion is valuable in determining the existence of a solid mass, such as a tumor, within an organ which is hollow; it is used to assess the relative amount of air or solid material which is present in the lung. Percussion is also an effective means of distinguishing the boundaries of organs or other body structures, such as bones, which differ in structural density. Borders of certain organs can

be traced by gradually comparing densities in the structure with those of surrounding tissues.

The sounds or notes elicited by percussion are designated and classified according to the qualities that describe their acoustic characteristics. *Resonance* refers to the clear hollow note which is the normal sound heard when percussing the lung. Although it is not loud, it is heard with ease and is low-pitched and well-sustained. *Tympany* is the note which sounds like the soft beating of a kettle drum. It is somewhat high-pitched, musical in character, clear, hollow-sounding, and well-sustained. A similar sound can be produced by filling the cheek with air and lightly tapping it with a finger. The tympanic note is heard when percussing over the stomach. *Hyperresonance* can be described as a cross between resonance and tympany. It is a well-sustained, intense sound which has a lower pitch than normal resonance, since it occurs when there is less density. A distinct feeling of vibration is sensed by the appraiser when a note is hyperresonant. *Dullness* is a sound which is high-pitched, short, soft, and thudding. There is no accompanying vibration. It occurs with increased density and solidness, and it is the sound which can be obtained by percussing over the heart when it is not covered by the inflated lung. *Impaired resonance* is the variation between resonance and dullness. It is sometimes also referred to as "slight dullness." The note can be produced normally over solid organs which are adjacent to the air-filled lung, such as the mediastinum and the upper portion of the liver. *Flatness* is a very short note which is high-pitched and nonmusical. It is absolute dullness and has no resonance or vibration. This note can be produced by percussing over solid tissue, such as the thigh.

The art of percussion necessitates striking or tapping the body surface lightly but sharply. There are two methods used to achieve percussion, direct and indirect. *Direct percussion* is achieved by striking the body surface directly with the fingers. The middle or ring finger is usually used, but the appraiser may prefer to substitute several partly bent fingers held closely together. This method is preferred for defining the cardiac border. *Indirect percussion* is used more frequently. This is a bimanual technique which is performed by placing the index or middle finger against the body surface with the palm and other fingers remaining off the skin, and using the tip of the middle finger of the other hand to strike the blow at the base of the distal phalanx.

To elicit undistorted sounds, a quick, sharp blow must be struck with the middle finger, holding the forearm stationary and making the striking motion with the wrist. Percussion should be gentle but firm, with equal pressure applied with each strike of the finger.

To learn percussion skills, the appraiser must practice the striking motion and become adept at detecting variations in the sounds produced. Practice on another person is essential, although there are some exercises that can be used prior to this. To learn to flex the wrist while keeping the forearm stationary, place the hand and forearm on a table and practice striking the surface of the table with the tip of the middle finger. Individual blows should be used so that the appraiser is certain that she is rebounding quickly to the flexed wrist position. Percussion of the thigh, in place of the table top, will provide the opportunity of experiencing percussion of a less firm surface.

Most of the percussion sounds described can be readily demonstrated on any normal individual. To produce resonance, percuss the lung at the right anterior portion of the third interspace. Repeat this following inhalation and impaired resonance will be heard. Then have the subject inhale as deeply as possible and the sound will become more resonant and possible slightly hyperresonant. Notes percussed at the fifth and sixth interspace will sound somewhat dull due to the underlying liver. At the seventh interspace, the note elicited should be flat because only the liver is present underneath. It is important to become thoroughly familiar with these normal percussion sounds before attempting to detect abnormalities and deviations.

The usefulness of percussion skills for the nurse is exemplified in the ability to detect mucus in the lungs of a postoperative patient and to specifically identify the lobe(s) in which its presence interferes with the exchange of air. Once these data have been gathered, the nurse can indicate and undertake nursing action to provide for adequate lung expansion.

AUSCULTATION. Auscultation is defined as the process of listening to sounds produced by the various organs of the body in order to detect deviations from normal. The lungs and the heart are the organs most frequently auscultated, but this technique is also useful in evaluating sounds produced in the abdomen, or by bruits, or by murmurs in the neck and abdomen. This is the physical appraisal skill which many consider most difficult to learn because it requires the appraiser to be able to distinguish the normal variations in sounds arising from body structures and to understand the basic principles of sound production in the body.

Auscultation can be achieved by direct or indirect methods. In using the direct method, the ear is placed directly on the body surface and the sounds are picked up by the unassisted ear. This procedure is used primarily when a stethoscope is not available. Indirect auscultation is achieved through the use of a stethoscope. A well-selected stethoscope, one which clearly picks up the sounds elicited, is crucial to effective auscultation. Many nurses who have learned ausculatory skills prefer to purchase their own stethoscopes to assure the quality of the instrument. A recent article by Littman (1972) highlights the several types of stethoscopes and their various characteristics.

As with other techniques of physical examination, each appraiser must develop her own approach to performing auscultation. Again, all areas should be auscultated symmetrically and systematically. Control of the environment is a crucial factor if noise is to be kept to a minimum so that accurate hearing and interpretation of sounds can be made. While background noise may not be noticeable during the interview, it may be significant enough to interfere with the low density sounds which must be detected on auscultation. As much extraneous noise as possible should be eliminated. It is also useful to explain this to the patient if he tends to talk during the examination.

Other sounds can be eliminated if the appraiser is deliberate about doing so. If a leak occurs between the chestpiece and the skin, a roaring sound will occur, making accurate perception of sounds difficult if not impossible. Any object touching the tubing or movement of the chestpiece over hair will produce confusing sounds. The appraiser will find it helpful to deliberately produce these sounds so that they can become easily recognized when they occur in the examination situation.

There are four characteristic sounds to consider in auscultation: frequency, intensity, quality, and duration. *Frequency* is the number of wave cycles which are generated per second by the vibrating structure. The pitch of the sound is determined by the frequency; the higher the frequency, the higher the pitch of a particular sound. *Intensity* relates to the height or amplitude of the sound wave. Vibration of low energy produces waves of low amplitude which in turn produce soft sounds; high energy vibrations produce loud sounds. *Quality* refers to the characteristic which distinguishes two sounds with the same degree of loudness and the same pitch, but coming from different sources. For example, although they may be of the same loudness and pitch, sounds coming from the heart and lungs can be differentiated. *Duration* reflects the number of continuous vibrations. The duration of vibrations coming from the internal organs of the body are reduced, or damped, by the soft tissue that covers them (Lehmann, 1972).

To be successful at auscultation, the appraiser must concentrate on what is being heard and tune out other distractions. Initially, the first level of discrimination is achieved, that of distinguishing normal from abnormal sounds. Later as more skill is gained, the appraiser will be able to discern the nature and significance of these auscultory findings. Some nurses, depending upon their roles, may seek only to achieve the ability to distinguish normal from abnormal. Others, for example those who are functioning in coronary care units, or functioning as primary care givers, may become exceedingly sophisticated in developing auscultation skills and in interpreting auscultatory findings.

Auscultation is a valuable assessment technique for the nurse. It can be used, for example, to detect the presence of breath sounds in the postanesthesia patient who may be suspected of needing ventilatory assistance, or the absence of bowel sounds in the patient whose abdomen is becoming distended.

## Processing the Data

Once substantial data have been accumulated, they must be translated into statements which identify the inherent problems which demand nursing action (nursing diagnoses). There is a significant cognitive step in the assessment process between the stages of data collection and nursing diagnosis. This step is comprised of cognitive activities which relate to classifying, analyzing, and synthesizing data, and lead to interpretation of their significance to the patient's health care situation.

The first step in processing data involves their *classification* into groups that establish relationships. Initially this may be done according to predetermined categories that comprise the assessment format being used; for example, data may be classified under such categories as social, emotional,

motor ability, nutrition, and so on. This is usually the stage at which assessment data are recorded. The recording should state data in definitive terms, but make no attempt at interpreting them at this point.

Following initial classification, other obvious relationships may become apparent, perhaps across categories, and data may be reclassified cognitively into groups from which differences can be distinguished, inferences can be made, and analysis facilitated. Less relevant data may be recorded and set aside for later use, if needed. This is an important function of classification as the total quantity of data available may be too massive to deal with initially. During this stage, it may become apparent that some data are missing or discrepant; if this occurs, the nurse may need to stop the classification process temporarily and seek additional data. This may also be necessary during the analyzing and synthesizing phases. The potential for collecting new data is present throughout, but the nurse must be cautious in deciding what is needed versus what is interesting but at the moment extraneous.

The classifying of data and activities relating to its *analysis* overlap. From the onset, the nurse is analyzing data to make decisions about its classification. This entails comparing data and recognizing patterns or trends. Data are compared to standards or norms to determine if there is a deviation, and if so, the extent of it. For example, the patient's weight is 198 pounds; the nurse compares this to the norm for a woman of the same height and body build, and notes that the patient is approximately 50 pounds overweight. During the analysis phase, the nurse draws heavily on her knowledge base; it is often necessary that she seek additional factual information from textbooks or other reliable sources to supplement this knowledge. Verification of data previously collected may also be indicated. Through analysis, data are manipulated so that they may be synthesized and applied.

According to Parker and Rubin (1966), the process of *synthesis* follows analysis and includes establishing connections, seeking similarities and differences, and deriving trends, hypotheses, and generalizations from the data. Once these have occurred, the nurse performs deductive and inductive analysis which leads to decisions about their relative significance, and to practice. Inductive analysis allows reasoning from the particular to the general; to infer that what is true of a sufficient

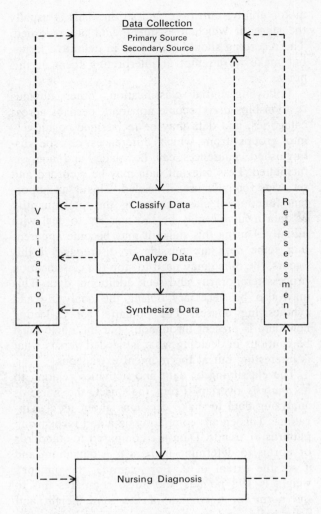

**Figure 2-2.** Schema of the nursing assessment process.

tion as well as on the nurse's knowledge and experience. It is useful in clinical decision making because it enables the nurse to understand, predict, and cope with situations by drawing conclusions that reflect interpretations beyond that which is possible on the basis of original data alone. Intuition may also serve a significant purpose in nursing practice. Inferences should be made consciously and cautiously, however, since they are made without conclusive evidence.

*Validation* is the process of seeking corroboration from other sources to reduce uncertainty about the completeness, quality, or perception of data. This is an essential component of the assessment process because it provides for affirmation of data collected as well as recognition of errors, inadequacies, and discrepancies. Validation may be achieved by verbal exploration with the patient or other significant persons; reference to an authoritative source, such as nursing texts; consensual agreement of a professional colleague or reference group; and testing to see if there is consistency with all else that is known about the situation.

The nursing assessment process, including its subprocesses of data collection; data classification, analysis, and synthesis; and nursing diagnosis, is depicted in the model shown in Figure 2-2. Optional interaction with the validating process is provided for in each step of the assessment process, as is the alternative for seeking additional data.

## Deriving Nursing Diagnosis

The nursing assessment process culminates in the formulation of nursing diagnoses. As noted previously, nursing diagnoses are statements of the patient's *functional disabilities* which in the nurse's judgment require specifically defined nursing actions; and, identified *functional abilities* which should be maintained and supported by nursing action. In addition, they provide the focus for nursing care planning, intervention, and evaluation. Nursing diagnoses are, according to the *Standards for Nursing Practice,* "related to and congruent with the diagnoses of all other professionals caring for the patient" (American Nurses' Association, 1973).

Nursing diagnoses differ from medical diagnoses in that they relate directly to patient care problems which necessitate and benefit from specifically defined *nursing* actions. They are complementary to

number of instances is true of all others. On the other hand, deductive analysis permits reasoning from the general to the particular; to infer that what is true of all instances will be true of another instance (Johnson, Davis, and Bilitch, 1970). Synthesizing activities lead the nurse directly to diagnosis; the decisions derived from inductive and deductive reasoning are, in fact, the nursing diagnoses.

There are two additional processes that are operational in processing assessment data: inference and validation. The *inference process* is conceptual and entails reflective movement from data to a premise and further, to other premises of increasing accuracy. An inference is an "educated guess" based on everything that is known about the situa-

the physician's diagnoses pertaining to disease and illness.

Nursing diagnoses should be clear, simple, specific statements which identify and communicate the problems inherent in the patient's situation. The implications for nursing intervention should be implicit within them. They should address not only the problems and needs of the patient, but also related needs of his family and other significant persons. Potential problems as well as actual problems should be included and specified as such. The patient's ability or inability to cope satisfactorily with a problem can be specified when appropriate. Each problem should be cited separately and concisely. Diagnoses are stated as the patient's problem, not as nursing problems or actions.

Nursing diagnostic statements overtly reflect the nurse's ability as an effective problem solver. They subject to professional scrutiny the nurse's scientific and clinical knowledge as well as her ability to use the assessment process effectively. Thus, the significance of the assessment process to nursing practice cannot be minimized.

## PLANNING

Planning constitutes the second major step in the nursing process. It logically follows assessment and nursing diagnosis, and focuses on formulating patient-centered goals and designing strategies, or nursing actions, for achieving these goals. Systematic planning, like systematic assessment, is essential if nursing care is to be comprehensive and individualized to meet the needs of patients and their families.

In planning the patient and the nurse interact at the decision-making level. To whatever extent possible, the patient and his family should be involved in making decisions that affect him and his plans of care. This is a basic concept which underlies nursing care planning. Too often, under the guise of "knowing what is best for the patient," nurses make unilateral decisions about ways for meeting patient needs and later wonder why carefully planned nursing measures were not successful. In some situations this may be warranted, for example, if the patient is unable to participate in planning because of the severity of his illness or if he is irrational. In such situations, family or other significant persons may substitute for the patient in making decisions about his care.

## Goals

The patient problems to be addressed in the planning phase are those reflected in the nursing diagnosis. The extent to which these problems are likely to be resolved forms the basis for deriving goals. Goals are the expected outcomes of nursing therapy. In other words, nursing goals indicate the specific behavior that the patient should be able to accomplish with the help of the nurse, within a predicted period of time, and under specific conditions. Such specificity of goals is applicable to some situations and not to others. In addition, the patient's influence upon goal achievement greatly affects the process and is not always predictable, despite the most careful assessment.

Goals emphasize desired changes in the patient's physiologic, psychological, or social behavior, and therefore are most appropriately written in behavior terms. The focus of the stated behavior is the patient's, not that of the nursing staff. For example, an appropriately stated goal might be: "Within two weeks, Mr. Lynch will self-administer Lente insulin, 40U, without error each morning before breakfast." This specific goal, jointly arrived at by nurse and patient, makes it clear behaviorally *what* Mr. Lynch will do (give himself Lente insulin, 40U), *when* he will do it (each morning before breakfast), and under what *specific conditions* (within two weeks and without error).

However, when working with a dying patient, it would be inappropriate to state a precise time for his expected acceptance of his approaching death. Rather it is important to recognize that patients' responses will vary, and that while the nurse can foster acceptance of death, achievement of this goal is difficult to predict and greatly dependent not only upon nursing intervention, but also upon the patient's emotional resources.

In addition to being behaviorally stated, goals must be realistic, achievable, observable, measurable, and acceptable to the patient. They must also be congruent with those of other health care professionals involved in the patient's care.

Once desired goals are determined, decisions are made about the nursing activities needed to achieve them. At this point in the nursing process, decision making centers on (1) hypothesizing possible approaches, (2) considering their consequences and the probability of their occurrence, and (3) choosing from alternative approaches those that will most likely achieve the goals. From this decision-making process emerges a statement of specific nursing activities or actions to be taken by those caring for the patient. To be complete, such statements should be clear, concise descriptions of nursing actions that leave little room for varying interpretations. It should be evident in the stated nursing action *what* will be done, *when* it will be done, *how* it will be done, and *who* will do it. An example of such a nursing action is: "The public health nurse will visit Mr. Lynch at home in two weeks to assess his ability to self-administer his prescribed insulin accurately and to determine whether or not further teaching is needed."

While it is often possible to state specific goals in behavioral terms, and while this approach is very useful, it is important to remember that not all aspects of human caring and of therapy can be so definitely and neatly specified. Thus a patient may unexpectedly show an increased acceptance of an illness as a result of support he receives and his own efforts. Such responses cannot be decreed by stating them as goals. They can be fostered by the sensitive, skilled nurse who recognizes that many developments toward health and well-being are still imperfectly understood but can be fostered by concern and support and by recognizing and respecting the health seeking forces within the patient.

Delineation of nursing actions facilitates the implementation phase of the nursing process. Implementation of care without the prior steps of assessing and planning would place nursing practice on a solely intuitive basis. While intuition is useful, a disciplined intellectual process which can be validated by others is essential.

## IMPLEMENTATION

Implementation of care involves interaction between the nurse and the patient and, often, other health team members. This interaction is directed toward assisting the patient to maximize his health capabilities and provides for his participation in activities related to his care. The implementation phase of the nursing process carries out the nursing care plan.

### Nursing Care Activities

A variety of terms has been used to describe the act of caring for patients. Some of the terms used interchangeably in nursing literature are: nursing care, nursing intervention, and nursing actions. The American Nurses' Association *Standards of Nursing Practice* characterize nursing actions as:

a) Consistent with the plan of care
b) Based on scientific principles
c) Individualized to the specific situation
d) Used to provide a safe and therapeutic environment
e) Employing teaching-learning opportunities for the patient
f) Including utilization of appropriate resources

Nursing care activities must be consistent with the nursing care plan as well as with the care given by other health team members. When inconsistency occurs, health team members may be working at cross purposes and in doing so, may jeopardize the achievement of patients' goals. The care plan should provide a point of reference for those who are concerned with the patient, so that the care given is comprehensive, consistent, and based on a systematic assessment of the patient's problems and needs and a logical plan for meeting these.

Nursing actions are founded on rationales which the nurse can justify through use of the nursing process. Care that emanates from a union of scientific knowledge and systematic assessment is not only justifiable by the professional practitioner, but it is also care which is individualized to meet the specific needs of the patient and his family. While care for patients with similar illness states may be similar in a number of ways, each patient's care should be unique, based on his specific situation.

During the implementation phase of the patient's care, nursing actions may involve directly caring for the patient; directing others in carrying out the nursing care plan; collaborating with physicians and other health care professionals; and/or making referrals on the patient's behalf to other agencies or resources. The activities carried out by the nurse reflect a combination of dependent, independent, and interdependent functions. Dependent functions are those which are prescribed by the physician or other health care professionals and are carried out by the nurse. For example, the physician orders an intramuscular antibiotic for the patient, and the nurse gives the injection according to the physician's directions. Independent functions are those which are both prescribed and carried out by the nurse within the context of the nursing regimen. For example, the nurse has observed that one of her patients, an elderly woman hospitalized for bronchitis, values independence but cannot walk safely unassisted. Judging that this woman could ambulate safely with the aid of a walker, the nurse prescribes the walker and assists her in learning to use it. Interdependent functions are those which are designed in collaboration with the physician or other health care professionals and may be carried out solely by the nurse or in collaboration with others. For example, a patient admitted to the community's free clinic for management of his hypertension is initially assessed by both the nurse and the physician independently; collaboratively they decide on a regimen of care. The nurse will manage the patient's ongoing care, monitoring his blood pressure and adjusting his low sodium diet as necessary. The physician will see the patient whenever fluctuations in his blood pressure indicate a need for changes in antihypertensive medications and/or when the patient or nurse seek his involvement for other reasons.

Nursing care activities vary according to a patient's particular problems and needs, but may include the following:

1. Caring for and comforting the patient in order to assist him in meeting his basic needs.
2. Curing activities—those related to alleviating disease and its symptoms.
3. Counseling the patient and his family in relation to their health-illness problems.
4. Providing anticipatory guidance in relation to biopsychosocial developmental tasks.
5. Teaching the patient and his family about promotion of health, prevention of illness, and management of health-illness problems.
6. Managing and manipulating the patient's environment to facilitate his well-being.
7. Intervening in crisis situations.
8. Assessing the patient's response to his care and adjusting the nursing care plan accordingly.
9. Coordinating the care activities provided by nursing staff and other members of the health team.
10. Referring patients to other resources (personnel and/or agencies) as these are needed.

**Recording.** Recording is another important activity which is included within the implementation phase of the nursing process. The patient's response to his care and progress toward expected outcomes should be recorded. This provides the basis for measuring whether or not goals have been achieved, and an ongoing means of communicating patient response and progress to others who are involved in his care. Recording formats vary among institutions and agencies. One system, called the problem-oriented record (POR), was designed to improve the adequacy and organization of clinical information for patient-centered care. It is used by nurses, physicians, and other health care professionals who are involved in a particular patient's care. It includes four basic components:

1. *Defined data base* which includes the physician's history and physical examination, the nursing assessment, and laboratory and other diagnostic reports.
2. *Master problem list* which contains a complete listing of the problems which have been identified, including those derived from the nursing assessment; they are numbered and titled and the list is attached to the front of the chart where it serves as an index to the rest of the chart.
3. *Initial plans for care* which are numbered and correspond to the problem list; patient-centered goals and nursing actions comprise the nurse's contribution to the plan of care.
4. *Progress notes* which are made up of narrative notes, flow sheets, and discharge notes; each note is numbered to correspond with the problem list and is recorded in a SOAP format (S = subjective data; O = objective data; A = assessment; and P = plan); all health care professionals who participate in the patient's care record on the progress notes.

The effective use by nurses of the problem-oriented method is predicated on acquisition of skills in assessment, problem identification, and problem solving. It demands collaborative participation of those involved with the patient's care, holding each health care professional accountable for his contribution. The basic components of the problem-oriented system closely parallel the activities inherent in the nursing process, providing a mechanism for their recording. Figure 2-3 illustrates the relationship between the nursing process and problem-oriented recording.

## EVALUATION

Assessing, planning, and implementing prescribed nursing actions are effective only if they enable the patient to progress toward goal achievement. Evaluation to determine such progress is an essential nursing activity. It is a major step in the nursing process, and involves appraising the quality and effectiveness of outcomes of nursing and health care in collaboration with individuals, families, peers, and other health care professionals.

The primary responsibility for evaluation rests with the nurse who assessed the patient's needs and planned his care. She is held accountable for the

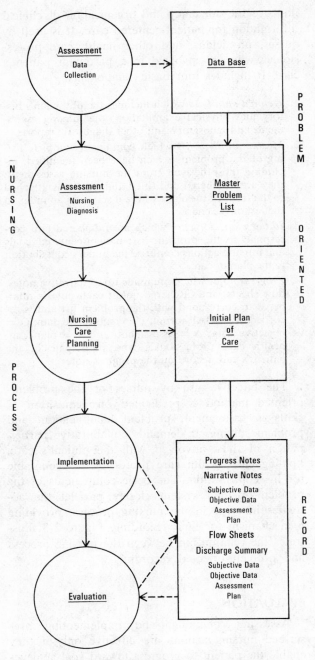

**Figure 2-3.** Model of relationship between the nursing process and the problem oriented record. (Adapted from Hegedus, Arleen H. *Nursing Process Module,* School of Nursing, The University of Michigan, Ann Arbor, Michigan, 1974. Mimeographed)

Lewis (1970) suggests that some aspects of the evaluation of nursing care are the mutual concern of all members of the health care team. The physician participates in the evaluation of those dependent nursing functions which he prescribed. In addition, in a collaborative relationship, he will participate with the nurse in evaluating independent nursing actions in terms of their contribution to the total care of the patient. The nurse, in turn, participates in the evaluation of the contributions of other health team members to the patient's care. Mutual concern of the nurse and the physician for evaluation is imperative since many nursing and medical functions are interdependent and are aimed at achieving common patient goals. This is also true of other health care professionals, such as social workers, physical therapists, dietitians, and occupational therapists, who may share common patient goals with the nurse.

The patient, too, should be an active participant in evaluating nursing actions and his own goal achievement. Feedback from the patient and his family should be solicited and heeded; in some aspects of evaluation of care, only the patient can supply the validating feedback.

What should the nurse consider in evaluating nursing care? She can judge the degree of success of the prescribed nursing care plan and subsequent nursing actions by monitoring and appraising the

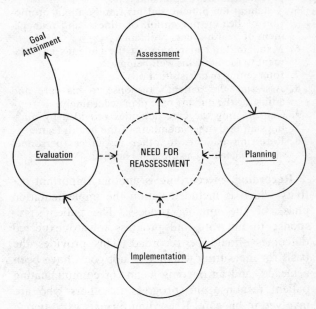

**Figure 2-4.** Model of relationship of reassessment to the nursing process.

evaluation process, while other nurses who care for the patient share in the evaluation. Each professional nurse is responsible and accountable for evaluating her own practice.

outcomes of care. Outcomes of care indicate the effectiveness of the care in meeting defined goals. Thus goals and the degree to which they have been met serve as the criteria against which to evaluate nursing care. For example, a stated goal for Mr. Lynch is that "within two weeks, he will self-administer Lente insulin, 40U, without error each morning before breakfast." To evaluate the outcome of the nursing actions aimed at helping him achieve this goal, the nurse must seek information about the regularity and accuracy with which he administers the prescribed insulin. This data may be obtained by talking with Mr. Lynch, by seeking validating information from his family, by monitoring the glucose level in his blood and urine, and/or by making one or several early-morning visits to his home to observe his insulin-taking behavior. Evaluation is carried out in consultation with the patient, who is aware of the process and of its purpose in helping him. If within two weeks the outcome is that Mr. Lynch is self-administering his insulin accurately according to the specified time dimensions, the goal has been achieved. If he is not performing according to the specified goal, for example, if he is taking the insulin at irregular times during the day, the situation demands reassessment and a revised nursing care plan.

**Reassessment.** Reassessment is an ongoing process which occurs throughout the nursing process. It involves reappraising the patient and his situation in light of the original baseline data included in the initial assessment. The patient's responses are assessed and the nursing care is evaluated. In addition, new sources of data may be sought. Additional data obtained through reassessment may supplement, validate, or invalidate judgments made in the original assessment. When new data obtained through reassessment indicate that the existing nursing care plans are no longer effective, nursing care is modified accordingly. If reassessment validates the current nursing care plan, the nurse proceeds with its implementation with increased confidence, remaining alert to new data which suggest the need for still further reassessment and evaluation.

While assessment is the first step in the nursing process and, therefore, provides data for planning care, reassessment may occur throughout all phases of the process, providing data for validating or modifying care as the patient's situation changes. Figure 2-4 illustrates the relationship between re-

assessment and the nursing process as a whole. It highlights the cyclical nature of the nursing process when this is warranted, while at the same time clearly indicating the potential termination of the process when patient care goals have been attained.

## REFERENCES AND BIBLIOGRAPHY

ALEXANDER, M., and BROWN, M.: Physical examination: The why and how of examination, *Nurs. '73* 3, 7:25-28, July 1973.

AMERICAN NURSES' ASSOCIATION: *Standards of Nursing Practice,* Kansas City, Missouri, prepared by Congress on Nursing Practice, American Nurses' Association, 1973.

BATES, B.: *A Guide to Physical Examination,* Philadelphia, Lippincott, 1974.

BOWER, F. L.: *The Process of Planning Nursing Care: A Theoretical Model,* St. Louis, Mosby, 1972.

BYERS, V. B.: *Nursing Observation,* ed. 2, Dubuque, Iowa, Brown, 1973.

CARLSON, S.: A practical approach to the nursing process, *Am. J. Nurs.* 72, 9:1589-1591, September 1972.

DAUBENMIRE, M. J., and KING, I. M.: Nursing process models: A systems approach, *Nurs. Outlook* 21, 8: 512-517, August 1973.

DURAND, M., and PRINCE, R.: Nursing diagnosis: Process and decision, *Nurs. Forum* 5, 4:50-64, 1966.

FOWKES, W. C., and HUNN, V. K.: *Clinical Assessment for the Nurse Practitioner,* St. Louis, Mosby, 1973.

FROEMMING, P., and QUIRING, J.: Teaching health history and physical examination, *Nurs. Res.* 22, 5: 432-434, September-October 1973.

GIBLIN, E. C. (ed.): Symposium on assessment as part of the nursing process, *Nurs. Clin. N. Am.* 6, 1:113-209, March 1971.

HEGEDUS, A. H.: *Nursing Process Module,* Ann Arbor, Michigan, The University of Michigan School of Nursing, 1974. Mimeographed.

JOHNSON, M. M., DAVIS, M. L. C., and BILITCH, M. J.: *Problem-Solving in Nursing Practice,* Dubuque, Iowa, Brown, 1970.

JUDGE, R. D., and ZUIDEMA, G. D.: *Physical Diagnosis: A Physiologic Approach to the Clinical Examination,* ed. 2, Boston, Little, Brown, 1968.

LEHMANN, J.: Auscultation of heart sounds, *Am. J. Nurs.* 72, 7:1232-1237, July 1972.

LEWIS, L.: *Planning Patient Care,* Dubuque, Iowa, Brown, 1970.

LITTLE, D. E., and CARNEVALI, D. L.: *Nursing Care Planning,* Philadelphia, Lippincott, 1969.

LITTMAN, D.: Stethoscopes and auscultation, *Am. J. Nurs.* 72, 7:1238-1241, July 1972.

LYNAUGH, J. E., and BATES, B.: Physical diagnosis: A skill for all nurses, *Am. J. Nurs.* 74, 1:58-59, January 1974.

MAYERS, M. G.: A search for assessment criteria, *Nurs. Outlook* 20, 5:323-326, 1972.

————: *A Systematic Approach to the Nursing Care Plan,* New York, Appleton-Century-Crofts, 1972.

McCAIN, R. F.: Nursing by assessment—not intuition, *Am. J. Nurs.* 65, 4:82-84, April 1965.

McCAIN, R., et al.: Systematic nursing assessment, Ann Arbor, Michigan, unpublished materials developed at the University of Michigan School of Nursing, 1969. Mimeographed.

NATIONAL COMMISSION FOR THE STUDY OF NURSING AND NURSING EDUCATION: *From Abstract Into Action,* Jerome P. Lysaught, Director, New York, McGraw-Hill, 1973.

PARKER, J. C., and RUBIN, L. J.: *Process As Content: Curriculum Design and the Application of Knowledge,* Chicago, Rand McNally, 1966.

SANA, J., and JUDGE, R. D.: *Physical Appraisal Methods: Nurse Evaluation of Patients,* Boston, Little, Brown, 1975.

VANDER ZANDEN, J. W., and VANDER ZANDEN, M. V.: The interview—what questions should the nurse ask? *Nurs. Outlook,* XI:743-745, October 1963.

WESSELING, E.: Automating the nursing history and care plan, *J. Nurs. Admin.,* 34-38, May-June 1972.

WOODY, M., and MALLISON, M.: The problem-oriented system for patient-centered care, *Am. J. Nurs.* 73, 7:1168-1175, July 1973.

YURA, H., and WALSH, M. B.: *The Nursing Process: Assessing, Planning, Implementing, and Evaluating,* ed. 2, Washington, D. C., The Catholic University of America Press, 1973.

# Caring for the Young Adult

## CHAPTER 3

## INTRODUCTION

In this chapter we shall discuss some aspects of normal development in the young adult, the developmental tasks he faces, and their implications for nursing care.

Before discussing physical development and developmental tasks, let us consider some of the broader aspects of caring for young adults today. What are some of the challenges, problems, and satisfactions?

The young adult has much working in his favor during illness. He is physically more resilient than the older person. Two days after an appendectomy he may be able to carry out activities which a middle-aged patient undergoing the same operation must postpone for a week. The young person often has an emotional resilience, too, which enables him to mobilize his energy quickly after a shock or a loss. This does not mean that he has necessarily dealt adequately with the experience inwardly. He may at a later time need to go back and re-examine the experience and its meaning to him.

The young person's resilience is enhanced by the support which his family and society offer him. During illness, he may receive emotional support from his family since he is more likely to have intact family relationships than is an elderly person. This may include ties with his parents as well as support from a wife and children of his own. In addition, social, educational, and health facilities and opportunities are usually more abundantly provided for young people than for those in middle and later life. For example, a convalescent teenager who receives a scholarship to a nearby college has a new world opened up to him—not only an educational world, but a network of contacts with other students and with teachers in a setting which emphasizes the development of his capacities.

The situation is different, though, for a 60-year-old widow who, in addition to the challenge of recovering from illness, must learn to support herself following the death of her husband. She is less likely to receive assistance with learning new skills, and she may have fewer opportunities to make new friends than the young person who is recovering from illness.

Because many young people have considerable support and assistance provided by others, it may be easy for the nurse to fail to notice the ways in which young patients require help. However, personal relationships do not take the place of the professional helping role of the nurse and other members of the staff. The nurse must guard against assuming that a young person (or a person of any age) who is surrounded by cards, flowers, and candy does not need her listening ear. Perhaps he does, and the nurse should offer him this opportunity.

The patient's resilience may, ironically, be another factor which deters the nurse from recognizing his need for a supportive listener. Nevertheless, it is important to help the patient to assimilate painful experiences. Too often family and friends discourage the patient from talking about the experience. They may be eager to forget the event which was also painful for them. At times like this, the nurse can help by showing a willingness to listen to the patient.

While young adults have the advantage of resiliency, they nonetheless face the emotional stresses of their age group. Young adults in our society are increasingly restless, dissatisfied with the status quo, and actively seeking participation in community affairs. Although being fed up with the hypocrisy of some of their elders is not new to young people, there is a growing outspokenness among the young, many of whom see no point in pretending to believe society's shallow contradictions. Although the young people who are the most openly nonconformist are in the minority, the search for involvement and for a chance to participate in righting social wrongs is widespread among youth. The search is not only for new outer experiences, but for new inner experiences as well. Some young people have turned to drugs, such as LSD, in their search for such experiences. There is also much emphasis upon separateness from the older genera-

tion—the jargon of the young is not just a sprinkling of slang, but also a vocabulary of its own. But the emphasis on separate vocabulary, styles of clothing, and so forth is sometimes accompanied by feelings of alienation and by a wish for meaningful communication with older people, and particularly with older people who have authority to effect change. Although some young people expend most of their energies demonstrating contempt for conformity and the "Establishment," many are eager to use their energies to work toward alleviating social injustice.

What implications has this for nursing care of young adults? The hospital is an environment where authority and hierarchy are much in evidence and where patients ordinarily have little voice in making the rules. If the young person is hospitalized for more than a brief period, the rigidity of rules and authority is likely to be especially irritating to him. He may find various ways to express rebelliousness, such as turning his radio up too loud, disregarding the physician's orders, and so forth.

However, in a medical-surgical setting, there is and has to be considerable emphasis upon order and predictability. Wounds require conditions which help them to heal, and this in turn necessitates a disciplined use of measures to eliminate pathogens from the environment. Sick people need opportunities for rest and quiet. Special diets and medications require meticulous attention to detail. No wonder then that the response of staff and other patients to a rather ebullient and somewhat disorderly young adult can be sharply critical, and in some instances even punitive. It becomes especially important to recognize that some of the attributes of the young person may be especially disconcerting and troublesome on a medical-surgical unit and that extra effort must be made to enforce necessary regulations and safety measures without being punitive.

To whatever extent possible, it is important to try to include the young patient in making decisions which affect him, and to make a special effort to interpret hospital rules to him. Even if the rules cannot be changed, they will be less galling to the patient who understands their purpose.

The physician and nurse can also provide the young patient with the experience of dealing with rational authority. Previously the patient may have viewed authority as essentially arbitrary and negative—something against which to pit himself. However, professional people, by the nature of their work, have many opportunities to emphasize the rational aspects of authority. The physician recommends bed rest, not to impose his will on the patient or to restrict his freedom, but because the patient's condition requires it. The nurse firmly encourages the postoperative patient to walk, not because she wants to inflict pain, but because walking will help him to recover. Emphasizing the reasons behind actions and decisions and avoiding arbitrary use of authority may help the young person to appreciate the fact that authority and discipline are not always negative and restrictive, but that they can also be positive forces enabling those with special knowledge and skill to exercise them for the benefit of others.

It is particularly helpful when working with long-term patients to try to initiate a discussion group which includes patients and staff. Regular meetings of the group can help patients to voice their questions and dissatisfaction with ward policies and can help the staff appreciate their patients' views. While all of the problems cannot be remedied, they can at least be discussed, and some of them can be solved. Maybe a record player can be obtained for the ward sitting room especially if it is located away from the rooms of the sicker patients. Maybe convalescent patients can have a kitchenette in which to prepare light snacks or be permitted to go to the hospital coffee shop.

Hospitalization can provide the young patient with the opportunity to have wider contact with adults outside the circle of home and school. The young person's contacts with his elders may previously have emphasized the distance between generations. The experience of illness and hospitalization brings out some very fundamental human problems, which cut across age differences and bring out the commonalities of human experience. The 20-year-old girl who is admitted to the hospital because of an impending miscarriage may find in her older roommate a source of strength and support. This young woman who may have prided herself on her separateness from older people may reach out to an older woman to share some of her intimate concerns and fears over losing her baby. By recognizing the ways that people of different ages can support one another, the nurse can avoid assuming that patients of similar age should automatically be placed together on the ward. While doing so fosters sociability of age-mates, it deprives

patients of contacts with those of different ages—contacts that are often lacking in the lives of young and old alike in our age-stratified society.

Idealism is one of the positive attributes of youth—idealism which can lend a glow and spark the effort and enthusiasm of older people. But inevitably the idealism of youth suffers some shocks as it comes up against reality. Being sick can increase the problem, because it brings the young person into close contact with many of the inadequacies of health care as he himself experiences them.

The nurse should allow the patient to talk about these discrepancies between reality and his expectations, and try not to respond defensively as she listens to him. Above all, she should avoid deceiving the patient. While it is not necessary to jump with him into an orgy of criticizing "the system," neither is it wise to say the system is faultless.

In contrast to some older persons who have scaled down their expectations of what life has to offer, and who accept, if not happily at least patiently, some of their misfortunes, many young people are especially impatient when they are sick. Illness or restriction may elicit a good deal of protest. While the nurse cannot personally provide an ideal situation for her young patient, she can serve as a sounding board as he voices some of his protest. His high expectations will present a challenge for those who provide health care. Along with some unrealistic demands, the young person often calls attention to situations which not only need to be changed, but can be changed. In so doing he may help improve the quality of his own care and that of others as well.

What of the nurse's own reactions to working with young adults? For the nurse who is herself in this age group there may be a particular tendency to identify with the patient; this can cause problems, especially if the patient has a terminal illness, such as leukemia—caring for a fatally ill young person is a stark reminder of the unpredictability of each person's life span. However, it is important for a young nurse working with patients her own age to keep her professional and social rules differentiated. The nurse may find herself relating to the patient as though he were a chum. As for the older nurse, she may carry over to the patient some of her own conflicts with her adolescent children and find herself responding to the patient in terms of problems she is facing with her own growing family. At times an older nurse will find that she is jealous of a patient's youthful resilience and attractiveness. Or she may become very protective of a young patient, perhaps treating him as she herself would like to have been treated when she was young. For nurses of all ages, the challenge in caring for young adults lies not only in providing the care which illness requires, but also in helping the patient move forward as much as possible with the developmental tasks of his age group.

## PHYSICAL CHANGES

Following the rapid changes of puberty, physical growth ceases in the period between 18 and 20. Thereafter a slow and barely perceptible decline in many physical abilities begins. At about 20 the body and general appearance no longer change quickly. The boy who always has longed to be tall may discover that he always will be short. The girl may have to accept being flat-chested or taller than is fashionable for a woman. A young person's physical powers may or may not coincide with opportunities for their optimal use.

**Visual Accommodation.** The ability of the eye to adjust to near and far vision is one of the reliable physiologic indicators of age. Children can see an object clearly when it is held almost at the tip of their noses. Even before puberty this ability begins to diminish gradually, and it continues to decline during most of adult life.

**Changes in Hearing.** Hearing changes also occur throughout life. Loss of ability to hear high tones begins in childhood. Hearing is most acute at about age 14; thereafter it declines gradually. So far as this faculty is concerned, a 20-year-old is already past his prime!

## DEVELOPMENTAL TASKS

**Autonomy and Authenticity.** One of the major tasks of young adults in our culture is to work toward self-determination and self-esteem—toward autonomy and authenticity. One aspect of achieving self-definition is to gradually differentiate oneself from one's parents by developing one's own values and making one's own decisions. Becoming independent does not mean breaking ties with parents but involves developing a different type of relationship with them, one in which the young person begins to accept the consequences of his own actions. Such a development does not take place

suddenly; indeed, it has its beginnings when the child is encouraged to make some decisions of his own. Young people whose parents have helped them gradually to assume more independence usually find this transition period easier than those whose parents continue to exert very strict control through late adolescence.

The development of authenticity and autonomy is also fostered by relationships with others who are honest in themselves, who live their own lives and have commitments and ideas of their own. As Friedenberg (1965) points out, too often the young adult deals with older people who so lack their own identity and are so preoccupied with adapting themselves to group norms that they do not convey a sense of being complete people. Their interaction with the young person may be filled with clichés about such values as good citizenship and getting along with others, but they lack a certain quality of firmness, individuality, and commitment which marks them as people whom one can genuinely interact with or even rebel against. Young people need to rebel to some extent in order to establish their own separateness and identity. Too often they find no one who will enter sufficiently into a real relationship with them to help them gain a sense of themselves and their own separateness.

**Occupation.** Along with independence from his parents, the young adult is expected to learn a trade or a profession and to begin to support himself. In our technologically advanced society, becoming proficient in a profession usually entails extended schooling and prolongs the young person's economic dependence on his parents well beyond the point at which physical maturity has been reached.

**Establishing a Home.** Among the responsibilities a young person may undertake are founding a home of his own, supporting it with his own money, marrying and having children. The need for extended schooling may make the achievement of some of these goals difficult. Marriage may be delayed, or the young adult may marry while he is still in school and will need to seek financial help from his parents. This is the time of life when, in addition to founding a home, the young person is encouraged to establish his own place in the community by taking a responsible part in community activities.

**Reality.** The adult is expected to face reality and to differentiate between it and fantasy. Progress in this task, as in the others, is achieved gradually throughout childhood and adolescence. Its accomplishment is of major importance in helping the young adult to sort out his own strengths and weaknesses and to set realistic goals for himself.

**Living with Conflict.** Each member of a family is striving to achieve his developmental tasks. At times family members are working toward similar goals; at other times the tasks which one member is trying to achieve are in conflict with those of another member of the family. Often an individual finds that there are conflicting demands made on him as he tries to achieve a variety of tasks, each of which may be important and worthwhile to him. For example, a young wife may find it difficult to remain active and interested in work outside the home if she is absorbed in establishing her home and family. A young husband may find that after a day filled with a variety of pressures at work he has little energy left for tackling problems which arise in relation to his son's schooling.

## NURSING CONSIDERATIONS

**Counsel and Encouragement.** Despite illness or handicap, the young individual is part of a world that values physical attractiveness, opportunities to develop one's own capacities, a chance to work and earn and to have one's own home. Obviously, many will be prevented by illness, as well as other factors, from achieving these goals. The nurse can help the patient to develop what he has to its highest potential. For example, the young paraplegic is often impotent as a result of injury to his spinal cord. He may be confined to a wheelchair. Recognizing these severe blows to his manly pride and the limitations that they have placed on his life, the nurse will avoid the common pitfall of treating a helpless adult like a child. On the contrary, she will recognize in every way possible the need of such patients for independence and privacy.

**Emotional Support.** Since illness or disability, whether emotional, physical, or both, complicates the process of maturation, it becomes particularly important to function with young people in ways which help them achieve their developmental tasks. The nurse should be truthful and honest in her relationship with the young person; she should not avoid unpleasant truths and attempt to sweep conflicts aside with an air of false sweetness. This does not help the young adult (who may be angry because illness is making it more difficult to achieve

maturity) to confront the issues which are troubling him. A nurse's unvarying sweetness may convey to him that he too should be "always nice" no matter how he feels.

Most people have been taught through their childhood years to control the expression of strong emotion. Before surgery, the child may plainly express his fear, giving those who care for him a chance to reassure and comfort him. The young adult may be no less frightened, but often shows his fear in less obvious ways. He, too, requires reassurance, but sometimes it is harder to recognize his need.

Because he is not yet sure of his own strengths, the young person may worry about the impression he makes on others. The hard job of working out how much dependence he can accept without interfering with his struggle for independence can make the patient irritable. He may retort angrily when he does not mean to. A response of anger by the nurse, although understandable, compels the patient to continue his anger to save face. Youth is a period of intense testing—of oneself and one's abilities, of the endurance of one's body, of one's influence on others. Being sick and in a hospital removes the individual from the opportunity to test himself in his usual environment.

A quick comment concerning a diagnosis or a manner of treatment may be the beginning, but it should never be the end of the efforts by physicians and nurses to help the patient to understand and cope with his illness. Understanding one's own illness is never a purely intellectual undertaking; it is a combined intellectual and emotional process that includes accepting what happened and planning what to do about it. For most patients the comment, "Don't worry" requires clarification. In subsequent conversations, the nurse may help the patient to see how in one area of his life, anxiety and tension might be contributing to his illness.

The nurse's role more often involves helping patients to recognize everyday situations that may contribute to illness or offering commonplace examples of ways in which they can follow the physician's recommendations. Such assistance is never insignificant, although it may seem lacking in drama. Movies and television notwithstanding, most people learn step by step, in seemingly small ways, to deal with stress.

**Respect for Privacy.** The young adult who is still developing his body image and working through his feelings about sex often finds illness particularly frightening. The bodily insults, such as lack of privacy or having needles forced into his skin and a thermometer pushed into his rectum, may be difficult to accept. Illness and surgery may mean to him that his ideal picture of a beautiful body cannot be his. Surgery on or near genitals can greatly intensify the fear of castration. Embarrassment—so easily brought on—is conscious, but the underlying thoughts may be subconscious. Providing maximum protection against unnecessary exposure and fully explaining what is going to happen before a procedure is started, and why it is done, lessen some of the tension. The very fact that the nurse shows concern about these things can convey to the patient that the hospital staff is not trying to manipulate him or increase his helplessness.

**Considering Special Needs.** Noncritically ill young adults often benefit when they are assigned beds near each other, because they often have similar interests.

Policies of the ward and the staff-patient relations should be geared to the special needs of this age group (as they should be adapted to the needs of each age group). A patient who is led to believe that his special likes and dislikes are important and heeded may be better able to face those problems for which there is less help available. At any age, success in coping with difficult problems can increase an individual's confidence in himself, as well as his skill in dealing with similar situations in the future. The dragons of pain, fear, loneliness, and anger reappear many times in the lives of most people. The young person who is helped to combat them during a personal crisis, such as illness, is girded for his future encounters.

However, it is also necessary to consider the reaction of older patients to having young people on the unit. In some instances an attractive young person becomes the darling of the ward, embodying as he does our culture's ideal of youth and good looks. It may be easier and more pleasant to spend time with him than with a worrisome older person. Anger at young people is common and often gets disguised by such reactions as criticism of hair styles. Friedenberg (1959) points out that some attributes of adolescents and young adults—loyalty, strong emotion, sexuality, and commitment—may be threatening to people in middle and later life, especially if these attributes have been rather deadened for the older person by societal pressures. Or

if the older adult feels that others consider him to be over the hill and expect him to abandon his own further achievements and ambitions in order to give place to the young, he may harbor exquisite resentment against young people. Thus, older patients may become resentful and complain of "those kids," especially if they feel that the nurse prefers giving care to younger patients. The nurse who recognizes this possibility can forestall much ill feeling by giving equal attention to older patients and showing recognition of their achievements.

**Creating a Positive Environment.** The young patient with a chronic disease or a permanent disability is in danger of missing the challenges and the learning appropriate to his age. The girl who is hospitalized for a long time does not meet many boys; studying in a hospital wheelchair is not the same as going to college. The nurse might search for ways in which she can change the patient's environment so that he has experiences that are more typical in our culture. Are there courses that the homebound or hospitalized adolescent can take? A party he can attend? Can transportation be provided to a church group? When parents, adolescents and nurses put their heads together and community resources are investigated, ways often can be found to provide the handicapped young person with the experiences he craves and needs.

**Working with the Family.** In addition to working with the young adult, the nurse has a role in working with his family. When illness strikes, families can be helped greatly by explanation and reassurance from the nurse. The nurse can allow them the opportunity to talk about the patient's illness and hospitalization and to express the shock they feel as well as their concern over whether the illness might, in some way, reflect lack of care or of awareness on their part. In the tension and conflicting demands of everyday life, many people experience twinges of regret and self-reproach for not having been, on one occasion or another, more perceptive of another's needs, or more generous in giving their time and attention. When sudden illness occurs, such feelings sometimes surge to the fore and may be expressed as "Is this partly my fault? Is there something I should have done to prevent it?" In such situations, the wise nurse will allow the family or friends to discuss the matter but will avoid any comment which implies blame. After the sudden shock of the illness and after the patient has received initial treatment, the nurse can assist the

CARING FOR THE YOUNG ADULT

family to recognize ways in which they can help to prevent similar problems or detect them promptly in the future.

**Encouraging Health Practices.** Helping young adults to maintain health and to promptly detect illness is an important function of the nurse, especially one who works in neighborhood health agencies or as an independent practitioner. Positive patterns of health care can be established or strengthened during young adulthood when, for example, a young woman learns the importance of regular gynecologic examinations and is assisted with family planning. Counseling can also assist young adults to deal with issues of child care, such as feeding problems, thus helping young families to build a healthful climate for child rearing. Early diagnosis is important in relation to health problems prevalent among young adults, and the nurse in her primary care role can assist patients to obtain needed treatment.

## Nursing Assessment

While flexibility is important, especially in relation to psychosocial and developmental aspects of assessment, certain guidelines may be useful. In relation to the short-term, acutely ill patient, assessment may include such factors as:

- **Level of activity. Since the young person usually has a great deal of energy, as soon as he begins to recover from acute illness or surgery he will need activities to help him channel his energy and to stay within the limits which will help him to recover.**
- **Peer support. It is important to encourage visits from the patient's friends. Too often the focus of the staff's concern for the patient's associates becomes limited to the parents, without sufficient regard for the important role which friends can play in providing support and companionship.**
- **Anxiety level. The young adult may be very concerned to "play it cool" and thus to enhance his own image as a person who is able to take stress. It is important to be especially perceptive and to give support in ways which do not undermine the patient's necessary efforts to cope with his emotions.**
- **The patient's environment. Often the most difficult aspect of being in a hospital is what one sees and hears. Serious illness and death, though commonplace to the staff, may be very upsetting to the young person who has never before had experiences with these aspects of life.**
- **Relationship with family members. Do they seem concerned about him? Do they visit? Does he seem glad to see them? Does he seem anxious when they leave?**
- **Interests and areas of developing competence.**

- **Appearance. Does the patient have the kind of physical attractivness so valued by young men and women? The style of dress the patient prefers is not at issue here; what is significant is the extent to which illness or disability interferes with the patient achieving the style he prefers .**

When one works with a patient over a longer time span, additional factors such as the following may be assessed:

- **Is the patient developing his own individuality and autonomy?**
- **Does the patient have social opportunities he needs in order to mature? (For example, opportunities to be part of a group and to relate to people of both sexes.)**
- **Is the patient developing greater independence of his parents?**
- **Does the patient have opportunities to develop his own competence—to learn to do some things well?**
- **Is the patient developing a feeling that his body is competent, through such activities as sports and dancing or hiking? This aspect of development may be seriously impaired by long-term illness or disability. It is important for the patient to develop his physical capacities as fully as is possible for him.**

These considerations by no means exhaust the possibilities for assessment of psychosocial and developmental needs of young adults. For example, the young adult with acute leukemia is faced with the issue of awareness of impending death and how to prepare himself for it. Your assessment will be concerned with how your patient is coping with this problem, rather than with his developing competence to prepare himself for work. The point made in Chapter 2 is re-emphasized here: the creative aspects of assessment must be dealt with individually by the nurse as she works with patients. Others can make suggestions and offer some guidelines, but rigid adherence to such suggestions can stultify the creativity of the nurse. This concern for flexibility need not detract from disciplined thinking. It is important to consider thoughtfully major areas of assessment in relation to the patient's stage of development and his psychosocial needs, as well as his particular illness.

## REFERENCES AND BIBLIOGRAPHY

BETTELHEIM, B.: To nurse and to nurture, *Nurs. Forum* 1:60, Summer 1962.

BRIGHT, F.: The pediatric nurse and parental anxiety, *Nurs. Forum* 4:30, 1965.

DUVALL, E. M.: *Family Development,* ed. 4, Philadelphia, Lippincott, 1970.

ERICKSON, E.: *Identity and the Life Cycle,* New York, International Universities Press, 1959.

FRIEDENBERG, E.: *The Vanishing Adolescent,* Boston, Beacon Press, 1959.

———: *Coming of Age in America,* New York, Random House, 1965.

GARRISON, K. C.: *Psychology of Adolescence,* Englewood Cliffs, N.J., Prentice-Hall Inc., 1965.

HAMMAR, S. L., and EDDY, J. K.: *Nursing Care of the Adolescent,* New York, Springer, 1966.

HOLMES, M., APPIGNANESI, L., and HOLMES, M.: *The Language of Trust,* New York, Science House, 1971.

JOSSELYN, I. M.: *Adolescence,* New York, Harper and Row, 1971.

KURTAGH, C.: Nursing in the life span of people, *Nurs. Forum* 7:298, 1968.

LORE, A.: Adolescents: People, not problems, *Am. J. Nurs.* 73:1233, July 1973.

MEYER, H. L.: Predictable problems of hospitalized adolescents, *Am. J. Nurs.* 69:525, March 1969.

MEYER, V. R.: The psychology of young adults, *Nurs. Clin. N. Am.* 8:5, March 1973.

NOWLIS, H.: Why students use drugs, *Am. J. Nurs.* 68:1680, August 1968.

ROGERS, D.: *The Psychology of Adolescence,* New York, Appleton-Century-Crofts, 1972.

ROSEN, S., et al.: Presbycusis study of a relatively noise-free population of the Sudan, *Ann. Otol.* 71:727, 1962.

SANKOT, M., and SMITH, DOROTHY W.: Drug problems in Haight-Ashbury, *Am. J. Nurs.* 68:1686, August 1968.

SMITH, DOROTHY W.: Patienthood and its threat to privacy, *Am. J. Nurs.* 69:508, March 1969.

TANNER, J. N.: *Growth at Adolescence,* Oxford, Blackwell Scientific Publications, 1963.

# Caring for the Patient
# Who is in Middle Life

## INTRODUCTION

The largest proportion of the population comprises those in middle life. In concern for the more dependent persons at the extremes of age, too little attention has been given to the study of this group. It is they primarily who maintain the nation's homes and businesses; it is they who care for the young and the old. When illness comes to a member of this age division, other lives are particularly likely to be affected. A man of 46 who has a heart attack may be concerned not only for his own welfare, but also for the welfare of his wife and children who, perhaps with his own parents, depend on him for support.

Middle life is the period when the individual's dependence is usually least acceptable, to the patient, to his close associates, and to those who care for him. For some people the middle years are more filled than any other period in life with opportunities for productivity and self-fulfillment and with responsibilities toward others. A change from the expected independence and productivity toward dependence and curtailment of productivity constitutes a major problem for the patient and for those who care for him. Before discussing this, let us consider some of the physical changes which occur during middle life.

## PHYSICAL CHANGES

**Strength.** Change in strength occurs continuously but so gradually that it is often not noticed. Nevertheless, a particular event can bring the change suddenly into sharp focus. For example, a man of 55 is driving along the parkway and has a flat tire. Through good luck and good management it has been years since he has had a flat. He begins the job of jacking up the car. All goes well until it is time to lift the spare tire into place. It is just too heavy. He realizes with a start that he is not as strong as he used to be. This fact is emphasized painfully when a lad of 20 stops to help him. With a cheery "Stand aside, sir," the younger man easily places the tire in position. The loss of strength which seemed to make its appearance in this man's 50's had actually been going on for two or three decades but had gone relatively unnoticed until an unusual event demanded the physical prowess that he no longer possessed. However, some of the loss of strength may be attributed to disuse atrophy, suggesting that regular exercise over a lifetime contributes to well-being. The middle-aged farmer and sailor note less loss of strength than the middle-aged man who has spent most of his time at his desk.

**Height and Weight.** There is a continuous increase in height and weight until about age 20. Height tends to remain constant until old age, when posture and settling of bones cause a slight decline. In contrast, weight continues to increase until about age 60. Commonly there is a lessening of exercise and slowing of metabolism without a corresponding decrease in caloric intake. If an individual has reached optimum weight during young adulthood, it is undesirable for him to continue to gain weight as he grows older. However, it is often difficult for him to stay slim.

**Aging.** During middle life there is a gradual slowing of metabolism and reaction time, as well as a gradual decline in visual and auditory perception. During this period early signs of aging make their appearance. Sometimes these early and obvious changes are traumatic for the individual in our youth-worshiping culture. In the Orient the wisdom of old age is regarded with reverence and respect, but in America, there is a particular tendency to deplore old age and to venerate youth. This attitude is reflected in the American preoccupation with cosmetics and youthful clothes.

**Pace and Exercise.** During middle life the individual gradually modifies his pace. This modification by no means indicates "sitting back," for these are usually the busiest years of life. However, there is a subtle change in the tempo of living, such as walking up steps more slowly instead of racing up two at a time, and shifting participation in sports from the most strenuous and competitive to those somewhat less demanding. A bank president seldom is obliged to run a race, or a lawyer to lift heavy weights. During active adult life many of the extremes of physical strength are not used, and their gradual loss is scarcely noticed.

Subtle but important cultural influences, as well as physical changes, cause a slow shift in activity at various ages, so that the older person often no longer seeks the more strenuous activities. Society shifts its expectations of what pursuits are considered appropriate for various age groups.

These shifts are not always consonant with desirable health practices, however. For example, in some areas of the United States little emphasis has been placed upon exercise for adults. Often it is expected that adults will merely be spectators, while exercise is left for the children.

Increasing recognition is being given to the ill effects of lack of exercise, particularly during middle and later life. Lack of regular exercise is believed to contribute to the development of atherosclerosis, one of the most prevalent and dangerous health problems of adults in this country. It also predisposes to obesity, lessened efficiency of the circulatory and respiratory systems, and decreased muscle tone and strength.

Rather than gradually slipping into a routine of too little exercise, persons in middle and later life should be encouraged to undertake regular activities that provide exercise as well as enjoyment. The type of exercise that is suitable and possible varies over the life span (for example, from football to golf) and from person to person. Brisk walking, swimming, gardening, and bicycling have been suggested as activities that can be engaged in by older persons who are in good health. Social pressures exert a not wholly desirable influence in the kind of activities older people feel free to undertake. Emphasis on conformity and on youthful glamor in sports attire discourage some older people from activities such as swimming and bicycling.

The middle-aged person who has neglected physical activity and who decides to begin a program of exercise is well advised to see his physician for a physical examination, and also to build up his exercise tolerance gradually. It is by no means unheard of for a middle-aged, sedentary person who decides to exercise in order to prevent a heart attack to suffer a myocardial infarction during an ill-considered burst of exercise for which he has not gradually prepared himself.

Changes in interests and activities occur gradually over the life span. Yet each age does have its own rewards. The boy playing football, the businessman taking his family for a drive, the retired gentleman cultivating his garden—each might bore the other; but each derives his own particular satisfaction.

**Menopause and Sexual Changes.** Menopause usually occurs in the decade of 45 to 55. The age at which menopause appears varies considerably among different women, just as there is wide variation in the age at which puberty is reached. Whereas puberty is marked by rapid growth, maturation of reproductive organs, and the development of secondary sex characteristics in response to the stimulation of sex hormones, menopause is characterized by shrinkage of reproductive organs due to the gradual reduction in sex hormones. Gradually ovulation and menstruation cease.

This period of life is often more difficult for women than for men. There is no physiologic climacteric or "change of life" among men, as there is among women, but rather a gradual decrease of sexual vigor. However, a proud new father at the age of 70 is by no means unknown. Contrary to popular belief, marked diminution in sexual response does not necessarily accompany menopause. Slowing down of sexual activity is a gradual and individual matter for both men and women.

**Eyesight.** The point at which loss of visual accommodation, called *presbyopia,* interferes with reading, sewing, and other close work usually starts between ages 40 and 50. The individual holds reading matter farther and farther from his eyes in order to see it clearly. This adjustment of position, known as the "tromboning effect," has given rise to many jokes about needing longer arms for reading. The person achieves artificial accommodation by using reading glasses for close work or by wearing lenses especially ground to provide for accommodation (bifocals, trifocals). In addition to changes for accommodation, there is a gradual decline in visual acuity; significant changes usually do not appear until about age 40. More light is needed for such activities as reading and sewing.

Many people are very sensitive about their eyesight. In their effort to disregard a decline in vision, they bring great discomfort to themselves and often to others, or they may needlessly curtail their activities. Successfully holding a job may depend on the ability to see well. Thus, it is important to help the older person to understand that change in vision is normal and that it happens to everyone. Wearing glasses is not a disgrace. For the individual who objects to wearing conventional eyeglasses, contact lenses may provide a solution.

**Hearing.** Hearing also gradually diminishes with age. Some persons, particularly in later middle life, find that the decrease is sufficient to interfere with their communication with others. Loss of hearing which occurs as a result of aging is called *presbycusis.*

In America loss of acuity in hearing is accepted with even poorer grace than decline in vision. Only gradually are people beginning to wear hearing aids without extreme self-consciousness. The fear that most people have of being less than perfect physically—an impossibility—makes them reluctant to call attention to a hearing defect by a visible aid. A person may attempt to conceal partial deafness if his job depends on normal hearing ability. The nurse may address an older man in her usual soft voice, only to find that he does not even look up from his newspaper. Rather than assuming that he is cranky, and ceasing further attempts at conversation, she may recall that hearing diminishes appreciably with age and repeat the greeting more loudly and distinctly. By speaking slowly and clearly, the nurse can avoid putting the patient with a hearing loss in the defensive position of asking, "What?" It is better to face the patient while speaking so that he can note lip movement and facial expression.

## DEVELOPMENTAL TASKS

In middle life the person is at the period in which society is making the greatest demands on him. He is responsible not only for himself, but also for the care of his children and often of his aging parents. It is at this time that the individual acquires most of his material possessions. Usually maximum earning power is reached during this period.

**Independence of Children.** Often it is difficult for middle-aged parents to accept their children's growing independence. The necessary changes in attitude may be especially difficult for the mother whose entire life has been devoted to her children and her home. The assumption that women should not work outside the home until their children have grown up is increasingly being challenged. However, for many women now in middle life, work outside the home means taking on a whole new way of life—something which is difficult for women in their 40's and 50's to do. For the woman who cannot make this transition to work or interests outside her home and family, this period can be extremely difficult. The menopause often coincides with these events, adding to the stress.

In contrast, her husband is usually still very much involved in his work and career; therefore, he often finds it less difficult to accept his children's growing independence. It is highly desirable for women to plan ahead for the period of perhaps 20 years when their children will be grown. Lack of planning and training often results in a woman being unable to find suitable employment, while the need for trained workers remains pressing. Seeking some opportunities for contact with her career, and for maintenance and upgrading of her skills while her children are small can help the woman in middle life to resume work outside the home and can help her deal with the change in her role which occurs as her children gain greater independence.

After their children have grown and established homes of their own, couples during middle life frequently turn more to each other for companionship and affection. During these years, after the pressures of child rearing have abated, they may find more opportunities to enjoy things together. A trip, a new and perhaps smaller home, or a hobby that interests them both are some of the joys which they can share.

**Dependence of the Elderly.** The increasing dependence of the elderly also presents strains on persons in middle life, not only financially, but also socially and emotionally. Apartments and homes tend to be small in modern urban society. They were planned to accommodate only the family of parents and children. Most people in our society prefer separate dwellings for each nuclear family. Some families manage very well, however, with a three-generation household. When families live together for economic reasons, even though they would prefer to live separately, strains and conflicts often result.

Because more people are living to very advanced age when the likelihood of physical and mental infirmity increases, their grown children become increasingly involved in care of older parents. (See Chap. 5 for further discussion of family and social problems in the care of the elderly.) However, in response to a social system that encourages the establishment of separate homes and families during early adult life, the individual by middle life often has transferred his primary loyalty to his wife and children. Such transfer is essential to the establishment of a new family unit with its own obligations to such responsibilities as child rearing and with its own pressures and changes, such as change of job location to a part of the country distant from the parental home. The needs of the parents, which become more pressing as time passes, revive the old problem of independence from parents. This time the problem is set in a new context, since now it is the child who is stronger and the parents who are weaker; the child who is richer, and the parents who are poorer.

Often the person in middle life feels squeezed by the conflicting demands of the young and the old. Both husband and wife may have to go out to work to provide sufficient income for their elderly parents as well as for themselves and their children. If there are very young children, the wife may understandably feel that she should not go out to work. The wife or the husband may rebel against supporting the spouse's parents, or additional problems may be created if all four parents of the couple depend on one breadwinner. With a longer life span, more and more old people live to be over 90. The very old are usually in the most difficult position because ordinarily they are the least self-sufficient. When they were young there were fewer retirement plans, and many are not covered by Social Security.

Problems may be lessened in families with enough money to enable the older person to maintain his own home and to secure, if necessary, such services as those of a housekeeper, home health aide, or practical nurse.

Such an arrangement enables the older person to remain in familiar surroundings and to maintain his feeling of independence longer than might otherwise be possible. However, many families do not have adequate financial resources for such an arrangement. If the parents become unable to care for themselves in their own homes, other arrangements must be considered:

- The parent shares the home of one of his children.
- One of the grown children returns to his parent's home to provide care.
- The parent resides in a home for the aged.
- The parent lives in a foster home.

Sometimes a change in living arrangements for the older person is precipitated by illness, and while the parent is in the hospital it is necessary to plan for his return to some home other than his own. If the family's decision is to have the older person share the home of his grown children, the hospital or public health nurse can often assist in making this transition as smooth as possible. Sometimes both the parent and his son or daughter need opportunities to talk over problems with an understanding listener. For example, the older person may express sadness or resentment at having to leave his own home. Friction may arise over the daily routine of the household. Two women in the same kitchen can create problems. Sometimes suggestions, made tactfully by the nurse, can help the family. Permitting the older person and his adult children as much privacy and freedom as possible is important. A room of his own and a place to keep treasured possessions makes the older person more comfortable. Opportunities for members of each generation to entertain their friends, though often overlooked, are also important.

If the family's decision is to provide care in a home for older persons, nurses can assist the family in choosing one where standards are high: where the menus are well planned, where there is enough well-qualified staff, where the building is safe, and where there are opportunities for rehabilitation. Care in a geriatric setting need not mean severing close family ties or terminating responsibility and participation in the care of one's parents. Many institutions utilize group programs to help grown children during the early period of their parent's residence in the institution. There are group discussions, led by the staff, and tours and observations of the activities. Grown children often feel guilty about placing their parents in an institution, even though it does not seem feasible for them to take the parent into their own homes. Their guilt often leads them to express anger and dissatisfaction toward the home and the care given. The reluctance that people often have in acknowledging the declining abilities of their parents presents problems in setting realistic rehabilitation goals. Grown children should be encouraged to discuss the problems they face in relation to their parent's care. Opportunity to express feelings of guilt and anger toward the institution and its staff is helpful. Tours of the home are useful, and the sons and daughters may be given the chance to observe and participate in the programs in such areas as the occupational and recreational therapy departments. Understanding the purposes of the various treatments, such as exercises, help to lessen the tendency of the grown children to view the home and its staff with dissatisfaction.

Observing the aging of one's parents is, for many people, a difficult experience. Changes that tend to occur with very advanced age—such as forgetfulness, loss of physical strength, and diminution of vision and hearing—may be very distressing. For a few people the experience of watching their parents age is so painful, particularly if the aging process is complicated by illness or marked impairment of function, that they find ways to withdraw from it. Sometimes, for example, they avoid visiting the parent or giving assistance that seems within their ability to provide.

Certain guidelines can be helpful in such situations. Remember that people vary in their ability to cope with certain kinds of stressful situations. Blaming the son or daughter for what appears to be neglect of his parents is usually ineffective in helping him to assume more responsibility. This approach may, in fact, make the son or daughter even more likely to avoid the situation, whereas an attitude of acceptance may help him to become better able to assist his parents. Helping the individual to learn of agencies and facilities that can help his parents may aid in reducing a seemingly overwhelming financial and emotional burden. Low-rent housing for the elderly, available in some communities, is an example of such assistance. Greater federal assistance, through such programs as Social Security and Medicare, also helps to ease financial burdens for the family as well as for the elderly individual.

Regardless of the attitude of the grown children, the nurse can be most helpful if she recognizes that the decision concerning the future care of the older person rests with the parent and the children, and not with her. The nurse's approach to the care of her own parents may be quite different. She should not attempt to impose her views on others but help them to find their own solutions. What she can do is help the elderly person and his family to see the alternatives open to them. Sometimes people see only one possible solution to a problem, whereas actually several other approaches may also be considered.

**The Concept of Time.** Some interesting changes occur in the way the person in middle life views time. He begins to be very much aware emotionally of something he has known intellectually for many years: time is not forever.

Changing time perspectives has some interesting and important implications. Time not only seems to be shorter, but it *is* shorter for the person of middle life. A man who feels himself to be in the wrong job and would like to enter another is aware that soon there will be no time left to make such a major change. The woman who has no children may feel that it will soon be too late to have any. The experience of seeing his parents age and his children mature is a further reminder of the mortal span.

**Satisfactions of Middle Life.** Just as young adulthood has its satisfactions as well as its stresses, so is middle life a mixture of the two. At this period the person has a chance to reap the harvest of his early struggle to found a home and to earn a living. Instead of dreaming of his own home, he may actually drive up to it. These lovely children are his. The "someday" for a trip abroad may have at last arrived. He may experience the satisfaction of achieving a respected place in his business and community—a feeling of usefulness and "neededness" greater than any he has felt before. At work he is important in getting the job done, and his years of experience have taught wisdom and skill that are highly valued by his company.

The process of finding a niche in a family and work and of becoming aware of the particular abilities a person possesses can be immensely satisfying. This aspect of middle life is often portrayed largely in its negative aspects, as assuming the burden of support of others, or as a closing of doors to various opportunities. The person in middle life who is perceptive of his own assets and of the ways in which he can utilize them for the good of his family, community, and society, as well as for his own self-development, can harness his energies to accomplish goals that to him are significant and worthwhile. He may be more able at this time of life than in his youth to differentiate what goals seem worth striving for, rather than attempting to meet a multitude of demands of society, some of which may be in conflict with one another. With a channeling and focusing of his energies may come additional time for enjoyment of the things he deems important. For one person this may be travel, for another study, gardening, or volunteer work.

Middle life makes an individual increasingly aware of choices. Some of the choices he has made himself; others have been made by circumstances.

If the direction of his life is recognized as essentially consistent with his values, middle life can be richly satisfying.

Of course, as at any period in life, all does not always go well. Nevertheless, it is during middle life that most people (if they are going to do so at all) bring their dreams and abilities to fulfillment. Inevitably, all the hopes are not fulfilled, and it is in late middle life that many people take stock, acknowledging, "While I have some things I've wanted, I haven't achieved others—and now I never will."

**Generation Gap.** Sometimes people in middle life seem to be an "in between" generation. Many of them were brought up with more restrictions and fewer choices than today's young. However, they are affected by current changes in values and life styles. Sometimes the way young people question the values of their elders becomes burdensome to the older generation, especially if they feel that they too would perhaps have liked to have more freedom in their lives, but feel constrained by work commitments, habit, lack of confidence, and responsibilities to others. Social pressures were different for them during their youth, with a far greater emphasis upon fulfilling society's expectations. A combination of feeling criticized by the young while at the same time being expected to carry heavy financial responsibilities as well as responsibilities for the care of others can lead those in middle life to feel resentful and, in turn, critical of young people.

**Social Pressures.** Unless the person in middle life finds greater satisfactions and opportunities for himself, resentment may grow when he notes that society begins to withdraw support from those of his age group, particularly during the fifth decade of life, when youthful attractiveness so valued in our country fades and signs of aging become unmistakeable. For the person who has not developed his own values and congenial life style, this can be a frustrating period of receiving constant reminders from magazines, TV commercials, and the like about how ugly it is to have wrinkles, gray hair, or a sagging figure. In work, too, resentment may develop. Unless the individual has been unusually successful, subtle changes in status become evident, with older workers sometimes stepping aside to a considerable degree before their actual retirement.

Such frustrating experiences are likely to be less troublesome to the individual in middle life who has developed competence as a person in his relationships with others and in his work, and who has earned recognition and satisfaction in his own achievement. The individual who has achieved a satisfying life style of his own is less vulnerable to the dictates and the rebuffs of society. If he has developed his own interests and tastes, he can pursue them with some measure of freedom from social pressures.

**Role of Women.** Women in middle life particularly lack society's support, and it is therefore especially important for them to develop their own competence as a way of coping with a rather pervasively negative attitude which stems from society's view that a woman's value lies in youth and physical attractiveness. Although the dilemma of women in middle life is often stated as more serious in the United States than elsewhere, Simone de Beauvoir (1972) indicates clearly that the problems of growing older are severe in many parts of the world. Her work is especially interesting because it discusses these issues with an unusual breadth in relation to various nations and cultures. The main theme of her book, brought out repeatedly in various contexts, is that the process of growing old is accompanied by pronounced withdrawal of society's support and esteem, and that older women are especially likely to be treated with avoidance, pity, and sometimes anger and derision. Such attitudes stem from viewing women largely in terms of reproductive capacity and physical attractiveness.

The woman's movement throughout much of the world, particularly in the United States, has been striving to counteract some of the negative forces which have constricted women's lives. The dilemma of women in our culture is strongly exemplified in the nursing profession, thus making the recognition of women as capable, intelligent members of society of particular interest to nurses.

**Seeking Fulfillment.** Despite the many problems, there are hopeful signs that people in middle life are offering more resistance to these constricting forces of society and age. They are making a greater effort to counteract the negative view of themselves and to seek broader, more satisfying lives. More and more women in middle life are realizing that their families are not helpless and are quite capable of assisting with household chores—and these women are seeking further education and work which interests them.

Nor is the issue wholly one of finding a second career or a more satisfying way of pursuing the same work. An important aspect of the second half of life as Jung (1953) points out involves developing inner resources and personal views about the meaning and value of one's life. For some people the realization that youth is over opens the door to discovery of other aspects of living which may have been previously ignored. Sidney Jourard's (1970) emphasis upon the necessity for many people to develop new ways of being, new projects, and new sources of satisfaction is especially relevant to people in middle life. He points out that people often become ill when their lives are no longer satisfying and meaningful and when others dispirit them by disconfirming them, reducing their hope, and diminishing the value they invest in their aims and purposes.

### Summary

Developmental tasks of middle life may be summarized as:

- Maintaining a satisfying family life; dealing with the growing independence of children and with the growing dependence of aged parents.
- Enhancing responsibility and contribution to work.
- Securing a home; building up financial resources.
- Assuming a greater role and more responsibilities in community activities.
- Coping with physical and emotional changes related to the aging process.
- Developing varied interests and relationships which can continue in later years.
- Moving toward individuation, such as by further definition of one's own values, life style, and religious beliefs.

## NURSING CONSIDERATIONS

A major problem confronting the individual who becomes ill during middle life is change of role and status, in his own eyes and in his relationships with others, from independence and productivity to dependence and curtailment of productivity. These changes also create problems at other age periods, but their impact is particularly severe during middle life.

**Encouragement and Emotional Support.** The patient in middle life, especially if his illness is life-threatening or disabling, is particularly likely to become anxious about incapacity. Concern about unmistakable signs of aging, while compensated for during good health, may surge forward with illness

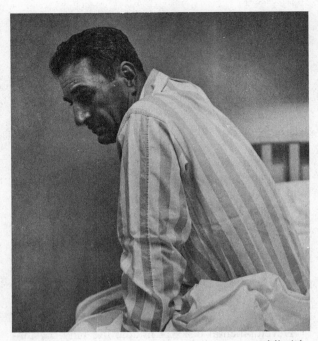

**Figure 4-1.** The experience of illness in middle life can precipitate thoughtful assessment of one's goals and values. Illness at this time of life may also spark feelings of discouragement and apprehension about the future. (Overlook Hospital, Summit, N.J.)

and be reinforced by a nonsupportive social environment (Fig. 4-1).

Jourard points out that many people who become ill with such conditions as myocardial infarction and peptic ulcer do so when their way of life and their social supports no longer sustain them, and they have been unable to develop new roles and new and more satisfying relationships with others. Nurses encounter many middle-aged patients for whom Jourard's comments seem especially relevant—a woman in her 50's with grown children who views her life as useless and who comes to the hospital because of recurrent migraine headaches.

Similarly, there is the man of 55 who is recovering from a myocardial infarction and says to himself, "It's going to be downhill from now on." This attitude may be subtly reinforced by his work colleagues who emphasize the need for rest and begin to leave him out of important decisions. Assuming (as is often the case) that the patient is able to participate fully in his work following the attack, he may face not only his own attitude of insecurity and self-doubt, but also a subtle condescension by colleagues who view him as no longer fully capable.

A great deal of stamina is required to combat a combination of attitudes such as these, and many people in middle life do not fully recover their accustomed level of functioning after illness, not because of physical incapacity, but because of their own loss of confidence which is reinforced by the condescension and doubts of others.

The nurse who is sensitive to these factors affecting patients in middle life can help her patients to continue their interests and perhaps also to develop new ones. She can by her own attitude encourage the patient to see his illness as temporary (if this is likely to be the case) and to plan for return to his usual activities.

Measures to combat discouragement and apathy should be initiated in concrete ways during hospitalization. Too often the routines of many hospitals reinforce feelings of incapacity, with their emphasis upon wearing nightclothes at all times, eating from a tray in bed, and bathing from a small basin. For patients in later middle life and old age such routines, suggestive of incapacity, can be especially devastating.

Thus, it is particularly important to use nursing approaches which foster the degree of independence of which the patient is capable.

For example, a 50-year-old man who is recovering from myocardial infarction must rest. He must stay in bed and allow the nurse to bathe him. Many patients in this predicament find it hard to rest; some of them, despite repeated instructions, get up to go to the bathroom and, in various other ways, do not follow the prescribed regimen. Reasons for such behavior vary with each patient, and it is important for the nurse to listen to her patient, so that she may better understand why he does not follow instructions. Frequently these patients express anger at curtailment of their activities and, particularly, at having decisions made for them. Many patients who suffer myocardial infarction are active, hard-driving people who are very much involved in their work. Suddenly, with the onset of infarction, the patient is reduced to the helpless physical dependence of an infant. If the patient expresses anger over the abrupt curtailment of his independence, one of the things the nurse can do is consider with him the areas where he can make decisions. Although he must be bathed, he can have some part in deciding when he will have his bath.

When the patient goes home, he should be encouraged to involve himself promptly in activities with others in order to regain his confidence and vigor. Particularly if the patient lives alone, planning and effort will be required to help him become involved and to feel that others are interested in him. For too long we have focused narrowly on the things a patient may not do and on hazards to avoid, without recognizing the importance of stressing what the patient can do and helping him to regain his zest for living.

**Relationship with Family.** While it is important to understand how devastating the problem of sickness and dependency can be to the patient in middle life, it is also important to recognize that the patient in this age group experiences equally distressing strains from other sources. This time of life is one of great stress, even without illness. In fact, a great variety of illnesses usually associated with emotional stress, such as asthma, peptic ulcer, and colitis, are common during this period. In a time of illness, a patient may be subjected to additional emotional pressures.

Aside from his own frustrations and discouragements, he must also deal with the reactions of his family and friends. In many instances, nurses assume that family and friends will respond sympathetically to the patient as a result of his illness. However, this is not always the case. Many times, the response is one of impatience and even anger because the patient cannot fulfill his usual role and responsibilities. More than at other periods of life, the individual carries considerable responsibility to others as well as to himself, and any extensive interruption in his ability to fulfill these responsibilities may elicit a considerable reaction from others, as well as from the patient himself. Colleagues may chafe at doing an extra share of the work to compensate for the patient's absence. Family members may feel strained, and sometimes angry, when they are called upon to carry additional financial and emotional burdens, and sometimes, to alter their own goals. The young man who longed to study medicine may be unable to do so after his father is disabled by a stroke. Instead of receiving financial help to further his education, he may have to go to work as soon as he finishes high school to help support the family.

If the nurse becomes aware of such feelings, she should not inject her own judgment into the matter, but should allow family and patient to air their feelings freely. At the same time, she must be careful not to pass judgment on a family situa-tion about which she may know very little. For example, if a patient has grown children who do not visit him frequently, the nurse must not jump to conclusions that the children are unsympathetic, and then condemn them accordingly. The situation affecting the patient's children may be completely unknown to the nurse. For instance, may be the son has a sick wife at home, and has all he can do to go to work and care for his wife and children when he gets home in the evening. Or perhaps the relationship between the patient and his children has never been close. Parent-child relationships during middle and later life are an outgrowth of those developed throughout the years.

The nurse should remember that a patient's view of his family is true as he sees it. She should let him express himself without taking sides, recognizing that she does not have all the facts and that even if she did, her role is to help both the patient and his family rather than to judge or condemn. Usually the members of the patient's family are doing the best they can within the limitations of a variety of emotional, social, and economic pressures.

Just as it is important not to assume that family and friends will react a certain way, it is also important not to expect that the patient is going to react in a stereotyped manner toward his family while he is sick and hospitalized. For example, there is a widespread expectation among nurses that the mother who becomes ill is more concerned about her children's welfare than her own, and that the father-provider who becomes ill is more worried about his family's welfare and support than he is about his own recovery. It seems likely that to some extent such statements reflect the expectations of nurses, rather than necessarily the reactions of patients. Some patients do respond to illness with greater concern for others than for themselves. However, a common response to illness, at any age, is increased concern for and preoccupation with one's own welfare, and diminished capacity to be concerned about the needs of others. Thus the nurse must be careful not to impose her own feelings on the patient. She may unwittingly convey her expectations to the patient by quickly introducing a question about his children's welfare, when the patient has voiced concern about his own condition and chances for recovery. To discuss the children at this moment may only make the patient feel guilty that he is concerned about himself when this is in fact a very legitimate and natural concern.

Yet it is very possible that the patient may be preoccupied with family considerations at this time. The modern independent small family consisting of parents and children encounters extra problems when illness strikes. If the mother becomes ill, there may be no one there to take over the housework and the care of the children. Employing someone to do this work is often difficult and unsatisfactory, even if the family can pay for it. And if the family cannot afford it, the patient may be forced to look to insurance or to public welfare for financial help —or even worse to suffer economic hardship rather than to admit that he needs money.

Recognizing that the individual's responsibilities and stresses are often numerous may help the nurse as she cares for patients whose illness is greatly affected by emotional strain. Illness can pose many profound questions concerning the meaning of life and death and, by providing a respite from the patient's usual activities, can afford him time for reflection (see Fig. 4-1). The nurse can help the patient by listening if he wishes to discuss some of these concerns. Unfortunately, the patient's concern with the "ultimate questions" is too often looked upon as morbid preoccupation with the self, and efforts are made to distract the patient by conversation about his flowers, the weather, and so on. By recognizing that the experience of illness can bring opportunity for growth, for confronting fundamental issues of life, and for greater depth of experiences and relationships in the future, the nurse can utilize more effectively the opportunities which she has to support the patient in his experience.

## Nursing Assessment

Because the assessment of psychosocial and developmental factors must be kept flexible, some suggestions made in relation to the young adult and to the elderly patient may be useful when assessing patients in middle life. The suggestions made in Chapters 3, 4, and 5 are not intended to be mutually exclusive but to be complementary to one another.

The following points may be used in assessing the patient in middle life:

- **To whom does the patient turn for help when he is sick? Family? Friends?**

- **How has the patient arranged for the interruption in his usual responsibilities toward work and family? Do these arrangements satisfy the needs of the situation, or is the patient under tension because his absence from home and work is not being adequately managed?**

- **What are some of the patient's assets and resources? Is he using them effectively?**

- **What are the effects of previous losses and previous illnesses upon the patient? (The experience of illness tends to reactivate feelings of loss and also to bring up previous illness experiences.)**

- **What are some of the patient's interests? It is important to consider vocational interests as well as hobbies. How can the patient be helped to maintain and possibly to expand his interests during illness?**

- **What are some areas of the patient's competence? How can he maintain his competence as fully as possible during illness?**

- **Has the patient been in good health previously? Has he kept his body in good condition through exercise, suitable diet, and avoidance of harmful substances such as tobacco?**

- **What are some of the patient's daily habits concerning such matters as sleep, elimination, diet, and personal hygiene? How may these affect plans for his nursing care?**

- **Is the patient's appearance attractive? Prematurely old? Unkempt?**

- **Does the patient have religious and philosophic beliefs which sustain him?**

- **Does the patient seem to be aware of his own feelings, and does he seem to act congruently with them?**

- **How is the illness affecting the patient's self-confidence?**

- **What does the patient know about community resources which can benefit him?**

## REFERENCES AND BIBLIOGRAPHY

AIKEN, L. H.: Patient problems are problems in learning, *Am. J. Nurs.* 70:1916, September 1970.

BRUDNO, J. J.: Group programs with adult offspring of newly admitted residents in a geriatric setting, *J. Am. Geriat. Soc.* 12:385, 1964.

DE BEAUVOIR, S.: *The Coming of Age,* New York, Putnam, 1972.

DUVALL, E. M.: *Family Development,* ed. 4, Philadelphia, Lippincott, 1970.

FRIEDMANN, E., and HAVIGHURST, R. J.: *The Meaning of Work and Retirement,* Chicago, University of Chicago Press, 1954.

HAVIGHURST, R. J.: *Human Development and Education,* New York, Longmans, 1953.

JOURARD, S.: Suicide: An invitation to die, *Am. J. Nurs.* 70:269, February 1970.

JUNG, C. G.: *Psychological Reflections,* JOLANDE JACOBI (ed.), New York, Harper and Row, 1953.

MURPHY, G., and KUHLEN, R.: *Psychological Needs of Adults,* Chicago, Center for Study of Liberal Education for Adults, 1955.

PARKES, C. M.: *Bereavement: Studies of Grief in Adult Life,* New York, International Universities Press, 1972.

PRESSEY, S., and KUHLEN, R.: *Psychological Development Through the Life Span,* New York, Harper and Row, 1957.

SAKOLYS, J. A.: Stages of adaptation to illness and disability: A psychosocial view, Chap. 29. Vol. III of *Current Concepts in Clinical Nursing,* M. DUFFY, et al. (eds.), St. Louis, Mosby, 1971.

SKIPPER, J., and LEONARD, R. (eds.): *Social Interaction and Patient Care,* Philadelphia, Lippincott, 1965.

SUTTERLEY, D. C., and DONNELLY, G. F.: *Perspectives in Human Development, Nursing Throughout The Life Cycle,* Philadelphia, Lippincott, 1973.

VINCENT, P. A.: Do we want patients to conform? *Nurs. Outlook* 18:54, January 1970.

# Caring for the Elderly Patient

## CHAPTER 5

## SOME FACTS AND MYTHS

A great percentage of medical-surgical patients, whether in general hospitals, nursing homes, or their own homes, are elderly people. Associated with physiologic changes of aging is an increased tendency toward illness and slowness in recovery from illness. To compound the problem, in our society many older persons are disadvantaged also in relation to family ties, income, housing, and opportunities to perform useful and respected work.

However, although these statements are true, they do not present the whole picture. Recent efforts to highlight the plight of the elderly have resulted in some exaggeratedly negative views. It is assumed, for example, that a large proportion of the elderly reside in institutions. Actually, only a small percentage of those over 65 are institutionalized, and it is likely that this percentage could be reduced if adequate facilities for home care (such as medical and nursing care and assistance with housekeeping) were available (Wahl, 1968).

The elderly are often portrayed as sitting on park benches, with little to do but feed the pigeons. This is true of some older people, but it does not accurately describe the majority. Interestingly, a significant proportion of the income of elderly persons comes from paid employment—much of it part-time (Wahl, 1968). This fact is all the more impressive when one considers that the labor market is becoming increasingly more resistant to employment of older persons.

Another common assumption is that the elderly are increasingly abandoned by their families. A contrast with "the good old days" is often made, nostalgically idealizing the large farmhouse which sheltered not only the nuclear family, but the older generation as well. While this was the case in some instances, there were other modes of responding to the issue of relationships between generations which are less widely discussed.

What about the young people who migrated across this continent, or from another land, leaving the older members of the family? In those days the leave taking was often final. Transportation facilities frequently did not permit a return visit to those who lived far away, nor was there telephone communication with them. Letters tended to become less and less frequent as family ties weakened due to prolonged separation. Sometimes the younger generation never knew what happened to their parents and other older relatives; certainly they could not assume continued responsibility for helping them in their declining years. This, too, is part of the way things used to be. Today, despite urbanization with its smaller living quarters and the tendency for each generation of adults to reside in separate homes, families have greater opportunity to keep in touch, by visits and telephone, and many families continue to do so, despite high geographic mobility.

We are often told that the problem of aging has been with us always, but that we are just not handling it as well as did our forebears. Actually the problem is not the same as it was. In years past the person who lived longer than 65 years was a rarity. Now it is possible for two generations of a family to be drawing social security: for example, one, age 65, and his parent, age 85. A young husband and wife may each have not only living grandparents, but great-grandparents as well. The problem is different, it is vastly larger, and it can no longer be viewed as the sole responsibility of families, but must be seen as a responsibility of society as a whole. The view that families alone are responsible for care of the elderly has brought some unfortunate results for individuals and, in the long run, for society. For instance, a couple in their late 50's may be continuing to support one or two older parents in a nursing home, at a time of life when they should be saving money for their own rapidly approaching retirement. When their retirement does come, they may be obliged to seek assistance through public welfare. Unmarried women in middle life are particularly vulnerable in this respect, as they are often expected to assume considerable

responsibility for care of the elderly. It is not infrequent for a woman in middle life to stop working in order to care for an older parent. When after some years the parent dies, the woman may find that she no longer possesses the skills and confidence to seek re-employment, thus becoming, herself, a candidate for public assistance. In these examples we see the way in which the problem of care of older people "backs up" as it were, when resources of the family are not adequate to meet the problem. Nor is the challenge only financial. It involves also the freedom of younger members of the family to marry and to seek education and satisfying work—in short, to move ahead with the multiplicity of tasks and responsibilities facing them, of which care of the aged is only one.

It is essential for nurses to view these problems broadly, over a long time span, and to recognize that the problem may significantly affect the lives of several members of a family, rather than just the older individual alone. It is also important for nurses to recognize their role in helping families make their own decisions in these matters, rather than making decisions for them or subtly influencing them about what course of action to take. The nurse must distinguish between her own values, in relation to care of her own elderly relatives, and the values which others may hold. The nurse who is too quick to recommend a nursing home, and the nurse who subtly implies that placing a relative in a nursing home is tantamount to abandonment, are both imposing their own values on others, rather than helping the elderly person and his family to consider alternatives and to decide what is best for them.

What are some other myths about the elderly—or views which, while once tenable, are so no longer? One is that they have so short a life expectancy that some therapeutic measures, which would be considered essential for a young person, are not worthwhile. Dentures, corrective glasses, provision of speech therapy, and psychotherapy may be neglected on the assumption that the patient has very few years in which to benefit from them. But many persons age 65 now live 20 and 25 more years! Views about care of the elderly must be reexamined in light of current life expectancy and also in light of values of the rights of individuals to health care, regardless of age.

Another view prevalent in our culture is that older people are useless. But is usefulness limited

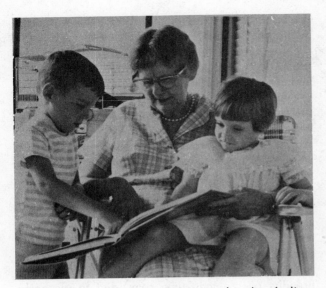

**Figure 5-1.** Babysitting gives grandmother feelings of usefulness and pleasure.

to being gainfully employed? What about the values to a family, a community, or a profession of having older members—members whose view has a different perspective and who can help those who are younger to be in touch with their own origins? (Fig. 5-1) What of the value to a youngster who has a close relationship with his grandfather who talks to him of family lore and of the way life used to be when he was a boy? What about the youngster who, through a grandparent who migrated to this country, is put in touch with his family's background in the "old country," and perhaps also has opportunity to learn a second language? In a fast-changing society, the elderly are an important link to past events and persons who have affected our lives.

The assumption is sometimes made that later life is synonymous with incapacity. One often hears an achievement of an older person received with astonishment, "Imagine, at *his* age!" Such responses are condescending and imply that the significant part of life is over once one has passed middle age.

But is it really? And even more important, does it *have* to be, or do our expectations sometimes make it so? The news that an elderly man and woman plan to marry is often greeted with a mixture of scorn and amusement, as though somehow the individuals are expected to have outlived their human need for closeness and companionship. Such views by the young are presumptuous and can undermine the confidence and resilience of many an

older person who senses that he is not expected to seriously seek new experiences, whether in work or personal relationships.

The process of aging brings many doubts and uncertainties: of ability to support oneself financially, to find companionship, and to do useful work. Attitudes of younger people, including those in the health professions, are especially important. Instead of "Why, at your age," they can convey "Well, why not?"

A great deal is heard about the losses of aging—and it is true that the elderly experience many losses—in personal relationships, income, health, agility, and opportunities to learn new things and to continue employment. However, it is necessary to view the losses not in the context of the values and goals of youth and middle life, but in the context of later life. For example, physical changes with aging are on the debit side. But what does it mean to the older person that his grip is weaker than when he was 40? It means that he must live somewhat differently and adapt to failing muscular strength. But how much of a disability is this to the older person who has gradually adapted his life style accordingly? Thus, even the stark reality of physical decline must be viewed in the perspective of the older person's life and not just in terms of measurements of how much he has lost in his youthful vigor and physiologic efficiency.

A great deal is also heard about the older person's disengagement: his lessened concern with daily events and increased preoccupation with his own thoughts. An increased concern with assessing one's life and accomplishments and one's relationships with others and with work occurs for many people during middle age and continues into later life. The older person often shows greater selectivity of involvement with certain people and with those aspects of his work which have most meaning and value for him. Whether or not this change constitutes loss depends upon one's values. In a society in which "business" and involvement with many individuals and groups is highly valued, and where little recognition is given to the importance of developing personal inner resources, these changes with age may be viewed as loss. However, if a high value is placed on development of the inner life, these changes with age are viewed as manifestations of personal maturation.

There is another aspect to the matter of disengagement: society's disengagement from the older person. There is, if you will, a reciprocal disengagement in which society withdraws from the older person much interest and support, and the aging individual withdraws some of his involvement with society. The older person whose services have been sought because of his skill and achievements at work may no longer be consulted by his colleagues after retirement. Younger family members are busily engaged in establishing their own homes and careers and may spend little time with older members of the family. Thus, the older individual has his tendency to disengagement greatly heightened by the disengagement of others from him and by the lack of opportunity to become involved in significant work and new learning.

Disengagement may thus be viewed as a psychological change in the aging individual and also as an aspect of society's reaction toward the elderly. The two processes together, along with physiologic changes of aging which result in decreased blood flow to the brain, sometimes result in a syndrome called *senility*. This word has unfortunate connotations of hopelessness; it is also frequently misused to label older people, resulting in further withdrawal of others from them and a resultant increase in the older person's symptoms. The word "senile" is used to describe older people who are forgetful and confused and who show feebleness and helplessness associated with advanced age. When the older person is helped to become involved with significant activities and with other people, his memory and orientation sometimes improve.

## PHYSICAL CHANGES

The average life expectancy at birth once was as short as 30 years. In some places in the world it still is 30 years. In the United States, however, the expectancy is around 70, with the result that the proportion of older persons has increased markedly since 1850; an even greater percentage of older people is expected in the next 50 years. Most human beings in the United States can expect to have the experience of growing old. The elderly seek more medical care than younger people because of the higher incidence of certain health problems among older age groups.

For example, the highest incidence of impaired vision and hearing occurs among older people. During later life certain prominent causes of illness and death, such as cancer, cerebral vascular accidents, and heart disease, also reach their peak. Several chronic diseases that have developed gradually often exist simultaneously in elderly people. Knowledge of normal physiologic changes which occur with aging can help the nurse plan her care of elderly patients and can enable her to assist patients and their families to cope with the aging process.

**Nutrition.**  There is a tendency for people to lose weight during old age and to suffer possible nutritional insufficiency. This may be related to lack of dentures, to boredom at eating alone, to lack of money, or to decreased gastric motility and diminished acuity of the sense of taste. While diet planning for the geriatric patient should limit calories to match lessened energy output, it should maintain weight unless the patient is obese. Many older people find that a light supper (perhaps of soup or cereal, bread and fruit) is sufficient for them at the end of the day when they are tired. Their heavier meal, then, comes at midday. Plans for helping the nonhospitalized aged receive adequate nutrition include provision of one hot meal a day, served either in the individual's own home or in a day-care center.

The older person continues to need fresh fruit and vegetables, milk, eggs, and meat. He should have enough fluid and roughage to encourage normal bowel function since chronic constipation may be a problem as a result of decreased peristalsis.

Since the sense of taste dulls with age, the diet should also include well-seasoned food. Serving unrecognizable pureed or ground foods insults the taste and the sensibilities of some older people. Offering foods in other ways, such as in stews, is more appealing, and can increase the older person's food intake.

Appetite also may increase when food is served in a way that enables the elderly person to help himself as much as possible—it is better to have the butter soft than to spread it for the patient; the patient who cannot feed himself the entire meal may be able to eat his bread without help. Eating is a social activity and should include pleasant conversation and companionship (Fig. 5-2).

**Position Sense and Speed of Reaction.**  Position sense and reaction time show gradual decline until the age of about 70, when the decline becomes rapid. The decline of these two faculties, together with diminished vision, is frequently a cause of accidents. It has been suggested that deterioration of the ability to make decisions and to formulate

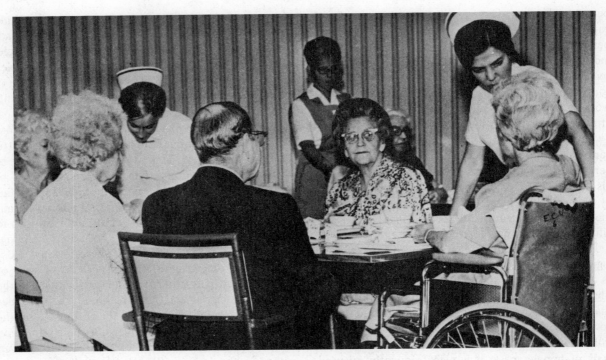

**Figure 5-2.** These older patients are encouraged to wear street clothes and to eat together in a dining room as soon as they are able to do so. (Overlook Hospital, Summit, N.J.)

judgments involving use of short-term memory are also important factors in causing automobile accidents among the elderly. Thus an older person may not comprehend quickly enough the variety of changes occurring in a traffic situation. He may fail to take account of a car emerging from a side street and fail to make a decision to stop even when his vision is adequate.

However, despite problems with vision, hearing, and decision making, older people in this country have achieved "safe driving" records which could be the envy of teen-age drivers. In light of their driving records it is apparent that many older people make realistic adaptations in their driving habits by driving only during daylight hours, avoiding heavy traffic and long fatiguing trips, and giving up their licenses when their waning abilities make this necessary. Because waiting for trains and buses is fatiguing, and since transportation is vital to the older person in maintaining his contacts with family and friends, it is important to counsel those older persons who require such guidance to promote safe driving.

Diminished agility, position sense, vision, and hearing also make older people prone to injury as pedestrians. Safety programs, then, should stress the need to watch for older people as well as chil-

dren. Older people should be encouraged to protect themselves by observing rules for pedestrian safety. Nighttime is especially hazardous when older people who are not alert step into the street without first surveying the traffic. Older people should be discouraged from walking unaccompanied at night. If they must walk alone after dark, they should be encouraged to use the best-lighted streets, and to be alert to the traffic.

A decline in position sense in older people frequently results in falls, a common cause of injury in this age group, especially women.

The susceptibility of older people to falls and fractures (their bones are more brittle and break more readily) should affect the planning of homes and apartments. Because of the increasing proportion of older people in the population, it is advisable to include basic safety factors in all housing and not to confine safety devices to units designed especially for older people: for example, stairs should not be too steep, should be adequately lighted, and should be provided with a handrail. Night lights and a sturdy handlebar near the bathtub or shower can be put up in any home.

**Skin.** Gradual changes in the skin and in the body's ability to adjust to heat and cold occur with age. The skin becomes drier and prone to wrinkling. In old age it may become thin, flaky and susceptible to irritation. The hair, also, becomes drier, thinner, and gray. Nails, particularly toenails, often become thickened and brittle as a result of diminished circulation to the extremities.

**Temperature Regulation.** During later middle life and old age the body gradually loses some of its ability to adjust to extremes of temperature. It is harder for an old person to keep warm in cold weather because his metabolism is slower, and he lacks physical vigor for the strenuous exercise that would help him to keep warm. In hot weather the older person does not dissipate heat as efficiently as a younger one, because his cutaneous vessels may not dilate as much and his sweating mechanism may not function as effectively as it once did. Now there are many welcome aids for keeping older people comfortable in very hot weather and in cold weather. Contrast the comfort of heated cars with a bulky lap robe. Modern heating that provides uniform warmth in the entire house is another boon. Air conditioning has made summers more comfortable for everyone.

The nurse can help by making adjustments to keep older people more comfortable and by remembering that they tolerate temperature changes poorly. If an older patient shares a room with younger people, fewer problems in regulating temperature may occur if the older patient is placed farthest from the window and is offered an extra blanket.

**Teeth.** Although the rate of formation of dental caries declines with age, neglect of the teeth during youth and middle life or the development of periodontal disease in middle and later life may make the wearing of dentures necessary in later years. Since considerable individual differences exist in the resistance of teeth to decay, some people lose their teeth as they grow old despite good dental care. Others have almost all their own teeth, and they can munch a raw apple as well as their grandchildren. The older person who needs dentures should be encouraged to obtain them, since his appearance and nutrition will benefit.

## Other Physical Changes

Changes in vision and hearing as age advances are discussed in later chapters. Other important physical changes include a considerable decrease in cardiac output, from 6.5 liters per minute at age 25 to 3.8 liters per minute at age 85 (Zorzoli, 1968). Since cardiac output affects circulation to all parts of the body, this change is of great significance. Vital capacity also diminishes markedly with age; there is decreased resilience of lung tissue due to thickening of the walls of the alveoli.

The elderly person has diminished ability to maintain homeostasis during stress; he has less "reserve" for dealing with the onslaughts of anxiety, exertion, infection, and fatigue. One example of the slowness of the homeostatic mechanism to adjust is illustrated by the fact that the body's ability to remove excessive glucose from the blood drops appreciably in old age (Zorzoli).

Physiologic response to exercise also changes with age; light exercise, which causes little change in the heart rate and blood pressure of young people, causes acceleration of heart rate and rise in blood pressure of older people. Thus, the circulatory system cannot respond as efficiently to the demands of exercise in later life; the heart and blood vessels cannot supply the increased demands of the muscles for blood as adequately as during youth.

Diminished effectiveness of circulation, related to such changes as atherosclerosis and arteriosclerosis, has serious and widespread effects—a lessened ability to heal a cut on the foot can cause an ulcer to form; decreased blood supply to the brain can result in loss of memory (particularly for recent events), in confusion, and in irritability.

The kidneys, too, are less efficient in old age. They cannot conserve water as effectively in situations (such as excessive sweating) where this is necessary. Urinary stasis, urinary frequency, and nocturia become more frequent with advancing age.

**Theories on Aging.** Despite knowledge of certain measurable changes in physiologic functioning, the basic causes of aging are not fully understood. There are numerous theories, only three of which will be briefly mentioned here: (1) One theory holds that loss of irreplaceable cells is the cause of aging. Some cells of the body do not reproduce themselves; they age, as the individual ages. When cells of this type (such as those of the brain) die, they cannot be replaced. (2) The autoimmune theory of aging postulates that the aging individual produces antibodies against substances normally present within his own body; changes thus produced in his body result in aging. (3) Another theory, put forth by Hans Selye, suggests that the gradual accumulation of calcium within the body and a shift of calcium from the bones to the soft tissues may be an important factor in the physiologic changes of aging.

## INTELLECTUAL DEVELOPMENT

### Teaching the Older Patient

Suppose that a 67-year-old woman has just discovered that she has congestive heart failure. The doctor has recommended rest, a low sodium diet, digitalis, and a diuretic. This woman has many new things to learn. Perhaps the most important of these will be the fact that she *can* learn. Older people themselves often have the false notion that ability to learn ceases at some point during life. Encouraging self-confidence in older people is the first big step in helping them to learn.

Unfortunately, the fact that older persons perform less well on some standardized intelligence tests (older people have particular difficulty, for example, with timed tests, since they perform more slowly than young people), has led some people to the dismal conclusion that a person becomes gradually less and less intelligent during middle and later life. It is more useful to consider these changes within the context of the individual's life than merely in terms of test results. Standardized intelligence tests are useful in predicting success of young people in school; but how useful are they, say, in predicting the success of a man in his 50's who is about to become president of his company? Many abilities, such as skill in leading others and wisdom in decision making, may be difficult to predict on the basis of intelligence test scores but may more readily be predicted from past performance at work. Qualities of wisdom, tact, patience, and understanding of self and others are not readily measured by standard intelligence tests. However, these are examples of abilities in which some older persons excel. The older person also has had many experiences to which he can relate new learning.

As she begins to teach the older patient, the nurse should convey to him her belief that he *can* learn. She should proceed more slowly than with her younger patient, to give the older person the extra time he needs to think about and respond to new ideas. She should speak slowly and distinctly to help the individual compensate not only for slowed reaction time but also for the hearing deficit so common among the elderly. If visual aids, such as graphs or pictures are used, she should allow the older person extra time to study them, and be sure he is wearing his glasses (if necessary) and that he has a good light. Visual materials which are large enough to be seen easily and which are clear and uncluttered should be used.

The nurse should find out about the patient's past experience and relate new material to it. Because older people have accumulated a vast store of experience, helping them to draw on it aids learning. She should always start with what the patient already knows and build on that. This precept means that at first the teacher listens to the patient. Only then can she know where to start. In the case of the 67-year-old woman with congestive heart failure, perhaps her husband was on a sodium-restricted diet many years ago, and she recalls how she prepared his meals. Can the patient obtain her digitalis when she needs more? What problems does she have, if any, in getting to the physician's office? Can she see the fine print on her vial of medicine? Perhaps she needs a magnifying glass to read it. How many stairs does this patient have to climb daily? Can groceries be delivered to her so that she does not have to carry them home? When can she rest during the day?

Learning is an important means of compensating for losses. For instance, the older person whose physical strength no longer permits him a career as an athlete may learn to be a manager or a sportswriter. Learning is also a means of reassurance that one still has the capacity to learn. Being able to master new knowledge and skill is important to self-esteem. Consider the blow which may come to the pride of a man in his late 60's who observes that the nurse is teaching his daughter how to administer his insulin injection without first evaluating whether he can learn this himself. Many times older people unnecessarily are denied the opportunity to learn new skills, thereby making it even more difficult for them to compensate for illness and disability and to continue their productive roles at work and in family life.

## PATTERNS OF AGING

Perhaps after a day of caring for several older people, some of whom have been cheerful and interesting while others have been cranky and tiresome, a young nurse has caught herself wondering what she will be like at that age. According to an old expression, as people grow older, they grow more like themselves. The old person who is cheerful and seems to be interested in everything probably has been that way for years; the person who views old age as an insuperable hardship may have found the problems of puberty and menopause insurmountable, too. Actually, preparation for later life is something that cannot be avoided. Whether planned or not, the attitudes and the abilities that individuals develop day by day will determine the kind of people they will be.

In spite of the deep truth in this statement, adults can learn and change. New opportunities and new experiences bring fresh insight to those who are alert and flexible enough to absorb them. One of the best ways to avoid the narrowness of view so often attributed to old age lies in maintaining a variety of interests and seeking new experiences.

Sometimes it is assumed that there is one successful pattern of aging. In our society continued active involvement in work and family affairs tends to be admired; therefore, those who adapt to aging in this way are especially likely to be considered successful. Others, however, adapt successfully by withdrawing somewhat from activities and relationships and investing more time and energy in solitary pursuits, such as gardening, reading, and reflection.

## DEVELOPMENTAL TASKS

Life does not cease making demands when the responsibilities of middle life have passed. In fact, some of the most difficult problems are reserved for the last part of life. Negative attitudes in our culture toward aging play a large part in aggravating the problems and decreasing the satisfactions of later life.

Society provides many educational opportunities for the young to learn to achieve the tasks set for the first half of life—tasks which are different from those of later life. For instance, during youth, emphasis is placed upon adapting to group norms, while in later life, the emphasis shifts toward development of greater individuation. Society places little emphasis on education for these significant tasks of later life. Some older people seek continued opportunities to learn and grow, through religious faith, psychotherapy, individual study and reflection, and their relationships with other sig-

nificant persons. But because some older people do not have plentiful opportunities for such enriching experiences, it is important for society to begin to develop educational programs for older people who wish help in adapting to physiologic and psychological changes and in dealing with the developmental tasks of later life.

**Dependence.** Many problems of aging revolve around dependence. People who live long enough (into their 80's and 90's) become, to some extent, dependent on others for companionship and often for financial support and physical care. Change from independence to dependence is usually gradual unless, for example, a sudden illness renders a previously self-sufficient person dependent.

Many older persons find dependence on others difficult to accept, even though they may recognize the necessity for it. Some of the elderly deny the need for any help, sometimes jeopardizing their own safety. Others readily become very dependent. Such older people tend to hang on to others, sometimes resulting in friction within the family as the demands for assurance exceed the capacities of others to meet them. Similar problems are observed in nursing homes in relationships between patients and nurses. In such instances the nurse should recognize the patient's needs for dependence and gradually help him to become more self-reliant. Ignoring the older person can cause him to redouble his efforts to gain the nurse's attention and support with a resultant increase of friction in the relationship. On the other hand, if the nurse shows interest and concern for the patient, the patient often begins to show interest in his progress also, initially to please the nurse, perhaps, and as a way of establishing a relationship with her, but later because he himself, with her help, has grown more self-reliant.

**Employment and Income.** One of the tasks of later life involves adjustment to decreased income. This is especially difficult, since in our society the degree of respect accorded a person depends to a great extent on his financial standing. Many factors are responsible for the economic plight of the elderly. Compulsory retirement is an important cause. Older people who are willing and able to work often find themselves at age 65 without any work to do and with a vastly decreased income. Physical decline also plays a part. Sometimes the individual's working life is terminated by an illness from which he never fully recovers. That more people are reaching old age means that the economic problems of this age group are multiplied many times.

That the attitudes of society have played a part in the problem is shown by the reluctance of employers to hire older workers. A popular stereotype characterizes the older worker as being prone to accidents and errors and frequently absent, slow, and unable to learn. There have been tendencies to emphasize the liabilities of age and to fail to recognize the assets which older workers possess. Studies have shown repeatedly that some aspects of this stereotype are not true and that others have been magnified beyond their true proportions. It is true, certainly, that the time needed for recovery from accidents or illness tends to increase with age. On the other hand, older workers tend to be careful, accurate, and dependable, although they are also likely to be slower than younger people and to have greater difficulty in adapting to change.

Employment opportunities for the elderly are lessening, not only because of prejudice against the abilities of older workers, but because of the need to provide jobs for younger workers. Due to technologic advances, increased leisure is apparently in store for all, and lack of paid employment among the elderly is, therefore, likely to increase.

To ease the problem of adaptation to increased leisure, some companies are helping workers plan for retirement and are initiating gradual rather than abrupt retirement. Under this type of plan the older worker may gradually work fewer and fewer hours until finally he stops working altogether. Such a plan gives the person more time to accustom himself to the changing pattern of work and leisure.

Attempts are being made to establish *more flexible retirement policies*. Older people who are able and willing to continue their work are being permitted to do so in some instances. Their work is re-evaluated periodically, and, when necessary, they may be transferred to less demanding types of work. However, there is little likelihood of widespread adoption of this approach, except in fields where there is a scarcity of trained personnel, because of the need to make jobs available for younger workers.

Much has already been achieved. Retirement and pension plans are more numerous than they were formerly. Yet resources continue to be meager for large segments of the population. Amounts of money available through pension plans and Social Security are often far less than is required for decent housing, food, and other necessities. The purchasing power of the dollar has declined precipitously, and many older people on fixed incomes lack the most fundamental necessities.

The type of work that an individual does has a bearing on his ability to continue it successfully into later life. Careers requiring great physical stamina, such as those in athletics, are notably short, whereas those which require many years of experience and personal contacts may be enhanced by added years. In the latter category might be listed such occupations as lawyer, salesman, physician, or clergyman. In contrast, unskilled laborers often experience decreasing income relatively early in life, since their work so largely depends on physical abilities.

Older people particularly need money to help them to overcome or to compensate for some of the infirmities of age. Medical expenses increase with age, and the older person is in need of services to carry out tasks now physically beyond his ability. Surely, wealthy older people are in a better position to cope with the physical decline of age than are the great majority of persons in this age group.

The enactment of federal legislation (Medicare) providing health benefits to the elderly has been an important advance in helping them to deal with the costs of health care. This program has also indirectly eased the burden for the families of some older people, since families often bore the entire cost of an elderly person's medical care.

Lack of money is not the only problem caused by retirement. Idleness, boredom, and loneliness often result, since work has absorbed so large a portion of most people's time and interest and has provided many contacts with other people. Because the ability to earn his way has been removed, a person may suffer from a loss of self-respect and feel that others are judging him as severely as he may be judging himself.

Retirement brings about a significant alteration (and in many instances) deprivation of social role. The individual's social role is linked to his occupation, be it bus driver, teacher, or salesman, and is an important factor in achieving social identity. Loss of the accustomed role requires a major shift in the individual's view of himself as he assumes a new role—that of a retired, rather than an active, worker. The individual who has developed interests and associations which are apart from his work and has developed a strong sense of personal identity is aided in coping with these changes.

**Time.** The problem of how to spend time looms large because the individual has so much free time. During his working life, the leisure after a day's work was highly prized because it was limited. Too much leisure may lead to feelings of futility and uselessness. Much has been written about the value of hobbies and interests in later life. However, older people tend not to develop new interests but to continue those they already have. There is an amazing continuity in interests throughout each individual's life. The interests developed throughout childhood and early adulthood tend to remain those of the later years. Of course, the manner in which he pursues them may change as time goes on. The boy who was interested in faraway places reads all the travel books he can find; later in life he may acquire the means and the opportunity to travel. Sometimes the added leisure of old age helps a person to develop dormant interests and talents—Grandma Moses picked up a paintbrush at 80. But most of us are essentially consistent in what we like to do. For instance, that man recovering from cirrhosis never has willingly read a book in his life. It is not likely that his enforced rest will turn him now into an enthusiatic scholar. However, he may be delighted to play cards with another patient.

When hobbies are developed during early and middle life, in later years they will be available to cushion the problem of too much spare time. Older women who have been housewives encounter less transition in this respect than do their husbands, whose retirement from work is often abrupt. The older woman continues her accustomed housekeeping duties, while her husband may feel out of place when he is at home all day.

For most people, however, hobbies do not provide a wholly satisfactory solution to the problems of increased leisure. Most individuals in our society have been taught that work is necessary, and that performing productive work is important in giving meaning to life. Hobbies are sometimes trivial; they may be merely measures to pass the time rather than to use time productively. The older person requires opportunities for meaningful, productive work and relationships—opportunities that are often lacking in various clubs for the elderly. The eager response of some older people to opportunities to serve, such as by helping disadvantaged children learn to read, underscores the need of older

persons to occupy their time usefully and productively.

**Loneliness.** The problem of loneliness is acute for most older people. Aside from losing contact with coworkers on the job after retirement, older people often suffer separation from family and friends. Inevitably, one spouse dies first. Since women live longer than men and tend to marry men somewhat older than themselves, there are more widows than widowers. Grown children often live at a considerable distance. Regardless of physical distance, the emotional and social distance between generations may be hard to bridge. The very old person outlives most of his contemporaries, and difficulties in travel make it hard for him to see old friends or to make new ones. Those who have developed interests and activities that they can enjoy alone are in a better position to cope with the problems of loneliness than those who have rarely undertaken any project or diversion by themselves. Being able to tolerate and to enjoy periods of being alone is an important asset at any age, but it is particularly important during later life. Like other abilities, it takes time to develop. It does not readily spring into being when one is old, but can be gradually acquired during youth and middle life.

The older person who has the capacity and energy to develop new relationships has an asset in dealing with loneliness. Some older persons seek situations, such as retirement villages, where they will have greater opportunities to meet people and form new friendships.

**Housing.** Housing is difficult for many older people from the standpoints of both money and companionship. Lack of money often forces them to find cheaper and less desirable accommodations. Usually, the new dwelling is smaller. The reduction in living space makes it necessary for the older person to part with many treasured objects accumulated over a lifetime, objects which he knows he will not replace. Older people sustain so many losses that they tend to cling to their possessions, sometimes hoarding objects that appear to others to be of little value.

Objects with which the individual must part may remind him of past accomplishments and relationships and, therefore, may be especially comforting to him. It is important that the elderly person be permitted to keep as many of his treasured possessions as possible, since they provide him with a link to his past and a comfortable feeling of "belonging here, among these things." Because being surrounded by familiar possessions provides environmental support, it is important to increase facilities for home care of the elderly and also to be as flexible as possible in permitting the older person to take some possessions with him if it becomes necessary for him to reside in an institution.

Efforts are being made to provide *more suitable housing* for older people at rents they can afford. Dwellings that emphasize safety and convenience offer fewer stairs, more handrails, wider doorways, and sometimes ramps to permit use of wheelchairs. Some small communities are being established for older people which combine a chance to live in apartments or small homes with such conveniences as an infirmary, shopping service, and recreational facilities.

Not surprisingly, the greatest need exists among those least able to pay for ideal retirement living. Their needs must be considered much more fully by the community, the state, and the nation. Some communities are establishing recreational and guidance centers for older people. Some centers serve a hot meal at noon, thus providing a place where older people who live in furnished rooms, with limited or nonexistent cooking facilities, may enjoy recreation and companionship as well as a good meal.

The plight of the elderly who live in meager furnished rooms is well publicized, and sometimes it is easy to generalize that this type of housing is typical of most older people. Actually, many older persons continue to live comfortably in homes or apartments of their own and to have the companionship of nearby family and friends.

Retirement communities and separate, smaller "retirement neighborhoods" made up of several housing developments for older persons have, despite their advantages, the disadvantages of limiting older people's contacts with younger people, and vice versa. People of different age groups seem to need contact with each other, and separate housing developments for the elderly seriously limit such contacts.

**Nursing Homes and Homes for the Elderly.** In response to the increasing number of older people, many more nursing homes and homes for the elderly have been established. Some of these are excellent, but others fall below adequate standards. Perhaps the most deplorable practice is that of placing indigent old people in publicly supported mental institutions simply because there is no other place for them to go or because symptoms of mental illness were not recognized and treated promptly. Older persons possess greater insight and flexibility than is generally attributed to them, and prompt psychotherapy could benefit many older persons and obviate their hospitalization.

Many older people, despite psychiatric diagnoses, such as depression or obsessive-compulsive state, can continue to live in the community, provided the environment is sufficiently supportive. Familiar surroundings, nearness of family, and opportunity to follow accustomed routines are examples of such support.

The tolerance of others for idiosyncrasies of behavior is another important factor in determining whether a patient is placed in a mental hospital. As age advances, some people become unmindful of social conventions. An elderly lady may wear ankle-length dresses and sneakers. If she is also inclined to ferret through trash left out for collection twice a week, her neighbors may decide she should be "put away." Differentiating between behavior which is eccentric, but not a hazard to oneself or others, and that which is hazardous or at least highly problematic for others, is difficult, and decisions may be quite variable, depending on such factors as the individual's socioeconomic status or where he lives (city or small town).

## Summary

In summary, the developmental tasks of later life include:

- Increasing self-knowledge; further integrating the facets of one's personality to a meaningful whole.
- Developing further one's spiritual life; recognizing and accepting life processes of growth and decline.
- Contributing experience and wisdom, gained through the years, to others.
- Maintaining a satisfactory home.
- Fostering close ties with family: spouse, grown children, aging siblings.
- Adjusting to retirement and (usually) to reduced income.
- Maintaining health as effectively and as long as possible; learning to live with diminished strength and vigor and sometimes with physical disabilities.
- Maintaining ties with the community: neighbors, friends, clubs, church.
- Adjusting to loss of spouse and friends of long standing.
- Facing death.

## SOME JOYS OF LATER LIFE

What about the joys of later life? For those whose lives have prepared them for it, there may be opportunities for many activities previously impossible because of the lack of time. In one sense older people have immense quantities of time at their disposal. In another sense they are nearing the end of their lives, and they realize the preciousness of the time left to them. Some older people with lively minds and eager curiosity take courses in subjects which have always interested them. Others rekindle interests in art, music, furniture refinishing, cooking or embroidery. Some older people experience gains during later life, stating that they are happier in many ways than they had been previously. Possibly the fact that most of the writing about the elderly is done by persons who have not yet reached this phase of life is relevant to the emphasis upon the negative aspects of aging.

As more older people are helped to live fuller and healthier lives, attitudes toward aging may become more positive. If young people have contact with older persons who are independent and active, their views about aging may become more optimistic. Nurses and physicians tend, by the nature of their work, to have considerable contact with elderly people who are in ill health and who are not coping well with the problems of daily life. Unless this is recognized as a possible influence on one's attitudes toward aging, physicians and nurses may, without being aware of it, develop rather pessimistic views.

The longer one lives the more time one has to know oneself and to understand others better. Of course, some people just live longer and learn little in the process. But older people have more opportunity to develop fine judgment and are able, thanks to experience, to make the knife-sharp distinction between the time to act and the time not to act. Whereas young people have a tendency to see things as black or white, the older person often has greater tolerance for ambiguity and, at the same time, a greater clarity about his own goals and strengths. An 18-year-old, of necessity, wastes time and energy in discovering the limitations of his own abilities. A 70-year-old can channel his energies better. He knows that he will never be a physicist, for example, and can be patient with the floundering of others. The older person has been through a career, marriage, expectations that failed to come true, and some ambitions that did. From this wealth of experience he may have achieved perspective that can only be envied by those younger than he.

## NURSING CONSIDERATIONS

**Attitudes.** Care of the elderly can evoke varied reactions within the nurse. On the one hand, it can be an unpleasant reminder that she too will grow old and die; it may remind her of troubling aspects in her own relationship with aging parents; or she may find the physical appearance of the elderly distasteful, since it does not exemplify youthful attractiveness. These reactions may lead the nurse to avoid older patients and possibly even to treat them with condescension.

On the other hand, the nurse may idealize the elderly person, perhaps in response to family teachings that older people are wise and have earned a place of honor and respect. The nurse who has idealized the elderly, viewing them as being benevolent and kindly and generously sharing their wisdom with the young, may also do an injustice to her older patients, by expecting them to exemplify her ideal of the elderly. Thus nurses who have a very negative or a very positive stereotype of older people may fail to take account of an individual patient's strengths and weaknesses.

One's views of aging can be made more realistic, perhaps, by remembering that the elderly are a disadvantaged group in our society. They are disadvantaged in relation to income, employment, housing, health, and companionship—to name but some of the important ways in which most older people do not share equally with those who are younger. While the disadvantaged may become more patient, tolerant, and generous, in many instances the reverse is true—they may become selfish, resentful, and demanding. The latter characteristics are sometimes attributed to older people on the basis of their age, whereas such characteristics, when observed, may actually reflect the individual's deprivations more than his chronologic age. In addition, some people simply are more pleasant to be with than others—a fact which is true during every period of their life.

**Physical Care.** Perhaps the older person's need to adjust to increasing physical limitations is the problem most familiar to nurses. Older people need gradually increasing amounts of help with self-care as their own ability to care for themselves diminishes. The thoughtful nurse will plan for this need, and she will help the patient's family to do so.

Many older people do not receive the kind of physical care they require. Sometimes it seems especially hard for others to carry out these measures. Neglecting the physical needs of the elderly is quite common in hospitals, too. It is not unusual for a nurse to say, "I can do these things for a baby. I expect him to be helpless. But with an old person—" Most people do not feel that the elderly have the appealing quality in their helplessness that infants possess. They do not seem to be cute or attractive, or perhaps no one expects them to be helpless. Nevertheless, if people live long enough (into the 80's and 90's), there comes a time when they need assistance with personal hygiene. Recognition of this necessity can help the nurse to plan for and to give this care and to teach family members to do so, too. Very old people become forgetful and unmindful of details, but it is not kind to allow them to have poor hygiene. Old people may develop severe scalp irritations, excoriated skin, and pressure sores which cause discomfort and pain.

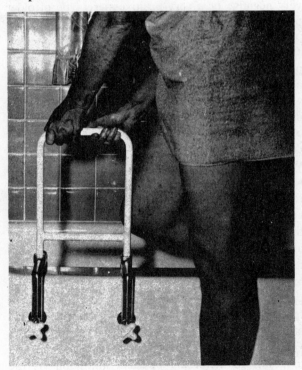

**Figure 5-3.** An attachable grab bar for bathtubs helps to prevent falls. (Bollen Products, Cleveland, Ohio)

Nurses who work in settings where many of the patients are very old and feeble sometimes experience feelings of anger and helplessness. Massive helplessness of patients can seem overwhelming and may be one reason why necessary nursing care is sometimes neglected. Not every nurse is equipped emotionally or interestwise to work with large numbers of geriatric patients, just as not every nurse can function comfortably in a pediatric ward. Awareness of her own particular assets and of areas in nursing where these can be utilized most effectively is essential to making the nurse's best contribution.

The prevention of physical discomfort is not the only reason for emphasizing the physical care of older people. It also helps them to maintain dignity and self-respect. Contrast the demeanor of the neglected old person with that of one whose snow-white hair is neatly coiffed, whose skin is clean and healthy, and whose dress is attractive. In speaking of self-respect the following point should be made clear: the nurse should make it a rule to call each patient by name. To address an older person by his own name, rather than as "Pop" or some other patronizing nickname, helps the older person to maintain his dignity and identity.

In addition to the general principles of personal hygiene which apply to anyone, certain other aspects of physical care are especially important for older people. The older person should be encouraged to care for himself as much as possible as long as he is able. Many devices are available to encourage self-help, such as tub seats, which enable the older person to take a tub bath without sitting all the way down in the tub, and handrails, which can be grasped by the older person as he gets in and out of the tub (Fig. 5-3). Ingenuity can suggest many similar devices.

**Skin Care.** Because circulation to the extremities is often poor in older people, care of the feet and the toenails is important. Lessened circulation may cause injuries or infections to heal poorly and even become gangrenous. Because the skin on the legs and the feet is usually very dry, cream or lotion should be used after bathing. Thickened, brittle nails should be trimmed carefully, a little at a time. Soften the nails first by soaking the patient's feet in warm water. Very thick nails that have been neglected may need the attention of a chiropodist. If an elderly person's feet are cold, bedsocks and extra blankets are a help. Hot-water bags and electric pads should be used cautiously because they may cause burns. The combination of diminished sensation and lessened circulation makes this danger more acute in the elderly.

Since the skin of older people tends to be dry and scaly, alcohol should not be used as a back lotion, because it is drying. Instead, cream or creamy lotion should be used. Frequent hot baths also tend to be drying. Instead of a daily tub bath, patients may have a partial bath on alternate days. It is important that all the soap be rinsed off the skin, since soap dried on the skin can be irritating. Friction from clothing and bedding should be minimized. For example, sleeves on the patient's gown should be kept down over his elbows to decrease irritation that can be caused by rubbing against the sheets.

Bath oil is helpful in overcoming dryness of the skin. However, when it is used, particular care must be taken to prevent the patient from slipping in the tub. A rubber mat is essential so that the older person does not step on a tub made slippery by bath oil.

A stall shower is desirable for use by the elderly, since it avoids the problem of stepping over the side of a tub, and lowering oneself into the tub. If the patient is weak and unsteady on his feet, a chair may be placed underneath the shower, making it possible for the patient to bathe while seated. The shower provides for the most thorough rinsing of soap from the skin, thus helping to minimize skin irritations so common in the elderly. Whatever method of bathing is used, particular care must be taken to insure privacy, since many older people are especially distressed when they cannot maintain their usual standards of personal modesty.

Older women sometimes have problems with slight incontinence of urine when they are coughing or sneezing (stress incontinence) or with vaginal discharge. Late in life the vaginal mucous membrane becomes thin and subject to infection. If the nurse or a family member notices that this problem exists, the physician should be consulted. He may recommend, among other treatments, a cleansing douche. Help the patient to keep clean through perineal care and use of disposable pads, if necessary.

**General Appearance.** Increased facial hair may be distressing to elderly women. It may be removed by careful cutting or shaving or by the use of a depilatory. Older men may need help with shaving. Tactful reminders and provision of enough clean clothing will help the patient to maintain his appearance. A predictable routine for changing clothing is helpful; for example, place clean clothes on the patient's bed for him to wear when he has finished bathing.

**Teeth.** Dentures require regular cleaning and brushing. If removed, they should be stored in an opaque covered jar. Instruct the patient not to roll them in tissues, because if they are so concealed they can be easily thrown away or lost. If helping the patient to clean his dentures, the nurse should put them in a small basin and take them to the sink to clean them. She should avoid holding them directly over the sink—they are easily dropped and broken.

**Elimination.** Elimination may pose particular problems in the elderly. Frequency of urination is not uncommon—many older men have hypertrophy of the prostate; older women often have relaxation of perineal structures with less efficient emptying of the bladder. Symptoms of frequent urination should be noted carefully and reported to the physician. At the same time care must be taken to prevent falls when the patient gets up during the night. Leaving a urinal or a bedpan within easy reach is often helpful.

Some older people have difficulty with constipation; this is likely to be especially troublesome to those who cannot get up and move around. Helping the patient to maintain adequate dietary and fluid intake and to have a regular time for evacuation may be the remedy. Sometimes enemas or mild cathartics are ordered by the physician. (See Chapter 6 for a discussion of the problem of incontinence which sometimes occurs in elderly patients who are deprived of significant human relationships.)

**Effects of Bed Rest.** Being confined to bed has adverse effects on older people. The decrease in activity causes a loss in muscle tone and frequently results in extreme weakness which is often difficult to overcome. Respiratory difficulties also may develop, since older people expand their chests less fully because of loss of elasticity of structures that increase and decrease the size of the thoracic cavity. Confinement to bed accentuates this problem and often leads to the development of hypostatic pneumonia. Decubitus ulcers are also common in the bedridden because of the lessened ability of the skin and subcutaneous tissues to tolerate pressure. Confinement to bed often intensifies the problem of decreased circulation which occurs in elderly people. Diminished circulation to the brain may cause disorientation.

In view of these complications, physicians usually permit elderly patients out of bed as soon as possible. As soon as he is able, the patient should be encouraged and helped to take a few steps and gradually to increase his activities. Older people, especially if they are weak from illness, have a tendency to stoop. It is important to encourage good posture at all times, whether the patient is in bed, sitting in a chair, or walking about. Providing a change of scenery by helping the patient to the sitting room or the porch is a boost to morale. When the nurse knows that the patient will be allowed up shortly, she should ask his family to bring his clothes, particularly his shoes. Paper slippers and long sashes on bathrobes may cause falls.

**Drug Reactions.** Elderly patients often have idiosyncratic reactions to drugs. For instance, barbiturates frequently cause confusion and disorientation rather than the relaxation and rest desired. Thus, it is very important that the nurse note carefully the elderly patient's response to drugs.

**Possessions.** Since older people tend to hoard things, it is sometimes necessary to help them sort out their treasures. The older person should participate and be consulted about things to be thrown away. Institutionalized older patients should have enough space to keep some of their possessions with them. In a busy general hospital, space often poses a problem, and the patient, stripped of all possessions but a few toilet articles, may begin to collect packets of sugar or wrappers that cover drinking straws! Rather than hastily cleaning out his stand, the nurse may persuade him to part with some of his possessions and to store others neatly in a small box. Helping the patient to feel more secure and at home in the hospital, as well as finding diversions that interest him, may decrease his tendency toward hoarding.

**Pace.** The older patient is slower in his movements and responses than a younger one. Attempts to make him hurry often result in confusion, irritation, and accidents. It is wise to plan nursing care so that the older patient has more time for his activities. For instance, since he eats slowly, serve him his tray first and collect it last. The thoughtful nurse will prepare everything the patient needs for self-care and then let him proceed at his own pace to complete those aspects of care that he can tend to

himself. Explanations of tests and treatments should be made slowly and, if necessary, repeated.

Even comparatively minor illnesses or injuries can have serious consequences for the older person, because they can tip the already precarious balance from independence to dependence. For example, if a 20-year-old student breaks her arm, resulting in some pain and inconvenience, her mother can cut her meat for her and help her dress, but her school work is hardly interrupted at all. If a 75-year-old woman breaks her arm, she may become somewhat confused and may be weak and tremulous for several weeks. If her husband is dead or also physically incapacitated, both may have to spend a few months living with relatives—a situation that can easily result in family tensions. Only after two or three months will the older woman be able to get about and care adequately for her husband and apartment.

This illustration emphasizes the need for helping the disabled older person to regain his independence as promptly as possible. Often, the older individual unnecessarily gives up some of his usual activities because others (and sometimes the patient himself) are too quick to assume that the patient will never be able to resume these activities.

**Safety.** The hospital environment presents certain hazards for the older patient. The high beds are a potential danger, since the elderly person may misjudge the distance to the floor and fall as he is getting up. Hi-lo beds, which are adjustable, are ideal in permitting the ambulatory patient to get out of bed easily. If high beds are used, a sturdy footstool should be put in place. It is wise to leave a dim light burning in the older patient's room during the night to enable him to orient himself more readily to his surroundings as he awakens, and to prevent him from falling if he gets up. Some older persons need side rails at night to remind them where the edges of the bed are and to discourage attempts at getting out of bed. If these are necessary, their use should always be explained to the patient, so that he does not feel imprisoned in his bed. His call bell should always be handy; otherwise, he may try to climb over the side rails to go to the bathroom.

Older people sometimes do not require as much sleep as younger ones. This may present a problem when a hospital room is shared with others. Keeping the patient awake and interested during the day often helps him to sleep better at night. If he awakens very early in the morning, some quiet diversion, such as reading, should be encouraged so that he does not waken his roommates. Whenever possible, it is preferable to encourage sleep by relying on general nursing measures rather than on drugs.

**Contact with Reality.** Even without the use of drugs, nighttime confusion and disorientation are common among the elderly and present a particular problem when an older person is moved away from his familiar surroundings to a hospital or nursing home. These episodes of confusion, which are especially likely to occur at night, are disturbing to the patient and to others and present a hazard to the patient's safety. The frequency and severity of these periods of confusion can usually be reduced by nursing measures, thereby lessening the stress of the hospitalization experience for the patient and others. Unfortunately, mismanagement of this problem is very common and can cause the patient to become more confused and disturbed. Initial attempts to control him and to lessen the noise he makes may take the form of scolding him and quickly closing the door of his room so that other patients are not awakened. Sometimes restraints are quickly applied before other measures are tried. These actions quite predictably increase the patient's agitation. If he becomes more agitated and confused, orders for sedation may be sought. The sedative itself sometimes exacerbates the problem. Often the use of restraints and sedatives can be avoided, if certain nursing measures are used to calm the patient.

If an elderly patient becomes noisy and confused, the nurse should go to him calmly, turn on a soft light (in addition to the night light, which should already be on), quietly explain where he is and who she is, and take hold of his hand as a further measure in establishing contact with him. (Occasionally, touching the patient leads to further agitation. She should note his reaction and guide her actions accordingly.)

Often these episodes are precipitated when the patient awakens from a dream and has difficulty distinguishing between reality and the dream. Sometimes the episode is precipitated by the patient's awakening because he needs to void. Still half asleep, he attempts to get out of bed to go to the bathroom, notes the side rails which, in the dim light, may make him feel "caged in." Unfamiliar surroundings, plus the urgency of the need to void, can add to his mounting fright. He may call out and become more confused and agitated. The more the nurse can do to help the patient orient himself to his surroundings and to her presence, the calmer he is likely to become. After initial measures to help the patient become calmer, she should ask him quietly what is troubling him. Usually the patient's agitation diminishes enough so that he can realize what the difficulty is—such as that he needs the urinal or that he had a frightening dream. If he speaks as though the dream *were* reality, such as by saying, "My son was just here," she can point out that it is the middle of the night and that his son was not there and ask him if perhaps it was a dream. Sometimes a glass of warm milk or a cup of tea has a calming effect and further assists the patient to reorient himself to the real world. Usually these nursing actions will result in the patient's being ready to go back to sleep. Before she leaves him, the nurse should remind the patient of the location of his call bell, of the fact that she will leave his door open and the night light on, and that he should press his call bell whenever he needs her.

Measures to help the patient maintain his contact with reality are, of course, necessary at other times as well and can serve to prevent somewhat the occurrence of episodes of acute confusion. When an individual is advanced in age or when illness has prematurely cut short what might have been productive later years, his disengagement from society (and of society from him) fosters preoccupation with fantasy, sometimes to the point where it is difficult for the individual to distinguish fantasy from reality, and past events and relationships from present events and relationships. Under such circumstances the nurse can help the patient strengthen his contact with reality by talking with him, and finding ways to stimulate his interest and participation in the environment so that he is not so isolated or detached. Rather than "routinely" bathing the patient, the nurse can encourage his observation and participation by asking whether the water is comfortably warm, whether his skin feels dry, and so forth. Since most older people have diminished vision and hearing, it is particularly important to see that they have their glasses and (if one is used) their hearing aid, to help them become tuned in to the environment. Turning up the volume on the TV set and obtaining books written in large print are examples of other measures which the nurse can take to help the patient maintain his sense of reality through contact with the environment.

The nurse's expectations have an important effect upon the patient. If the nurse expects her elderly patients to be disoriented and forgetful, they are more likely to be so. In contrast, the nurse who converses with her elderly patients in a way which shows she expects them to be capable of responding and remembering is likely to foster this behavior. Much depends, of course, on the patient's capacities; it is essential to evaluate his abilities and to gear expectations realistically.

The nurse who speaks slowly and distinctly and who presents one suggestion or request at a time, rather than a rapid barrage of instructions, is facilitating the older person's ability to respond and is showing that she considers him capable of doing so. There is no quicker way for an older person to lose ability to care for himself than to be in a situation where he is treated as though this capacity has already been lost. The older person senses that he is no longer considered capable of managing such tasks as storing his dentures safely in the jar on his stand or cleaning them himself; he gives over these self-care functions, which help him maintain some privacy, independence, and contact with reality. A vicious circle may ensue, in which the members of the staff grow more impatient with the elderly person's detachment and less inclined to talk with him or to encourage his participation. He, in turn, turns more and more to his inner world of fantasy. Meaningful relationships are an important measure in helping the patient to maintain contact with reality; thus, the relationship with the nurse can be significant.

**Group Participation.** Of equal significance, if not more so, is the patient's relationship with others, especially other patients and older people. Patient interaction through group experiences can significantly reduce the patient's isolation and help him to maintain his contact with reality. Through group discussions patients can discuss common health problems, such as constipation and poorly fitting dentures, and can learn how to deal with them. They can encourage one another to seek medical care as needed and to follow prescribed treatment. Carrying out treatment requires hope, and group support is one way of giving the patient a sense of hope.

Even disoriented patients can be helped by group interaction. Through group participation, some patients previously quite disoriented gradually become more attuned to reality. The support of the leader and the group members, plus the stimulation of contact with the group, serve as a magnet to pull these patients toward reality. As they become better oriented, they find greater opportunities for participation and greater willingness of others to interact with them.

A focus on physical care to cope with the effects of disorientation and loss of social skills can lead to overreliance on such modalities as bibs, restraining sheets, and so forth, to the neglect of the powerful effects of group support and participation in helping the older person revive some of his social skills and his orientation to reality.

Of course, group discussions among older people can be conducted by nurses in many settings, other than the hospital. A nurse may regularly conduct such a group once or twice weekly among older residents of a housing development, at a golden age club in the community, or in a nursing home. The focus of the meetings may be on daily problems of living and can provide opportunities for socialization and contact with reality. Topics of concern may include coping with bureaucratic procedures to obtain Social Security checks and health benefits, dealing with loneliness, finding ways to occupy one's time, protecting oneself from crime, getting along with grown children, coping with the loss of a spouse, facing death. Contacts made in the group may also foster the members' ability and interest in helping one another at times other than the scheduled meetings. For example, one group set up a system for telephoning other older people living alone in their community. These calls, made on a daily basis or more often if necessary, helped the recipients to feel someone's concern for them and provided friendly, predictable contact and the offer of help when needed. These older people gave each other companionship and some feeling of security. They also saved several lives by calling an ambulance when the person they were telephoning failed to answer and was subsequently discovered at home having suffered a cerebral vascular accident, a myocardial infarction, or diabetic acidosis. Those who did the telephoning had the satisfaction of helping others and participating in very useful work.

## Summary

Caring for older people can be interesting and satisfying. Because they have lived so long, they have had experiences very different from ours. The passage of time and the changes in our civilization make it unlikely that we shall ever have these experiences ourselves, but through association with older people we can share their experiences. Most of us have never chased rattlesnakes off the front porch or fought in World War I. These and countless other experiences can come alive for us through the reminiscenses of older people.

Some nurses believe that the elderly should not talk about the past but, instead, must be engaged in conversation solely about present and future events. For many elderly persons, however, daily events are relatively insignificant in comparison with events in the past. Is it any wonder that a retired archeologist may sometimes prefer to reminisce about his explorations in far-off lands, rather than sticking to conversation about card parties held in the nursing home? One need of the elderly involves assessing past events, achievements, and losses and integrating these life experiences. The nurse who insists that the patient talk only of the present and future interferes with this task, in the mistaken belief that she is "keeping him from living in the past." The patient requires opportunities to talk about past, present, and future in ways that are useful to him. Sometimes nurses discourage patients from talking about death; nevertheless, this is a major life experience which the elderly face. Is it any wonder some of them wish to talk about it?

Finally, it is important to remember that older people give a sense of continuity and stability amid the rapid changes of modern living. Because they are likely to adopt changes more slowly and cautiously, they can provide a balance for the impatience, the shortsightedness, and the eagerness of youth. If we recognize that the older person has something valuable to contribute at home, at work, and in the community, we can have a part in helping him to maintain his health and to continue to make his unique contribution as long as possible.

## NURSING ASSESSMENT

As mentioned previously, the sections on assessment in Chapters 3 and 4 may be useful in assessing all patients, old as well as young. The following suggestions may be especially relevant in the assessment of the elderly patient:

- What are the patient's physical capabilities? Consider particularly: vision, hearing, teeth, balance and position sense, physical agility, speed and coordination in such activities as walking, dressing, and eating; tolerance for exercise.

- Are his habits conducive to maintaining health? Consider exercise, diet, care of teeth and dentures, bowel hygiene, sleep, consideration for personal safety.
- Does he seem well-oriented psychologically? Friendly toward others? Does he remember recent events well? Does he seem interested in what goes on in the world? Does he find enjoyable and useful ways to occupy his time?
- How does the patient compensate for physical decrements? Glasses? Hearing aid? Dentures? Cane? (The ability and resourcefulness of the patient in compensating are very important.)
- If the patient has such disabilities as loss of memory or a tendency to lose himself in fantasy, how does he counteract them? (A small notebook in which he writes necessary daily information helps; making a schedule for his day, including such activities as taking walks, time to chat with others, and daily tasks, can help control a tendency to withdraw into fantasy.)
- Who are the patient's close associates? It is essential to think flexibly and not just in terms of conventional family ties. Does the patient live with a friend? Have pets? Does he have friendly neighbors? Does he have close family?
- Does the patient have ways of exercising his competence and usefulness? Does he receive recognition of his competence? It is important to think broadly and not just in terms of paid employment.
- Does the patient seek help readily when he needs it? Does he call the doctor? Go to the clinic? Ask friends for help?
- Does the patient have religious and philosophical beliefs which support him and help him find meaning in his life?
- Are the patient's financial resources adequate? Is there enough money for a pleasant, safe place to live, for food, recreation, for health care?
- Does the patient have opportunity for varied social contacts?
- Does the patient have opportunities to give and receive affection?

## REFERENCES AND BIBLIOGRAPHY

BROWN, L. J., and RITTER, J. I.: Reality therapy for the geriatric psychiatric patient, *Perspec. in Psych. Care* X, 3:135, 1972.

BURNSIDE, I. M.: *Psychosocial Nursing: Care of the Aged,* New York, McGraw-Hill, 1973.

CARLSON, S.: Communication and social interaction in the aged, *Nurs. Clin. N. Am.* 7:269, June 1972.

CONTI, M. L.: The loneliness of old age, *Nurs. Outlook* 18:28, August 1970.

CULBERT, P. A., and KOS, B. A.: Aging. Considerations for health teaching, *Nurs. Clin. N. Am.* 6:605, December 1971.

CUMMINGS, E., and HENRY, W. F.: *Disengagement,* New York, Basic Books, 1961.

DE BEAUVOIR, S.: *The Coming of Age,* New York, Putnam, 1972.

HAHN, J., and BURNS, K.: Mrs. Richards, a rabbit, and remotivation, *Am. J. Nurs.* 73:302, February 1973.

JENNINGS, M., et al.: Physiologic functioning in the elderly, *Nurs. Clin. N. Am.* 7:237, June 1972.

KURTAGH, C.: Nursing in the life span of people. *Nurs. Forum* 7:298, 1969.

LANE, H. C.: Protecting and supporting the elderly, *Nurs. Clin. N. Am.* 7:253, June 1972.

LARSON, L.: How to select a nursing home, *Am. J. Nurs.* 69:1034, May 1969.

LEVINE, R. L.: Disengagement in the elderly—its causes and effects, *Nurs. Outlook* 17:28, October 1969.

MCFARLAND, R. A., et al.: On the driving of automobiles by older persons, *J. Geront.* 19:190, 1964.

MOSES, D. V.: Reality orientation in the aged person, *Behavior Concepts and Nursing Intervention,* C. E. Carlson (ed.), Philadelphia, Lippincott, 1970.

_____: Assessing behavior in the elderly, *Nurs. Clin. N. Am.* 7:225, June 1972.

NEUGARTEN, B. L.: Biological and psychological aspects of aging, in *Selected Readings in Aging,* St. Louis, Gerontological Society, 1968.

ROBERTS, J. M.: Loneliness, *Perspec. in Psych. Care* 10:227, December 1972.

ROSEN, S., et al.: Presbycusis study of a relatively noise-free population in the Sudan, *Ann. Otol.* 71:727, 1962.

ROSS, E. K.: *On Death and Dying,* New York, Macmillan, 1969.

SCHWARTZ, D., et al.: *The Elderly Ambulatory Patient,* New York, Macmillan, 1964.

SHANAS, E.: *The Health of Older People,* Cambridge, Harvard University Press, 1962.

_____, et al.: *Old People in Three Industrial Societies,* New York, Atherton Press, 1968.

STONE, V.: Give the older person time, *Am. J. Nurs.* 69:2124, October 1969.

TALLMAN, M., et al.: Disengagement and the stages of aging, *J. Geront.* 24:70, January 1969.

TAYLOR, J., and GAITZ, C.: Obstacles encountered in the rehabilitation of geriatric patients, *Nurs. Forum* 7:64, 1969.

UJHELY, G. B.: The environment of the elderly, *Nurs. Clin. N. Am.* 7:281, June 1972.

WAHL, A.: Who are the elderly? In *Selected Readings in Aging,* St. Louis, Gerontological Society, 1968.

WEISS, A.: *Nurses, Patients, and Social Systems,* Columbia, Missouri, University of Missouri Press, 1968.

WILKIEMEYER, D. S.: Affection: Key to care for the elderly, *Am. J. Nurs.* 72:2166, December 1972.

YALOM, I., and TERRAZAS, F.: Group therapy for psychotic elderly patients, *Am. J. Nurs.* 68:1690, August 1968.

ZORZOLI, A.: Biomedical factors in aging, in *Selected Readings in Aging,* St. Louis, Gerontological Society, 1968.

# Nurse-Patient Relationships

## CHAPTER 6

An awareness by the nurse of the diverse effects that illness can have on the patient and his family affects the atmosphere that she creates on the ward. A manner that is warm, but not prying, and that shows willingness to let patients be themselves can help a patient to cope with his problems, whether or not he chooses to discuss them. An environment in which there is flexibility in applying rules and encouragement of participation in diversional activities helps patients to feel less restricted and less helpless. The nurse can create an atmosphere which at least does not make the problem worse.

Consider the following statements which a nurse made in one day: "You can't stand in the hall. Patients are not allowed in the hall." "I smelled smoke in your bathroom. You must have sneaked a cigarette." "Visiting hours are OVER. Can't you see that it's five minutes past?" "There's to be no card playing in this room. You're too noisy when you play cards." These approaches not only are rude; they are dehumanizing. People can cope with their worries better when they are treated with respect.

The restrictions imposed by hospital life are harder to bear when the nurse gives the impression that the routine is more important than the person, and that her control of the ward counts more than the patients' feelings. It would have been more helpful in the above example to allow, even to encourage, the patients to play cards and to socialize, recognizing that this can alleviate tension and boredom. Imposing needless, and sometimes trivial, restrictions can increase feelings of frustration and anger, particularly in patients who have already been denied many freedoms usually taken for

63

granted, such as freedom to come and go, to conduct business, and to live with their families. If, in the course of the card game, the patients become noisy it would be preferable to discuss this with them, helping them to recognize the need to lower their voices, or if possible, finding them a place to play away from the sicker patients.

## THE NEEDS OF THE MEDICAL-SURGICAL PATIENT

There are numerous ways in which general knowledge about nurse-patient relationships can be adapted to the particular requirements of medical-surgical patients.

- In most instances the medical-surgical patient has sought care for some physical condition; this condition may, of course, be aggravated by emotional stress or even be caused by it. Usually, however, the patient's attention and the focus of his treatment are on his bodily ailment. Keeping in mind that the patient's attention is usually on his physical condition and that he is not primarily concerned with seeking personal counseling will help you set the tone for your relationship with him. Your ability to give emotional support and counseling will be enhanced by recognition of the patient's view of why he is seeking treatment (e.g., to control the bleeding of his peptic ulcer).
- Caring for medical-surgical patients requires a high degree of ability to consider both the physical care of the patient and his emotional reactions to illness and treatment. Often you will be able to combine these two aspects of care, particularly as you gain more experience. You will find that you can listen to the patient while you bathe him or make his bed, as well as during the times when you sit down to talk with him. Also, the way that you provide physical care constitutes an important aspect of your relationship with the patient. Is your touch rough or gentle? When you assist him out of bed, do your motions convey firmness and support or are they gingerly and hesitant?
- Remember that others, too, may be giving the patient emotional support. Keeping this in mind will help you to maintain perspective about your relationship with the patient, so that you are less likely to conclude that supporting him emotionally is solely up to you. This is rarely the case. Particularly in the general hospital, many patients keep in touch with relatives, clergy, and friends, as well as with a personal physician. In long-term and geriatric settings the patient is likely to be more isolated from contact with other significant persons. Usually, however, you are one of the people to whom a patient may turn with emotional problems. If he turns to others primarily, it is by no means necessarily an adverse reflection on the care you give. If you interpret it as such, you may interfere with the patient's relationships with others at a time when he particularly needs to maintain his ties with them.
- Frightening and painful procedures are common on medical-surgical units. Although at first you are a stranger to the patient, the stress of experiences such as undergoing surgery can lead the patient to rely on you more quickly and more fully for emotional support than would be likely if he were not faced with these experiences.
- Medical-surgical patients are often more outwardly poised than is likely to be the case among pediatric, geriatric, or psychiatric patients. One of your challenges in working with this group of patients will involve not only helping them maintain poise in stressful circumstances (when the patient shows that to do so is important to him), but also encouraging expression of personal feelings.
- Care of medical-surgical patients involves a good deal of physical contact. Be alert for the slight tensing of muscles which enables you to feel, rather than see, that the patient does not welcome being touched. If you notice this reaction, be especially deft and quick in your ministrations. Avoid leaning over him as you bathe him and make the bed. People vary in the amount of physical closeness they can tolerate without discomfort. If a person is up and about, he can step back when others stand too close. However, the patient confined to bed must rely on others' perceptiveness of his reactions.
- There is enormous variety among medical-surgical patients: variety of age, diagnosis, and degree of illness—to name but three variables. Some patients will be completely helpless; others will seem able to care for themselves. Your approaches to these groups of patients will be different.

## OVERVIEW

You may be better at one mode of care than others. Working with a patient who is relatively self-sufficient may be more satisfying than working with a patient who is comparatively helpless. Or perhaps it is the other way around. The most important thing is that you know in which situation you are most comfortable. The more realistically you are aware of your own needs, the better care you will be able to give to all your patients. How you function with patients will depend largely on the goals you set for yourself in nursing. You can be an angel of mercy, but you may be a frustrated one (and therefore less effective) if you imagine yourself flying through the wards, relieving all suffering as you go. If you see yourself coddling and mothering patients, know that there are times when a patient needs coddling and mothering more than anything else; but the next day or week that same patient may need to do things for himself. Will this change threaten your need, your self-concept so much that you cannot do justice to his new requirements? If you prefer to think of yourself as an adviser to patients who are able to care for themselves physically, will you also have the tender touch for the patient who is totally dependent on your care? The change from the dependence of illness to the relative self-sufficiency of convalescence may be difficult for the patient—and for you as well. Will you be able to adjust the relationship between you in response to the patient's changed state?

Eventually, you will be able to choose the work in which your own goals and needs are met best. In the meantime you have to function in all kinds of situations. The more flexible you can be, the more service you will be able to give your patients, and the more satisfaction you will have from a job well done.

The following points provide some basic guidelines for nurse-patient relationships applicable in any setting:

- **Be yourself.** You can borrow techniques from someone you admire, but do not try to imitate someone else. Sick people are perceptive, anxious, and suspicious, even if they do not show it. If they feel your genuineness, they will be better able to trust you.

- **Small points of care are important to the sick.** Reactions to something as personal as illness are not always logical and rational. The big fact of recovering may be lost in the little annoyance of being served cold coffee. But if the patient feels your interest in him, your concern for his welfare and comfort, he is less likely to become angry.

- **Size up the situation between your patient and yourself.** Do not rush in with too many busy activities at once, unless they are of vital necessity to the patient. Learn early in your career to get the feel of your patient. What is his general condition? What is he expressing? Is he in pain? Does he seem to be resigned or apprehensive? What does his attitude do to you? Can you accept it, or do you feel a need to change it? If a patient looks as if he were sinking because he has slipped down in bed, of course you will want to change this position by lifting him up. However, if he is angry or whiny, can you accept this mood and not deny him his feelings?

 Sometimes it helps to start the day's relationship by an objective, bland phrase like "How did you sleep?" Do not use terms suggesting values, such as "It is a nice day," or "You are looking better now." He may be furious that it is a nice day outside and he is tied down to his bed for another six weeks with a broken leg. Maybe he is afraid of what will happen when he gets out of the hospital, and your statement that he is looking better only frightens him more. If you discuss your problems, you give him an opportunity to misinterpret what you are saying. If you tell him how busy you are because another nurse did not come to work, he probably will conclude that you are too busy to bother with him.

 A question like "Well, how are things going?" will give the patient an opening, and if you quietly wait or in an unbusy fashion go about your business at the bedside, he may start talking to you. Don't expect to be reassured by the patient. If he says, "Fine," but does not look as if he meant it, do not say, "Good," because again you would be cutting him off from expressing how he really feels. It often helps to repeat the patient's statement or to summarize it. This response will give him an opening to say more, if he wishes. To put your patient in the position of having to say what he thinks is expected of him is undesirable, because this might not correspond at all to his true feelings. It is all too easy to indicate to a patient what he should feel, and he will often parrot back what he thinks the nurse wants to hear.

- Guard yourself from another very common pitfall. Suppose the patient says that he feels "terrible." You may not know what to say next. You do not want him to feel terrible, and you are there to help him, but you do not know what to do about it. Accept the statement that he feels terrible. You might reflect, "You don't feel well today?" If you try to talk him out of the way he feels, to cheer him up, he will have a new problem besides his original difficulty. He may feel guilty for not having lived up to the nurse's expectation. Learn from the beginning that if a patient is unhappy and says he is unhappy, you, personally, do not have to solve all of his problems. You may be able to help him, but your assistance will consist of helping him to help himself. Let him know that you have this confidence in him. Do not decide your patient's goals for him. Help him to attain the goals he sets for himself.

- Besides giving the expert technical care that gradually you will learn to give, there are several ways in which you can help your patient by the relationship you establish with him. One is to help him gather as many facts as possible about his situation so that he can make reasonable decisions. Another is to teach him new skills with which he can help himself either to live with or to recover from his illness. And, particularly important, you can support him as he goes through the various stages of illness and recovery (Fig. 6-1).

- If the patient asks no questions and discusses none of his feelings with you, do not pry; but do not assume that he understands all, or that he has perceived nothing of what is going on around him. If it appears that he wants to know, explain treatments and tell him what to expect, so that he can use the information to orient himself to his new surroundings. But do not urge discussion on the unwilling patient. The wise

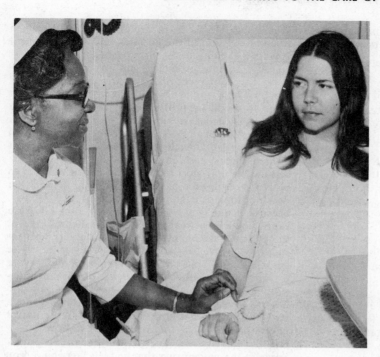

**Figure 6-1.** The nurse is helping this young woman to cope with the anxiety over pending surgery. (Overlook Hospital, Summit, N.J.)

nurse realizes that respecting privacy and pride can prevent a patient from feeling that he has been forced to exhibit his fears and doubts, possibly regretting the revelations later. Most people have a need to appear poised and to present themselves well to others, specially to strangers. To the majority of patients, most of the hospital staff are strangers.

- Such trivial reassuring clichés as "Don't worry" and "Everything will be all right" mean the same thing to a patient as "I don't want to hear about your troubles." They tell the patient that you do not know how to help him examine his fears. They may make him suspect that you and the doctor are keeping horrible things about his condition from him, and they may even lead him to conclude that you are not quite bright. If your patient says that he is worried or does not feel well, he has opened the door to expression of his feelings. If the nurse unperceptively pushes aside his remark by saying something like "Everything will be fine," she shuts the door, thus avoiding involvement but leaving the patient to cope with his feelings alone. This patient needs to be given the opportunity to express doubts. Trying to allay doubts only makes him more unsure. This is false reassurance, which implies that the patient's feelings are not to be trusted, and it says to him that he should not pay attention to them either.

- Do not hesitate to discuss other pertinent topics which may concern the patient. For example, many patients worry about whether and when they may resume sexual activities. While such questions are often left unasked by married patients, unmarried people may be especially reluctant to bring up the subject. It does not help an unmarried teenager who has had sexual relations if the staff assumes an attitude that implies that this aspect of life exists only for those who are married. If the patient initiates some discussion of sex, avoid implying that he is shameful to talk of such a matter, or that he ought not have a sexual self. Instead, listen to him. An openness of what the patient may be experiencing and a readiness to listen to his concerns can alleviate much anxiety and also supply factual information. A patient who has had a myocardial infarction, a venereal disease, or a gynecologic operation can benefit from a factual discussion of the effects his recovery will have on sexual activity.

- It is not uncommon for patients to ask for advice after they already know what they are going to do and could not possibly follow the advice they know they will get. Do not fall into this trap. Ask the patient what he thinks, what is possible for him. Encourage him to talk. Perhaps behind his questions are deeper anxieties. One of the important things to know is the difference between the patient's asking a qustion because he wants to know the answer and his asking a question because he wants reassurance, or because he wants to test the relationship between the nurse and himself.

- Accept every patient as an adult who perhaps momentarily must be cared for physically as a baby. But never talk down to a patient. Just because a man is lying in bed instead of standing up is no reason to resort to the use of patronizing expressions, particularly the "we" which is notorious in the nursing profession. ("Now we're going to have a bath.")

- At the same time be generous with gentle ministrations. A patient needs to feel that someone cares about him.

- Never smother a patient with the kind of attention that retards his ability to do as much for himself as he can.
- When a patient is angry, let him be. He may not be angry with you, even though it is you he is scolding. Although crankiness is hard on others, it is often better for the patient than swallowing his anger and getting indigestion or worse from it. However, this depends on the patient and on the situation. Some people are more comfortable when helped to preserve their aplomb. To perceive these differences is a difficult but important part of nursing.
- Your relationships with patients will be affected not only by your concept of yourself as a nurse, but also by the patient's image of you as a nurse. When he enters the hospital, whether or not he has been hospitalized previously, he has some preconceived expectations about you. Based on stories he has heard, his reading, television, and his own past experiences, he may think of nurses in a stereotyped way, considering them to be cold and heartless, or sweet and giving, ministering angels, or otherwise. To a surprising extent the patient's reaction to the hospital will be governed by such notions. The newly admitted patient who expects the nurse to be gentle with him and take good care of him will behave differently from the patient who thinks of the nurse as a maid in a white uniform; both will act differently than the patient who expects the nurse to ignore him.

## EMOTIONAL CONSIDERATIONS

Patients experience a wide range of feelings, including anxiety, frustration, anger, conflict, and grief. These terms are so commonplace that most people use them rather loosely. However, a clear understanding of the meaning of each of these words can help the nurse deal more effectively with the patients she cares for.

### Anxiety

Anxiety at times is confused with fear. However, there is a difference between them. The person who is afraid usually can identify the cause of his fear—his knees may tremble after a narrow escape from an auto crash (trembling and a pounding heart are natural reactions to danger). In anxiety the external circumstance is not as easily identified. Often the patient feels uneasy, or he has a general feeling of impending unpleasantness or disaster but is unable to explain why he feels this way. The patient is usually not aware of the underlying cause of his anxiety, although he may be aware of situations which precipitate it. Because the patient is often unable to identify the cause of his anxiety, he frequently feels helpless and overwhelmed.

A patient may be anxious without realizing that the anxiety is masking concern over desertion by his family or dread that the operation will result in bodily mutilation, making him less a man or her less a woman. A patient may be anxious because he believes that his disease was self-caused, or he may have the misconception that his wicked neighbor willed him ill. (Belief in this form of the "evil eye" is surprisingly prevalent, even now.)

Anxiety has been defined in various ways: as an energy and as an emotional response without a specific object; as a response to threats to one's self-respect and to the respect in which one is held by others. Threats to survival, whether physical survival or survival as an integrated personality, elicit profound anxiety. Thus patients with certain diseases, such as emphysema or coronary artery disease, may suffer severe anxiety.

The levels of anxiety vary from mild (1+) to panic level (4+). In mild anxiety the individual's ability to observe is heightened; this ability is reduced in moderate and severe anxiety, and the individual tends to focus on details. In mild anxiety the individual's ability to perceive relationships between events is enhanced; as anxiety becomes more severe, he progressively loses this ability. Ability to learn is enhanced by mild anxiety but is impaired in moderate and severe anxiety. In panic-level anxiety the individual may describe feelings of "disintegrating" or "being swept away." It is important to realize that, whatever the individual's physical capacities, he is helpless while in the grip of this degree of anxiety and requires assistance to reduce the anxiety to more manageable levels. Staying with him is one measure which is useful. Listening to him is another. He may speak of one detail and this in distorted fashion. As the nurse listens and as the patient becomes somewhat less anxious, he begins to "put together" in a more coherent way what he is trying to communicate, thus enabling the nurse to respond. A severely anxious person is sometimes helped by concentrating on a detail, such as counting, or by carrying out some physical activity, such as walking or rocking.

We know that when a person is very anxious he cannot see all aspects of a problem. He tends to see and to magnify only a single detail or a few details, and sometimes he makes the wrong connections. An anxious person often becomes confused and unable to follow directions or the explanation given to him about a treatment.

The nurse should avoid cutting off her patients when they begin to talk. Although verbalizing does not in itself relieve anxiety, it can be the beginning of understanding. Letting a patient talk opens the way to understanding and dealing with problems. Sometimes a patient can recognize the need for further, more expert help.

The competent nurse knows when not to pursue the matter, as for example, when her skills are not adequate for the amount of help the patient seems to need (in which case she assists him to find someone who is sufficiently skilled to help him) or when other factors, such as the patient's physical condition, make further discussion of anxiety-producing matters unwise at that time. A patient who has just suffered myocardial infarction may, as he speaks of his recent close encounter with death, experience an increased pulse rate and restlessness and may show signs of increasing ventricular irritability on the ECG monitor. In such circumstances the wise nurse will not encourage the patient to explore the problem further, but will suggest that the patient save further discussion until later. (After saying this, it is important for the nurse to make herself available to the patient later, when his physical condition has improved, so that "talking later" does not become a way of avoiding listening to the patient.) In the situation just described, administration of a "p.r.n." order for sedation may also be appropriate, in order to alleviate physiologic manifestations of anxiety which are particularly hazardous to a patient who has experienced recent myocardial infarction.

When a patient has a life-threatening physical need and is also terrified, attention must be given first to the physical need; psychological needs can be considered after the emergency is over. Thus, when a patient hemorrhages, all concentration must be directed first toward stopping the flow of blood. The competence with which the nurse acts will aid the patient to control, if not to understand, his fear. When a patient is in pain, the pain should be relieved, if possible, before consideration is given to how he reacts to it. Attention to physical needs is one way of communicating support to the patient. Ignoring physical needs, even such simple ones as giving fresh water or lowering the bed to a more comfortable position, is a way of telling the patient that no one cares and of increasing his anxiety. Words should not be used in any situation in which action is more appropriate.

The nurse should recognize that she is a stranger to the patient. He is not likely to discuss all his thoughts with her; nor should he. Talking about some problems can help the patient to feel less alone with the other problems—often the main ones—that he does not talk about. Frequently, it is erroneously assumed that the patient is revealing his innermost thoughts, but this assumption is not always true, particularly when the relationship between the nurse and the patient has been brief.

Some patients prefer not to discuss their emotional problems with the nurse, in which case she should respect their wish for privacy. The nurse's need to help should be tempered by an understanding of what will bring relief to the particular patient. Some patients find it most helpful for the nurse to give support in nonverbal ways; others are benefited if they are encouraged to talk about how they feel.

Sometimes, because the patient's anxiety is so great, he bursts out with a flow of emotion-laden personal concerns even when the nurse's contact with him has been relatively brief. The patient may later worry over telling so much about his personal life. The nurse should stay with him and listen supportively during his period of distress, but avoid questioning him or encouraging him at this time to go on. When the patient is calmer and has had a chance to think over what he has told her, he will be better able to assess what topics (if any) he wants to pursue. Under such circumstances the patient may seem embarrassed when he sees the nurse later. She should let him bring up the subject of his outburst if he wishes, but should not initiate the discussion. She should show, by the way she cares for him, that she thinks none the less of him because of the incident.

**Dealing with Your Own Anxiety.** What are some of the things you can do when you become anxious? If you can, leave the situation for a moment to collect yourself and think it through. However, there are times when you cannot leave, such as when the patient is bleeding. Try to concentrate on some concrete, helpful thing you can do. Hold a compress in place, or empty the emesis basin, or take the patient's pulse. These actions give you time to think what to do next.

Merely learning to recognize when you are anxious often will keep you from being helpless in the grip of anxiety. When you know you are anxious —except in an emergency—stop! Think the situation through. Find help; do not race blindly ahead with what you are doing. At such times the patient may get the wrong medication or the side rail may be left down, so that he falls out of bed. Every person who deals with helpless people has the responsibility to stop work when he is unable to function. Extreme anxiety can keep one from functioning and can make one a hazard. So can physical illness or excessive loss of sleep. None of these "excuses" is accepted legally if a patient is harmed.

Knowledge and competence are an insurance against anxiety. On the other hand, do not expect too much of yourself. As you learn new things, you will have moments of insecurity. Just as the patient who is anxious concentrates on smaller and smaller details, you, too, will find that your ability to perceive the whole situation narrows with anxiety and grows with the increase of knowledge and capability.

## Frustration and Anger

What happens in frustration? A person sets a goal, but some barrier prevents its fulfillment. The result is frustration, which is made up of feelings of helplessness and anger. The amount of frustration one feels is dependent on how important the goal was, what similar past experiences the person has had, and how he handles feelings of helplessness and anger. If a nurse's goal is to see her patient well, she is thwarted when he gets sicker. If she thinks to herself that this patient's recovery is a test of her worth as a nurse, and he gets sicker in spite of everything she does, she will become more frustrated than if she had never set up this unrealistic test. A patient who fails to walk well on his new artificial leg will be frustrated. We do not always know what goals another has set for himself. Therefore, we cannot assume that the failure that does not frustrate one person will not frustrate another. One patient may be thrilled to find that he can walk around his bed; another may be dismayed to find that he will be barred from entering an athletic contest.

Frustration ends in anger. It is important to be aware of anger when it exists so that it can be traced to its origins. If anger stems from frustration, both the goal and the barrier can be evaluated. Perhaps the goal will be lowered (make the patient comfortable instead of trying to cure him), the barrier modified (assist in research on new methods of dealing with that disease), or new skills developed to circumvent the barrier.

If a person becomes angry and does not acknowledge it, the anger can become subconscious. This happens when a person may feel the need to hide from himself the fact that he is angry—the anger may be too painful to face; it may interfere with the picture the person has formed of himself. Unknown anger that is still present as psychic energy is harder to handle because one does not know of its existence. Suppose the nurse's frustration at having the patient get sicker rather than better is what has made her angry; but to be aware of her anger would hurt her view of herself as a gentle person. She may be angry with the patient for not responding to her ministrations; or with herself for setting up an unattainable goal; or at the existence of incurable illness; or with the head nurse, whose assignment to this patient has led to frustration. She may take a great dislike to the patient for reasons which appear to her to originate in him. For instance, she may disagree with his outlook on life, she may blame his decline on his lack of will to live, or she may become irritated by the tone of his voice. She is trying to set up a logical reason for her anger. She is rationalizing her anger and projecting its cause from herself to the patient. Rationalization is a common mechanism which we all use at times.

The nurse may ask the head nurse not to assign her to this patient. Instead of solving the problem she is withdrawing from it. Or she may unreasonably blame herself for not being the good nurse she thought she was, even going so far as to think that it was her fault that the patient had to die. She is turning her subconscious anger inward.

The trouble with feelings and reactions of which we are not aware is that they complicate and obscure the situation without offering a rational solution to the problem. Acknowledge to yourself that you are angry, when you are. Sometimes anger has a perfectly legitimate basis, and at such times the expression of it is justifiable. The more realistically you can accept anger in yourself, the better you will be able to accept it in your patients. If you can say, "I'm furious, and it's all right to feel that way," you will be more able to say, "He's furious, and it's not bad to feel that way." Then you can proceed to handle the anger-provoking situation more rationally and realistically.

Patients have many reasons for being angry. Just being sick is frustrating. Restriction of activity, such as that imposed by an illness or disability, is frustrating. Being unable to control the most ordinary daily routines, such as getting a hot cup of coffee, brushing one's teeth or urinating, is frustrating. The confinement to a room or a small space in a ward makes smaller and smaller details more and more important.

As a result, a patient may become angry with you. The anger from his frustration may be projected to you, so that he may disagree with your outlook on life, blame his decline on your lack of care, and bristle at the tones in your voice. You are taking the brunt of the patient's unrecognized, subconscious anger at being ill, disabled, or helpless. All of us prefer to be treated kindly rather than gruffly, to be liked and appreciated. It is hard not to be hurt by anger, even if we suspect that its cause is elsewhere or that it is a cover for fear.

As you attend various staff conferences, you may notice that patients' fear and anxiety are usually more frequent topics of discussion than patients' anger. Possibly it is more difficult for nurses to recognize and deal with angry patients than with those who express fear, thereby tending to elicit a supportive response from the nurse. The angry patient is often labeled "difficult," "demanding," or "uncooperative"—which of course merely avoids considering the patient's anger and trying to find out what the difficulty is.

What can you do about such a situation? Hostility is often met with hostility. The patient is angry with you, and so you get angry with him. This reaction does not lead to any constructive end. What else can you do? You can accept the emotion, and perhaps your acceptance of it will lead the patient to accept it himself. Act as a mirror for the expression of his feelings. Let him talk. Help him to talk. If he feels angry, he has a reason for it, and it is often better for all concerned for him not to simmer silently, but to talk about what bothers him. If he is angry but does not show it outwardly, it does not mean that the anger has gone away. You can say, "Do you want to tell me about it, Mr. Johnson?" The angry patient may try to line you up on his side against a physician or another nurse. Avoid taking sides, but do not avoid the patient's feelings.

Some of the things about which the patient expresses anger can be remedied. Try to see that he receives hot coffee if cold coffee is one of the things which makes him angry. Many of the main causes of anger, however, cannot be remedied. If the patient must remain in traction for six weeks, and

therefore misses a long-awaited trip, there is nothing he or anyone else can do about changing the situation. In addition to giving your patient opportunities to express his anger, help him to find activities to help use up the excess energy mobilized by anger. Physical activity is especially beneficial. The patient with a lower limb in traction can still exercise his arms; these exercises can be useful not only in preparing him for crutch-walking, but also in using some pent-up energy engendered by anger, thus helping him to relax.

There may be times when you will become angry with a patient. It is nothing to be ashamed of. You are human, too. Even a superior nurse will lose her temper occasionally. When it happens, accept it in yourself and talk it over with someone else. What frustrated you? What touched off your hostility? Are your goals too high? Is there some way to get under, around, through, or over the barrier? Work your way out of the trouble spots by being aware of your own feelings.

## Conflict

The medical-surgical patient is often confronted with making decisions which have far-reaching consequences, and often he is expected to arrive at his decision promptly. Such situations set the stage for conflict—a situation in which the patient feels torn between opposing goals. It is not uncommon for patients to have to choose "the lesser of two evils;" sometimes neither alternative is really desirable, and the question revolves around which choice has the most assets. Often the situation is complicated by the fact that no one can predict, for certain, just what the outcome of a particular treatment will be. Nevertheless, the patient must reach a decision.

The nurse's role in such situations is to act as a sounding board while the patient expresses his conflict and considers the alternatives. When a patient is in conflict, it is important to help him get the necessary information to help him in decision making. It is also important not to try to make the decision for the patient. Realistic time pressures of course do exist. However, the time pressure should not be intensified beyond what is required by the situation.

## Grief

Grief is a reaction to loss of someone or something significant to the individual—loss of spouse, job, a body part, or a capacity.

Engel (1964) has described stages through which an individual moves during normal grief. First is the stage of shock or disbelief. A woman whose husband has just died may hold a straw to his lips and tell him to sip the water. Her actions deny the truth of the situation, which is too hard for her to bear. The next stage involves gradual awareness of the reality of the loss. The individual experiences the pain of bereavement, anger (at oneself, at others, and at the lost person for his departure), crying, and withdrawal of interest in other people and in the surroundings. Often there are feelings of emptiness, listlessness, and lack of appetite. The final stage is of restitution or recovery, when the individual renews his interest in other people and in his work and feels a resurgence of vigor and sense of purpose in his undertakings. The duration of the grief process is variable, from a few weeks to as long as a year. Its duration and severity depend on such factors as the significance and magnitude of the loss for the individual, his capacity to deal with it, and the resources he has to sustain him during crises, such as job, family, and friends.

Think of patients you have cared for who have lost functions or body parts and see whether you note similarities to the process just described. Crying is a usual reaction following removal of a breast, for example. Unless one considers the fact that the patient has come up against a serious loss, her tears may be ascribed to babyishness or to inability to tolerate pain.

What can you do to help patients who are experiencing grief? Remember that the patient cannot be hastened through the various stages, nor can he skip over them. In fact, premature efforts to help him see the bright side and to move ahead with rehabilitation may only make him feel more alone and more despondent. If, instead, you can recognize the stage of grief that your patient is in and support him as he experiences it, you will be more likely to help him move on to the next stage. For instance, a patient with partial aphasia following a stroke may be seething with frustration and anger over impairment of his ability to speak. The nurse's approach which emphasizes, "Come now, buck up and try harder," can make such a patient more convinced that others do not understand, more angry, and more likely to withdraw from others and from efforts at speech rehabilitation. In contrast, the nurse who is sensitive to the patient's reactions

will be concerned when the patient bangs down his book of speech exercises and, instead of ignoring the behavior or giving him a lecture, will take the time to listen and try to understand what the patient is attempting to communicate. Allowing him to express the frustration and anger and acknowledging that he is confronted with a frustrating experience will help the patient to feel less alone and to move on through the remaining stages of grief.

Not all patients move through grief successfully. Some become immobilized, as it were, in one stage of grief and are unable to move forward and utilize the abilities and opportunities which are open to them. It is important for the nurse to recognize when a patient seems to be reacting this way and to discuss her observation with the physician. Often such patients require the help of a psychotherapist to aid them in dealing with the problem.

Do not expect your patients to move smoothly forward through stages of grief, however. Progress is usually uneven; this in turn adds to the patient's discouragement. Sometimes, after a day of feeling his strength and interest in recovery returning, he will revert to an attitude of hopelessness. Recognize that this does not necessarily signify defeat, and help the patient to realize that the process of recovery from any significant loss is usually uneven.

Society has certain expectations about what warrants grief and how much grief is appropriate. It is considered appropriate for a woman to grieve many months after the death of her husband, but a reaction of similar length and intensity following the death of her dog may be viewed as foolishness. Remember that the patient grieves for what is important to him and for those he loves, regardless of the yardstick society uses to measure the appropriateness of his reactions. Losses have very personal meanings to the individual who experiences them.

The patient's reaction is also affected by the magnitude of other serious losses in his life, how well he has recovered from them, and his personal resources and assets. For the elderly lady who has outlived all of her relatives and close friends, the death of a beloved pet during her hospitalization may be overwhelming, while for a patient with family and friends and a challenging career, the death of a pet, although painful, may not constitute a major loss. Likewise, one patient may seem withdrawn and apathetic for months following removal of a gangrenous toe, while another patient may, a few weeks following amputation of his leg, begin learning to use his artificial limb and start making plans to return to work.

## CRISIS

Considerable emphasis has been given lately to concepts concerning crisis and crisis intervention. Although space does not permit lengthy discussion here, some of these concepts will be discussed briefly, since they are especially relevant to medical-surgical patients. The reader is referred to the bibliography for some excellent materials on this topic.

Crisis has been defined in different ways. For some, crisis means an experience during which one's coping methods seem inadequate for the situation. Another view states that a crisis presents a challenge—an opportunity or a turning point. Sudden illness, bereavement, loss of job and income, failure at school, are all examples of unpleasant crises. However, a feeling of crisis can arise also from welcome events. The birth of a baby or the start of a new job with greater responsibility may develop into a crisis if a person feels unequal to the new demands.

Whatever the basis of the crisis, several outcomes are possible: the person may develop new ways of coping as a result of the crisis and emerge stronger and better prepared for future crises; he may resume functioning at his previous level; or he may function from then on at a lower, less effective level.

**Helping the Patient to Deal with Crisis.** For the medical-surgical patient, crisis may occur in various contexts, such as discovering that one has diabetes or that a serious operation is necessary. The experience of hospitalization constitutes a crisis for many people.

In helping the patient deal with the situation, the nurse and other members of the health team can maintain frequent contact with the patient and let him know that they are available to be called at other times, should need arise. They can help the patient to learn about and to utilize resources, helping him take an active part in making decisions so that he feels less powerless. If convalescent care presents a problem, the social worker can describe the various facilities available and then allow the patient to decide which one is best for him (rather than deciding for him).

The nurse can help the patient cope with the crisis by talking with him and helping him to deal with each stage as it arrives. Learning what diabetes is, learning about his diet and how to give himself insulin, coping with the anger at having this serious illness and with the anxiety over what complications may arise are all steps to be taken.

The nurse can also assist the patient to keep in touch with others, if this is helpful to him. She can have a telephone placed at his bedside, if he wishes, show him where to mail letters, welcome his visitors, call the clergyman if the patient wishes to see one and arrange for the patient to attend religious services at the hospital chapel.

It is important to find out what supports a patient has and to help him to use them. Patients often have many more resources than the staff realize. For the patient who enjoys music, a small radio may bring much comfort and easing of tension. For the patient who typically copes with problems through cognitive skills, it is important to help him learn about his condition and treatment.

The important thing to remember is that a patient is helped to deal with crisis by developing a feeling of mastery and competence from successfully managing difficult tasks. Too often, however, the popular stereotype of patienthood is one of helplessness. Of course, some patients are helpless, either physically or psychologically, or both. However, by far the largest proportion of medical-surgical patients have considerable means of helping themselves, but they are often so awed by the hospital and so unsure of themselves in this strange environment, that they feel unnecessarily helpless. Unfortunately, many aspects of hospital care reinforce feelings of inadequacy. The much-mocked, too short hospital gown so destructive of human dignity, the lack of information, the restriction of one's living space all contribute to this feeling.

It would be extremely helpful, if patients were permitted to help themselves and each other, yet few aspects of care on many medical-surgical units have been so neglected as this. The following suggestions, then, are aimed at encouraging patients to help themselves and each other.

• **Introduce patients admitted on the same day. Invite all who are not acutely ill to come to the lounge for a brief informal discussion of hospital policies and helpful information, such as the various services available. In the process new patients can meet one another and some of the staff.**

- Talk with patients in small groups about concerns which they all share. Teaching preoperative patients in a group of four or five provides some group support as well as the necessary instruction. Patients quickly begin learning who else is about to have surgery and often develop an informal network of their own for encouraging one another throughout the experience. The importance of friendly interest and concern for one another among the patient group is vastly underestimated. Gestures of help, such as bringing the newspaper and dropping in for a brief visit, can lead patients to feel less helpless and less dependent on the staff.

- Encourage patients to be together and to help one another. A ward snack nook and lounge where patients can go to fix themselves light refreshments can foster friendliness among patients. Convey to patients that you enjoy seeing them visit one another. Too often medical-surgical patients are placed in a room, possibly shared with a very ill patient, and given little opportunity for contacts with others at a time when they are frightened and lonely.

   However, it is important to remember that not all patients seek contact with other people when they are ill. Some may prefer not to deal extensively with other patients. Others, whose care requires rest and quiet, may be burdened by too many interpatient relationships. The patient's preference and his requirements in terms of physical and emotional well-being should be the deciding factors in determining whether or not to encourage contacts with other patients.

- Encourage patients to ask questions. Provide information readily. If this is not possible, help the patient to find answers to his questions from others. Avoid conveying the expectation that patients will meekly follow instructions without asking what is happening to them.

- Listen to your patient when he complains. Try to find out what the problem is and try to solve it with the patient (not for him, unless he is actually powerless to deal with it).

- Encourage physical self-sufficiency as fully as possible. Suggest that a patient wear comfortable clothes rather than nightclothes whenever he is able.

- Utilize group discussions as well as individual talks with patients to help them express their feelings (Fig. 6-2). This is especially helpful in dealing with feelings which seem socially unacceptable. For instance, many postoperative patients are angry because of the physical pain and bodily intrusion they have experienced. Expressing some of this anger in a group can help patients cope with it. Knowing that others also experience anger can help patients who chide themselves that they should be experiencing only gratitude.

- Talk with family and friends who visit encouraging their questions and recognizing their concern for the patient. Listen to their suggestions.

- Encourage the patient to discuss problems with the staff member who is most able to help. Questions concerning the physician's plan of care are best addressed to the physician, who can then explain his rationale for therapy and also experience, firsthand, the patient's questions and worries. The patient is likely to have a greater sense of satisfaction from talking with the person who has the authority to deal with the situation. He may feel less helpless and less fearful of the physician's awesome "omnipotence." Likewise, questions concerning his nursing care are

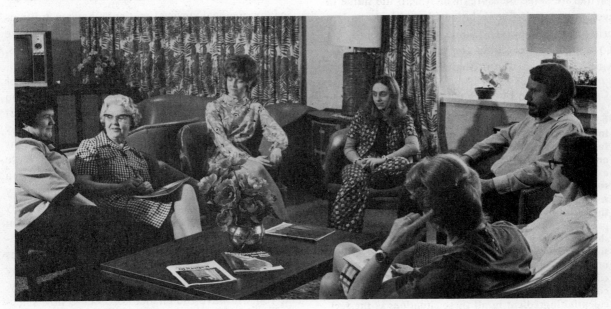

**Figure 6-2.** These convalescent patients are discussing with the nurse (sitting farthest to the right) their experience with illness and their plans for going home. (Overlook Hospital, Summit, N.J.)

best addressed to the nurse, rather than to the aide or the cleaning lady. The nurse can help the patient by helping him to find out who is the appropriate person to consult on various matters.

## BRIEF NURSE-PATIENT RELATIONSHIPS

As you work with medical-surgical patients you will find that your contact with some of them is limited to one 10- or 15-minute period. Your first reaction may be that 10 or 15 minutes do not count for anything in a relationship. Think about it again. Have you ever had an experience in which the brief response of another person was very important to you, even though you never saw the person again? Suppose there has been a car accident. The way the policeman responds to the people who are involved is important to them at that time, and it may also affect their reactions to future situations in which they must call for help.

The patient who enters the emergency room terrified of the bleeding and pain of a scalp laceration may remember years afterward the nurse's calmness and skill, her sureness as she touched the wound, and the way she helped him gather his own strength. The nurse who can establish this kind of relationship with a patient not only helps him over the immediate crisis, but fosters his ability to respond to others who care for him later.

What are some measures which help the nurse to develop a supportive relationship with a patient during a brief period? (Some of these points are also applicable to caring for patients during diagnostic and therapeutic procedures.)

- **Concentrate on what the patient is going through. Avoid social clichés which are not only meaningless but often offensive in such situations, because they imply denial of the stressful experience the patient is facing. At such times the patient needs to focus his energy on the situation at hand; he should not be expected to divert some of it into an effort to be sociable. For example, if a nurse is helping care for a patient following an automobile accident and sees that the physician is about to carry out a painful procedure, such as cleaning the wound or suturing, she may say to the patient, "Now look at me, and squeeze my hand hard. It's going to hurt for a minute." Or a patient may be helped by being asked to count aloud, thus giving him something specific to concentrate on when he is anxious and in pain. The essential ingredient in all these situations is the feeling of support and encouragement which the patient receives from the nurse.**

- **Establish some physical and eye contact with the patient. Gently placing your hand on the patient's shoulder may be more appropriate and more effective in some instances than verbal reassurance. (Occasionally your patient will show that he does not welcome physical contact, in which case it should be kept to a minimum.)**
- **Have your equipment handy, neat, and in good condition. You cannot concentrate on the patient if you are frantically hunting for a sterile syringe of the proper size. Also, remember that an environment which is orderly and clean can increase the patient's confidence in his care.**
- **Perform your technical skills with as much confidence and dexterity as possible. If some of them are new to you, practice away from the patient until you gain proficiency.**
- **Be alert to the patient's physiologic, as well as his emotional, reactions. Are his lips becoming cyanotic? Did his pulse rate just increase by 20 beats?**

You may ask, "But how can anyone attend to so many things at once?" You will find that, with experience, you can carry out and observe many things almost automatically. You don't have to tell yourself, "Check the pulse; observe skin color." You will just *do* these things, and as you become more quickly responsive to various indices of the patient's condition, you will find that you are more alert to danger signals in the patient's physiologic and emotional state.

## SUSTAINED NURSE-PATIENT RELATIONSHIPS

Many medical-surgical patients have conditions which require extended care. Frequently these patients, many of whom are in the older age groups, receive initial care in the general hospital and subsequent care in their own homes, nursing homes, or some other type of extended-care facility. If you work in a clinic serving patients with chronic heart disease or peripheral vascular disease, you may care for some of the same patients for many months or years. You will become acquainted with these people in a way which is not possible during a short-term relationship. You will have opportunity to observe how their conditions are affected by other events in their lives. The patient's condition may improve markedly after the birth of a grandchild and deteriorate when the young family moves to a distant part of the country. You will have many opportunities to teach the patient and his family, and you will have the chance to observe how effectively they use your instruction. Does the patient with varicose veins continue to appear at the clinic wearing round garters, or is she now using a garter belt? If the former is true, how can you revise your approach so that she will be more likely to accept your suggestions?

Working with long-term patients provides many satisfactions; it also poses some problems. While you have the satisfaction of seeing some of your patients improve, others for various reasons will remain unchanged or even get sicker. You will be called upon to continue working with the patient and family during extended periods often marked by exacerbations and remissions of the illness.

Maintaining a professional role with the patient presents additional challenges. Because you have known him for a long time, it may be difficult for you to differentiate between a professional role and a social role. There is also greater likelihood, because of your familiarity with family problems, of becoming a protagonist for one family member or another, rather than helping the family to assess problems and deal with them.

Long-term patients in the general hospital often get lost in the shuffle. The acutely ill surgical patient, for example, or the accident victim claims the staff's time and attention in a way that an elderly man with chronic congestive heart failure may not. As you work in the general hospital, be alert to the special requirements of long-term patients. Are there activities on your ward in which they can participate, such as using library material, playing cards and so on? Is there a place where the patient can eat his meals out of bed, with others, if he is able? Most important, do staff members spend time talking with these patients, or is their care delegated largely to the nonprofessional staff because it is considered "routine"?

As you work with these patients, avoid reminding them that others are sicker and require more of your time. Spend the time with them that you can spend wholeheartedly, showing that you feel they deserve your concern. The long-term patient typically has significant problems in adapting to the restrictions imposed by his illness. Listening to these patients and their families and helping them take stock of their situation are an important part of your role.

The care of long-term patients highlights the importance of faithfully carrying out care every day, even though there is no quick improvement. Sometimes there is no improvement at all, and one realizes that treatment is serving only to hold ground which might otherwise be lost, rather than to provide improvement. The very sameness of the care, day by day, can be discouraging to both nurse and patient. Almost anyone can perceive the drama of bringing a patient out of anaphylactic shock, but not every nurse is attuned to helping an emphysema patient do his breathing exercises daily and to feeling joy when the patient blows out one more candle today than he did yesterday.

The relationship which the nurse has with the long-term patient is especially important since many of these patients have few ties with their families and friends. Because other significant relationships are so often lacking, what the nurse provides as a listener and as one who is concerned about the patient's welfare is especially important. Some aspects of care frequently handled by families of short-term patients become the concern of the nurse: helping the patient to find recreational activities, requesting visits from the chaplain if the patient wishes it, seeing that he has necessary clothing and toilet articles—all may become concerns of nursing staff. Nurses can show their interest and support of patients by attending to the daily matters which help the patient toward greater freedom and mastery of his situation, aiding him to use the abilities which he has and assisting him to keep in touch with those who are important to him. Wheeling the patient to the phone booth and helping him get the necessary change to call his family can be just as significant aspects of nursing, particularly for this group of patients, as rubbing their backs or providing adequate fluid intake.

## THE QUIET PATIENT

The facial expression assumed by a patient is not necessarily a good indication of what is happening inside him. Cheerfulness can be a mask behind which lurk fears and anger of a most urgent nature. The quiet person deserves your attention as much as the noisy one. The need of the quiet person to talk may be as great, and it may be even harder for him to express himself. It is usually not healthy to be too obedient or cooperative. The cooperative patient is the one who is the popular patient. His popularity is his bargaining point for security. But the patient who pleases the staff may do so at the expense of his own health. One patient was such a good sport that he told no one about the pain he was experiencing until his peptic ulcer perforated.

## THE PATIENT WHO FREELY EXPRESSES EMOTION

Certain patients by their behavior may make it hard for nurses to accept them. For instance, some grown-up patients act like uninhibited children. They demand more service than anyone could give. They cry. They are stubborn, not doing what was ordered by the physician. They do not act as persons of their age usually do. Such patients sometimes cause anxiety in the nurse, because they do not meet her expectations. However, the nurse should remember that the patient who seems to be willful and obstinate may be trying to maintain his own integrity and his will to fight. The patient who acquiesces in every demand may have given up.

There may be another reason for the nurse's difficulty in tolerating patients who do not act in a grown-up way. They may remind her of parts of herself which she has learned to control, traits which she now regards as unacceptable in her standards of good behavior. If she does not like these characteristics in herself, it is only natural that her first reaction to them in others will be one of distaste. Or she may simply fear that in the same circumstance she would behave in a similar manner.

Some patients may lose control completely, either physically or emotionally. They may soil themselves, laugh and cry at the same time, scream or climb out of bed. These patients may arouse the nurse's long-forgotten memories, which are kept out of the forefront of awareness because they are associated with too much pain. Those who were severely punished during their toilet training sometimes feel a special revulsion toward people who are incontinent. Those who as little children had to control any show of emotion for fear of punishment may be upset by a free flow of emotions from others.

Some adults may be ashamed of their behavior when it becomes childish; but when they are sick and forced to depend on the care of others, they cry and complain more easily. If a patient is embarrassed by his behavior, the nurse can point out to him the temporary nature of his dependence. Nurses see people *in extremis*, with their defenses badly shaken. A matter-of-fact "This is not unusual" acceptance of the situation may help to convey to the patient recognition of the temporary nature of the circumstance and a subtle tone of support. When people are temporarily shorn of their usual poise and self-control, the nurse can help them to maintain their dignity.

There are times when it is natural for a patient to lose emotional control and cry. It may be a great compliment to your relationship that the patient feels emotionally secure enough with you to cry. A flow of tears can relieve tension. At such times, it is well to let the patient cry. The compassion of acceptance may allow a man to cry in the nurse's presence without feeling less manly because he did. The nurse who says to a patient, "Don't cry," may mean, "Don't cry in front of me, because it makes me feel uncomfortable." She might say instead, "It's all right to show how you feel." A nurse has to be able to stand the discomfort of another's tears, because the tears may help to relieve the patient's tension. As long as the nurse can recognize her own reaction to the tears of others, she can let the patient cry without feeling overly anxious herself. If the nurse disapproves of crying, perhaps she should not cry herself; but it is not a part of good nursing care to impose one's own standards on others.

It is important to assess the patient's capacity for control at a given time and also to consider some possible reasons for his behavior. While it is useless, and possibly harmful, to demand that a patient show greater control than is possible for him, it is important to establish a plan of care which enables the patient to maintain the self-control which he can muster. For example, if a patient with multiple sclerosis spills water on the bed each time he tries to drink and bursts into tears of frustration as a result, the nurse can place a half-full glass with a flexible straw on the over bed close to the patient. The patient can then draw the table toward him when he wants to drink and sip the water without having to handle the glass. A patient who is incontinent at night may be able to avoid soiling himself if the urinal is left where he can reach it.

This approach is not likely to be effective if the patient is soiling himself to get attention. Sometimes the nurse's reaction to such a patient is one of further rejection, cleaning him up in the most perfunctory manner possible and avoiding him the rest of the time. Medical-surgical patients who behave in this manner are often elderly people who are severely lacking in meaningful relationships with others. Eventually the patient regresses to a childish way of seeking attention which is distasteful to others and serves only to isolate him further. This in turn leads to more soiling. The patient and nurse become victims of a vicious circle while he suffers more humiliation, isolation, and regression and she is harassed with additional work which at first glance appears wholly unnecessary. It is the nurse who must break the circle by recognizing how her own actions are aggravating the situation and by giving more attention to the patient than that associated with changing him.

Many of the medical-surgical patients who lack emotional control have some neurologic impairment, such as results from cerebral vascular accidents and multiple sclerosis. Others lack control primarily because of anxiety. In either instance it is important to remember that the patient has diminished capacity to perceive and respond to the subtle cues relied upon extensively in social interaction. When you must set limits with a person whose ability to perceive the nuances of social interaction is diminished, it is essential to use a very forthright approach, devoid of ambiguities. This does not imply that you speak brusquely or that you are unkind, but it does mean that you speak with an honesty and clarity often not permissible in a purely social interaction. By using a direct approach you help the patient avoid missing your comment altogether or misinterpreting its meaning.

While it may seem to others that a patient lacks emotional control, it may seem to the patient that he is using extraordinary control to deal with emotions of overwhelming intensity. The surge of anger felt by a patient suddenly stricken with coronary occlusion may be so intense that he thanks Providence that he has controlled it sufficiently not to strike out at anyone. To others, however, this patient may seem to control his anger poorly, because he sometimes makes sarcastic remarks about his care. As you give patients opportunity to verbalize some of their emotions, you may wonder at the degree of control which some of them have, in light of the urgency of their feelings.

## THE PATIENT FROM A DIFFERENT CULTURE

The nurse may find herself shying away from a patient for reasons other than personal behavior. He may speak a different language, or his customs may be so strange that the nurse feels that there is no common meeting ground for communication. A black student may find it strange to bathe a white patient. The customs of a patient newly arrived from the Orient may seem strange to the American student.

A Puerto Rican man can be expected to be especially modest, and the nurse should understand that having a female nurse bathe him may be embarrassing to him.

Many of us have a tendency to shy away from the unfamiliar, because it usually provokes more anxiety than the familiar. We may be uncertain what to do or say. Because we do not know what to expect next, we feel uneasy. Yet there is a certain sense of adventure in exploring the unknown. What are the thoughts and feelings of a person different from us in background or age? As the unknown unfolds, we find that we have grown, and that our own perspectives have been enriched.

At the same time we must be aware that different cultures are governed by different standards. Not all cultures view cleanliness in the same way. Most Europeans do not consider themselves clean without frequent cleansing of the rectal and genital regions, especially after a bowel movement. There are people in other groups who do not believe in a daily bath. If a patient enters the hospital with nits clinging to the shafts of his hair and black lines under his fingernails, will his condition color your feelings about him as a person? If your answer is "Yes" (and it may well be), try to draw a distinction between a person's standards of hygiene and the person as an individual.

## EMOTIONAL INVOLVEMENT

You may become attached to some patients, especially if you have cared for them a long time. They like you, and you like them. They are *your* patients. You may be unwilling to relinquish them to their families or to death. Although you should not be afraid to like your patients, emotional involvement with a patient does not mean the same thing as emotional involvement with an old friend, a family member or your fiancé. Relations with patients are more temporary. You are a professional person maintaining a tacitly understood relationship based on service. Usually, you do not call your patient by his first name; you do not display your personal life to him; you are not coy. Within the professional relationship you can be warm and express your interest in a different fashion. You show a patient that you like him by taking him as he is, by perceiving his needs and meeting them promptly. The tender touch at just the right moment, the word of encouragement when he is feeling low will bring satisfaction to both of you.

The more you understand what comforting the patient means to you, the more free you will be to do it well.

If a man misinterprets your ministerings, idealizing your relationship into something more personal than you intend, you may occasionally have to side-step a pass or two. He may build up your relationship beyond his actual scope to give himself a feeling that he has someone to lean on while going through a trying illness. When a patient, any patient, identifies with those who can help him, he feels less helpless. Although it might not be unnatural for you secretly to smile at his behavior, your professional attitude will be maintained by reminding yourself that his needs and judgments are different when he is sick. Sometimes it is preferable to speak very plainly, particularly when the patient is highly anxious, or has some neurologic problem. For instance, an elderly man who had no family or friends repeatedly made passes at the nurses, with the result that they avoided him. One nurse who encountered the problem said firmly but kindly, "I don't want you to do that." The patient never used the behavior again with that nurse. The nurse brought the matter up in a team conference, where the question was raised of whether the patient's behavior could be due to extreme loneliness. The patient responded well when all the nurses straightforwardly voiced their objections to his "wandering hands," and, in addition, spent more time with him and encouraged him to join in ward activities.

## THE SUICIDAL PATIENT

The depressed patient bears watching; he may be thinking of suicide. Signs of depression are: lack of enthusiasm, prolonged insomnia, listlessness, reluctance to speak, neglect of appearance, withdrawal, lack of interest in anything, and feelings of worthlessness. It may be difficult to get the patient to say anything. Suicide in the nonpsychotic patient is often an attempt to escape from an overwhelming situation, which frequently is the loss of love. Hostility is often a factor, too. Anger at self, the wish to hurt those close to him who have hurt him—usually such influencing factors are unrecognized by the patient. In some instances it is possible to avert suicide if the patient thinks that one person in the world will listen to him and is concerned for him. That one person can be a nurse. The background leading to suicide is a long, complicated web of events and feelings. The nurse is expected to recognize depression and protect the patient by reporting her observations promptly to the physician. Obvious hazards, such as a razor in the patient's stand, can be removed quietly.

If a patient threatens suicide, pay attention to him. He may mean it. Do not leave the patient alone. Communicate with the physician. Alert the rest of the nursing staff. Chart your observations. Where pain, incurable disease, crippling disability, and impending death are present—as they may be on any general hospital floor—suicide, like fire, is an ever-present possibility.

## THE COMPLAINING PATIENT

Some patients continually complain about pains and aches or the service of the hospital. These patients are often disliked, particularly by the nursing staff. Perhaps complaints about which little can be done leave the nurses feeling helpless. What is it that lies at the root of the patient's bitterness and continual complaints? Has anyone tried to find out? Is this the only way the patient can get any attention? In the course of this patient's day does he have any warm human contact? Any opportunity for a feeling of accomplishment or satisfaction? A patient, because he is a patient, is cut off from his family and friends, his work, and his own fireside. His habitual sources of satisfaction are usually not available in the hospital, where his sore toe and his elevated leukocyte count may receive attention while his own self is starved for human contact. A nurse, even though she may fumble some in the trying, can delight this patient by alleviating his loneliness.

The all-too-prevalent practice of calling patients who complain frequently (and some who do not) by such terms as "crocks" reveals eloquently the lack of perception and understanding in the speaker. Perhaps nurses label patients as a way of putting distance between themselves and the patients who make them anxious. The subconscious reasoning may be that a patient who is labeled as "uncooperative" is so unworthy that nurses are excused for avoiding him. A patient who does not meet the nurse's expectations, one whom she has not the knowledge and the competence to deal with, may make her anxious. By stereotyping and labeling him she in a sense dismisses him. Stereotyping can be done by a whole group, with disastrous effects on the patient. The night nurse reports to the day staff, "He's uncooperative," and sets up the climate and expectations. Once a patient is labeled as uncooperative, he probably will not disappoint anyone. He will be uncooperative.

Who are the "good" patients? Many nurses think that submissive patients are "good," and by bestowing approval on the quiet ones they force patients to hide their feelings. Often the behavior expected of patients is made evident to them subtly but very clearly. "Ms. Glenn is a wonderful patient, Doctor. She's always smiling." Therefore, Ms. Glenn must go on smiling, even if it kills her. Her ulcer may grow bigger, but she's smiling. If one morning she might frown or cry, perhaps the nurses would not approve of her and therefore not take care of her.

Some patients do not complain because they are at the mercy of the nurse. They dare not antagonize her, or the physician, or the orderly. A patient lying in bed, sick and in pain, depends on the hospital staff. He is in a vulnerable position, and the danger of being ignored—psychologically and physically—is a real one. A patient may be afraid to complain, no matter how miserable he feels, because he may observe that the more cranky patients are left thirsty and in wet beds. But fear of expressing feelings is not a stepping stone to health.

## THE PATIENT WHO IS PHYSICALLY UNAPPEALING

Our culture places heavy emphasis upon cleanliness, pleasant odors, and attractive appearance. The patient who has had radical head and neck surgery for removal of cancer is badly disfigured; the patient with infected skin lesions has an unpleasant odor; the patient with tuberculosis or staphylococcal infection can transmit the condition to others.

Try not to expect yourself to be impervious to unpleasant sights and odors, and do not be afraid to discuss your reaction to these problems. Having been brought up in a society which places emphasis upon the elimination of body odor, for example, you will quite naturally be unaccustomed to and, at times, distressed by, unpleasant odors. Gradually you will learn how to handle yourself in such situations, how to deal as effectively as possible with the problem (such as by lessening odor), and you will begin to accept that nursing, like all kinds of work, has some aspects which are more difficult or less pleasant than others.

As you work with patients whose physical condition is unappealing to you, try, as far as possible, to be aware of your reactions toward the patient. If you really feel slightly nauseated or want to excuse yourself on some pretext, acknowledge to yourself that this is the case. You will then be more likely to be aware of your interaction with the patient and better able to control the response you convey to him.

It is also helpful to ask someone else (such as your teacher) to observe unobtrusively as you give care to the patient, and to let you know afterward her impression of your interaction with the patient. Sometimes you will be unaware of how your facial expression or gestures come across to another person, and a candid impression from someone else can alert you to trouble spots, as well as help you become aware of your strengths. Another important barometer of your approach is the reaction of the patient. Of course, if he shows embarrassment or withdrawal, it may be entirely due to his own reaction to his situation; it may, however, be an indicator that he perceives that you do not accept him.

Accepting the patient definitely does not mean accepting disarray of the surroundings and inattention to the patient's personal hygiene. One nurse entered the room of a patient with an infectious disease. The door was closed and when she opened it, she found three left-over meal trays, a bedpan which needed to be emptied, and an irritable, resentful, disheveled patient. The first step in relating to him involved concrete measures to help improve his situation, not with an air of "Oh, what a mess you are" but, "You look uncomfortable; let's see what can be done about it."

If you have questions about whether a patient's condition is infectious, ask and find out what measures you must take to protect yourself. Having made sure that your knowledge is adequate, you will find it easier to use a sure touch, rather than a gingerly one.

## THE "SELF-CARE" PATIENT

A good many medical-surgical patients are described as "self-care." Some are on general wards; others are on separate units designed especially for them. These patients present no less of a challenge than the more physically helpless patients, in the establishment of the nurse-patient relationship, but the challenges are somewhat different.

Because physical care is so important an aspect of working with medical-surgical patients, nurses (and patients too) are sometimes at a loss concerning establishment of their relationship if the patient does not require physical care. One may hear at the morning assignment conference, "Mr. Brown—oh, you don't have to do anything for him. The aide makes his bed and he does everything else for himself."

What, then, of the nurse-patient relationship with "self-care" patients? It is important for the nurse to consider how she can relate helpfully to this group of patients and to recognize that her role is not confined to administration of medicines, scheduling various diagnostic tests, and acting as a hostess. Among the "self-care" patients are many who are undergoing diagnostic tests. Frequently the patient has a good deal of free time; in fact some patients describe the experience as one of interminable waiting: waiting to go to scheduled appointments, waiting for test results. Frequently the waiting is accompanied by anxiety. Until a diagnosis is made, the patient has no concrete "enemy" to grapple with. Instead, he may have many vague fears about what may be wrong and a general feeling of powerlessness. One patient said, when she learned her diagnosis, "Oh, I feel so relieved. Now at least I know what it is, and I know what I have to do about it."

One important aspect of care of these patients involves explaining diagnostic tests to them and helping the patient understand the results. Both should be done in close collaboration with the physician. If you find that a patient is scheduled for some test or procedure about which he seems to know nothing, bring this to the physician's attention. Maybe the patient's preparation for the test has escaped the physician's notice. If so, it is appropriate for you to mention it, just as you would expect a colleague to remind you if you left a side rail down. On the other hand, the patient may have been so anxious that he understood none of the physician's explanation. This is important to notice, if it is the case, since it means that, unless it is a dire emergency, time must be spent with the patient to discover what is troubling him, before the procedure is undertaken.

Patients need opportunities, too, to review with the nurse the results of their tests, the diagnosis the physician has made, and the treatment which he has prescribed. Often, after the physician has given the patient the information, the patient wants a chance to talk about it again—to review what was said, to clarify terms, and the like. Often there is an element of psychological shock involved in hearing a diagnosis for the first time. The patient may re-

spond with, "Oh, I can't need an operation." Gradually as he reflects upon it and talks about it, he begins to face the fact that he does need an operation and then wants to review what is entailed and what results he can expect following surgery. Often it is necessary to refer the patient's questions to the physician at this stage. Usually the patient has forgotten or become confused about what the physician told him initially. Opportunity to discuss this again with the physician is helpful to the patient once the first shock of the diagnosis has diminished. If the situation is very threatening to the patient, he will require repeated opportunities to talk with the nurse and physician in order to prepare himself for treatment.

Do not encourage the patient in brooding over "What if it's ____?" If no one really knows what is wrong, it is best not to engage in a type of conversation with the patient which, under the guise of "instruction," really provides "worry data." Instead, encourage the patient to occupy himself with ward activities and, when you talk with him, encourage him to concentrate on the specific measures the physician has ordered, such as how to prepare himself for diagnostic tests.

Although this discussion has concentrated on preparing patients for diagnostic tests as an illustration of how the nurse can relate helpfully to a patient who does not require physical care, many other examples could be given. The main point is that the nurse assess the situation in which the "self-care" patient finds himself, and that she consider ways in which she can, by her relationship with him, help the patient cope with his situation.

## THE PATIENT WHO IS UNCONSCIOUS

Your first thought may be that if the patient is unconscious, there can be no relationship. However, the nurse does not turn off her reactions because a patient is unconscious. Sometimes imperceptibly, the patient who appears comatose begins being aware of the nurse. In any case, she is aware of him.

Some nurses find it very difficult to care for a patient who cannot respond in some way; others may find it a relief not to have to relate verbally to the patient. For some nurses, unconsciousness may signify the epitome of helplessness so that they prefer to avoid caring for these patients because it evokes too much anxiety. The nurse must try to avoid, on the one hand, treating the patient as though he were an object, rather than a person, and on the other hand, feeling overwhelmed by the seriousness of his condition. As you care for these patients try to think of concrete, individual nursing needs which you observe and plan ways to meet them. Is the skin on the patient's sacrum redder? How can you position him to promote good body alignment and prevent pressure sores? Has he shown any sign of returning consciousness—the flicker of an eyelid? Concentrating on such practical and individualized observations will help you avoid being overwhelmed by the gravity of the patient's condition and also to avoid thinking of the patient as an object.

Care of an unconscious adult, particularly if he is heavy, is best undertaken by two nurses working together. The physical and emotional burdens for the nurses are made lighter when they are shared. Each can encourage the other in how best to give mouth care, prevent obstruction of catheters, and so on. However, it is essential to keep in mind that the patient may hear you, even though he cannot respond. Make it a rule never to say anything in your patient's presence which you do not want him to hear.

As you work with the patient, if there seems to be any possibility of returning consciousness, speak to him slowly and gently, saying what you are about to do. Occasionally you will observe someone shouting at an unconscious patient—or slapping his face brusquely. Such actions are never warranted and may reflect the nurse's anxiety over working with an unconscious patient.

Just as the experienced nurse seeks help when moving a heavy person to avoid straining her back, she will also seek help with situations (whatever their nature) which are emotionally overburdening. Talk with your teachers and supervisors about your reactions to very ill patients as an aid in helping you understand these reactions and deal with them.

## THE DYING PATIENT

Please see Chapter 12 for discussion of this topic.

## THE PATIENT WHO REFUSES
## HIS TREATMENT

A teacher, lawyer, or salesman is, upon admission to the hospital, expected to "take orders" unquestioningly. A host of indignities surround him.

No matter how necessary these may be from the standpoint of running the hospital, they can be galling to the patient. The abrupt change from being in charge of his own affairs to acquiescing to directions of others is difficult for many patients. Anxiety over the diagnosis and its implications plays a part in patients' refusal to follow treatment. The patient may refuse treatment because he cannot acknowledge that he could be sick enough to need it. When a patient refuses treatment, he places the nurse in a difficult position. The nurse is expected to see that prescribed treatment is carried out, whether this involves taking medication, staying in bed, or keeping within a prescribed diet.

Frequently the nurse assumes more responsibility than she can handle in such situations, and her frustration may then get in the way of effectively dealing with the patient who refuses treatment. What nurse has not been reminded, for example, that it is *her* responsibility to see that the patient stays in bed, sticks to his diet, or whatever. Yes, it is the nurse's responsibility, but it is not hers alone, as is often implied. It is also the patient's responsibility to follow his treatment, and, except in unusual circumstances when he is unable to make his own decisions, it is basically a matter for the patient to decide, once he has acquired the necessary facts. It is also the physician's responsibility to see that his patient has necessary information concerning the treatment, and encouragement to follow it.

Keeping these factors in mind will help you maintain perspective concerning your role and your responsibility. By concentrating on what your responsibility really is and recognizing the limits of your authority, you will be less likely to feel overwhelmed by the situation and more able to concentrate on what you can do to help the patient. For example, suppose you are informed during morning report that a coronary patient refuses to stay in bed and that it is your job to see that he does. If you do not think it through, what are you likely to do? You will probably approach the patient bristling with authority and begin scolding him. You have been placed in an untenable situation, and you are ready to vent your indignation on the patient. Suppose, instead, that you think about the situation this way: the patient is twice as strong as you; there is no way that you can physically force him to do anything. The entire responsibility for seeing that he remains in bed does not rest solely on your shoulders, nor will it be "all your fault" if he keels over during one of his trips to the bathroom. You do, however, have a responsibility to do all in your power to help the patient follow his treatment. With your responsibility cut down to more manageable size, how will you approach the patient?

Start by thinking of his situation. What may be some reasons for his not staying in bed? Did his physician explain the need for bed rest fully, and did the patient understand the explanation? Is his call bell answered promptly, or does he feel that he must choose between wetting the bed and getting up to go to the bathroom? Does the thought that he has had a coronary make him so anxious that he does everything possible to deny his illness? These are among the possibilities. How can you find out what is troubling the patient?

If you scold him, he is likely to tune you out. Instead, try starting to give his care, and then gently asking him what makes it so difficult for him to stay in bed. Listen carefully to what he says and avoid cutting him off. The most important reason may not be mentioned until some of the lesser ones have been expressed. Avoid giving the patient a lecture on the pathophysiology of myocardial infarction and of the possibility of dire consequences if the order for bed rest is not followed. Most patients are already only too well aware of the seriousness of heart attacks. Emphasizing this is likely to frighten the patient further and make him more prone to deny his condition.

As you listen to the patient, keep attuned not only to underlying fears which he may express, but also to his recounting of daily annoyances. Often these patients, in their frustration and anger at being suddenly stopped in the midst of a busy life by a serious illness, start out by complaining that coffee is served cold, that no one wants to empty the urinal, and so on. Let the patient know that you will do what you can to remedy these problems. When the patient senses your concern about his daily frustrations and notices that you are interested in seeing what can be done about them, he may be more likely to confide other concerns to you.

One crucial consideration, when working with a patient who refuses his treatment, is acknowledgment that the patient (except under unusual circumstances which are dealt with in literature on the legal aspects of nursing) has the right to refuse his treatment. The nurse who proceeds with this realization will do so with a more realistic assessment of the patient's role and of her own. It is then the nurse's job to help the patient make the best possible decisions for his own welfare, rather than to place herself in the false position of deciding for him what he may and may not do.

## FAMILIES

You may find yourself jealous and resentful of the patient's relatives. It is an understandable reaction. When you have carefully nursed a patient through a crisis, you may feel possessive and resent a wife or husband, children or parents as intruders. Examine your goals again. You are the professional nurse and not the mother, the wife, or the husband. Find satisfaction for your personal needs outside of the work situation, and you will be of better service to your patients and their families. We are not saying that it is wrong to find satisfaction in a job well done. We are saying that if the total satisfaction of a nurse's life comes from work, she may have a tendency to hold patients too close.

Nurses have specialized knowledge and skills that help patients to recover. But a loved member of the family can make many contributions to the peace of mind and the comfort of a patient that, because of the closeness of the relationship, is beyond even the most skilled tongue and hands. When it is appropriate, capitalize on what the family can do for the patient; do not exclude them. Help the family to encourage the patient in the hard things that he has to learn. Is he walking better? A word of praise from a loved one may mean more to the patient than the applause of the entire hospital staff. Is a patient worried about his new diet? Let his wife show him how she will fit it into their daily lives. Perhaps a patient will eat better if his wife brings some food from home. With permission of the physician and the physical therapist, encourage the family to participate in the rehabilitation program in speech and exercises.

It may not be easy for a daughter to sit passively by while others care for her mother. The illness alone makes her uneasy, and her inactivity may make her feel even more powerless. Action is a good antidote for this kind of feeling. Instead of allowing her to feel left out, suggest that her mother might be cheered by the evening paper, or ask her to encourage fluids (if the patient needs fluids). Say something like this: "Your mother will probably take the fluids better if you give them to her."

Feelings of guilt about illness are common and often irrational. A son might think, "If I had spent more time home, Father would not have had this heart attack." A wife may think, "If I had gone on that trip with John, he wouldn't have been in this car accident." That these thoughts may be irrational does not lessen their sting. Being able to participate in the care of the patient may help the family to feel in some small measure less guilty. The nurse should provide opportunities for the family to talk about the experience, if they wish.

Visitors should be made to feel welcome. They are the patient's contact with his usual life. Show them how to cheer the patient without tiring him. Is the visitor standing at the bedside, awkwardly clutching his coat? Draw up a chair for him; show him where to hang his coat. Share with close relatives important aspects of the patient's care. Point out to them how much better the patient feels when his wife or his daughter or mother helps to care for him, if this is the case.

Several other challenges must be considered when working with patients' families, particularly in long-term illness. (Although the terms "relative" and "family" are used here, remember that what is really meant is those persons closest to the patient. For some patients this is a close friend.) It is easy for nurses to view family members only in their role of helping the patient and to disregard their other responsibilities. In an acute illness, it is common for relatives to discontinue other responsibilities temporarily in order to help the patient. If illness continues, however, the patient's family must begin to resume other obligations. As you talk with the patient's relative, try to consider the situation which that person faces. One aspect of it, to be sure, is the patient's illness. However, do not close off other topics of conversation, if the family member wishes to introduce them. As you listen to some of his other concerns, such as the fact that one of his children has cerebral palsy or that he belongs to a union that is now out on strike, you will gain greater appreciation of his situation and you will have less tendency to consider him solely in the role of the patient's helper.

Society sets certain standards concerning responsibility when a family member is ill. Perhaps nowhere are these standards so forcefully upheld as in health care institutions. At morning reports and team conferences one frequently hears rather negative comments about patients' families: they do not take the patient home; they do not visit, and so on. This criticism is understandable, as health personnel must rely on families to fulfill their role in helping the patient. When families do not meet these expectations, not only does the patient lack the support and encouragement that he needs, but also the work of physicians and nurses is made more difficult. Remember that not all families can meet your expectations in helping the patient for a variety of reasons, many of which may remain unknown to you. For example, some family members are not emotionally stable enough to cope with prolonged illness and dependence of another person. Others may have conflicting obligations— to other family members, work, and so on. As you work with the patient's relatives, be alert to their attitudes and to their resources for helping the patient, rather than establishing, according to your values, what the family should do. The former approach will enable you to help the family use the resources they do have. What questions do they have about the patient's care? What community resources may be of help to them?

Long-term illness, particularly, is likely to bring about changes in family relationships. The woman who ordinarily consulted her husband about business matters may turn instead to her son-in-law for this advice, after her husband has had a stroke. In general, try to help families to retain their usual patterns of relationship during the illness period. Encourage the young mother with congestive heart failure to continue to participate in the aspects of her children's care of which she is capable, rather than turning it over entirely to a relative or a housekeeper.

Evaluate your own intervention with family members. Do you, without meaning to, encourage a family member to withdraw from her usual relationship with the patient? Suppose you are teaching the patient's wife how to irrigate and dress his colostomy. In your emphasis on the procedure, and your zeal to help her perform it correctly, are you losing sight of the fact that you and she are beginning to talk as though she were another nurse rather than the patient's wife? The family member, particularly if he or she is well informed about medical and nursing matters, may have a tendency to substitute a highly "clinical" approach for the personal relationship with the patient if the illness poses problems affecting this relationship. For instance, although the patient's wife may spend a great deal of time at the hospital, most of it may be focused on concern for her husband's diet, his dressing, the condition of the skin around the stoma, and so on. Such an approach may be one indication of failing to deal with the implications of the husband's illness for their personal relationship.

Although a relative's reluctance to learn to care for the patient is usually quickly noted, an overly "clinical" approach may not attract attention, since it fits in with the staff's expectations. If you notice that a relative is beginning to speak of the patient's care almost as though she were the "assistant nurse," perhaps you can spend some time talking with her—other than the time you have allocated to teaching her the various procedures. By showing interest in her and in her concerns, rather than just in her ability to carry out her husband's care, you may make it possible for her to talk over some of her personal reactions with you. No matter how well informed a patient's wife may be about her husband's condition, she is still his wife and not another nurse. Do not allow your conversations with her to focus exclusively on the techniques of her husband's care, but show your concern also for her reactions and her comfort. Far from working to the patient's disadvantage, this approach may be a help to him. After his wife has had a chance to talk about some of her own worries about the effect of her husband's colostomy on their home life, she may be more likely to talk with him about how things are going at home, how the children are doing in school, and so on. Although the nurse and the patient's wife may not notice, at first, the fact that she has dropped such topics from the conversation in favor of more clinical ones, the patient is often acutely aware that his role has suddenly shifted exclusively to that of a patient in his wife's eyes.

Keep in mind that illness, such as cancer or heart disease, in a family member is a powerful force in mobilizing the anxiety of relatives. They may show their anxiety in various ways: by withdrawing, by becoming too "clinical," by talking about the patient rather than to him, or even by ascribing whatever difficulties the family may be having to the patient's illness. The more you can recognize that anxiety plays a part in such reactions, the better able you will be to help the family care for the patient.

The transition from hospital to home can be a stressful experience for the patient and his family.

Particularly if the patient has been away from home for an extended period, he often has a tendency to idealize his relationship with his family. During the long months of hospitalization he may have sustained himself by thinking about how wonderful it will be to be home again and how warmly his family will welcome him. Even in devoted families, some tarnishing of this ideal is likely to occur, as the patient returns home to real family life. The imperfections of his relatives, which he may have forgotten during hospitalization, are still there—as are his own shortcomings as a participant in family life.

Another and more difficult discovery which is by no means uncommon among long-term patients is that their families have formed other relationships which supplant or, at least, lessen their ties to the patient. Before you conclude that this is crass disloyalty, remember that it is natural for people to turn to others for companionship when a person who has been fulfilling this need is no longer able to do so. Both the patient's reaction of idealizing his family while he is in the hospital and the family's turning to others for roles which he customarily filled are natural and understandable. Often it is possible for the patient to re-establish his ties with family and friends when he returns home. Sometimes it is not, and the patient must recognize that the place he had filled in the lives of others, to which he was so eager to return, no longer exists and that he must begin all over again to develop new relationships. As you work with patients who are making the transition from hospital to home, your appreciation of these factors will help you to assist the patient's family to assess the situation realistically.

## ASSESSMENT

Assessment of the nurse-patient relationship involves not only the patient's participation, but also the nurse's interaction with him. Although assessment in this area is not as measurable as, say, the amount of urine output in an hour, nevertheless it is important to assess the usefulness of the relationship in helping the patient during his experience of illness.

Such assessment may be carried out in many ways. The nurse can notice her own response to the patient. Is she genuinely interested in his progress? Annoyed with him? She can notice also the patient's response to her. Does he seem to brighten up when she comes into the room? Does he begin to share with her some of his personal concerns? Does he show emotion, such as anger and sorrow? Reviewing tape recordings of talks with the patient can be helpful to the nurse in assessing her relationship with the patient, as can videotapes and written notes. These methods are especially helpful when shared with a teacher or a group of peers who give their views and suggestions.

Various written guides and rating scales are also available to assist in assessing the nurse-patient relationship. One of these has been developed by Aiken and Aiken (1973). They provide a scale which includes five important ways in which the nurse can facilitate a therapeutic relationship with the patient: (1) empathetic understanding, (2) positive regard, (3) genuineness, (4) concreteness, and (5) self-exploration. Within each category are descriptions of behavior ranging from ineffective to effective. Such a rating scale is useful in helping the nurse evaluate the effectiveness of her interaction with the patient in assisting him to recognize and express his feelings, view himself as a worthwhile human being, respond genuinely, communicate clearly and specifically, and explore the meaning and impact of events in his life.

## REFERENCES AND BIBLIOGRAPHY

AIKEN, LINDA, and AIKEN, JAMES L.: A systematic approach to the evaluation of interpersonal relationships, *Am. J. Nurs.* 73:863, May 1973.

AMACHER, NANCY JEAN: Touch is a way of caring, *Am. J. Nurs.* 73:852, May 1973.

AQUILERA, D. et al.: *Crisis Intervention: Theory and Method,* St. Louis, Mosby, 1970.

BELL, N. W., and VOGEL, E. F. (eds.): *The Family,* rev. ed., New York, The Free Press, 1968.

BLAKER, K. P.: Systems theory and self-destructive behavior, *Perspec. in Psych. Care* 10:168, October-November 1972.

CARLSON, CAROLYN E.: *Behavioral Concepts and Nursing Intervention,* Philadelphia, Lippincott, 1972.

ENELOW, A. J., and SWISHER, S. N.: *Interviewing and Patient Care,* New York, Oxford University Press, 1972.

ENGEL, G. L.: Grief and grieving, *Am. J. Nurs.* 64:93, September 1964.

FRANCIS, G., and MUNJAS, B.: *Promoting Psychological Comfort,* Dubuque, Iowa, Brown, 1968.

GLASER, B. G., and STRAUSS, A.: The social loss of dying patients, *Am. J. Nurs.* 64:119, June 1964.

GOLDIN, P.: Therapeutic communications, *Am. J. Nurs.* 69:1928, September 1969.

GOLDSBOROUGH, J. P.: On becoming non-judgmental, *Am. J. Nurs.* 70:2340, November 1970.

GREGG, D.: Reassurance, *Am. J. Nurs.* 55:171, 1955.

———: Anxiety—a factor in nursing care, *Am. J. Nurs.* 52:1363, 1952.

HARDMAN, M. A.: Interviewing? Or social chit-chat? *Am. J. Nurs.* 71:1379, July 1971.

HARRIS, T. A.: *I'm OK—you're OK,* New York: Harper and Row, 1969.

HITCHCOCK, J. M.: Crisis intervention—the pebble in the pool, *Am. J. Nurs.* 73:1388, August 1973.

JOHNSON, M. A.: *Developing the Art of Understanding,* New York, Springer, 1967.

KING, J. M.: The initial interview: Basis for assessment in crisis intervention, *Perspec. in Psych. Care* 9:247, November-December 1971.

LEVINE, M. E.: The intransigent patient, *Am. J. Nurs.* 70:2106, October 1970.

LIDZ, T.: *The Person: His Development Throughout the Life Cycle,* New York, Basis Books, 1968.

MALONEY, ELIZABETH M.: The subjective and objective definition of crisis, *Perspec. in Psych. Care* 9:259, November-December 1971.

MAY, R.: *The Meaning of Anxiety,* New York, Ronald, 1950.

MENNINGER, K. A.: *Man Against Himself,* New York, Harcourt, 1956 (section on Suicide).

———: *The Vital Balance,* New York, Viking, 1963.

PARAD, HOWARD: *Crisis Intervention,* New York, Family Service Association of America, 1965.

PARKES, C. M. *Bereavement: Studies of Grief in Adult Life,* New York, International Universities Press, 1972.

PEPLAU, H. E.: *Interpersonal Relations in Nursing,* New York, Putnam, 1952.

———: Professional closeness . . . as a special kind of involvement with a patient, client, or family group, *Nurs. Forum* 8:343, 1969.

QUINT, JEANNE C.: *The Nurse and the Dying Patient,* New York, Macmillan, 1967.

ROBERTS, J. M.: Loneliness, *Perspec. in Psych. Care* 10:227, December 1972.

ROGERS, C.: Carl Rogers describes his way of facilitating encounter groups, *Am. J. Nurs.* 71:275, February 1971.

SHNEIDMAN, E. S.: *Essays in Self-Destruction,* New York, Science House, 1967.

SHNEIDMAN, E. S.; FARKEROW, N. L.; and LITMAN, R. E. (eds.): *The Psychology of Suicide,* New York, Science House, 1970.

SMITH, DOROTHY W.: Patienthood and its threat to privacy, *Am. J. Nurs.* 69:508, March 1969.

SPIEGEL, J.: *Transactions,* New York, Science House, 1971.

SULLIVAN, H. S.: *The Interpersonal Theory of Psychiatry,* New York, W. M. Norton, 1953.

THALER, O. F.: Grief and depression, *Nurs. Forum* 5:9, 1966.

THOMAS, M. D. et al.: Anger: a tool for developing self-awareness, *Am. J. Nurs.* 70:2586, December 1970.

TRAVELBEE, J.: *Interpersonal Aspects of Nursing,* Philadelphia, Davis, 1971.

UJHELY, G. B.: *The Nurse and Her Problem Patients,* New York, Springer, 1963.

_____: *Determinants of the Nurse-Patient Relationship,* New York, Springer, 1968.

_____: Basic considerations for nurse-patient interaction in prevention and treatment of emotional disorders, *Nurs. Clin. N. Am.* 1:179, June 1966.

_____: Grief and depression—implications for preventive and therapeutic nursing care, *Nurs. Forum* 5:23, 1966.

_____: What is realistic emotional support? *Am. J. Nurs.* 68:758, April 1968.

VINCENT, P. A.: Do we want patients to conform? *Nurs. Outlook* 18:54, January 1970.

WILLIAMS, FLORENCE: Intervention in maturational crises, *Perspec. in Psych. Care* 9:240, November-December 1971.

WOLFF, I. S.: Acceptance, *Am. J. Nurs.* 72:1412, August 1972.

# Concepts of Health and Illness—Fundamental Physiologic Processes

Nursing, as one of the health professions, is concerned with helping people to obtain and maintain optimal health as well as with preventing disease and caring for those who are ill, or who require rehabilitation to promote optimal functioning.

Health and illness are relative states. Constantly in flux, they depend on the satisfaction of biologic, psychological, and sociologic and cultural needs and the ability to make suitable adaptations to stresses affecting these needs as they arise from within or without the individual.

James (1968) has suggested that disease should be thought of in four stages:

Stage 1.  Disease foundations and predisease factors such as heredity, smoking, habitual overeating.

Stage 2.  Presymptomatic disease, such as the early stages of cancer and tuberculosis when the stricken person may feel and appear healthy; or the period of fairly effective psychosocial functioning prior to situational crisis with which the person with impaired personality development is unable to cope.

Stage 3.  Onset of symptoms—that time in the natural history of the disease when patients require treatment or help from the physician.

Stage 4.  Rehabilitation to the fullest extent possible; or the period of management of incurable conditions.

In the past, most of the patients nurses contacted were at Stage 3 or 4 but today with more research and greater emphasis on Stages 1 and 2, nurses participate in the care of clients so that disease might be prevented or lessened in severity.

## HISTORIC VIEWS OF DISEASE

Historically, the concepts of man's health and illness have evolved from an early emphasis on cellular pathophysiology to a more integrated approach which views health and illness as involving man's psychological and sociocultural dimensions as well as his biologic makeup.

Many early leaders in medicine and public health believed the major cause of disease was germs. The germ theory had as its contributors such scientists as Purkinje, Schleiden, Schwann, Pasteur, and Koch. Efforts to combat germs by destroying them through sterilization or neutralizing their toxins became the major protection against disease. Yet, René Dubos (1963), who has spent much of his life studying tuberculosis, has said, "The more I study the tubercle bacillus, the less I think it has to do with tuberculosis."

In the late 19th century a French physiologist named Claude Bernard shifted the emphasis in disease theory from anatomic or cell structure to physiologic function when he studied the internal environment of the body, or the "milieu interieur." He recognized that germs were a necessary but not a sufficient cause for some diseases and that many diseases did not involve germs as major causes. Bernard wrote in 1878 that a healthy being is "a piece of constancy living and moving in a world of variables," but the internal variables, such as oxygen and pH have very narrow limits. When man is not able to maintain the dynamic constancy within these limits, he becomes ill.

In 1932 Walter Cannon, an American physiologist, again brought forth this long-neglected concept of the constancy of the "milieu interieur" and renamed the dynamic state of equilibrium "homeostasis." To maintain homeostasis, man must be able to balance the components of his internal environment such as endocrine secretions, water, electrolytes, proteins, vitamins, and oxygen. He must obtain the materials needed and convert or eliminate what is in excess. Thus pathology can arise from deprivation such as vitamin deficiency, or from excess such as sodium ions. Endocrine disturbances can arise from deprivation as well as excess of hormones.

Though Cannon's work emphasized material components of the body, the later work of scientists such as René Spitz (1954) showed that deprivation of psychological and social factors could provoke serious disease and even death though physical needs were met.

## CONCEPT OF STRESS

Another derivative from the concept of homeostasis is the concept of stress. Stress, according to Engel (1953), can be "any influence, whether it arises from the internal environment or from the external environment, which interferes with the satisfaction of basic needs or which disturbs or threatens to disturb the stable equilibrium."

Hans Selye, a contemporary Canadian physician-physiologist studying the integrative functions of the neuroendocrine systems, found that the constancy of the internal environment can be maintained only when external variations are not excessive in degree or too sudden in onset. Stress tolerance, or the ability to adapt to stressors without a breakdown in homeostatic mechanisms, is an individual thing based on heredity, environment, intelligence, and the experiences of growth and development.

In Selye's theory (1956), stress is a specific physiologic condition manifested by a general adaptation syndrome. No matter whether a stressor be biologic, such as surgical trauma or bacterial toxins; psychological, such as worry, fear, rage; or sociologic, such as a new job or increased family responsibilities, the same non-specific general adaptation syndrome results if the stressor is excessive in degree, ill-timed, or too sudden in onset.

The general adaptation syndrome consists of three stages: the alarm reaction, stage of resistance, and stage of exhaustion or death. Most stressors evoke the first two stages of response. An individual goes through these defensive stages a great many times during life. They are purposeful homeostatic reactions.

The general response to a stressor is accomplished through the coordinate efforts of the endocrine and nervous systems. Acting through the nerves, stressors produce adrenalines and acetylcholine in nerve endings; and a few nerve filaments go directly to the adrenal medulla. Also, through the endocrine system, stressors stimulate the pituitary to secrete adrenocorticotropic hormone (ACTH), which then stimulates the adrenal cortex to produce predominantly anti-inflammatory corticoid substances or glucocorticoids, namely cortisone and cortisol. Glucocorticoids tend to be inhibitory and catabolic.

The adrenal cortex is also stimulated to produce proinflammatory corticoids or mineralocorticoids, namely aldosterone and desoxycorticosterone. Mineralocorticoids tend to be stimulative and anabolic.

Selye found that imbalances between these two types of hormones as well as an excess of ACTH can be responsible for disease through their effect on certain "target organs." These include the thymus and lymphatic system; joints and connective tissue; blood vessels; the liver, kidney, pancreas, and gastrointestinal tract.

The adaptive hormones of the pituitary-adrenal system appear to be necessary to maintain life during the alarm reaction of the general adaptation syndrome when large tissue regions are under stress. The body then gains the time necessary for the development of specific local adaptive phenomena in the directly affected region.

During the stage of resistance the directly affected region can cope with its local task without the help of adaptive hormones.

At times, when the body uses one organ system repeatedly to cope with a threatening situation, disease can result from its disproportionate excessive development, or from its eventual breakdown due to wear and tear. Specifically, Selye uses the term "diseases of adaptation" to refer to those maladies resulting from an excessive or insufficient amount or an improper mixture of adaptive hormones. Nephritis, nephrosis, peptic ulcer, keloid formation, hypertension, arthritis are among those so classified.

A broader consideration of man's adaptive processes suggests, however, that all diseases are processes in adaptation. Man is constantly reacting to the stressors of the internal and external environment. Biologic mechanisms for survival come into play when a peritoneal inflammation is walled off by the omentum as well as when a soldier is prevented from going forth to possible death through the development of an hysterical paralysis. The metabolic process is always creating shifts in the internal milieu and normal adaptive response strives for survival.

As the psychiatrist Leonard Cammer writes (1962), "In order to survive, each organism seeks to express its greatest potential through physiologic adaptation. As part of this physiologic process, the psychologic activity of the adaptive mechanisms emerges, in all its complexity, and relates the person as a total unit, to his culture and environment."

Stress is obviously not an entirely negative concept. Inherent in each individual's growth and development are markedly stressful situations which, if mastered, give zest and fullness to life. In the oyster the pearl is produced in response to a stressor. One needs stress to live. At each stage of development there are stressful tasks to be learned and mastered which ready one for the next stage of development, whether this be toilet training for the toddler, developing sound heterosexual relationships for the adolescent, or entering the nursing profession as a young adult.

The person who subjects himself to the stress of physical conditioning involved in a daily two-mile run gradually increases the efficiency of his cardiovascular system. This is beneficial compared to the person who limits his exercise to changing the channels on his television set.

Trying something for the first time, whether it be a new job, a new skill, or a new role in life, is often a stressful experience. But as one perseveres and grows in ability and confidence, the apprehension diminishes and life is enriched because one made the effort to continue to learn and grow.

Presently, tangible components of the stress response are being identified in chemical and physical terms. During the stress reaction the following are some of the changes that occur:

1. Blood and urinary levels of 17-hydroxycorticoids rise, indicating increased production of glucocorticoids.
2. The eosinophil count drops, indicating that the anterior pituitary is secreting greater than normal amounts of ACTH, causing an increased production of glucocorticoids.
3. Urinary excretion of aldosterone is increased, which mediates increased sodium retention and potassium excretion.
4. There is increased urinary excretion of catecholamines (epinephrine and norepinephrine).
5. The basal metabolic rate is increased.
6. There is increased breakdown of liver and muscle glycogen, with increased urinary nitrogen loss due to gluconeogenesis.

Though Selye's stress theory is not the final answer to disease causation, it represents a more comprehensive approach to health and illness than any heretofore. It takes into account the biologic, psychological, and sociologic and cultural stressors involved in an individual's internal and external environments, the meaning that the stressors have for the individual, and how he deals with stress in an attempt to maintain homeostasis.

For example, a middle-aged male patient who sustains an acute myocardial infarction or a female patient who undergoes radical mastectomy for breast cancer both sustain cellular damage. Psychologically, each has new and different changes and deficits to adjust to by acquiring a different concept of self. Sociologically, the participation of each in his or her social roles, whether as parent, spouse, employee, or any other, will be altered temporarily at least, and perhaps permanently. Patients with the same diagnosis differ in the state of equilibrium they reach after illness because their adaptive responses on the biologic-psychological-sociologic levels are different.

Biologically, the individual's mode of adaptive responses is limited by genetic endowment as well as by morphology and physiochemical structure. Psychological adaptation also depends on genetic endowment plus one's relationships to significant others, finite and the Infinite. Though individuals have greater latitude sociologically for new adaptive modes, inertia and cultural tradition often impede the development of new coping mechanisms, particularly if they contradict old values. For example, a woman who was raised in a social atmosphere of sexual mystery may be experiencing much distress from symptoms, but be too embarrassed or ashamed to undergo examination and early treatment for cancer of the cervix.

The body, with its marvelous capacity for coping with large variations in the assaults of various stressors sometimes reaches a point when quantitative excesses cannot be compensated for and symptoms result. Symptoms represent the evidence of damage or the defense reaction to excessive stress. Though symptoms have been categorized classically as mental or physical, each disease process involves all tissues of the body, directly or indirectly and in varying degrees.

Though symptoms may indeed reflect an organic disturbance, cellular pathology may not necessarily have initiated the symptom complex. Disease is usually the result of multiple factors. A female diabetic patient, well controlled with diet and insulin, may be looked upon as being in a state of equilibrium. But the social and psychological stressors of her husband's sudden death may be sufficient to provoke acute symptomatic illness. Organic disorders are concomitants in the complex of biologic, psychological, and social patterns of adaptation, and illness should be looked upon as a breakdown in total living. Good treatment, then, emphasizes the function of the individual in all his dimensions.

## NURSING AND STRESS

How does nursing fit into this more comprehensive view of health and illness? Examining some of its dimensions, nursing care involves:

1. Preventing, modifying, reducing, or removing stressors.

Nurses can anticipate the adaptive tasks facing an individual through a knowledge of the developmental needs and tasks facing him at his particular stage in the life cycle. The prevention of illness at crisis points in life is enhanced when individuals are prepared for new adaptive tasks. Nurses can assist in the maintenance of homeostasis by participation in programs of health education. Participating in immunization programs, encouraging routine Pap smears, or speaking to members of a Golden Age Club on the prevention of falls are other ways.

In the hospital, the nurse who cares for the patient with an acute myocardial infarction monitors his ECG continuously to detect the added stressor of dangerous cardiac arrhythmias and prevent it from interfering with the heart's effective function and healing.

2. Supporting the adaptive processes utilized by the patient in his attempt to establish a new state of equilibrium.

To support adaptive processes one must know the nature of such processes. Nurses study such subjects as anatomy and physiology, pathophysiology, psychology, and cultural anthropology so that they can understand patients' modes of adaptation, assess where they may need assistance, establish priorities, and intervene appropriately.

During illness, support of the patient's natural defenses and adaptive processes can be accomplished while working with the physician and other members of the health team. Management of the internal environment through such activities as the control of pain with drugs, the administration of fluids and electrolytes, or antibiotics and other medications offer specific kinds of help.

Understanding the mental mechanisms patients use to cope with threats to their integrity enables the nurse to be supportive. Just nonjudgmentally listening to the patient as he confronts his weaknesses, identifies his strengths, and attempts to reassess the direction of his life relieves the patient's autonomic nervous system of the burden of carrying this load internally. The nurse who listens supportively may help the patient to deal with an amputation although she cannot prevent the amputation. Nor can she solve the patient's problems for him. She can assist him to identify what the problems are and where she and the other available resources can be of assistance.

Management of the external environment is often necessary to promote rest, a major treatment for many illnesses. Nursing activities which promote rest include arranging for a comfortable room temperature, providing a cotton instead of a wool blanket for the allergic patient, controlling noise, providing a pleasant, appropriately cheerful environment, and spacing nursing activities for the benefit of the patient rather than for the convenience of hospital departments.

Using good judgment regarding the number of visitors and the length of visitation assists the patient in his attempt to regain equilibrium. The elderly lady might greatly benefit by having the rules relaxed and her daughter near at hand most of the time whereas the active businessman might need to be protected from the oversolicitude of his office associates. Respecting the patient's usual ego and cultural supports by permitting him to assist in planning his care or arranging for his desired clergyman's visit are other ways that permit the patient to concentrate his adaptive resources on the task of healing.

3. Recognizing that applying stressors is a necessary part of the treatment process and that, in moderation, stress is necessary for life.

Nursing should not add to the patient's illness through ignorant or sympathetic neglect or inflict iatrogenic diseases upon him.

Patients have optimum stress tolerance levels. These need to be accurately assessed so that patients are guided to use their adaptation energy at a rate and in a direction appropriate to the capacity of their minds and bodies.

The patient in shock has very limited and only essential physical activity so that his metabolic demands are minimized.

The nurse who encourages the postoperative cholecystectomy patient to cough up secretions introduces another stressor, but minimizes its effect by splinting the incisional area. Stress is also minimized by teaching the patient to cough properly preoperatively when he is apt to be more comfortable. Letting the patient know what is expected of him, commending his often heroic efforts, and giving him pain medication as warranted after he has performed his task are ways of supporting him through this stressful experience. Introducing minimal stress through coughing and deep breathing exercises prevents the major stress resulting from atelectasis and hypostatic pneumonia.

Though bed rest is a treatment designed to reduce stress in many illnesses, it can be hazardous in itself. The nurse who uses good judgment in encouraging deep breathing, in turning and properly positioning her bed-rest patient prevents more stressful complications. Providing the usually very active business executive on enforced bed rest with diversional material of his preference reduces his discomfort and promotes his adaptation.

When the nurse attempts to teach a diabetic patient how to inject himself with insulin, she indeed may introduce a stressor. His normal emotional response may result in trembling, pallor, or profuse diaphoresis.

Thus, the diabetic should learn self-care after he has some control of symptoms and he is not in severe disequilibrium. The judgment that comes from knowledge and experience enables the nurse to determine how much stress is appropriate for the individual patient, when to apply it, and when to lessen or remove it.

## MORBIDITY AND MORTALITY

Illness can devastate a person's plans and hopes. A person with chronic heart disease, tuberculosis, or arthritis may be unable to finish school, earn a living, run a home, have an active social life, or make his contribution to community and world affairs.

Almost any disease can occur at any age; newborn babies die of cancer, and grandfathers catch chicken pox; but many diseases are characteristic of certain ages. For example, appendicitis is more

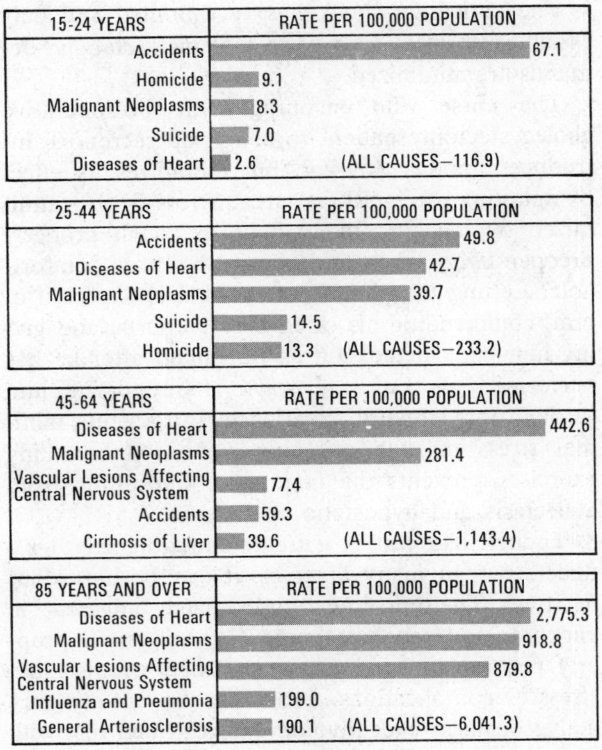

| 15-24 YEARS | RATE PER 100,000 POPULATION |
|---|---|
| Accidents | 67.1 |
| Homicide | 9.1 |
| Malignant Neoplasms | 8.3 |
| Suicide | 7.0 |
| Diseases of Heart | 2.6 (ALL CAUSES—116.9) |

| 25-44 YEARS | RATE PER 100,000 POPULATION |
|---|---|
| Accidents | 49.8 |
| Diseases of Heart | 42.7 |
| Malignant Neoplasms | 39.7 |
| Suicide | 14.5 |
| Homicide | 13.3 (ALL CAUSES—233.2) |

| 45-64 YEARS | RATE PER 100,000 POPULATION |
|---|---|
| Diseases of Heart | 442.6 |
| Malignant Neoplasms | 281.4 |
| Vascular Lesions Affecting Central Nervous System | 77.4 |
| Accidents | 59.3 |
| Cirrhosis of Liver | 39.6 (ALL CAUSES—1,143.4) |

| 85 YEARS AND OVER | RATE PER 100,000 POPULATION |
|---|---|
| Diseases of Heart | 2,775.3 |
| Malignant Neoplasms | 918.8 |
| Vascular Lesions Affecting Central Nervous System | 879.8 |
| Influenza and Pneumonia | 199.0 |
| General Arteriosclerosis | 190.1 (ALL CAUSES—6,041.3) |

**Figure 7-1.** Leading causes of death, according to age group, both sexes, in the United States, 1967-Con. (*The Facts of Life and Death,* Washington, D.C.: U.S. Department of Health, Education and Welfare, 1970.)

common in people under 45, whereas diabetes occurs most often after 45. Some diseases are a major cause of disability at every adult age level (Table 7-1). For example, cardiac disease is a problem of great magnitude at every age, and in the United States it ranks first as the cause of death of those over 45 (Fig. 7-1).

**Table 7-1. Main Illnesses and Handicapping Conditions in the United States (Estimated)***

| | |
|---|---|
| Diseases of heart and circulation (including cerebrovascular diseases) | 28,200,000 |
| Mental disorders (including alcoholism) | 20,000,000 |
| Arthritis and rheumatic conditions | 16,000,000 |
| Hearing impairments | 8,549,000 |
| Mental retardation | 6,000,000 |
| Visual impairments | 5,390,000 |
| Diabetes mellitus | 4,000,000 |
| Epilepsy | 1,000,000-2,000,000 |
| Other neurologic disorders | 2,300,000 |

* *Facts on The Major Killing and Crippling Diseases in the United States Today,* The National Health Education Committee, Inc., New York, 1971.

*Morbidity* means sickness. It usually is expressed as a rate in relation to population. If 39 people are ill in a population of 1,000, the morbidity rate is 39 per 1,000. *Mortality* means death. If 25 people die in a population of 1,000, the mortality rate is 25 per 1,000. An *acute* condition is one in a rapid state of change. Usually it appears rather suddenly and produces effects dramatically. The common head cold is an example. The word *acute* can be misleading to patients and their families. It does not refer necessarily to the seriousness of disease; rather it describes the rapid nature of the onset and the progress. In contrast, the term *chronic* describes the lengthy, sometimes endless persistence of a condition without much change for the better. Nor does this term necessarily indicate degree of danger. A chronic skin rash could be more discouraging than deadly; a chronic kidney disease is often a serious threat to life.

The seriousness of the problem is graded as *severe, moderate,* or *mild.* A stage of the disease may be described as *early, late,* or *terminal. Terminal* usually means a stage preceding death. *Terminal pulmonary insufficiency* would describe a state in which the patient is approaching death from inadequate lung function.

A disease may be described also as *primary* or *secondary.* A *primary* condition is assumed to have developed independently of any other. A subsequent disorder that develops as a result of an original illness is called *secondary.* A common example of secondary disease occurs in patients with heart disease: when the heart fails, there can be secondary impairment almost anywhere in the body; kidneys, lungs, and liver frequently become involved. In secondary disease there are multiple problems to be diagnosed and treated simultaneously, and each detracts from the body's capacity to deal with any condition effectively.

## DISEASE TERMINOLOGY

**Hereditary Conditions.** Heredity can be an etiologic (causal) factor. From the moment of conception the destiny of thousands of traits is decided. Some of these inherited traits can impair the function of the body, and the individual is born with hereditary disease or a tendency to develop it. Hemophilia and color blindness are disorders transmitted by the genes from parent to child. Many hereditary diseases are carried in the genes as recessive traits and are not manifested in every generation.

**Congenital Defects and Diseases.** Although they are often confused with hereditary conditions, congenital diseases are not necessarily the same. Although congenital disease is present at the time of birth, it is not always transmitted by the genes. It can result from some unfavorable event or unfortunate environmental condition experienced by the fetus during the period of pregnancy. For example, drugs and radiation can affect the developing fetus. The mother can transmit an infection of her own, such as syphilis, to the fetus, and at birth the child has congenital syphilis. An illness of the mother, such as German measles, may impair normal development of the fetus, and the resulting defects would be termed *congenital*.

The etiology of the congenital defect may be unknown. Until it is known, it is difficult to take steps to prevent it. The cause of congenital heart disease is obscure in most instances. The congenital irregularity may be a serious threat to life, as when a baby is born missing a vital organ; or disfiguring, as in polydactylism (more than the usual number of fingers or toes); or so slight as to escape notice completely. One woman lived for 76 years with a congenital diaphragm across her duodenum before it caused her enough trouble to have a roentgenogram taken. Any part of the body, inside or outside, can be anomalous (deviating from the usual).

Few, if any, people are born perfect. The flaw may be tiny, a mole or the deviation of a minor blood vessel; or the defect may be important to appearance or health. The thought of being deformed is troublesome to most people. Through the ages such persons as dwarfs, whose anomalies were evident, have been objects of morbid curiosity, social ostracism, and fear of ill omen; and the present is not entirely free of this attitude. Those with obvious major deformities have the constant reminder before them of their imperfection, their "wrongness." The experienced nurse can come across the grossly deformed person and show no surprise, shock, or curiosity, but instead an acceptance of the patient as a fellow human being.

**Trauma.** The term *trauma*, meaning injury, applies to both physical wounds, such as those a person suffers in an automobile accident, and to psychic wounds, such as those suffered in the loss of a loved one. Trauma accounts for a major portion of morbidity and mortality. In 1968 injuries

in and about the home alone caused more than 28,000 deaths in the United States, and many more were hurt but did not die. This toll is 28 times the mortality from aircraft major catastrophes. A more detailed discussion of trauma is to be found in Chapter 13.

**Deficiency Diseases.** Disorders resulting from the lack of essential dietary substances required by cells for their normal function and maintenance are deficiency diseases. Some specific deficiencies can produce clear-cut disorders; for instance, lack of vitamin C causes scurvy—historically, the disorder that affected seamen on long voyages without fresh foods. It was found that citrus fruit, commonly limes or lime juice, prevented the disease, and the world had a treatment for scurvy long before its etiology was understood. Today, except for the deficiencies producing certain anemias, it is more common to see mixed deficiency diseases, the result of general malnutrition rather than a deficiency of one particular element alone.

**Dietary Excesses.** The body is harmed not only by the deficit of materials that it requires, but also by the excess. Too many calories produce obesity, and overdoses of certain vitamin and mineral preparations can be harmful.

**Hypoxia.** Hypoxia (insufficient oxygen) produces dramatic effect, for all body cells require an adequate uninterrupted supply of oxygen. Mental impairment often quickly follows hypoxia and anoxia (lack of oxygen). The cells of the central nervous system are damaged by an oxygen deficiency most easily. The tissues responsible for the control of heart rhythm are readily affected by hypoxia. Insufficient oxygenation of these tissues can lead to cardiac arrhythmia and arrest.

Local areas may receive insufficient oxygen while the rest of the body is properly supplied. Such a problem results from a decrease of local blood flow (ischemia). Among the more frequent causes of ischemia is the plugging of an artery with material that either forms there, as in thrombosis, or is delivered there by the circulation (embolism). Ischemia can be produced accidentally by applying an encircling bandage or cast too tightly on a limb.

Ischemia may damage nerves irreparably. Less sensitive tissue, like muscle, also can undergo damage. If the ischemia is relieved and has not been too severe or prolonged, healing may occur in time. However, serious and long-continued ischemia can cause necrosis (death) of the involved tissues. Decomposition of the necrotic tissue begins, and gradually the area darkens to purple and eventually to black. This massive death of tissue is called *gangrene*.

When an area of tissue is deprived of blood supply long enough to become necrotic, the affected tissue is described as an area of *infarction* (Fig. 7-2).

**Neoplasia.** This term refers to the new formation of abnormal tissue. Such growths are called *tumors*. A *benign tumor* is one usually similar to the tissue in which it originates, and it is covered by a capsule of fibrous tissue. It may have little activity except local growth, or it may carry on the processes characteristic of the tissue from which it started. Benign tumors of endocrine glands can produce the hormone of the gland. A certain benign tumor of the pancreas is capable of making insulin. Benign tumors typically stay within their capsules and do not spread to other sites.

A benign tumor may cause trouble for several reasons. In certain locations it is disfiguring. In other cases it grows to occupy too much space and crowds the normal structures so that they cannot function properly. A hormone-producing tumor may function outside of the organized body commands, secreting the hormone in excess or at inappropriate times.

Once located, benign tumors usually can be excised and will not regrow. However, while benign tumors usually are viewed as not so dangerous as cancer, they can prove to be just as deadly. A benign tumor in the brain or the spinal cord that grows in an inoperable site can be fatal.

*Malignant tumors* (collectively called *cancers*) grow and act in total disregard of body order. Their cells may differ considerably from those of the tissue of their origin. They tend to spread (metastasize) to other parts of the body. To track down all the metastatic "seeds" of a malignant tumor may be impossible. The malignant tumor can invade, crowd and weaken normal structures. For example, bones become fragile, and blood vessels break open. The tumor can absorb nutrients so greedily that normal tissue is malnourished in its presence. Some cancers arising from endocrine glands may secrete hormones and produce additional disorder. So great is the capacity of cancer for causing destruction, pain, and ultimately death, and so difficult is the control of many of the malignant neoplasms, that cancer is one of the most dreaded of all diseases. For further discussion of cancer, see Chapter 17.

**Infection.** Many species of plant and animal parasites are offensive to living cells in the human being. These organisms, classified as protozoa, yeasts, molds, bacteria, rickettsiae, and viruses, can harm human cells by growing within them or producing *toxins*.

Infection is invasion of the body by an organism that produces harm (called a *pathogenic organism*, or *pathogen*). Each organism must live in an environment suited to its needs, and not all tissue sites appeal to it. For example, the bacillus that causes typhoid fever thrives in lymphoid tissue. The organism of tetanus cannot survive in oxygen; hence, to multiply and produce the toxins of its serious disease it needs to live deep in a wound. Viruses live inside cells and may be very selective as to which kind of cell they will inhabit. The polio virus inhabits selectively the anterior horn cells of the spinal cord.

Because we do not live in a sterile environment, we are constantly bombarded by organisms, but we are not always sick. Becoming infected depends on several factors: (1) the number of invading organisms, (2) how virulent they are, and (3) the resistance of the host.

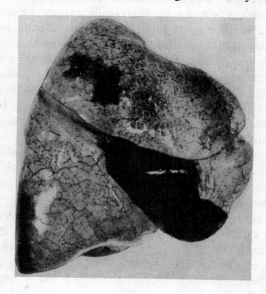

**Figure 7-2.** A blood clot has prevented adequate circulation to the middle lobe of the lung, and destruction of tissue (infarct) has resulted. (Hardy, J. D., *Pathophysiology in Surgery*, Baltimore: Williams and Wilkins)

As a rule, foreign material, dead or alive, is tolerated poorly by the tissues. Whether the organisms consume nutrients needed by the cells, invade them and disturb their structure or activity, or in some other unknown way offend the tissue, they do produce injury and death of body cells. The group of organisms finds food in the host, adapting its enzymes to the chemical compounds in the host. This is the incubation period, and during it the host is usually unaware of the organisms and may be symptomless. The organisms thrive on the food, and they multiply. The host may become a patient. (See pp. 108 to 111 for a discussion of the body's response to infection.)

**Idiopathic (Unknown) Etiology.** Though they are being extensively studied, cancer, diabetes, and rheumatoid arthritis are diseases of unknown origin. The effects of aging are apparent, but *why* these changes take place is not clear. There are many other disorders of obscure etiology. For some of them there is a satisfactory treatment. As a general rule, cure must await knowledge of cause, but this order is not always true. Recall the case of scurvy.

## WATER AND ELECTROLYTE REGULATION

### Normal Functioning of the Body Fluids

The human body is 60, 70, sometimes 80 per cent liquid, depending upon age, sex, and body fat content. This liquid, our *body fluid,* consists largely of water and electrolytes. Body fluid can be divided into two major compartments—*cellular fluid* (often called intracellular fluid), contained within the billions of body cells, and *extracellular fluid,* which comprises plasma and interstitial fluid, the "bath water" that surrounds and bathes the cells. Usually regarded as interstitial fluid are lymph and cerebrospinal fluid. Another class of body liquid, neither cellular nor extracellular fluid, includes the secretions (e.g., gastric juice) and the excretions (typified by urine). Secretions and excretions are derived from extracellular fluid, although they differ greatly from this fluid in composition; nevertheless their depletion depletes extracellular fluid and, ultimately, cellular fluid.

The great mission of body fluids is to maintain the body cells in a constant healthy state. In this, body fluids really serve as agents for the body homeostatic mechanisms. As the primary step in accomplishing this mission, the extracellular fluid (Claude Bernard's "internal environment") is maintained within the narrow bounds required for health. Then, through a never-ceasing to and fro movement of essentials and waste products between the extracellular and cellular compartments, via the cell membranes, the precise chemical composition for optimal cellular health is maintained. (Picturesquely and accurately, Bernard termed cellular fluid the "environment of life.")

The proper functioning of body fluids demands a host of intra- and inter- compartmental exchanges of water and electrolytes, accomplished by a bewildering yet ever-logical interplay of physical and biologic forces. These include osmosis; diffusion; filtration; active transport (accomplished with the help of energy from adenosine tri-phosphate, or ATP) in which substances necessary for cell growth are "carried" through the cell membrane; passive transport; and pinocytosis, the process whereby very large molecules, such as proteins, are engulfed by the cell membrane into the interior of the cell. The complex mechanisms of these essential processes lie within the realm of basic physiology, and the learner is referred to specialized textbooks for further study or review.

**Measurement of Electrolyte Activity.** The electrolytes of the body fluids are active, dynamic chemicals. In searching for a unit that would measure chemical activity (as opposed to mere weight), chemists long ago discovered the milliequivalent (mEq.). One mEq. of any electrolyte possesses the chemical combining power of 1 milligram (mg.) of hydrogen. A given number of mEq. of any cation (positively charged electrolyte such as sodium $[Na^+]$) will unite chemically with the same number of anions (negatively charged electrolytes such as chloride $[Cl-]$). The mEq. of an element or compound (combination of elements behaving as 1 ion, e.g., bicarbonate $[HCO_3-]$ is determined by taking the millimole (mM.), which is the atomic or molecular weight of the element or compound in mg. and dividing by the chemical valence. In substances having a valence of 1, 1 mM. = 1 mEq. In substances with a valence of 2, 1 mM. = 2 mEq., and so on.

**Tonicity of Body Fluids.** Tonicity of a body fluid refers chiefly to the concentration of electrolytes. Normally this is 155 mEq. of cation and 155 mEq. of anion for extracellular fluid. When these values are present we say the fluid is *isotonic.* If the value rises above 155 we say the solution is *hypertonic;* if it falls below 155 we say the fluid is *hypotonic.*

Similarly, fluids for parenteral administration are classified as isotonic, hypotonic, or hypertonic, according to their respective electrolyte concentrations. In some situations, however, glucose and other substances which are not electrolytes can affect tonicity.

**Composition of Body Fluids.** Each body fluid has its own peculiar composition. Cellular fluid contains large amounts of potassium, magnesium, and phosphate. Extracellular fluid, on the other hand, comprises large quantities of sodium, calcium, and chloride.\* Plasma and interstitial fluid manifest this striking difference: plasma boasts large amounts of proteinate, interstitial fluid almost none, proteinate serving as a sponge that prevents certain ingredients of plasma from seeping into the interstitial space.

**Intake.** How are water and electrolytes gained for the body fluids? Water alone is acquired by drinking distilled water and through oxidation of foodstuffs and body tissues. Softened water, well water, mineral water, and most city water supplies provide both water and electrolytes. Food supplies these and, in addition, other nutrients. Hospitalized patients may gain water and electrolytes via nasogastric tube, intravenous needle, or rectal tube.

**Output.** In health the body loses electrolytes via the lungs in breathing, through the eyes in tears, through the kidneys in urine, through the skin in perspiration, via the intestines in feces. Insensible perspiration, which never ceases, accounts for removal of water alone. In illness or injury additional losses occur: burn or wound exudate, hemorrhage, vomiting, and diarrhea help deplete the body of both water and electrolytes. So, of course, does rapid breathing. Suction via gastric or intestinal tube, enterostomy, colostomy, and cecostomy also cause great losses of water and electrolytes. Drainage from surgical operations or from abscesses contains both water and electrolytes, as does fluid extracted via paracentesis.

In the healthy adult, the volume of urine excreted is about equal to the volume of fluid ingested as fluid, and normal losses of water through the lungs and skin and in the stool approximately equal the water derived from solid food and from chemical oxidation in the body. Thus, on a volume basis, gains approximately equal losses. The body homeostatic mechanisms (i.e., kidneys, lungs, pituitary gland, parathyroid glands, heart, and adrenal glands) alter the chemical composition of body excretions according to the needs of the body by retaining those electrolytes that are needed and excreting the rest. Thus, in health, the volume and chemical composition of the body fluids remain within the narrow limits of normal.

During illness, however, homeostasis may become upset. Intake of food and fluid may cease or diminish, while normal losses continue, so that losses exceed gains. In addition to normal losses, abnormal losses may occur, further upsetting the precarious balance between gains and losses. Or, gains may be greater than losses, as when the kidneys are not functioning properly. In either case, the normal volume and composition of body fluids may be altered so that a fluid imbalance occurs.

## Disturbances of the Body Fluids

Body fluid disturbances pose a major problem in illness. Indeed, every seriously ill patient is a candidate for one or more of them, and they may even develop in patients who are only mildly or moderately ill. Since cellular and extracellular fluid are in intimate contact constantly, an imbalance in either will ultimately affect the other. However, since extracellular fluid is available to us for examination (as plasma) and cellular fluid is not, body fluid disturbances are usually thought of in terms of the extracellular fluid.

There are some 16 fundamental imbalances that can affect the extracellular fluid. These are best presented by using the clinical picture approach first introduced by Moyer and later expanded upon by Snively and Sweeney. In this approach, each imbalance is presented as a clinical picture, with its own set of causative mechanisms; its own symptoms, both *subjective and objective;* and its own laboratory findings.

The first two clinical pictures involve changes in the volume of extracellular fluid. They result from any condition that causes a decrease or increase in both the water and electrolytes of extracellular fluid in approximately the same proportions as would be found in the normal state.

The next four clinical pictures describe the imbalances known as acid-base disturbances. These

---

\* Geologists tell us that the composition of the cellular fluid harks back to that remote era, two billion years ago, when single cell organisms first appeared on our planet; the composition of extracellular fluid reflects that of the Cambrian Seas, of a mere three hundred million years ago, when vertebrate life first ventured ashore.

involve changes in the concentration of hydrogen ions in the extracellular fluid, which is determined by the ratio of carbonic acid to base bicarbonate, normally 1:20.

Recall that the pH scale ranges from 1 to 14; 7 is neutral, below 7 is acid, and above 7 is alkaline. The normal pH of extracellular fluid ranges from 7.35 to 7.45 (slightly alkaline).

## Fundamental Imbalances Affecting Extracellular Fluid

### VOLUME CHANGES IN EXTRACELLULAR FLUID

| | HISTORY | SYMPTOMS | LABORATORY FINDINGS |
|---|---|---|---|
| Volume Deficit | decreased water intake; diarrhea; draining fistula; intestinal obstruction; systemic infection; vomiting | acute weight loss—in excess of 5 per cent; body temperature drop; dryness of skin and mucous membranes; longitudinal wrinkles or furrows of tongue, oliguria or anuria | packed cell volume or hemoglobin increased; red blood cell count increased |
| Volume Excess | congestive heart failure; excessive adrenocortical hormones; excessive ingestion of sodium chloride; hyperaldosteronism; parenteral infusion of isotonic solution of sodium chloride; renal disease | acute weight gain—in excess of 5 per cent; edema; edema of tissues at operation; moist rales in lungs; puffy eyelids; shortness of breath | packed cell volume or hemoglobin decreased; red blood cell count decreased |

### COMPOSITION CHANGES OF MAJOR EXTRACELLULAR ELECTROLYTES

| | | | |
|---|---|---|---|
| Sodium Deficit | excessive sweating plus drinking plain water; gastrointestinal suction plus drinking plain water; inhalation of fresh water; parenteral electrolyte-free solution; potent diuretic; water enema | abdominal cramps; apprehension; convulsions; finger-printing on sternum; oliguria or anuria | plasma chloride below 98 mEq./L.; plasma sodium below 136 mEq./L.; specific gravity of urine below 1.010 |
| Sodium Excess | decreased water intake; diarrhea; excessive ingestion of sodium chloride; inhalation of salt (ocean) water; tracheobronchitis; unconsciousness | dry, sticky mucous membranes; flushed skin; oliguria or anuria; thirst; tongue rough and dry | plasma chloride above 106 mEq./L.; plasma sodium above 147 mEq./L.; specific gravity of urine above 1.030 |
| Potassium Deficit | burn after third day; diabetic acidosis; diarrhea; draining fistula; parenteral potassium-free solution; potent diuretic; ulcerative colitis; vomiting | anorexia; gaseous distention of intestines; silent intestinal ileus; soft, flabby muscles; weakness | electrocardiograph shows low voltage, flattened T wave, depressed ST segment; plasma potassium below 4 mEq./L. |
| Potassium Excess | adrenal insufficiency; burn, early; excessive parenteral administration of potassium; massive crushing injury; mercuric bichloride poisoning; oliguria or anuria; oral intake of potassium exceeding renal tolerance; renal disease | diarrhea; intestinal colic; irritability; nausea | electrocardiograph shows high T wave, depressed ST segment; plasma potassium above 5.6 mEq./L. |
| Calcium Deficit | acute pancreatitis; excessive administration of citrated blood; massive infection of subcutaneous tissues; parenteral administration of calcium-free solution; primary hypoparathyroidism; recent correction of acidosis; sprue | abdominal cramps; carpopedal spasm; muscle cramps; tetany; tingling of ends of fingers | plasma calcium below 4.5 mEq./L.; Sulkowitch test on urine shows no precipitation |
| Calcium Excess | excessive administration of vitamin D; hyperparathyroidism; multiple myeloma; parathyroid tumor; pathologic fracture; prolonged immobilization; renal disease | bone cavitation; deep bony pain; flank pain; kidney stones; muscle hypotonicity | plasma calcium above 5.8 mEq./L.; Sulkowitch test on urine shows heavy precipitation |

## COMPOSITION CHANGES OF MAJOR EXTRACELLULAR ELECTROLYTES (CONTINUED)

| | HISTORY | SYMPTOMS | LABORATORY FINDINGS |
|---|---|---|---|
| Protein Deficit | burn after third day; decreased food intake; decubitus ulcers; fracture; loss of whole blood; severe trauma; wound drainage | chronic weight loss; emotional depression; pallor; ready fatigue; soft, flabby muscles | plasma albumin below 4 Gm./100 ml.; packed cell volume, hemoglobin, or red blood cell count decrease (significant only if iron stores are adequate) |
| Magnesium Deficit | chronic alcoholism; diarrhea; enterostomy drainage; impaired gastrointestinal absorption, medical or surgical; parenteral administration of magnesium-free solution; vomiting | Chvostek sign positive; convulsions; disorientation; hyperactive deep reflexes; positive therapeutic responses to magnesium sulfate; tremor | plasma magnesium below 1.4 mEq./L. |

## CONCENTRATION (pH) CHANGES IN EXTRACELLULAR FLUID OR ACID-BASE IMBALANCES

| | | | |
|---|---|---|---|
| Primary Base Bicarbonate Deficit of Extracellular Fluid (Metabolic Acidosis) | decreased food intake; diabetic acidosis; ketogenic diet; parenteral infusion of isotonic solution of sodium chloride; renal disease; salicylate intoxication (not early); systemic infection | deep, rapid breathing (Kussmaul); shortness of breath on exertion; stupor; weakness | plasma bicarbonate below 25 mEq./L. in adults, below 20 mEq./L. in children; plasma pH below 7.35; urine pH below 6. $P_{CO_2}$ (mm. Hg.) below 35 arterial, below 40 venous |
| Primary Base Bicarbonate Excess of Extracellular Fluid (Metabolic Alkalosis) | excessive adrenocortical hormones; excessive ingestion of sodium bicarbonate; gastrointestinal suction; parenteral potassium-free solution; potassium deficit; potent diuretic; vomiting | hypertonicity of muscles; tetany; depressed respiration | plasma bicarbonate above 29 mEq./L. in adults, above 25 mEq./L. in children; plasma pH above 7.45; urine pH above 7; plasma potassium below 4 mEq./L. $P_{CO_2}$ above 38 arterial, above 41 venous |
| Primary Carbonic Acid Deficit of Extracellular Fluid (Respiratory Alkalosis) | anxiety; early salicylate intoxication; extreme emotion; fever; hysteria; intentional overbreathing; oxygen lack; rapid breathing (not Kussmaul) | convulsions, tetany; unconsciousness | plasma bicarbonate below 25 mEq./L. in adults, below 20 mEq./L. in children; plasma pH above 7.45; urine pH above 7. $P_{CO_2}$ below 35 arterial, below 40 venous |
| Primary Carbonic Acid Excess of Extracellular Fluid (Respiratory Acidosis) | asthma; barbiturate poisoning; breathing excessive carbon dioxide; emphysema; morphine poisoning; occlusion of breathing passages; pneumonia | coma; disorientation; respiratory embarrassment; weakness | plasma bicarbonate above 29 mEq./L. in adults, above 25 mEq./L. in children; plasma pH below 7.35; urine pH below 6. $P_{CO_2}$ above 38 arterial, above 41 venous |

## POSITION CHANGES OF WATER AND ELECTROLYTES OF EXTRACELLULAR FLUID

| | | | |
|---|---|---|---|
| Plasma-to-Interstitial Fluid Shift of Extracellular Fluid | acute occlusion of major artery; burn, early; intestinal obstruction; massive crushing injury; perforated peptic ulcer; severe trauma | cold extremities; low blood pressure; pallor; tachycardia; weak to absent pulse; weakness | packed cell volume or hemoglobin increased; red blood cell count increased |
| Interstitial Fluid-to-Plasma Shift of Extracellular Fluid | burn after third day; excessive infusion of large molecular solution (plasma, dextran, etc.); fracture; loss of whole blood | air hunger; bounding pulse; cardiac dilatation; engorgement of peripheral veins; moist rales in lungs; pallor; ventricular failure; weakness | packed cell volume or hemoglobin decreased; red blood cell count decreased |

## NURSING ASSESSMENT AND INTERVENTION

In the clinical picture approach, a systematic assessment of the patient's history, symptoms, and laboratory data not only allows one to recognize body fluid disturbances, but often makes it possible to anticipate or even prevent their development.

## Taking the History

The nurse who understands the sequence of events that precedes development of body fluid disturbances is in an excellent position to anticipate them, to alert the physician to potential or actual problems, and to institute preventive nursing measures. In assessing the patient's history, one should keep the following questions in mind: (1) What homeostatic mechanisms are impaired? (2) Has the patient been taking medications that may alter fluid balance? (3) Has intake of food or fluids been altered? (4) Has the patient suffered any unusual losses of fluids? (Charts that list the composition of the various secretions and excretions are available in most physiology texts. Reference to them provides valuable clues as to what imbalances might be expected to follow unusual losses of the various fluids.)

## Using Symptoms as a Guide to Assessment

The nurse is perhaps in a better position than anyone else to observe the patient for symptoms of body fluid disturbances. When significant symptoms appear, the nurse can relay them to the physician, thus facilitating early diagnosis and treatment. The ability to sort out observations demanding urgent action develops with a working understanding of fluid balance and application of this knowledge. Observations important in the early detection of fluid imbalances are body temperature; pulse, in terms of rate, volume, regularity, and ease of obliteration; respiration, in terms of rate, depth, and regularity; blood pressure; condition of peripheral veins; condition of skin and mucous membranes; phonation, in terms of quality, content, and formation of speech; fatigue threshold; facial appearance; behavior; condition of skeletal muscles; sensation; and desire for food and water.

## Evaluating Laboratory Data

In some specialized units (e.g., renal dialysis and coronary care), the nurse may order some laboratory tests. This is also the case in some nursing homes or outpatient situations where the nurse is the primary care therapist. For example, the nurse who works with chronic congestive heart failure patients needs to monitor the effects of potassium-depleting diuretics or a low sodium diet. Nurse specialists in the health management of diabetic patients may decide when a blood glucose is necessary.

However, minimal proficiency requires that the nurse be able to recognize abnormal results of tests ordered and alert the physician. Variations in laboratory values for individuals of different ages are important considerations when evaluating the results of laboratory tests. Normal values for the red cell count, hemoglobin, packed cell volume, and plasma bicarbonate differ in infants, children, and adults. This is true not only for average values, but normal values as well.

In addition to the nurse's role in assessment, there are several nursing skills that are particularly concerned with fluid balance.

## Intake and Output Records

Accurate intake-output records provide a basis for medical and nursing judgments. Indeed, the physician should be able to use the nursing intake-output records as a major tool in diagnosis, as well as in the formulation of fluid replacement therapy. Unfortunately, neglect in keeping accurate nursing intake-output records is widespread, even though it is not technically difficult to measure fluid intake and output or to record the measurements. In view of the importance of accurate intake-output records, the nurse should:

- **Learn the volumes of glasses, cups, bowls, and other fluid containers used in the hospital.**
- **Remember that intake includes any intake and that output includes any output.**
- **Make sure that the patient, his family, and everyone involved in the patient's care knows that intake-output records are to be kept. If the patient's condition permits, he can help by keeping track of what he drinks and by measuring his urine. Ambulatory patients should be cautioned not to discard urine before it is measured.**
- **Measure all fluids amenable to direct measurement— guesses should be reserved for fluids that cannot be measured directly.**
- **Record measurements at the time they are obtained.**
- **Estimate the amount of fluid in uncaught vomitus, incontinent urine, incontinent liquid stools, wound exudate, and blood, and record it as an estimate. It is better to make a guess than to give no indication at all as to the amount.**
- **Describe the amount of clothing and bed linen saturated with perspiration.**
- **Check intake-output records for completeness before leaving the unit.**

## Body Weight

Because intake-output records are so frequently inaccurate, some authorities recommend body weight as the most reliable guide to fluid loss or gain. Weights taken before the patient eats breakfast are the most accurate. The patient should empty his bladder before being weighed, and he should be weighed on the same scales and should wear the same or similar clothing each time the weight is checked.

## Forcing Fluids

It is important to encourage fluid intake during preoperative and early postoperative periods, unless contraindicated by the type of surgery (e.g., on the gastrointestinal tract) or by the patient's concomitant illnesses, should there be any. Postoperative orders should indicate whether the patient may have fluids, what kinds, how much, and when. If the amount is to be unusual in any way, the physician will specify this on the order (e.g., "encourage fluids to 2,000 ml.," or "restrict fluids to 750 ml. per day"). Forcing fluids helps to regulate the patient's water and electrolytes and reduces the need for prolonged intravenous therapy.

Fluids are usually best tolerated when given frequently in small amounts. In the elderly patient, thirst is often diminished, so that he may not drink liquids that are simply set before him. Such a patient will frequently drink them if the nurse sits and talks for a few moments—not because he feels thirsty, but because drinking becomes a pleasant social event. When a patient's preferences for certain fluids do not conflict with the physician's orders, giving him the fluids that he likes will usually increase his intake. The choice of liquids offered may be planned around the patient's needs for other nutrients. For example, milkshakes may be offered to the patient who needs additional calories and protein; or, if he needs potassium, orange juice or cola may be offered.

Sometimes the fluids offered are directed toward correcting certain conditions. For example, Lytren (a commercial multiple-electrolyte preparation that, when diluted according to instructions, is hypotonic in relation to body fluids) is frequently used to replace water and electrolytes in postoperative patients or in those with diarrhea. Small sips of ginger ale or cola in ice chips may relieve nausea. On the other hand, giving liquids to a nauseated patient may induce vomiting and further deplete water and electrolytes. When this occurs, the nurse should withhold all food and fluids from the patient, administer antiemetics as ordered, and in collaboration with the physician when necessary, develop a plan of care to be effected when nausea diminishes so that nutrients will not be withheld longer than necessary.

## Irrigation of Body Cavities

Isotonic solutions (i.e., those having a similar osmolality with body fluids) should be used for irrigation of body cavities. When hypotonic solutions such as water are used for irrigation, electrolytes from the extracellular fluid diffuse into the irrigating solution and are subsequently withdrawn from the body via the suction tube.

## Care of the Edematous Patient

Edema may be relieved by flotation pads, alternating mattresses, or similar devices. Edema fluids may be redistributed and the blood supply to the area increased by *gentle* rubbing of the skin. Vigorous rubbing may cause cellular damage.

Gravity aids the flow of liquids; the edematous patient is positioned with this principle in mind. For example, elevating the head of the bed for a patient with pulmonary edema will allow fluids to flow away from the lungs; elevation of an edematous extremity increases venous return and reduces capillary pressure. Frequent changes in position prevent fluids from pooling in a dependent part. For example, the sacrum is a dependent area when one is supine, and this area is highly susceptible to formation of decubitus ulcers. The male patient may benefit from a scrotal support. When the patient is in the sitting position, placing his feet on a stool will reduce pressure on the popliteal area. A small, soft pillow placed between the thighs will help accomplish equalization when a patient is in the side lying position. Shoes, if worn, should be nonconstrictive, soft, and supportive.

Absorption from edematous tissues is poor, so such areas should be rejected as possible sites for injections.

## The Nurse's Role in Parenteral Fluid Therapy

Every day, intravenous solutions are administered to hospitalized patients the world over to maintain daily requirements, to replace losses, and to serve as vehicles for drugs. It is extremely important, therefore, that the nurse know the purpose, physiologic effect, and possible complications of fluid therapy. Familiarity with the solutions used in the hospital is absolutely essential for skillful monitoring of infusions (Fig. 7-3).

**Preparing the Patient.** The nurse finds out what the patient's attitude to intravenous therapy is. He may think of it as a last measure resorted to by desperate doctors. Allowing him to express his thoughts and explaining to him that it is merely another way of eating may help to lessen his fear. If preoperatively the patient sees others getting intravenous fluids, the nurse can tell him that he also may get some fluids this way after his operation.

**Starting Intravenous Infusions.** The legal status of the nurse in starting parenteral fluids varies not only among states, but also among hospitals. Large institutions may require residents or specialized IV teams to start an infusion, while small hospitals may offer specialized preparation for a nurse to perform this role. It is the nurse's professional responsibility to assess her own knowledge and skills and to know the rules of the institution and the law before assuming this role.

The administration of intravenous infusions should not interfere with other aspects of nursing care. If the arm is supported carefully in the correct position, the patient can be turned without dislodging the needle or intracath. The arm is kept well splinted and the tubing loose while turning the patient.

**Adding Medications to Intravenous Solutions.** The nurse's role in adding medications to solutions or injecting a medication directly into the vein also varies from one place to another. Nurses, physicians, pharmacists, and administrators collaborate on policy decisions, considering the legal issues as well as the safety and therapeutic needs of the patient. The nurse has a responsibility to evaluate and take on what she is prepared for and discuss her professional competencies with other health team collaborators. One important factor for the nurse to consider is how closely she can observe the patient after an IV injection.

Strict aseptic technique is essential. It is safer when two persons check the medication and dosage. The bottle must be clearly labeled as to *all* contents of the solution. As more types of parenteral fluids and a greater number of drugs are given intravenously, incompatibility becomes an increasing hazard. The pharmacist is an excellent source of information concerning incompatibility.

**Determining the Desired Flow Rate.** One of the most important considerations in administering fluid therapy is the rate of flow. Ideally, the physician should specify the desired flow rate. When he does not, the nurse should request this information. In actual practice, however, there are times when the nurse assumes this responsibility, such as for the postoperative patient. To do so intelligently, one

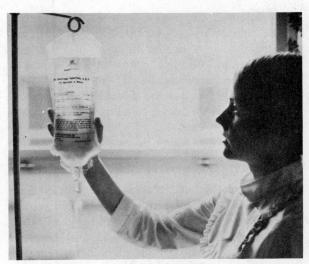

**Figure 7-3.** Nurse carefully checks solution label on Viaflex® plastic parenteral solution container. (Courtesy, Travenol Laboratories.)

must consider several factors, including body surface area, condition and age of the patient, and composition of the fluid.

In general, the larger the individual, the more fluid and nutrients he requires and the faster he can utilize them. The usual infusion rate is 3 ml. per m.² body surface area per minute. Nomograms are available to determine body surface area.

The heart and kidneys play a vital role in the utilization of infused fluids. In the elderly patient, these two systems are often impaired, and a rapid infusion may result in pulmonary edema. In determining the desired flow rate, it is essential to consider what and how homeostatic mechanisms are impaired.

Generally, the desired infusion rate is slower if the solution serves as a vehicle for administration of drugs. The drug effect, recommended infusion rate, and possible complications should be considered. For example, too rapid infusion of a solution containing potassium can result in cardiac arrest.

Infusion rates may be faster if the intended effect is diuresis. Glucose, for example, if given faster than it can be metabolized, will accumulate in the bloodstream, increase the osmolality, and act as a diuretic. If, on the other hand, glucose is given for its caloric effect, a slower infusion rate would be in order.

Amino acid solutions such as protein hydrolysate (Amigen) may be ordered to promote cellular repair in conditions involving prolonged malnutrition.

These solutions are administered slowly to prevent nausea and feelings of warmth. IV hyperalimentation therapy involves the infusion of hypertonic solutions of glucose plus a protein hydrolysate or crystalline amino acids directly into the superior vena cava in order for the patient to achieve and maintain positive nitrogen balance. Hyperalimentation therapy is indicated in conditions of severe protein loss such as major burns, malnutrition, after major gastrointestinal surgery, or in cancer patients receiving radiation or chemotherapy resulting in gastrointestinal upsets. Nurses caring for patients receiving this form of intravenous therapy require special preparation (Colley and Phillips, 1973).

Plasma (blood minus red blood cells) may be given in emergency situations when there is no time to type and cross-match whole blood. In cases of severe hemorrhage, the plasma would be administered rapidly.

Fat emulsions, because of their many untoward reactions, must be started very slowly, then speeded up only as the patient's reaction allows.

Alcohol may be administered in lieu of glucose since it supplies a greater number of calories (6 to 8 per Gm.). It must be given slowly according to the patient's tolerance.

**Monitoring the Flow Rate.** Not only is it important to determine the desired flow rate initially, it is necessary to maintain the correct flow rate. Several mechanical factors can affect the rate of flow, including height of the bottle, amount of solution in the bottle, size of the needle, drop size, temperature changes, plugged vent, trauma to the veins, change in position of the needle, and clot in the needle. Factors to be considered are:

The higher the container, the greater the flow. Lowering or raising the bed will change the height of the container (if IV standard is not attached to the bed) and thus will alter the flow rate.

The greater the volume of solution in the bottle, the greater the flow. As volume decreases, the flow rate slows. Therefore, the rate of flow must be adjusted periodically.

The size of the needle also affects flow rate. The larger the lumen, the greater the flow since there is less resistance to blood flow by the walls of the needle. Some find it surprising to learn that a shorter needle, even though the lumen is smaller, may provide a faster rate of flow than a longer needle. Again, this is because there is less resistance from the walls of the needle.

The number of drops in a ml. of fluid varies with the manufacturer and type of IV set. It may range from 10 to 60 gtt. The nurse should become familiar with the product used in her particular situation.

Cool solutions (e.g., blood) may cause vasoconstriction and thus alter flow rate. A warm towel placed proximal to the infusion site will offset this reaction.

A plugged air vent in the infusion flask will stop the flow rate, as air must flow freely into the flask to replace fluid.

Phlebitis or thrombosis decreases the size of the lumen of the vein, thus decreasing the flow.

A change in the position of the needle may alter the flow rate. The bevel may become lodged against the vessel wall. A change in position of the patient's arm or elevation of the needle with a piece of cotton may re-establish flow.

Any stoppage of the flow, as may occur when there is a delay in changing bottles, will allow a clot to form within the needle. Increased venous pressure may likewise allow a clot to form. Leaving the patient's arm in a dependent position or taking a blood pressure on the same arm as the infusion site are two common causes of increased venous pressure.

## Complications of IV Therapy

Incompatibility has already been mentioned. Other frequently encountered complications include the following:

**Circulatory Overload.** Overloading the circulatory system with excessive intravenous fluids may cause increased venous pressure, venous distention, increased blood pressure, coughing, shortness of breath, increased respiratory rate, and pulmonary edema with severe dyspnea and cyanosis. The nurse should be particularly alert for this reaction in patients with cardiac decompensation. Should it occur, the nurse should stop the flow and put the patient in the high Fowler's position. The physician should be notified immediately. Oxygen therapy may be necessary as well as other measures for relief of pulmonary edema.

**Speed Shock.** Too rapid administration of solutions containing drugs may induce a systemic reaction called speed shock. The bloodstream is flooded with the drug, and toxic concentrations are supplied to organs such as the heart and brain; syncope and shock may occur. Symptoms vary with the offending drug. The flow must be stopped immediately; a small bottle of the same clear solution can be used to keep the vein open until the physician (who should be immediately contacted) gives further orders.

**Local Infiltration.** The needle may become dislodged and allow fluids to perfuse into the subcutaneous tissues. Certain medications, especially norepinephrine (Levophed), will cause necrosis and sloughing of tissues if allowed to infiltrate. Swelling, blanching, and discomfort at the infusion site, significant decrease or complete stop in the flow rate, and failure to get blood return into the tubing when the bottle is lowered below the needle are indications that infiltration has occurred. The infusion must be terminated and restarted at another site.

**Thrombophlebitis.** Hypertonic solutions and many medications are irritating to the vein and may result in thrombophlebitis. Thrombophlebitis at an infusion site may be manifested by pain along the course of the vein, redness and edema at the injection site, and, if severe, systemic reactions to the infection (tachycardia, fever, and general malaise). The infusion should be terminated at that site. To prevent thrombophlebitis, some institutions require that the site of the infusion be changed periodically. Cold compresses followed later by warm wet dressings may be ordered to relieve pain and inflammation.

**Air Embolism.** Air embolism usually occurs when blood is given under pressure, but the danger is present in all intravenous infusions. Small amounts of air are not always harmful, yet as little as 10 ml. may be fatal in some patients. The presence of air embolism is manifested by sudden vascular collapse, with symptoms of cyanosis, hypotension, weak rapid pulse, venous pressure rise, and loss of consciousness. Immediate measures include stopping the infusion, putting the patient when possible on his left side with his head down, administering oxygen and notifying the physician.

**Pyrogenic Reactions.** Contamination of equipment or parenteral fluids may precipitate a febrile reaction. Symptoms include an abrupt temperature elevation and chills, which begin approximately 30 minutes after the infusion is started; headache; backache; general malaise; and nausea and vomiting. Vascular collapse with hypotension and cyanosis may occur when the reaction is severe. To prevent pyrogenic reactions, one should use strict aseptic technique in every procedure involving the infusion. Equipment or solutions with broken seals must never be used. All solutions should be checked for clarity and those that are cloudy discarded. When symptoms of pyrogenic reaction occur the infusion is terminated but the container and contents kept for culture. Vital signs are taken and the physician is notified immediately.

**Blood Incompatibility.** Whole blood is given when the patient needs both red blood cells and plasma. Incompatibility may occur from inaccurate cross-matching or (most frequently) from careless administration of the wrong blood. *Prevention* is the best treatment for this condition. *Two* persons should check the full name of the patient; the medical order; the hospital number on the chart, on the blood bottle, and on the patient's identification band; and the blood type on the chart and on the blood bottle.

Because an acute hemolytic reaction becomes evident during transfusion of the first 20 to 100 ml. of blood, it is highly desirable that the patient be carefully observed during this part of the transfusion. The blood should be discontinued immediately if sudden sharp back pain, chills, dyspnea, and cyanosis occur. The blood bottle and set must be saved and refrigerated so that further incompatibility tests may be made. All urine is saved and observed for discoloration. (Hemolysis of red blood cells occurs and liberates hemoglobin into the plasma. This hemoglobin may discolor the urine as it is excreted. More dreaded is that the hemoglobin may precipitate in the renal tubules, leading to necrosis and urinary shutdown.)

**Allergic Reactions.** Blood from a donor with food or drug allergies may cause itching, erythema, urticaria, chills, wheezing, bronchospasm, and angioneurotic edema; severe allergic reaction may produce anaphylactic shock. Appearance of any of these symptoms is an indication to immediately stop the transfusion. Severe reactions require treatment with an injection of 0.5 to 1.0 ml. of 1:1000 solution of epinephrine, or with adrenal steroids. Less severe reactions are treated with antihistamines.

The following case histories illustrate how the nurse can reach a correct tentative nursing diagnosis by using the clinical picture approach:

CASE 1

Mr. G., age 40, was recovering from subtotal gastrectomy. A Levin tube connected to low continuous suction had been inserted. Since the patient complained of dry mouth and excessive thirst, the physician permitted him to suck small quantities of ice chips. But Mr. G. demanded more and more, and by the second day, his intake amounted to more than 1 L. per 24 hours. When the nursing staff attempted to withhold ice chips, he became angry and agitated. On the third day, he appeared lethargic and disoriented. He complained of headache and cramping pain and expressed feelings of anxiety. Respiration became shallow and irregular and decreased to 10 per minute. The nurse reviewed Mr. G.'s symptoms and the events of the preceding 48 hours, then made a tentative nursing diagnosis of sodium deficit with probable potassium deficit and base bicarbonate excess (metabolic alkalosis). Laboratory tests, ordered after consultation with the physician, corroborated the nurse's impressions. The lab studies revealed decreased sodium and potassium and elevated bicarbonate. Urine pH was 8.0.

CASE 2

Ms. K., age 80, was brought to the hospital emergency room suffering from orthopnea and dyspnea. Her face and eyelids were puffy, and the extremities revealed 3+ pitting edema. Family members stated that Ms. K. had experienced nausea and vomiting for the past 24 hours. The physician tentatively diagnosed her condition as congestive heart failure and admitted her to intensive care, where she received nasal oxygen and morphine sulfate. Because of oliguria and edema, she was also given a potent diuretic intravenously, along with a digitalis preparation. A Foley catheter was inserted, and an intravenous infusion of 5 per cent dextrose in water started to keep a vein open. The oliguria persisted, so the physician ordered repeated doses of furosemide to be given every 12 hours. Profuse urination occurred after the second dose; nevertheless, the furosemide was continued. After 72 hours, Ms. K. developed nausea and extreme weakness and became uncooperative and disoriented. Examination revealed her muscles to be soft and flabby. After reviewing the preceding events and current status, the nurse made a tentative nursing diagnosis of potassium deficit with possible sodium deficit. Plasma

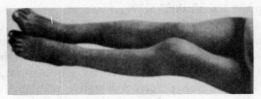

**Figure 7-4.** Atrophy of the muscles of the left leg. The knee is infected with tuberculosis. (Bailey, H., and Love, M.: *A Short Practice of Surgery*, ed. 14, Philadelphia, Lippincott)

electrolyte studies ordered after consultation with the physician revealed a plasma potassium of 2.5 mEq. per L., and plasma sodium, 135 mEq. per L.

The community health nurse, the nurse who works in an HMO, or as a primary therapist in an ambulatory care setting or a nursing home must be prepared to assess the fluid balance and electrolyte status of patients, especially elderly ones, in order to avoid the need for crisis care. Patients on low sodium diets, potassium-depleting diuretics, those with renal or respiratory deficiencies, with bouts of diarrhea or constipation, or with acute infectious processes such as influenza are particularly prone to fluid or electrolyte imbalance.

## BODY DEFENSES
### Sources of Body Protection

The body maintains many reserves. When a blood vessel fails, often the body can replace its function with the development of other vessels to the stricken part (collateral circulation). Oxygen cannot be stockpiled, but the body does have a supply of minerals, vitamins, food, and fluid beyond immediate requirements. There is a reserve capacity for many vital functions of the body. For example, there is more lung tissue than is normally required. There are two kidneys, although one could provide satisfactory renal function. There is reserve liver function, and dual organs of sight and hearing.

**Hyperplasia.** This extra growth of normal tissue is a mysterious body asset resulting in *hypertrophy* (enlargement). We do not always know how the body commands this extra growth, but it occurs in certain tissues in time of extra need. If one kidney is removed, the remaining kidney may enlarge, increasing the amount of available kidney function. Other examples in endocrine glands, muscles, heart, and lymphatic tissue are common.

At times hyperplasia can occur when no apparent need for it exists. There may be hyperplasia in the thyroid gland, with such excess secretion that it is toxic to the body.

(With disuse some tissues and organs decrease in size and in capacity to work [*atrophy*] (Fig. 7-4). In a limb confined for a long time in a cast, bone as well as muscle may show this effect. Atrophy from disuse usually reverts to normal with the return of normal demand on the involved structure. Atrophy can occur without evident reason, and it may resist reversal to normal.)

**The Autonomic Nervous System.** Another source of body protection is the organized provision for *adjustment* through the autonomic nervous system. If a normal person stands up, the momentary rush of blood toward the lower limbs causes immediate orders from this system to constrict the blood vessels in the lower body. Since there is no room in the constricted vessels for an undue proportion of the body blood, a fair share is ensured for distribution to other parts of the body, particularly the brain, where arterial flow is not aided by gravity.

Orders through the autonomic nervous system regulate sweating, alter the size of the pupils of the eyes, speed and slow heart rates, and direct many other adjustments in the body that are beyond voluntary control. Moment to moment, whether human beings are awake or asleep, the autonomic nervous system is making adjustments in response to the ever-changing environment around and inside them.

**Provisions Against Hazards.** Externally, the skin shell, with its superficial layer of dead cells, is a relatively impermeable covering. As long as it remains intact, it is the major protection of the body from invasion by organisms. The outer layer of the skin prevents soaps, lotions, perfumes and other chemical irritants from coming in contact with living cells.

Openings into the body are not without protection. Hydrochloric acid in the stomach creates an environment in which bacteria do not thrive. The reflexes of blinking and sneezing guard the eyes and the respiratory tract. Secretions in these areas have antimicrobial activity. The unprescribed use of washes, gargles, douches and irrigations often do not offer as much protection as the natural material they wash away. Body openings have a rich blood supply and abundant lymphatic tissue to serve the cells of the area, if they are invaded by organisms.

The hard bony skull is protection for the delicate tissues of the brain. The rib cage is protection for the thoracic organs. A whole series of defensive barriers protects the lungs from infection by organisms of the air and the teeming bacterial population of the nose and the throat, through which every breath passes. Tears and mucus wash away particles of dust and microorganisms. Tiny cilia beat against foreign matter to hasten its exit from the body.

**Major Internal Defenses.** These are the highly organized reactions called forth when the body is threatened. These reactions can originate in the endocrine glands, through their chemical messengers, the *hormones*. For example, in times of sudden, urgent distress everyone has experienced the sensations of a large dose of epinephrine (Adrenalin). When the sympathetic division of the autonomic nervous system orders this hormone released from the adrenal medulla, it enters the bloodstream and produces a massive bodywide reaction. The alert state of the body produced by epinephrine has been described as preparation for "fight or flight."

A second hormonal reaction can occur when the pituitary gland orders the adrenal cortex to discharge its adrenal cortical steroid. Hydrocortisone constitutes a major part of the substance released. (A study of this material, which we have available as a drug, can be found in Rodman and Smith, *Clinical Pharmacology in Nursing,* Lippincott, 1974.) Blood pressure, water and electrolyte regulation, the membranes covering cells, and the metabolism of glucose are only a few of the structures and the mechanisms affected. Particularly during periods of prolonged stress the hormonal activity of the adrenal cortex provides a key to the widespread reaction that defends the body. (See beginning of this chapter.) Hormones also regulate many processes to maintain a normal cellular environment. The hormones help to avoid the harm that could follow those occasions when excess fluid, sugar, or salt ingestion otherwise would upset radically the normal environment of the cells.

## The Inflammatory Response

A wound is a break in the continuity of tissue, caused by physical means, such as a knife or burns. How does the body handle the problem of injury or necrosis, in which some special attention is required that is not routine for the rest of the body? First, there must be some way for the injured area to signal its distress. There must be provision for the removal of dead cells, and some kind of replacement must fill in the defect left behind.

In Selye's theory of disease causation, tissue death and inflammation characterize the local adaptation syndrome (LAD) which is greatly influenced by the general adaptation syndrome. The extent of the local reaction is dependent upon the balance between pro-inflammatory and anti-inflammatory hormones secreted by the endocrine glands in response to alarm signals sent off by the stressor itself.

*Inflammation is the body's response to damage of cells.* Regardless of the cause, whether a cut, a burn, a bruise or a pinch, the reaction is similar. The signal that starts the reaction may be the release from dead or injured cells of some of their internal substances, such as histamine. These substances have a profound effect on the capillaries they contact. The capillaries dilate widely and thus bring greatly increased amounts of blood to the area. If the action takes place in the skin or in tissues close under it, the redness produced by this flushing is visible. This site is warm to touch, because it has a greater supply of blood than the tissue around it.

Not only do the capillaries dilate, but the "mesh" of their walls also is opened. Normally, capillaries are permeable to the passage of water and electrolytes, but in this situation they permit extra fluid and some protein of the plasma to escape. This extra content in the tissue spaces produces swelling. Often the swelling is sufficient to stimulate the receptors for pain. The blood vessel changes are responsible for the *cardinal symptoms of inflammation: swelling, pain, redness, and heat.*

The patient is made uncomfortable by the throbbing often felt in the part. The tense tissues of the damage-area no longer cushion the impact of the heartbeat in the vessels. The jolt is transmitted by the nerves, and the patient feels the throb of each heartbeat.

Among the substances released by the injured cells is one which attracts leukocytes. They pass through the capillary walls into the damaged tissues. When there is extensive tissue damage, with consequently great release of the substance that attracts leukocytes, this material may be absorbed and circulate in the blood. It appears to stimulate the production of more white blood cells. A blood count taken at this time will demonstrate an increase in the white cells of the blood far beyond normal (leukocytosis).

Each of the various kinds of white cells has a different function. The *neutrophil,* the most numerous type, engulfs small particles, particularly bacteria. It can digest 15 or 20 before it dies. The *monocyte* engulfs large-sized bacteria or debris. The ability of cells to take into themselves organisms or particles of other matter is called *phagocytosis;* the cells that have this ability are called *phagocytes. Lymphocytes* are associated with immune bodies

that the body manufactures to destroy foreign organisms and to neutralize their toxins. Although *eosinophils* are increased in number in many allergic diseases, their function is obscure. The function of the *basophil* also is obscure.

*Fever often accompanies inflammation.* How inflammation influences the temperature-regulating center is not clear. Possibly a substance absorbed from the injured cells is the signal that stimulates this response.

These effects of inflammation might prove to be beneficial. The protein escaping into the damaged tissue tends to gel and impede movement of materials within the site. Swelling and pain encourage the individual to keep the injured part at rest, which prevents activity from dispersing the contents of the injured area. Bacteria or an offensive substance, such as a foreign chemical, could create additional harm if distributed beyond the local tissue. Fever may be beneficial by speeding the rate of chemical reactions, thus bolstering the chemical defenses.

Inflammation attracts attention. The patient feels its effects, and the doctor relies on its features to help to locate and to identify the place and the type of body injury. By watching the sequence of symptoms it is possible to decide whether the body is overcoming its problem successfully or needs help to master it.

At times it is desirable to combat inflammation by countering the vascular dilatation. For example, cold compresses may be prescribed for a sprained ankle, because there is no apparent benefit from the painful swelling, and no microorganism needs to be isolated. The removal of necrotic tissue still takes place, although at a slower pace because of the vasoconstriction induced by the cold. Sometimes the doctor prescribes cold compresses for the first 24 hours to impede swelling, and then warmth to increase blood supply and to hasten the removal of waste.

In summary, important effects of inflammation include:

- The capillaries dilate to bring more blood to the part, and in the blood more oxygen, nutrients, leukocytes and heat.
- Swelling occurs as fluid escapes from blood vessels into tissues.
- Pain is felt because these changes cause pressure on nerve endings.

## Tissue Repair

As damaged tissue is being cleared of its debris, the signal for repair is given. One of two types of repair follows: replacement with tissue identical with that destroyed or replacement with scar tissue.

When there is a break in tissue, cells bordering the defect multiply and fill it. However, if the defect is large, the ability to re-establish identical cells is diminished or lost. To encourage repair with normal or near-normal structures, the sides of identical tissue are brought together. The surgeon lines up each of the surfaces of tissue he cuts through at the time of operation. The sutures hold the tissues firmly in this position and allow the patient reasonable freedom of movement without worry that the wound edges will shift.

In a surgical wound in which no infection or undue stress on the incision separates the properly sewn tissues, healing will occur with some normal cells and a small amount of scar tissue filling the defect. The patient will have a narrow line of scar cells the length of the incision. This ideal healing—the surgeon's goal—is called *healing by first intention* (Fig. 7-5).

Skin and certain tissues of the intestine heal very rapidly, but other areas usually require between two and three weeks to unite. Bone repair takes even longer. Because of the difference in the rate of healing in different tissues, various suture materials are used in different sites during an operation. Some suture material is absorbed; some is not. The time of removing nonabsorbable stitches varies according to the amount of time required to unite firmly the structures that they join.

The higher the specialization of the tissue, the less chance it has of replacing itself with cells close to those of the original structure. The central nervous system cannot repair itself with the kind of tissue destroyed. There will be material in the space where cells were lost, but it will be scar tissue.

Scar tissue also fills large defects that occur elsewhere in the body. Sometimes the edges of a traumatic wound are so far apart that they cannot be pulled together satisfactorily. Sometimes the debris of infection separates the surfaces of tissues. Rather than leave such debris to accumulate under closed skin, the surgeon keeps the wound open. He expects the wound to fill in with scar tissue rather than with normal tissue. The open skin provides a way of escape for dead cells and other debris that must be removed from the area before regrowth can be

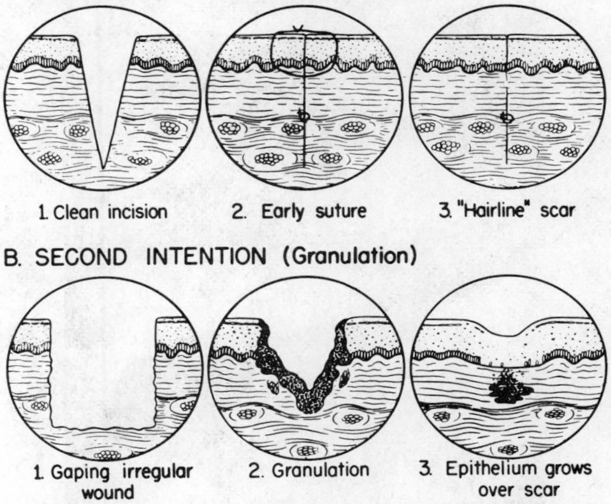

**A. FIRST INTENTION (Primary union)**

1. Clean incision    2. Early suture    3. "Hairline" scar

**B. SECOND INTENTION (Granulation)**

1. Gaping irregular wound    2. Granulation    3. Epithelium grows over scar

**Figure 7-5.** First and second intention wound healing. (Rhoads, J. E., et al.: *Surgery-Principles and Practice*, ed. 4, Philadelphia, Lippincott.)

completed. The body can absorb the debris in time, but the more rapid drainage of the open wound permits an earlier healing. To maintain such drainage, packing may be placed in a crevice to keep it open. As the wound closes in from the bottom, less and less packing is left in it. Finally, when scar tissue has filled the defect, the skin is sewn shut or allowed to grow over it. This process is called *healing by secondary intention*. In *third intention healing* a large gaping wound is filled in with granulation tissue.

The scar mass is formed by cells called *fibroblasts*. These cells locate throughout the protein gel and start to extend little fibrils or threads from the cell body. As the threads weave and intertwine, a network is formed from side to side. To nourish the working cells in this area, otherwise deprived of circulation, capillaries from normal tissue bud out and crisscross the defect. They give a pink or bright-red appearance, and at this stage the tissue being formed is called *granulation tissue* (Fig. 7-6).

Granulation tissue is delicate and very vascular. Great gentleness should be used when changing dressings to avoid damaging newly forming tissues, as well as to prevent unnecessary discomfort to the patient. Packing or gauze that adheres to the tissues should be moistened with sterile saline before removal, to avoid pulling the delicate tissues apart.

When the union of tissues is satisfactory, a signal stops further work by the fibroblasts. In the weeks

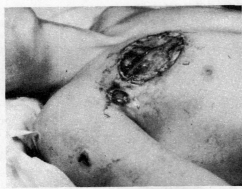

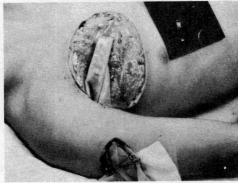

**Figure 7-6.** Gunshot wound of arm and anterior thorax. The wounds were débrided, and adequate drainage was established. A graft was required to close the chest wound. Note the granulation tissue in the second picture. (Hardy, J. D.: *Pathophysiology in Surgery*, Baltimore, Williams & Wilkins)

of the reasons for attempting care that allows healing with a minimum of scar formation.

The scar is as strong at three weeks as it ever will be, but it continues to change for a long time. With contraction, the scar squeezes out the capillaries that once richly infiltrated its network. It begins to blanch, and over months and years it becomes colorless.

*Blood flow is the key to healing.* Healing is poor where there is normally a poor supply of blood. The anterior portion of the lower leg is such a site, and injuries there heal slowly (Fig. 7-7). Because adipose tissue has poor vascularity, it heals slowly. The surgeon knows extra care and time will be required for healing in an obese person in whom great pads of fat have been joined together within the wound. Circulation must never be impaired by carelessness. Tight garments or dressings on or above a wound should not pass without notice. When there is a leg wound, the patient must be encouraged to move from an unfavorable position, such as crossed legs.

Excessive tension or pulling on wound edges can delay healing. The nurse observes for any signs of impaired circulation, such as swelling, coldness, absence of pulse, pallor, or mottling, and reports them. A dressing, particularly one applied to an extremity, should be not so tight as to impair circulation.

## BODY RESPONSES TO INFECTION

### Inflammation

The inflammatory defense in infection is usually greater than that in which no pathogen is involved. The patient with a necrotic area of heart muscle

to follow their fibrils tend to harden and contract. The drawing tight of the network of tough fibrils can cause deformity. The pull of a contracted scar is strong enough to tilt the head or keep an entire limb in a contorted position. This problem is one

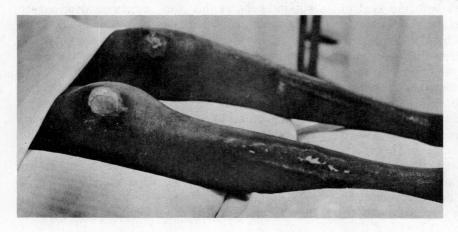

**Figure 7-7.** This patient's legs are paralyzed. He came into the hospital with these decubitus ulcers. Daily dressings, scrupulous cleanliness to prevent infection, and encouragement of circulation coaxed the ulcers into healing. It took 18 months.

due to a myocardial infarction will have an inflammatory response: a slight fever and a slight leukocytosis; whereas in infection the leukocytosis is usually pronounced. Infection also influences the kinds of white blood cells that will appear. In viral disease the response may not be characteristic, or there may be little response. However, in many bacterial infections rapid changes occur that demonstrate how the body is handling the infection. When a physician suspects that a patient may have an early appendicitis, he can watch the white blood cell counts, taken a few hours apart. If there is a growing inflammation and infection, the white cells increase in number.

An infection that has not spread is said to be *localized*. A white, thick exudate of dead cell debris develops inside an outer shell. This material is pus, and a pocket of pus is called an *abcess* (Fig. 7-8). A furuncle (boil) is an abscess of the subcutaneous layers of skin. Around its edges the fight between leukocytes and bacteria continues and adds to the pus accumulation. The pressure of the pocket of pus causes pain.

When the infection is conquered in the tissue surrounding the abscess, the surgeon may drain the abscess safely. If a rim of a furuncle reaches the skin surface, the abscess may rupture spontaneously. A liver abscess may rupture and evacuate its contents into the abdomen. The abscess can join two surfaces with a channel between them (fistula). For example, a gonococcal infection of the vagina can invade the adjoining tissue of the overlying bladder, resulting in a fistula between vagina and bladder. Urine then would not stay in the bladder but would seep through the fistula and drain from the vagina.

Infections caused by certain organisms localize more readily than do others. The streptococcus, for example, can produce products that tend to break down the confining protein gel of the inflammatory exudate. Therefore, its ability to spread in the tissues and to invade lymphatic channels is greater than that of some other organisms. Wide tissue

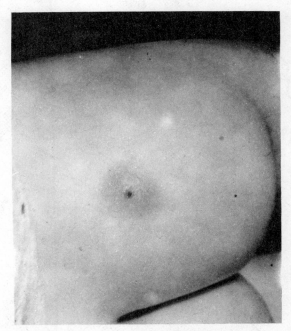

**Figure 7-8.** This painful abscess followed an intramuscular injection. Note the swelling and the redness. (Medichrome—Clay-Adams, Inc., New York, N.Y.)

inflammation without pus is characteristic of its infection (Fig. 7-9).

The infection caused by the staphylococcus tends to become walled off. The organisms can multiply rapidly inside the walls, but they have less chance to extend into surrounding structures.

The lymphatic system has nodes at frequent intervals (Fig. 7-10). These nodes are a defense against infection, but sometimes they become infected themselves. Inflammation of the lymph glands is called *lymphadenitis* (Fig. 7-11). The swelling in the lymph gland at the node produces a tender, firm lump—a signal that organisms have reached this point. If the organisms are sufficiently numerous and virulent, they may resist destructive forces in the lymph channels and pass through node after node. Eventually, the lymph glands drain into the veins, and bacteria are deposited in the blood-

**Figure 7-9.** Streptococcal infection of hand and arm. There is no localization. (Rhoads, J. E., et al.: *Surgery-Principles and Practice*, ed. 4, Philadelphia, Lippincott.)

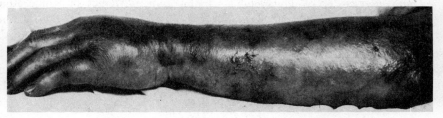

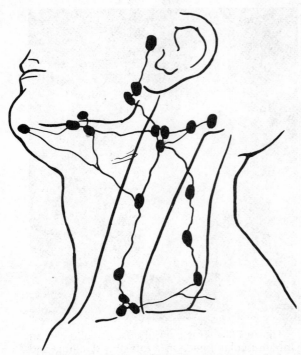

**Figure 7-10.** Lymph nodes of the neck help to prevent spread of infection from a primary site in the head or neck to the rest of the body.

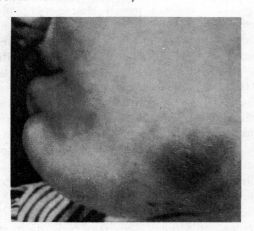

**Figure 7-11.** Infected laceration of lip with purulent lymphadenitis caused by *Staphylococcus aureus.* In this instance a lymph node itself became infected. (Rhoads, J. E., et al.: *Surgery—Principles and Practice,* ed. 4, Philadelphia, Lippincott)

stream. When infective organisms circulate in the blood, the condition is called *septicemia.* Although organs such as lung, spleen and liver are rich in lymphatic tissue traps, septicemia threatens by

blood-borne delivery every tissue in the body in which the organism might find living conditions suitable to its taste. Once in the blood, although defensive forces continue to wage war, the organisms may spread throughout the body to infect many tissues.

*Fever is a cardinal sign of infection.* It is almost always present when there is septicemia. The temperature may increase as the infection grows. A very sudden high fever is not uncommon in infection. The superficial blood vessels constrict to avoid loss of warmth from the blood. Sweating stops, and circulation is diverted to the deepest, most protected blood vessels. The patient feels cold. Muscles begin to contract in uncontrollable shivering and shaking. Heat is being produced by the activity of the chill. Suddenly the patient feels extremely hot. Sweating and vasodilation occur. Fever at this time can be dangerously high. It tends to subside gradually over a period of hours, but in some patients the new excessive temperature level remains relatively unchanged hour after hour.

A chill often is a signal that the body is responding to microorganisms that have entered the bloodstream. It is, therefore, an opportunity to identify the organisms. If the patient is in the hospital his physician should be notified so he can draw blood for culturing if he wishes.

A severe chill is both uncomfortable for the patient and frightening. The chattering of his teeth and the shaking of his body—movement that he cannot control—may be so violent that the whole bed shakes with him. He can stop only after his skin is warmed. He may need several blankets over him. Hot-water bottles and heating pads may help especially at the feet. A physician's order may be needed before these are applied. External heat may help, but the chill ceases in response to the internal mechanism of the body. Antipyretic-analgesic drugs are useful for reducing temperature and making the febrile patient more comfortable.

As soon as the chill is over, some of the covers from the patient should be removed. Sudden extremes of temperature should be avoided, but too much covering will increase the patient's temperature unduly. Since a chill is a result of peripheral blood vessel constriction, it is not infrequent for a patient to have a fever of 103° and be shaking with the cold he feels. His TPR should be checked every 15 minutes, or as ordered. A patient who has experienced a chill should have his temperature taken at least every hour until the temperature is stable. The patient may be drenched in sweat as the temperature starts to drop. To prevent too rapid cooling and to lessen discomfort, his gown should be replaced with a dry one and any damp bed linen changed.

Hospitals present a problem in infection because they have a high population of pathogens donated by patients whose infections release billions of organisms of proved virulence. These pathogens become resident organisms on the skin and the mucous membranes of hospital personnel. They also live on the hospital floors and equipment. When such numbers of available virulent organisms come in contact with many vulnerable hosts, such as the patients debilitated by other diseases or those with wounds, infection can become extremely common. Many organisms, especially staphylococci, have developed resistance to certain antibiotics. Because of these known hazards, infection control committees have been developed to govern practices in the hospital, such as isolation procedures, wound cultures, housekeeping standards, operating room activities, and to investigate the sources of nosocomial (hospital-acquired) infections with the objective of preventing their recurrence. In essence, all the rules apply the principle that in a hospital the only way to avoid infection is to separate the organisms from the potential hosts.

## Immunity

Two reactions to infection may occur—the basic response of inflammation and the response related to immunity.

The body reacts to any substance not normal to it. Some of the reactions are common to all people while others develop from each individual's experience. The response depends on material called *immune bodies*. They are capable of altering the nature of foreign material (*antigen*). Immune bodies can produce many kinds of alterations, but the successful outcome is the destruction of the antigen. The immune bodies that destroy organisms are called *antibodies*. The immune bodies that destroy toxins are called *antitoxins*.

Human beings are born with some immune bodies. The tissue of other animals and of other people, when present in a person's body, usually is destroyed by native immune bodies. In addition to natural immunity, the body responds to some foreign substances by producing antibodies and antitoxins to destroy them. When an antigen is introduced into the body for the first time, the lymphatic tissue begins to manufacture an immune body. Sometimes the original experience with a specific antigen is so profound that the tissue can pour out antibodies at any time for the rest of the person's life. This state is *permanent immunity*. *Temporary immunity* requires the renewed stimulus of antigen to produce antibodies.

Killed organisms or those that are alive but attenuated (lacking in virulence) are made into a vaccine, which can be injected to stimulate the body to produce antibodies against that organism. When a virulent form of the organism subsequently invades the body, the defense has already been prepared. In a similar way, modified toxins (toxoids) can be injected to stimulate the body to make antitoxin. This kind of immunity is *active immunity*.

If another individual or animal has become actively immune to an organism or a toxin, a special preparation of the serum from that person or animal can be given a threatened individual to provide some defense, even though the recipient has played no part in producing it. If the use of this serum is protective, the individual is said to be *passively immunized*. When the donated serum disappears, the individual has no immunity left. His own lymphatic cells have not been stimulated to produce antibodies.

## SUMMARY

The homeostatic processes by which the body protects and defends itself are constantly in use, and most of the time they are impressively successful. Their activity is noticeable only when they are severely challenged. If the defenses are weakened, inhibited or destroyed, the body can be an easy victim of unfavorable influences that a normal individual could be expected to counteract without difficulty. In general, the very young, the old and the poor are an especially easy prey to complications. Malnutrition and fatigue lower body defenses. The smooth, methodical healing of a bone can be slowed by an attack of pneumonia, and vice versa. One disease almost always makes another worse, in itself a compelling reason for the avoidance of secondary complications by every known nursing measure.

When the patient's adaptive responses, time, or therapy falter, one complication can follow another. Then the struggle between health and death is on in full force, and the attention to nursing details can make all the difference to the patient.

## REFERENCES AND BIBLIOGRAPHY

AULD, M., et al.: Wound healing, *Nurs. '72* 2:36, October 1972.

BAHRUTH, A.: Keeping track of I.V. injections, *Nurs. '73* 6:51, June 1973.

BURGESS, AUDREY: *The Nurse's Guide to Fluid and Electrolyte Balance,* New York, McGraw-Hill, 1970.

CAMMER, L.: *Outline of Psychiatry,* New York, McGraw-Hill, 1962.

CANNON, W.: *The Wisdom of the Body,* New York, W. W. Norton and Co., 1932.

COLLAGENASE: *Nurs. '73* 3:35, October 1973.

COLLEY, R., and PHILLIPS, K.: Helping with hyperalimentation, *Nurs. '73* 3:6, July 1973.

DICKENS, M.: *Fluid and Electrolyte Balance,* ed. 2, Philadelphia, F. A. Davis Co., 1970.

DUBOS, R., in LIEF, H., LIEF, V., and LIEF, N.: *The Psychological Basis of Medical Practice,* New York, Harper and Row, 1963.

EGAN, A. P.: Perfecting I.V. piggyback techniques, *Nurs. '74* 4:28, January 1974.

ENGEL, G.: Homeostasis, behavioral adjustment and the concept of health and disease, *in* Grinker, R. (ed.): *Midcentury Psychiatry,* Springfield, Ill., Thomas, 1953.

*Facts on the Major Killing and Crippling Diseases in the United States Today,* The National Health Education Committee, Inc., New York, 1971.

FOSTER, M.: *Claude Bernard,* Longmans, 1899.

GLADSTON, I. (ed.): *Beyond the Germ Theory,* New York, Health Education Council, 1954.

GUYTON, A.: *Textbook of Medical Physiology,* ed. 4, Philadelphia, Saunders, 1971.

HARDY, C.: Infection control: What can one nurse do? *Nurs. '73* 3:18, August 1973.

HART, S. E.: An overview of health—Health: A conceptual model, No. 52-1472, NLN Publ. 2, 1973.

HEATH, J.: A conceptual basis for assessing body water status, *Nurs. Clin. N. Am.* 6:189, March 1971.

I. V. sets, product survey, *Nurs. '72* 2:28, October 1972.

JAMANN, J.: Health is a function of ecology, *Am. J. Nurs.* 71:970, May 1971.

JAMES, G., in TALCO, P., and REMENCHEK, A.: *Internal Medicine Based on Mechanisms of Disease,* St. Louis, Mosby, 1968.

KEE, J.: Fluid imbalance in elderly patients, *Nurs. '73* 3:40, April 1973.

McGILL, D.: Giving I.V. push, *Nurs. '73* 3:15, June 1973.

METHENY, N., and SNIVELY, W.: *Nurses' Handbook of Fluid Balance,* ed. 2, Philadelphia, Lippincott, 1974.

MOORE, V.: I.V. fluids, product survey, *Nurs. '73* 6:32, June 1973.

PLUMER, A.: *Principles and Practice of Intravenous Therapy,* Boston, Little, Brown, 1970.

SEYLE, H.: *The Stress of Life,* New York, McGraw-Hill, 1956.

SNIVELY, W., and BESHEAR, D.: *Textbook of Pathophysiology,* Philadelphia, Lippincott, 1972.

SNIVELY, W., and DICK, R.: Computer approach to diagnosis of body fluid disturbances, *J. Ind. State Med. Assn.* 59:233, March 1966.

SNIVELY, W., and ROBERTS, K.: The clinical picture as an aid to understanding body fluid disturbances, *Nurs. Forum* 12, No. 2, 1973.

SPERO, J.: An overview of health—Health: A community systems model, No. 52-1472, NLN Publ. 9, 1973.

SPITZ, R.: Unhappy and fatal outcomes of emotional deprivation and stress in infancy, *in* Galdstone, I. (ed.): *Beyond the Germ Theory,* New York, Health Education Council, 1954.

STROM, J.: Improving I.V.'s, *Nurs. '73* 3:24, November 1973.

VODA, A.: Body water dynamics—a clinical application, *Am. J. Nurs.* 70:2594, 1970.

WU, R.: *Behavior and Illness,* Englewood Cliffs, N.J., Prentice-Hall, Inc. 1973.

# Interrelationships of Mind, Body, and Social Systems

## THE CONCEPT OF PSYCHOSOMATIC ILLNESS

Psychosomatic connotes more than a kind of illness; it is a comprehensive approach to the totality of an integrated process of transactions among many systems: somatic, psychic, social, and cultural. It deals with a living process that is born, matures, and develops through differentiation and successive stages to new forms of integration of parts and other wholes. It deals with stresses, strains, and adjustments, with acute emergency mechanisms, disintegrations, and chronic defensive states or disease. In fact "psychosomatic" refers not to physiology or pathophysiology, not to psychology or psychopathology, but to a concept of process among all living systems and their social and cultural elaborations (Grinkler, 1973).

The concepts expressed by Grinker convey a broader view of psychosomatic illness than the traditional one of a certain problem leading to a particular symptom, such as anger leading to a headache. However, this dimension of psychosomatic illness is not negated by Grinker's definition; rather it is broadened to consider the individual as a system, who is in turn part of larger interactive systems such as the family, a work group, and a community.

Von Bertalanffy (1968) describes individuals and groups in relation to general systems theory. The individual is a system of interrelated physiologic and psychic functioning. He is affected by transactions with other individuals and groups, and they are affected by him, in a process of mutual interaction.

Within this process stress, if it is not overwhelming, can provide opportunities for learning and for the growth of individuals and groups. But severe stress, either temporary or permanent, can overwhelm coping abilities, thus crippling the individual's maturation, or leading to regression and personality disorganization (Von Bertalanffy, 1968). If it does not exceed coping resources, stress may be confined within one part of a system; but if the resources of that part are not adequate to deal with it, it will extend to others parts (Grinker, 1973). This concept can be illustrated physiologically and psychologically in relation to the individual, and also in the relationships among individuals.

For example, if a small amount of bleeding occurs as a result of a finger prick, the physiologic consequences of blood loss are negligible. If a larger amount of blood is lost due to severe injury, the physiologic effects are far-reaching, and are manifested by tachycardia, a fall in blood pressure, and so on. When the blood supply to such vital organs as the brain and the heart is insufficient, the damage may be so great that death follows.

In another example, a woman experiences menopausal symptoms. She seeks medical advice and is given a prescription for Premarin. The drug controls her physical discomfort. She continues effectively in her work and in her home life. But another woman undergoing menopause becomes markedly depressed and irritable. Because her coping abilities are overwhelmed, the stress not only cripples her own living, but is passed on to other individuals and systems of which she is a part. Her relationships with coworkers and with her family suffer, and as a result they experience stress. Relationships within her family have been problematic; her husband is very dependent on her to be strong, to make decisions. When she is unable to fulfill this role due to her own distress, he becomes anxious and belligerent, is frequently absent from work, and is in danger of losing his job. Thus, the circle widens to affect *his* work associates, who, in their angry response to him, further increase his anxiety and his belligerence.

Thus when the nurse works with patients whose illness is termed "psychosomatic," it is helpful to recognize that the illness may result from a complex web of factors within and outside the individual in his transactions with others. This view can help the nurse to work effectively with the patient, with an attitude of openness and inquiry into the many facets of his life which may contribute to his symptoms, and with an awareness that the patient's symptoms can affect others, such as family and friends, whose responses in turn affect him. Recognition of these interacting systems can help the nurse to respond helpfully to the patient and also to intervene effectively in relation to the system. For example, in relation to the menopausal patient, the nurse may work with the physician and the psychologist to help both the woman and her family to deal with the various distressing responses.

Thus it can be seen that the psyche (mind) and the soma (body) continuously interrelate. Rest and enjoyable activity can bring a sense of zest and rejuvenation reflecting mental and physical well-being, while fatigue, disappointment, and frustration can lead to physical symptoms, such as indigestion and insomnia. Drugs (cortisone for example) can lead to mood changes. Physical illness or surgery can lead to a surge of anxiety over one's competence in various roles, such as professional and family roles. Everyday experiences, like developing a headache after a quarrel, or urinary frequency before an examination, attest that the organism responds as a whole, rather than as strictly psyche or soma.

This complex interweaving between mind and body is expressed by B. Stokvis as follows:

> Within the scope of the modern totality conception both the psychic and the physical factor can be simultaneously cause and effect. There exists, in fact, no essential separation between the mind and the organism, since the psychic condition may be determined by the state of the organism, and conversely. What happens is a process which is simultaneously psychic *and* somatic (Jores and Freyberger, 1961).

In the past, emphasis was placed upon developing personality profiles related to various illnesses, such as coronary artery disease and hypertension. Such profiles have been developed by H. F. Dunbar, among others (Dunbar, 1947). However, more recently emphasis is being placed upon the complex interactions of mind, body, and social systems, as defined by Grinker at the beginning of this chapter. It has been observed that illness and death occur with far greater frequency following stressful experiences, such as the death of a spouse, loss of job, or a move to a new part of the country. A study done by Dr. L. Ruch and Dr. Thomas Holmes and their associates illustrates the increased risk of illness and death in the period following life crises (Ruch and Holmes, 1971).

## Contributing Factors

*Anxiety* is a contributing factor to many psychophysiologic changes. Sometimes the circumstances leading to disturbed physiologic states are hard to pinpoint, as may be the case with a patient who has had hypertension for many years. On the other hand, the relationship of symptoms to these circumstances may be clear, or may become clear as the patient is assisted to observe the relationship between them, his feelings, and his symptoms.

Physical symptoms, such as palpitation, tachycardia, sweating, or disturbance of sleep, which may reflect anxiety, often occur over a prolonged period. The symptoms may seem mysterious and threatening, because the patient is unaware of their cause. The patient whose heart beats more rapidly and forcefully as a manifestation of anxiety may report this symptom to his doctor, and that he feels something is wrong with his heart. Often the patient is not aware that he is anxious. He knows only that his heart keeps pounding for no apparent reason.

Almost any symptom can have its origin in emotional stress. Some patients almost invariably have the same symptom when they become anxious. One may have diarrhea, another asthma, and a third may develop hives or eczema. Some people develop two or several different symptoms, which are often experienced in an alternating fashion. One man was troubled with colitis and eczema. When his eczema was severe, his colitis subsided. When his colitis was severe, his eczema subsided.

*Prolonged anger* can contribute also to psychosomatic illness. For example, one theory of the relationship between anger and hypertension postulates that unrecognized and unrelieved anger results in structural changes in blood vessel walls. The autonomic nervous system is stimulated to constrict the arterioles, thus raising blood pressure. The heart beats faster to push the blood through the narrowed lumen of the vessels. Respiratory rate increases as blood passes more quickly through the lungs. These changes prepare the person to fight, to flee, or otherwise to take action. They are reversed after action has been taken, and the emotion has been relieved. The theory states that when anger is subconscious, unrecognized, and undischarged for a period of years— as it might be in a person who, having to live with an anger-producing situation, has no adequate avenues of expression for his feeling—the physiologic changes become structural and permanent. According to this theory, the arterioles lose their elasticity, and the blood pressure is elevated permanently.

How psychic events may lead to gastritis is suggested by a man known as Tom. When Tom was 9 years old, his esophagus was burned so badly that no food ever passed through it again. An opening was made into his stomach (gastrostomy), and he ate by inserting food into his stomach through the opening. It was possible for physicians to make direct observations of Tom's stomach over a period of time and to relate changes in his stomach to the emotions that he was experiencing. It was found that the amount of gastric secretion, motility, and blood flow to his stomach changed in response to Tom's emotions. When he was sad or withdrawn, the blood supply to his stomach was lessened, gastric secretions were depressed, and his stomach was relatively inactive. When Tom was angry, the mucous membrane of his stomach became red and engorged. Blood flow to the stomach increased, as did gastric secretions and motility. The picture was one of gastritis (Wolf and Wolff, 1943).

The stressful situation may be prolonged, or it may cause the patient so much anxiety that symptoms persist. Disordered functioning can lead to structural changes in the affected organs. A feeling of epigastric discomfort may become more than a disagreeable sensation. The patient may develop a peptic ulcer and organic change, which may be brought about by psychic or emotional stress. One theory states that stress stimulates the autonomic nervous system to produce more hydrochloric acid in the stomach than is needed for digestion. The increased acidity irritates and finally erodes the lining of the stomach.

Emotional stress can lessen the body's resistance to disease, and it is one of several factors that can lead to illness. For example, a patient may develop bronchitis when under intense emotional stress. Skin tests may reveal that he has an allergy to dust and feathers. However, when the patient is relaxed, he may show few or no symptoms of bronchitis, even when he is exposed to dust or feathers. Emotional strain often intensifies allergic symptoms and also may play a part in causation of infectious diseases by decreasing the body's resistance.

It is not clear why a patient who expresses anxiety in a bodily illness does so with certain symptoms and not with others. The particular organ that manifests symptoms may be especially susceptible to disordered functioning, perhaps due to hereditary weakness, or the symptom itself may have particular meaning for the patient. For example, it has been suggested that the wheezing, labored respirations of an asthmatic may be a substitute for weeping in a patient who does not feel free to cry out loud.

Sometimes a person subconsciously develops an illness as a way of handling *a desperate need,* such as that for affection. The only real cure is to satisfy the primary desire. An example is a woman who has pain in her heart, not because of organic heart disease, but because the symptom is a way of gaining, if only temporarily, the love and the attention for which she longs. Her husband cannot leave her when she is so sick; her children are concerned. Her pain is just as severe as if it were the result of a physical cause.

> No one really wants to be sick. But these . . . [people] may want something else so badly that sickness is brought upon them. If it helps achieve the desired end, it is welcome for what it brings, not for what it is. If it fails, as it so often does, it becomes a double tragedy (Dunbar, 1947).

## THE REALITY OF PSYCHOSOMATIC ILLNESS

Many people, including the families of patients and members of the health professions, believe that the influence of emotional stress on physical illness makes the latter less real or wholly imaginary. But psychosomatic illness is real. Acknowledging the reality of the patient's illness is important; it is the first step in helping him.

A patient who develops bronchial asthma, whether in response to psychic factors, allergy, infection, or a combination of all three, has constriction of bronchi and production of copious, stringy respiratory secretions. His breathing becomes labored. Respiration becomes so impaired that the vital functions of inhaling oxygen and exhaling carbon dioxide are inadequate for the body's needs. The patient may develop cyanosis. Regardless of what caused these symptoms, the patient is acutely ill and may die.

The patient with psychosomatic illness is often neglected. The same staff who give excellent care to patients whose illness does not carry the stigma of the word *psychosomatic* not uncommonly ignore, scorn, or ridicule the patient whose illness is believed to be related to emotional stress. One possible reason for the stigma may be the use of the term *psycho* as a prefix, which may convey the idea that the patient is mentally ill, and thus subject him to the contempt and

avoidance so often the lot of the mentally ill. Another reason may be that the patient is considered a weakling. Or prejudice may be due to a belief that the patient is feigning illness in an attempt to get attention or favors.

In the latter instance, a patient with psychosomatic illness is often confused with a malingerer, one who deliberately shams illness to achieve some secondary gain, such as financial compensation or excuse from work. The essential difference between psychosomatic illness and malingering is that the malingerer feigns symptoms. It is a conscious process in which he is aware that he is pretending to be sick. The patient with psychosomatic illness develops *real* symptoms as a manifestation of largely unconscious psychic conflicts.

Condemnation of the patient with psychosomatic illness can persist despite intellectual understanding of theories about the causes of the illness. The patient can sense immediately whether those who care for him are trying to help him, or whether they are belittling him.

The patient with psychosomatic illness is in a difficult position. Sometimes his therapy consists of being told to go home and forget it. He often detects veiled contempt behind the ministration of physicians and nurses. Frequently, his symptoms are ignored by those who care for him. "Keep his mind off it" may be the ward's watchword in dealing with him.

Because the patient does not understand how his symptoms come about, he often feels helpless. He feels sick, but no one seems to believe him. He may begin to wonder whether he is imagining the symptoms. Or he may long for the concreteness of an underlying physical cause. The patient knows that a diseased appendix can be removed, and that an infection can be cured by drugs. But what can be done for symptoms that seem to have their origin in emotional stress?

## TREATMENT OF PSYCHOSOMATIC ILLNESS

The first step in helping the patient is to accept and acknowledge his illness. The cause of his symptoms must be found, and measures must be taken to relieve them and to prevent their recurrence. Thorough examinations are essential. It is not unknown for a patient whose illness is considered psychosomatic to be found later to have cancer or some other disease. The thorough search for physical causes of the symptoms helps to gain the patient's confidence. He knows that his condition and welfare are being taken seriously. If no organic basis for his complaints is found, he usually will find this news easier to accept when he knows he has had a thorough examination.

Finding no physical cause for the disorder points the way to understanding the patient's condition. What is the cause? Is it emotional stress? If so, what kind? What are the problems which are upsetting the patient? Knowing that it is only "nerves" does not help the patient, because it does not help him to learn what to do about it.

By carefully listening to the patient and by observing his responses, the nurse can learn about the emotional difficulties the patient is experiencing and help him to see the possible relationship between his symptoms and emotional stress. Until the patient himself begins to see this relationship, the relief of symptoms is transitory and random. When he begins to understand the cause-and-effect relationship, he may begin to find other ways of handling his emotional problems. Almost any example is an oversimplification, because the situations have many diverse and subtle aspects. Perhaps the patient will be helped by learning to express some of the anger he feels, as well as by beginning to modify some of the situations that make him angry.

At times referral to a psychotherapist is necessary, to assist the patient in coping with his life situation, and thereby alleviate the anxiety. Some hospitals have separate units for the care of psychosomatic patients, where emphasis is placed on both the emotional and the physical components of the illness.

Sometimes psychotherapy is carried on individually; sometimes, in groups. One of its objectives is to help the patient to become aware of the deep-rooted and often unconscious causes of his anxiety. Another objective is to assist the patient to cope more effectively, and with less stress, in the daily life situations encountered at home and at work.

Nevertheless, the patient's physical discomfort should not be ignored. While the emotional factors responsible for his illness are being studied, he needs to feel that others are concerned about his symptoms, and that he will be helped to be more comfortable. Moreover, he should be helped to understand that such treatment can offer only temporary relief and cannot be relied on if emotional problems are neglected. The relief of symptoms may involve the prescription of a wide variety of drugs, such as antacids, antidiarrhetics, and antipruritic lotions for itchy, inflamed skin.

The patient's symptoms indicate the type of treatment that may provide relief. Sometimes sedatives or tranquilizers are prescribed to lessen the patient's anxiety, thus helping to relieve his physical symptoms. However, these drugs do not provide a substitute for the patient's understanding of the relationship between his symptoms and stress situations.

There is no easy cure for psychosomatic illness. Discovering the causes of the patient's illness and helping him to understand and to find more satisfactory ways to cope with his problems are challenges to all who work with the patient. Frequently, the process takes many years. Some patients are unable to accept the idea that their symptoms originate in emotional conflicts; therefore, they cannot begin to move toward identification of their emotional problems. These patients may continue to be treated symptomatically by such measures as diet and medication. As some future time it may be possible for them to recognize a relationship between their physical symptoms and their emotional conflicts.

The necessity for careful assessment of the patient's emotional and physical status, and for collaboration by members of the health team, cannot be overemphasized. Psychosomatic disorders sometimes mask more severe disturbances of personality (Grinker, 1973). It is especially important that the patient's emotional responses be monitored while his physical symptoms are being treated. With relief of physical symptoms his emotional disturbance may be more clearly manifested.

## NURSING CONSIDERATIONS

Nursing care of the patient with psychosomatic illness requires much tact, insight, and judgment. The patient needs someone to listen to him, to be concerned about his symptoms, and to respect him. Prying or attempting to force him to acknowledge a relationship between his symptoms and emotional problems may make him more anxious, with intensification of his physical symptoms and resistance to any later suggestion that he receive psychotherapy.

Often the nurse makes observations that seem to show a relationship between the patient's physical symptoms and other events in his life. These observations are important. Do symptoms "come and go," leaving the patient free of discomfort for part of the day, or do they persist throughout most of the day and night? What things tend to relieve the symptoms? Medication? Diversion? Often this relationship is the first tangible evidence of the connection between the patient's symptoms and his emotions. For many patients, recognition of this relationship is the first step toward accepting this connection. One woman with colitis was unable to see the link between attacks of colitis and other circumstances in her life until one day, while she was talking to her doctor, she said "I never have colitis in the summer when I'm away at the beach." At that moment she herself began to see the relationship between the symptoms and situations in her life.

As the nurse gradually develops a relationship with the patient, she can listen with greater sensitivity to his concerns, and during this process, she can often find opportunities to help the patient understand the relationships between his symptoms and his life experiences. Helping him to see such relationships is an important aspect of nursing care of the patient with psychosomatic illness.

The nurse should avoid stereotyping the patient as soon as she learns his diagnosis. Patients with psychosomatic illnesses cannot be neatly separated and labeled. All patients have some anxiety, and each patient is an individual. The nurse should let her patient show her what he is like.

Opinions differ greatly about the role of the emotions in the causation of various illnesses. For example, one article states that rheumatoid arthritis is due to repressed hostility. Another says, just as emphatically, that it is due to allergy or infection. When many different possible causes are listed for an illness, its etiology remains uncertain. It is also possible that an illness may have primarily physical causes in one person and primarily emotional causes in another.

The nursing of all patients, including those whose illnesses have been diagnosed as psychosomatic, includes considerations of both physical and mental comfort. For example, if an antacid has been prescribed for such an illness, it should be administered without any words or actions that would convey to the patient, "You really don't need this, but here it is anyway."

**Use of Placebos.** Sometimes the physician prescribes a placebo (a medication given not for pharmacologic effect but for the relief which may result from suggestion). A sugar pill or an injection of sterile water is sometimes used for this purpose. Administration of any drug carries with it expecta-

tion of relief, as well as tangible assurance of the physician's and the nurse's interest in lessening the patient's discomfort. These effects are enhanced by a statement from the person administering the drug concerning the benefit that may be expected.

Some patients are more likely to be relieved by the placebo action of a drug than others. The fact that help is obtained from a placebo does not mean necessarily that the patient has a psychosomatic illness. One man with cancer was kept comfortable for several weeks by injections of sterile saline. Later he required narcotics for control of pain. His physician's comment was, "We'll use the placebos as long as they'll help him. When they don't, we'll start using narcotics." The patient was spared temporarily some of the undesirable side effects of narcotics, including tolerance to the drug and the consequent need of larger doses.

Whether or not the patient's symptoms can be relieved by a placebo is sometimes a clue to the cause of his illness. The nurse should observe and report whether the symptoms have subsided and for how long.

Suggestibility is a complex phenomenon. It can be a most useful therapeutic tool, even extending to the use of hypnosis as an anesthetic. The various factors in suggestibility are not fully understood, but it has been noted that anxious patients are especially likely to have good results from placebo therapy. Demonstration of interest in the patient's treatment and progress is believed to enhance the success of placebo therapy.

Placebos, like any medication, are prescribed for a definite purpose—either to relieve certain symptoms or to aid in diagnosing their cause.

**Let the Patient Talk.** It may be the nurse to whom the patient turns to talk over the physician's findings that his illness is due primarily to emotional rather than physical causes. Frequently, the patient initiates the conversation after he has undergone a series of tests and examinations. He may find it upsetting that he has no physical disorder curable by such measures as drugs, diet, or even surgery. He needs time to think this fact through, as well as help and support. If psychotherapy has been recommended, this thought, too, may be very disturbing. The nurse should let the patient talk about his thoughts on the subject. She should convey to him that he is not odd because he has physical symptoms as a result of emotional stress. Many people reflect emotional stress in physical symptoms. If he is doing so to the extent that he is often uncomfortable, it is merely an indication that he needs treatment.

People are under more stress than most of us realize. Our culture emphasizes presenting a brave, smiling face. Even close friends and members of the same family are often unaware of the degree of stress other members are experiencing. Psychosomatic illness is understandably very common.

Because the effects of emotional stress on physical symptoms are being studied in relation to such a wide variety of diseases, this aspect of study will be described throughout this book.

## THE DELIRIOUS PATIENT

Delirium is a state of disorientation and confusion caused by interference with the metabolic processes of the neurons of the brain. The condition is usually temporary and reversible. Delirium usually clears when its cause has been removed.

The delirious patient is disoriented as to time and place and may have illusions and hallucinations. An *illusion* is an inaccurate interpretation of stimuli within the environment. The patient may think that his sister is calling him, when actually the nurse is calling him. *Hallucinations* are subjective sensory experiences that occur without stimulation from the environment. The patient may hear a voice calling him, when no one is calling him.

The delirious patient is restless and confused. He has defects in memory and judgment. He often behaves impulsively and acts on incorrect interpretations of his environment. For instance, he may believe that a window is a door and attempt to escape through it. Often delirium develops suddenly; it can subside equally quickly. A patient may seem well oriented at bedtime but be delirious an hour later. Symptoms are usually worse at night. Often the patient becomes quite anxious, because he senses that his ability to cope with his environment has lessened.

Nursing care of the delirious patient involves protecting him and others from harm and helping him (as far as possible) to minimize the disorientation and confusion. The basic cause (drug intoxication, fever, alcoholism) is treated medically. In the meantime the following nursing measures can help to lessen the patient's confusion and to protect him from harm:

- **Keep sensory stimuli to a minimum. The room should be quiet. Avoid unnecessary conversation.** Chatter, especially if it concerns abstract subjects, is likely to confuse the patient further. Be concrete and repetitive in your conversation. For example, repeating, "You're in the hospital, and I am your nurse," can help the patient to orient himself to his environment. Keep explanations brief and simple, such as "Here is your soup" or "I'm going to wash your back." Try not to reflect the patient's restlessness and agitation. Feelings can be contagious. Speaking quietly and slowly may help to lessen the patient's apprehension.

- **Keep the patient's room softly lighted during the night.** Soft light will help to prevent the increased disorientation that usually occurs when the patient is left in a darkened room, and it will contribute to his safety by enabling others to observe him.

- **Protect the patient from harm.** If he tries to act on his illusions, he may fall out of the window, thinking it a stairway and an escape route from the danger that he perceives around him. Most hospitals require a physician's order before restraints can be used. If the delirious patient has such an order, be sure that the restraints in no way impair circulation, and that they give the patient as much movement as is compatible with safety. Many people, delirious or not, react to physical restraints with anger; the delirious patient may be made more excited by them. Remove the restraints whenever there is adequate supervision so that the patient can move about. If he has been pulling against them, his skin may be reddened—or worse, broken—where he was restrained. Help him to sit up as much as possible, if he is permitted to do so.

- **The delirious patient usually is incapable of feeding himself.** Feed him slowly and allow him to assist, if he is able. Encourage fluid intake, unless the physician has left orders to limit fluids.

- **Side rails can help to keep the patient in bed.** Try to help the patient to understand their purpose, so that he is prevented, if possible, from considering the rails a confining cage from which he must escape. A patient who is physically strong enough can climb over side rails.

- **Having someone remain with the patient, assuring him that he is being cared for, can help greatly to lessen his agitation and to prevent him from hurting himself.** Sometimes a family member can stay with the patient, if shortage of staff makes it impossible for nursing personnel to do so.

- **Keep objects with which the patient could harm himself away from him.** For instance, a paper drinking straw should be used instead of a glass one and a paper cup instead of a water glass. Cigarettes and matches should not be left within reach.

- **Remember that the patient cannot control his behavior. Scolding him is both inappropriate and ineffective.**

Delirious patients require extensive nursing care. Their unpredictable behavior often interferes with the goals of those caring for them. For instance, the patient may spill a glass of water on the bed just after you have changed it. Do not show impatience or anger to the patient, although it is important to recognize that you are annoyed, if you are. As far as possible, modify the environment and the plan of care to help to prevent incidents that can upset the patient and those around him. For instance, it is better to hold the glass for the delirious patient than to allow him to hold it himself.

## NURSING ASSESSMENT

Flexibility is essential, and assessment must be individualized for each patient. The following questions are suggested to guide the process of assessment of the patient with a psychosomatic disorder:

- **How does the patient describe his symptoms (sensations he experiences, timing, and so on)?**
- **Under what circumstances does the patient experience symptoms? Has he noticed any events of circumstances which seem to trigger his symptoms?**
- **What measures relieve the symptoms?**
- **Is the patient awakened from sleep by his symptoms?**
- **What is the patient's home situation? (Ask him to describe a typical day at home; to tell you who shares his home; to describe his relationships with them.)**
- **What is the patient's work situation? (Ask him to describe a typical day at work including his relationships with his coworkers.)**
- **Does the patient experience anxiety: i.e., is he aware of feeling anxious? If so, under what circumstances?**
- **Does the patient have other symptoms, or other diagnosed illnesses, besides the one for which he now seeks help?**
- **What emotions does the patient convey as he talks? Anger? Sadness?**
- **Is he experiencing the symptoms while he is talking with you? Are there times while he is talking about himself that the symptom appears, or grows worse?**

Seek this information in an unhurried manner with clearly communicated concern for the patient, and convey an approach that allows the patient to elaborate on points that seem significant to him. Avoid a "cut and dried, question and answer" approach; instead, bring up significant questions, listen carefully, and notice what other points the patient brings up, in relation to these questions. Because seeming digressions can yield valuable information, it is important to allow enough time to listen to them.

## NURSING INTERVENTION

The nurse intervenes both independently and as a colleague of other health team members. She also functions dependently, when carrying out the phy-sician's orders for medical therapy. A few guidelines for nursing intervention:

- **Listening emphatically, thereby helping the patient become more aware of his feelings, and of circumstances under which he experiences symptoms.**
- **Interacting with the patient's family and friends to become increasingly aware of the patient's role in various systems and the possible relevance of relationships with other "significant persons" to his symptoms.**
- **Studying data, and devising plans for nursing action based on the data.**
- **Conferring with other health professionals.**
- **Assisting the patient to find resources, i.e., individuals and groups, who can help him to cope with stress.**
- **Teaching the patient useful concepts and health practices that may alleviate and control his symptoms.**
- **Administering physical comfort measures and controlling the environment to promote recovery.**
- **Administering prescribed medical therapy.**
- **Assisting the patient to plan his day to maximize opportunities for recovery.**

## REFERENCES AND BIBLIOGRAPHY

BARNARD, M. et al.: Psychosocial failure to thrive, *Nurs. Clin. N. Am.* 8:557, September 1973.

BUCHAN, D. J.: Mind-body relationships in gastrointestinal disease, *Canad. Nurse* 67:35, March 1971.

CHAVIGNY, K.: Psychosomatic illness and personality, *J. Psychiat. Nurs.* 7:261, November-December 1969.

DUNBAR, F.: *Mind and Body: Psychosomatic Medicine,* New York, Random House, 1947.

————: *Emotions and Bodily Changes,* ed. 4, New York, Columbia University Press, 1954.

EVERSON, T. C., and COLE, W. H.: *Spontaneous Regression of Cancer,* Philadelphia, Saunders, 1966.

FORRERR, G. R.: The therapeutic use of placebo, *Mich. Med.* 63:558, 1964.

FRANK, I., and POWELL, M.: *Psychosomatic Ailments in Childhood and Adolescence,* Springfield, Ill., Thomas, 1967.

GARNER, H. H.: *Psychosomatic Management of the Patient with Malignancy,* Springfield, Ill., Thomas, 1966.

GOODWIN, D. W.: Psychiatry and the mysterious medical complaint, *JAMA* 209:1884, September 22, 1969.

GRINKER, R. R.: *Psychosomatic Concepts,* rev. ed., New York, Jason Aronson, 1973.

JORES, A., and FREYBERGER, H. (eds.): *Advances in Psychosomatic Medicine: Symposium of the Fourth European Conference on Psychosomatic Research,* New York, Basic Books, 1961.

KIMBALL, C. P.: Conceptual developments in psychosomatic medicine: 1939-1969, *Ann. Intern. Med.* 73:307, 1970.

KISSEN, D. M., and LESHAN, L. L. (eds.): *Psychosomatic Aspects of Neoplastic Disease,* Philadelphia, Lippincott, 1964.

LAZARUS, R. S.: *Psychological Stress and the Coping Process,* New York, McGraw-Hill, 1966.

LEWIS, H. R., et al.: *Psychosomatics,* New York, Viking, 1972.

MENNINGER, K. A.: *Man Against Himself,* New York, Harcourt, 1956.

_____: *The Vital Balance,* New York, Viking, 1963.

MOWCHENKO, G.: Care of patients with G.I. diseases that have a psychological component, *Canad. Nurse* 67:38, March 1971.

NODINE, J. H., and MOYER, J. H.: *Psychosomatic Medicine,* Philadelphia, Lea, 1962.

PEPLAU, H. E.: *Interpersonal Relations in Nursing,* New York, Putnam, 1952.

PRICK, J. J., and VAN DE LOO, K. J.: *The Psychosomatic Approach to Primary Chronic Rheumatoid Arthritis,* Philadelphia, Davis, 1964.

RUCH, L., and HOLMES, T.: Scaling of life change, *J. Psychosomatic Res.* 15:221, June 1971.

SELYE, H.: *The Stress of Life,* New York, McGraw-Hill, 1956.

_____: The stress of life: New focal point for understanding accidents, *Nurs. Forum* 4:29, 1965.

_____: The stress syndrome, *Am. J. Nurs.* 65:97, March 1965.

SHAPIRO, A. K.: Etiological factors in placebo effect, *JAMA* 187:712, March 7, 1964.

SHOCHET, B. R., et al.: A medical-psychiatric study of patients with rheumatoid arthritis, *Psychosomatics* 10:271, September-October 1969.

SPIEGEL, J.: *Transactions,* New York, Science House, 1971.

VON BERTALANFFY, LUDWIG: *General System Theory,* New York, George Braziller, 1968.

WAHL, C. W. (ed.): *New Dimensions in Psychosomatic Medicine,* Boston, Little, Brown, 1964.

WARSON, S. R., et al.: The role of intentionality in recovery: Operational concepts, *Psychosomatics* 10:225, July-August 1969.

WENAR, C., et al.: *Origins of Psychosomatic and Emotional Disturbances,* New York, Hoeber, 1962.

WITTKOWER, E. D., et al.: A global survey of psychosomatic medicine, *Int. J. Psychiat.* 7:499, January 1969.

WOLF, S., et al.: *Life Stress and Essential Hypertension,* Baltimore, Williams & Wilkins, 1955.

WOLF, S., and WOLFF, H. G.: *Human Gastric Function: An Experimental Study of a Man and His Stomach,* London, Oxford, 1943.

# The Patient with Allergy

## PATHOPHYSIOLOGIC THERAPEUTIC CONSIDERATIONS

Most patients use the word *allergy* to denote their own exaggerated reaction, such as sneezing, respiratory embarrassment, itching, or skin rash, to substances, situations, or physical states that are without comparable effect on the average individual. The word allergy is often used to designate *immunologic* reactions whereby the body is injured in the course of its immune response to substances recognized as foreign to it. In this sense the allergic reaction is an immune reaction which is *altered* from being protective to being injurious to the host. Reactions other than immunologic which are exaggerated or adverse in certain individuals are better termed *intolerant*, *idiosyncratic*, or *functional* reactions.

To best care for patients with diseases in which exaggerated reactions are an important part of the illness and to care for all patients in which there is risk of such reaction to treatment, particularly medication, a rudimentary knowledge of the nature of both immunologic and nonimmunologic adverse reactions is required.

### Immunologic Reactions

*Immunogens*, *antigens*, or *allergens* are nearly synonymous terms used to describe substances such as microbes, drugs, pollens, danders, foods, and even body tissues or organs, capable of stimulating the host to produce cells and antibodies which specifically recognize the foreign substance and initiate its elimination from the body. The cells which recognize and respond to immunogens are of two lymphocyte types. B type lymphocytes (bone marrow derived and dependent; equivalent to bursa dependent lymphocytes in the chicken) respond to immunogen stimulation by clonal proliferation and transformation into plasma cells which produce antibodies. Antibodies are contained in the gamma globulin fraction of serum and are called immunoglobulins. The basic structure of immunoglobulin is shown in Figure 9-1. Five classes of immunoglobulins have been recognized: IgG, IgM, IgA, IgD, and IgE. The T lymphocytes (thymus dependent) respond to immunogens directly and through release of mediators called lymphokines to attack invading microbes, neoplastic cells, or transplanted organs.

The nature and magnitude of the immune response the host produces to foreign substances is determined in part by the route and dose in which the substance enters the body and by the genetic constitution of the individual. Immunologic reactions injurious to the host have been conveniently categorized by Gell and Coombs (1968) into four types.

**TYPE I—Anaphylactic Reactions.** Anaphylactic reactions, also referred to as *immediate*, *atopic*, or *reaginic hypersensitivity*, are capable of producing a spectrum of disease ranging from mild local reactions at the site of interaction with the allergen, such as the sneezing, itching, and watering of eyes and nose of "hay fever," to systemic reactions such as hives and giant swelling of the skin, to respiratory distress from bronchospasm and even to shock and death from vascular collapse (fatal anaphylaxis).

The patient who is "allergic" in the sense of being susceptible to a Type I reaction has formed a specific antibody of the IgE class of immunoglobulins to allergens to which he has been exposed. Certain individuals and families tend to form these IgE antibodies (reagins) on natural exposures to many substances such as tree, grass, and weed pollen grains, animal danders, constituents of house dust, mold spores, and occasionally foods. These individuals frequently, but not invariably, have childhood eczema, hay fever, or asthma and have been called atopic individuals. All normal people have some IgE antibody. Large amounts of IgE antibodies are produced in the normal immune response to parasitic infestation without apparent harmful effect on the host. A few individuals will develop IgE antibody following their first treatment with drugs such as penicillin, and are at risk of having an anaphylactic reaction on subsequent exposure to the drug.

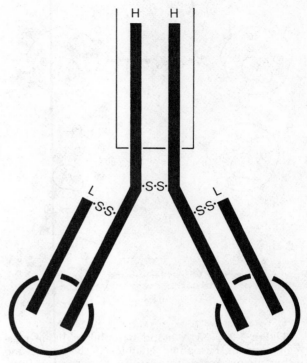

**Figure 9-1.** Diagram of an immunoglobulin molecule. The molecule consists of two long or heavy (H) and two short or light (L) chains of amino acids held together by disulfide bonds (S-S). Circles indicate that portion of the molecule which combines with antigen. IgE antibodies fix to mast cells and complement attaches to IgG and IgM complement-fixing antibodies at that portion of the molecule indicated within the box.

Anaphylactic reactions involve a chain of events leading to tissue changes. These are shown in schematic form in Figure 9-2A. Basophils and tissue mast cells of the anaphylactically sensitized individual are coated with specific IgE antibodies. When the specific allergen comes in union with adjacent corresponding IgE antibodies, a series of intracellular enzymatic steps is initiated which leads to secretion of the chemical mediators histamine, the slow-reacting substance of anaphylaxis (SRSA), and the eosinophil chemotactic factor of anaphylaxis (ECFA) from the large basophilic storage granules of the cell. This reaction is called a *cytotropic* reaction in that the basophil or mast cell changes but is able to survive and reconstitute its mediators, as opposed to a *cytolytic* reaction in which the cell dies. Histamine increases vascular permeability, allowing tissue edema formation, and constricts certain smooth muscles. The effects of histamine are blocked

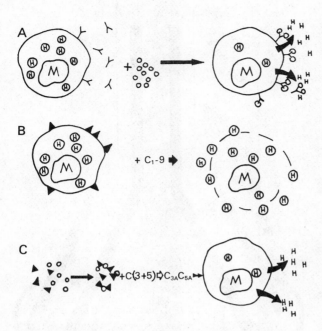

**Figure 9-2.** (A) A blood basophil or tissue mast cell contains basophilic granules of histamine and other chemical mediators (H). The Y's are anaphylactic antibodies (IgE) and the open circles are antigen. Union of antigen bridging adjacent antibody molecules results in the release of the histamine and other chemical mediators. (B) A red blood cell (RBC) with surface antigenic markers (triangles) is represented. The Y's are complement-fixing (nonanaphylactic) antibodies which on combination with antigen fix the complement components and lead to disruption of the cell membrane. (C) Soluble antigen (triangles) upon union with complement-fixing antibodies (Y's) form soluble immune complexes which circulate and activate the complement components with release of the anaphylatoxins $C_{3a}$, $C_{5a}$.

by the antihistamine drugs. SRSA also constricts smooth muscle, such as that in the bronchial tree; this effect is not blocked by antihistamines. ECFA attracts eosinophils from the bloodstream and bone marrow to the site of allergen-antibody union. Other chemical mediators including serotonin and platelet aggregating factor are less important in human anaphylactic reactions.

The extent and severity of an anaphylactic reaction are determined by the location and amount of chemical mediators released which in turn are dependent upon the number of mast cells and basophils degranulated by interaction with allergen. In "hay fever," (a misnomer in that grass or weed pollen rather than hay is the usual allergen and fever is not a part of the syndrome), allergens from airborne pollen lodge in the eyes and nose of the allergic individual and combine with IgE antibodies on mast cells in the mucous membranes allowing mediator release which leads to the itching, watering, and tissue swelling typical of this syndrome. In some patients with both anaphylactic sensitivity and imbalance of autonomic control of the bronchial tree, aeroallergen exposure may lead to the symptoms of both hay fever and bronchial asthma (see below). If an allergen enters the bloodstream (e.g., penicillin given by mouth or parenterally, or injected bee venom) in an individual anaphylactically allergic to the substance, the simultaneous, relatively massive release of chemical mediators from basophils in the bloodstream and mast cells in all body tissues may lead to systemic manifestations of anaphylaxis including urticaria, angioedema (see Plate 1), bronchospasm, cardiac arrhythmia, vascular collapse, shock, and death.

**TYPE II—Cytotoxic or Membranolytic Reactions.** Certain diseases result from the formation of antibodies to foreign or altered cells or tissue membranes. These antibodies are usually of the IgG or IgM class and may have the capability of activating the complement system, further amplifying the reaction leading to lysis of the cell or tissue membrane to which the antibody has attached. A schema of this type of immunologic reaction is shown in Figure 9-2B.

The *complement system* consists of more than 10 serum proteins. When complement-fixing antibodies bind to membrane antigens, the first component of complement attaches to the antibody and initiates a cascade of reactions including the successive activations of the other complement components. Parts of these components attach to the cell membrane producing structural damage in the form of tiny holes in the membrane which disrupt function of the membrane and eventually lead to dissolution of the membrane.

Examples of Type II reactions include hemolytic transfusion reactions and drug induced hemolytic anemia. In these examples red blood cells or drugs adherent to red cells are recognized as foreign by host antibodies. In major hemolytic transfusion reactions, the recipient has preformed natural or acquired antibodies to the transfused red blood cells. Upon intravenous infusion, the donor cells are attacked by the recipient antibody and complement resulting in cell lysis with intravascular release of hemoglobin and pyrogens, thus the hemoglobinemia, hemoglobinuria, and fever of an acute transfusion reaction. In the hemolytic drug reaction, the antibody combines with the drug absorbed to the red cell membrane, and fixes the complement leading to cell damage or lysis.

Examples of altered tissues to which the host may produce antibodies are the basement membranes of the lung and the kidney in Goodpasture's syndrome (hemoptysis with nephritis) and kidney in post-streptococcal glomerulonephritis. In the latter instance the antibody to streptococcal antigens may cross-react with glomerular basement membranes to initiate the kidney injury.

**TYPE III—Immune Complex Reactions.** When relatively large quantities of antigen (in contrast to Type I reactions which require only minute amounts of antigen) gain entry into the bloodstream and evoke an antibody response, soluble complexes of antigen and antibodies may be formed and the complement system activated. A schema of this type of immunologic reaction is shown in Figure 9-2C. When the soluble complexes are filtered through the kidney or the microvasculature of the skin and joints, there may be sufficient accumulation of complexes and complement components to produce an inflammatory reaction. Activation of the complement system results in the release of the fragments $C_{3a}$ and $C_{5a}$ from the respective complement components. These are mediators which increase local vascular permeability and are chemotactic for eosinophils and neutrophils. Attracted neutrophils ingest the antigen-antibody complexes and may release proteolytic enzymes which further intensify the inflammatory process.

Human serum sickness is an example of a Type III immunologic reaction. The administration of heterologous antiserum such as horse tetanus antitoxin initiates an immune response in the human recipient of the foreign protein. After 10 to 14 days of circulation of the foreign protein in the bloodstream, the recipient has mounted a sufficient antibody response to start the formation of antigen-antibody complexes. These complexes are trapped in the microvasculature of the skin, joints, and kidneys and produce the clinical syndrome of fever, urticaria, arthralgias, and in some instances, acute nephritis. As a greater proportion of the population has received prophylactic active immunizations and as human antiserums have replaced horse antiserums, human serum sickness has become a relatively rare disorder.

Type III immune reactions account for part of the pathophysiology of several naturally occurring human diseases. In infectious hepatitis, hepatitis-B antigen-antibody complexes in the bloodstream account for the transient skin rashes and arthralgias seen in this disorder. When there is persisting circulation of hepatitis-B antigen-antibody complexes, the clinical syndrome of polyarteritis nodosa may develop. In human systemic lupus erythematosus, nuclear constituents, ordinarily sequestered from the host's own immune system, are released into the bloodstream and recognized as foreign by the body. This disorder often is called an *autoimmune* disease in that antibodies to the host's own tissues are formed and circulating antigen-antibody complexes produce renal, skin, and other system diseases. Circulating immune complexes probably play a role in other diseases in which there is vasculitis, including some instances of rheumatoid arthritis.

**TYPE IV—Cellular Reactions.** Immune reactions in which lymphocytes recognize the foreign antigen and attempt to eliminate it from the body require 24 to 72 hours for full manifestation and are dependent upon lymphocytes and macrophages for their expression. For these reasons, this type of immune reaction has been called *delayed,* or *cellular, hypersensitivity.* The typical example of such reaction is the skin response to tuberculin testing. An individual who has had exposure to *Mycobacterium tuberculosis* and has developed sensitized T-lymphocytes, responds at 24 to 72 hours following the skin test with local induration and redness at the test site. This reaction depends on the presence of a few specifically sensitized T-lymphocytes which release several *lymphokines,* mediators including macrophage inhibition factor, cytotoxins, transfer factor, interferon, and others which account for the histopathology and effectiveness of the reaction.

Cellular immune reactions are the body's main defense against mycobacteria, fungi, viruses, neoplasms, and transplanted tissues. When drugs, radiation, or antiserums are used to suppress cellular immune response to allow survival of a tissue or organ transplanted from a nonidentical donor, the patient's defense against normally harmless infective agents is impaired, and he may experience severe infection due to these organisms. Protective isolation is used to help prevent such infection. In some instances the patient's inability to mount an effective cellular immunologic reaction to neoplastic cells

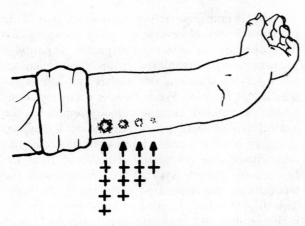

**Figure 9-3.** Positive skin tests indicative of anaphylactic hypersensitivity. Reactions are characterized by a wheel surrounded by erythema. The severity of reaction frequently is described as ranging from 1+ to 4+.

may allow proliferation and metastases of these cells accompanied by further impairment of the cellular immune response to the point of unresponsiveness or *anergy.*

The most common cellular immune response which is interpreted as harmful by the patient is *contact dermatitis,* a manifestation of cellular reaction to poison ivy, certain metals, cosmetics, and a wide variety of other substances (Fig. 9-3).

## NONIMMUNOLOGIC EXAGGERATED REACTIONS

In contrast to immunologic reactions which can be well categorized because laboratory methods are available to detect antibodies and sensitized cells, nonimmunologic exaggerated reactions have generally not been as well characterized as to underlying mechanism. Reactions to drugs account for approximately 5 per cent of hospital admissions and are experienced by approximately 15 per cent of patients receiving drugs. Many of these adverse reactions occur in normal patients and reflect overdosage, side effects, or the interaction of multiple drugs. Adverse reactions to drugs and other substances occurring in only a few susceptible patients may occur on an immunologic basis or may reflect *intolerance* or *idiosyncrasy.* For lack of better understanding, otherwise unexplained exaggerated reactions are often termed *functional* reactions; many of these reflect exaggeration of autonomic function.

**Intolerance.** Certain individuals are unusually sensitive in a *quantitative* sense in that they experience undesirable toxic effects from amounts of substances, particularly drugs, well tolerated in the normal population. If these toxic effects are manifest through the autonomic nervous system they may be labeled as *functional,* though the patient will think he is *allergic.*

Certain individuals find they can tolerate only small portions of foods such as strawberries or citrus fruits without breaking out in hives or other skin rashes. Rapid intravenous injection of radiopaque dyes, particularly those used for intravenous pyelography, provoke urticaria and occasionally hypotension in a few individuals. Frequently these same individuals will tolerate the same amount of dye if it is administered over a longer time interval. Reactions to strawberries and intravenous dyes may closely mimic a Type I immunologic reaction, as these substances provoke release of histamine from basophils and mast cells, but by a mechanism apart from that initiated by IgE antibodies. As histamine is the main mediator of these reactions, antihistamines are helpful in preventing or controlling such reactions.

Certain individuals are unduly susceptible to expected side effects from drugs. Examples are extreme and prolonged somnolence after administration of sedatives, tranquilizers, and antihistamines; unexpected jitteriness, agitation, or palpitation following administration of stimulants including caffeine in coffee; and a tendency to nausea or vomiting following usual doses of aspirin or other gastric irritants.

**Idiosyncratic Reactions.** An idiosyncratic reaction is a *qualitatively* different reaction to a food or drug based upon a biochemical alteration in the way the patient handles the substance administered.

Individuals who lack intestinal lactase are unable to split the disaccharide lactose, the main carbohydrate in milk and milk products, into monosaccharide which is absorbable by the gut. Accumulation of lactose in the intestine leads to formation of gas and intestinal cramping which the patient interprets as an *allergic* reaction to the milk.

Approximately 10 per cent of the American black population have a deficiency of the enzyme glucose-6-phosphate dehydrogenase (G6PO) and are susceptible to shortened life span of their red cells on exposures to oxidant drugs, such as the antimalarial drugs primaquine and quinine, analgesics including aspirin and nitrofurantoin, sulfa, and chloramphenicol antibiotics as well as others. In a broad sense these patients might be considered *allergic* to these medications.

In some patients, particularly the very young and very old, barbiturates produce excitement and even delirium rather than the depression and somnolence expected. The basis for this reaction is not clearly biochemical, but it is idiosyncratic in the sense of being altered in a qualitative sense.

**Functional Reactions.** The autonomic nervous system automatically coordinates physiologic processes and compensates for the multitude of stresses the body encounters. It consists of the neurons, ganglia, and plexuses that provide innervation to most of the glands of the cutaneous and mucosal surfaces and to heart and smooth muscle.

Functional reactions frequently are exaggerations of autonomic responses which produce symptoms some patients interpret as being *allergic*. For example, the patient with an exaggerated gastrocolic reflex who experiences intestinal cramping leading to bowel movement after eating particular foods or most foods may interpret his symptoms to be a "food allergy." The gastroenterologist is more likely to diagnose this patient as having a functional gastrointestinal disorder.

The individual who notes nasal congestion and watering on exposures to dampness, cold, or modest amounts of irritant fumes or cigarette smoke may well state that he is "allergic" to the respective precipitating factor. In these instances the term vasomotor rhinitis can be applied.

Bronchial asthma is a disorder in which there is enhanced bronchial responsiveness to a variety of stimuli. Contraction of bronchial smooth muscle and hypersecretion of mucus from the bronchial mucosa account for the majority of symptoms and signs. Many patients with asthma find that exercise, irritant fumes, laughter, or other emotional upset can evoke episodes of asthmatic symptoms. If the asthmatic individual also has the potential for a Type I immunologic reaction to airborne allergens, he may experience asthmatic symptoms in addition to hay fever symptoms on exposure to the allergen to which he has IgE antibodies.

## DIAGNOSIS

The key to diagnosis of any allergic state is a careful history to elicit past experiences of exaggerated reactions. The health history of patients with rhinitis, asthma, urticaria, or eczema will often list those factors which initiate, aggravate, or perpetuate the disorder. The nurse participates in the collection of relevant information in the collaborative effort of members of the health team to develop a data base. The process of gathering information should include a careful query for history of food or drug reaction. For drugs this history should be obtained both at the time of initial patient evaluation and by repeated query for a specific new drug prior to its administration.

Nurses who work with allergists, and physicians who specialize in the detection of immunologic reactions, learn how to apply and interpret skin tests for Type I and Type IV immunologic reactivity. All nurses have a responsibility for checking with the patient regarding possible drug allergy before administering any new drug to the patient.

Skin tests for anaphylactic (Type I) reactivity are begun with minute amounts of the suspected allergen applied to scratches on the skin or injected intradermally in very dilute solution. This lessens the danger of a severe reaction in a highly allergic individual. There have been reports of serious anaphylactic reactions from intradermal injection of penicillin in persons suspected of having penicillin allergy. Positive skin reactions are characterized by the appearance of a wheal surrounded by erythema after 10 to 20 minutes following application of the skin test. The severity of reaction is frequently described in a scale of 1+ to 4+ as shown in Figure 9-3. If the scratch or dilute solution of intradermal test is negative, more concentrated extracts of allergen are used for subsequent testing at 15 to 20 minute intervals by intradermal injections. Observation of the patient undergoing skin testing is not limited to the skin, as signs of systemic anaphylaxis such as generalized itching, sneezing, difficulty in breathing, pallor, faintness, or sweating may appear during the testing. Similar anaphylactic type reactions may occur following the administration of medications, particularly penicillin. It is essential to ask a patient to remain under observation for 20 minutes following administration of pencillin by any route to make certain that there has been no anaphylactic type reaction. Nurses carry a major responsibility for observing patients following procedures which carry risk of allergic response, such as skin testing, desensitization therapy (see below) and administration of drugs such as penicillin.

Skin tests for cellular hypersensitivity (Type IV) entail the intradermal injection of 0.1 ml. of the test material such as PPD (purified protein derivative of *Mycobacterium tuberculosis*), coccidioidin, histoplasmin, or agents such as *Candida albicans* or mumps vaccine used to detect the normal presence of delayed cutaneous hypersensitivity. When there is question of contact dermatitis, suspect materials are applied to the skin and are covered with patches to insure continued presence of the material on the skin for 48 to 72 hours. Caution must be taken in patch testing to make certain that the individual has not had a delayed hypersensitivity reaction to the occlusive tape dressing, particularly adhesive tape. Both intradermal and patch tests are read at the end of 48 hours for induration and erythema. Intradermal tests are considered positive if an area of induration greater than 10 mm. in diameter has appeared.

## TREATMENT

**Avoidance.** When it is feasible, avoidance is the surest and safest method of preventing a recurrence of any type of allergic reaction.

For individuals who have illnesses such as eczema, urticaria, hay fever, and in some instances asthma, in which anaphylactic type immunologic reactions have been suspected by history and confirmed by skin tests, avoidance alone often results in appreciable improvement in the patient's symptoms. Avoidance of animal danders and foods are examples.

Total avoidance of airborne pollens, house dust, and mold spores may not be feasible. If symptoms are mild, antihistamines may control the symptoms and avoidance may not be necessary. If the anaphylactic potential is strong or if the allergen exposure is great, additional measures may be required. For individuals who are sensitive to house dust, steps can be taken in the household to limit dust exposure (see below).

**Hyposensitization.** *Hyposensitization* or *immunotherapy* can be undertaken for relief of symptoms due to allergens which cannot be avoided. This entails repeated injections of the substances to which the individual has shown positive skin tests. There is appreciable risk in this treatment as one is administering the substance to which the individual is anaphylactically hypersensitive. Errors in dosage, or administration of solutions prepared for another individual, may result in a systemic anaphylactic reaction. Hyposensitization is usually started three to four months before the expected pollen season for pollen allergic individuals and thereafter continued on a yearly basis. Hyposensitization with house dust

can be given at any time of year. Hyposensitization injections are given twice a week or weekly as the dose is gradually increased and maintenance doses are given at one to six week intervals. Hyposensitization has been found to be most effective in patients with seasonal allergic rhinitis (hay fever) and of some value to patients with other diseases in which anaphylactic hypersensitivity is important.

As in skin testing, the risk of anaphylactic reaction is always present following hyposensitization injections. Doses are measured in one ml. syringes to an accuracy of 0.01 ml. and administration is subcutaneous, usually in the arm so that a tourniquet can be applied above the level of injection. Patients must remain under the observation of the nurse for at least 20 minutes after injection so that if anaphylactic reaction occurs the physician can be immediately notified and treatment can be administered immediately.

The appearance of the signs of *systemic anaphylactic reaction* constitute a medical emergency necessitating immediate treatment. Administration of subcutaneous epinephrine 1:1,000, 0.25 ml. for adults, and 0.10 ml. for children under 12 years of age should be a standing order to the nurse who administers skin tests or hyposensitization injections or who administers medications when a physician is not immediately available. Additional resuscitative efforts, including administration of intravenous fluids, vasopressor drugs, oxygen, antihistamines, and corticosteroids may need to be undertaken. Therapy involves a collaborative effort by the physician and nurse in an effort to reverse the dangerous train of physiologic events.

Treatment of cellular hypersensitivity reactions frequently entails the use of systemic or topical corticosteroids and occasionally the use of immunosuppressive drugs or antiserums. These drugs need be used judiciously, because they have side effects and because they suppress the cellular immune response. Prolonged administration of these agents requires careful assessment of the patient's response by the nurse and the physician.

For mild drug tolerance, frequently a smaller dose of the drug may have pharmacologic benefit with an acceptable level of adverse reaction. Patients who have experienced severe *idiosyncratic* drug reactions, as well as patients who have had *systemic anaphylactic* drug reactions, must absolutely avoid the medication to which they have had serious reaction. Thus, it is essential for the patient to be informed of his drug allergy. In these instances, the patient should alert medical personnel by wearing a medallion which indicates his potentially fatal drug allergy. Such medallions can be obtained through most pharmacies and several companies. In addition, through instruction, the patient is prepared to discuss his allergy with health personnel.

**Management of Functional Reactions.** The management of *functional reactions* often provides a difficult challenge to patient, nurse, and physician. Frequently the patient's psychological interpretation of these reactions determines their significance to him. In these instances, the nurse and physician need an extra degree of empathy in order to help the patient cope with his reaction. The nurse can be helpful to the patient in reaffirming the physician's assurance that such reaction reflects an exaggeration of a normal automatic body function rather than a serious underlying disorder such as infection or neoplasm. Drugs which alter autonomic function, including tranquilizers and anticholinergic and sympathomimetic drugs, may be helpful in controlling the symptoms of exaggerated autonomic function. Caution against overuse of these drugs, such as the frequent overuse of sympathomimetic nasal decongestant sprays or drops, must accompany their prescription.

Helping the patient to understand cause-and-effect relationships between his symptoms and stresses in his life can help him to cope more effectively and thereby to diminish or eliminate his symptoms. Helping the patient to deal with stress is important also in dealing with symptoms of allergy, which can be intensified by such factors as anxiety and fatigue.

## NURSING ASSESSMENT AND INTERVENTION

We shall consider nursing assessment and intervention of the patient with allergy in relation to the following factors:

> cognitive factors
> emotional factors
> age and developmental level
> socioeconomic factors
> physical factors

### Cognitive Factors

The patient and his family must learn what substances he should avoid, or, if this is impossible, how to mitigate their harmful effects. For example, the patient with an allergy to cat dander should avoid exposure to cats, or if that is not possible or acceptable, he may take medication, such as antihistamine drugs, to relieve symptoms. An asthmatic patient who begins to experience respiratory distress may sometimes abort a full-blown attack by prompt use of medication, such as isoproterenol, and by quickly avoiding further exposure to environmental factors which exacerbate the symptoms.

To take these measures quickly, the patient must know when an attack is imminent. Difficulties often arise because the patient does not heed beginning warning signals, such as slight tearing of the eyes or slight itching of the palate. This is particularly true when he is absorbed in interesting activities or when he denies the significance of the symptoms. Sometimes it is necessary for him to experience an attack several times before he becomes fully aware of these signals. When the patient's allergic response is severe or life-threatening, he may respond with such measures as promptly injecting epinephrine and quickly contacting his physician or going to an emergency room. Thus the primary responsibility for prevention and early treatment of allergic symptoms rests with the patient himself, or, if he is unable to fulfill it, with his close associates. Specific and carefully planned instruction is therefore a primary responsibility in caring for the patient with allergy.

### Emotional Factors

Experiencing allergic symptoms often provokes anxiety, and symptoms of allergy are frequently intensified by emotional stress, thus causing a vicious cycle. The patient's apprehension at seeing large hives spread over his body can intensify the reaction and make the itching worse. The asthmatic patient's breathing may become more labored as his fear of being unable to breathe intensifies. In such situations an important aspect of relieving the symptoms is the patient's ability to control and reduce his anxiety, and the ability of others to assist him to do so. If the stress exceeds the level of his coping ability, professional counseling may be beneficial.

In a long-term view, the patient's overall anxiety level frequently affects his susceptibility to allergic symptoms. Thus, a student may have an upsurge of symptoms during final examinations, without additional exposure to the offending allergens. Chronic anxiety over such concerns as job security, money, and family relationships can cause intensification of allergic symptoms.

The nurse can assist the patient to control his anxiety during acute symptoms by staying with him, calling his attention to what is being done to provide relief and the rationale for these measures, and, in a calm, reassuring manner, conveying her concern for him. In long-term situations where the patient's relief involves helping him to understand the cause-and-effect relationship between his symptoms and his anxiety, the nurse whose education and experience have prepared her for this role may assist the patient, by group or individual counseling, to understand this relationship. The goal of such understanding is to help the patient find ways of coping with stressful situations more effectively and with less anxiety.

### Age and Developmental Level

The young adult often experiences unaccustomed stress as he develops his life style from one of dependence to independence and interdependence. Thus new and varied work experiences, the birth of a child, and having a home of his own can cause stress which in turn may intensify allergic symptoms. Attacks may also be precipitated by travel to different regions where the young adult is exposed to unaccustomed environmental factors. However, young adults are often quick to learn, and when provided the opportunity, can make rapid progress with cognitive and emotional aspects of learning which help them to deal with allergic symptoms.

Social stigma is an important factor, as young adults are often hurt by peer rejection. For example, it is not uncommon for a patient with asthma to encounter rejection from peers who condescendingly state, "It's all in his head" or "He brings it on himself." Such half truths, resting upon a perception of the frequent relationships between symptoms and anxiety, when brought to the patient's attention in a destructive manner, can lead to his isolation from those whose support he needs, and consequently to greater anxiety and lessened ability to cope with his condition.

Denial of illness is common in this age group. This is a period of intense concern with body image and with physical capacities.

Similar considerations apply to the adult in middle life. However, during this period the patient often has the advantage of having a more settled life style, with greater predictability of the types of allergens to which he is exposed. While he may be slower to learn, he may offset this by his greater life experience and maturity which can be channeled toward coping with allergic symptoms. He may also be better able to withstand peer pressure and rejection, should it arise, than is the young adult.

The elderly patient may require considerable assistance with self-care, which may include measures to control allergic symptoms. Allergic responses seem to be less frequent and less severe among the elderly than among younger people.

### Socioeconomic Factors

Dealing with allergic reactions can be expensive. Air conditioners for home and car as well as electronic furnace filters are often prescribed for patients with allergies to pollen. The cost of such appliances is tax deductible, if a physician certifies that they are necessary to the patient's health. But health care is expensive for most people in the United States, and although tax deductions are helpful, cost is still a major concern for those of low and moderate income. Allergy treatment is typically long-term. Expense can range from a modest expenditure for medication and occasional visits to a physician or clinic, to high costs for care in emergency rooms and intensive care units, and for frequent outpatient visits over an extended period. Those with low incomes and minimal health insurance who are least able to bear the cost are most likely to experience stress related to this expense and to receive inadequate care. They may also do without other desirable aspects of life, such as a summer vacation, to pay for health care.

Nurses can help patients to deal with these problems by assisting them to find out about benefits for which they are eligible, such as Medicaid and veterans' benefits, and by helping them to cope with high prices of medication. For example, a medical-center pharmacy which serves clinic patients may charge much less for a prescription than a neighborhood pharmacy.

Although moving to a different climate is less frequently suggested now than previously, due to more effective therapy, this may occasionally be necessary and result in social and economic problems. Allergies to substances in the new environment may also develop.

Time may be lost from work due to symptoms of allergy; however, with effective therapy and education of the patient, work absence can often be minimized or avoided.

Stress within the family may occur when one member must spend a disproportionate amount of the family income for health care, or when one member's inability to travel or to undertake various new activities curtails the opportunities of the rest of the family for such experiences.

## Physical Assessment

In assessing the patient's physical condition, consideration must first be given to the body systems which are affected. Here we shall consider two systems commonly affected by allergy, and indicate physical assessment for each.

RESPIRATORY SYSTEM

*When the patient has allergic rhinitis*
Observe the following:
- Profuse watery nasal discharge, sneezing
- By use of nasal speculum, pale, edematous mucous membrane lining nasal cavity, swollen turbinates interfering with sinus drainage

Related signs and symptoms:
- Watery discharge from the eyes, redness of the eyes, facial edema, cough

Subjective symptoms:
- Itching of the nose, eyes, and sometimes of the palate
- A feeling of nasal congestion, sometimes including pain in the region of the sinuses, particularly the maxillary sinuses

*When the patient has bronchial asthma*
Observe:
- Labored breathing characterized by a wheezing, gasping sound and by a prolonged phase of expiration
- Use of accessory muscles of respiration, such as by raising the chest with shoulder muscles, in an effort to expand the chest and get more air
- Production of thick, stringy, white mucus, coughed up with difficulty
- Assumption of a sitting posture in an effort to facilitate breathing
- Symptoms of anxiety, such as pronounced restlessness

Subjective symptoms:
- Tightness and constriction in the chest, difficulty in breathing, a feeling of suffocation, and related severe anxiety over interference with normal breathing

INTEGUMENTARY SYSTEM

Observe such symptoms as:
- White raised lesions surrounded by redness of the skin (urticaria)

- Reddened, edematous areas of skin, or red rash on skin, which may be in contact with particular substances, such as cosmetics, clothing
- Thickening and scaling of the skin, development of brownish, leathery-looking areas on the skin, as occurs in chronic eczema

Subjective symptoms:
- Itching of the skin; a feeling of dryness and tension in the skin
- Distress and embarrassment over the appearance of the skin
- Pain in a lesion, which may occur, for example, if scratching leads to infection

## Other Aspects of Nursing Assessment and Intervention

In addition to physical assessment, it is important to consider the patient's environment, because factors in the environment may precipitate or exacerbate symptoms. Such factors as molds in damp areas, smoke and dust are important to note, as are the presence of vegetation and animals. The foods the patient has eaten or drugs he takes and the relationship between ingestion of these substances and the onset or aggravation of symptoms are also important.

## Goals of Nursing Care

Goals of nursing care of the patient with allergy include:

- **Helping the patient to understand his condition and factors which cause and exacerbate symptoms; how to avoid or minimize contact with these factors; how to follow his prescribed treatment regimen (drugs, hyposensitization); and how to recognize warning signals of the need for immediate treatment and indications that previously effective therapy is no longer effective and requires revision.**
- **Helping the patient to maintain his health in a state which lessens his vulnerability to symptoms of allergy. Adequate rest, dealing constructively with sources of anxiety, enjoyable exercise, stimulating companionship, opportunities for giving and receiving affection, a feeling of acceptance and esteem from family, friends, and colleagues, and the opportunity to engage in stimulating, useful work are all examples of factors which enable the patient to maintain health. Prompt treatment of respiratory infections is an important aspect of health maintenance.**
- **Helping the patient to relieve symptoms and achieve as much comfort as possible when symptoms occur. Severity of symptoms ranges from the occasional distress of itching urticaria, to chronic and sometimes life-threatening symptoms of bronchial asthma. (See Chapters 30 and 56 for detailed discussion of nursing intervention in these conditions.)**

## Specific Measures in Nursing Intervention

Certain measures are especially important in the nursing care of patients with allergy.

When the patient is experiencing symptoms, at home, at work, or in the hospital, it is essential to remove from the environment any substances which may aggravate the symptoms. For example, the custom of sending plants and flowers to hospitalized patients, while an indication of concern, may aggravate allergic symptoms in susceptible people. To find ways of solving this problem, the nurse may initiate a discussion among the patients involved. Shaking linens and dusting furniture with a dry cloth increase dust in the air; such practices should be avoided in the care of all patients.

Smoking, by the patient, his roommates, or visitors, is a frequent factor leading to increasingly severe allergic symptoms. Education concerning the effects of smoking, and limiting the areas where smoking is permitted, can alleviate the problem.

Bedding used in hospitals should be of the type least likely to cause or aggravate allergies. For example, Dacron pillows should be used instead of feather pillows. Woolen blankets should be avoided.

Environmental considerations for patients at home include: the type of bedding used in relation to factors causing allergy, methods of house cleaning (vacuum cleaning is preferable to sweeping; damp dusting is preferable to dry dusting), availability of air conditioners if needed, the presence of pets, and so on.

It is especially important to help the patient make changes in his home environment after considering the factors involved, rather than having the nurse decide and then try to convince the patient to follow her decisions. Helping the patient to notice cause and effect is often the most effective way to initiate change, and persistence is often required to effect enough change to reduce symptoms.

Discussing with the patient in a detailed, systematic way, his usual habits and any unusual exposure which preceded symptoms of allergy is important. For example, the nurse inquires about foods the patient usually eats, medications he takes, and any new substances to which he has been exposed. Among hospitalized patients it is especially important to note the drugs the patient is taking in relation to the appearance of allergic symptoms.

## Nursing in Relation to Drug Therapy

It is important for the nurse to teach the patient about side effects of prescribed drugs. For example, the drowsiness which may accompany use of antihistamines can be an advantage when the drugs are used at night, but may present a hazard during the day, especially if the patient drives. By checking with the physician, it may be possible for the patient to change the antihistamine to one which causes minimal or no drowsiness.

Epinephrine, ephedrine, and related drugs also cause side effects such as tachycardia and nervousness. It is important for the patient to understand that these effects are transitory. If symptoms are severe, it is essential for the patient to refer the problem to the physician rather than to adjust the dosage or avoid using the medication as prescribed. Sometimes it is necessary for the nurse to teach family members how to administer epinephrine subcutaneously and how to use nebulizers. In both instances it is essential for the patient to use the medication promptly and to administer it correctly at the onset of symptoms.

Corticosteroids, when used systemically for more than a brief period, may produce dangerous side effects. Their use with allergic patients is usually restricted to the period of most severe symptoms. The nurse should observe the patient for such effects as change in mood (e.g., euphoria), appearance of easy bruisability, "moon face," weight gain, and so on. Because corticosteroids mask symptoms of infection, it is especially important to note any slight early symptoms of infection and to discuss these observations promptly with the physician. (For a more detailed discussion of corticosteroid therapy see Chapter 49.)

The nurse may work with a physician at his office in the care of patients requiring hyposensitization, or at a clinic. It is important to observe the patient carefully after he has received the dose of antigen. The patient is asked not to leave before at least 20 minutes have elapsed. The nurse should observe as unobtrusively as possible any sneezing or tearing, itching or urticaria near the site of the injection, respiratory difficulty, pallor, nervousness, or feelings of faintness. If the patient shows any of these symptoms, the nurse should alert the physician immediately and work with him to alleviate the symptoms. Such severe reactions are unusual, but it is important to be alert for their occurrence. Nursing care of patients in anaphylactic shock involves frequent assessment of blood pressure, pulse, level of consciousness, amount of urinary output, color and temperature of the skin. Treatment must be quick and carried out in a reassuring manner. The nurse's ability to work smoothly and collaboratively with the physician is of utmost importance. Detailed attention must be given to the effective administration of such agents as intravenous fluids, oxygen, and drugs.

Other situations in which there is considerable risk of severe allergic response involve administration of penicillin and the use of intravenously injected dyes during intravenous pyelography. The patient whose response to penicillin has not been fully evaluated should always be observed for at least 20 minutes following an injection of this drug. This consideration is especially important when medications are administered in the patient's home, where staff and emergency supplies are not quickly available to him and the family.

## REFERENCES AND BIBLIOGRAPHY

BACH, F. H., and GOOD, R. A. (eds.): *Clinical Immunobiology,* Vol. 1, New York, Academic Press, 1972.

BEESON, P. B., and McDERMOTT, E. (eds.): *Cecil-Loeb Textbook of Medicine,* ed. 13, Philadelphia, Saunders, 1971.

CRANEN, R. F.: Anaphylactic shock, *Am. J. Nurs.* 72: 718, April 1972.

FEINBERG, S. M.: Allergies and air conditioning, *Am. J. Nurs.* 66:1333, June 1966.

GELL, P. G. H., and COOMBS, R. R. A. (eds.): *Clinical Aspects of Immunology,* ed. 2, Philadelphia, Davis, 1968.

GOOD, R. A., and RISHER, D. W. (eds.): *Immunobiology,* Stamford, Conn., Sinauer, 1971.

KINTZEL, K. GORMAN (ed.): *Advanced Concepts in Clinical Nursing,* Philadelphia, Lippincott, 1971.

LANDRUM, F. L.: Nursing in an allergist's office, *Am. J. Nurs.* 58:677, May 1958.

LESTER, J.: Nursing intervention in anaphylactic shock, *Am. J. Nurs.* 72:720, April 1972.

MATHISON, D. A., STEVENSON, D. D., TAN, E. M., and VAUGHAN, J. H.: Clinical profiles of bronchial asthma, *JAMA* 244:1134-1138, 1973.

McGOVERN, J. P., and KNIGHT, J. A.: *Allergy and Human Emotions,* Springfield, Ill., Thomas, 1967.

MOHNEY, S.: Some important clues to adverse drug reactions, *RN* 36:48, March 1973.

MOODY, L.: Asthma: Physiology and patient care, *Am. J. Nurs.* 73:1212, July 1973.

MULLER-EBERHARD, H. J.: The molecular basis of the biological activities of complement, The Harvey Lecture Series, 66, New York, Academic Press, 1972.

NAYYAR, R.: A night of panic in the High Sierras, *Am. J. Nurs.* 73:1218, July 1973.

PATTERSON, R. (ed.): *Allergic Diseases, Diagnosis and Management,* Philadelphia, Lippincott, 1972.

RODMAN, M. J.: Drugs for allergic disorders, *RN* 34: 63, June 1971.

————: Drugs for allergic disorders, *RN* 34:53, July 1971.

RODMAN, M. J., and SMITH, D.: *Pharmacology and Drug Therapy in Nursing,* Philadelphia, Lippincott, 1974.

SADAN, N., et al.: Immunotherapy of pollinosis in children, *New Eng. J. Med.* 280:623-627, 1969.

SAMTER, M. (ed.): *Immunological Diseases,* ed. 2, Boston, Little, Brown, 1965.

SHELDON, J. M., LOVELL, R. G., and MATHEWS, K. P.: *A Manual of Clinical Allergy,* Philadelphia, Saunders, 1967.

VAUGHAN, J. H., BARNETT, E. V., and LEDDY, J. P.: Immunologic and pathogenetic concepts in lupus erythematosus, rheumatoid arthritis and hemolytic anemia, *New Eng. J. Med.* 275:1426 and 1486, 1966.

# The Patient in Pain

## CHAPTER 10

## PAIN: SOME CHARACTERISTICS

"Physical pain is not a simple affair of an impulse traveling at a fixed rate along a nerve. It is the resultant of a conflict between a stimulus and the whole individual" (Leriche, 1968).

Pain is a universal but very private and very complex biopsychosociocultural phenomenon. It is usually described as a disagreeable sensation elicited by a potentially harmful stimulus. Its purpose is mainly protective. Pain is the symptom that most often prompts the seeking of medical help. The relief of pain and provision of comfort are viewed by the lay public as among the major functions of the nurse.

The destruction that can occur in the absence of pain demonstrates its value. Some cancers are painless until they have become well entrenched and have spread to adjacent areas. A patient whose legs are without sensation owing to a spinal injury will not feel the pain of an overheated hot-water bottle, and severe burns may result.

The possibility of pain is a means of judging the safety of the environment; for example, one avoids touching potentially hot objects or approaches them with great caution. Pain can also be an instrument of power and control over others.

Pain is accompanied by an affective quality of suffering, misery, anguish, punishment, or torture. In the suffering of pain there can also be for some a source of satisfaction or pleasure.

The suffering of pain can be induced by the perception of real, threatened, or imagined injury. For example, a person fearful of cancer can experience abdominal discomfort. But pain is real whether or not injury is;

it exists whenever an individual says it exists. Physicians and nurses do not deal directly with pain, but with the patient's statements or reports about his pain.

Prolonged, sudden, or severe pain is a stressor which interferes with the maintenance of homeostasis. Nursing intervention in pain is based on a careful assessment process which involves collecting as much data as possible about the pain which the patient is experiencing, the possible underlying processes, and ways in which the patient attempts to deal with his pain. Nursing goals include the relief of pain to the extent possible and helping the patient cope with pain while he experiences it.

Sudden and severe pain, because it is so disabling, requires prompt intervention even before a full assessment is carried out. For example, a person walking up a ramp who experiences severe chest pain is placed immediately at rest before any further assessment is carried out.

## NEUROPHYSIOLOGY

### Stimuli

Pain generally occurs whenever tissues are being injured. Pain receptors may be stimulated by chemical, thermal, electrical, or mechanical agents. (Even minor stimuli, such as a too tight cast or taut drainage tubes, stimulate pain receptors.) Pain can be expected following surgery, trauma, infarct or ischemia, which can be termed noxious stimuli. However, because of individual variations in pain perception and response, pain may be absent in the presence of injury and present in the absence of injury.

### Receptors

Pain receptors exist as free or naked nerve endings almost everywhere in the body. They are widespread in the superficial layers of the skin, but the concentration varies. For instance, the insertion of a needle in the back of the hand hurts more than in the upper thigh, since the former structure is more richly supplied with nerve endings. The more nerve endings in an area, the more precisely the area of pain can be localized. Pain arising from cutaneous receptors is called *superficial* or *surface* pain. That arising from deeper structures, such as muscles and joints, is referred to as *deep* pain, while pain arising from the viscera is referred to as *visceral*.

Internal tissues, such as the periosteum, the arterial walls, and the joint surfaces, are well supplied with pain receptors. There are comparatively few pain receptors in the viscera; some structures, such as the alveoli, are completely insensitive. Organs such as the stomach and uterus can be incised or the cervix cauterized with little discomfort to the patient because this is a localized type of injury.

Because of the relative scarcity of receptors compared with the body surface, the quality of deep and visceral pain differs from that of superficial pain. It tends to be duller, of longer duration and less localized. A patient with a ruptured gallbladder may experience pain over the entire abdomen, not just in the upper right quadrant. However, a stimulus that causes diffuse irritation of pain nerve endings throughout a viscus, such as the occlusion of blood supply to a large area of the bowel, can produce severe pain. Nerve endings in diffuse areas of deep tissues and viscera are stimulated by tissue ischemia, distention of a hollow viscus, spasm of the smooth muscle in a hollow viscus, stretching of ligaments, or chemical damage. Examples are angina pectoris, gas in the colon, stones in the ureter, bile duct spasm, and childbirth. The lining of the stomach is sensitive to chemical irritation from excessive hydrochloric acid. Peptic ulcers cause intense burning pain when gastric acids reach pain fibers in the ulcer crater.

### Transmission of the Pain Stimulus

Much is unknown about the neurophysiology of pain and presently advocated theories do not adequately explain all sensations of pain. However, understanding what each theory contributes can be helpful in planning appropriate relief measures.

**Specificity Theory.** The classical theory of pain postulates a direct line communication system between the stimulus, pain receptors, pain fibers, and pathways in the spinal cord to a "pain center" in the brain. This theory explains why surgical procedures for intractable pain such as cordotomy are successful. It does not explain the marked individual variations in response to comparable painful stimuli.

It is hypothesized that pain impulses in the peripheral nerves are transmitted from receptors via specific groups of myelinated and unmyelinated nerve fibers. The former group (A delta fibers) conveys impulses more quickly than the latter group (C fibers) does.

If a blow on the skin is suffered, the immediate sensation is a sharp, blinding pain (A delta transmission). Then after a slight delay there follows the slow, dull, and burning pain that is conducted by the unmyelinated group (C fiber transmission).

The nerve fibers feed into the dorsal ganglia of the spinal cord and ascend to the thalamus. It is here that awareness of pain occurs; but not until the impulses are conveyed to the cerebral cortex can the pain be analyzed, its location identified, and its intensity evaluated.

The route by which deep-pain impulses are conducted to the central nervous system differs from that of superficial impulses, and it is more complicated. True visceral pain is transmitted to the central nervous system via sensory autonomic fibers. The sensations of pain are *referred* to surface areas of the body often far removed from the painful organ. Sensations from the parietal peritoneum, pleura, or pericardium are conducted directly through skeletal nerves to the spinal cord, and the sensations are usually localized directly over the painful area.

**Referred** pain is that in which a pain within the body is translated into a false superficial location. For example, pain caused by air under the diaphragm is felt as pain in the shoulder or scapula. The location of referred pain on the surface of the body depends on the original derivation of the visceral organ in the embryo (Guyton, 1971).

Although the exact process by which this referred pain occurs is not completely understood, one opinion is that when visceral pain fibers are stimulated intensely, pain sensations from the viscera spread in the spinal cord into some of the neurons that normally conduct pain sensations only from the skin. The individual gets the feeling that the senations actually originate in the skin itself.

**Pattern Theories.** Pattern theories of pain support the concept that a code that provides the information that there is pain results from patterning of the nerve impulses generated by receptors (McCaffery, 1972, p. 32).

**Gate Control Theory.** Melzack and his associates (1968) propose that the transmission of pain signals from the body to the spinal cord and brain is a dynamic rather than a fixed process, one capable of modulation. According to the theory, part of the pain signaling system is a gatelike mechanism embedded in the cells of the *substantia gelatinosa* which extends the length of the spinal cord. The gate may be open, partially open, or closed so that, at times, signals from injured tissues may never get to the brain.

According to Melzack, modulation of pain signals can occur in several ways. When stimulated, large fibers in the sensory nerves running from the body's surface to the central nervous system tend to "close the gate" and thereby diminish the level of pain perception. Excitatory signals of small fibers in the same nerves tend to open the gate and produce increased pain. The gating mechanism sums up the net excitation-inhibition impulse and conveys this net result to the brain.

Other pain inhibiting components of the gate control system include a central biasing mechanism in the brain stem and a central control system in the thalamus and cerebral cortex which can also act to close the gate to further incoming pain signals. Portions of the reticular formation in the brain stem can send blocking signals through fibers that descend to the spinal cord or through fibers that connect to other transmission areas in the brain to inhibit the perception of pain.

Fibers that descend from the cerebral cortex, the seat of memories of cultural experiences, expectations, suggestion, anxiety, and other psychological processes can close the gate and decrease the level of perceived pain.

More specifically, mechanisms in the cerebral cortex control afferent input in terms of its meaning to the individual. A *sensory-discriminative system* gives information about space or location of pain, time, and intensity. A *motivational-affective system* contributes the quality of unpleasantness, mobilizes internal defenses, and triggers action aimed at stopping the noxious stimulation. A *central control* or *cognitive system* evaluates and analyzes input in terms of past experiences, probable outcome, and meaning of pain.

Thus, the gate control theory takes into account the influence of psychological, social, and cultural factors in the neurophysiology of pain in viewing pain as a complex, individual, perceptual experience. In addition, the gate control theory provides a theoretical base for the efficacy of massage, scratching, back rubs, application of menthol rubbing agents, and electrical stimulation of large cutaneous fibers in pain relief. There is thought to be a relationship betwen gate control theory and acupuncture, but the relationship is not entirely clear (see p. 145).

## THE PAIN EXPERIENCE

The pain experience is a subjective one and consists of two components: pain perception and pain reaction.

### Pain Perception

Pain *perception,* or the threshold for recognition of pain, is thought to be localized in the thalamus. Pain perception arises when different impulses from pain receptors that have been stimulated result in the awareness of the pain sensation.

There is marked uniformity among people in the perception of pain. If a pin is pressed against the skin of 100 people, the amount of pressure necessary to cause pain (i.e., to reach the pain threshold) would be practically similiar in every case. However, the individual responses to pain would vary widely.

The intensity, frequency, and duration of the afferent impulses influence the severity of the pain sensation perceived. However, the intensity of pain is not always a reliable index of the seriousness of the condition. The pain of appendicitis is ample warning of rapidly approaching danger. On the other hand, the excruciating pain of tic douloureux (see Chap. 23) seems to be out of proportion to the actual pathology. If an injury occurs that is sufficiently serious to destroy the nerve endings (as in an electric burn), pain will be absent in the affected area.

### Pain Reaction

Afferent impulses perceived as pain in the thalamus are transmitted to the cerebral cortex where the sensation of pain is mentally interpreted by the patient in terms of his previous experiences. Pain *reaction* involves motor, autonomic, and psychic responses.

**Motor Response.** Reflex skeletal muscle activity stimulates a person to withdraw from external pain sources. Visceral and deep pain stimulates the reflex tightening of muscles over the affected area. This is called "guarding."

Voluntary muscle responses which persons employ in seeking pain relief include pacing the floor, clenching the fists, rubbing, scratching, drawing the knees up to the chin or assuming unusual postures, writhing, or tossing about restlessly.

**Autonomic Response.** The stress of pain results in altered sympathoadrenal activity.

Surface pain stimulates the sympathetic nervous system into a series of reflex actions. Adrenalin is poured into the system; blood pressure, pulse, and respiratory rates rise; and blood is drained from the brain, the skin, and the gastrointestinal tract and flows into the muscles. This is the "alarm" reaction which, physiologically speaking, readies the patient for action to fight against or flee from the cause of the pain. On the other hand, deep pain is more likely to cause failure of the defense reaction. The patient feels week and nauseated, and he may vomit or faint, have diarrhea or vertigo. He may be very tense or restless. Hypotension, bradycardia, pallor, and sweating occur. These signs are frequently observed in patients with such conditions as acute myocardial infarction or perforations of abdominal viscera when homeostatic mechanisms fail. Severe pain may cause shock and even death. Continued pain can result in added damage to the body organs because of the prolongation of physiologic reactions.

**Psychic Response.** Reflex responses to pain are influenced by cognitive, emotional, and sociocultural factors.

The psychic reaction to pain is far more subtle than reflex reactions. Following comparable degrees of pain stimuli, the reactions of individuals vary tremendously. The way an individual responds to pain depends on many factors. His physiologic and psychological state and his adaptive resources, his cultural background and beliefs, his previous pain experience, the location of the pain, and the response of the people around him all influence his reaction.

COGNITIVE FACTORS. Understanding and consenting to a painful experience makes the experience more tolerable though still painful.

The same person may react differently in different situations, depending on what he has at stake, the degree of anxiety present, his state of health, and the distractions that are (or are not) present. A woman who may tolerate the pain of childbirth gladly because she wants the baby may be less willing and able to tolerate a gallbladder attack. Older people may view pain as a prelude to death. When a person is fatigued or in poor general health, he may endure pain less quietly than when he is rested and well. A toothache may be more tolerable than a pain in the chest, because the patient knows that the ache in his mouth does not endanger his life.

Distractions make a vast difference. A small wound received while playing basketball may scarcely be noticed. The same amount of pain caused by a needle being injected into a vein seems to be much more severe, because the patient focuses all his attention on the procedure. Nurses sometimes find that a patient experiences pain more acutely at night and during early morning hours, when his mind and body are unoccupied by the activities of the day. According to the gate control theory, the decrease in sensory input leaves the gate more open to increased pain firing signals thereby increasing the patient's experience of pain.

EMOTIONAL FACTORS. Emotions such as anxiety and fear enhance the perception of pain (keep the gate open for more pain signals), and intensify the pain response. The intense sensation of pain further increases anxiety, thus setting up a vicious cycle. High levels of anxiety also augment both the motor and autonomic reactions to pain. Nursing interventions that reduce anxiety or fear such as staying with the patient, or explaining to him what is going to take place decrease the level of perceived pain.

SOCIOCULTURAL FACTORS. Pain has many meanings. To one it may be a symbol of punishment for real or imagined sins; to another it may mean a test of strength. A person with deep religious faith may be able to tolerate conditions that usually result in severe pain because his suffering has a spiritual purpose.

A patient's cultural background contributes to the way in which he reacts to pain. Some groups have a greater tendency to hide overt expression, whereas others show a freer flow of feelings. One person complains loudly and emotionally, whereas another suffers in silence. Upbringing, sex, age, and circumstances affect response. Parents have taught their children when to complain and how loudly.

While studies have shown that there are general cultural components in response to pain (Blaylock, 1968; Zborowski, 1969), the nurse must avoid stereotyping patients according to their cultural background since even within the same culture individual variations can differ markedly.

The patient in pain who does not complain shows discomfort by other means. He may curl up in bed or assume an abnormal posture, such as kneeling, or toss about. His pulse is often elevated, and he may perspire. Facial expression is revealing; those in pain will look tense, with taut muscles, clenched teeth, fixed eyes, and a drawn expression. Some express pain covertly through such mechanisms as focus on detail, demandingness or argumentativeness. Behavior reversal such as unusual quietness or hostility from a usually placid person may also be manifestations of pain.

## NURSING ASSESSMENT

When possible, data gathering through interaction with the patient as well as observation and examination is advocated for an accurate assessment of the patient's condition before attempting to intervene. However, in situations of sudden and severe pain, assessment and intervention are often concurrent. Pain must be relieved to avoid shock or a situation so physiologically compromised that the patient's condition is worse than need be. Putting a patient with chest pain at rest, immobilizing a fractured part, or giving medication for severe trauma are examples of intervention carried out before a complete assessment can be made.

When pain is recurrent the patient can be taught to gather some of the data to assist in analyzing his pain experience so that he can better participate in his treatment plan. The following are major points to consider in pain assessment.

### Subjective Data

- **Nature (sharp, prickling, dull, burning, aching, knife-like, squeezing, deep, pulsating, gnawing, pressing, throbbing, cramping, nauseating)**
- **Intensity (mild, moderate, severe)**
- **Location and site of origin (left lower abdomen, inner aspect of right upper midthigh, entire left chest)**
- **Onset (occurred suddenly, slowly, slowly building up to present intensity, similar to pain that the patient had at home, first occurrence); what precipitates it**
- **Duration (intermittent, returning at 5- to 6-minute intervals and lasting about 30 seconds; persistent since 3:30 A.M.; brief, lasting 15 minutes)**
- **Spread (radiates down left arm, extends from groin to knee)**
- **Relation to circumstance (before or after eating, as the patient turns to the right side, when the patient moves his foot)**
- **Control (apparently relieved by elevation of the limb; patient reports that pain stops when he lies still)**
- **Emotional response (e.g., feelings of anxiety, anger)**

### Objective Data

- **General appearance including indications of emotional state**
- **Motor reaction (position assumed, guarding, activity such as pacing, gritting teeth)**

- **Autonomic reaction (blood pressure, pulse, cardiac arrhythmias, vomiting, respiration, perspiration, pallor, dilation of pupils)**
- **Psychic reaction including anxiety level, symbolic meaning of the pain or mental associations of the pain with past experiences; nonverbal responses; reactions of others to the patient's expression of pain, and situational triggering circumstances.**

Sometimes pain is relieved or intensified by a change in the course of the disease. The severe pain of acute appendicitis suddenly vanishes when the appendix ruptures. The sudden absence of pain is both a dangerous symptom and an important observation to make. On the other hand, an increasing amount of pain under a cast after the fracture has been reduced means that something is wrong. Changes in pain should be discussed with the physician.

Because of the subjective nature of pain, it is best to report only what is actually observed and what the patient says. For example, on one chart the nurse wrote: "10:15 A.M.: Patient complained of severe colicky pain in his entire lower abdomen. Said pain started suddenly about 10 minutes ago. Patient was observed rocking on his knees in bed. Pulse 132, respiration 40. Profuse diaphoresis. Vomited 120 ml. of undigested food."

### Inferences about the Pain Experience

Whatever the patient's response to pain, there are no rights or wrongs about it. A person who complains loudly may antagonize a nurse who admires stoicism more. On the other hand, a patient who silently suffers may neglect to call attention to a serious condition; therefore, he may fail to get medical attention. The nurse does not judge how severe pain *should* be, nor how much the patient should show his suffering. The nurse does need an understanding of the cultural components involved in the wide variations in patients' responses to pain as well as an awareness of her own responses and views about pain so that she can be more open to the experiences of others.

It is also necessary for the nurse to know what the usual kind of pain experience associated with a particular condition is. For example, severe abdominal pain five days after an appendectomy is atypical, and assessment of the patient must ensue.

In reviewing the data the nurse considers the following questions: Is this an atypical experience for this patient? What is his anxiety level? What environmental factors could have influenced the pain experience? Did earlier nursing interventions give pain relief? Is the patient maintaining homeostasis? What are the probable causes of his pain?

## NURSING INTERVENTION

### History

The nurse may participate in relief of pain in many ways. Initiating the nursing care plan begins with a history of the patient's pain experience and his coping mechanisms. The patient may think his ways of helping to achieve pain relief may be unacceptable to health personnel but these should be elicited and respected.

Some coping mechanisms patients may employ are complete inactivity or the assumption of unusual body position; very strenuous work or play or purposeful diversion to distract; verbal methods such as prayer or the repetition of verses, phrases, or exercises; ritualistic behavior such as pacing or clenching fists; focusing attention by counting objects in the environment; daydreaming; seeking out others or isolating oneself.

A baseline level of the patient's vital signs, body position, usual affect, and activity should be obtained when he is not in pain, for later comparison.

### Environmental Factors

The patient in pain is preoccupied and unable to respond to people and events in the same way as he does when he is not in pain. Small talk not only does not distract him, but is an added burden. Pain makes noise especially bothersome and tires the patient. The nurse can help visitors to understand the patient's need for quiet and his inability to respond to them in his usual manner, while assuring them that all possible is being done to help the patient to become more comfortable.

### Timing and Planning

Because movement usually increases pain, the patient often tries to remain as still as he can. However, measures to prevent complications frequently require movement. For example, postoperative deep breathing, turning from side to side, and ambulation may increase the immediate discomfort of the patient. The nurse should explain why these measures are necessary. She should talk to the patient before surgery so that he knows what to expect. If the patient is forewarned to expect pain, he may be helped to understand it as necessary and transitory, and this knowledge may help him to relax and feel less worried and tense. Frequently, painful dressings can be timed so that they are undertaken after the patient has had an analgesic. The nurse should organize the patient's day so that periods of necessary activity are followed by rest periods.

## Movement

Some patients are able to find ways to move that hurt them the least. The patient in pain should be consulted before he is moved. One may wish to roll over unaided, while another can tell the nurse where to place her hands.

Other patients in pain, however, need not be burdened with the additional decision making involved in movement. Rather, they need the gentle but firm, sure motion of a nurse or a team who explains first what is about to happen. Asking the patient when and where it hurts as he is moved and positioned can give the kind of information needed to retain the approach or try a different method.

Splinting a painful part often helps. This can be accomplished with an abdominal binder, manual support of a limb, or holding the operative site when coughing after chest surgery. Supporting the joints helps to move a painful limb in one piece and is far more comfortable than allowing a part to lag. A limb may be moved on a pillow, or the whole body on a turning sheet. The nurse should move slowly and steadily, stopping when the patient requests it. Jerky and swift motions increase pain. In one instance a woman was surprised to discover that, although she could not move her mother's recently paralyzed arm without an outcry from the patient, there was never a complaint when the nurse repositioned the arm. The nurse showed the daughter how to cup her palms under the wrist and the elbow and move ever so slowly and steadily, pausing for a moment when there was the slightest muscular resistance.

## Control of Anxiety

Reducing anxiety or preventing it from mounting plays a major role in the control of pain. Keeping the patient informed and educating him about his condition reduces fear of the unknown and helps the person to direct his attention toward problem-solving approaches to achieve comfort. Just staying with a patient permits him to "borrow strength"

until medication can take effect. In addition encouraging him to discuss whatever is bothering him helps reduce anxiety to more tolerable levels.

## Comfort Measures

Sometimes pain can be lessened to a tolerable level by the presence of a nurse who takes care of small but important details. The patient who is alone in a room can be comforted by a nurse who expresses a word of encouragement or sympathy, massages tenseness from an aching shoulder, rests a sore muscle by supporting it with a pillow, elevates an edematous hand, gives a refreshing mouthwash, cools bed-weary feet with an alcohol sponge, or tightens a rumpled sheet. In some instances heat, cold, ultrasonic therapy, oxygen, or physical therapy technics may be more effective than drugs in relieving mild or moderate pain.

Patients in a hospital or nursing home often derive comfort from their own possessions and these should be permitted whenever possible.

## Drug Therapy

Analgesics should not be used to replace nursing care and never to quiet a patient because the nurse is weary of his complaints. When they are ordered, they should be used as necessary to keep the patient comfortable. No patient ever should be allowed to suffer needlessly. Nor should any word or expression be conveyed to the patient of impatience at administering the drug.

Sometimes, when pain is severe, such as in acute myocardial infarction, a patient may be hesitant to accept narcotics for a physiologic or a psychosocial reason. Recognizing his stoicism, the nurse explains the rationale for the ordered medication and plans with him to discuss his reaction at a later time when pain relief has been obtained. The patient who absolutely refuses narcotics should not have them forced upon him. The matter should be promptly discussed with his physician.

The development of sound judgment in giving prescribed drugs for the relief of pain is one of the finer points in nursing. Three important points to remember in drug administration are:

1. Pain is relieved more readily before it becomes too severe. An analgesic should be given before the pain has developed completely.

2. A drug can mask symptoms that the physician may need to observe to establish a diagnosis. Analgesics are given only for the pain for which they are

ordered, not for another pain. For instance, if the patient has an order for aspirin for headache he should not be given aspirin for a pain in the calf of the leg.

3. If the patient with acute pain does not obtain relief from the drug within the time of its predicted effective action, the physician should be notified. The patient should not be expected to wait until the next ordered dose without other measures for his comfort.

The very act of giving medication is proof to the patient that someone cares that he is uncomfortable, and that there are measures available to help him. The action of a drug can be reinforced by a patient's faith in it. In administering a drug for pain the nurse should inform the patient of the expected effect, because the power of suggestion will be valuable in itself.

After the medication for pain has been administered, the patient should be left undisturbed. If he is awakened from the sleep that follows the administration of morphine, he may be unable to recapture relaxation. Pain is wearing, and rest is hard to come by. The patient should not be awakened to have his temperature taken (unless specifically ordered at this time), for routine housekeeping chores or for a social call on the telephone. The necessary nursing interventions that will help him to rest should be given before he receives the medication.

Relief of pain often brings better physiologic functioning (for example, pain can decrease renal efficiency) and these changes should be recorded. Accurate reporting may help the physician to adjust the drug dosage. Perhaps he will wish to increase or decrease the amount given, add another drug for potentiation of effect, or change the drug if the pain is unrelieved.

Grouped according to pharmacologic action, drugs may (1) counter the cause of the pain (example: antacids), (2) block peripheral pain impulses (example: procaine) or (3) modify the central reception of pain (example: morphine) (Wang, 1963).

**Placebo.** A placebo is an inactive substitute given instead of a medication. Relief of pain by a placebo is in no way synonymous with malingering. The patient indeed has pain. But since pain is an integrated experience of perception *and* reaction, "the response to a placebo is a pharmacologic effect whose site of action is the affective reaction (psychic processing) to stimuli from any source" (Keats and Lane, 1963). Pain relief by a placebo is neither

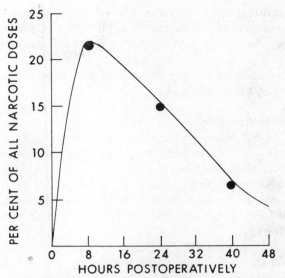

**Figure 10-1.** Average time course of pain following major abdominal surgery expressed as the frequency with which narcotics were administered for pain in the postoperative period. (Keats, A., and Lane, M.: Symptomatic therapy of pain, *Disease-A-Month*, June, 1963; by permission of Year Book Medical Publishers, Inc.)

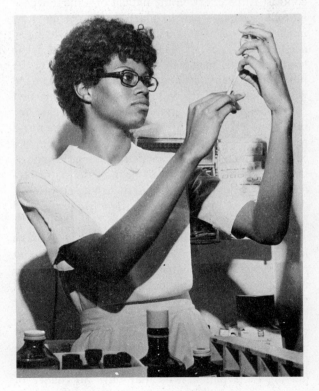

**Figure 10-2.** Having reviewed her patient's need with the instructor and nursing team leader, a nursing student promptly prepares medication for pain.

consistent nor predictable. The affective response is influenced as well by the "placebo" effect of a trusting relationship with the nurse, physician, or other persons, distraction, suggestion, environmental factors such as privacy and noise, and spontaneous changes in painfulness.

### Nursing Attitudes

Many nurses and patients are overly concerned with the threat of addiction when using narcotics in short-term illnesses. Studies have borne out two authors' thought that "refusing to administer medication to prevent addiction is akin to refusing to give food to prevent obesity" (Francis and Munjas, 1968).

It is important for the nurse to avoid the attitude that she must stand guard between the patient and his medication. This is especially important in such illnesses as cancer, in which pain is usually severe and of long duration. An attitude that conveys to the patient that he will not be left unaided to endure pain which he finds unbearable often results in his experiencing less pain because he is less fearful. In contrast is the effect on the patient of a nurse whose attitude seems to say to him: "I will decide how much pain you have. I will decide if and when you need (deserve) relief." Usually, this patient is so fearful that his pain will be underestimated by the nurse, and so anxious about being left alone to cope with something which to him is overwhelming, that he makes more and more frequent demands for relief, and because of their very frequency the nurse refuses. A struggle between nurse and patient results: he demanding, and she withholding. Emphasis instead should be placed on helping the patient to feel that his nurse is *with* him, and that she will not desert him when pain renders him frightened and helpless.

A patient who exhibits his discomfort may make a nurse feel helpless. She may feel thwarted and react by ignoring the patient. The more skill she develops in making patients comfortable, the less will be her need to run from a situation that she feels she cannot handle. Sometimes a nurse grows weary of a patient with chronic severe pain. This is a difficult problem, requiring maturity on the nurse's part and ability to sustain her standards of nursing for a patient who may have no chance of recovery.

Group nursing conferences or interdisciplinary conferences can provide for ventilation of feelings and peer support of the nurse, increase self-awareness, and afford an exchange of suggestions for more effective patient management.

Groups of patients with chronic pain can also benefit from meeting together with a prepared leader who can help them to share, learn, and support one another in their efforts to cope with long-term pain.

Various types of systemic relief-giving drugs such as sedatives or tranquilizers also are sometimes helpful in the management of pain by reducing the anxiety component of the pain experience.

General anesthesia gives absolute temporary relief from pain, but it is not practical and carries too high a risk for use except in such procedures as operations or the setting of certain bones. Local anesthesia sometimes is applied to remove pain from a single part. Sprays, ointments and the injection of an analgesic, such as procaine, into a local nerve group (nerve block) are used to relieve pain. When analgesic ointments are ordered, their application is restricted to the specific area, because the larger the surface (especially when denuded) to which they are applied, the more systemic absorption there will be.

### Evaluation

The effectiveness of pain relief measures should be evaluated objectively in terms of changes in the motor, autonomic, and psychic reactions noted during the initial assessment, and subjectively in terms of the patient's expressions of relief. If the patient does not feel relief, then his pain is not relieved and more data gathering and reassessment of nursing diagnosis and intervention is necessary. Reassessment often involves collaborating with the physician who reviews medical assessment data and the medical plan of care.

The nursing process components in relation to the patient's problem of pain become part of the patient's record. Successful approaches become part of the nursing care plan if pain is a continuing problem.

## MANAGEMENT OF CHRONIC PAIN: GENERAL CONSIDERATIONS

### Intractable Pain

Intractable pain is pain that is not managed easily. The term usually is applied to chronic pain. Acute pain is different from chronic pain in some important ways. When a man crushes his finger in a car door, he is aware of the emergency nature of the situation and expects that the pain will end in the foreseeable future. There is no such time limit to the severe pain associated with such conditions as disseminated cancer and advanced chronic pancreatitis. Patients with these conditions often have days so filled with intense pain that all other thoughts are excluded from consciousness. Pain demands an almost exclusive concentration on itself, and almost every other consideration becomes secondary or nonexistent. The patient's family or associates become frustrated at the inability of medical treatment and their own efforts to relieve the patient's suffering.

Some patients with chronic pain say that it seems senseless to them, and that this is its most difficult aspect. Renal colic calls attention to a pathologic condition and serves as a warning, but the repetitious pain of arthritis seems to them to have no purpose. Meaningless suffering is damaging to the integration of personality. So the patient with chronic pain makes endless efforts to control his reaction to it and to maintain a sense of himself.

Nurses may be able to help such patients to build defenses against pain. It is necessary for the nurse to think first about her own reaction. If severe pain so frightens her that she avoids the patient, cannot listen to what he has to say, and thinks only of sedating him, her helpfulness will be diminished. Religious counselors can be a great comfort to both the nurse and the patient.

A patient can be helped to maintain his dignity by minimizing his helplessness as much as possible. He should be provided with as much decision making and activity as the situation will warrant. For example, the homebound woman with arthritis can be assisted to find ways to continue some of her homemaking responsibilities during those times when she is able to move about. In the hospital, efforts should be made to find something for the bed patient to do, when he is able, that truly interests him, so that he does not spend relatively pain-free time just lying there, waiting for the pain to become more severe. The patient will be groping for both an answer to the question "Why?" and a way to behave that is acceptable to him in the very difficult circumstance of pain in the present and the promise of pain in the future.

If it is not time for his medication and the patient is in pain, staying with him and giving attention to comfort measures often is effective in lessening his distress and helping him to wait until medication can be given safely.

When the patient is dying slowly and in pain, the physician may be able to regulate the dosage of narcotics so that increasing tolerance does not rise so rapidly that the drug is no longer effective. Addiction is unlikely when a narcotic is given for only a few days, but addiction becomes more likely as the drug is given for longer periods. The nurse and the physician work together to try to keep the patient comfortable without giving the narcotic so frequently that its effectiveness is lost, and the patient is left with no help for his pain.

The patient in continuous, severe pain may be contemplating suicide. If he has intractable pain due to some incurable disease, he may worry about becoming a burden to his family, and he may dread the future, fearing that the time will come when narcotics will relieve his suffering no longer.

Additional aspects of the nursing management of patients with chronic pain are presented in other sections. See, for example, the chapters on cancer, arthritis, and vascular diseases as well as Chapter 6 on crisis intervention.

Surgery

Sometimes intractable pain can be eliminated by cutting the nerves that transmit it. There is usually a price to pay in disability, numbness or less control over a function, but relief from pain is usually worth it to the patient. Surgery to relieve pain may be performed when the patient has distress in a localized area from cancer. Pain that is widespread throughout the body cannot be eliminated by neurosurgery. More rarely, surgery may be performed for continuing pain following herpes zoster, frequent gastric crises in tabes dorsalis, continuing painful phantom limb following an amputation and neuralgia after peripheral nerve injury.

A *cordotomy* is an interruption of the pain-conducting pathways in the spinal cord. After the operation there will be loss of temperature sensation (attended, therefore, by a danger of burning the skin) and of pain on the affected side, but no loss of tactile sensation. In addition, there may be some weakness of the limb on the side opposite the operation. If a bilateral cordotomy is performed, the patient's legs may be so weak that he is unable to walk. Difficulty in bladder control is to be expected as well as impaired sexual function in the male.

Because this operation is most often done for patients with uncontrolled cancer, the relief of severe pain for the remaining days of the life of the patient is usually more important than mobility or bladder continence. When several roots are severed, the patient has a loss of position sense.

A *rhizotomy* is division of a sensory root just as it enters the spinal cord, an operation that may be used for patients with cancer of the lungs. It may cause loss of position sense and numbness below the level of the incision.

Both standard cordotomy and rhizotomy involve a laminectomy, and the postoperative care of the patient is similar to that of a patient operated on for a herniated disk or a tumor of the spinal cord (see Chap. 24).

*Percutaneous cordotomy* involves the insertion through the skin of a spinal needle into the antero-lateral tract. An electrode is then directed into the tract, stimulated to insure proper position and the tract is then coagulated with diathermy. Pain as well as temperature sensation is affected. Since it is a relatively innocuous procedure which is well tolerated by patients, percutaneous cordotomy can be performed on those too debilitated to withstand laminectomy. Postoperative care involves appropriate neurologic observations and supportive care.

Sometimes a second cordotomy is necessary, especially if the patient had general anesthesia during the first cordotomy and could not describe his sensations during the operation. For this reason observing and recording the exact location of any postoperative pain is important.

A *tractotomy* is division of the pathways in the brain stem, eliminating the senses of pain and temperature, but leaving the sense of touch and other sensations undisturbed. A *neurectomy* is an interruption of peripheral or cranial nerves to eliminate localized pain by cutting the nerve fibers (rather than the roots). Movement and position sense are affected.

Because there usually is diminished sensation below the level of the interruption of the nerve pathways extra care must be taken to prevent ischemic ulcers. An alternating air-pressure mattress may be used. Back care should be given several times a day, and the patient should be repositioned at least every two hours. Muscular weakness and a loss of position sense may make the patient lie more quietly in bed than he should. A footboard is used to prevent outward rotation of the feet and the legs. Exercises

should be done several times a day. When the patient gets out of bed, he may need a walker or a cane.

If bladder and bowel sensations are diminished, the patient will need to be taught to regulate these functions. For example, he will feel no longer the usual signs of needing to defecate. He may be able also to learn to void regularly. Tidal drainage may be used initially to help to re-establish bladder tone.

Cerebral surgery such as a *prefrontal lobotomy* may be performed as a desperate last resort. This operation will not affect the perception of pain; rather, it diminishes the anticipation and the dread of it. A prefrontal lobotomy interferes with the interpretation of pain that transpires in the frontal lobe. The patient who has repeated or continuous excruciating pain becomes emotionally and physically exhausted. Following a prefrontal lobotomy he still feels the pain, but he becomes less responsive to it. He also becomes less reactive to almost everything else, including the feelings of others. He may become rude, apathetic, and incontinent. His sensitivity is blunted.

The neurosurgeon will discuss the expected outcome with the patient and with his family as well. It is important that all anticipate the results realistically to avoid a loss of rapport between the patient and the medical personnel at a time when the patient desperately needs to have faith in the people around him. The patient has already suffered much, his pain threshold by this time is lowered, and the recovery from surgery is long and difficult. Even if the patient's pain is relieved, he may be irritable, angry and in need of much gentle attention.

Other cerebral procedures such as *thalamotomy* which destroys the thalamic nuclei by thermocoagulation thus altering the perception of pain are in the experimental stage.

## Electrical Stimulation

A relatively new method of chronic pain relief which gained impetus from the gate theory involves electrical stimulation of peripheral nerves which is thought to stimulate the gating mechanism and close the gate to pain impulses. Stimulation can be performed through the skin (percutaneously), through a wire inserted near a nerve (percutaneously), or through implanted devices. The peripheral nerve implant involves the attachment of an electrode to a sensory nerve, connection of the electrode wire to an implanted radio receiver, and the use of an external transmitter whose antenna is placed on the skin over the receiver by the wearer who sends an impulse to the nerve to block the pain impulse. The dorsal column stimulator operates on the same principle but the electrode is attached during laminectomy to the dorsal column of the spinal cord at a level appropriate to the location of the pain.

Patients are carefully screened for these procedures which have been helpful in such conditions as phantom limb pain, cancer, sciatica, and arthritis. In addition to pain relief, withdrawal from drugs and increased physical activity are treatment goals (Goloskov, 1974).

## Acupuncture

Acupuncture analgesia is an old Chinese practice whereby long fine needles are inserted into selected points of a person's body often resulting in dramatic relief of pain. Acupuncture stimulation takes place by twirling the needles or sending electrical stimulation through them. According to gate control theory, acupuncture stimulation may activate the brain stem and trigger the nervous system to close the gate on pain signals. Pain perception and response during acupuncture is also thought to be diminished by the lessening of anxiety resulting from the patient's faith in the cultural acceptability of the procedure and his response to the suggestibility of success. Lessening of anxiety also increases the efficacy of conventional analgesic drugs sometimes given prior to acupuncture treatment (Melzack, 1973).

## Psychogenic Pain

Pain is not either organic or psychogenic. Psychological and organic elements are involved in all pain. However pain may be experienced with little or no input from peripheral receptors and may be generated or modified in the brain itself.

A child's early socializing experiences may predispose to the use of pain to meet psychological needs in adulthood. Demonstrations of suffering and complaints of pain can be unconsciously used to control others. Pain may be a means for a person to express conflict, relieve guilt, or control aggression, or it may be a manifestation of unverbalized fears.

Pain can be viewed as a continuum with organic and psychological factors playing a greater or lesser role. When psychogenic factors predominate, treatment of this aspect is required; however, analgesics may also contribute to pain control. Depending on the underlying problem, the nurse can help by estab-lishing a trusting relationship with the patient and offering opportunities for him to verbalize thoughts and feelings. However the nurse should recognize that the patient may require more expert help such as a clinical nurse specialist, a psychologist, or a psychiatrist to cope with his response to pain and in some instances may become free of his pain by resolving the psychological problem.

Help may also be obtained through group psychotherapy, pain clinics, hypnosis, operant conditioning or behavior modification techniques, or biofeedback and autogenic training (Pain and Suffering, 1974).

## Pain and Suffering

The experience of pain with its concomitant suffering has elements of fear, anxiety, loneliness, and the unknown. One can never comprehend the extent of another's suffering. But it is in the effort to comprehend it that much relief of the patient's pain and the loneliness that accompanies it can be found. The way the nurse gives a medication, and the other relief measures she uses, can be as helpful to the person in chronic pain as the medication itself.

It is not an easy task of nursing to stand by in the face of another's pain. But it is unrealistic to assume that technically competent, compassionate, collaborative nursing care can eliminate all suffering. The nurse who assists the patient to best cope with his unrelieved pain in his own way makes a significant contribution toward the alleviation of suffering.

## REFERENCES AND BIBLIOGRAPHY

BILLARS, K.: You have pain? I think this will help, *Am. J. Nurs.* 70:2143, October 1970.

BLAYLOCK, J.: The psychological and cultural influences on the reaction to pain: A review of the literature, *Nurs. Forum* 7:262, 1968.

BRENA, S.: *Pain and Religion: A Psychophysiological Study,* Springfield, Ill., Thomas, 1972.

BRUEGAL, M. A.: Relationship of preoperative anxiety to perception of postoperative pain, *Nurs. Res.* 20:26, January-February 1971.

CARTER, B.: Comparison of individual pain reactions to injections of distilled water and normal saline, *ANA Reg. Clin. Conf.,* p. 219, 1967.

CASEY, K. L., and MELZACK, R.: Neural mechanisms of pain: A conceptual model, in *New Concepts in Pain and Its Clinical Management,* E. L. Ray (ed.), Philadelphia, Davis, 1967, pp. 13-31.

CASHATT, B.: Pain: A patient's view, *Am. J. Nurs.* 72:281, February 1972.

CHAMBERS, W., and PRICE, G.: Influence of the nurse upon effect of analgesics administered, *Nurs. Res.* 16:228, Summer 1967.

CLEMENCE, SR. MADELEINE: Existentialism: A philosophy of commitment, *Am. J. Nurs.* 66:500, March 1966.

COPP, L.: The spectrum of suffering, *Am. J. Nurs.* 74:491, March 1974.

DAVIS, L., and PENDLETON, S.: Nurses' inferences of suffering, *Nurs. Res.* 18:100, March-April 1969.

DIERS, D., et al.: The effect of nursing interaction on patients in pain, *Nurs. Res.* 21:419, September-October 1972.

DRAKONITIDES, A.: Drugs to treat pain, *Am. J. Nurs.* 74:509, March 1974.

FINNESON, B.: *Diagnosis and Management of Pain Syndromes,* ed. 2, Philadelphia, Saunders, 1969.

FRANCIS, G., and MUNJAS, B.: *Promoting Psychological Comfort,* Dubuque, Iowa, Brown, 1968.

GAUMER, W.: Electrical stimulation in chronic pain, *Am. J. Nurs.* 74:504, March 1974.

GOLOSKOV, J., and LEROY, P.: Use of the dorsal column stimulator, *Am. J. Nurs.* 74:506, March 1974.

GUYTON, A.: *Textbook of Medical Physiology,* ed. 4, Philadelphia, Saunders, 1971.

KEATS, A., and LANE, M.: The symptomatic therapy of pain, *Disease-a-Month,* June 1963.

KEOUGH, G.: The neuropacemaker-relief for patients with intractable pain, *RN* 35:ICU 1:September 1972.

LERICHE, R.: Surgery of pain, in *Familiar Medical Quotations,* M. Strauss (ed.), Boston, Little, Brown, 1968, p. 356.

LIPTON, S.: The relief of intractable pain by cordotomy, *Nurs. Times* 69:755, June 14, 1973.

MAC BRYDE, C. M., and BLACKLOW, R.: *Signs and Symptoms,* ed. 5, Philadelphia, Lippincott, 1970.

MCBRIDE, M. A.: The additive to the analgesic, *Am. J. Nurs.* 69:974, May 1969.

MCBRIDE, M. A., et al.: Nurse-researcher: The crucial hyphen, *Amer. J. Nurs.* 70:1256, June 1970.

MCCAFFREY, M.: *Nursing Management of the Patient with Pain,* Philadelphia, Lippincott, 1972.

_____: Intelligent approach to intractable pain, *Nurs. '73* 3:26, November 1973.

MCLACHLAN, E.: Recognizing pain, *Am. J. Nurs.* 74:496, March 1974.

MASTROVITO, R.: Psychogenic pain, *Am. J. Nurs.* 74:515, March 1974.

MELZACK, R.: How acupuncture works: A sophisticated Western theory takes the mystery out, *Psychol. Today* 6:28, June 1973.

MELZACK, R., and WALL, P. D.: Gate control theory of pain, in *Pain,* proceedings of the International Symposium on Pain organized by the Laboratory of Psychophysiology, Faculty of Sciences, held in Paris, April 11-13, 1967, ed. by A. Soulairac and others, London, Academic Press, 1968, pp. 11-31.

Pain and Suffering. Special Supplement, *Am. J. Nurs.* 74:489, March 1974.

PILOWSKY, I., et al.: Pain and its management in malignant disease, Elucidation of staff-patient transactions, *Psychosom. Med.* 31:400, September-October 1969.

RODMAN, M.: Drugs for pain problems, *RN* 34:59, April 1971.

STARNBACH, R.: *Pain: A Psychophysiological Analysis,* New York, Academic Press, 1968.

SIEGELE, D.: The gate control theory, *Am. J. Nurs.* 74:498, March 1974.

STORLIE, F.: Pain, describing it more accurately, *Nurs. '72* 2:15, June 1972.

THERRIEN, B., and SALMON, J.: Percutaneous cordotomy for relief of intractable pain, *Am. J. Nurs.* 68:2594, December 1968.

TURNBULL, F.: Pain and suffering in cancer, *Canad. Nurse* 67:28, August 1971.

WANG, R. I. H.: Control of pain, *Am. J. Med. Sci.* 246:590, 1963.

ZBOROWSKI, M.: *People in Pain,* San Francisco, Jossey-Bass, 1969.

# Dependence on and Abuse of Tobacco, Alcohol, and Drugs

## CHAPTER 11

## AN OVERVIEW

When the topic of drug dependence is discussed, one tends to think first of narcotics. But alcohol, which is frequently regarded as a beverage and not as a drug, has potent pharmacologic effects, and dependence on alcohol is common. Dependence on nicotine is also often overlooked as an example of use of a harmful substance.

In this chapter we shall discuss dependence on the following agents known to have harmful effects on the body: nicotine, alcohol, amphetamines, LSD and other hallucinogens, marihuana, barbiturates, nonbarbiturate sedative-hypnotics and minor tranquilizers; and potent narcotic analgesics (opium derivatives).

But before considering each substance, we shall discuss some of the dynamics of drug dependence in general. It must be remembered that the implications of dependence differ for each of these substances. For example, it is illegal to take narcotic drugs without a physician's prescription, and to do so leads to complex economic and social problems. Excessive use of alcohol, although not in itself illegal, may lead to arrest if one is driving while intoxicated. Smoking, on the other hand, is socially acceptable, despite the fact that it is discouraged for health reasons. Nor is smoking usually connected with such personal and social problems as divorce and poverty, as are alcohol and narcotics. It does not impair one's judgment nor interfere with personal relationships or achievements at work.

Nevertheless, dependence on all of the drugs mentioned in this chapter has the following factors in common:

The substances are all harmful; discontinuing the use of these substances is difficult.

## Brief Historical Background

For years drugs obtained from plant substances were used in the United States by the American Indians to produce altered states of consciousness. But drugs were not used in this country for other than medical purposes until the 1840's when Chinese laborers were brought over to help build the transcontinental railway. As one of their "employment benefits" they were given opium which was widely available and accepted in their culture.

Opium use increased during the 1850's with the introduction of the hypodermic syringe and morphine became more prevalent during the Civil War when morphine was widely used for analgesia. At this time medical personnel were unaware of the potential for physical and psychological dependence caused by prolonged and excessive use of morphine. This dependence became evident after the war and became known as "soldier's disease." It was to become even more prevalent following World War I, and by the end of World War II heroin, which was first used in the United States as a substitute for morphine in the treatment of addicts, was widely abused.

Thus we can see that the first 50 years of this century saw the steady introduction of new substances into this country which are major factors in our present drug problems.

## Drug Abuse

While drug dependence is the more precise designation, the term drug abuse is found frequently enough in the literature to warrant some discussion here. This term is used to designate the use of a group of drugs that can alter mood and behavior in ways that are defined either by social norm or by statute as undesirable or harmful (Glasscote et al., 1972). The drugs may be illegal, such as heroin, LSD, and marihuana, or legal, such as alcohol or nicotine, in which case they are said to be "abused" if the amounts of or purposes for use are other than that intended. Other drugs which are frequently abused are barbiturates, methadone, and amphetamines.

## Characteristics of Dependence

In varying degrees, according to the agent and the individual, dependence on nicotine, alcohol, and other drugs includes a strong need to continue taking the agent, ambivalence toward it, and withdrawal symptoms when it is withheld.

**The Need.** Understanding the urgency of the need is difficult for the nondependent person. Many of those who are dependent require daily consumption. They are victims of their own need, and everything in life becomes secondary to it.

For example, to their own amazement, smokers in countries where both food and cigarettes were scarce after World War II found themselves forgetting long-established manners and morals, not for bread and meat, but for a cigarette. A suburban housewife hides a bottle of alcohol to keep her family and friends from knowing how much she drinks. The person dependent on narcotics frequently commits petty crimes to secure money to buy the next dose of drugs. In such instances, the comfort and safety of others are ignored in the face of the need. The need defies usual social sense.

**Onset of Dependence.** Drug dependence takes time to develop. There is no clear-cut point at which the person who drinks changes from a social drinker to an alcoholic who can no longer control his drinking. There is no warning that a person will be unable to stop smoking, or that heroin will become more important than family or job. By the time the person realizes that he is dependent, he has changed. He has lost control over the habit before he knows that he has. It may take ten years for alcoholism to develop fully, and several more years before it is identified as a problem by the patient. Cigarette smoking may also take months or years to become a problem. However, dependence on narcotics may occur within a few weeks.

**Ambivalence toward the Habit.** At first the intake of the agent has a pleasant effect. Heroin, alcohol, and tranquilizers can reduce tensions, perhaps making an unbearable world seem less difficult. A cigarette can make a 15-year-old feel manly, competent, and poised.

Later a craving for the agent is noticed at odd moments—on a bus, in a theater, during reading. Finally, the dependence is fully established. Work is planned around the break that allows a smoke or a drink. Social activities where there will be no drinking or smoking are avoided.

Yet now the intake of the drug is accompanied by anxiety as well as pleasure. A drink is downed or a narcotic hastily injected not for pleasure, but as a relief from tension. This factor of diminishing pleasure seems to operate more fully in some persons than in others. For some who stop taking the drug, the loss is intense, and it may be compounded by the person's inability to find a satisfactory substitute.

Regardless of increased anxiety, approaches which stress practical considerations such as cost and physiologic effects are often ineffective in stopping the habit. For example, despite the increased cost of cigarettes, anti-smoking campaigns, and awareness of health hazards, Americans spent more for cigarettes in 1970 than in 1964.

**Tolerance.** Tolerance buildup is a major problem in drug dependence. When tolerance develops, the dose that was previously effective no longer gives relief, and an increased dose is necessary to obtain the original effect. As dependence progresses, the alcoholic can indulge in heavy drinking without getting drunk, the cigarette smoker increases his daily consumption, and the person dependent on narcotics requires higher and higher doses. Although this tolerance can increase, it is limited and can be exceeded, in which case signs of acute toxicity may appear. For example, the alcoholic may be able to consume several drinks and show no ill effects, but downing a bottle of whiskey in an hour can render him stuporous. Over a period of time such excessive intake can lead to profound and serious physical effects, such as delerium tremens (DT's) and cirrhosis of the liver. As another example, the youthful smoker may begin with a few puffs and gradually increase to two or three cigarettes a day. If he exceeds this tolerance, he may experience pallor, nausea, and perhaps vomiting. But as time passes his tolerance rises, and eventually he may level off to a pack or more a day.

It should be noted that the shorter acting the substance, the more the potential for abuse. That is, there are few known addicts to phenobarbital which is a long-acting preparation. There is, however, increasingly widespread dependence on short-acting preparations such as secobarbital. The reason is clear: short-acting drugs provide an immediate pleasurable effect. Therefore, the more pleasure obtained from a drug, the more the potential for physical and/or psychological dependence.

**Withdrawal Symptoms.** If a strong psychological and physiologic dependence on the substance is established, the patient suffers psychological and physical symptoms when the drug is abruptly discontinued. Withdrawal of narcotics, alcohol, nicotine, or other drugs produces symptoms peculiar to that particular drug and will be discussed later.

## Theories of Cause

For years attempts have been made to explain the causes of drug dependence. While the physical and social sciences have made important contributions to our knowledge of individual and social behavior, much in the way of prevention, treatment, and research has been fragmented. For example, more popular explanations have centered on physiologic, psychological, or social and environmental grounds. These explanations tend to place both the blame and the responsibility for the dependence on the afflicted individual. More recently, however, drug dependence has been recognized as a complex problem involving or influenced by a multiplicity of interrelated variables, such as availability of the drug, affluence, alienation and peer pressure, values and beliefs concerning drug use, social and economic deprivation, boredom, rebellion, and the relationship between the drug use and the total life experience of the individual. It is recognized that drug dependence like other human behavior has no single cause. As a health problem it is interwoven with other human problems now existing in society. Thus a more appropriate therapeutic approach would be a combined multidisciplinary effort which would focus on the complex relationships between the drug dependent individual and his environment.

## Incidence and Economics

Dependence on drugs is increasing and has become a major health problem. There are between 90 and 100 million users of alcohol in the United States alone, 9 million of whom were considered alcoholics in 1973. Yearly cigarette production has increased from 4.2 billion in 1900 to 583 billion in 1970, and cigarette consumption has increased despite known health hazards (Brecher, 1972). In March, 1973, the Bureau of Narcotics and Dangerous Drugs set the addict population at 560,000. However, it is felt that for every known drug user there are probably three who are unknown, and the number of drug users not involved with addictive drugs who become casualties of their drug use is undetermined.

Drug use and subsequent dependence has spread rapidly among young people between the ages of 10 to 25 (Van Dusen and Brooks, 1970). Experimentation with drugs now stretches from grammar school through junior high and senior high school into college and adulthood. In addition the socio-economic spread of drug use is greater now than ever before. What was once a slum problem has now become both an urban and a middle-class suburban problem. And while the more affluent may be better able to minimize detection, they are still subject to numerous pressures which, though unlike those of lower income groups, may be as influential as the latter in initiating drug use as an attempt to escape stress.

Drug dependence is as expensive to the individual as to society. The drug dependent individual and his family may experience loss of income due to loss of time from work, inefficiency at work, illness or disability, and premature death. The cost of drugs is another factor to consider. The cost of those available legally, alcohol and nicotine in particular, has been rising steadily, partly as a result of increasing taxes. For the person whose income is meager, expenditure for drugs may mean that other important needs are neglected.

The person dependent on illegal drugs is placed in an impossible financial position. He depends on the pushers who sell them, and has no recourse if the price is exorbitant, if he does not have the money, or if the drug he buys is diluted. Many soon find themselves without funds, and their stealing is directly related to their need for the drug.

As we can see the economics of drug consumption is complex. On the one hand, many people derive income from the legitimate drug industry, and taxes on purchases of alcohol and tobacco form an important source of government revenue. On the other hand, higher levels of governmental expenditures are for health and illness problems related to drug use, including education, training, and research. For example, in December 1970 the Comprehensive Alcohol Abuse and Alcoholism Prevention, Treatment, and Rehabilitation Act was passed (P.L. 91-616) providing funds for research and training programs related to alcohol dependence. At both federal and local levels funds have been made available for both inpatient and outpatient treatment facilities and personnel.

## Treatment

**Phases.** Treatment comprises two phases. Initially, it is aimed at alleviating the physical symptoms caused by withdrawal of the drug and giving psychological aid to help overcome the acute sense of loss that the patient suffers. After physiologic adjustments have been made, psychological craving and/or the physiologic craving remain and require continued, long-term consideration.

Although craving is not fully explainable, it is accepted by some authorities as a phenomenon that is present for some time, probably months, after discontinuation of drug use, along with anxiety and depression. The desire to be relieved of this triad —anxiety, depression, craving—may explain the relapse among those who were dependent, and serve as a rationale for establishing long-term treatment programs. Treatment and nursing care that ignore the long-term rehabilitative aspects of a therapeutic program are doomed to fail.

Unless the contributing personal and social problems of the dependent person are dealt with there is a great likelihood of recurrence. It is usual for the alcohol and nicotine dependent person to discontinue drinking and smoking many times only to return, perhaps during moments of stress. There is also the likelihood that other drug dependent persons may experience relapse during periods of stress. In 1970 the relapse rates among attenders at 17 smoking clinics were reviewed, and it was found that at the end of 48 months more than 80 per cent of those who had stopped were smoking again. Other withdrawal clinics (among them some funded by the American Cancer Society) have reported success of 30 per cent after a year as compared with 15 to 20 per cent seven years ago.

However well-intentioned, the efforts of others to help the patient are useless unless he himself recognizes the problem and wants help with it. Pleading with or scolding him often results in increased drug use because he feels misunderstood, angry at the invasion of his privacy, and rejected by others. Drug dependence of any sort cannot be cured merely by confronting the patient with the problems his habit is creating for him and for his family. Usually, he is already painfully aware of these, and self-blame and blame from others does not constitute treatment. He may be helped more by being informed of the availability of such services as those provided by professionals, paraprofessionals, or ex-drug users. Frequently law-enforcement personnel are helpful in identifying treatment settings for drug users who have been arrested.

**Facilities and Programs.** Availability of treatment facilities for persons who wish to end dependence on a drug has only recently improved, and condemnation by society in general and sometimes by health personnel complicates the treatment. For example, some hospitals refuse to admit alcoholics for treatment. In others the alcoholic may be discharged as soon as he has "sobered up," even though further treatment may be needed. Hospital and outpatient treatment for narcotic dependence is quite limited, but has increased with the aid of federal funding. Although smoking usually is not condemned, it is only beginning to be recognized that many persons who wish to stop smoking require assistance to do so.

Overcoming physical dependence on drugs is sometimes the beginning, but never the end of the patient's struggle to overcome his drug dependence. There are three major forms of treatment, although there are variations of these and comprehensive programs which combine all three. They are: detoxification (administering decreasing doses of the same drug taken by the user or one that is cross dependent with it); methadone maintenance (a controversial treatment approach for heroin dependence); and residential programs or therapeutic communities. The individual may be offered individual or group psychotherapy, a buddy system (such as that used in AA) or community-based follow-up clinics (which are becoming more available, and are frequently staffed by ex-drug users and professionals).

Sometimes patients may be unaware of existing resources. Helping patients to find facilities and communities to develop them are a part of creative nursing that can mean the difference between health and disease. Consulting the telephone directory and writing to national organizations are two ways in which the nurse may discover existing local resources. She can then learn their location, the range of services offered, the nature and cost of treatment, who is responsible for services, and the availability of long-term or short-term treatment or both. Armed with this knowledge she can share information with interested groups concerning early detection, referral, and treatment methods currently being used in the community. By talking to interested groups, such as PTA's, sending letters to newspapers, and serving on hospital committees she may help to create facilities where they are needed.

## SMOKING

### Harmful Effects

Tobacco smoke contains more than 200 known chemical compounds, including nicotine, and at least seven others which are known to cause cancer (carcinogens) in laboratory animals. Cigarette smoke also contains a number of cocarcinogens, such as phenol, which when repeatedly applied to tissue after a carcinogen has been applied, markedly increase the number of cancers produced.

While the effects discussed here primarily concern the smoker, studies have shown that when nonsmokers are exposed to a "smoking environment" measurable effects occur as follows: increase in heart rate, in both diastolic and systolic blood pressure and in $CO_2$ level in the blood. In addition non-

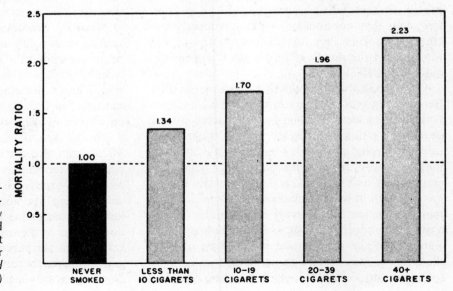

**Figure 11-1.** Mortality ratios: total deaths. Mortality ratios for total causes of death by number of cigarettes smoked daily at the time of enrollment in study. (American Cancer Society: *Cigarette Smoking and Cancer*, New York, The Society)

smokers may complain of irritation of the eyes and nose, sore throat, cough, headache, hoarseness, nausea, and dizziness.

**Cellular Changes.**   In the upper respiratory tract, ciliary activity and a mucous sheath are protective; in the lower tract macrophages (which ingest foreign particles, including tobacco tars), the lymphatic system, and possibly the fluid lining of the alveoli are protective. Repeated inhalation of cigarette smoke decreases the efficiency of these mechanisms and may destroy them. The cellular changes that occur in the epithelium of the trachea and the bronchi of smokers include thickening, the presence of atypical cells, inhibition of ciliary activity, decrease in the number of ciliated cells, chronic inflammation, rupture of alveolar septa, impairment of alveolar stability, thickening of the walls of arterioles and small arteries, decreased efficiency of phagocytes and slowed mucus flow (The Health Consequences of Smoking, 1971). The more cigarettes smoked, the greater the cellular changes, some of which may be precancerous.

**Lung Cancer.**   The increase in cigarette smoking has been paralleled by an increase in deaths from lung cancer. Studies reveal that there is an increased risk of developing lung cancer related to the number of cigarettes smoked per day and the duration of smoking. The mortality rates for women who smoke are lower than for men who smoke but have been steadily increasing. This may be due to the fact that women smoke fewer cigarettes per day, use filtered or "low tar" cigarettes, and have lower levels of inhalation. Pipe smokers and cigar smokers who usually do not inhale develop lung cancer more frequently than nonsmokers, but less frequently than cigarette smokers. Pipe smokers are especially prone to cancer of the mouth (The Health Consequences of Smoking, 1971).

**Chronic Obstructive Pulmonary Disease (COPD).** Besides lung cancer, cigarette smoking is an important factor in morbidity and mortality from chronic obstructive pulmonary disease. COPD is characterized by chronic obstruction to air flow within the lungs, as seen in chronic bronchitis, pulmonary emphysema, and bronchial asthma. It causes breathlessness both at rest and on exertion, decreased pulmonary function, and as every heavy smoker knows, a chronic, productive cough, with or without dyspnea. Paralysis of the cilia caused by smoking prevents the clearing away of foreign particles, such as those found in tobacco smoke, which are then deposited on the epithelium. In addition the pathology seen in chronic bronchitis (increase in the number of goblet cells, hypertrophy, and hyperplasia of bronchial mucous glands) can be caused by smoking. Smoking has not been as clearly identified as a cause of emphysema, but the rupture of alveolar septa and the fibrosis caused by smoking seem to be related to this disease, and it is known that the risk of developing or dying from COPD is much greater in the smoker than in the nonsmoker. In a group of smokers who coughed, more than 70 per cent of those who stopped smoking showed a decrease in coughing, whereas among those who continued to smoke, less than 5 per cent improved (The Health Consequences of Smoking, 1971). The symptoms of bronchitis and emphysema tend to be progressive, especially in smokers, and may result in respiratory crippling to the extent that the patient is unable to work or even to walk because he cannot breathe adequately.

**Cardiovascular Disease.**   Cigarette smoking is a significant risk factor in the development of coronary heart disease, and is greater than the risk due to pipe and cigar smoking. Because of the effect of cigarette smoking in altering peripheral blood flow and peripheral vascular resistance, it appears to be a factor in aggravating peripheral vascular disease. It has been shown frequently that cessation of smoking aids in partial or complete remission of symptoms in peripheral vascular disease.

## Dependence on Nicotine

Cigarette smoking is for most smokers a dependence on the drug nicotine.

**Nicotine Poisoning.**   Excessive or too rapid smoking can result in nicotine reaction, particularly in novice smokers. The person may have a burning mouth, giddiness, headache, photophobia, weakness, cardiac irregularities (such as tachycardia), nausea, and vomiting. Heavy smokers may experience some of these symptoms chronically.

**Physiology.**   When a cigarette is smoked, about 90 per cent of the 1 to 3 mg. of nicotine in it is deposited in the smoker's lungs. His heart rate at rest and after exercise is faster than that of the nonsmoker, and his blood pressure also increases, resulting in detectable ECG changes. Smoking causes constriction of the smaller blood vessels in his limbs, resulting in thromboangiitis obliterans, a condition which seldom occurs in nonsmokers. In addition, smoking retards healing of peptic ulcers. In short, the overall mortality rate from all disease is greater for the smoker than for the nonsmoker.

Cigarettes are said to be stimulating when one is tired and soothing when one is excited. One explanation is that the dependent smoker who consumes a pack and a half or more a day does so to maintain a high level of nicotine in his brain (Russell, 1971). Besides the pleasure obtained from the act of lighting, mouthing, and handling a cigarette, smoking satisfies different needs at different times. But it also lessens the senses of taste and smell. Thus increased appetite and consequent weight gain commonly accompany cessation of smoking.

## Stopping Smoking

Attempting to help people who wish to stop or to decrease smoking is a part of nursing. In such attempts, a clear understanding of the fact that the problem is one of nicotine dependence is crucial, especially when the nurse is caring for hospitalized patients whose illnesses are worsened by smoking. In this situation, as in any nursing situation that involves teaching about health, the nurse contributes by cooperating with others, such as the physician and the psychologist. Perhaps she will also talk to community groups about health practices, be in contact with workers in industry, or be employed in a clinic or a school.

**Withdrawal Symptoms.** When a nicotine dependent person stops smoking, he may experience such physical signs and symptoms as nervousness, drowsiness, lightheadedness, headaches, fatigue, constipation and diarrhea, insomnia, diaphoresis, tremors, and palpitations (Guilford et al., 1966). Chest pain, anorexia, and hunger have also been reported. In addition, it is not uncommon to have impaired concentration and memory, anxiety, distorted time perception, restlessness, and great irritability. The craving is so urgent that the person engages in some remarkable mental gymnastics, as to why he should have a cigarette immediately.

**Helping the Patient.** Decreasing the number of cigarettes smoked a day may be the most satisfactory solution for some people. But it is important to support the patient in whatever method he finds useful rather than to persuade him to adopt different measures, however helpful these may be to other individuals. Listening to the patient can help the nurse to recognize his views about why he wants to stop smoking. Supporting him as he seeks goals which are important to him is more likely to be effective than trying to persuade him to change his goals. Thus, helping a woman maintain her resolve to stop smoking is more likely to succeed if the nurse recognizes and respects the fact that the woman is more concerned about her baby's care and her own pride in mastering her craving than she is about the danger of lung cancer.

The attitudes of those in contact with the person who is attempting to become an ex-smoker are of prime importance. Although the nurse may be in a position to inform the patient about the dangers of smoking, fear techniques and preaching are known to fail. Such approaches may instill fear but not change the habit—an undesirable psychological situation. The decision and the action must lie with the patient, with the nurse supporting him. Otherwise, he may feel that the nurse is trying to manipulate him and reject her message.

Relapses are to be expected. The nurse should respond to these by helping the patient realize that he is not weak-willed because he failed in his resolve this time, but that each time he stops, it can become easier to do so.

Among the measures which the nurse can take to help patients stop smoking are: conducting group discussions which provide information and group support; helping patients to become familiar with various techniques, such as delaying the first smoke and gradually increasing the delay until smoking has stopped; using a dummy cigarette; planning for the period when smoking will be stopped, to try to make circumstances as favorable as possible for success; considering the issues of whom to tell and how to deal with the problem of being around others who continue to smoke. Having someone to talk with who will give support when the urge seems overwhelming is important. Interrupting usual cues to smoking (such as lighting a cigarette when talking on the telephone, or after a meal) may be helpful. Some individuals find that restricting the places where they may smoke helps them to decrease cigarette use. Clients who become especially tense during the process of giving up smoking may be treated by their physicians with mild sedation until the most acute discomfort subsides. Nurses can be instrumental in setting up antismoking clinics in hospital outpatient departments, in industry, and in schools. For example, a ward which serves cardiac patients might have a regularly scheduled group meeting which is available to all interested patients to help them stop smoking.

## Prevention

Because it is so difficult to stop smoking, it is logical to pay attention to its prevention. Studies indicate that teaching 5th and 6th graders may be more effective than trying to reach high school students, because by that age it is probably too late to begin the necessary preventive education. This finding places a special responsibility on school nurses to provide children with information about the health hazards associated with smoking so that fewer children will become smokers.

A survey done in 1968 and again in 1970 showed that in the two-year interval teen-age smoking increased for both sexes and at every age level from 12 to 18. Parental smoking and smoking of older brothers and sisters influences the smoking behavior of teenagers (Fig. 11-2). This should be recognized as a difficulty in trying to promote effective prevention programs.

Other measures that may lessen the health dangers of smoking include:

- Explaining the nature and development of nicotine dependence.
- Making cigarettes less easily available. Some cafeterias, especially those serving young people, have removed their cigarette-vending machines.

- Changing what is smoked from tobacco to some other substance, such as papaya leaf. Palatability, acceptance, finding a nonharmful substance, and enjoyment replacement are a few of the problems here.
- Effective filtration. What is to be filtered out of the hundreds of components of smoke is a problem. One hundred per cent filtration would result in smoking hot air.
- Restriction of smoking in public places.
- Increased taxation on tobacco products.
- Restriction of advertising of cigarettes.
- Labeling packages for tar and nicotine contents, and placing a warning on each pack of cigarettes.

The last two measures have already been implemented in the United States, as well as in other countries.

More attention is being given to community education about nicotine dependence with particular emphasis upon young people. The nurse can play an important role in these programs and in such programs to help people stop smoking as the American Cancer Society's IQ (I Quit) campaign which was started in 1972 and was designed to give recognition to those who have stopped for at least one month. She can also help to promote acceptance of measures such as the labeling of cigarette packages, and the removal of cigarette-vending machines from areas used primarily by young people.

The areas where a person may smoke are becoming more and more restricted. For example, the Federal Non-Smokers Relief Act provides for separate seating of passengers on all interstate buses. Nonsmokers are exerting pressure on lawmakers to assist them to preserve their right not to inhale cigarette and pipe smoke, while maintaining the rights of smokers. Members of organizations such as the American Public Health Association and the American Nurses' Association have agreed to abstain from smoking during sessions of national meetings.

## DEPENDENCE ON ALCOHOL

Only a small percentage of alcoholics live in the skid-row sections of our cities. Ninety-five per cent are ordinary people in homes, offices, and schools (Fort, 1973). They come from all occupational and social groups—rich or poor, executives or laborers—and they are scattered throughout the community.

Many efforts have been made to differentiate excessive drinking from alcoholism, but as yet there are no wholly-agreed-on criteria. One definition states that an alcoholic is any individual who relies on alcohol to meet the ordinary demands of living,

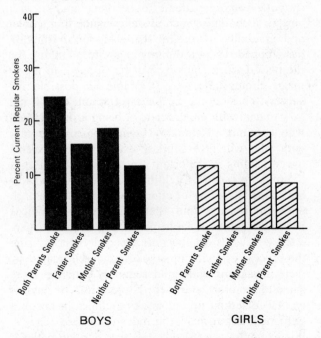

**Figure 11-2.** Teenage smoking is related to parental smoking. (U.S. Department of Health, Education and Welfare, National Patterns of Cigarette Smoking Ages 12 through 18 in 1968 and 1970)

even after alcohol has brought him difficulty in family and job relationships (Biers, 1962).

Drinking patterns vary widely. Some alcoholics maintain themselves most of the time in a state of intoxication that dulls their reactions to personal problems and interferes with judgment and human relationships, but that permits them to perform some routine tasks. Other alcoholics alternate periods of sobriety with drinking sprees during which they drink until they are unconscious.

Regardless of the manifold problems associated with alcoholism, many alcoholics have an amazing ability to maintain themselves in the community. They manage to continue working and, sometimes, to conceal their disability from all but their families and closest friends. Often the condition continues with varying degrees of severity for a large part of the individual's life.

Women as well as men become alcoholics, although they are less well accepted by society than are men alcoholics. However, because women typically confine their drinking to their own homes, sometimes the mistaken assumption is formed that alcoholism is largely a man's disease. Although the effects of a woman's drinking are less noted in public places, the effect of a woman alcoholic on her family is devastating. She is more likely to be protected by family and friends and therefore less likely to seek help.

The alcoholic may stick to one drinking pattern, or he may vary the pattern at different periods of his life; no one pattern invariably characterizes his behavior. However, one person who is developing alcoholism often feels the need to drink regularly during the day, and often he drinks furtively and alone. Another may drink heavily in the evening but abstain during the workday. Later the individual usually finds that he must drink also during working hours. He sneaks drinks and gulps them as fast as he can.

Hangovers increase in severity; nausea, vomiting, weakness, and headache are the typical symptoms. The patient misses work more and more frequently, and he has blackouts (amnesia).

Whatever the definition, there are certain characteristics associated with this form of drug dependence which are consistently predictable:

1. Alcoholism is present when the individual loses the ability to control his drinking patterns.
2. Unhappiness, tragedy, misery, and suffering are the hallmarks of the alcoholic life.

3. Alcoholism and/or uncontrolled drinking are responsible for at least half of all traffic fatalities.
4. Life expectancy for alcoholics is 12 years shorter than the average.
5. The alcoholic loses at least one month a year more from work than does the nonalcoholic.

## Assessment of Patients for the Possibility of Alcoholism

The nurse as primary care giver has an important role in assessing patients in relation to the possibility of alcoholism. The American Medical Association suggests the following considerations.

1. **Increasing consumption of alcohol, whether on a regular or sporadic basis, with frequent and perhaps unintended episodes of intoxication**
2. **Drinking as a means of handling problems or relieving symptoms**
3. **Obvious preoccupation with alcohol and the expressed need to have a drink, especially if habitually repeated**
4. **Surreptitious drinking or gulping of drinks**
5. **Tendency toward making alibis or weak excuses for drinking**
6. **Refusal to concede what is obviously excessive consumption and expressing annoyance when the subject is mentioned**
7. **Frequent absenteeism from the job, especially if occurring in a pattern, such as following weekends and holidays**
8. **Repeated changes in jobs, particularly if to successively lower levels or employment in a capacity beneath ability, education, and background**
9. **Shabby appearance, poor hygiene, and behavior and social adjustment inconsistent with previous levels or expectations**
10. **Persistent vague somatic complaints without apparent cause, particularly those of insomnia, gastrointestinal difficulties, headaches, anorexia**
11. **Persistent marital and family problems, perhaps with multiple marriages**
12. **History of arrests for drunkenness or drunken driving**

Additionally, alcoholism should be considered if the physical examination reveals the following:

1. **Coarse, unexplained hand tremors**
2. **Poorly explained contusions and abrasions in various stages of healing, except in the elderly**
3. **Gastritis or duodenal ulcer which fails to respond to usual therapy**
4. **Palpable, nontender liver**
5. **Evidence of premature organic brain deterioration, such as forgetfulness, disorientation, emotional lability**
6. **Obvious evidence of inappropriate use of alcohol, such as in the hospital or before an appointment**

## Physiology

Alcohol is absorbed directly from the stomach and small intestine into the bloodstream, without digestion. The rate of absorption is slowed by the presence of food in the stomach. However, when alcohol is taken on an empty stomach, its effects are felt quickly, and reach a peak in about 20 minutes.

**Effects on the Central Nervous System.** Alcohol acts directly on the central nervous system. It is a depressant with sedative-hypnotic, analgesic, and even anesthetic properties. The highest intellectual functions, such as judgment, are the first to be impaired, and the vital physiologic functions such as breathing, which are under control of the brain stem, are the last to be affected. Thus, the inebriated individual may lose his life due to an error in judgment while driving, although the same level of alcohol intoxication would not jeopardize his vital physiologic functions such as respiration.

Alcohol is not a stimulant, although many persons regard it as such because an inebriated person may feel or act stimulated due to lessening of inhibitions.

The effects of alcohol on the central nervous system are related to the level of alcohol in the blood and brain (Table 11-1). When alcohol enters the capillaries, it diffuses into all body tissues. The tissues which have the best blood supply have a particularly rapid accumulation of alcohol. For example, the level of alcohol concentration in the brain quickly comes into balance with that of the blood. Later, alcohol is taken up by tissues with lesser blood supply, thus drawing some alcohol away from the brain. However, the most important factor in reducing brain levels of alcohol is oxidation of alcohol by the patient's body.

Between 90 to 95 per cent of alcohol is metabolized to carbon dioxide and water. Most of the rest is excreted unchanged in the breath and urine. The first steps in metabolic breakdown of alcohol occur in the liver. Later, metabolism occurs in all cells of the body, where the acetate derived from alcohol is fed into the cellular system for obtaining energy from food (Krebs' cycle).

Energy is produced in the process of oxidation of alcohol to carbon dioxide and water, and in this sense alcohol is a food. Alcohol produces seven calories for every gram oxidized. However, alcohol does not contain essential nutrients such as vitamins and amino acids.

**Effects on the Liver.** There is evidence that prolonged, excessive consumption of alcohol has the ability to produce striking changes in the liver, even in the absence of dietary deficiencies. Because of this, effective treatment of alcohol-induced liver in-

Table 11-1. Effects of Intake of Increasing Amounts of Alcohol

| BLOOD CONCENTRATION OF ALCOHOL PER CENT | AMOUNT INGESTED OUNCES | EFFECTS |
|---|---|---|
| 0.05 | 2–3 | Uppermost level of brain depressed: centers of inhibition, restraint, judgment. Person feels euphoric, confident.* |
| 0.1 | 5–6 | Lower motor areas of brain depressed. Loss of digital dexterity, muscular coordination, auditory and visual discrimination and tactile perception. Speed of motor responses decreased. Pulse and respiration increased. Speech slurred. |
| 0.2 | 10 | Midbrain affected. Constricted pupils. Pale skin. Mental confusion, emotional instability. Tends to lie down. |
| 0.3 | 16 | Stuporous. Temperature below normal. Pulse weak. Sphincter control gone, reflexes going. |
| 0.4–0.5 | | Coma. Reflexes gone. |
| 0.6–0.7 | | Centers that control respiration and heartbeat markedly depressed. Death occurs when these centers become paralyzed. |

* The dangerous time for taking the wheel of a car has already arrived. Reaction time and muscular coordination are beginning to be affected, restraint and judgment are not normal, and yet the drinker feels more confident. This is the worst possible combination for handling a car.

Source: Rodman, M. J., and Smith, D. W.: Clinical Pharmacology in Nursing, Philadelphia, Lippincott, 1974.

jury necessitates control of alcohol intake; maintaining an adequate diet will not suffice. Alcohol has adverse effects upon the liver and leads to fibrosis and to fatty infiltration which gradually impair the functioning of the liver.

**Effects on Other Parts of the Body.** Alcohol affects other parts of the body besides the central nervous system and the liver. It can irritate the mucosa of the mouth, the throat, and the stomach leading to hoarseness and gastritis. Moderate intake of alcohol has little effect upon the heart; in fact the sedative and analgesic effects of alcohol may help relieve the pain of coronary insufficiency. Prolonged excessive alcohol intake, however, can lead to myocardial damage.

The ingestion of alcohol makes the individual feel warm, and he therefore frequently goes out in winter weather without adequate clothing; the problem of exposure is made worse when the individual lies for hours out of doors in a stupor. Alcoholics often smoke heavily and have a high incidence of chronic bronchitis and emphysema. These conditions are exacerbated during periods of stupor when the alcoholic fails to cough up respiratory secretions. Recently it has been noted also that those who have an excessive alcohol intake have an increased incidence of cancer of the mouth and throat, and that the combination of heavy drinking and heavy smoking heightens the risk of cancer. Hypostatic pneumonia is a frequent complication of severe drinking bouts, due to the individual's prolonged immobility, shallow breathing, and failure to cough up secretions. Pulmonary tuberculosis is also common among alcoholics.

Korsakoff's psychosis is a condition resulting from prolonged toxic effects of alcohol on the brain. The individual shows memory loss, particularly for recent events. The prognosis for recovery is poor, and peripheral neuropathy is common among alcoholics. Damage to motor and sensory nerve fibers leads to numbness, tingling, and weakness of the extremities. The nerve damage is not due to the direct action of alcohol, but is believed to be caused by multiple vitamin deficiencies resulting from the alcoholic's inadequate diet.

## Effects on the Family

The alcoholic's spouse may suffer from lack of money and attention as the need for drink takes up more and more of the partner's thought, time, and earnings. There may be many nights when the spouse does not come home at all. If the alcoholic is a man, his wife may try to shame him into stopping, but he may be so ashamed already that he will only drink more. She will threaten to leave him, and sometimes she will.

In some instances the wife's behavior may foster the patient's alcoholism in various and subtle ways of which she may not even be aware. For example, she may seek as a marriage partner someone whom she can dominate and hold in low esteem.

In many instances the patient's wife is able to help her husband overcome the condition. However, the strains on the marital relationship are severe, and divorce is common.

Often the effect on children in the home is disastrous. Relationships between their parents are strained, and the alcoholic parent's reactions to his children are unpredictable. He may be kind and affectionate when sober, but harsh and violent when drinking. In such a situation it is difficult for children to obtain the consistent affection and security they need, and to develop trust in the alcoholic parent. The expectancy of future alcoholism among these children is high.

The family tends to grow more and more isolated because of shame and the difficulty of maintaining ties with friends and relatives. After numerous social occasions when the alcoholic embarrasses everyone, his family tends more and more to refuse invitations and to avoid inviting others to the home. The unpredictability of the alcoholic's behavior is a major problem for his family. Every day may be filled with anxiety over how the alcoholic will act, what difficulties or accidents he may become involved in, and which neighbors may see him staggering as he walks.

Because alcoholism is socially unacceptable, the family usually makes every effort to conceal the problem from others. They are thus cut off from the kind of help and support they might receive if the condition were more acceptable.

Problems in family relationships often are compounded by the way in which alcohol affects the patient's behavior. For example, gross neglect of the usual standards of dress and of personal cleanliness during intoxication tends to lower the esteem of others and himself, as do his angry outbursts.

Perhaps the most difficult aspect of all for the family is the fact that the patient cannot be treated successfully until *he* seeks treatment. In their desperation the family may find many community resources for treatment, but they are useless to the patient unless he himself decides to use them. Often the patient does not seek this help until he has hit bottom—perhaps he has lost his job and alienated his family. Experiences like waking up in a jail or a hospital with no recollection of how he got there may shock the patient into being able to admit the need for help and into beginning to seek it.

## Withdrawal Symptoms

About 4 per cent of alcoholics with an eight- to ten-year history of heavy drinking have brief episodes of mental disorder called *delirium tremens*, or the DT's. The onset of delirium tremens is sudden, although before it an alcoholic is often restless, anxious, and sleepless. DT's are especially likely to occur when the patient cannot maintain his usual high alcohol intake. Gastrointestinal disturbance, hospitalization, or imprisonment are examples of circumstances which may precipitate delirium tremens because the patient is temporarily unable to drink alcoholic beverages. Characteristics of DT's are tremors that may shake the whole body and hallucinations. The patient sees—and less frequently hears—things that are not there. Most commonly he sees fast-moving animals or grotesque shapes and colors. Some patients see small people running over the floor or climbing on the chair. Restless, violent, unceasing activity that may take the form of running from the animals accompanies DT's. The activity is so great that it may lead to death from heart failure or exhaustion, especially if the patient is malnourished.

The patient experiencing DT's is in the throes of extreme anxiety. He knows who he is, but he may misidentify other people or objects. He may understand that he is having hallucinations, but this realization does not make the animals go away. He perspires, and therefore dehydration and electrolyte imbalance are further increased. Respiration, pulse, blood pressure, and often temperature are elevated. If DT's come when the body has an added strain, such as pneumonia, the body's resistance to alcohol poisoning is decreased.

## Treatment

The patient brought to the hospital with acute alcohol poisoning is highly agitated, and he may have or soon develop DT's. His blustering, noisy behavior may be part of his defense against feelings of utter helplessness and fear. The nurse must protect him from injury. Physical restraints should be avoided whenever possible, because they often aggravate the condition by making the patient feel fettered and more helpless. The nurse must use her ingenuity to provide maximum protection with a minimum of direct physical restraint. Closing and locking the window and placing side rails on the bed are examples of measures that can help to protect the patient. The presence of a nurse or a nursing assistant who is calm, firm, and watchful helps to protect the patient from injuring himself and lessens his extreme agitation.

**Drug Therapy.** Drug therapy for acute alcohol poisoning includes:

- Vitamins, especially the vitamin B group. Alcoholics usually suffer from vitamin deficiency; vitamin B deficiency may be so severe that the patient develops pellagra.
- Paraldehyde which is often used as sedation during periods of acute agitation.
- Tranquilizers which are widely used to lessen the patient's restlessness and agitation. Some, such as chlorpromazine (Thorazine), also help to relieve nausea and vomiting. Meprobamate (Miltown, Equanil) is another tranquilizer commonly administered.

Phenothiazine-type tranquilizers must be administered cautiously, however, because they potentiate the depressant and hypotensive effects of alcohol. Tranquilizers are also used to control withdrawal symptoms, such as nervousness and tremulousness, when the patient is being helped to abstain from alcohol. Continued use of these drugs presents hazards, however, as alcoholics are likely to become dependent on tranquilizers and sedatives, such as phenobarbital. Medical supervision of drug therapy is essential for alcoholics, who so readily transfer their dependence on alcohol to other agents.

Intravenous fluids and electrolytes may be given until anorexia, nausea, and vomiting are controlled sufficiently to permit the adequate intake of oral fluids. Encouragement of a nutritious diet is essential as soon as the patient can tolerate it.

After the acute phase has passed, the patient requires long-term treatment. Disulfiram (Antabuse) is a drug sometimes used as an adjunct to other kinds of therapy for chronic alcoholism. The drug causes no apparent effects when given alone, but the ingestion of even small amounts of alcohol by a patient taking Antabuse causes flushing of the face, nausea, vomiting, diarrhea, rapid pulse, fall in blood pressure, palpitation, and sometimes collapse. The patient must consent to the use of Antabuse and be fully aware of the symptoms he will experience if he takes a drink. The use of this drug is not without danger: If the patient is unable to resist the temptation to drink, he will become seriously ill.

Antabuse is given orally. Usually the patient takes 500 mg. a day for the first few weeks, and then he is placed on a daily maintenance dose of 125 to 500 mg. daily. The rationale underlying the use of Antabuse is that it will deter the alcoholic from drinking because he knows the alcohol will make him very ill.

Citrated calcium carbimide (Temposil; CCC) is another drug which is used to deter drinking. CCC takes effect more rapidly than Antabuse, but its action is of relatively short duration. It is reported to produce a lower incidence of side effects, such as gastric distress, headache, and drowsiness, than Antabuse.

**Some Ways of Assisting the Patient.** Because many alcoholics try to hide their condition, it is especially important to show sensitivity when dealing with them. Illness and accidents associated with drinking are occasions when alcoholism comes to the attention of nurses and physicians, and are opportunities for the patient to acknowledge his problem and to seek help. Unfortunately, the alcoholic is often rebuffed by health professionals, and the opportunity to assist the patient to acknowledge and to deal with his drinking is lost.

The alcoholic is particularly perceptive of the attitudes of others toward him. Because of unfortunate past experiences, he often expects to be treated with scorn and condescension, and he may be ready to defend himself in a demanding, restless manner. Such behavior may be a cover for feelings of helplessness, anxiety, and self-loathing. By her kindness, patience, and tact the nurse can show him that she considers him a worthwhile individual. By her actions and words she can convey to him that she regards him as a sick person who needs treatment, that her relationship with him is based on helping him toward recovery, and that she believes recovery is possible.

Often this period, when he wonders how he got into this predicament, is a time of great remorse for the patient. The nurse can help him to begin moving from remorse and self-blame to thoughts of how he can help himself, and allow others to help him. It is important that the patient not be pushed

at this time, nor given the feeling that a treatment program has been mapped out for him. Lecturing, and advice giving should be avoided. Instead, emphasis should be placed on acceptance of him as he is and opportunities should be provided for him to talk about his situation and his feelings, without the nurse prying or giving advice. It is not likely that she can give him advice that he has not heard already many times.

Another important aspect of caring for the alcoholic involves setting limits. This has nothing to do with punishment or feeling superior to the patient. It means simply that the nurse must keep the patient's demands within limits that she can reasonably fulfill and that are consonant with his treatment. This rule holds for any patient. However, the alcoholic patient may present a particular challenge in this aspect of nursing.

It is helpful for the nurse to state how much time she can spend with the patient. Often such a statement helps to avoid misunderstanding later.

Consistency is important, because it helps the patient to feel more secure. The nurse should not be punitive in the way she enforces hospital rules. She should let the patient know what is expected and be consistent in these expectations. For instance, if a patient is not allowed to smoke in bed, he should not be permitted to do it one day and scolded for it the next. Instead, the rule and the reason for it should be explained.

The patient should never feel that he is being coerced. He should always be approached in ways which safeguard his freedom of choice. For example, talking to him about Alcoholics Anonymous may make him think, "Oh, here come those sermons. Now they're after me again." Placing a few pamphlets about AA where the patient can read them if he wishes to may be more effective in helping him to learn about the organization.

When symptoms of acute poisoning subside, the patient needs assistance in passing the tedious hours. The occupational therapist can be especially helpful. If there is no occupational therapist, the nurse should make a particular effort to find out what the patient's interests are and to help him to continue them.

Often those who are going through a similar experience can help one another in ways that no one else can. Who can better understand the terror, the aches, and the nausea than one who has just experienced them? When the patient recovers from symptoms of acute poisoning, he may be ready to help a new alcoholic who has just arrived. His gesture of friendly concern, like sharing the morning paper or bringing fresh water, and a comment like "I know how it is; I just went through it myself" can open the way to mutual help that may continue after both patients have left the hospital.

### Rehabilitation

Some hospitals have carefully planned programs of follow-up care for their alcoholic patients. For example, the patients may come back to the hospital one evening a week for group discussions shared with other alcoholics. During these meetings, the hospital dietitian may lead a discussion on planning an adequate diet, and a member of Alcoholics Anonymous may talk with the group about the work of that organization. Others who may be invited to participate in this type of discussion are physicians, clergymen, nurses, and social workers.

Psychotherapy may help the patient to gain greater insight into the emotional problems that have led him to dependence on alcohol. Psychotherapy may be carried out individually or in groups.

It may be helpful to include family members in some of these sessions. This reinforces the belief that the patient is not entirely to blame for the problem, and recognizes the importance of the interrelationship of the patient and significant others in the problem.

**Alcoholics Anonymous** (AA) is an organization composed of and run by alcoholics who by helping each other find that they themselves have been helped. The organization has been notably successful. Often it has helped people who have failed to be helped by other means. It is the acknowledged prototype for other groups that have been organized since to help people with various kinds of problems.

The philosophy of AA is disarmingly simple. It is expressed in a prayer its members use, "God grant me the serenity to accept the things I cannot change, courage to change the things I can, and the wisdom to know the difference."

AA stands ready to help the alcoholic, but it will not seek him out, even though entreated by the patient's family to do so. AA believes that until the patient shows that he wants help by seeking it, he cannot be helped.

Handling the problems of each day as they come instead of looking for a permanent solution brings alcoholism (and many other problems, too) down

to a manageable size. The AA member who has achieved relative sobriety turns around to help others and finds to his surprise that what he has already achieved looks like a mountain to another not as far advanced. His new status helps his badly damaged self-esteem and his loneliness.

**The National Council on Alcoholism** is not a part of AA, but works in cooperation with it. This Council is the national voluntary health agency in the field of alcoholism. Its functions include education to inform the public about alcoholism, research into causes of alcoholism, and service. It finds community resources, such as physicians who specialize in the treatment of the disease, hospital beds, interested clergy, and local chapters of AA. It then coordinates the need of the alcoholic with the available resources by giving information and counseling. The Council itself gives no treatment but is a bridge to treatment.

Organizations for the treatment of alcoholism are listed in the telephone directory. The address of Alcoholics Anonymous is, P.O. Box 459, Grand Central Annex, New York, N.Y., 10017. A letter to the New York City office of the National Council on Alcoholism at 2 East 103rd Street will bring an answer regarding resources for treatment of alcoholism in a specific community. There are family group discussion meetings for the families of the alcoholic. Information about these groups may be obtained by writing 40 East 40th Street, New York, N.Y., 10017. For example, wives of alcoholics can find assistance through Al-Anon, by which they may be helped to overcome their loneliness and shame and learn ways of helping their husbands to overcome their dependence on alcohol. Alateen is the name given to similar groups for the adolescent children of alcoholics. Such groups as Alateen are important in helping to prevent the development of alcoholism and other problems among adolescents who have an alcoholic parent.

## ABUSE OF OTHER SUBSTANCES, SUCH AS LSD, HEROIN, AMPHETAMINES, MARIHUANA

As the nurse becomes more involved with the community, the problems of abuse of these drugs becomes more significant in nursing practice. Not many years ago most nurses' involvement with drug dependence and abuse was confined largely to such problems as the care of terminally ill cancer patients who became addicted to narcotics as a result of therapy with these potent pain-relieving drugs. But as nurses become more active in caring for teenagers and young adults in school health services and community mental health centers, and, as public health nurses, in caring for families in their homes, they become increasingly aware of the problem of drug abuse and dependence.

The student nurse has a particular professional stake in this matter. She may feel loyalty to the youth-culture which encourages drug use, and at the same time an identification with a profession which seeks to limit use of potent and hazardous drugs without medical advice, and whose members, regardless of age, tend to be viewed as authorities on matters affecting health. The consequences of being known as a drug abuser can be very serious for members of the health professions whose work requires a high degree of responsibility in adherence to laws concerning drug use, and also provides easy access to certain types of drugs commonly used in therapy. Thus, the student nurse is faced with the problem not only of delineating her own values in relation to drug use, but also considering the implications of these values for her future career.

Whatever her personal beliefs, the nurse must convey to young people her concern, interest, and willingness to talk frankly with them about the problems of drug use. Nurses in high school and college health services have an especially important role in helping young people to make decisions based on factual knowledge, rather than on ignorance. The nurse can also promote and participate in educational programs to help young people learn about drugs. One of the tragedies of the current situation is that young people tend to turn to each other rather than to nurses and physicians for information. An attitude of silent avoidance on the part of health professionals is not useful. Silence does not prevent young people from knowing about and using drugs, but it does keep them from gaining accurate information, and from obtaining the emotional support in thinking through the problem that a concerned adult can give.

## Dependence on LSD and Other Hallucinogenic Drugs

Lysergic acid diethylamide (LSD) is a semisynthetic derivative of ergonovine which was synthesized in 1938 by Stoll and Hofmann. However, it was not until five years later that the tremendous power of this substance was realized. This occurred when Hofmann ingested a small amount of LSD, and discovered the only constant of the drug—its totally unpredictable nature.

LSD was originally employed to study the properties of schizophrenia mimicked by the chemical. However, it was quickly determined that LSD caused a schizophrenic-like reaction, and that the preliminary symptoms were not helpful as far as the anticipated studies were concerned.

Today LSD is medically used only in a strictly controlled research setting. Although its general popularity has declined since the mid-1960's, the problem of clandestine manufacturing makes LSD readily available outside the strict research guidelines.

Other hallucinogens have been available for a longer period. For the past 150 years peyote has been used by Indians in the Southwestern United States and Mexico in their religious rituals and the ceremonies of the Native American Church. Such use rarely, if ever, leads to dependence. This dried top of cactus is moderately available. Psilocybin and dimethyltryptamine (DMT) are relative newcomers to the illicit drug trade. The former is obtained with difficulty, but the latter is less difficult to obtain, and is readily available in some areas.

### Pharmacology

In addition to LSD, there are the following hallucinogenic drugs: the seeds of some morning glory varieties ("Oloiuqui," Riviea corymbosa; Ipomoea violaceus), the active principle of which is closely related to LSD; mescaline, a phenethylamine present in the buttons of a small cactus (mescal, peyote, lophophora williamsii); psylocybin, and indole found in a mushroom ("teonanacatl," Psilocybe mexicana); and DMT, a synthetic indole, also found in seeds of a South American plant (Piptadenia peregrina). All are highly potent, with LSD being one of the most potent drugs now available. Tolerance to hallucinogens develops rapidly, but usually is lost in two or three days. Some users have built up their LSD doses to 1,000 micrograms or 2,000 micrograms over a period of days. The average dose is 200 micrograms to 400 micrograms.

Further, there is cross-tolerance among LSD, psilocybin, and mescaline, although tolerance to mescaline develops more slowly than to the other two. Paradoxically, some users report a state of increased sensitivity to LSD once they have lost their tolerance. Relapse simulating the drugged state has been reported without ingestion of additional LSD.

LSD in crude form is relatively simple to synthesize, given a supply of lysergic acid or one of the ergot alkaloids. Lysergic acid, in turn, can be produced by deep fermentation processes with only moderate difficulty, provided there is suitable equipment and knowledge. The synthesis of lysergic acid however, is accomplished only with great difficulty. Since lysergic acid has been brought under federal control, DMT, a relatively new synthetic with a somewhat shorter and more "harsh" action than LSD, has appeared on the illicit market. An LSD "trip" or "experience" usually lasts about 12 hours and the onset is said to be fairly "gentle," whereas a DMT trip lasts about two hours and has a sudden or "rough" onset.

## Complications

A variety of complications has been reported in the medical literature, but three appear to be the most prevalent.

1. Reappearance of the hallucinated, disorganized state without further ingestion of an hallucinogen is one type of complication. This has occurred in subjects within two months after a series of relatively few exposures. It also has occurred more than 12 months after a series of more than 200 exposures that had extended over a period of years.
2. Panic is a frequent complication. Hospitalization may be sought by the user or his companion, neither of whom can cope with the sense of terror.
3. A third relatively common complication is the development of an extended period of psychosis, sometimes after a single exposure, and usually involving a person who was prepsychotic or had a history of current or previous psychosis.

## Treatment

In the acutely intoxicated state, the patient should have an immediate trial with phenothiazine medication, preferably administered intramuscularly. The phenothiazines tend to block the action of LSD. Dosage will, of course, vary with the severity of the intoxication. Barbiturates also may be found useful in lieu of, or in addition to, phenothiazines. Caution about the additive effects of these drugs must be observed if they are used in combination. Once the period of intoxication is over, and if symptoms of mental illness are apparent, medication should be prescribed on the same basis as for a similar type of mentally ill person who has not been involved with hallucinogens.

Because the hallucinogens do not cause physical dependence, there are no physical complications of withdrawal. Those caring for the patient, however, must determine at the onset of treatment whether other drugs are being taken simultaneously which require careful withdrawal management.

## LSD Flashbacks

Flashbacks may occur many months after ingestion of any hallucinogenic drug. They are most commonly seen after taking LSD and frequently are enjoyed as a "free LSD trip" or experienced with minimal discomfort. Horowitz estimated that one out of every 20 LSD users experiences flashbacks, mostly perceptual distortions. Only the most severely distressing reactions are brought to treatment.

**Definition.** Flashbacks are spontaneous recurrences of the original LSD experience long after the acute effects have worn off. They may occur suddenly and unexpectedly with full intensity, although more typically they are brief and attenuated. They usually last for only a few minutes but may last several hours. Patients may experience flashbacks after a single LSD trip, but usually flashbacks recur after many LSD ingestions. They may recur occasionally or as frequently as several times per day.

Shick and Smith (1970) divide flashbacks into three categories: perceptual, somatic, and emotional. Perceptual flashbacks are the most common, and somatic and emotional flashbacks are the most distressing. They almost always are accompanied by an acute panic reaction. The perceptual flashbacks are most often visual although any sensory modality may be affected. Visual phenomena include intensification of colors, visual illusions such as halo effects, shimmering, pseudohallucinations (the appearance of geometric forms and figures which the patient realizes are not really there), and occasionally true hallucinations of insects or animals. Patients may experience frequent spontaneous visual imagery.

Somatic flashbacks are less common but much more disturbing. They consist of feelings of depersonalization in which the patient's body or body parts may feel unnatural, unreal, or foreign to him and may be accompanied by numbness, parathesias, or pain. Emotional flashbacks are often most upsetting and consist of a recreation of very distressing emotions originally associated with the acute LSD reaction. These emotions include loneliness, panic, or depression and may be so intense that the patient may become suicidal.

**Diagnostic Assessment.** Flashbacks resulting from ingestion of LSD or other hallucinogenic drugs must be differentiated from prolonged LSD psychoses, from schizophrenic reactions, and from organic brain disease. Flashbacks occur long after the acute effects have worn off. They may occur spontaneously or be precipitated by smoking marihuana. They are usually fleeting, although the onset is sudden. Patients are asymptomatic during the intervals between flashbacks. In contrast, the chronic LSD reaction consists of prolonged psychosis or severe depression continuous with the original LSD experience. Neither the onset nor the cessation of symptoms occurs suddenly, as in the case of flashbacks. Patients with chronic LSD reactions or with schizophrenia are more likely to have a significant history of emotional disturbance prior to ingesting LSD, and their illnesses tend to be unremitting. Patients with organic brain disease may initially have symptoms resembling flashbacks, but they eventually present a more severe organic brain syndrome with disturbance of judgment, orientation memory, intellect, and emotions.

**Treatment and Nursing Care.** LSD flashbacks are usually self-limiting and tend to diminish in frequency, intensity, and duration with time. The patient should be reassured. If he is very anxious or panicky, he should be treated like the patient experiencing an acute panic reaction. He should be taken into a quiet room and reassured in a calm, confident tone. Medication is usually unnecessary, but diazepam (Valium), 10 to 20 mg., orally, may be given to allay the patient's anxiety. He may take Valium, 5 mg., orally, at the first sign of recurrence. He should be cautioned against taking any hallucinogenic substance, including marihuana, as these substances may precipitate flashback reaction.

If flashbacks persist or become more intensive, the patient should have a thorough psychiatric and neurological evaluation to determine if he has any additional underlying organic or emotional pathology. Since stress may play a very important part in precipitating flashbacks, psychotherapy is frequently helpful.

Advocates of self-administration of LSD emphasize its "consciousness-expanding" properties and its use in providing extraordinary experiences. They stress the greater perceptiveness, and the emotional growth and insight which they attribute to LSD.

These are goals which others seek through psychotherapy and through religious experience. The question which must be raised is whether the seeking of quick results in expanded consciousness through use of LSD can be justified, in view of the serious hazards involved in use of this drug. In light of current evidence concerning its hazards, the drug is still restricted to research use with psychiatric patients.

The marked variability of response to LSD makes the problem of its abuse more difficult. One person may have a "good trip," and recommend it in glowing terms to a friend, who then experiences panic followed by a period of psychosis requiring hospitalization. Young people, especially, are understandably bewildered when hearing such varied accounts of the drug's effects. The nurse can make an important contribution by helping young people appreciate the hazards and the variability in effects of LSD, and by helping them to consider other safer ways of expanding their consciousness and insight. The nurse who takes seriously a young person's search for meaning, insight, and heightened awareness is in a better position to guide the youth to seek these experiences in safer ways than the nurse who scorns the young person for searching for new dimensions of experience which have, by various means, been sought throughout the ages of human existence.

## Amphetamines

Amphetamines are central nervous system stimulants. They are misused in efforts to increase alertness and wakefulness, particularly during fatiguing and stressful experiences, for example, when taking examinations or driving long distances. The slang expression for these drugs is "speed."

This category of drugs includes such preparations as benzedrine, dexedrine, and other salts and isomers of methamphetamin sulfate. The major difficulty in treating patients with complications from using central nervous system stimulating (CNS) drugs is the initial recognition and diagnosis of the problem. Unless in a state of withdrawal, the patient usually manifests a remarkably alert, restless wakefulness. He may appear talkative and emotionally enthusiastic. Some tremulousness, anxiety, irritability, and hostile aggressiveness may be noted. In addition, these patients may be highly overactive and at times unable to sit still.

It is not unusual for these patients to experience hallucinations and delusions of the paranoid type when suffering psychotic reactions to high dose intravenous use of central nervous system stimulants. Additionally, a physical examination will reveal an excessively dry mouth, dilated pupils, brisk reflexes, and tremors.

Clearly, the complications associated with the paranoid psychosis are the most widely-known phenomena in the chronic amphetamine user. There has been much debate as to whether a true physical and psychological dependence is developed with long-term use of central nervous system stimulants. To solve the problem one need only refer to the World Health Organization's description of addiction. Continued use of central nervous system stimulants is marked by increased tolerance (*need to increase dose to achieve desired results*), and well-defined physical withdrawal upon abrupt cessation of use.

Once the diagnosis of amphetamine psychosis is established and the patient no longer is receiving the drug, a series of behavioral changes will be noted. Visual hallucinations will subside within 24 to 48 hours. The delusional content will decrease markedly over the next 7 to 10 days. Usually within 24 hours of the last illicit dose the patient will begin to sleep for increased lengths of time. It is not uncommon for such patients to sleep 18 to 20 hours at a time. Extensive dreaming will be noted. At these times the patient often resembles a narcoleptic in that he or she is half awake and half asleep and verbalizing dreams. Just prior to the sleep stage the patient may be irritable and/or depressed. Depression may continue and indeed increase in intensity over the next two weeks. Suicidal ideation is not uncommon, and the patient may appear apathetic and uninvolved.

## Management of Amphetamine Withdrawal

**Medication.** This author (Hickey) found that initial treatment with moderate doses of haloperidol and gradual withdrawal of this drug within the first four days of treatment often alleviates much of the agitated state seen on admission. This, however, is often replaced by depression which can be treated with tricyclic antidepressants. In fact, antidepressant medication can be started even while the patient is still on haloperidol. Antidepressant medication often aids in avoiding a period of three to four weeks of chronic apathy and fatigue combined with depression. It is usually not necessary to continue the antidepressant beyond a month following withdrawal. Perhaps one of the more important aspects of the inpatient psychiatric care of amphetamine withdrawal is allowing the patient to sleep.

**Nursing Care.** Nursing care during this period of hypersomnia should emphasize avoiding disturbing the patient's sleep, which is necessary to his recovery.

Later, during the first two weeks of withdrawal, it is important to set the stage for subsequent treatment of the underlying personality problems and disabilities. Establishment of a strong therapeutic relationship during this phase can often carry the patient over the rough spots during the ensuing months. It is wise to explain to the patient the expected depression, apathy, and lack of initiative that will tend to wax and wane over the next two to four months and that these symptoms have a direct relationship to the previous extensive drug use and not just to situational or intrapsychic processes. This is also the time to describe to the patient that many individuals feel an intense desire to return to use of amphetamines and that more than likely he will at some time ask for supplies of amphetamines "to tide him over." It is extremely important to be aware of the intense pressures, including suicidal threats, that amphetamine abusers will exert. Occasionally experienced clinicians allow themselves to fall into a pattern of rescuing the patient with amphetamines instead of appropriate use of tricyclic antidepressant medication.

Finally, during this early period of treatment, it is wise to establish urine checks as an expected continuing regimen so that later one does not become engaged in the usual argument with the patient about whether the therapist trusts him or not. Establishment of other components of the long-term therapeutic regimen is, of course, dependent upon the local resources available.

## Dependence on Barbiturates

The barbituric acid preparations have the opposite reaction of central nervous system stimulating drugs. Just as the latter increase the biologic functioning of the body, barbiturates depress or slow these functions. Central nervous system stimulants can kill by overstimulating the cardiovascular and pulmonary systems, while barbiturates and sedatives kill by depressing these systems.

Contrary to widespread opinion, heroin is not the most difficult to deal with from a dependence status. There is little conclusive evidence demonstrating that heroin is physiologically damaging. To date all biologic deterioration is usually associated with, and a direct result of, a poor life style and self-neglect. Barbiturates do cause damage to several body systems including the brain and cardiovascular networks.

**Management of Barbiturate Withdrawal.** Unlike the heroin addict, the barbiturate addict must undergo withdrawal in a hospital setting. Decreasing doses of phenobarbital over a two- to three-week period are usually indicated. The progression of barbiturate withdrawal is highlighted by the following symptoms: anxiety, sleep disturbance, nausea and vomiting, irritability, restlessness, tremulousness, postural hypotension, seizures, withdrawal psychosis, hyperpyrexia, and death. Table 11-2 is a recommended detoxification schedule for a barbiturate addict taking an average of 1,500 to 2,000 mg. per day (Hickey).

**Table 11-2. Recommended Detoxification Schedule for Barbiturate Addict (1,500 to 2,000 mg. per day)**

| DAY | 6 AM (MG.) | 12 NOON (MG.) | 6 PM (MG.) | 12 MIDNIGHT (MG.) | TOTAL DAILY DOSE (MG.) |
|-----|-----------|---------------|-----------|-------------------|------------------------|
| 1 | 100 | 132 | 132 | 200 | 564 |
| 2 | 100 | 100 | 132 | 200 | 532 |
| 3 | 100 | 100 | 100 | 200 | 500 |
| 4 | 100 | 100 | 100 | 164 | 464 |
| 5 | 64 | 100 | 100 | 164 | 428 |
| 6 | 64 | 64 | 100 | 164 | 392 |
| 7 | 64 | 64 | 64 | 164 | 356 |
| 8 | 64 | 64 | 64 | 132 | 324 |
| 9 | 32 | 64 | 64 | 132 | 292 |
| 10 | 32 | 32 | 64 | 132 | 260 |
| 11 | 32 | 32 | 32 | 100 | 228 |
| 12 | 32 | 32 | 32 | 100 | 196 |
| 13 | 0 | 32 | 32 | 100 | 164 |
| 14 | 0 | 0 | 32 | 100 | 132 |
| 15 | 0 | 0 | 0 | 100 | 100 |
| 16 | 0 | 0 | 0 | 64 | 64 |
| 17 | 0 | 0 | 0 | 32 | 32 |
| 18 | 0 | 0 | 0 | 0 | 0 |

Phenobarbital is commonly available in 100 mg. capsules; 16, 32, and 64 mg. tablets.

The dosage of phenobarbital to be given daily is calculated by substituting 30 mg. of phenobarbital for each 100 mg. of the short-acting barbiturates the patient reports using. Hickey allows two days for switching from short-acting barbiturate to phenobarbital before beginning withdrawal. In spite of the fact that many barbiturate addicts exaggerate or minimize the magnitude of their dependence, the patient's history is the best guide in initiating therapy. If the magnitude of the addiction has been grossly overstated, toxic symptoms (slurred speech, sustained nystagmus, or ataxia) will occur during the first day or so of treatment. Usually this problem is easily managed by omitting one or more doses and reducing the daily dose by 50 per cent.

Should withdrawal signs or symptoms (tremors, muscular weakness, hyperreflexia, or postural hypertension) appear at any time, an intramuscular injection of 200 mg. of phenobarbital is given, and the daily dose is increased. After stabilization is achieved on the phenobarbital, the total daily dose is decreased by 30 mg. per day as long as the withdrawal is proceeding smoothly.

Should toxic symptoms be present, one dose, or one-fourth of the daily dose, is omitted. Having the dosages divided this way is additional protection for the patient.

This technique has been applied in the treatment of over 50 barbiturate dependent individuals. Its success can be measured by its capacity to provide safe, relatively comfortable, and easy treatment of the physical dependence. It is emphasized however, that the treatment of physical dependency is only the first stage in rehabilitation of an individual who has based his life style on the abuse of barbiturates.

Most barbiturate dependent individuals are brought into therapy only by outside legal or social pressure. Unlike the heroin addict—who frequently seeks therapy on his own because he is tired of the daily routine required to raise money for his habit—the barbiturate addict is usually not under financial pressure. A large habit of 2,000 to 3,000 mg. per day could be maintained at a maximum cost of $10 to $15 per day—more typically $5 to $10 per day.

The combined services of nurse, physician, vocational rehabilitation counselor, and psychological support in the form of an individual or preferably, group psychotherapy, are strongly indicated. A long-term (six months to one year) residential treatment center should be considered, especially if the individual has used barbiturates for more than a year, or has demonstrated intentional or subintentional suicidal behavior. Unfortunately, "soft" drug residential facilities are rare.

For many barbiturate addicts, completely drug-free existence is not possible unless the individual is in a very supportive environment. His alcohol consumption needs to be closely monitored, as many addicts switch to alcohol to lessen anxiety, depressive symptoms, or to again experience intoxication.

Some barbiturate addicts may need to be treated with long-acting antianxiety agents, or antidepressants. Others can better learn to control their anxiety through hypnosis, medication, or progressive muscle relaxation exercises.

## Dependence on Opiates: Heroin, Methadone, and Related Drugs

Many professional nurses will come in contact with opiate addicts who are admitted to a hospital with a primary medical diagnosis with opiate addiction being a secondary complication. There are increasing numbers of nurses becoming involved directly in drug rehabilitation programs as nurse counselors. This increased demand for nurses in rehabilitation programs is due in part to the mandate of federal regulations under which the programs must operate, and also to some nurses' increased skill in such measures as individual and group counseling.

The consistent administration of a powerful analgesic, can allow pain from another disease to go unrecognized and therefore untreated. Whenever an addict requires treatment for any disease, it is essential that physicians and nurses know that he is an addict. Addicts usually require larger doses of premedication and anesthesia for surgery. Because he is engaged in an illegal activity, an addict often will hide the fact that he is addicted; yet this information is important to the anesthesiologist. The observation of constricted pupils, which may mean that the patient is addicted to opiates, would be a most valuable observation to make. Because the addict's technique may not be sterile, he may develop complications like local infections or hepatitis from the use of unsterile syringes and needles.

### Withdrawal Sickness

Withdrawal sickness, a self-limiting but extremely uncomfortable illness, occurs when addicts do not take the narcotic to which they are addicted. The symptoms of withdrawal from narcotics begin to become severe about 24 hours after the last dose, and they reach their peak in 36 to 72 hours, after which they taper off. The patient feels sick and apprehensive. Soon his eyes tear, and his nose becomes congested. Withdrawal from morphine causes repeated yawning. The patient perspires and feels hot and cold flashes. "Goose bumps" are raised on his skin. He feels anxious and restless. Temperature, blood pressure, and pulse are elevated. Vomiting, diarrhea, anorexia, headache, muscular aching and twitching, and severe abdominal cramps follow. Coma and collapse are possible. The patient is most comfortable lying on his side in a flexed position, and he will naturally assume this position. Keep a blanket over him, even on hot days. Because cigarettes are distasteful to him, he will refrain from smoking while withdrawal symptoms persist.

It is important to differentiate between *physical* withdrawal and psychological dependence. Physical withdrawal symptoms are of a few days' duration, but psychological dependence, and the craving for the euphoria produced by the drug, can last for years even when the patient is prevented from obtaining the drug during that prolonged period. This emphasizes the need to focus on helping the addict deal with his psychological craving which can lead him to seek narcotics.

It is important for the professional nurse to have some understanding of the personality disorders manifest in the addict. Without this understanding, she will become quickly frustrated, and as a result, she may withdraw from the patient. In general, addicts have learned to be manipulative and masters of the con. As hospital patients they are concerned about going into withdrawal. Many addicts will not admit to opiate use upon entering the hospital for fear of legal ramifications. When an addict is an inpatient, there is the danger of inadvertent overdose, even when the staff is aware of the fact the patient is an addict. It is not uncommon for these patients to continue receiving drugs while hospitalized. The usual route of supply is through visitors. The supply of outside drugs may potentiate the effects of medication administered by hospital personnel.

Thus, it is important for the nursing staff to clearly outline the rules and regulations of the hospital to the addict patient. In addition, it is essential for physician and nurse to work together in setting limits and in noting the possibility that visitors may have to be restricted. An attitude of firmness and concern for the patient is most effective.

It is important not to assume that a demanding, negative attitude on the part of the addict is a personal or professional affront. The less the nurse personalizes this behavior, the more effective the patient's care is likely to be.

Several national studies have described certain demographic characteristics of heroin addicted individuals. Male—75 per cent; black—66 per cent; Puerto Rican or other Spanish-speaking people—8 per cent; under 21 years of age—29 per cent; 21 to 25 years of age—42 per cent; over 25—29 per cent; blue-collar workers—61 per cent; unemployed—19 per cent; used drugs less than nine years—12 per cent; 9 to 10 years—35 per cent. At least 40 per cent of all addicts seeking treatment had done so on several occasions.

## Rehabilitation Programs

Since the middle of the last decade hundreds of drug rehabilitation programs have opened across this country. These programs can be classified according to modality:

1. Residential therapeutic community
2. Inpatient hospital
3. Outpatient, drug free
4. Outpatient, chemotherapeutic substitution
5. Detoxification

Most of these programs are supported financially by federal grants. Additional support is gained through private donations and fund-raising campaigns. The federal government through the Special Action Office for Drug Abuse Prevention and the National Institute on Drug Abuse has established prorated annual treatment costs allowable in each modality. Current figures are:

1. Residential therapeutic
   communities      $ 5,000 per year
2. Inpatient hospital      $40,000
3. Outpatient, drug free      $ 1,800
4. Outpatient, chemotherapeutic
   substitution      $ 1,800
5. Detoxification—Depending on
   whether outpatient or not

These cost figures are expressed in patient years. (A hospital treating ten addicts continuously for one year could be eligible for $400,000.00 from the federal government.)

**Therapeutic Communities.** Therapeutic communities are organizations which, for the most part, have been initiated by former drug addicts; others, such as Synanon of California, were started by former alcoholics; and still others, like Odyssey House of New York, by professionals like Dr. Judianne Densen-Gerber, a psychiatrist and lawyer.

Most are staffed by former addicts and run essentially on an eclectic psychiatric model. The daily routine for residents in these groups usually involves assuming responsibility for care of the living quarters and encounter groups.

It has been difficult to monitor the effectiveness of these programs due to their very closed and cloistered nature. A successful completion of treatment usually takes at least 6 to 18 months. Data available indicates that many patients entering treatment leave against advice before completing the program.

**Outpatient Drug Free Programs.** Outpatient drug free programs are usually loosely knit and poorly organized community-based intervention centers. The mainstay of these programs is usually some counseling. Unfortunately, patients' contacts may be sporadic, thus limiting the usefulness of such clinics.

**Outpatient Chemotherapeutic Substitution.** Clearly the most widespread form of treatment is with chemotherapeutic substitutions for heroin, of which methadone is the best known and most controversial. Methadone as a potential agent for treating heroin addicts was first postulated by a British psychiatrist. Working in Canada in 1958, Dr. Robert Halliday began to dispense methadone in decreasing doses on an outpatient basis. Initially he dispensed methadone in a tablet form. Because the addicts continued to inject the drug by dissolving the tablets, Dr. Halliday then began to dispense methadone dissolved in a high glucose base solution which made injection impossible.

In 1963 Drs. Vincent Dole and Marie Nyswander, a husband and wife team at Rockefeller University, discovered what is now known as the *Dole-Nyswander blockade*. They determined that in each addict a dose of methadone between 40 to 120 mg. blocks the effect of heroin. At that dose an addict could inject heroin and realize no euphoric reaction. To find the blockade level in each addict is a matter of titration. Additionally, since tolerance to methadone develops more slowly than heroin, the blockade dose does not incapacitate the addict as does heroin, and the dose of methadone could be gradually reduced without the untoward effects of withdrawal. It is this philosophy which makes methadone maintenance the most common form of treatment for heroin addiction. The theory is that heroin addicts can be maintained on methadone and undergo a process of social reintegration concurrently.

The success of methadone is as yet unknown. Its abuses are widespread. Methadone is far more toxic than street heroin. However, Dr. Frances Rowe Gearing of Columbia University has proven through epidemiological research that addicts who remain in methadone treatment at least 12 months have an 80 per cent likelihood of staying off drugs.

Methadone therapy may have a beneficial effect on this nation's addiction problem; however, we must learn to use it more judiciously. The problems of methadone addiction became so widespread that the federal government was forced to amend the Controlled Substances Act and severely curtail the availability of methadone in March, 1973. Today physicians generally can no longer prescribe or dispense methadone, and community pharmacies can no longer stock this drug. Addicts must go to clinics which are certified by both federal and state governments, in order to obtain the drug.

## Marihuana

Without doubt, marihuana is the most controversial drug available today. It has been used by civilized man since 3500 B.C. for many and varied reasons. In 1898 cannabis sativa was described in a text on pharmacognacy as an effective, mild, tranquilizer. Estimates of marihuana users in the United States range up to 24 million. In 1972 there were 188,000 arrests for marihuana violations. Some of those convicted have been sentenced to life in prison (Texas) while others have been given $5.00 fines (Michigan).

**The Expected or Usual Effects of Marihuana.** Effects of marihuana include:

1. Euphoria, elation, relaxation, well-being, dreaminess, self-confidence, jocularity, laughing, silliness
2. Feelings of detachment, clarity, cleverness, wittiness, disinhibition, depersonalization, thinking changes-irrelevant thoughts, disturbed associations, altered reality testing, decreased concentration and attention span, altered sense of identity
3. Sensory novelty and increased awareness of stimuli —vivid images, illusions and hallucinations—both auditory and visual
4. Speech changes—rapid, impaired, talkative, flighty, demonstrating some difficulty with sequential thoughts and poor immediate memory
5. Altered concepts of time and space
6. Suggestibility
7. Wish to transmit insight
8. Rapidly changing emotions
9. Altered sexual feelings
10. Increased appetite and thirst, slight nausea

11. Heaviness and pressure in the head, dizziness
12. Sleepiness
13. Lightness, numbness, and weakness of limbs, sensations of floating, parathesias, changes in body sensations and body image, restlessness, ataxia, tremor, dry mouth, tachycardia, urinary frequency, injected conjunctiva, some paranoid, anxious or panicky feelings, or precordial distress, and tightness in chest
14. Recently there has been some evidence of change in brain waves of experimental animals who smoke marihuana.

It is very unusual to see a patient presenting a serene reaction to marihuana at a hospital, because the drug is usually used in a social setting which has significant impact upon the reaction. One question must be considered carefully: Why do we consider a person who consumes alcohol specifically to get drunk a possible alcoholic and not put the marihuana user under the same scrutiny? The sole purpose of ingesting marihuana is to alter the state of consciousness.

## SUMMARY: PATTERNS OF DRUG USE

Patterns of drug use can be summarized as follows:

A. Prescriptive: The legal and legitimate use of a drug to solve a problem for which the drug is intended. Such drugs are obtained through a professional diagnosis and recommendation.
B. Experimental: Almost everyone may fit this pattern at one time or another. It is usually associated with youthful risk-taking behavior. Individuals in this pattern of use may become casualties of their experimentation. For example, the LSD user who has a psychotic reaction after using the drug once or twice; the marihuana experimenter who is arrested.
C. Episodic: A person from time to time "ties one on," perhaps at the office Christmas party. This style of use becomes potentially dangerous when the episodes are tied to problem solving (*like getting drunk after a family fight, or after losing a job.*)
D. Social-reaction: This style of drug use is widespread, and includes such common practices as the enjoyment of wine with meals, of coffee and tobacco during the traditional coffee break. More recently the use of psychotomimetic drugs during a rock concert has become common. This pattern of use becomes more dangerous when the drug is used as a facilitator. ("*I can't dance until I have a few drinks.*")
E. Compulsive: The person's life is centered around the use of a drug, which determines where he or she lives, what to do for a living, and with whom to associate. The drug of choice will be taken on a daily basis, usually several times a day. The person is physically or psychologically dependent. This style of drug use is always a problem.

## PREVENTIVE NURSING MEASURES

Addiction to drugs of a person with severe, long-term pain is a tragedy. Use of narcotics to relieve the pain of such conditions as arthritis and peripheral vascular disease usually is avoided for this reason. Some patients, such as those who require relief from severe pain due to terminal cancer, cannot obtain relief by any other therapy. If addiction to narcotics occurs in such instances, it is viewed as an unavoidable complication during treatment of an acutely painful terminal illness. In most hospitals narcotics must be reordered by the physician at frequent intervals (such as every 48 hours), thus bringing to the attention of the physician the question of whether the patient should continue to receive the drug. If the nurse observes that a patient seems to be relying on narcotics, she should consult the physician. Above all, she should never use narcotics ordered by the physician for the relief of pain merely to quiet a patient who is making difficult demands on the staff. Instead, she should consider the reason for the patient's behavior, and in consultation with the physician develop a plan for dealing with the patient's discomfort.

Correct interpretation of orders and exercise of judgment in the use of medication orders, particularly p.r.n. orders, is essential. Frequently, nursing measures may be used quite effectively in alleviating discomfort, for example, change of position; adjusting dressings; increasing activity within defined limits. A soothing back rub or a glass of warm milk (if permissible) may be helpful at bedtime.

Any person who regularly receives narcotics for whatever reason can become addicted. Addiction is *not* limited, as is commonly supposed, to those who are socially and educationally disadvantaged.

Physicians, nurses, and pharmacists have a special responsibility in prevention and early detection of drug addiction, because they are the ones who handle narcotics as part of their work. Destroying disposable syringes and needles before discarding them to prevent their possible use later by addicts is an example of something nurses can do to help to combat the problem. Keeping the medicine closet locked is another. Those whose work involves handling narcotics are especially vulnerable to addiction. Honest recognition of this possibility has helped many a professional person to avoid the pitfall of taking unprescribed drugs with the idea that it will be all right "just this once."

## NURSING ASSESSMENT IN RELATION TO DRUG DEPENDENCE

Key points to remember:

- **There is no "typical" drug user. Users may be found in all age groups, all socioeconomic groups, all ethnic groups, all occupational levels, and among both males and females.**
- **The person dependent on drugs may show no signs if he is getting the drug regularly. If he is not getting the drug regularly, signs of withdrawal may occur between 4 to 24 hours after the last dose.**

**The Interview.** The first contact with the person usually provides some opportunity for the collection of baseline data. It is important at this initial meeting to establish a trusting relationship; therefore, the nurse should be aware of her own thoughts, feelings, and attitudes in relation to drug dependence. These are readily revealed in interactions with people in clinics, schools, homes, or hospitals through such behavior as the language used in the interview, punctuality, or lack of it, in keeping appointments or treatments; names used in referring to patients, and the responsibility entrusted to patients.

**Family History.** Some knowledge of parent and sibling use of drugs may add to an understanding of the patient's use of drugs. The family is recognized as an important institution for forming responsible citizens. Both family and peer group influence cannot be underestimated. Parents may abdicate their responsibility, or relate to their children in destructive ways. On the other hand, family authority may be strong and supportive to the patient and should be further supported by health team members. Peer groups are important, especially so for adolescents. Their influence may be positive or negative in relation to drug use. An important aspect of the nurse's assessment involves noting the patient's strengths, and the positive relationships which he has, and respecting and supporting these whether or not they conform to her own ideas of the "ideal family." For some young people, the greatest support and guidance comes from teachers; for others, a particular sibling or a particular pet may be especially loved and may provide companionship and affection.

Nurses can talk informally or formally with parents (or guardians) concerning the indiscriminate use of medications and about discussions with their children of their own medication use. This form of drug education for parents can take place at meetings of organizations, PTA meetings, churches, clinics, doctors, offices, and health centers.

**Social History.** Assessment should include information about the client's living conditions, work situation, and economic status. He is asked about his use of alcohol, tobacco, or other drugs, the use of sedation and/or stimulants, or vitamins. The nurse can get an idea of the context within which the person uses drugs, the regularity with which they are used, and the reasons for their use.

Frequently individuals may self-report drug use, or friends or relatives may provide this information. As part of the initial assessment, especially when drug use is confirmed, it is important to learn what was taken, when it was taken, and in what amount. This is crucial since appropriate intervention varies with each drug used.

**Past History.** Eliciting information about the person's past drug problems and complaints for which medications were sought is mandatory, particularly when such problems as insomnia or vague physical complaints are reported. It is also helpful to have the person describe his usual activities, both activities of daily living and recreation; how he responds to stressful situations; what his social activities usually are and note any changes over time. Looking for changes in behavior over time may give cues to possible drug use.

OBJECTIVE CUES. Among the objective cues which may be used by the nurse are the following:

**General appearance—Note any change in grooming habits**

**Eyes—Red, watery; pupils may be either dilated or constricted**

**Motor status—Lack of coordination; tremors**

**Level of consciousness—Drowsiness; decreased alertness**

**Verbal ability—Distortion in mood and thought patterns**

**Appetite—Extremes—either anorexia or craving for food, particularly sweets**

**Vital signs—Temperature, pulse, respiration, blood pressure (Table 11-3)**

**Gastrointestinal complaints—Abdominal pain; nausea; vomiting; constipation or diarrhea**

**Other signs—Skin: needle marks; tracking**

Continuing assessment is crucial, particularly with inpatients, to avoid accidental overdose by giving a prescribed tranquilizer, sedative, or narcotic to a person who may have been given a drug by a relative or friend. Accidental overdose has also occurred in emergency rooms in certain instances where drugs were given to a person with a history of drug use unknown to the health team. Hospitalization or institutionalization does not automatically cut the drug user off from his or her source of supply.

## Goal of Treatment

The nurse understands that she is part of a team the leadership of which varies as the individuals within the team bring their expertise to bear on the multifaceted problem of drug dependence. The team members should be clear on the goals of intervention which may vary from decreased drug use to abstinence, and may include improvement in functioning, vocational training and work, changing life style, increased level of wellness, and decreased involvement with legal authorities. Whatever the goal, it should be realistic, and may not initially include cure or immediate, total recovery.

**Table 11-3. Guide for Physical Assessment in Relation to Dependence on Harmful Substances**

| DRUG | EXPECTED EFFECTS | WITHDRAWAL SYMPTOMS |
|---|---|---|
| Nicotine | Increased pulse, heart rate<br>CNS stimulant<br>Relaxation<br>Increased alertness | Palpations, nervousness<br>Drowsiness, light-headedness<br>Fatigue<br>Headache<br>Insomnia<br>Constipation and/or diarrhea<br>Tremors |
| Alcohol | Drowsiness<br>Euphoria<br>Impaired reaction time and judgment<br>Impaired coordination | Delirium tremens<br>Insomnia, restlessness<br>Anorexia<br>Anxiety, fear<br>Terrifying hallucinations<br>Temperature elevation |
| Amphetamines | Elevated pulse and blood pressure<br>Elevated temperature with high doses<br>Dilated pupils<br>Feeling of excitement and increased energy and alertness<br>Euphoria<br>Decreased appetite<br>Insomnia; decreased fatigue<br>Tremors; dry mouth | Severe depression<br>Lethargy<br>Suicidal tendencies |
| Marihuana | Reddened eyes<br>Drowsiness<br>Increased appetite<br>Euphoria, increased sensory awareness<br>Clumsiness, ataxia | |

**Table 11-3. (Continued)**

| DRUG | EXPECTED EFFECTS | WITHDRAWAL SYMPTOMS |
|---|---|---|
| LSD | Distortion of sensory perception<br>Visual hallucinations<br>Dilated pupils<br>Increased BP and P<br>Tremors<br>Lack of coordination | Anxiety<br>Suicide potential<br>Dilation of pupils<br>Panic<br>Tachycardia<br>Possible flashbacks;<br>visual hallucinations |
| Heroin | Drowsiness<br>Euphoria<br>Decreased pulse and respiration<br>Pinpoint pupils | Increased TPR<br>Diaphoresis<br>Abdominal cramps<br>Muscle cramps<br>Diarrhea<br>Running eyes and nose<br>Restlessness;<br>insomnia<br>Dilated pupils<br>Yawning; sneezing<br>Nausea and vomiting<br>Tremors |
| Barbiturates | Sedation; relaxation<br>Dilated pupils<br>Decreased anxiety<br>Impaired judgment and memory<br>Lack of coordination<br>Euphoria<br>Sluggishness;<br>slowed reflexes | Insomnia; restlessness<br>Nervousness<br>Irritability<br>Hyperreflexia<br>Weakness<br>Tremors<br>Anorexia<br>Nausea and vomiting<br>Convulsions<br>Death |

# REFERENCES AND BIBLIOGRAPHY

Addicts treated with contract therapy, *Am. J. Nurs.* 73:1794, October 1973.

AMERICAN MEDICAL ASSOCIATION: Manual on Alcoholism, Chicago, American Medical Association, 1972.

BARBEE, E. L.: Marijuana—a social problem, *Perspec. in Psych. Care* 9:194, September-October 1971.

_____: The pros and cons of methadone maintenance, *J. Psych. Nurs. and Ment. Health Serv.* 11, 6:18-21, November-December 1973.

BIER, W. C. (ed.): *Problems in Addiction,* New York, Fordham University, 1962.

BLANE, H. T.: *The Personality of the Alcoholic,* New York, Harper and Row, 1968.

BLOCK, M. A.: *Alcohol and Alcoholism: Drinking and Dependence,* New York, Wadsworth, 1970.

BLUM, R. H., et al.: *Horatia Alger's Children: The Role of the Family in the Origin and Prevention of Drug Risk,* San Francisco, Jossey-Bass, 1972.

_____: *Society and Drugs: Social and Cultural Observations,* San Francisco, Jossey-Bass, 1969.

_____: *Students and Drugs,* San Francisco, Jossey-Bass, 1970.

BOWERS, M. D., and FREEDMAN, D. X.: "Psychedelic" experiences in acute psychoses, *Arch. Gen. Psychiat.* 15:240-248, September 1966.

BRECHER, E., and the editors of Consumer Reports: *Licit and Illicit Drugs,* Boston, Little, Brown, 1972.

BRILL, L., and LIEBERMAN, L.: *Major Modalities in the Treatment of Drug Abuse,* New York, Behavior Publications, 1972.

BRINK, P. J.: Nurses' attitude toward heroin addicts, *J. Psych. Nurs.* 11:7, March-April 1973.

CAMERON, D. C.: Narcotic drug addiction, *Am. J. Psychiat.* 119:793, February 1963.

CHAFETZ, M. E.: New federal legislation on alcoholism—opportunities and problems, *Am. J. Pub. Health,* LXIII, 3:206-208, March 1973.

CHAFETZ, M. E., et al: *Frontiers of Alcoholism,* New York, Science House, 1970.

CHAFETZ, M. E., and DEMONE, H. W., JR.: *Alcoholism and Society,* New York, Oxford University Press, 1962.

DOLE, V. P.: *Management of the Opiate Abstinence Syndrome. A Treatment Manual for Acute Drug Abuse Emergencies,* Washington, D.C., National Clearinghouse for Drug Abuse Information, Publication #16, 1974.

DOLE, V. P., et al.: Methadone treatment of randomly selected criminal addicts, *New Eng. J. Med.* 280: 1372, June 1969.

Drug abuse; everybody's problem, *Social Health Papers,* New York, American Social Health Association, 1973.

EINSTEIN, S., and GARITANO, W.: Treating the drug abuser: problems, factors and alternatives, *Int. J. Addictions* 7, 2:321-331, 1972.

FISHER, G., and STANTZ, I.: An ecosystems approach to the study of dangerous drug use and abuse with special reference to the marijuana issue, *Am. J. Pub. Health,* LXII, 10:1407-1414, October 1972.

FOREMAN, N. J., and ZERWEKH, J. V.: Drug crisis intervention, *Am. J. Nurs.* 71:1736, September 1971.

FORT, J.: *Alcohol: Our Biggest Drug Problem,* St. Louis, McGraw-Hill, 1973.

_____: *The Pleasure Seekers: The Drug Crisis, Youth and Society,* Indianapolis, Bobbs-Merrill, 1969.

GEARING, F. R.: *Methadone Maintenance Five Years Later,* Proceedings, Third National Methadone Conference, Napan, New York, 1971.

GLASSCOTE, R., et al.: *The Treatment of Drug Abuse: Programs, Problems, Prospects,* Washington, D.C., Joint Information Service of the American Psychiatric Association and the National Association for Mental Health, 1972.

*Guidelines for Drug Use Prevention Education,* Washington, D.C., Bureau of Narcotics and Dangerous Drugs, United States Department of Justice, January 1972.

GUILFORD, J. S., et al.: *Factors Related to Successful Abstinence from Smoking: Final Report,* Pittsburgh, American Institutes, 1966.

GOODE, E. (ed.): Marijuana, New York, Atherton Press, 1969.

HAGUE, SR. BETSY: In San Francisco's tenderloin, *Am. J. Nurs.* 69:2180, October 1969.

HARDY, R. E., and CULL, J. G.: *Drug Dependence and Rehabilitation Approaches,* Springfield, Ill.: Thomas, 1973.

HUEY, F. L.: In a therapeutic community, *Am. J. Nurs.* 71:926, May 1971.

HUNT, W. A. (ed.): *Learning Mechanisms in Smoking,* Chicago, Aldine, 1970.

JAFFE, J. H., SCHUSTER, C. R., SMITH, B. B., and BLACHLEY, P. H.: Comparison of acetylmethadol and methadone in the treatment of long-term heroin users, *J. Amer. Med. Assn.* 211:1834-1836, March 1970.

KEUP, W. (ed.): *Drug Abuse: Current Concepts and Research,* Springfield, Ill., Thomas, 1972.

KLEBER, M. D.: The New Haven Methadone Maintenance Program, *Int. J. Addictions* 5:449-463, September 1970.

KIMMEL, M. E.: Antabuse in a clinic program, *Am. J. Nurs.* 71:1173, June 1971.

KING, S. H.: *Youth in Rebellion, Drug Dependence,* Washington, D.C., National Institute of Mental Health, July 1969.

KNOTT, D. H., and BEARD, J.: *Diagnosis and Therapy of Acute Withdrawal from Alcohol; A Treatment Manual for Acute Drug Abuse Emergencies,* Washington, D.C., National Clearinghouse for Drug Abuse Information, Publication #16, 1974.

KOLANSKY, H., and MOORE, W. T.: Effects of marihuana on adolescents and young adults, *J. Psych. Nurs. and Ment. Health Serv.* IX, 6:9-16, November-December 1971.

KREPICK, D. S., and LONG, B. J.: Heroin addiction: A treatable disease, *Nurs. Clin. N. Am.* 8:41, March 1973.

LEWIS, P.: The role of the nurse in a drug crisis center, *J. Psych. Nurs. and Ment. Health Serv.* XI, 6:14-17, November-December 1973.

LONG, B. L., and KREPICK, D. S.: New perspective on drug abuse, *Nurs. Clin. N. Am.* 8:25, March 1973.

LOURIA, D. B.: *The Drug Scene,* New York, McGraw-Hill, 1968.

————: Lysergic acid diethylamide, *New Eng. J. Med.* 278:435, February 1968.

MANDEL, W., GOLDSCHMIDT, P., HICKEY, R. F., SCRIGNAR, C., and O'CONNOR, G.: *Inter-Drug: An Evaluation of Treatment Programs for Drug Abusers,* Baltimore, Johns Hopkins, 1973—O.E.O. Contract B2C-5409.

MILLSOP, M.: Occupational health nursing in an alcohol addiction program, *Nurs. Clin. N. Am.* 7:121, March 1972.

MORGAN, A. J., and MORENO, J. W.: Attitudes toward addiction, *Am. J. Nurs.* 73:497, March 1973.

MUELLER, J.: Treatment for the alcoholic: Cursing or nursing, *Am. J. Nurs.* 74, 2:245-247.

MUELLER, J., and SCHWERDFEGER, T.: The role of the nurse in counseling the alcoholic, *J. Psych. Nurs. and Ment. Health Serv.* 12, 2:27-31, March-April 1974.

NELSON, K.: The nurse in a Methadone maintenance program, *Am. J. Nurs.* 73:870, May 1973.

NYSWANDER, M. E., and DOLE, V. P.: Rehabilitation of heroin addicts after blockade with Methadone, *N.Y. State J. Med.* 66:2011-2017, August 1, 1966.

————: A medical treatment for diacetylmorphine (heroin) addiction, *J. Am. Med. Assn.* 193:646-650, August 23, 1965.

PILLARI, G., and NARIES, J.: Physical effects of heroin addiction, *Am. J. Nurs.* 73:2105, December 1973.

RANDALL, BROOKE PATTERSON: Short-term group therapy with the adolescent drug offender, *Perspec. in Psych. Care* XI, 3:123-128, 1971.

RUSSELL, M. A. HAMILTON: Cigarette smoking: Natural history of a dependence disorder, *British J. Med. Phys.* 44:9, 1971.

SHEFFET, A., HICKEY, R. F., LAVENHAR, M. A., WOLFSON, E. A., DUVAL, H., MILLMAN, D., and LOURIA, D. B.: A model for drug abuse treatment program evaluation, *Prevent. Med.* 2:510-523, 1973.

SMITH, D. E., and WESSON, D. R.: Diagnosis and Treatment of Adverse Reactions to Sedative-Hypnotics, National Institute on Drug Abuse, HSM-42-73-177, 1974.

*The Health Consequences of Smoking. A Report to the Surgeon General: 1971,* Washington, D.C., Department of Health, Education and Welfare, Public Health Service, Health Services and Mental Health Administration, 1971.

VAN DUSEN, W., and BROOKS, H. B.: Treatment of youthful drug abusers, *Mod. Hosp.* pp. 74-76, July 27, 1970.

WESTMAN, W. C.: *The Drug Epidemic,* New York, Dial Press, 1970.

WORLD HEALTH ORGANIZATION: *WHO Expert Committee on Addiction-Producing Drugs,* 13th Report, Technical Report Series No. 273, 1964.

YOLLES, S. F.: The drug scene, *Nurs. Outlook* 18:24, July 1970.

ZWICK, D., and BROWN, M.: Workshop on drug abuse, *Nurs. Outlook* 19:476, July 1971.

# Care of the Dying Patient

## CHAPTER 12

Care of the dying patient is a topic which has been long neglected by all health professionals. However, it is now receiving more attention, and the reader is referred to the bibliography at the end of this chapter for references on this important subject. Space limitation permits only a brief discussion here.

There are many indications that death has been a taboo subject in our society, much as sex was a taboo topic in the Victorian era. For example, euphemisms are widely used in place of the word "death," and great effort and expense are often employed to prepare and show the body of the deceased in a way which makes it appear that death has not occurred.

Many people have little contact with death occurring naturally in the home. Frequently death occurs among awesome equipment and busy physicians and nurses who may feel that the death of a patient signifies their failure as healers. In the hospital environment, death is seldom viewed and discussed as a natural and universal experience. The role of health workers in supporting the patient and his loved ones during this experience is often de-emphasized by the stress placed on details of therapy which, though necessary and important, do not convey human caring, and are often carried out in an impersonal and dehumanizing way.

It has often been noted that, although physicians are usually accorded the primary and sometimes the sole responsibility for deciding what and when the patient should be told about his illness, they may have severe problems in dealing with this aspect of patient care, due to their commitment to saving life.

Recently there has been renewed interest in providing hospices for care of dying patients, where emphasis is placed upon physical and emotional support of the patient during the experience of dying rather than upon cure, which is no longer a realistic goal.

## AWARENESS CONTEXTS OF PATIENT-STAFF INTERACTIONS

Greater concern is now being expressed about the patient's rights to know the truth, if he wishes to know, as well as the family's right to participate in decision making about what and how much to tell the patient (Elder, 1973).

Attitudes of falseness and denial interfere with provision of supportive care for the patient and his family. The patient whose illness is terminal is often dealt with by evasion and a false and superficial cheerfulness which he is usually quick to detect. Glaser and Strauss (1965) have described varied awareness contexts of patient-staff interaction:

- A closed awareness context, in which the staff knows the diagnosis and prognosis but the patient does not
- A suspicion context, in which the dying patient suspects the truth, while the staff acts as if recovery is anticipated
- A pretense context, in which patient and staff are aware of both the truth and each other's knowledge of impending death, but continue to act as if recovery will occur
- An open awareness context, in which patient and staff are aware of the impending death and discuss it openly

Family members often have little opportunity to discuss their feelings with nurses and physicians, and frequently they become involved in the suspicion and pretense contexts as a result of their own discomfort and lack of preparation for coping with death. Deception and pretense are potent stimulators of anxiety in human relationships, and the dying patient, because of his frailty and his need for emotional closeness, is especially vulnerable to anxiety arising from a sense that others are deceiving and evading him. He frequently perceives the fact of his approaching death, but must deal with it alone, further burdened by the falseness of others' communications with him.

Thus one of the most important contributions that the nurse and others can make is providing the opportunity for honest, open relationships. Not all patients, families, and staff are capable of such relationships; nevertheless, as in any crisis, the possibility of growth exists.

The nurse may avoid talking with the dying patient in any but a very superficial way, because she is uncertain about how she will respond when he asks The Question. Tension over this increases when the nurse (usually unrealistically) views herself as the only one to whom he can turn for help in dealing with his illness. Often the patient gradually recognizes clues in the behavior of others toward him that indicate that his illness is terminal. Thus the view of the dying patient as thoroughly unaware and seeking a disclosure from the nurse is often incorrect, and it greatly interferes with the nurse's relationship with him. When given the opportunity, dying patients often disclose awareness of their own approaching death by a remark about plans for providing for their children, leaving gifts for their families, and so on. When they reflect the patient's realistic assessment of his situation, such comments should be accepted rather than refuted. Sometimes no verbal reply is necessary, as acceptance is expressed nonverbally in the nursing care.

Although it is important for staff to communicate with one another in behalf of the patient, it is also important for individual staff members to establish their own unique relationships with dying patients. These relationships are often impeded by a preoccupation with finding out what others have told the patient and what others think the patient knows. As a result, receptivity and spontaneity toward the patient are often blunted by the suggestions and admonitions of others, making it impossible for the nurse to respond humanly and warmly to the patient.

Frequently conflict arises among those working with the patient, concerning what he should be told. For example, a clergyman may favor telling the patient, while the physician insists he not be told, and the family is undecided about which approach is preferable. It is usual for the nurse to be viewed primarily as carrying out the wishes of others, rather than as a member of the health team who contributes to making such decisions.

This situation is changing, however, as greater emphasis is placed upon sensitivity to the patient and upon the nurse's responsibilities as a professional. Sometimes the patient will openly state that he knows he is dying; sometimes he will convey this by making indirect statements which relate to his perception of his condition. For example, an elderly patient looked out at the trees during winter, just after an ice storm. He spoke sadly, saying that the trees were old, and that the weight of the ice was too heavy for them, and that they would soon break. He made no direct reference to his own situation. The nurse listened, sensing a sadness in the old man whose strength was waning.

Responsive communication with the dying patient must flow with what he is expressing. Thus, it is essential that professional persons caring for the patient and his family and friends respond in ways which are helpful to the patient. Elizabeth Kübler-Ross (1973) points out that patients will indicate what they know, what they want and are ready to be told, and from whom they seek help. When the old man spoke of the heavily burdened trees, the nurse planned to spend more time with him, because she heard his expression of feeling burdened, sad, and frail. The professional nurse's responsibility for her own actions in such situations is very great, and must be handled with skill and sensitivity. Her interventions must be guided by her level of skill and her experience.

Although death can occur in any clinical setting, it occurs most frequently on medical-surgical units and, of course, in geriatric services. In the past, most people died at home; death in the hospital was primarily the lot of persons who were destitute or without family to care for them.

## THE NURSE'S ROLE IN THE CARE OF THE DYING PATIENT

In this chapter we shall consider the nurse's role in the care of the dying patient, and some ways in which she can help him and his family during this significant experience. We shall consider the nurse's role primarily in relation to:

• Herself
• The patient
• Other patients on the ward
• The patient's family

### The Nurse's Understanding of Death

Because it is less usual in our society for neighbors and friends to gather round when death occurs —providing lodging and food for visitors, and companionship and support for the family—many persons have their first experience with death in the highly charged emotional situation of the death of a close relative.

Thus it is essential that the nurse consider her own views about death, and recognize that many of her patients and their families come to this experience quite unprepared to deal with it. For example the person whose only experience with death has been a visit to a funeral parlor, where someone has explained, "See, he is not dead; he is sleeping" is ill prepared for the reality of the change which occurs with the cessation of breathing and the sudden stillness of the patient who crosses the threshold between life and death.

The development of an individual's philosophy and religious beliefs concerning death, and of his ability to accept the reality of death is a lifelong process of personal growth. The individual who thought he understood his views on death may find that he has really hardly begun this process when confronted by the sudden death of his young wife. And, as he grows old and the time of his own death draws near, he is again challenged.

For the nurse and for all persons in the health professions, this process of personal growth is enhanced by their care of dying patients and their families. The nurse's ability to help dying patients and their families is based upon her own understanding and inner growth, and upon her own humility, recognition, and acceptance of death as part of life. Emphasis is upon recognition of what this experience means to the patient and to those close to him, upon helping them to express their thoughts and feelings, and upon supporting them as they pass through the various stages of the experience.

### Caring for the Dying Patient

Elizabeth Kübler-Ross (1973) has identified the following stages in the period preceding death: denial, anger, bargaining, depression, acceptance. However, not all patients have the emotional resources to pass through all these stages, and sudden death, of course, precludes a period of preparation for both the patient and those close to him. A supportive, close emotional relationship with at least one other person can aid the patient to make this transition.

Ronald Koening (1973) presents a different viewpoint. He believes that the issue of approaching death is less significant for many patients than the progressive loss of life as their disease progresses, and such experiences as pain, sleeplessness, anxiety, and depression take away the enjoyment of living. Koening stresses the importance of measures to preserve comfort and opportunities for enjoyment. His view of the period just prior to death is that it is usually less a stage of acceptance than one of emotional and physiologic bankruptcy: a point where there is nothing to be added, and nothing of significance left to be taken away. He believes that an important aim in the care of the patient is to postpone the arrival of this stage as long as possible.

The emphasis upon control and order, and the denial of nonrational and nonintellectual aspects of living so prevalent in our culture, further impedes work with dying patients. Too often dying patients are expected to conform to a model of passivity and gratefulness, when their grief, anger, and rebellion cry out for expression. Many of them turn inward, preoccupied with their thoughts and recollections. Kübler-Ross (1973) points out that a common "gut" reaction of staff when faced with a dying patient is "I hope he doesn't die on me." Thus, isolation due to the withdrawal of others from him is one of the most poignant problems of the dying patient.

The patient often indicates preference for certain staff members and certain "significant others" to be close to him when he is dying. His preferences should be respected. A particular nurse's aide, or a particular friend, may be the person toward whom he turns for closeness.

Three important aspects of nursing care of dying patients are: (1) supporting the patient as he begins to consider his approaching death; (2) fostering communication with the patient so that he does not face this experience in increasing isolation from others; and (3) talking with family members and with others who care for the patient, such as the physician and clergyman, concerning observations about the patient and plans for his care.

**Physical Comfort.** The patient requires thoughtful attention to his physical comfort: to position change, sips of fluids, if he is able to tolerate them, a quiet restful environment. Primarily, he needs consideration as a human being, in all the varied ways that this can be demonstrated through thoughtful care. He requires particularly to be protected from the routine, impersonal care which is typified by large numbers of health workers who arrive to take his temperature, provide a water pitcher, and so on.

Because the dying patient tends to become isolated from others, it is particularly important to spend time with him which is over and beyond that required for physical care and treatments. During this time the primary objective is listening to him and supporting him as he comes close to death.

**Spiritual Concerns.** It is also important to be sensitive to the patient's spiritual concerns and to help him obtain the religious counseling and rites which he wishes. If the patient is too ill to express his wishes, his family should be consulted concerning his spiritual care.

It is preferable for the clergyman to have the opportunity for contact with the patient over a period of time, rather than only at the time of death. Particularly when death approaches suddenly, it is helpful to remember that many clergymen will minister to any person during this crisis, not just to those of their own faith. Although each denomination has its own doctrines, it is also important to remember that patients respond individually to death. Thus, stereotyping a religious approach by saying, "This is the way Jewish people view death" denies the patient's individuality in the way he responds to his faith and to other factors which influence his response to approaching death.

The patient can grow as a person when he approaches death. His philosophical and religious views may mature; he may develop a broader view of his life as part of the cosmos, and his death as a natural event in the ebb and flow of life. He may experience a tenderness and closeness toward family and friends which he has not felt before. On the other hand, he may become progressively disengaged from others as death approaches. If so, his close associates may need help in understanding this change.

**The Need for Familiar Possessions.** Often the patient has a particular need for familiar and treasured possessions. It is especially important to keep such possessions near him. Pictures of loved ones and articles which are gifts from people he cares for may be especially precious to the patient at this time.

## The Other Patients on the Ward

Frequently the dying patient is placed apart from other patients. If there is no private room, he may be wheeled into a treatment room, or even into a hallway. Although such measures are often undertaken in the belief that the patient and his roommates will be more comfortable, this is not necessarily the result. It is preferable to discuss with the roommates their reactions to having the dying patient with them, and also to talk with the patient himself about moving him, if he is still aware of his surroundings and able to respond, rather than to move him suddenly without explanation or discussion. Such sudden transfers can arouse anxiety, both in the person who is moved and in his roommates. If the other patients are ambulatory, they often can be observed tiptoeing past a treatment room or hallway, looking in to see what is going on and how the ex-roommate is faring. Such actions showing concern, curiosity, and anxiety may be met with an abrupt pulling of the curtain by the nurse caring for the dying patient. Sometimes after death has occurred, all doors to patients' rooms are closed, without explanation, as the stretcher on which the deceased person is being wheeled to the morgue passes down the corridor. Patients' questions about what has occurred are often met evasively. When patients are quite certain what has happened, and ask the whereabouts of the patient when they see his bed is empty, it is preferable for the nurse to say calmly that he has died, and to make herself available to patients who want to discuss the fact that death occurred on the ward.

The important question for the nurse to consider is: "Do these approaches make the dying patient and other patients on the ward more comfortable and less anxious?" Responses are highly individual, and no one approach is suitable in all situations. If a dying patient's roommate is disturbed because of the patient's condition, or because of the frequent presence of visitors, it is best for him not to share a room with the dying patient. If, on the other hand, a close relationship has been developing between the two, both may prefer to continue sharing a room. Considerable support and comfort may be offered to the dying person by his roommate who, in turn, may grow in the process of offering such support.

### The Patient's Family

Families of dying patients particularly need the support that a nurse can give. Often their own process of grieving begins when they learn that the patient's illness is terminal. Some family members begin to withdraw emotionally from the patient at this time because they find the experience too painful. Others draw closer, realizing the shortness of the time left with the loved one. The family's feelings do not conform necessarily to others' idealized views of what these feelings should be. For instance, a family member may feel anger that the patient is about to leave

him. The more he can express his feeling to an understanding listener, the better, because it helps him to recognize the emotion, and to consider whether it is one which would be beneficial to share with his dying relative. He can thus avoid burdening the patient and he can free himself to relate as constructively as possible to the dying patient.

The possible harm from direct expression of feelings between relatives and the dying person is often overestimated. Family members may be so cautioned against showing any but cheerful feelings that they assume an air of false cheerfulness when visiting the patient, who, in turn, senses the "mask" and feels isolated from those to whom he turns for closeness. When the family member finally can no longer keep up the pretence, but shows grief, both the relative and the patient often experience relief at the honest communication between them. Of course this does not mean that it is helpful for family members to burden the patient again and again with their grief, or with their refusal to let him go when death is near.

Thus, a major problem among family members of dying patients in our culture seems to be the inability to communicate frankly with the dying person. The regret at tenderness unexpressed, and thereafter unable to be expressed, is one of the most poignant problems of grieving relatives. The nurse who can accept direct, straightforward communication from families can help them be more direct with the patient, thereby assisting them to have this enriching experience.

Perhaps nowhere is the stereotyped expectation of what the family *should* do and how it *should* react, so strong as it is toward relatives of dying patients. As a result, family members may have their opportunity to experience this significant event in their lives impaired by the expectations of others. The nurse should notice how the patient's relatives respond, and what they seem to want and need.

For example, one patient's husband may want to sit quietly with his dying wife most of the day. To argue with him that he should "get more rest" may be useless and irritating both to him and the nurse. Instead, it would be more helpful for her to provide him with an easy chair, encourage him to visit the coffee shop for nourishment, and help him to feel comfortable and accepted as he does what he shows he wants to do: remain with his wife. On the other hand, another husband may show that short visits are best for him, or may be all that is possible for him in light of responsibilities to others and to his work. It is important for the nurse to help him and his wife to have these short visits free of other interruptions: she should make a special effort not to schedule treatments during the husband's visit and to avoid conveying to him any attitude of "It's about time you came," or "Where have you been?" Some family members will openly express their grief—and it is helpful if they can do so to the nurse, in a private room or office. Others seem to need a "stiff upper lip" to cope with the experience. In either case it is important that the nurse respect the way the relative is dealing with the situation.

It is important for family to have some room near the ward where they can go and have privacy to talk with other relatives, to cry, and to rest. Such facilities are extremely limited, and often family members are seen standing for long periods in the corridor (while one or two relatives remain with the patient). Use every effort to find a place where they can have some privacy, and can be seated comfortably. Make frequent visits to them if they show they wish this contact. Just sitting with them for a short time and expressing concern for their comfort and welfare, and listening to some of their concerns, can bring comfort. The family frequently worries about how much the patient is suffering. It is helpful to explain that, as life ebbs, so usually does awareness of pain and discomfort. Thus, as the patient's death draws near, he may seem "detached," very often he slips into unconsciousness. It is then that the family's suffering is likely to be acute, although the patient's suffering is lessened.

Helping family members to express their emotions and, as much as possible, to understand what is occurring can help them bear their grief after the patient's death, and to recover from it. The nurse has many opportunities to gently assist the family to deal with the reality of death. For instance, if the patient's wife keeps calling to her husband who has just died, and trying to rouse him, the nurse can gently lead her away to a private room and stay with her. Often, after some brief agitation and denial, the relative will burst into tears, with the support of the nurse and her comforting presence.

When death has occurred, it is usual for the relatives or friends to leave the hospital at once. However, some may wish to remain for a time with the body of the deceased, and it is important to provide them a period of privacy before postmortem care is given. Particularly if only one friend or relative is present at the time of death, it is important to offer to stay with him for a time, before he leaves the hospital. If the individual seems very upset, it is important to suggest that he stay for a time until he feels calmer, or that he call a relative or friend to accompany him when he leaves the hospital.

## SUMMARY: ASSESSMENT AND INTERVENTION

Assessment of the dying patient includes such factors as:

- **His readiness to acknowledge that death is approaching**
- **His supports: for example, his religious views, his close ties to others**
- **His life situation: whether he is responsible for care of others, such as children; whether he has adequate income to provide for his own care, and, if necessary, for others who survive him**
- **His physical condition: for example, skin, hydration, appetite, sleep, pain**
- **His emotional response: for example, depression, anger, acceptance**
- **His family's (or other significant person's) response to his approaching death**
- **The response of the health team to the patient, and the effect of this response upon the patient (i.e., closed awareness; open awareness)**

Nursing intervention includes such considerations as:

- **Relief of pain**
- **Adequate provision of fluids and other nourishment**
- **Provision for elimination, possibly involving care of urinary catheter, use of suppository or enema**
- **Provision of a quiet, supportive environment**
- **Cleanliness, skin care, prevention of decubitus ulcers**
- **Responding to the patient in ways which help relieve his anxiety, lessen his loneliness, and help him to cope with the experience**
- **Assisting family members to deal with their own relations and also to support the patient**
- **Collaborating with others on the health team in behalf of the patient, and assuming professional responsibility for one's own actions in relation to physical care, communications, and dealing with family**
- **Recognizing the patient's preferences concerning who is with him, and facilitating the presence of these people with the patient**

## REFERENCES AND BIBLIOGRAPHY

AVORN, J.: Beyond dying, *Harper's Magazine* 246, 1474:56, March 1973.

BROWNING, M. H., and LEWIS, E. P.: *The Dying Patient: A Nursing Perspective,* New York, Am. J. Nurs. Co., 1972.

BURNSIDE, I. M.: You will cope, of course, *Am. J. Nurs.* 71:2354, December 1971.

DAVIS, B. A.: Until death ensues, *Nurs. Clin. N. Am.* 7:303, June 1972.

DOMMING, J. J. et al.: Experiences with dying patients, *Am. J. Nurs.* 73:1058, June 1973.

DRUMMOND, E. E.: Communication and comfort for the dying patient, *Nurs. Clin. N. Am.* 5:55, March 1970.

ELDER, R.: Dying in the USA, *Int. J. Nurs. Stud.* 10, 3:171, August 1973. Condensed and Reprinted in *Nurs. Digest* 2, 5, May 1974.

ENGEL, G. L.: Grief and grieving, *Am. J. Nurs.* 64:93, September 1964.

FEIFEL, H. (ed.): *The Meaning of Death,* New York, McGraw-Hill, 1959.

FLETCHER, J.: Ethics and euthanasia, *Am. J. Nurs.* 73:670, April 1973.

FRENCH, J., and SCHWARTZ, D. R.: Terminal care at home in two cultures, *Am. J. Nurs.* 73:502, March 1973.

GLASER, B. G., and STRAUSS, A. L.: *Awareness of Dying,* Chicago, Aldine, 1965.

HENDIN, D.: *Death as a Fact of Life,* New York, W. W. Norton, 1973.

HISCOE, S.: The awesome decision, *Am. J. Nurs.* 73:291, February 1973.

KASTENBAUM, R., and AISENBERG, R.: *The Psychology of Death,* New York, Springer, 1972.

KAVANAUGH, R.: Helping patients who are facing death, *Nurs. '74* 4:35, May 1974.

KOENIG, R.: Dying vs well-being, *Omega* 4, 3:181, 1973. Condensed and Reprinted in *Nurs. Digest* 2, 5, May 1974.

KÜBLER-ROSS, E.: Letter to a nurse about death and dying, *Nurs. '73* 3:11, October 1973.

_____: Dying with dignity, *Canad. Nurse* 67:31, October 1971.

_____: *On Death and Dying,* New York, Macmillan, 1969.

_____: What is it like to be dying? *Amer. J. Nurs.* 71:54, January 1971.

KUTSCHER, A. H. (ed.): *Death and Bereavement,* Illinois, Thomas, 1969.

MEAD, M.: The right to die, *Nurs. Outlook* 16:20, October 1968.

MITFORD, J.: *The American Way of Death,* New York, Simon and Schuster, 1962.

PARKES, C. M.: *Bereavement Studies of Grief in Adult Life,* New York, International Universities Press, 1972.

PEARSON, L. (ed.): *Death and Dying,* Cleveland, The Press of Case Western Reserve University, 1969.

QUINT, J. C.: *The Nurse and the Dying Patient,* New York, Macmillan, 1967.

QUINT, J. C., STRAUSS, A. L., and GLASER, B. G.: Improving nursing care of the dying, *Nurs. Forum* 6:369, 1967.

RAMSEY, P.: *The Patient As a Person,* New Haven, Yale University Press, 1970.

SCHOENBERG, B., et al.: *Loss and Grief: Psychological Management in Medical Practice,* New York, Columbia University Press, 1970.

SHUSTERMAN, L. R.: Death and dying—a critical review of the literature, *Nurs. Outlook* 21:465, July 1973.

SOBAL, D. E.: Death and dying, *Am. J. Nurs.* 74:98, January 1974.

SPITZER, S., and FOLTA, J.: Death in the hospital—a problem for study, *Nurs. Forum* 3:85, 1964.

WALKER, M.: The last hour before death, *Am. J. Nurs.* 73:1592, September 1973.

WEBER, L.: Ethics and euthanasia: Another view, *Am. J. Nurs.* 73:1228, July 1973.

# Nursing in
# Accident and Disaster

The nursing care of the patient who has sustained an accident or has been a victim in a disaster involves the same process as that involved in the care of patients with any other condition—assessment, inference, nursing diagnosis, goal setting, intervention, and evaluation.

There are notable differences, however. Because care needs arising from accident and disaster are often urgent, the mental operations of the nursing process must be performed rapidly, and intervention must be swift and sure to avoid further trauma or delay. Often the setting for action is lacking in support equipment, materials, and personnel, and improvisation becomes a factor in the problem-solving approach. Jurisdictions for practice are blurred also; it is in the interest of the patient and community that the best trained, most competent persons on the scene administer first aid or emergency care until such time as the patient can be transported to a hospital or physician's office for further assessment and care. Firemen, policemen, and other trained paramedical rescue workers, together with nurses and physicians, form an emergency care team for the benefit of the individual and the community.

A major role of the nurse in accident and disaster is in the assessment of hazardous situations and in taking action to prevent the occurrence of personal or community accidents or disasters.

## INCIDENCE OF ACCIDENTS

Deaths from accidents in the United States are exceeded only by deaths from the major cardiovascular diseases and cancer.

It is estimated that in the United States in 1972, accidents took over 117,000 lives. Of these, over 56,500 were killed in automobile accidents, others at home or at places of employment (*Statistical Bulletin,* January, 1973).

Notably, almost one-half of all accidental deaths involved motor vehicles. For all ages combined the death rate in 1969 due to motor vehicle accidents among white males was 40.0 per 100,000 in the United States as compared with 14.6 for white females. The death rate from motor vehicle accidents reaches a peak in the age range 15 to 24; with advancing age, motor vehicle accident deaths diminish; among the elderly falls become the leading type of accident fatality (Table 13-1) (*Statistical Bulletin,* June 1973).

**Table 13-1. Mortality from Leading Types of Accidents by Age and Sex in the United States, 1969**

| TYPE OF ACCIDENT | DEATH RATE PER 100,000 UNITED STATES* | | | | | |
|---|---|---|---|---|---|---|
| | ALL AGES | UNDER 15 | 15-24 | 25-44 | 45-64 | 65 AND OVER |
| **MALE** | | | | | | |
| Accidents—All Types | 77.4 | 29.2 | 115.4 | 75.9 | 82.0 | 172.8 |
| Motor vehicle | 40.0 | 11.9 | 82.0 | 42.7 | 36.0 | 55.0 |
| Falls | 8.6 | 0.9 | 2.0 | 3.5 | 10.1 | 65.3 |
| Drowning† | 4.5 | 4.9 | 8.3 | 3.1 | 2.7 | 2.9 |
| Industrial type | 5.5 | 1.7 | 5.6 | 7.5 | 8.5 | 6.5 |
| Fires and flames | 3.4 | 2.1 | 1.4 | 2.5 | 5.5 | 11.5 |
| Water transport | 1.5 | 0.4 | 2.0 | 2.3 | 2.0 | 1.3 |
| Poisoning by solids and liquids | 1.6 | 0.4 | 2.8 | 2.0 | 1.7 | 2.8 |
| Poisoning by gases and vapors | 1.1 | 0.2 | 1.7 | 1.5 | 1.5 | 1.4 |
| Firearms | 1.8 | 1.1 | 3.5 | 1.7 | 1.7 | 1.3 |
| **FEMALE** | | | | | | |
| Accidents—All Types | 29.8 | 16.7 | 28.3 | 20.1 | 29.9 | 120.6 |
| Motor vehicle | 14.6 | 7.9 | 23.1 | 13.1 | 15.3 | 24.7 |
| Falls | 6.3 | 0.5 | 0.3 | 0.7 | 3.6 | 70.9 |
| Fires and flames | 2.0 | 1.7 | 0.6 | 1.2 | 2.9 | 6.6 |
| Poisoning by solids and liquids | 0.9 | 0.3 | 0.5 | 1.2 | 1.8 | 1.2 |
| Drowning** | 1.0 | 1.8 | 0.7 | 0.5 | 0.6 | 0.8 |
| Poisoning by gases and vapors | 0.3 | 0.1 | 0.6 | 0.3 | 0.4 | 0.5 |
| Industrial type | 0.5 | 0.6 | 0.2 | 0.3 | 0.5 | 1.2 |
| Water transport | 0.1 | 0.1 | 0.2 | 0.2 | 0.1 | 0.1 |
| Firearms | 0.2 | 0.2 | 0.4 | 0.2 | 0.2 | ** |

* White population.
† Exclusive of deaths in water transportation.
** Less than 0.05.
Source: Reports of the Division of Vital Statistics, National Center for Health Statistics, June 1973.

One point of view among those who are studying accidents is that accidents are not an inevitable penalty of life or necessarily due to bad luck or chance. Investigators are applying epidemiologic research

attitudes and techniques to the problem in the search for prevention. Many accidents are caused by taking a chance "this once"—running the speedometer to 70, balancing on a rickety chair just a moment to hang a picture, going out in a sailboat without a life jacket. Why are these "just once" chances taken? Why are seat belts installed but not used? What are the many factors that make an automobile crash? Why do people fall?

Accidents do not stem from a single cause. Usually, they are the outcome of many complicated interrelated factors, which may include environment, relationships between people, and an individual's emotional state.

The many and complex factors contributing to accidents are only beginning to be understood. Some of them are subtle. An individual does not have to be in the grip of obvious anxiety or conflict to permit unsafe conditions to exist which, intellectually, he knows are hazardous. For example, a nurse who was very concerned about safety in hospitals permitted an electric cord to stretch across the center of the floor in her apartment. Such reluctance on the part of an individual to consider his own vulnerability to harm may be one aspect causing accidents.

Some feel so hopeless that efforts to prevent accidents do not seem worthwhile. For example, the community health nurse may be shocked to discover that some poverty-stricken families allow hazards to exist that they could easily rectify. However, the feeling of rejection by society, the pressure of poverty, and the lack of opportunity can be so oppressive that people become apathetic.

## SAFETY IN THE HOME

Nurses can help to increase the awareness of dangers at home and to recommend safer living conditions. More accidents occur at home than anywhere else. The National Safety Council and other governmental agencies have focused attention on accidents related to home components, those features attached with a relative degree of permanency to a building. Injuries are most frequently associated with stairs, and in descending numbers with tubs/showers, nonglass doors, windows and glass doors, and burns from hot water in bathrooms (*A Design Guide for Home Safety,* pp. 1-2).

Suburban living has its own hazards, particularly since the advent of the "do-it-yourself" movement.

A rotary power lawn mower sends a rock through the air like a lethal missile. A man falls off a ladder while he is painting his house. A person, ignorant of electrical matters, tries to fix faulty wiring and receives an electric shock or starts a fire.

The nurse gives counsel on ways to avoid accidents. For example, nurses are called upon to teach proper precautions in relation to medications kept at home, to prevent small children from getting hold of them, and to prevent mistakes by adults. Similarly, advice on the storage of potentially dangerous household chemicals can be provided by nurses. Examples of other areas of accident prevention include:

- Prevention of severe lacerations from glass doors, either storm doors or shower doors. The nurse should be able to point out the need for special safety glass in these doors and should be able to supply the name and address of a dealer who can furnish them.
- Proper design of basement stairs. Today, many have an angle of 45 degrees, inadequate handrails, and steps that are too narrow. As a result, many falls result in serious or fatal injuries. Nurses can help educate the public on the need for a moderate slope, wide steps, and adequate handrails.
- Safeguards in the use of home electrical appliances and proper grounding of home power tools to prevent electrocution.
- Improving safety of bathtubs and showers with nonskid surfaces and adequate hand grips.
- Provision of safe toys for children.

## Falls

Stairs should be well lit, have adequate banisters, and be free of such obstructions as children's toys. In order to see better where he is going when he is carrying a bundle up or down stairs, a person should rest it on his hip rather than hold it in his arms. Scatter rugs should have nonskid pads under them, and floors should not have such a high polish that they are slippery. Nonslip pads in bathtubs and handrails nearby help to prevent skidding with wet feet. A night light or a flashlight should be available within an arm's reach of every bed. Frills on aprons are dangerous in small kitchens. Sharp tools, especially kitchen knives, should be in racks to avoid cutting fingers reaching into a drawer.

These precautions are particularly important when there are persons in the home over 65. Elderly people, who tend to have poor neuromuscular coordination, lapses in memory, poor vision and hearing, are more prone to accidents in the home than younger adults. A new pair of glasses may help to prevent a fatal accident.

## Fire

Smoking presents a special hazard, and each year many fires are started by the careless use of cigarettes and matches. Smoking in bed is dangerous, especially after drinking. In addition to other common-sense precautions, every home (and car) should be equipped with strategically placed fire extinguishers.

## Gas Poisoning

Gas poisoning is another major domestic hazard. Carbon monoxide, a colorless, odorless, and tasteless gas resulting from incomplete combustion of carbon and its compounds, is the major cause of home gas poisoning. It is dangerous in concentrations of more than 0.06 per cent. This gas is produced wherever internal combustion engines are operated, and it is given off by cooking-gas flames and all devices, such as heaters and lanterns, that burn gasoline or kerosene.

Gas poisoning can be prevented by the use of properly installed and maintained equipment. Soot, rust, and gum should be removed from all gas-burning appliances. Flues in coal or oil-burning heaters should be checked regularly to make sure that they are not clogged. Kerosene room heaters should not be used without chimney connections. The exhaust system in cars should be checked regularly for defects. Adequate ventilation in both cars and rooms should be available in all weather. A window should be open a little at all times. The motor of a car should not be run in a closed garage. Some automobile accidents are believed due to carbon monoxide seeping into a moving car and affecting the driver's reflexes, alertness, and judgment.

Because carbon monoxide has a much greater affinity for hemoglobin than does oxygen, it replaces oxygen in the bloodstream, which then becomes oxygen-poor. There is considerable variation in individual response to the accumulation of carboxy-hemoglobin; the patient may simply lose consciousness, or he may complain of headache, dizziness, muscular weakness, and visual disturbance before the loss of consciousness. He may appear pale or cherry-red in color. Activity increases the demand for oxygen, thus further endangering the patient. Coma and death may follow.

The patient should be moved to fresh air, and if he is not breathing, mouth-to-mouth resuscitation should be started. Since the inhalation of pure oxygen speeds the release of carbon monoxide, an inhalator for administering oxygen should be obtained. A mixture of oxygen and 5 per cent carbon dioxide is helpful, since the carbon dioxide stimulates the respiratory center. Hyperbaric oxygen therapy may be used. The patient should be kept quiet to avoid further depletion of his oxygen supply. In cases of severe poisoning, the patient is hospitalized for observation. Dizziness, headache, muscular weakness, sensory disturbances, disorientation, restlessness, and paralysis may be symptoms. Since some of these may be delayed, the patient should be watched carefully. There may be residual cerebral disability due to insufficient oxygen to the brain.

## Chemical Poisoning

Carbon tetrachloride, a common household and industrial chemical, is extremely poisonous. Any concentration high enough to be smelled is dangerous. It produces severe and even fatal liver damage and should not be kept in the home or garage at all. Cleaning agents and fire extinguishers containing carbon tetrachloride should be avoided or eliminated. Hydrogen sulfide, the gas which gives rotten eggs their smell, is extremely dangerous in high concentrations and has killed sewer workers in a matter of seconds. Oxides of nitrogen, found sometimes in silos, have resulted in the death of several farmers and those trying to rescue them. A single deep inhalation can produce fatal lung injury. Farmers should know about the dangers of silo gases and if one is overcome in a silo, rescuers should not enter unless they are wearing special gas masks; ordinary respirators and gas masks are not adequate. Benzene is another dangerous chemical which should not be used in or near homes. Its fumes can cause severe and fatal blood disorders as well as other disorders. Insecticides, pesticides, herbicides, and other gases and vapors which are sprayed can be highly dangerous and should only be used by those trained in the proper procedures, and with adequate safeguards against contaminating others as well as the operator. In general, any foreign material should be considered potentially toxic and excessive inhalation avoided. Even hair sprays have produced serious lung illness in hairdressers and women who used them to excess.

## GENERAL PRINCIPLES OF FIRST AID

First aid is not the amateur practice of medicine; it consists of measures that keep the patient alive and prevent further damage until definitive medical treatment can be initiated.

The right kind of first aid depends on the situation; judgment in an emergency is made after a systematic rapid assessment of the patient in the particular situation. The ability to make accurate judgments and perform appropriate interventions under stressful circumstances develops after acquiring knowledge, applying it, and evaluating one's performance as an individual and team participant in a number of similar situations.

Suppose a man's entire left leg, back, and hands are burned. What is done depends on where the accident happened and on the availability of medical care and hospitalization.

If the above-mentioned patient was burned at a gasoline station in the middle of town, the approach would be to summon an ambulance and prevent contamination of the burns or further trauma; if the accident took place deep in the woods on a camping trip the approach would be to apply pressure dressings (clean and, if possible, sterile), encourage the patient to drink an electrolyte solution (one teaspoon of table salt and one-half teaspoon of bicarbonate of soda or baking soda to one quart of water), prepare a makeshift stretcher, and transport him.

Important general principles of first aid deal with physiological priorities:

- Bleeding is stopped.
- An airway is established and cardiopulmonary resuscitation is initiated after assessment of need.
- A sucking wound of the chest is covered at once and kept sealed though sterile materials are not available —even the hand can be used. Seconds can make the difference between life and death.
- Medical help is obtained as rapidly as possible. If there is to be a long time lag before the patient will be treated by a physician, decisions and techniques may be necessary that usually are in the medical domain. But after first aid and stabilization measures are completed, the patient should be transported to a medical facility as rapidly as is consistent with safety. Many communities have first aid or rescue squads; some have mobile emergency hospital units with radio and telemetry systems that allow for medical consultation while enroute to the hospital. Some states have enacted laws which permit paramedical personnel to administer therapies enroute as ordered by the physician. The police can always be called for assistance or direction.

A patient is not moved unless he is further endangered by staying put (for example, if he is on a cliff, in danger of falling, or if he is on a railroad track that may be used). A minor injury can become a major one when the patient is moved incorrectly. The rule is to keep the patient lying flat but with an open airway until he is seen by a physician, or until a plan to move him has been evolved on the basis of the nature and the extent of his injuries. If the patient must be moved immediately, he is handled as gently as possible, with his body kept as straight as possible. Any injured parts are handled as little as possible. Enough help should be obtained to ensure the patient's and the rescuer's safety. Sometimes, in the excitement of the moment, people forget others are around, and they try single-handedly to move a heavy person.

A systematic assessment for injuries is made after stopping the patient's bleeding and establishing respiration and circulation. A very dangerous wound may be tiny and hidden by clothing. There might be a small puncture wound in the chest that penetrates to the pleura. An abdominal wound or hidden bleeding also could be present.

Almost all emergency conditions entail some degree of shock, so chilling should be avoided. The patient should not become overheated because excessive heat can increase shock.

Each injury is considered as maximum. If one sees blood, one thinks of hemorrhage. If one suspects a sprain, it is splinted as a fracture. If the patient feels faint, he is treated as if he were in shock. Nothing is lost by caution, and an injury actually may be more serious than it looks.

The patient is not given anything to drink or to eat until the full extent of his injuries has been diagnosed by a physician. This rule can be broken if there is a long delay between the time of injury and the medical attention. However, an unconscious person is never given anything to drink, and an injured person is never given an alcoholic beverage. Alcohol acts as a vasodilator, so that heat loss from the body is increased, thus increasing shock; and vasodilation increases bleeding.

The patient is attended until a physician or ambulance arrives, unless there are a large number of casualties who must also receive help.

Further injury is prevented by transporting the patient flat and carefully, and by a trained person taking command over untrained persons who might harm the patient.

- The physician is told concisely and accurately what happened, what injuries are suspected, and what first aid was given. This information can be written if necessary, and the note attached to the patient in such a fashion that it cannot be missed, such as by pinning it on the patient's shirt, coat, or dress. If pencil and paper are lacking, imperative facts can be written on the patient's forehead with lipstick. "T 3:30" would warn the physician to look for a tourniquet, and it would tell him what time it was applied.

Every emergency is psychologically traumatic. The very suddenness of becoming a casualty is shocking. A sense of security is conveyed to the victim by the manner of rescue workers who may not feel calm but who demonstrate calmness. Fear and con-

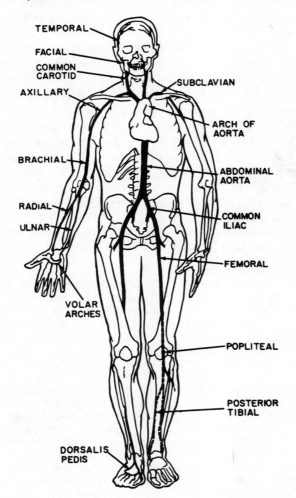

**Figure 13-1.** Arteries that may be palpated (except the aorta and the common iliac) and compressed. The dotted line on the left leg indicates that the arteries travel along the back of the leg.

TEMPORAL
FACIAL
COMMON CAROTID
AXILLARY
SUBCLAVIAN
ARCH OF AORTA
BRACHIAL
ABDOMINAL AORTA
RADIAL
ULNAR
COMMON ILIAC
FEMORAL
VOLAR ARCHES
POPLITEAL
POSTERIOR TIBIAL
DORSALIS PEDIS

fusion can be minimized by a sense of teamwork; the patient is directed how to help with specific directions, for example, "Don't try to move your leg. I'm going to put a splint on it. The ambulance is on its way, and I'll stay with you until it comes. You'll soon be in the hospital where the physician can find out exactly what is wrong." A patient or bystander is not told what the diagnosis might be, but the message is conveyed to him that the situation is under control.

The principles of crisis intervention in psychological emergencies are described in Chapter 6 (Nurse-Patient Relations).

## FIRST AID IN VARIOUS EMERGENCIES

### Hemorrhage

The bleeding source is located and stopped quickly. Most people can tolerate the loss of a pint of blood, but losing a quart or more leads to shock. A patient can hemorrhage to death in less than one minute from a large artery that is severed, but most bleeding can be stopped by pressure and elevation. To control bleeding, direct continuous pressure is applied on the wound, which usually will stop the hemorrhage. A sterile bandage, a clean handkerchief, a piece of cloth, or bare hand if necessary can be used. Or, pressure is applied on a major artery leading to the wound. The artery is pressed against the bone. The part is elevated (Fig. 13-1 and Fig. 13-2).

The American Medical Association advises that a tourniquet should be applied only for an amputated, mangled, or crushed extremity. It is tightened enough to stop the bleeding. A note is written stating that a tourniquet has been applied. The tourniquet should be loosened every 20 minutes to allow blood to flow to the part. Since a tourniquet may mean the loss of the part distal to it because of reflex arterial spasm, one is applied *only* when all other measures have failed to stop the hemorrhage, and only when the arm or leg already is missing, crushed, or mangled.

### Cessation of Respiration

This condition may be due to drowning, electric shock, carbon monoxide or other gaseous poisoning or to disease. Treatment must be begun at once.

Mouth-to-mouth breathing is the most effective method of resuscitation. Properly performed, it can maintain in good physiologic condition a patient

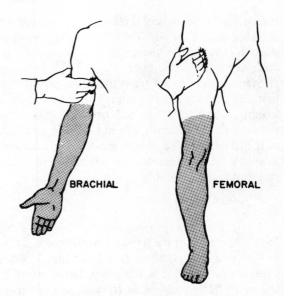

**Figure 13-2.** Methods of occluding the brachial and femoral arteries to control bleeding from injuries in the shaded areas. Pressure is applied to artery and bone behind it.

who is not breathing for himself. Speed in initiating the procedure is important.

The airway is cleared. An obstruction in the mouth, the trachea, or the bronchi will prevent ventilation of the lungs. The inside of the patient's mouth is wiped with a handkerchief. If it is necessary, the victim is turned on his side and sharply slapped on his back. This procedure may dislodge an obstruction in a bronchus. The tongue must not obstruct the airway.

The patient's nose is pinched so that the air blown into his mouth does not escape.

The rescuer takes a breath, and blows into the patient's mouth until the chest rises. A rush of expired air is heard while the rescuer takes his next breath. The relaxation of the chest wall is observed. The patient's lungs are reinflated as soon as his expiration is complete. About 12 respirations a minute are given.

If some air is being blown into the stomach it can be expelled by turning the patient's head to one side and exerting gentle pressure just below the diaphragm. The rescuer must be careful not to take such large breaths that he becomes dizzy, because artificial respiration may be necessary for hours. Breaths are just deep enough to inflate the patient's lungs. There is enough oxygen in such breaths for victim and rescuer. Artificial respiration is continued until the patient breathes for himself or is declared dead by a physician. When the patient does start to breathe for himself, he is watched continuously for at least one hour.

Many people recoil from this close physical contact, and more so if the patient is old or looks unkempt. A thin cloth placed between the rescuer's mouth and the patient's will not impede ventilation.

If a double-ended plastic airway (Resuscitube) is available, it can increase the efficiency of artificial respiration considerably.

## Shock

The patient is kept lying flat with his feet 8 to 12 inches higher than his head (unless there is dyspnea in this position). If there is a head injury, the patient is kept flat. He is not permitted to exert himself at all. He should be as still and as quiet as possible. Excessive heat induces vasodilation which can increase shock so the patient is kept warm, not hot. Hot-water bottles are not used and sweating is not produced because valuable electrolytes and water are lost in perspiration. Nothing is given by mouth unless there will be a long interval between the time of injury and the time of medical attention. If this is the case, the patient may be started on sips of water unless vomiting occurs. If sips of water are tolerated, an electrolyte solution made up of one teaspoon of table salt and one-half teaspoon of bicarbonate of soda (or baking soda) to one quart of water may be given. Fluids are not given to an unconscious patient, or to one with a head injury or an abdominal wound, or to any patient who will receive medical attention within two hours.

## Electric Shock

When a person is in contact with a live conductor of electricity, another can become a part of the circuit while attempting to rescue him. The rescuer should avoid standing on a wet surface and a dry, nonconducting object—for instance, loose clothing or a piece of wood—should be used to push or to pull the person away from the conductor. The skin of the victim is not touched directly; otherwise, the rescuer may become a victim.

A severe electric shock results in cardiac arrest from ventricular fibrillation. The only definitive treatment for this is electric defibrillation. If a defibrillator is not immediately available, the patient must be given mouth-to-mouth respiration and closed chest cardiac compression while being transported to the nearest treatment facility.

## Wounds

Unless a sterile bandage is available, most wounds should be uncovered and left exposed to the air until they are treated surgically. Clothing is cut away so that threads do not fall into the wound; the patient is exposed as little as possible. The wound is not washed or cleansed with antiseptic, or anything else. If the patient has to be transported, the wound is dressed with a sterile bandage until it can be seen by a physician. A chest wound should be assumed to communicate with the pleural cavity, and it should be covered with an airtight seal. If no adhesive tape is available, the wound is covered with the hand. If tape is available, a sterile gauze or a clean handkerchief can be placed between the wound and the tape. Evisceration of intestine through an abdominal wound should not be pushed back inside the abdominal cavity. The wound is covered with a wet gauze or handkerchief (sterile, if it is available, or as clean as possible).

If there are several casualties, the patient with a penetrating abdominal wound receives first priority in removal to a hospital. If a physician arrives at the scene, his attention should be directed to this patient first. If the patient with an open wound will not be seen by a physician for many hours, the wound can be flushed with sterile water and covered with a dry sterile dressing.

## Snakebite

In the United States there are several types of poisonous snakes. Some (rattlesnakes, copperheads, cottonmouths and water moccasins) are classified as pit vipers; the other is the coral snake. Pit vipers have a deep pit between each eye and nostril. Coral snakes in this country have brilliant red, yellow, and black bands that encircle the entire body. They can be distinguished from nonpoisonous snakes by noting that their red rings are always bordered on both sides by yellow, and by remembering this ditty,

*Red to yellow kill a fellow;*
*Red to black venom lack.*

If a patient has two small puncture wounds close together, it can be assumed that he has been bitten by a poisonous snake. If in doubt, first aid should be given as if the snake were poisonous, and the snake identified (or at least described). Its size, color, design, and the shape of its head are noted.

Even an apparently dead snake can bite, and most have enough poison to harm a second victim, so care should be used in handling or examining the snake.

Persons bitten by snakes native to the United States usually recover, but the bite may be fatal, depending on the size and the type of snake and on the amount of venom that has been injected into the patient. Ten to 35 per cent of snakebites are fatal (Hornibrook, 1956). In all likelihood the person who is bitten will be extremely apprehensive.

First aid is directed toward removing as much of the venom as possible and preventing the spread of the venom throughout the patient's body. A tourniquet is applied above the wound (Fig. 13-3). This tourniquet should be tight enough to occlude venous and lymphatic circulation, *but it should not be so tight that there is no pulse.* Speed is important; the quicker the tourniquet is applied, the less venom will be circulated throughout the patient's body. Every 10 or 15 minutes the tourniquet is moved up just above the progressively swelling area. With a razor blade or other clean sharp instrument, a crisscross incision is made into the wound. The incision should go through the skin but not the underlying muscle. The wound is suctioned by syringe or suction cup, if available; otherwise, by mouth. Venom is not toxic when it is ingested (but what is suctioned by mouth is spit out); this technique is not dangerous unless the rescuer has a cut on his lips or mouth. Suctioning is continued until nothing more can be extracted from the wound. Then the patient is transported to a physician, Poison Control Center, or other medical care facility.

Contrary to popular opinion, whiskey is not "snakebite medicine." Antivenom is the only specific medication. Because it is made from horse serum, many people are allergic to it. The physician also will give an antitetanus injection.

Snakebite kits include a tourniquet, suction cup, razor blade, antivenom powder, iodine, a vial of sterile water, and instructions. One should be taken on camping trips in snake country and high boots should be worn in areas inhabited by snakes.

## Animal Bites

Bites from any warm-blooded animal must be regarded as potential rabies threats and must be reported at once to a local health officer who will specify the treatment to be used. As a first aid meas-

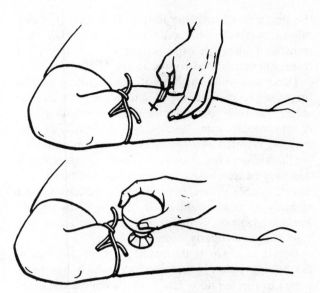

**Figure 13-3.** First aid for a poisonous snake bite. A tourniquet is applied proximal to the wound, a crisscross cut is made into it, and suctioning is instituted. A suction cup such as this one is included in snakebite kits.

ure, thorough washing with either tincture of green soap or benzalkonium chloride solution (1:100 or 1:1,000) *but not both* is helpful. There should be a predetermined policy at each emergency room for handling animal bites.

## Poisoning

There are so many agents that are poisonous that it is impossible to discuss all of them here. The nurse should be familiar with the location and operation of the local Poison Control Center and call promptly when she needs advice. Such centers are usually associated with the emergency room of a centrally located general hospital. Exhaustive up-to-date files are kept on many poisonous household products and other poisonous agents. A wide range of appropriate therapeutic agents are kept ready for emergency use by specially prepared staff. If the necessary information is not available at the local center, the physician can call a regional office or the National Clearing House for Poison Control Centers and obtain vital information in a matter of minutes.

**Food Poisoning.** Food poisoning can be caused when food is contaminated with such organisms as *Staphylococcus aureus, Clostridium botulinum,* and *Clostridium perfringens.* The toxins produced by the organisms cause the illness. In infection transmitted by food, the food serves as a vehicle that transfers pathogenic organisms (such as *Salmonella*) from a contaminated source to the victim.

Food poisoning may be of nonmicrobial origin, for example in cases of contamination by insecticides. Naturally toxic plants, such as certain strains of mushrooms, some berries, and some wild plants, may be ingested through accident or ignorance.

*Clostridium botulinum* produces a neurotoxin that may cause nausea and vomiting, headache, lassitude, double vision, muscular incoordination, and inability to talk, swallow, or breathe. This organism, an anaerobe, is found most often in foods that have been improperly canned at home.

Botulinus toxin is destroyed by heat just below the boiling point; therefore, food which has been boiled in the previous few hours is considered safe. However, the *spores* of botulinus are not killed by boiling, even for hours. Therefore, food which is boiled and then kept in closed containers for several days can be lethal. Botulism can also be acquired from improperly cured sausage and fish. Ordinarily, this bacterium doesn't grow in a highly acid medium, so most fruit preserves are quite safe. Any can which is swollen or seems to contain gas should be discarded unopened. Foods suspected of being contaminated should not be tasted. There have been some deaths from a single taste. Smoking, salting, marinating, and drying food do not necessarily kill the spores of *Clostridium botulinum*.

Botulism is treated with antitoxin, a positive-pressure respirator, and intravenous therapy. Early treatment is important; the mortality rate is about 65 per cent. Death often is due to respiratory failure (Dolman, 1964).

Staphylococci grow in food, especially creamed food that has not been sufficiently refrigerated. Symptoms may include weakness, diarrhea, nausea, vomiting, and abdominal cramps that develop a few hours after ingesting the contaminated food and last for a day or two. Death is rare. Food poisoning may not be recognized until the food is absorbed, and the patient has symptoms, usually diarrhea and vomiting. The patient is kept quiet, and medical help obtained as quickly as possible. Parenteral fluids and sedation may be given. To prevent food poisoning, nurses should teach the importance of cleanliness in food preparation, and of prompt and adequate cooking and refrigeration. For example, in preparation for a picnic, the arrangements must include refrigeration. Sometimes food such as potato salad is prepared in large quantity and left out of the refrigerator for hours before it is consumed because of lack of room on the shelves. This is a dangerous practice.

**Drug Poisoning.** Drug poisoning in adults results sometimes from suicide attempts, from drug abuse, and sometimes from the theory that if one pill is good, several must be better. Drug poisoning may or may not be recognized promptly. It is important to discover what the patient ingested. If the patient is conscious, he is asked or the container is located, the label is read, and its antidotal instructions, if any, are followed. Burns on the mouth suggest a corrosive acid or alkali. If the container is not found immediately, an attempt is made to dilute the poison by giving the patient (if he is conscious) as much milk or water as possible. Rapid action is important.

Vomiting is induced unless the poison is ammonia, or a strong acid or alkali (which burn tissue on contact), or any petroleum product, such as gasoline, lighter fluid, or kerosene. Vomiting is not induced in these instances because of the danger of aspiration. Vomiting should not be induced if the patient is already comatose or convulsing. If the patient complains of severe pain or a burning sensation in his mouth and throat, vomiting is not induced.

The breath is smelled for fumes. If no burns and no fumes are noted, vomiting is induced by putting a finger down the patient's throat or by making him drink copious amounts of water to which has been added several tablespoonfuls of bicarbonate of soda. The patient's head is turned to one side while he is vomiting; every precaution is taken to avoid aspiration. After he has vomited, more antidote is given (if it is known), or (if it is not known) four egg whites in a glass of milk, or two teaspoonfuls of flour or any other starch in a glass of water or milk may be given. Alcohol is not given.

Transportation to a hospital is arranged. If the container is found, it should be saved. If not, a specimen of the patient's vomitus is saved. If the patient urinates, a specimen is obtained for analysis. The observation of vital signs and the prevention of chilling are important first aid measures.

If the poison has been absorbed, the first aid is suggested by the symptoms. For instance, if the patient is not breathing, mouth-to-mouth breathing is started. If he is convulsing, the aspiration of saliva must be prevented and the patient kept free from further harm. If an overdose of barbiturates has been taken, the patient should be kept aroused; however, any exertion that may tire him unnecessarily must be avoided. Black coffee can be given to the patient if he is conscious. He should be transported to the hospital as rapidly as possible. Urinary amount, if any, is estimated. The patient who develops kidney shutdown may be placed on dialysis (see Chap. 64). If the drug poisoning is due to a suicide attempt, it is not usually helpful to discuss this with the patient, nor to try to reassure him by saying, "Everything will be all right." He should be assured that the nurse is interested in caring for him, and that she is taking adequate steps for his safety. After the patient is in the hospital, he needs to be attended constantly, for he may attempt suicide again.

A form of poisoning which is becoming more common is due to a combination of alcohol and sleeping pills (usually barbiturates). Moderate amounts of the two taken close together can be fatal. Patients with prescriptions for barbiturates should be warned not to take alcohol and barbiturates within two hours of each other.

**Gas Poisoning.** When gas poisoning is suspected, the patient is removed from the area of the fumes. If he is overcome at home, windows are opened and the patient removed from the room. If he is not breathing, mouth-to-mouth resuscitation is started while awaiting an ambulance with oxygen and resuscitation equipment. The patient must be hospitalized as rapidly as possible.

## Exposure to Temperature Extremes

**Heatstroke (Sunstroke).** In this disorder, the body's normal responses to increasing temperature are not functioning. The patient feels dizzy, weak, and nauseated, and he may have a headache, but but there is no perspiration. The skin is red, hot, and dry to the touch. There may be convulsions or collapse. Without treatment the patient probably will die.

The immediate first aid measure is to cool the patient. He is removed from the sun and sponged with cool water. If he is conscious, he may have cool drinks. If ice is available, it can be put in packs and placed on forehead, axillae, and around the body and the legs. Cold water can be poured on the patient, or he can be fanned or put into a cool tub. The temperature is taken frequently, and cooling is continued until his fever is down to about 101 degrees F. Sustained high fever will result in brain damage. These patients need hospitalization even if they respond to first aid measures. The patient may have a lifelong problem with heat regulation after an episode of heatstroke, possibly necessitating a move to a cooler climate or the regulation of his life so that he is not exposed to heat for long periods of time.

**Heat Exhaustion.** This disorder is characterized by circulatory disturbances brought about by an excessive loss of salt and water by prolonged sweating. The patient feels dizzy and faint, and he may have headache, muscle cramps, and nausea. In contrast with heatstroke, the skin is pale and damp. Uncorrected, the condition leads to collapse, but it usually is possible to rouse the patient.

Heat exhaustion is treated as if it were shock, except that it is necessary to cool the patient. Water with one teaspoon of table salt in each glass is given. To relieve muscle cramps, firm pressure is applied against the muscle with the flat of the hand. Heat exhaustion often can be prevented by taking adequate salt and water during a time of excessive exposure to heat and by observing such common-sense precautions as avoiding strenuous exertion and wearing suitable clothing. At times, patients may have a combination of heatstroke and heat exhaustion, and the physical signs may not be as distinct as descriptions suggest.

**Overexposure to Cold.** The patient is warmed as quickly as possible. Gradual warming is not necessary.

**Frostbite.** Severe cold causes injury to tissues; frostbite is a degree of cold injury. There is extreme vasoconstriction and thrombosis, as well as direct injury to the walls of the blood vessels and the cells. Exudate escapes from the damaged vessel walls, resulting in edema. There is ischemia of the tissues, and the skin blanches. The frostbitten part becomes numb and stiff. As it warms, it turns a bright pink and blisters.

Experience in World War II and the Korean War showed that the previously common practice of slowly warming a frostbitten part causes more tissue damage than rapid warming.* The affected part is bathed in comfortably warm water for 10 minutes. The temperature of the water must be com-

---

* Bureau of Medicine and Surgery Syllabus of Lesson Plans for Teaching First Aid, NAVMED P-5056, Under the Authority of the Secretary of the Navy, Washington, D.C., 1957.

fortable for the patient. The patient tests it; water that may feel warm to normal skin may feel hot to frostbitten skin. After bathing, the skin is blotted dry and a dry sterile dressing is applied using sterile gauze to separate skin surfaces. The part is elevated. It is not rubbed with snow or anything else, and cold water or cold air is not permitted to touch it. Hot-water bottles and heat lamps should not be used. If legs or feet are involved, the patient should not walk. Frostbitten fingers or hands can be wrapped in warm covering, such as wool, or placed in the patient's axillae while he is being transported.

When the patient arrives at a treatment center, therapy includes rest with the part elevated. Debridement and grafting may be necessary. Because deep circulation is less affected than is superficial circulation, this surgical treatment usually is effective.

The degree of injury varies in severity. In mild cases, recovery is complete. In severe cases, amputation may be necessary. Patients who have been severely frostbitten may, for years afterward, experience numbness and tingling when the affected part is exposed to cold. Patients are advised to protect the affected part in the future from injury or exposure to cold.

Prevention of frostbite includes:

- Avoiding skin contact with the $CO_2$ in fire extinguishers.
- Avoiding constricting clothing, such as shoes and socks that are too tight, or the use of circular garters in cold weather—these further impair blood supply to the part.
- Keeping the entire body as warm and dry as possible when in extreme cold.
- Teaching persons likely to be affected, such as skiers, to exercise legs, feet, arms and fingers if they are in a situation likely to cause frostbite.
- Teaching persons vulnerable to frostbite to observe each other's skin for the development of yellow-white patches (on the ear lobe for example) and to heed such sensations as pricking or pain, which may herald frostbite.

## FIRST AID IN MINOR EMERGENCIES

### Fainting

A momentary deficiency in cerebral oxygenation causes fainting. It can be distinguished from other forms of unconsciousness by its temporary nature. Usually, the patient regains consciousness as soon as he has attained a horizontal position.

If a person feels faint, he should lie down flat, without a pillow. Tight clothing is loosened around the neck and the waist. Falling must be prevented when possible, since the injury sustained by the fall may be far more serious than the faint. If the patient cannot lie down, he should sit down and put his head between his knees. He should be seen by a physician to determine the cause of the fainting.

### Sunburn

A first-degree burn may be soothed by cool compresses. The skin is handled gently to avoid further trauma. Blisters should be dressed with sterile gauze. They should not be punctured. If the burn is extensive, medical treatment must be obtained.

### Bites and Stings

**Ticks.** A tick is killed with a few drops of turpentine, or touched with a hot needle to make it release its hold. Then, using tweezers, it is removed very gently from the skin. A tick is not crushed since this could transmit to the patient virulent pathogenic microorganisms which some ticks carry. Excessive force is not used in trying to remove a tick. The area is scrubbed with soap and water.

**Bees, Wasps, Hornets.** The stinger is removed with a sterile needle or tweezers (only honey bees shed their stinger). An icebag and baking soda compress (one tablespoon per quart of water) is applied to reduce the swelling and the itching. If the person is allergic to the sting of that insect, the sting may be fatal. Any symptoms of allergy after a sting demand immediate medical attention.

**Poisonous Spiders, Tarantulas, and Scorpions.** Death of a healthy adult from spider bite or scorpion sting is rare, but the symptoms can be extremely painful. Deaths have occurred in children and in adults in a weakened condition. The best known toxic spider is the black widow, which secretes a neurotoxin. This spider is a shiny black color with a red to orange hourglass on its *ventral* surface.

A less well-known spider is at least as dangerous. The brown recluse spider originally was reported in Missouri but seems to have spread throughout the continental United States. It is somewhat smaller than the black widow, and ranges from light tan to dark brown in color. It has a banjo-shaped spot on its *dorsal* surface. The brown recluse is a shy animal and is usually hidden from view. It bites when it feels trapped. Unfortunately, it sometimes lives in old clothing or shoes kept in a garage or basement. When a person tries to put these garments on, the spider, presumably in self-defense, bites. The initial bite is seldom painful and often is unnoticed. The toxin, however, contains an extremely potent digestive enzyme, and after a few hours, it destroys a large amount of tissue, leaving an open wound which may not heal for many months. Secondary infections can ensue. For this reason, a report of a spider bite must be taken seriously, even if there is no pain, and no initial evidence of toxicity. If possible, the spider should be identified. If this cannot be done, any person bitten by a spider of unknown species should be referred to a physician for immediate observation and definitive management. A spider bite should not be incised by a first aid worker (as is done with snake bites). The incision is likely to do little good, if any, and may cause a serious infection. For temporary relief, cold applications to the bitten area are helpful, but freezing of tissues must be avoided. There are specific medical treatments for black widow spider bites, including the intravenous injection of calcium gluconate and the use of an antivenom. Thus far, there is no antivenom available for brown recluse spider venom, but one may be developed. The part should be kept lower than the rest of the body for several hours.

The tarantula, a giant spider of fearsome appearance, has venom of such low toxicity that it poses no danger to human beings. Unfortunately, the appearance of the spider, and its use in several movies and television programs as a symbol of great danger, may produce undesirable psychologic effects in someone who has been bitten. The victim, who may have seen even the valorous James Bond cringe before a tarantula, is not likely to accept the nurse's reassurance that he is in no danger. Accordingly, in such situations, the use of some harmless procedure to relieve the patient's concern or terror is advisable. A paste made of bicarbonate of soda and water placed over the bite can be reassuring. The patient is in much greater danger from his own fear than he is from the bite. The nurse, aware of this, should show concern and attention to the bite and its treatment but avoid communicating her own fear, which she may have, to the patient.

Scorpion stings are often painful, but the scorpions found in the United States can rarely produce lasting harm to an adult. Cold applications are helpful until the patient is seen by a physician.

## Hiccups (Singultus)

Hiccups are caused by recurrent spasms of the diaphragm. They can usually be cured by breathing into a paper bag, accumulating carbon dioxide (but *not* a plastic bag). Sometimes, drinking water while holding the nostrils closed will stop the attack. If hiccups persist more than 30 minutes after these maneuvers have been tried, a doctor should see the patient.

## Other Emergencies

Other emergencies are discussed throughout this book and include:

Acute Alcoholism. See Chapter 11.
Allergy. See Chapter 9.
Burns, See Chapter 65.
Cardiovascular. See Chapters 34, 38, 61, and 62.
Convulsions. See Chapter 23.
Diabetic Acidosis and Insulin Reaction. See Chapter 50.
Epistaxis. See Chapter 28.
Insects in the Ear. See Chapter 27.
Foreign Bodies in the Eye. See Chapter 26.
Fractures. See Chapter 19.

## SAFETY IN THE COMMUNITY
### Automobile Accidents

Motor vehicle accidents have killed more people in America than have all the wars we have fought since the Revolution. Over 5,000,000 people are injured every year by motor vehicles. Proper use of seat belts would save many lives. The belts should be worn whenever the car is moving. Most fatal accidents occur within a 50-mile radius of the victim's home and at relatively low speeds. The lower belt should be snug over the bony prominences of the pelvis; the upper belt diagonally across the chest. Both are needed. Over 70 per cent of the injuries are to the head and face (Perry, 1964). Chest injuries are the next most common, then abdominal, and then limb. Sixty-six per cent have multiple injuries.

Because of the numbers of serious accidents and deaths to children riding in automobiles, it is recommended that postpartum patients be educated *before* leaving the hospital on the proper automobile transportation of infants and children. Children should *never* be held on the driver's lap. A sudden stop or minor collision can throw the driver's body forward, crushing the child against the steering wheel.

Presently, the lap-shoulder combination seat belt is the best restraint system available. One regional study showed that this combination significantly reduces maternal injury and consequently fetal death because ejection from the car, which is the greatest threat to both mother and fetus, is virtually nonexistent. Thirty-three per cent of ejected women and 47 per cent of fetuses died, whereas when mothers were not ejected maternal deaths occurred in only 5 per cent of cases and fetal deaths in 11 per cent. (*Emergency Medicine,* October 1972).

Authorities have found that the frequency of injury was reduced from 75.5 per cent to 29.9 per cent with the use of seat belts (Braunstein, 1957). If the person is thrown out of the car, the chance of death is 5 times greater than if the person stays inside (Money, 1961). Other preventive measures include: properly designed and approved child safety car seats, knowledge of and compliance with traffic regulations, adequate locks on all car doors, unobstructed vision, a well-padded dashboard with no projecting objects, no driving after drinking, and defensive driving.

## Other Community Safety Needs

Nurses are expected to exercise leadership in community action to reduce the toll of accidents and disasters. The particular problems will vary with the community, and some examples are:

- Adequate tornado and hurricane warning systems.
- School design to provide safe shelter to students in the event of a tornado.
- Safer roads.
- Keeping concentrations of explosive and inflammable materials at a safe distance from schools, homes, and other areas where there are many people.
- Safe use of farm equipment.
- Promotion of driver education courses.
- Adequate sanding of icy streets and sidewalks.
- Appropriate safety precautions for swimming pools, lakes, and rivers. With the increase in home swimming pools there has been an increase in broken necks and paraplegia in vigorous adults from dives into too shallow water.

At the national level, nurses, as individual citizens and as members of their associations, should give effective support to laws and regulations designed to reduce the toll of accidents and disasters. Examples include regulations on automobile design, safer highways, gun control, hurricane and tornado warning networks, tornado-resistant construction of public buildings, and safe transportation of inflammable, explosive, and poisonous materials.

Industrial nurses can help to locate health hazards and to educate employers and workers in the use of safety practices and devices; school nurses are in an excellent position to teach children about safety — crossing the street, not playing with matches, and washing before eating. School nurses have multiple opportunities to work with parents, both in individual conferences and in groups. Any nurse can be called on to consult with groups interested in making their environment safer.

Perhaps a nurse is asked to speak at a club or a fraternal group meeting or to instruct boy scouts, girl scouts, 4-H clubs or community action groups. Some resources that may be helpful are:

- Life insurance company publications on various aspects of accident prevention
- Publications of the National Safety Council and American Red Cross
- The local Community Nursing Association
- Various local official bureaus, such as the Health Department, the Department of Sanitation, and the Fire Department, and university Cooperative Extension Divisions
- The handbook, *Control of Communicable Diseases in Man,* American Public Health Association, New York, 11th edition, 1970

### Medic Alert

Nurses can foster safety also by participating in health education programs that help patients learn self-care and what to do in an emergency. Community agencies can be better prepared to help in an emergency if they have vital information. For example, a patient with a hidden medical problem that should be known in an emergency, such as an implanted pacemaker, allergy to penicillin or tetanus antitoxin, diabetes, or Addison's disease can become a member of the MEDIC ALERT Foundation International, Turlock, California 95380, for a small fee. The patient wears a MEDIC ALERT emblem on a bracelet or neck chain which has on it the Central Answering File telephone number and the patient's major problem(s).

## NURSING DURING DISASTER
### The Problem

Many of the problems of a natural disaster (flood, hurricane, and so on) are identical with the problems of a man-made disaster (fire, war, and so on). In both types of catastrophe, a sudden, unexpected event leaves behind it injured people and animals, damaged property, and overall confusion. Also, each type of disaster has its own special hazard, sometimes foreseen and sometimes not. In flood, there is danger of typhoid; in fire, of burns; in nuclear war, of radiation sickness. Because of the sudden and heavy strain on existing medical facilities, advance preparation and planning are necessary to avoid needless death and suffering. In any type of disaster there may be more wounds than there are bandages to bind them; there may be more victims dying of asphyxia than there are first aid workers to resuscitate them; there may be more shock than there are physicians or nurses to treat it.

In this country more than 1,500 persons died during 1972 in catastrophic accidents (i.e., accidents taking five or more lives), and thousands received injuries. The loss of life was due to mainly natural disasters such as hurricanes, tornadoes, and floods, accidents in mines and quarries, railroad and civilian aviation accidents, fires, and motor vehicle accidents (*Statistical Bulletin,* January 1973).

Disaster nursing includes the care of others besides the injured. For example, Hurricane Agnes, which in June 1972 raged up the eastern coast and caused the most extensive floods in the nation's history, caused 122 deaths, but thousands lost their homes and possessions and were forced to live in emergency shelters for considerable periods of time. This living in temporary quarters created health problems in which nursing services were essential for the welfare of these people.

Some rules for survival that apply to any type of disaster are:

- Preparation—planning what to do if and when the event occurs
- Forewarning—recognition that danger is imminent
- Prevent secondary disaster, when possible, and further casualties—past secondary disasters have included epidemics, crashes of rescue vehicles, and fires
- Communication—coordination of disaster units
- Application of disaster plans
- Transportation—making it possible for essential equipment and personnel to move quickly and efficiently
- Continued care for the injured after the emergency is over
- Proper care of the dead
- Restoration of normal living conditions

## Principles of Disaster Nursing

One of the largest problems of the nursing profession in any disaster is how to make the most efficient use of both skills and time. There probably will be more casualties needing immediate attention than the number of trained medical personnel will be able to care for—more casualties than available time, equipment, and facilities can handle. Even under normal circumstances, one severely burned patient admitted to a surgical or an emergency ward can tie up supplies and personnel for hours. In a major disaster, hundreds or thousands of patients will be classified as urgently injured.

The following principles apply to all types of disasters: floods, fires, hurricanes, earthquakes, tornadoes, and war.

- The most efficient possible use must be made of each person's hands, feet, brains, energy, and time. There will be limited personnel and many casualties, and therefore every movement must count. Nonessential work, such as putting the room in order, or rescue work that lesser prepared individuals can do, should be delegated.
- The unexpected can be anticipated. There will be noise, and probably confusion, lack of absolutely essential supplies and facilities, despair and panic.
- Supplies must be utilized economically. When they run out, the basic principles of sterile technique, anatomy, physiology, and first aid must be considered as improvisations are made. For example, if no commercial splints are available, anything that is stiff enough and long enough can be used.
- Nothing should be done to make a casualty less able to care for himself.
- The three cardinal rules of first aid apply to disaster nursing: establish respiration, stop hemorrhage, and care for shock. Also, in order of importance are these principles: save life, preserve function, give comfort, preserve cosmetic appearance.
- Nursing will be performed under unfamiliar circumstances. The specific details may have to be changed from nondisaster hospital nursing, but the basic principles will remain the same. In a major disaster, nurses may have to make decisions and carry out techniques that usually are in the province of physicians, such as delivering babies, dressing wounds, and immobilizing fractures.

Perhaps the most difficult adjustment nurses have to make in major disasters is a change of nursing philosophy from "first priority of attention to the most seriously ill" to "first priority of attention to those most likely to benefit from treatment." This philosophy means that nurses must steel themselves to give their time to the patients with a chance for survival instead of attending the sicker patients who unfortunately probably will die anyway.

The decision as to which category a patient falls into is made by the most experienced skilled health worker present. Even then, it is impossible to be correct in every case, and some patients with a good chance of survival if operated upon may be placed in the group which is given a low priority—the "expectant" group. A nurse placed in charge of such a group must always be on the alert for evidence which would justify a patient's reclassification. If she encounters such evidence, it is her responsibility to notify the senior team member at once.

- Although speed in disasters is important, haste should not make nursing practice unsafe. Actions should be timed at an efficient rate. Priorities are acted on—putting out a fire, controlling hemorrhage, isolating the patient with symptoms of infection.
- If not wearing a uniform, a nurse should improvise an alternative form of identification.
- Other potential sources of danger such as buildings about to crumble, a leaking gas line, fire about to break out, or shattered glass nearby should not be overlooked.
- All patients should be tagged with the following information: the name, the address, the location of the casualty during the disaster, the medications given, and the type of injury. Tags can be made from paper or adhesive tape.
- Those who can care for themselves, but not for others, should be moved rapidly out of the confusion and away from the casualties who need care, preparatory to transport to a welfare center. The elderly should be kept out of the chaos as much as possible, since they tend to become confused. Separating young children from their parents should be avoided. Older children, perhaps eight years and up, may be put to work if there is adequate supervision for them. Although they cannot carry stretchers and should not be asked to do tasks that require judgment beyond their years, they may be valuable, for example, in running errands, carrying supplies back and forth, and serving drinks to workers and selected groups of casualties.

## Triage

This is the name given to the sorting of casualties so that the greatest number will receive the best care possible. Triage allows for the most efficient use of time, personnel, and supplies. Suppose there are five injured people, one physician, and one nurse. The injured are:

Mr. A has over 85 per cent third-degree burns.
Mr. B has 35 per cent second- and third-degree burns.
Mr. C has multiple lacerations without hemorrhage.
Mr. D has a fractured clavicle.
Ms. E has a traumatic amputation of the leg and is bleeding badly.

How can the two do the most for this group? To save lives, in what order should first aid be applied?

Who should be given priority for transport to a hospital? The grouping of the patients may be as follows:

- *The immediate treatment group* includes those patients who need and will respond to immediate treatment. This group, which receives first priority of attention, includes patients with reversible shock, respiratory defects, hemorrhage, severe lacerations, compound fractures, and burns of 15 to 40 per cent of the body surface. Ms. E and Mr. B belong in this group.
- *The minimal treatment group* includes those who, after receiving treatment that requires minimal time, can return to work or can care for themselves. Mr. D would be in this category. So would other patients with simple fractures, and those with 10 per cent or less burns of the skin, but not of face or hands.
- *The delayed treatment group* includes those casualties who will not die if treatment is delayed (although their wounds may become infected). This group includes patients with long bone fractures, moderate lacerations without hemorrhage, second-degree burns on less than 30 per cent of the skin and third-degree burns on less than 20 per cent, and noncritical central nervous system injuries. Mr. C would qualify for this group.
- *The expectant group* includes those who are so severely injured that only with prolonged and complex hospital care is there any chance for survival, if then there is a chance. Included in this group are patients with irreversible shock, severe burns, and critical injuries of the central nervous system and the respiratory system. Although these patients receive lowest priority for surgery and transport, there may be time not to neglect them entirely. With a minimum expenditure of time, they can be made as comfortable as possible. Mr. A would be in the expectant group. If he is not already unconscious from shock, perhaps he would be given morphine to relieve pain, but he would be given no other treatment.

Such groups are not stable. The classification is a continuing process, dependent on alterations in the availability of physicians, supplies, operating rooms, and time, and on the changing status of the patient's condition. The first reasonably healthy person on the scene makes decisions about first aid. In the example of the five casualties, the highest priority should be given to controlling Ms. E's hemorrhage. The first physician on the scene makes the decision about immediate treatment and the order in which the patients should be transported. If there is no physician, a nurse may have to decide. At aid stations and again at hospitals the casualties are re-evaluated and reclassified.

Another aspect of triage is the grouping of similar types of casualties. For example, placing patients with burns in one group and fractures in another simplifies care and is economical with regard to both time and supplies.

## Psychological First Aid

*Disaster fatigue* is a term that may be used to describe the psychological disorders resulting from a major disaster. For anyone directly involved in a catastrophe, preoccupation with self, disbelief in the situation, weakness in the knees, sweating, and transitory suspension of the usual adult functions are expected and not abnormal responses. In addition, every person will react according to his own past experiences, his preparation and practice in meeting emergency situations, his personality patterns, and what he has at stake during the emergency.

In any disaster it is important for those who are still able to function to recognize the types of psychological reactions that the shock can cause. The following are fairly common reactions:

- Depression. The depressed person seems to be numb, slowed, stunned, unable to talk, to take action, or to assume responsibility for himself. This kind of apathy is the most common reaction to disaster.

    Depression often is a first stage in a syndrome of reaction, followed by a period of suggestibility, gratitude for help, but low efficiency. This second stage may last several days. The third stage is characterized by a feeling of euphoric brotherhood between the sufferers, and enthusiasm for making plans for rebuilding. In the fourth stage, there is a sense of loss and dissatisfaction with the handling of the disaster (Garb and Eng, 1969).
- Hyperactivity. This person responds to extreme anxiety by talking too much, moving too fast, joking too loudly (without real humor). He is unable to resist distractions, and he jumps from task to task. He is incapable of listening to the ideas of others or of taking directions.
- Panic. This is highly emotional behavior caused by the belief in an *immediate,* severe threat, resulting in actions that increase rather than decrease the danger for the individual and for others. Panic results from the following conditions:
    1. Belief in a danger in seconds or minutes.
    2. A limited number of escape routes.
    3. Belief that the escape routes are closing but not yet closed.
    4. Absence of effective leadership.

    Panic must be distinguished from fright, which is usually a rational protective action.
- Hysterical conversion. This is a psychiatric term meaning a reaction in which the casualty subconsciously converts his anxiety into a physical symptom. Examples are blindness, deafness, and paralysis. The

patient is unaware of the process of conversion. He knows only that he cannot see, hear, or move, and he assumes that he has physical injuries.
- Disaster fatigue cases may be classified according to their severity:
    1. Mild. These are the people whose self-concern interferes with effective action.
    2. Moderate. These people have decreased ability to communicate verbally, and they are unable to concentrate and to carry through on a job.
    3. Severe. These people are out of contact with reality.

Experience with previous disasters suggests that there will be a ratio of 10 to 25 fatigue casualties to every 100 physically injured. Of these fatigue casualties, 50 to 75 per cent are likely to be mild, 30 to 40 per cent moderate, and 1 to 3 per cent severe (Am. Psychiat. Assoc.). In the less severe degrees, disaster fatigue will respond to first aid; in severe degrees, further treatment will be necessary in a clinic or perhaps in a psychiatric hospital. The object of the first aid is to help those who are mildly or moderately affected to return to effective action promptly, and to make those who are severely affected as comfortable and as safe as possible until more comprehensive care can be arranged.

A first step in psychological first aid is talking to the affected person. He should be asked what happened—to provide data useful in planning care and to give him an opportunity to share his feelings. If only three minutes are available to a person, those moments should be his alone. A drink of water, a rest, and a chance to talk things out are helpful. A question about his usual occupation may give a clue to what he can do to help. As he starts to function again, he helps himself. A job at which he can have success may increase his ability to become self-directing, more confident, and more in control. This first aid may make the difference between a person who is so upset that he requires care and a worker who is contributing his skill and energy.

Some general principles of psychological first aid for disaster fatigue are:

- Factors such as level of anxiety, denial of reality, confusion should be assessed.
- Nonverbal communication is often more important than what is said.
- An individual's limitations should be accepted as real. It is ineffective and a waste of time to have the attitude, "Why should he act so distressed when we are all in the same boat?"
- The *panicky* individual must be quickly identified and segregated because panic is contagious. He

should know that a prompt recovery is expected. A way should be found to utilize his abilities. If this technique fails, he should be kept segregated by assigning one or two other people to stay with him, and made as comfortable as possible until he can be transported to a destination where he can receive medical attention.

- Contact should be established with the *overactive* person. His attention can be gained by listening briefly to his ideas, and steering him into a useful job.
- The *depressed* patient needs an interested helper who will encourage him to do simple tasks that may help to restore his sense of purpose.
- A person who has *hysterical conversion* can be provided comfort and safety until he can be transported. If he is able to work, jobs that he can do are beneficial to him and others.
- Pity should not be shown for casualties suffering with disaster fatigue, no matter how pitiable the situation is, because sensing this emotion in others will only confirm a victim's fears of inadequacy.

Nurses have limits of physical and emotional stamina. There will be more to do than any one person can do; urgent things must receive attention but goals unrealistically high should not be set.

Provision must be made for rest and rotation of all workers, including nurses.

## Supervising Others

The registered nurse will have many others, less well-trained, working under her supervision. The proper selection of tasks to be performed by each is very important, and expectations of each person should be clearly defined. This is a key to good supervision. The untrained but eager worker frequently functions best when he is assigned one task rather than many.

## SAFETY IN THE HOSPITAL OR EXTENDED-CARE FACILITY

Many factors contribute to making hospitals and other inpatient facilities less safe than most industrial plants. There are weak and disabled people, oxygen, an unusual concentration of pathogenic organisms, radiation, and waxed floors with people hurrying over them. When the staff is aware of these dangers, accident rates fall. More accidents are caused by unsafe acts than by unsafe conditions.

The following points of safety are among the most important:

- In one study 29 per cent of all accidents to nurses comprised lacerations, bruises, and burns (Carner, 1952). A dustpan and broom should be used to re-

move glass slivers from the floor. The hands should be protected with gauze when breaking ampuls, and broken glass should be wrapped in paper toweling before it is discarded, to prevent cutting anyone who may handle the trash.

- Lifting is the greatest cause of injury in hospitals (Mammen, 1964). Lack of adherence to principles of body mechanics and insufficient help for the task are contributing factors.
- A footstool should be used when a patient is helped out of bed if the bed cannot be lowered. If the patient is elderly or tends to become disoriented, especially at night, side rails are kept on, for he may try to get up alone, forgetting how high the bed is. All patients should be observed frequently on evening and night shifts. An elderly patient may be sleeping soundly one moment, and the next he may be climbing over the side rails in the dark to get to the bathroom. A Hi-lo bed is kept in low position when the patient is allowed up or has a tendency to get up, and a night light is kept on. When the patient is in bed, casters on the bed and the bedside stand should be locked, so that the bed and the stand do not separate if the patient reaches for something. When a patient is being moved to or from a stretcher, it must be held securely against the bed, so that the patient does not slide down between it and the bed.
- Patients must be protected from falls. Porters should wash and wax one side of a hallway or ward at a time, always leaving a dry path. Nonskid wax should be used. Handrails in the halls are helpful. Patients in wheelchairs should be taught to use the brake. Stairs should be well lit and have nonskid abrasive strips. Long electrical cords should be positioned so that they are not a tripping hazard.
- "Busy" signs instead of locks on hospital bathrooms are indicated. A patient in trouble (faint, in pain, and so on) in the bathroom should not be locked inside. Call bells should be in easy reach.
- Stretchers are narrower than beds, and the patients on them may not be well-oriented. They should be strapped on, and they should be covered by a blanket to prevent chilling from the drafts of the hallways. Arms and legs should be under the blanket, so that they do not get caught in the elevator door or squashed between the stretcher and the bed.
- Trying to muddle through with an unfamiliar piece of equipment can be dangerous. For instance, if the nurse does not know how to use a Hoyer lift correctly, the patient may fall. If the nurse does not know the purpose of various dials on a respirator, the pressure applied to the lungs may be too great.
- The proper use of equipment is mandatory. This includes thorough orientation of all personnel who will use it as well as availability of the manufacturer's instructional materials.
- Hot-water bottles should be tested for leaks, the temperature of the water should be measured before filling, and the cap should be safely secured.
- Patients and visitors should be cautioned not to manipulate dials on equipment unless they have been

specifically instructed. When heating equipment, such as lamps or inhalators, is used, safety precautions must be explained to the patient.

- Metal beds should not be placed against metal radiators, because if the light socket is defective and the patient touches the light switch, he may receive a fatal electrical shock.
- All defective electrical equipment should be reported immediately. All electrical equipment should be checked regularly and be properly grounded, preferably through the use of a 3-prong plug. The "cheater" adaptor, a device used to make a 3-prong plug fit into a 2-blade socket, is of no use as an effective ground unless the little pigtail ground wire is connected to the outlet face plate.
- For precautions against radiation injury see Chapter 18, Nursing Management in Radiotherapy.

## Fire

Time is vital when a fire starts. A suggested order of action is: remove the patients nearest to the fire; call the operator, report the location of the fire or if there is a firebox, set the alarm; close doors and windows, turn off the electrical, the oxygen, and the ventilating equipment; remove the helpless patients from the area; try to put out the fire, using the fire extinguishers or wet blankets or linen; remove wheelchair patients from the area, then ambulatory patients, then staff.

If the fire is still a small one, such as a sheet just starting to smolder, douse it with water and put the fire out before doing anything else. Turn off oxygen (oxygen does not itself burn, but it supports combustion). A special fire extinguisher is necessary for electrical fires.

Rapid enough evacuation of patients may not be possible, especially in older buildings in which the construction aids rather than deters the progress of the fire. It takes healthy children three minutes to leave a three-story school building, but in an uncontrolled fire, dangerous smoke conditions can be created in two to seven minutes. How long would it take to remove patients from a hospital? Some cities require that new hospital and nursing home buildings be equipped with an automatic fire detection system, in which a bell is sounded when sufficient heat is created, and a sprinkler system, which also is activated by heat. Sprinkler systems are advised for all hospitals and nursing homes. All nurses should be familiar with the fire plan of the hospital in which they work.

Nurses should also be aware of potential fire hazards in the construction and maintenance of hospitals, and as a professional responsibility, should insist absolutely that all hazardous conditions be corrected or eliminated immediately. Some older hospitals may be legally exempt from the laws regarding fire safety, but they are not exempt from fires.

In addition to correction or elimination of all fire hazards, realistic, frequent fire drills are needed in all hospitals, and nurses should insist on having them.

Detection, containment (of smoke, heat, and flame), and extinguishment are the main principles of fire control. Closing doors and windows helps to contain smoke as well as flames—an important

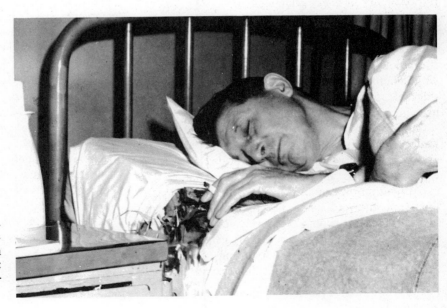

**Figure 13-4.** The sedated patient who smokes without supervision may doze off and cause a fire, as this patient did. (Ahl, V.: A visual aid for a fire safety program, *Am. J. Nurs.* 57:209)

197

point because of the damaging effects of inhaled smoke. Most deaths in fires come from smoke inhalation.

Smoking in the hospital must be limited to those areas where it is permitted. This applies to everyone —patients, staff, and visitors. An aide who smokes in the linen room is inviting disaster.

As noted above, oxygen does not burn but it does support combustion. Therefore, matches, lighted cigarettes, pipes, or cigars, and electrical appliances are excluded from the area where oxygen is being used or stored to minimize fire hazard.

Patients who smoke in bed are a major cause of fires in hospitals (Fig. 13-4). If the patient is allowed to smoke, he must have an adequate ash tray. Furtive smoking is hazardous; the patient can quickly crush a lit cigarette in a wastepaper basket or a bedside paper bag full of tissues. Patients must be attended if they smoke after they have had sedation, but a punitive attitude is unwarranted; rather, someone should stay with the patient if he wants a cigarette.

Decorations, such as those for Christmas, may be a fire hazard. They should be without electrical attachment, and they should be fireproof. Trash that collects also may be a fire hazard, and it should be removed. Appliances that give off heat such as steam inhalators, heating pads, and lamps should be used with appropriate fire and burn precautions.

Knowledge of the location and the operation of the fire extinguishers on each unit and the type of fire each extinguisher is designed to put out is the responsibility of every staff member.

Because ether is highly flammable, it is never used near flame; for example, adhesive marks should not be cleaned off a patient's skin while he is smoking. A patient who has been anesthetized with ether exhales combustible fumes for a considerable time postoperatively. Lighting a match near him is hazardous.

The operating room has its own special hazards. Many anesthetics are combustible: for example, cyclopropane, ether, and ethyl chloride. A tank of explosive gas is never put by the radiator. To avoid igniting the combustible gases, clothing made of silk, rayon, wool, nylon, and plastic never is worn in the operating room, because a spark from the static electricity that these materials generate could ignite one of the gases. All operating rooms have protective rules which must be known and adhered to by staff members.

## Reports

Reporting accidents in writing is standard procedure in hospitals. The purpose of this is not to fix the blame on individuals but to identify the causes and to prevent repetition of the accidents. Many hospitals have established safety committees to study the reports and to provide safer working conditions.

## EMERGENCY NURSING IN THE HOSPITAL

Some large hospitals have emergency wards with triage areas in which patients stay during the first hours or days of an acute disorder. Thus, an emergency ward in a large hospital might have the following patients in one evening:

A woman in cardiac failure
A woman recovering from diabetic coma
A woman being prepared for the operating room for treatment of multiple injuries sustained in an automobile accident
A man from the same accident, in coma from head injuries
A man with severe burns
A fireman with smoke poisoning
A man in coma due to an overdose of barbiturates

When the emergency is over, the patients are transferred to regular hospital wards, where their treatment is continued or some may be discharged or transferred. Hospitals without emergency wards use the regular wards or the intensive care unit to treat the patients having acute difficulty.

Any illness can become severe enough to require emergency care, and nurses caring for the patient should be prepared to recognize a developing emergency and intervene at the earliest possible moment, for example, by obtaining more data, such as vital signs or an ECG, administering oxygen, or calling a physician.

For example, a man recovering from a herniorrhaphy may have a myocardial infarction; a woman who seemed to be doing very well on a Sippy diet may suddenly hemorrhage from her peptic ulcer; a patient who seemed to be moody when he was admitted may try to jump out the window.

Many principles of emergency nursing apply to any nursing situation in the hospital—on the ward, in the clinic, in the emergency ward itself. For example:

- Emergencies can be anticipated. Enough should be known about each patient to recognize when his illness becomes serious. This involves knowing the diagnosis and what the danger signs are. For example, the nurse must know not only what the general symptoms and signs of insulin shock (reaction) are, but what symptoms of hypoglycemia are characteristic for a particular patient. Does he become irritable? Drowsy? Dizzy? An important part of good emergency nursing involves recognizing impending disaster and knowing when to intervene.

The nurse may be the first person to see a patient in an emergency. Whether the patient is hospitalized or comes into the nurse's care from the street, the principles of first aid apply.

The nurse must move fast to aid respiration, or stop the bleeding. Her report to the physician must be as accurate as it is prompt. She must move quickly enough to take care of what needs to be done, and yet not in such a manner as to add confusion to the scene.

- Since the nurse is often the first one to greet the terrified patient and his family, she must not, in her haste, neglect the kind word of encouragement. And because her contact with the patient may be brief, she must relate to him quickly, perceive his feelings, and respond to them. The right word at the right moment, the touch on the arm, the chair offered, the assurance that the physician is on his way, the deft application of a dry sterile dressing—all can help to make the patient and his family feel secure in the knowledge that he will be cared for at the time when he desperately needs help.

- The patient is supported in every way possible. The priest, minister, or rabbi is called if the patient so wishes. If the patient seems apologetic for what he now considers a foolish accident, an offhand remark by the nurse that he was wise to come for treatment, or that the accident is a common one, may help him to feel less embarrassed. Providing competent treatment and concentrated care often helps to allay anxiety. On the other hand, the extent of the patient's injuries should realistically be explained by the physician, so that the patient will not imagine that his injuries are more or less serious than they actually are. The patient should be encouraged to discuss what happened and his reactions to it; ignoring this aspect does not help him to assimilate the traumatic experience. The nurse should be especially observant for symptoms which seem in excess of the injury, or for denial of the injury, and know when and how to intervene. They can signal extreme anxiety.

- Legal implications of the situation should be kept in mind. Provisions should be made for the patient's valuables to be collected carefully and sent home with a relative or deposited in the hospital safe. Clothing should be handled with care, even if it is bloody or soiled. A patient who sees health workers handle his clothing as if it were repugnant considers himself rejected. If the clothing must be cut, a seam is cut when it is possible, so that it can be repaired.

The nurse may work with the police to help to establish the identity of an unaccompanied, helpless person. For example, if the patient is unable to sign a consent for surgery, his family must be located.

- The nurse functions in relation to others on the emergency care team, and delegates responsibility accordingly. An acute emergency demands smoothness, with each member of the team contributing his share of efficiency. The nurse should anticipate the information that the physician will want. For instance, if the patient is bleeding or in shock, she should gather nursing assessment data and share this information with the physician when he arrives.

- Supplies must be ready for use. Such emergency equipment as defibrillator, cardiac pacemaker, etc. are of no value unless they are operational when needed. Responsibility to make certain that the equipment and the supplies are in functioning condition must be clearly assigned. It is every nurse's responsibility to know where the emergency supplies and equipment for her work area are, and how to use them.

- Instructions in regard to follow-up care must be clear and complete. Because patients and their families tend to be anxious, verbal instructions are easily confused or forgotten. Did the physician say to take the pill every four hours for two days, or every two hours for four days? *Instructions must be written down.* Referral to social service or to the community nursing agency may be indicated. For example, a patient who has attempted suicide should be referred for psychiatric evaluation and care rather than discharged home without a plan to attempt to discover and treat the cause of his depression. The elderly patient who is admitted for the third time because of a home accident may benefit from a referral to the community nursing agency for home visits to review ways to prevent further accidents.

Emergency nursing requires knowledge, judgment, timing, alertness, and a high level of technical skill. There is no substitute for knowing the basic principles of physiology, behavioral concepts, sterile technique, and first aid so well that when the pressure is on nursing intervention is of high quality. It is a necessary learning experience for both the individual nurse by herself and all the members of the emergency team in a group to critically review the emergency situation after the event to see where improvements can be made.

## REFERENCES AND BIBLIOGRAPHY

Accidental death toll higher in 1972, Metropolitan Life Insurance Company, *Stat. Bull.* 54:10, January 1973.

AHLES, SR., M. A.: Disaster nursing . . . death to ideals? *Cath. Nurse* 10:50, June 1962.

AMERICAN MEDICAL ASSOCIATION: *First Aid Manual,* Chicago, The American Medical Association, 1962.

AMERICAN RED CROSS: *Disaster Handbook for Physicians and Nurses,* rev., Washington, D.C., 1966.

ARENA, J.: The treatment of poisoning, *Ciba Clin. Symp.* 18:3, January, February, March 1966.

BAER, E.: Civil disorder: mass emergency of the 70's, *Am. J. Nurs.* 72:1072, June 1972.

Basic concepts of the mass-casualty disaster plan, *RN* 35:OR/ER 15, May 1972.

BEATTY, C. J.: Guess who's dying at dinner, *RN* 35:52, November 1972.

The bite of man and beast, *Emerg. Med.* 5:112, February 1973.

BOYD, D. R.: Open wounds, *Emerg. Med.* 3:100, September 1971.

BRAUNSTEIN, P. W., et al.: Preliminary findings of the effect of automobile safety design on injury patterns, *Surg. Gynec. Obstet.* 105:257, September 1957.

CARNER, D. C.: Safety saves nurse, *Am. J. Nurs.* 52:1477, 1952.

COLE, W. H., and PUESTOW, C. B.: *First Aid: Diagnosis and Management,* ed. 6, New York, Appleton-Century-Crofts, 1965.

COSTELLO, D., and ELLIMAN, V. B. (eds.): I, Emergency nursing; II, Disaster nursing, *Nurs. Clin. N. Am.* 2 (complete volume), June 1967.

COWAN, L.: Emergency! *Am. J. Nurs.* 64:123, April 1964.

A Design Guide for Home Safety, Washington, D.C., U.S. Dept. of Housing and Urban Development, 1972. (Stock Number 2300-00201, U.S. Government Printing Office, $1.50.)

DIAMOND, E. F.: Emergency care of acute poisonings, *RN* 36:OR/ED 8, June 1973.

*Disaster Fatigue,* Washington, D.C., American Psychiatric Association Committee on Civil Defense, 1956.

Distinguishing the deadly scorpion's sting, *RN* 36:OR/ED 14, June 1973.

DOLMAN, C. E.: Botulism, *Am. J. Nurs.* 64:119, September 1964.

The driving risks in common medications, *Patient Care* 6:69, November 30, 1972.

FLINT, T., and CAIN, H.: *Emergency Treatment and Management,* ed. 4, Philadelphia, Saunders, 1970.

GARB, S., and ENG, E.: *Disaster Handbook,* ed. 2, New York, Springer, 1969.

HADDON, W., et al.: *Accident Research,* New York, Harper, 1964.

HERSHEY, N.: The nurse who works alone, *Am. J. Nurs.* 62:91, December 1962.

———: When the nurse is injured, *Am. J. Nurs.* 67:1458, July 1967.

HORNIBROOK, J. W.: Snakebites, *Am. J. Nurs.* 56:754, 1956.

Insect stings. Emergency therapy for severe reactions, *Patient Care* 6:46, May 30, 1972.

KESNER, B. J.: Accident control for nursing personnel, *Am. J. Nurs.* 51:565, 1951.

MAHONEY, R.: *Emergency and Disaster Nursing,* ed. 2, New York, Macmillan, 1969.

MAMMEN, H. W.: The need for employee health services in hospitals, *Arch. Environ. Health* 9:750, 1964.

McQUILLAN, F. L.: Accidents are about to happen—unless patients are trained in safety attitudes, *Mod. Nurs. Home* 26:43, June 1971.

MONEY, R. A.: The medical aspects of road safety and traffic accidents, *Med. J. Aust.* 48:655, 1961.

Mortality from accidents in the United States and Canada, *Stat. Bull.* 54:9, June 1973.

PERRY, J. F., and McCLELLAN, J.: Autopsy findings in 127 patients following fatal traffic accidents, *Surg. Gynec. Obstet.* 119:586, 1964.

Phone triage by R.N.'s means better ambulance service, *RN* 35:OR/ER 21, October 1972.

Quick action for possible poison, *Patient Care* 7:107, October 1, 1973.

RIEHL, C. L.: *Emergency Nursing,* Peoria, Ill., Chas. A. Bennett Co., 1970.

SHERMAN, J. W.: Electrical safety for coronary patients, *Hospitals* 45:72, May 1, 1971.

THOMPSON, R. E.: Static electricity—causes and controls, *AORN* 12:81, October 1970.

Those critical first minutes, *RN* 35:46, June 1972.

Two belts for the road, *Emerg. Med.* 4:141, October 1972.

When an insect sting becomes an emergency, *Nurs. Update* 4:14, May 1973.

# UNIT TWO

## Care of the Patient Who Undergoes Surgery

# Preparing for the Patient's Surgical Experience

Modern surgery is a far cry from the era of the barber-surgeons of medieval times, and even from that of the mid-20th century. Since the advent of anesthesia and the improved techniques and equipment from the related fields of biomedics and engineering, veritable miracles are happening in surgical services. This chapter will discuss the concept of surgical intervention and the process of nursing care as it proceeds in both the nursing unit and the surgical suite. Emphasis is on the physical setting and the sequence of the operative phase, whether the operation is an emergency or an elective (nonemergency) procedure. Chapters 15 and 16 deal in greater depth with the specific nursing responsibilities in the preoperative and postoperative phases of the patient's experience.

## THE CONCEPT OF SURGICAL INTERVENTION

Before proceeding to specific details, a definition of the concept of surgical care will be discussed. It is important to realize that every patient experiences essentially the same basic components of care, whether his is a relatively simple, uncomplicated examination or a highly complex operative procedure. Every patient is more likely to receive the quality care he has a right to expect when each individual involved in his care understands the specific requirements at any point along the continuum from the beginning of illness to rehabilitation. When surgery is considered to be the method of choice for treating the patient's condition, a complex process is activated. The patient, as well as the surgeons, anesthesiologist, and nursing team, contributes to the

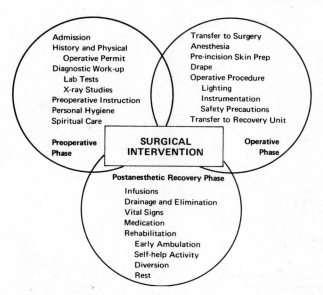

Admission
History and Physical
Operative Permit
Diagnostic Work-up
Lab Tests
X-ray Studies
Preoperative Instruction
Personal Hygiene
Spiritual Care

**Preoperative
Phase**

Transfer to Surgery
Anesthesia
Pre-incision Skin Prep
Drape
Operative Procedure
Lighting
Instrumentation
Safety Precautions
Transfer to Recovery Unit

**Operative
Phase**

**SURGICAL
INTERVENTION**

**Postanesthetic Recovery Phase**

Infusions
Drainage and Elimination
Vital Signs
Medication
Rehabilitation
Early Ambulation
Self-help Activity
Diversion
Rest

**Figure 14-1.** The phases of care of the surgical patient. The preoperative phase, the operative phase, and the postanesthetic recovery phase are interrelated and interdependent.

outcome. How can such a complex process be understood?

Figure 14-1 is one way to think about it. This diagram shows the interdependence of the phases of the surgical process. Within each phase certain essential facts are brought together and serve as the basis for decision making. The surgeon, usually in consultation with the internist, radiologist, and anesthesiologist, formulates his plan for surgical intervention. This means that with the best available information and technical resources the surgeon hopes to bring about effective therapy or to establish a definitive diagnosis upon which further therapy may be based. Surgical intervention is the central event of this therapeutic process, preceded by careful diagnostic preparation, sustained by physiologic and psychological support, and followed by immediate and long-range care and rehabilitation.

**Nursing Responsibility**

An important consideration for nursing is that the process of care requires careful, detailed planning and coordination, and accurate assessment of the patient so that he is given the maximum benefit of competent technical and personal care. Everyone involved shares in the legal and ethical considerations governing the rights and duties of persons during the restoration of bodily health. Such matters as informed consent and bodily integrity are under-

stood against a background of medical jurisprudence of which no practitioner may plead ignorance (Sarner, 1968).

On the nursing unit the professional nurse keeps informed by communicating with the surgeon and other colleagues as well as with the patient and his family, so that the plan of care is understood by everyone involved, and progress is made to achieve the desired outcomes of patient safety and comfort. In the operating and recovery rooms too, the nursing staff is informed of the required surgical intervention so that there is a minimum of delay and no oversight of detail that could interfere with competent and safe care for the patient.

The efficiency with which the process of care is carried out depends upon an understanding of the physical setting, responsibilities and relationships of medical and nursing personnel, the management of supplies and equipment during the sequence of events surrounding surgical intervention, and adequate assessment of the patient.

Assessment of the Patient

Assessment of the patient involves such considerations as:

- **His level of anxiety and his ability to cope emotionally with the stress of surgery.**
- **His understanding of the surgery to be performed, of the anesthesia to be used, and of his own participation necessary in the pre- and postoperative periods.**
- **Whether he has given written informed consent for the procedure.**
- **His physical status: for example, nutrition, hydration, presence of other illnesses.**
- **Factors which may complicate pre- and postoperative care: for example, denial of the implications of the surgery or presence of arthritis which will make postoperative ambulation difficult.**
- **His supports in the crisis of surgery: friends, family, work to return to, adequate income, interests which help him tolerate the time he must be away from his usual pursuits, religious and philosophical beliefs which sustain him.**
- **Resources and plans for convalescent care. Has he someone to help him at home? Will he require care in a convalescent home?**

**THE PHYSICAL SETTING**

As a rule, surgery of any degree of complexity is performed in a hospital. Some patients may go to a physician's office or an outpatient clinic for the removal or repair of superficial lesions, or for simple diagnostic measures which are of minimal risk. For example, an injury sustained at work or in a street accident may require only the application of a few sutures or a plaster cast. The emergency room of any well-equipped hospital provides the physical facilities needed to render effective service for initial treatment of trauma. Outpatient services in a general hospital provide for minor treatment and follow-up visits of patients undergoing surgical care.

In a general hospital, the operative service, called the surgical suite, is an area specially designed and constructed to provide an environment that is convenient and safe for both patients and personnel. The surgical suite may consist of many individual operating rooms efficiently arranged near lounge areas, clerical stations, and recovery room services. It is set off from the main flow of traffic in the hospital. To assure maximum environmental safety from microorganisms, the suite is air conditioned and separated by an interchange area for authorized personnel to change from street clothes into clean cotton clothing (Fig. 14-2). Communications into the suite are made through the clerical station by using the intercom system or the telephone. Inside the suite, a specially constructed flooring and electrical system are used to assure patient safety in potentially hazardous atmospheres where flammable anesthetic agents are used. For atmospheric control of human-generated static, the air supply ventilating the surgical suite is humidified. During the operative procedure, conductive footwear is worn by the surgical team to prevent the accumulation of electrical charges. This footwear may be either specially constructed shoes with conductive soles or disposable conductive boots applied over street shoes (Fig. 14-2).

An operating room, whether in the emergency service or obstetrical unit, or within the surgical suite, has essentially the same characteristics. A surgical specialty may add unique features, such as built-in roentgen-ray equipment in a neurologic or urologic unit. The essential characteristics of an operating room are illustrated in Figure 14-3.

## THE PREOPERATIVE PHASE

Initially, the patient sees his physician in the office or at the clinic, or he is seen by a surgeon called in consultation after the patient is hospitalized. When surgery is decided upon, the surgical suite at the hospital is notified in advance so that an operating room will be available. The patient's admission to the hospital sets the preoperative phase into motion.

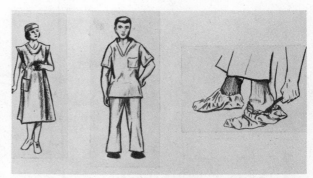

**Figure 14-2.** Cotton clothing worn by men and women in the surgical suite. (American Hospital Supply Corp., Evanston, Ill.) Conductive shoes are worn, or conductive shoe covers are used. (Will Ross, Inc., Milwaukee, Wis.)

In the admitting office, the patient's preadmission medical history form is used to minimize delay in preparing hospital records. The fact sheet of the patient's chart carries significant information that is used by all team members throughout the patient's hospital stay.

It is very important that the admitting record be accurate, especially in specifying the site of operation. This is particularly true if the designation "right" or "left" is used because this record is the basis for all future considerations for the patient in the hospital.

An identification bracelet is applied to the patient's wrist to assure safe administration of medications and treatments and to prevent misidentification of the patient in the operating room.

**Permission for Operation.** The consent form, or operative permit, is part of the admitting record. The patient is asked to sign the consent form showing that he agrees to have the surgery performed, or stating exceptions if he has any to make. This form implies that the patient understands the nature of the treatment. He usually is asked to sign a consent for diagnostic procedures, such as cystoscopy and bronchoscopy, as well as for major surgery. If the patient has more than one such procedure or operation during his hospital stay, he signs a permit for each of them separately. The signed consent protects the patient, the hospital, and the physician. The patient is protected from having surgery to which he has not consented, and the hospital and the physician are protected against claims that unauthorized surgery has been performed.

For the consent to be valid, the person giving it must be alert and understand what he is doing. He should not be allowed to sign a permit after he has

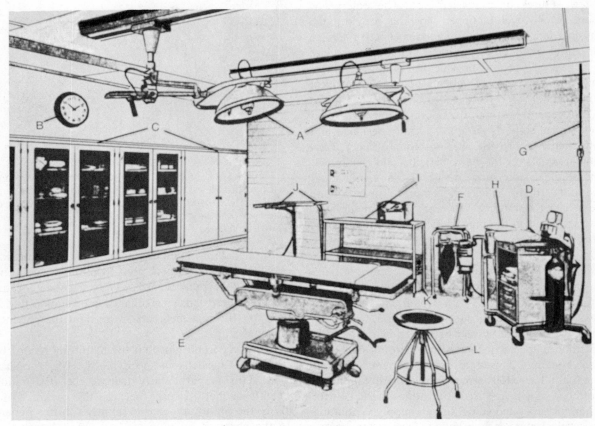

**Figure 14-3.** Essential characteristics of an operating room: (A) overhead lights; (B) wall clock; (C) storage cabinets; (D) anesthetic machine; (E) operating table; (F) sterile basin; (G) gas supply tubing; (H) nonsterile water basin; (I) instrument table with portable suction unit; (J) mayo tray stand; (K) kick bucket; (L) anesthetist stool. (Ohio Medical Products, Madison, Wis.)

received preanesthetic medication or if he has not understood an explanation concerning the anticipated surgery. If he is intoxicated, mentally incompetent, or otherwise incapable of understanding, a relative or guardian must sign for him. A child who is too young to understand the procedure or its consequences may not legally consent to have an operation. One of his parents or his legal guardian must sign the permission for him. It is customary to require the signature of a parent if the patient is under 21 years of age. To save the patient's life, it may be necessary in emergencies to obtain verbal consent by telephone from a responsible relative.* Two surgeons in consultation (which is recorded on the patient's record) may proceed with surgery in an extreme emergency if the patient is unconscious and if there is no one to give consent.

Any person who has the ability to understand the consequences of his own actions may refuse consent for surgery or any other treatment, even after the physician has explained the reasons and recommended treatment.

**Admission to the Nursing Unit.** When the patient is admitted to the nursing unit, he is welcomed by the nurse responsible for his care who interviews him and records pertinent data, thus initiating the history-taking aspect of assessment. She introduces him to other staff members assigned to care for him. The nursing assessment along with the medical plan is then worked into an initial program of care.

Initial instructions to the patient will be influenced by how much and what kind of information the patient's physician has given to him and to his family. Baudry and Weiner (1968) have stated some

---

* For further information concerning consent for surgery and other treatments, see Sarner, H.: *The Nurse and the Law.* Philadelphia, W. B. Saunders, 1968.

general principles of what they call "family management" that can help the nurse to relate effectively with the persons involved in this admission phase.

The physician and nurse develop an initial working plan, which is individualized for each patient. The nurse explains to the patient that his physician has been notified of his admission. She carries out the important initial procedures and gives appropriate information to the patient, while he, in turn, has the opportunity to give her information that she can incorporate into the plan of nursing care. Such matters as the degree of self-help ability, any physical handicaps, and personal preferences or strong dislikes that he has may be noted.

For most people, entering the hospital for surgery is a crisis. Usually patients are in the hospital only a day or two prior to surgery; therefore, the focus at this time should be on matters which are of primary concern to them, for example, the type of anesthesia, the surgery itself, and measures for self-help.

Accurate recordings of the patient's vital signs, blood pressure, weight, and physical appearance are made so that there is a basis for comparison throughout the phases of his care. Such diagnostic tests as the electrocardiogram (ECG) and the additional laboratory studies of the blood and urine or of body organs by means of x-rays or isotopes will be explained when and as they pertain to the patient. Whenever possible, depending on his ability to understand, the patient is encouraged to participate in his own care or, at the very least, to have the information which helps him feel more secure and which enables him to cooperate intelligently with the physician, the nurse, and the technologists.

In addition to careful assessment of the patient's physical status, the nurse should be alert to his psychological needs. (See Chapter 15 for a detailed development of effective nursing in the preoperative phase.)

**Personal Hygiene.** Most patients who enter the hospital for surgery are able to care for their own personal needs, but they need instruction and encouragement while they prepare for the experience of an operation. The nurse provides assistance for those patients who require it or whose personal hygiene habits are poor.

The patient should bathe thoroughly either the evening before or the morning of surgery. If surgery is scheduled very early in the morning, it is best to have the patient bathe the evening before. If surgery is scheduled late in the morning, the patient should be allowed to sleep later than usual. There will still be time to complete his care, and he will be spared many anxious hours of waiting. Most patients are up and about before surgery and can take a tub bath or shower using a bacteriocidal preparation for thoroughly cleansing the skin. For those who are able to use them, these facilities are preferable to a sponge bath from a small bath basin. Not only is the patient's bath facilitated, but he is spared being made dependent on others before this is necessary.

Most patients who are able to shampoo their hair before coming to the hospital, because they will be unable to do so for a time after surgery. If the patient has been hospitalized for some time preoperatively, he may, if he is able, have a shampoo at the hospital.

These preparations, along with the specific preoperative measures that each operation requires, take place before the patient is transferred to the operating room. (See Chapter 15 for a detailed analysis of these measures.)

### In the Operating Room

While these preliminary considerations are taking place, another sequence of events is going on within the surgical suite. Recall that when the decision for surgical intervention was agreed upon between physician and patient, the hospital surgical service was notified. To understand better the process of surgical intervention, perhaps a brief discussion of how the surgical suite is organized will help.

Surgery is not only an event in the patient's life, it involves a place and the people who contribute to the surgeon's plan of care once the operation is scheduled. Depending on the nurse's understanding of the setup and relationships within the surgical suite and recovery room, she can help allay the patient's fears. In some hospitals, clinical specialists in surgical nursing are members of the health team who promote continuity of care between the operating room, the nursing unit, and the recovery or intensive care unit.

### Scheduling the Operation

The operating room schedule is a predetermined plan which serves as a guide for the efficient use of rooms, time, and personnel. The basis for planning

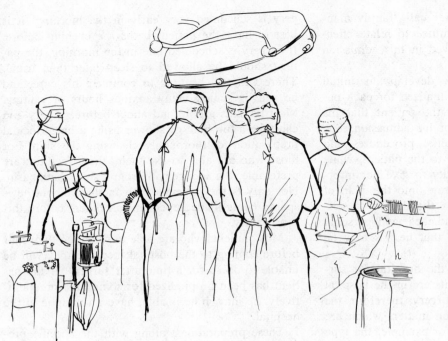

**Figure 14-4.** An operation is in progress. The scrub nurse is standing in such a position that she can pass instruments easily to the surgeons. She keeps her tray in order and anticipates what will be needed next. The basin (right) is sterile, and it is used to rinse instruments as they become soiled. The circulating nurse, just beyond the anesthesist's head, takes care of unsterile equipment and keeps the sterile tables supplied.

the schedule is the procedure performed by each surgeon. Scheduling is a continuous process, but for any given day the work for the following day is printed on a form that may be distributed to the nursing units and hospital departments so they may plan their work schedules in relation to the surgery schedule. This form indicates the room assigned, the time of operation, the surgeon, the operative procedure, the patient, and his age, and room number, and the type of anesthetic. Each of these pieces of information has meaning for the staff concerned with the responsibility for safe patient care.

The steady flow of events planned for an operative procedure depends on the understanding each person has of the interdependence of people, supplies, and equipment and the coordination of information necessary to accomplish the procedure safely and efficiently. Planned surgery affects the patient, the surgeon, and the hospital service. For example, a mother who has been told that she must have her gallbladder removed must make adjustments at home. This may include making arrangements for someone to stay with her children, someone to look after her husband's meals, and someone to care for her after she returns home. The surgeon schedules the procedure and plans his work, meetings, and rounds to other hospitals accordingly.

Hospital services, especially surgical, are costly. Lack of foresight which results in delays, unused operating time, or overtime spent for late-hour surgery that could have been prevented contributes to increased costs for hospitalization.

Effective performance by the team members is best assured when assignments are made in advance on the basis of the operating room schedule, unless, as in some services, the unit is so large that some of the nursing staff are permanently assigned to the orthopedic, urologic, cardiovascular, or eye services respectively. In any case, the schedule provides the basis for the nursing and anesthesia staff to know in advance their individual responsibilities. The surgery schedule is an important device used for planning the utilization of rooms and the assignment of personnel.

### The Surgical Team

The surgical team consists of surgeons and assistants, the anesthesiologist or nurse anesthetist, the professional nurse, and practical nurses or technicians (Fig. 14-4). Nursing assistants, clerical staff, and housekeeping aides all contribute a vital part to the whole effort with their supporting services.

In general, the functions of the team members may be defined as follows:

*Surgeon.* A physician who has specialized in the practice of surgery. He makes the decisions concerning the kind of surgery necessary and performs the operations.

*Anesthesiologist.* A physician who has specialized in the administration of anesthetics. He works with the surgeon in determining the type of anesthetic to be used, and he administers anesthetics.

*Anesthetist.* One who has specialized in the administration of anesthetics, usually not a physician. Some nurses become anesthetists.

*Instrument Nurse.* A nurse who, after scrubbing and donning sterile gown and gloves, assembles and prepares sterile supplies and assists the surgeon during the operation by anticipating the supply and instrument sequence as required.

*Circulating Nurse.* A nurse who prepares and assembles supplies before and during the operation. Both the instrument nurse and the circulating nurse count the sponges used during the operation to make sure that all sponges have been removed from the patient before the incision is closed.

*The Professional Nurse.* The professional nurse may also function as a circulating nurse during the patient's operation. She is responsible for the planning, coordination, and administration of nursing care of a group of surgical patients scheduled into the surgical suite. She is assisted by other registered nurses, practical nurses, technicians, and aides.

Team members proceed through precision movements with attention to detail, safety, and speed. Effectiveness of personnel and of their organization as a team insures that the operative procedure will be done quickly and safely. Inadequate facilities slow down the process. Speed is important and is related to safety. For example, the period of time that the patient is anesthetized should be limited to the interval necessary to minimize the time he must stay in the recovery room. Thus, poor organization can result not only in inconvenience for staff and delay for other patients, but also in diminished quality of care for the patient who is experiencing surgery. Experienced personnel and necessary facilities, supplies, and information can minimize friction, irritation, and frustration before the procedure begins.

## Plan of Procedure

The procedure the surgeon plans will determine the equipment required. Every surgical service maintains an index of surgeons' preferences in what might be called a procedure card file or index. The preference card indicates the usual setup required for a given case with instructions for special supplies and instruments, equipment, suture routine, position, table accessories, and presurgical prep routine. These details have meaning for the surgical nursing staff who have related them to the

anatomy and to an understanding of the surgical techniques that surgeons are specially educated to perform.

## THE OPERATIVE PHASE

The immediate preoperative preparation of the patient takes place on the nursing unit. A nursing assistant from the operating room presents a written "call slip" on the unit to obtain permission to take the patient, with his chart, to surgery. At this time, the nurse on the unit and the nursing assistant from surgery use a preoperative checklist to be sure that each task required for safe patient care has been carried out. This is the same list used for organizing the assignment of care in the preoperative phase. Preoperative checklists vary with the policies of particular hospitals. They consist of a list of observations to be made and tasks to be carried out just prior to surgery (see p. 230). Typical items include making sure that the operative consent has been signed and that the patient has voided. When these tasks have been performed with careful attention and due consideration for the patient and his family, both the patient's nurse and the assistant from surgery help the patient onto the stretcher, and together they take him to the operating room.

While the nursing team prepares the setup and the surgeons are preparing to put on the sterile attire that constitutes part of the sterile field, the anesthesiologist is preparing the patient for the anesthetic. Some general principles that briefly explain this aspect of the procedure may be helpful.

### Administration of Anesthetics

Anesthetics are drugs that block the patient's perception of pain. Those agents that act systemically to produce loss of consciousness and inability to feel pain are general anesthetics. Local or regional anesthetics act locally to block nerve fibers for pain insensibility and do not cause loss of consciousness. A spinal, caudal, brachial, or pudendal block is accomplished by the injection of a liquid drug, such as lidocaine (Xylocaine), into a region of these nerve fibers. Anesthetics may be administered by intravenous infusion, inhalation, or topically, or by a combination of these methods.

### Methods of Administration

The anesthesiologist selects the most suitable method and agent for each patient depending upon such factors as the age of the patient, his physical condition, and type of surgery being performed.

**Intravenous Infusion.** Drugs injected into the vein by intravenous infusion, e.g., sodium pentothal, are added to commercially prepared solutions, such as dextrose in water or physiologic saline. Infusion is accomplished through the use of a sterile disposable needle and tubing set. This is the most common method of induction. The intravenous setup used for induction of anesthesia is manufactured so that blood may be added to this same set if blood transfusion is indicated later during the operation.

Sometimes the patient's condition is so critical that a small incision is made (after local anesthesia has been accomplished) to expose the vein, and a sterile cannula is inserted to assure adequate flow of the infusion. A surgeon makes the incision using a sterile cutdown set and appropriate-sized cannula. Patients who are receiving prolonged infusions or who are positioned so as to hazard dislocation of the needle require the use of a cannula which may be inserted through the skin by means of a percutaneous injection of a needle-carrying cannula.

**Inhalation.** Gases such as mixtures of nitrous oxide–oxygen or cyclopropane are administered by inhalation using such methods as open drop, the mask technique (the oropharyngeal blower), closed rebreathing, or the endotracheal technique. Agents used for intravenous induction provide only superficial loss of consciousness. Gases are used to accomplish deeper levels of anesthesia.

ENDOTRACHEAL ANESTHESIA. In selected cases, gaseous anesthetics are given by the endotracheal route. Usually the patient is given general anesthesia first. When he loses consciousness and his muscles relax, a long tube is inserted into the tracheobronchial passage. Anesthesia is given through this tube during the rest of the operation. By means of the tube the anesthetist can "breathe" for the patient—that is, he can control not only the amount of anesthetic reaching the lungs, but also the amount of air and oxygen reaching the lungs and the carbon dioxide leaving the lungs. Bronchial secretions can be aspirated through the tube with a catheter.

The use of endotracheal anesthesia has greatly facilitated many newer types of surgery. For example, it is particularly useful in chest surgery. When endotracheal anesthesia is used, it is possible to open the chest without collapsing the lungs because the anesthetic and the oxygen can be administered directly to the lungs, causing them to expand and contract even when the chest wall is open and the normal pressure relationships are temporarily interrupted. Because there is negative pressure within the thoracic cavity, when the chest is opened, air is sucked in, collapsing the lungs. Unless gases are being carried to the lungs by a tube, respiration could be seriously impaired.

**Spinal Anesthesia.** Dramatic improvements in spinal anesthetics have made it possible, in some cases, for the surgeon to operate on patients who might not otherwise survive. Patients in advanced age or precarious clinical status, who might not tolerate the insult of inhalation anesthesia and the shock of surgery, benefit from the use of better technique and improved drugs for spinal anesthesia.

For the administration of a spinal anesthetic, the patient is positioned either sitting up or on his side to insure injection of the drug into the correct site. The anesthetist depends on his knowledge of anatomy, performing the injection aided by palpation and anatomical measurements. This type of anesthetic, like the general anesthetic, is administered before the patient's skin is prepared for the incision. The patient may remain awake or doze off and on during the procedure. It is extremely important to limit conversation during the procedure and to avoid discussing anything that would alarm the patient. This is obviously true in the case of the conscious patient, but reports indicate that even the patient who has received a general anesthetic, though apparently oblivious, hears and is affected by conversation around him (Marx, 1967).

**Topical Anesthesia.** Topical application of solutions, ointments, jelly, or powder to body surfaces also produces local anesthesia. These agents are administered after the patient is positioned, the skin is prepared, and the patient is draped. No other anesthetic is administered so the patient is conscious, although he may be sedated.

**Regional Anesthesia.** A variation of a local anesthetic is the injection of a drug into the nerve center of a body region. This is also called a regional anesthetic. This highly desirable technique requires skill in administration to insure adequate effect and to prevent nerve damage.

A *brachial block* results from the injection of an anesthetic drug into the network of lower cervical and upper dorsal spinal nerves supplying the arm, forearm, and hand.

A *caudal block* is an injection into the cauda equina, the nerve endings at the end of the spinal cord. This injection affects nerves in body regions lower than those nerves affected by a lumbar spinal injection.

A *pudendal block* affects the pudendal nerve posterior to the ischial spine, affecting also the femoral and the ilio-inguinal nerve. This type of local infiltration is used in selected cases for childbirth or minor operations on the perineum of a female patient. The student is referred to pharmacology texts for a discussion of anesthetic agents.

Possible Complications of Anesthesia

Two major hazards associated with the administration of anesthetics are the danger of static or electrical spark in the presence of explosive gases, and the danger of cardiac arrest. Incidents occurring from both of these hazards are less frequent since practitioners have become better acquainted with their causes and the factors that prevent their occurrence.

During the 1950's, surgeons revised their approach to the problem of cardiac arrest from a drastic chest-opening technique for heart massage to that now widely employed—closed chest massage and mouth-to-mouth artificial resuscitation. Determination of the causes and prompt institution of a program of definitive action are the hallmarks of successful resuscitation whenever cardiac arrest occurs. Readiness of personnel and equipment in the operating room is important in counteracting the unforeseen effects of drugs or gases on the central nervous system.

**Electrostatics Cause Anesthetic Explosions.** As more effective agents are developed to replace anesthetic gases, it may be possible to eliminate entirely the hazards associated with these agents. But until that time comes, the controls for prevention of explosion must be understood and enforced for patient safety. For a complete understanding of the details, the student is encouraged to refer to the sizable literature on this subject.

The problem exists because gaseous anesthetic agents, to be effective, must be soluble in the lipid membranes of the brain. Such agents are also flammable. Mixtures of agents, such as cyclopropane and ether, with oxygen are commonly used. Even though halothane substances appear to provide suitable anesthetic properties without the explosion hazard, the use of these agents has not yet completely replaced the effective but flammable anesthetics such as ether and cyclopropane.

Three factors combine to cause an explosion: a flammable mixture, an ignition source, and carelessness. The anesthetic mixture can be confined to the anesthesia machine and the patient's respiratory passages by using a closed technique of administering the gas. If it effectively controls leaks, such a system limits the spread of flammable vapors. Some anesthetic agents are present in the liquid state and are subject to spilling. Most gaseous mixtures are heavier than air and settle toward the floor where friction from movement of objects and electrical potential between objects is registered on contact.

Two principles are involved in the control of the electrostatic hazard, or the ignition source. A spark occurs as a result of a difference between the electrical potential in objects. It is necessary on the one hand to prevent a rapid buildup of the potential, and on the other hand to provide a conductive pathway over which the inevitable accumulation of electrostatic charge can leak away.

Hence the program for control of explosion hazards rests on the education of all personnel who participate in these atmospheres and on the restricting of traffic within the area which is properly structured and equipped to provide the safety features. Essentially, the use of conductive flooring provides the electrical pathway interconnecting everything and everyone in the room. Safe furniture is made of metal or electrically conductive material. Contact of the furnishings and equipment is established through conductive casters, tires, or leg tips. Personnel are electrically conductive with the floor through the correct application of specially designed shoes, slip-ons, or shoe covers (see Fig. 14-2) which maintain body contact and are kept free from insulating accumulations of dirt and debris, such as wax or grease. A conductimeter to determine the presence of electrical conductivity is used by surgeons, anesthesiologists, and nursing staff before they enter the operating room. In addition, all persons are instructed to stay away from the anesthetic machine. For those who must come close to it, slow and deliberate motions become a matter of habit so that the rate of generation of static does not exceed its rate of dissipation.

**Resuscitation from Cardiac Arrest.** The condition known as cardiac arrest (standstill) requires a closely coordinated, swiftly executed plan of action for successful resuscitation. The causes of cardiac

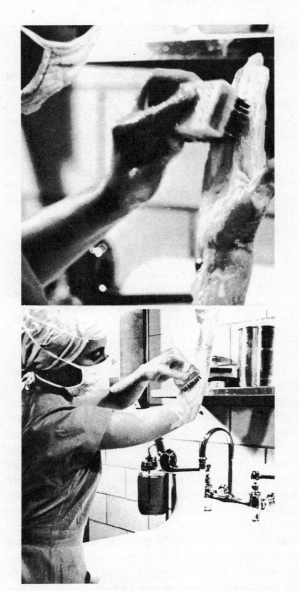

**Figure 14-5.** Although scrubbing procedures and routines vary from one hospital to another, the basic principles of aseptic practice remain the same. Notice that the nurse holds her hands higher than her elbows, and that no skin areas are left untouched. (Ethicon, Inc., Somerville, N.J.)

arrest are now better understood and it is possible to detect them so that preventive measures can be instituted (see Chap. 61). If cardiac arrest occurs, circulation of oxygen must be accomplished within a minimum of three minutes to prevent permanent damage and loss of normal brain function. Establishment of a patent airway and restoration of heart action are the goals of the cardiac resuscitation pro-

gram. Each surgical service has its own specific plan of action. New staff members learn the details of the program in order to respond quickly in concert with the anesthesiologist and other team members to institute prompt return of heart action and circulation of oxygenated blood.

## The Surgical Intervention

Team members who are to work within the sterile field carry out a clearly defined technique for handwashing called the scrub routine (Fig. 14-5). Improved detergent-germicides that effect adequate skin disinfection are used along with a handbrush or polyurethane sponge saturated with the germicide. In one such routine the hands and arms are scrubbed with providoneiodine (Betadine) for ten minutes. Before scrubbing starts, the nails are cleaned with an orangewood stick. During the scrubbing process the hands are held slightly higher than the elbows, so that the water will run off the elbows rather than back over the hands and forearms.

When the team is gowned and gloved and the patient is anesthetized, positioned, prepped, and draped, the surgical procedure progresses through a sequence of steps based on the surgeon's objective and the anatomy of the human body. For this reason, everyone who assists the surgeon should have a basic understanding of gross anatomy and the relationship between tissues and organs of the body. These specific details are used for planning and organizing the supplies and equipment and the use of instruments throughout the operation. Although the procedure differs according to the surgeon's objective, every operation consists of essentially the same activities. Most of the instruments used by the surgeon are variations of implements used for dissection, retraction, or manipulation of tissues, followed by repair or approximation of the dissected tissues.

The operative procedure can be described as a process with more or less distinct phases: exposure, isolation of the defect, and reconstruction or closure.*

**Exposure.** Depending on the site of operation, the exposure phase is more or less prolonged. In a simple superficial incision, the exposure may be identical with the incision. If scar tissue or adhesions are present, the exposure may be difficult and

---

* The material describing the phases of the surgical procedure is adapted from Hoeller, Sr. Mary Louise: *The Operating Room Technician*, ed. 2, St. Louis, Mosby, 1968.

time consuming. During this phase, tissues are separated (by sharp or blunt dissection) and retracted, blood vessels are clamped and ligated, and organs are walled off and retracted. Careful identification of all the structures is vital to avoid unintentional injury.

**Isolation, Removal, or Repair.** With adequate exposure, the surgeon carries out the main purpose of the procedure, which involves isolation, removal, or repair. When the diagnosis is confirmed and reveals the exact location of the pathology, tumor, or defect, the blood supply is clamped, divided, and ligated. If necessary, adjacent organs are sutured to remaining structures and the specimen is delivered from the wound (Fig. 14-6). The surgeon replaces the organs, being careful to avoid twisting or malpositioning. Then he begins the wound closure or reconstruction. It is at this point that the first closing sponge count is made.

In some cases the operation consists of the repair of a defect, congenital (present at birth) or traumatic. The surgeon's plan should be understood so that equipment and supplies are on hand. Repair of the defect may involve reconstruction with tissue transplants or synthetic implant materials. When these are required, advance planning assures a sufficient and safe supply to minimize delays.

**Reconstruction or Closure.** Each layer of the wound is identified and approximated carefully. The cells of each tissue layer begin immediately to reconstitute themselves in the complex process known as healing. When the operation takes place inside a cavity, the membrane lining is closed first, followed by the muscle layer, its membrane (fascia), and finally the subcutaneous layer and the skin. The primary suture line is sometimes supported by a secondary line, called a retention suture, which is used to reinforce the primary closure during delayed healing. It is important to remember that these steps in wound closure provide the logical and chronological arrangement of the suture sequence. Suture size, needle size, and the order of their use are determined by the tissues the surgeon is dissecting and repairing.

## POSTANESTHESIA RECOVERY

The recovery room (PAR or RR) is usually a very large room with accommodations for a group of patients to be under the continual surveillance of highly skilled personnel. Patients usually are in

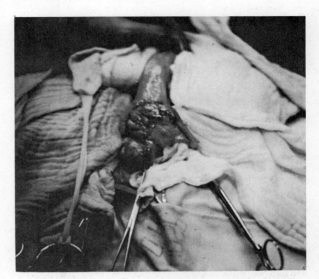

**Figure 14-6.** The removal of an appendix, which is lying on the gauze (*center*). Note that sterile sponges encircle and protect the operating site. (Dr. Martin E. Silverstein)

cubicles which can be curtained off during nursing procedures or examinations, in consideration of the patient's need for privacy, and the needs of other patients who are nearby. Equipment at each bedside and at the nursing station is available for immediate application in case of need. Recordings of vital signs are made at frequent intervals and the progress of the patient's recovery from the anesthetic is charted on the patient's bedside record.

As a rule, the endotracheal tube is removed by the anesthesiologist before the patient leaves the surgical suite. A complication which can arise during this critical time is *laryngospasm*. The natural respiratory response to noxious gases is a forced expiratory grunt as the thoracic and abdominal muscles tense into a protective shield. The same reflex can be stimulated by action on nervous structures of the body, notably, the rectal or perineal muscles, the periosteum, and a pulling action on abdominal viscera. Too light a plane of anesthesia allows this protective reflex to narrow the laryngeal space, resulting in high-pitched inspiratory stridor. This condition requires that the patient be assisted with respiration manually, along with being supplied a slightly higher oxygen content than ordinary air. An oropharyngeal airway (see Fig. 16-1) is inserted to prevent the tongue from obstructing the air passage during this phase of the patient's recovery from anesthesia. This airway is left in position until the patient begins to regain consciousness, giving evidence of the return of the swallowing and cough reflexes. Even then, the patient is so positioned that vomitus or secretions will not be aspirated into the tracheobronchial passages. If necessary, suction is used to promptly remove vomitus and secretions so that the patient will not aspirate them.

When the patient is fully reacted and there is no evidence of complications, he is prepared to return to the nursing unit. The length of time varies, but an average duration of the postanesthetic period is about one and one-half to two hours. If the surgery is of such a nature that intensive nursing care is required, the patient may be sent to the intensive care unit. In this unit, measures similar to those in the recovery room are taken to foresee and prevent critical complications. Some aspects of these complications are discussed in later chapters.

### Nursing Responsibilities

The chief responsibilities of the nurse during the immediate postoperative recovery period are (1) to assure a patent airway, (2) to help maintain adequate circulation, (3) to prevent or treat shock, and (4) to attend to proper positioning and the function of drains, tubes and intravenous infusions, (5) to reassure the patient by her presence and to help him orient himself as he recovers from the anesthesia, (6) to relieve pain, and (7) to provide prompt information to family or friends who may be waiting by informing them that the surgery is over and that the patient has arrived in the recovery room. (Such information may be given via the nursing staff on the patient's unit or directly by the RR nurse if there is a waiting room adjacent to the recovery room.)

**Positioning and Skin Care.** Positioning the patient is an important measure in preventing interference with circulation; normal body alignment should be maintained. Precautions are taken to prevent displacement of the infusion needle because maintenance of the infusion is important to adequate circulatory function. If the patient is in one position for any prolonged period, measures are taken to prevent pressure over bony prominences and delicate tissues like the ear. A skin surface that rests against another is protected to prevent excoriation. A patient with a cast is observed closely to detect interference with circulation either because of swelling or a malposition. Change in the color of the skin (cyanosis or blanching) with either hyper-

emia or loss of heat would necessitate careful checking and, if necessary, splitting or trimming of the cast. The physician should be notified at the onset of these symptoms or in the event that the patient's complaints of persistent pain are not relieved by nursing measures.

The patient usually is kept flat in bed for six to twelve hours after the surgery. Unless the physician has ordered otherwise, the patient may be turned from side to side.

**Pain Relief.** As the anesthesia wears off, the patient will begin to have sensation in the anesthetized parts. Often he describes this as "pins and needles." He also will begin to experience pain in the operated area; analgesics usually are ordered to relieve the pain.

Medication for pain relief or sedation is ordered by the surgeon. The recovery room nurse exercises judgment in administering the first postoperative medication. Judgments in this matter are based on knowledge of the drugs used for anesthesia and their effect on the action of drugs used for pain relief. The physician is guided by these considerations when ordering analgesics for postoperative patients.

**Recovery from Spinal Anesthesia.** Patients who develop headache may have to remain flat for a longer period. There has been so much discussion about "spinal headache" that patients sometimes think it an inevitable sequel to spinal anesthesia. The nurse should remember not to contribute to this impression by the power of suggestion. A statement like "I'll keep your bed flat so you can doze" is preferable to "I'll keep the bed flat so you won't get a headache."

Nursing care and observation are important after spinal anesthesia, although the fact that the patient does not lose consciousness simplifies some aspects of postoperative care. Even though the patient is conscious, it is important to remember that he usually has had medications that may make him dizzy and confused. When the nurse leaves the patient, she should make sure that the side rails are in place and that the call bell is handy. Later, when she observes that he is sufficiently alert, she may lower the side rails.

At first the patient's lower extremities will feel numb and heavy. Even though an explanation of this feeling was made before surgery, it is important for the nurse to repeat the explanation that numbness is usual and will subside in a short time. Many patients become apprehensive because of this symptom, and fear that the anesthesia has resulted in paralysis of their legs.

**Shock and Fluid Therapy.** The pattern of the vital signs gives the nurse a clue to the degree of shock. Postsurgical shock due to blood loss, fluid shifts, and neurogenic factors is usually mild and amenable to therapy.

Intravenous fluids are regulated to prevent overhydration but are specified in amount and rate of flow to treat dehydration. The kind and specific amount of intake for fluids and blood depends on the patient's requirements and the kind of surgery performed. The rate of flow is carefully determined at the start and checked frequently to keep it flowing at the required number of drops per minute.

Intravenous fluids are usually administered throughout the operation and into the recovery phase until the patient's blood pressure is stabilized. This is a routine precaution that is desirable in the event of sudden reaction which might precipitate shock. Maintenance of adequate circulation is essential for prompt treatment of vascular collapse even in a mild form. If the surgical procedure is a major one, fluids are needed to maintain nutritional status until the patient is able to resume oral nourishment. The rationale for fluid replacement is summed up by Halasz (1967) in terms of the three essential parameters that affect body-fluid homeostasis. Included in the order of their importance are: (1) assessment of the circulating volume as the first and most immediate consideration, (2) correction of major pH disturbance (especially sodium or potassium) to restore vascular tone, and (3) correction of specific electrolyte abnormalities as determined in laboratory findings.

**Care of Drainage Tubes.** The number and kinds of drains and tubes vary with the surgical intervention. Specific details of the use of drains in surgery are discussed in relation to those procedures that require them. What is essential is that the nurse determines the adequacy of drainage so that when drains are not functioning properly, measures may be instituted to correct the malfunction. To prevent further complications and delayed healing, indwelling drains must be kept in proper position and in working order. Catheters and tubes must be checked to prevent kinking or clogging that interferes with adequate drainage of urine or bile. Calmness, patience, and if necessary, repeated explanations will be required to help the patient understand these drains and tubes. This is much more difficult to do in the postoperative period if adequate explanation has not been included in the preoperative instruction, according to the patient's level of understanding.

## Transfer to the Nursing Unit

Just as the nursing unit was notified when the patient was received in the recovery room from surgery in order that the family would know of the patient's progress, the recovery room nurse informs the unit of the plan to return the patient to his room. A complete report of care given and of his condition are relayed. A nurse, aided by a nursing assistant, returns the patient to his unit.

## SUMMARY

The patient who consents to have surgery, particularly when this involves taking a general anesthetic, renders himself completely dependent on the knowledge, the skill, and the integrity of those who care for him. In accepting this trust, members of the surgical team have an obligation to make the patient's welfare their first consideration during the period when they are ministering to him. The handling of the patient should be as gentle as possible; every effort should be made to prevent injury. The patient should not be left alone until he has recovered from the anesthetic. The most meticulous attention is given to preventing infection and other complications, such as hypostatic pneumonia. It is the conscientious attention to each detail and the teamwork and concern of all who care for the patient that translate knowledge of modern techniques into a miracle of healing.

## REFERENCES AND BIBLIOGRAPHY

AMA News: Is your anesthetized patient listening? *JAMA* 206:1004, October 1968.

ATKINSON, L. J.: The circle of patient care, *AORN* 16:45-50, September 1972.

BALLENGER, WALTER F., et al.: *Alexander's Care of the Patient in Surgery,* St. Louis, Mosby, 1972.

BAUDRY, F., and WEINER, C.: The family of the surgical patient, *Surgery,* 63:416-22, March, 1968.

BERNZWEIG, J. D.: *Nurse's Liability for Malpractice: A Programmed Course,* New York, McGraw-Hill, 1969.

BRODIE, S. F.: Surgical operating suites of the future, *AORN* 9:33, January 1969.

BURGESS, M. G.: Nursing care plan for the postoperative patient in the recovery room and intensive care unit, *Nurs. Clin. N. Am.* 3:499-502, September 1968.

CARNES, M. A.: Postanesthetic complications, *Nurs. Forum* 4:46-55, 1965.

CONVERSE, M. C.: Preanesthetic physical examination, *Hospitals* 42:42, September 1968.

DODGE, J. S.: What patients should be told: patient's and nurse's beliefs, *Am. J. Nurs.* 72:1852-54, October 1972.

EGBERT, L. D.: Psychological support for surgery patients, *Int. Psychiat. Clin.* 4:37-51, February 1967.

HALASZ, N. A.: Fluid and electrolyte balance in the poor risk patient, in Lorham, P. H. (ed.): *Anesthesia for the Poor-Risk Patient*, International Anesthesia Clinic, vol. 5, pp. 725-33, Boston, Little Brown, 1967.

HOELLER, SR. MARY LOUISE: *The Operating Room Technician*, ed. 2, St. Louis, Mosby, 1968.

JACOBS, R. H.: Prototype designs reflect innovations in operating room planning, *Hospitals,* 43:1240, June 1969.

JOHNSON, J. E.: The influence of purposeful nurse-patient interaction of the patient's postoperative course, *ANA Regional Clinical Conferences,* 2:16-22, 1965.

LEONARD, P. F., and GOULD, A. B., JR.: Dynamics of electrical hazards of particular concern to operating room personnel, *Surg. Clin. N. Am.* 45:817-28, August 1965.

LINDEMAN, C. A., et al.: Effect of preoperative visits by O R nurses, *Nurs. Res.* 22:4-16, February 1972.

MARX, G. F.: Pain and awareness during surgical anesthetic, *N.Y. State J. Med.* 67:2623, October 1967.

MEYERS, B. L.: Patients in an O R corridor, *Am. J. Nurs.* 72:284-5, February 1972.

NEUMAN, B. M., et al.: A model for total person approach to patient problems, *Nurs. Res.* 21:264-69, May-June 1972.

PLEITEZ, J. A.: Psychological complications of the surgical patient, *AORN* 15:137-8, August 1972.

RAMSEY, M. A.: A survey of preoperative fear, *Anesthesia,* 27:396-402, October 1972.

SARNER, H.: *The Nurse and the Law,* Philadelphia, Saunders, 1968.

TITCHENER, J. L., and LEVINE, M.: *Surgery as a Human Experience,* New York, Oxford University Press, 1960.

WHITE, J. J., et al.: The comparative effectiveness of iodopher and hexachloraphene surgical scrub solutions, *Surg. Gynec. Obstet.* 135:890-92, December 1972.

WILBUR, S. A., and DERRICK, W. S.: Physiological monitoring during anesthesia and surgery, *Biomed. Sci. Instrum.* 3:197-206, 1967.

WINSLOW, E. H., and FUHS, M. F.: Preoperative assessment for postoperative evaluation, *Am. J. Nurs.* 73, 8:1372-4, August 1973.

ZEPERNICK, R. G.: New trends in anesthesia, *Nurs. Forum* 4:41-45, 1965.

# The Preoperative Patient:
# Nursing Process

As discussed briefly in Chapter 14, improving the quality of patient care requires that nurses, surgeons, and anesthesia personnel work together to facilitate the most effective care necessary for optimal well-being throughout the patient's surgical experience. Ideally, communication can also be established by using preadmission sources (the physician, community health nurse, clinic, or emergency service involved in the patient's illness) to obtain basic data needed for patient assessment. Initial information developed with sufficient clarity, accuracy, and brevity provides a basis for ongoing assessment of the patient's needs, problems, and resources.

## PREOPERATIVE ASSESSMENT

Assessment is "the initial and continuing determination of why a person should be under nursing care" (Orem, 1971). Just as the physician obtains data from a careful history, laboratory tests, roentgen examinations, and consultation of specialists to assess the patient physically and biologically, so the nurse gathers information which provides indications for initial evaluation and serves as a basis for planning ongoing nursing care and reassessment as conditions change. The efforts of nurse, physician, and other staff are measured by the accomplishment of goals appropriate for the patient.

For the patient undergoing surgery, the concerns of the nurse are twofold: (1) assuring adequate physical and psychological preparation so that the experience of the unknown or the unexpected may be of minimum discomfort and (2) assuring that the patient will be re-

217

stored to optimum performance following the operation. Attainment of these goals is facilitated by the nurse's understanding of the nature of the surgery, the medical regimen, the patient's level of understanding, and the means available to assist the patient to resume daily living following hospitalization.

Besides providing basic nursing care, the nurse contributes her understanding of the patient's needs, problems, and resources. She assesses the total care situation and skillfully applies psychosocial principles to help the patient and his family deal with the surgical experience. Since an operation invariably causes some degree of crisis for the patient, certain insights based upon the concept of crisis intervention will be useful to the nurse as she assesses and cares for the surgical patient.

**Crisis Intervention**

For many patients and their families, a surgical experience is a crisis. Each patient's psychophysiologic reactions will vary, depending on such factors as his coping ability, the nature and course of the illness, the surgeon-patient and the nurse-patient relationships, and the hospital environment. The psychological response to surgery may range from considerable confidence to high anxiety. Thus the nurse should apply her knowledge of behavioral cues in developing her understanding of the patient's response to the experience.

How the patient comes through the crisis depends largely on the patient himself, on others closely associated with him and his world, and on the related aspects of environmental support. In planning her support, the nurse can discover from the patient's past history how he usually handles crises and how well he is able to cope with stresses of separation and threats to wellness. From this, she can determine what support the patient will need and the resources he has to sustain him during the threat of the operation.

At the same time, through her observations of family members, visitors, and the patient's conversation, the nurse can begin to assess the extent to which the patient is supported by other significant people in his life. She will also be alert to his knowledge of available community resources, the support they offer, and the method of obtaining their services and if necessary, be ready to supply this information. She should also be aware of other facets of the patient's situation, such as his role in the home, the state of his finances, and the prospects

he faces for recovery and return to work. The nurse will utilize this information along with the values of the patient in developing goals with him.

The peak crisis period is relatively brief for most patients. The immediate preoperative period may range from several days to a few weeks prior to operation, while the immediate postoperative period covers the initial 48 hours to a few days recuperation in major operations. The patient should be cautioned, however, that full recovery does not necessarily coincide with the healing of the wound. He will need adequate rest to recover from the onslaught of the anesthesia, the trauma to deep tissues which require a longer period of healing than does the skin, and the psychological stress. Even after the period of hospital convalescence, discharge and return to previous surroundings often present new crises, depending on the demands upon the patient or those surrounding him. Adequate preoperative learning through purposeful instruction should be begun well before the operation in order to help the patient deal with the long-range aspects of the experience as well as the immediate effects. Careful nursing intervention in the early preoperative phase promotes recovery and minimizes complications.

Objectives in Crisis Intervention

During crisis it is essential to provide for frequent, open significant communication between the patient and the nursing staff. Patients do not get well just by medicines. They need to want to get well, to be hopeful, and to feel that others care about them.

Objectives in crisis management are to intervene quickly and skillfully in order to help the patient identify his fears, to notice and to use his assets, to think logically, to come to decisions which are right for him, and to learn to use the help and resources available to him.

In assisting the patient to accomplish these objectives, the nurse must have sufficient knowledge of the dynamics of behavorial motivation, language, and nonverbal communication. She must also be able to examine her own assumptions, expectations, beliefs, and inhibitions as well as those of the patient and his family.

**NURSING INTERVENTION**
**Emotional Support**

The nurse who believes that patients should be encouraged to express their fears and to ask questions will reveal this in her manner. For example, if a patient says, "I'm a little nervous," the nurse may respond, "You're a bit uneasy." Thus she shows that she understands what the patient means, and she leaves the way open for him to discuss it further if he wishes. On the other hand, if the nurse believes that patients should accept quietly all that is done for them "for their own good," she may reply, "Oh, there's nothing to be nervous about." Such a statement implies that the patient's feelings are foolish or unnecessary, and it prevents further discussion of the matter.

Of paramount importance is the nurse's attitude toward the patient. If she really cannot stand the patient's expression of fear or doubt, she may convey this disapproval by gestures or facial expressions, even though she replies "correctly."

What fears may the surgical patient have? Consider the woman who is to have breast surgery. Fear of the diagnosis probably looms large. She may fear mutilation; amputation of the breast would alter her appearance irrevocably. (Even though a prosthesis may be worn that keeps others from realizing she has had surgery, the patient will experience a change in body image.) She may be very concerned about her husband's reaction to her changed appearance. The possibility of cancer—and of major surgery—may arouse fears of pain and death. The thought of being unconscious and unable to know or in any way control what is happening to her is disquieting. Fear of unrelieved pain after surgery is often a source of apprehension.

Patients differ in their emotional reactions to surgery. Just as some people have a particular fear of speaking before a group, some have an extreme fear of surgery. It is most important to recognize these reactions for the sake of the physical and emotional welfare of the patient.

Patients who are extremely frightened respond poorly to surgery; they seem to be particularly prone to complications like cardiac arrest and irreversible shock. Unless the operation is an emergency, many surgeons defer surgery if the patient is very frightened. If the patient has been extremely fearful before surgery, he may show unusual behavior afterward, perhaps not recognizing changes in his body that have resulted from surgery, or withdrawing from others and seeming very depressed. Thus the nurse should be alert for symptoms of unusual emotional reaction during the preoperative period and should report them carefully. Baudry

and Weiner (1968) point out that the task of preoperative instruction is a dual one—giving information and correcting misconceptions. Throughout preoperative instruction, the nurse recognizes mechanisms of defense as part of a process that does not necessarily imply pathology or illness in the personality.

## Preoperative Instruction

Preparation for elective surgery (surgery to improve the patient's health, not emergency surgery) begins well before the day of operation. A careful, clear explanation by the surgeon of the reason for the surgery and of the results to be expected is necessary. It is important for the nurse to talk with the physician, so that she knows what his plan of care is for the patient. When the team knows what information the physician has given, nurses are in a better position to help the patient understand any points that are not clear or overcome any misconceptions he or his family may have.

After the physician has discussed the surgery with the patient, the nurse explains the plan for preoperative and postoperative nursing care and ways in which the patient can participate in helping himself to recover. For example, she explains the purpose of the deep-breathing exercises and that turning and range of motion exercises are prescribed. She might say, as she demonstrates the deep-breathing exercises, "After your surgery, we want you to take deep breaths, like this, so you can get rid of sputum or mucus so that your lungs can expand fully." Then she lets the patient practice the exercises and praises his successful efforts.

Often patients are admitted to the hospital one or two days before surgery. Because of the shortness of the time available to work with the patient before he goes to surgery, it is essential that teaching be planned carefully. Although certain aspects of admitting the patient, such as care of valuables, may be delegated to nonprofessional personnel, it is the nurse who must assume responsibility for assessing the patient's reaction to his impending operation and for supporting him and teaching him what he can expect, and how he can help himself during the surgical experience.

Before surgery the patient usually is alert and free of pain. During the immediate postoperative period he is drowsy from medication and anesthesia, and often has pain. Pain and sleepiness interfere with learning. The nurse should apply this understanding by teaching her patients during the pre-operative period. Repetition and review will be necessary postoperatively, but by then the patient will be better able to participate, because he knows what to expect. The nurse should remember that the patient probably is anxious and that anxiety may interfere with learning. For this reason, she should learn to recognize defenses, such as denial or forgetting, and plan her explanations in accord with the patient's readiness and ability to receive instructions. Planned use of simple, factual explanations that are adjusted to the patient's ability and needs are an essential part of the nursing care plan. A patient who is helped to understand what he can do to help himself is prepared to cooperate with the health team.

In one study patients who had had the opportunity to explore the meaning of surgery and to ask questions of the nurse concerning the surgical experience were compared with a control group who had received only routine care limited largely to the physical aspects of preparation for surgery. A far lower incidence of postoperative vomiting occurred in the first group than in the second (Dumas and Leonard, 1963). The implication is that the nurse's skilled attention to the patient's emotional needs can lessen the likelihood of postoperative vomiting, with its discomforts and dangers. It is also undoubtedly true that preoperative patients who are helped to understand and to cope emotionally with the surgical experience are spared much anxiety, the effects of which can influence recovery—even after the patient has gone home.

While vomiting is obvious, many of the other effects of preoperative anxiety are more subtle, and all too often they are ignored in practice. Modern nursing practice is becoming better informed of the meaning of behavior and the significant cues to which the health team can respond. If the nurse recognizes anxiety and knows how to respond, she also learns to seek the assistance of other persons skilled in health care. She discusses with the physician the patient's behavior patterns which the observations of an alert staff bring to the nursing care conferences. The preoperative phase is a crucial time to assist the patient to begin his journey to recovery or to work at his postoperative limitations of rehabilitation. For some situations, a psychiatric consultant or a clinical specialist in psychiatric nursing works with the nursing unit team during the pre- and postoperative phase (Kelouch, 1968).

**Group Teaching.** While individual teaching and the opportunity for the patient to talk with the nurse about his concerns are always indicated, group teaching may be supplemented. This offers the patient an opportunity to share some of his concerns with others who face surgery and to gain support from the group as well as from the nurse. It has particular advantages for some shy patients, who may benefit from hearing discussion elicited by questions of others—questions they would like to raise, if they could summon the courage.

Since group teaching is not appropriate for all patients, it is important to evaluate the patient's readiness for it before inviting him to participate. For example, a patient who denies that he is about to have surgery should be worked with individually by the nurse; placing him in a group of persons about to have surgery is likely to cause him greater anxiety and greater withdrawal from the reality of his imminent surgery. After some individual teaching, he may profit from joining a group discussion.

The patient who shows high anxiety by talking a great deal and expressing much fear also requires individual work with the nurse before joining a group. Such a patient is likely to communicate his anxiety to others, thus increasing their anxiety. In addition, the very anxious patient usually cannot use the group discussion effectively until his own anxiety level is lower, enabling him to attend to what others in the group are expressing and to the instruction that is being given. The patient experiencing moderate anxiety may, however, find group discussion helpful if the group is supportive of him. Patients can derive considerable help in dealing with their own anxiety from being part of a group whose members are all facing similar problems.

All patients who, before surgery, participate in group discussion and demonstration of such procedures as deep-breathing and coughing require the nurse's individual attention afterward, to assess what they learned in the group, to provide an opportunity for questions and concerns which they did not feel free to bring up with others present, and to clarify aspects of the group discussion which may have been confusing to or misinterpreted by them. In reviewing the group discussion, it is preferable to ask the patient what he remembers and what he considers were the significant points brought up in the group, rather than to ask if the discussion was clear to him. The latter question may be answered simply by the word "yes" and may obscure much misunderstanding and apprehension about the surgical experience.

### A Guide for Demonstrating Procedures for Postoperative Patients

This guide may provide a basis for demonstration to a group of patients, and a return demonstration by them of each of these steps.

1. Breathe deeply. Expand chest fully. Inhale. Exhale. Rest.

2. Cough deeply, holding the place where your incision will be. Rest.

3. Exercise your legs while lying on your back. Do this exercise one leg at a time. Flex knee; draw it up toward chest. Then extend knee, lower leg onto mattress. Rest. Extend and rotate foot. Point toes as far away from you as possible; then toward you as far as possible. Tighten leg muscles. Rest.

4. Getting out of bed, and back into bed
   a. The nurse will place your bed in "low position" close to the floor.
   b. She will assist you to sit up and place your legs over the edge of the bed. (Demonstrate, with nurse and patient.)
   c. Place your feet firmly on the floor. With assistance of the nurse, stand up and walk to the chair.
   d. The nurse may place a folded sheet snugly around your abdomen the first few times you get up. This, like holding your incision when you cough, lessens pain. Sometimes a "binder" is used for this purpose. (Demonstrate.)
   e. After the first time or two, begin to concentrate on standing up straight when you walk and on gradually increasing the number of steps you take.
   f. When getting back into bed, sit slightly over "halfway" toward the head of the bed. Gently and slowly swing your legs up onto the bed. The nurse will adjust the head rest for your comfort. She will not leave the knee rest up, because this places pressure behind your knee.

5. Turning in bed
   At first, the nurse will help you. Here is how to turn in bed, with her help. (Demonstrate.) When you are turning yourself, lie on each side and on your back. Alternate your position frequently.

The nurse will help you with all these procedures, designed to help you recover quickly from your surgery, the first few times you do them and whenever you need her assistance. Soon you will be doing more and more of these kinds of activities on your own.

While it is wise to demonstrate procedures to preoperative patients, it is important that group teaching not focus exclusively on procedures such as coughing, deep breathing, and leg exercises, but that time be allowed for patients to express some of their concerns and questions. Unless group teaching is handled with sensitivity to the responses of patients, it can become a stereotyped period of information giving, which can leave them feeling alone and bewildered by the welter of new information they are expected to acquire.

### Diversional Needs

If the patient's preoperative preparation is extended over several days or weeks, diversion is important to make the time pass more quickly. The patient may enjoy reading, watching television, or painting. As with medication (see below, Preoperative Medication), diversion should not replace but should be used in conjunction with careful psychological preparation. Other patients, as well as staff members, affect the patient's attitude toward surgery and the whole experience of hospitalization. An attempt should be made to place the patient among other patients who are cheerful and recovering rather than near those who are very ill, depressed, or bitter. A patient who discusses his own treatment in gory detail, with resentment and anger, should have his interaction channeled toward the staff rather than with newer patients, who may be frightened by his remarks.

The best nurse-patient relationship can be marred if the nurse seems confused and disorganized in carrying out physical aspects of preoperative care, or if her lack of knowledge and technical skill jeopardizes safe preoperative preparation. Because it is especially important to appear calm and well-organized, even during a first experience in preparing patients for surgery, the nurse should make a list of important points and carry it in her pocket the first few times she prepares patients for the operating room. It will free her from excessive concern over forgetting important details, and enable her to concentrate more on the patient's reactions and special needs.

### Family Considerations

Family members need to understand what measures are necessary to prepare the patient for surgery, so that they can participate intelligently in his care and provide him with further explanation and encouragement. Sometimes the patient can accept the necessity for surgery better if it is explained further to him by a relative whom he loves and trusts. Many family members want to be near the patient and to help in any possible way to prepare him for surgery. Their presence helps the patient to feel less alone and assures him of his family's concern and interest.

The nurse who believes that family members have a right to be with the patient and that their presence can be helpful will reveal this attitude in her manner toward the family. On the other hand, if she believes that the family is in the way or likely to upset the patient, she will behave in a way that will create unnecessary tension.

Patients and families whose needs have been ignored often later, in their anxiety and uncertainty, ask many questions and make many small requests. They are likely to be very upset over minor changes, and they then may be labeled "difficult" or "uncooperative." For example, if a nurse denies her patient the comfort and the reassurance of her husband's unhurried presence, his visits may be hasty and furtive, because he is made to feel that he is interfering with his wife's care. The lack of explanation about his wife's care may establish the basis for worry and even doubt about the quality of care that she is receiving. Could this lack on the nurse's part indicate that she is more comfortable in avoiding the genuine care and concerns as well as insightful professional service that would benefit both the patient and her husband?

## Religious Considerations

It is generally accepted among professional practitioners that each patient's religious beliefs are respected, including his right to disbelief. Since religious faith is a source of strength and courage as well as of spiritual consolation, for many patients, every effort should be made to help the patient to maintain ties with his church, either through the services of his own clergyman or through the hospital chaplain. This is especially important during a crisis, such as a pending operation. Most hospital administrations make adequate provisions for patients to secure the services of their chosen clergy. Nursing personnel at the patient's bedside may pass on a request to see a chaplain, rabbi, or minister, or notice of the patient's admission may have been sent to the pastor.

Sometimes, in the desire to protect the patient's belongings and to keep his bedside stand neat just before surgery, a nurse strips him of religious articles that can be a solace to him. Despite the usual rules about not taking personal possessions to the operating room, it is often possible to modify these rules so that a patient may take a religious medal with him. In this case everyone must be alert to prevent loss of the article during surgery. A small medal can be taped to the wrist. This method of fastening it is safer than pinning it on the gown, since the gown may need to be changed quickly, and the medal might be thrown into the laundry.

## Emergency Surgery

The patient who enters the hospital for an emergency operation must be prepared for surgery as quickly as possible. However, even in this situation the nurse's manner can convey to the patient and the family a sense of calmness and a feeling that the patient is in good hands. Even though explanations must be brief, they should be given if the patient is aware enough to understand them.

With the current emphasis on the value and necessity of adequate physiologic assessment of the trauma patient, there is growing evidence that, even in an emergency, the concepts of a nursing practice theory can be implemented. In an integrated system of coordinated emergency service where measures taken to control critical life-threatening injuries at the scene assure a modicum of physiologic stability, the nurse interrelates her initial assessment with the information relayed by the ambulance personnel and that obtained immediately following the patient's arrival at the hospital. The nurse's skill in reducing the patient's anxiety (as well as her own), when applied in an emergency contributes to adept management of the patient's initial well-being and provides a basis for effective interventions beyond the immediate contact.

Careful research into the information about the accident and injury has brought into focus the psychosocial factors associated with trauma (Haddon, 1964). Motivation to get well or to remain sick is influenced chiefly by two factors: (1) the emotional state of the person and (2) the reaction of others who are significant to the patient. For example, from a study of chronic asthmatic patients it has been shown that the overanxious and overprotective attitude of others, including physicians and nurses, has frequently led to increased disability and influenced the acceptance or rejection of continued medical, nursing, and rehabilitation efforts. As soon as emergency measures have been carried out, it is especially important to spend time talking with the family, helping them to understand what has happened. When the patient recovers sufficiently, extra thought and attention should be given to helping him to understand the illness or accident that has overtaken him.

## PREOPERATIVE MEDICATION

Barbiturates, such as phenobarbital and sodium pentobarbital, often are given the evening before surgery to help the patient to sleep. Sometimes tranquilizers, like meprobamate, are given for a day or two before surgery to help the patient to remain calm. About an hour before surgery a narcotic, such as morphine or meperidine hydrochloride (Demerol), usually is administered to relieve apprehension. (Because morphine depresses respirations, some doctors prefer to use Demerol preoperatively.) Most patients who enter the hospital for surgery are unaccustomed to taking sedatives and narcotics. Elderly people particularly may become restless and confused after the administration of barbiturates. Often another type of sedative, such as chloral hydrate, is ordered for them.

If a general anesthetic is to be given, atropine often is administered with the narcotic to lessen respiratory secretions, thus decreasing the likelihood of respiratory complications resulting from aspiration of secretions. If a patient receives atropine, he should be told that it will make his mouth feel dry.

To make sure that the maximum effect is obtained, the nurse will plan the work so that there is no delay in giving a preoperative medication. The optimum time for the medication is 30 to 45 minutes before surgery.

It should be explained to the patient that the preoperative injection will make him very sleepy. He should be asked to stay in bed, once the drug has been administered, and to call the nurse if he needs anything. The importance of not smoking after the medication has been given should be stressed, since the patient is likely to fall asleep, drop the cigarette on his bed, and suffer severe or fatal burns. If he feels he must smoke one last cigarette just before surgery, someone should stay with him while he is smoking. When the patient is left alone, side rails are put up into position and the call button is left where he can reach it. He should be instructed to stay in bed and advised that the medication will be in effect about 20 minutes after it is given. A sense of drifting, some perceptual distortions, and fear of loss of control due to the effects of the drug often require the nurse to offer calm reassurance and to stay with the patient until he is asleep.

On the day of surgery the patient's care should be planned in such a way that he need not be disturbed after the narcotic has been given, so that the medication can exert its beneficial effect. He need not be left entirely alone, if someone's quiet presence would make him feel more secure. While the patient is resting in bed or in the operating room suite, he should not be approached with social chit-chat that serves to keep him alert and awake. If he has been carefully prepared before the narcotic is given and is not disturbed afterward, he will go to sleep after the narcotic has been administered. Although often he may awaken when he is taken to the operating room, the medication dulls his awareness of the experience and makes it easier for him to relax and to take the anesthetic.

Drugs should never be used as a substitute for explanation and reassurance. It has been noted that sedatives administered without any attempt at reassurance or explanation make the patient drowsy but not necessarily calm. Opportunity to talk with a professional person about the surgery the patient faces has been shown to be effective in allaying anxiety. A patient may put on his call light repeatedly during the night before surgery, making numerous small requests, such as having the window raised or lowered and otherwise making apparent his loneliness and apprehension. Instead of calling the physician at once for an order for additional sedation, the nurse should stay with the patient for a little while, and let him talk with her. He probably has many questions and worries concerning the anticipated surgery. The nurse who can sit down and listen will usually find that the patient will begin to relax and, with the help of the sedative given earlier, soon will go to sleep. Straightening the bedding, adjusting ventilation, and giving a back rub are other measures used by skillful nurses to help patients to relax and to rest. These comfort measures are a way of telling the patient that someone knows and cares. In this way, skillful assessment and effective intervention combine human compassion with intelligent understanding of the usefulness of prescribed medication.

| NAME: _____ | | | |
|---|---|---|---|
| ROOM NO: _____ | NURSING CARE PLAN | | |
| Blood Pressure and Pulse: | | | |
| Day of Surgery: | Daily: | POINTS TO CONSIDER | TEACHING AND APPROACH |
| TPR: | O₂: Liter Flow: | | |
| Cough and Deep Breathe: Times: | | | |
| Dressing: Type: | Times: | | |
| Foley Cath: Changed: | Check Voiding: / Due to Void: | | |
| Intake: | Output: | | |
| Bath — Type: | | | |
| Perineal Care: | Weigh: | | |
| Exercise: Time: | Type: | | |
| Oral Hygiene: | Dentures: | | |
| Change Position — Time: | | | |
| Activity — Time: | | | |

Figure 15-1. Sample form for a nursing care plan used by the nursing team during the immediate postoperative period.

## PHYSICAL PREPARATION AND HOSPITAL PROCEDURES

Preoperative preparation may extend over a period of several weeks and may include many tests, x-ray studies, and laboratory procedures, as well as education of the patient and the family. The nurse plays an important part in explaining the necessity for preoperative tests and in carrying out the preparation for them. For instance, she may have the patient fast until blood specimens have been drawn, or she may give enemas prior to x-ray studies of the gastrointestinal tract.

Preoperative patients have their medical histories taken and a complete physical examination performed. In addition, certain laboratory tests such as urinalysis, complete blood count, and hemoglobin determination are usual. These procedures are carried out to discover any pre-existing disease that might alter the patient's response to surgery or his recovery from it. For instance, urinalysis may suggest the presence of diabetes mellitus or chronic nephritis. In many hospitals a routine chest roentgenogram is taken to make certain that the patient has no unsuspected pulmonary disease such as tuberculosis. If unsuspected disease is discovered, the operation may be delayed while measures to treat or to control the condition are instituted.

Often surgery must be undertaken despite the presence of other illnesses. The patient with multiple sclerosis may require surgery for a broken leg, or a patient with heart disease may have to have his appendix removed. These long-term illnesses affect plans for medical and nursing care. The surgeon often consults the patient's physician concerning the management of the coexisting disease. For instance, the patient with heart disease may require daily doses of digitalis, as well as a low sodium diet. The patient with multiple sclerosis may need considerably more assistance with the activities of daily living than would most surgical patients. A diabetic patient needs special treatment before, during, and after surgery. These needs have to be considered in planning nursing care.

As preparations are made for the patient's surgery, the plan of nursing care is coordinated with the surgeon's plan of care. The patient and the family have the benefit of the advance planning that the surgeon, anesthesiologist, and nursing team do. Evidence of these plans is recorded on each patient's chart. Progress of the plans, including information that has been communicated to the patient, and future goals are projected so that the team members share in the goals set by the team leader who assesses patient needs and defines the aims of nursing care in the light of the surgeon's plan of care. Specific provisions of these plans are discussed in the chapters describing patient needs in particular surgical interventions.

A design for organizing some of the information that serves as a basis for nursing care conferences is illustrated in Figure 15-1.

### Immediate Preoperative Care

Immediate preparation for surgery usually starts the afternoon before the patient is to have his operation.

**Skin Preparation.** The purpose of skin preparation is to make the skin as free of microorganisms as

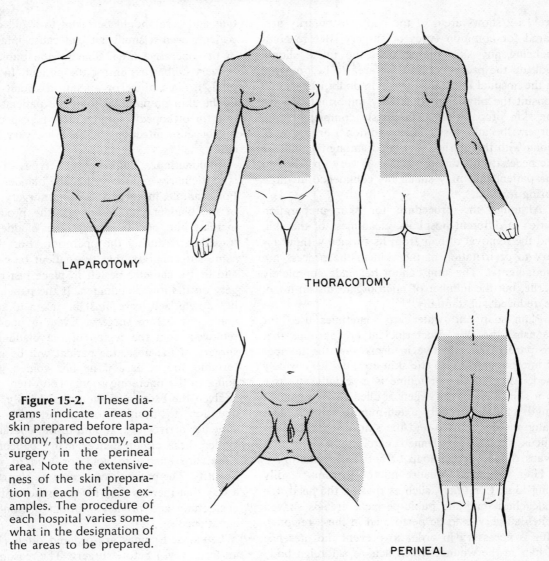

LAPAROTOMY

THORACOTOMY

PERINEAL

**Figure 15-2.** These diagrams indicate areas of skin prepared before laparotomy, thoracotomy, and surgery in the perineal area. Note the extensiveness of the skin preparation in each of these examples. The procedure of each hospital varies somewhat in the designation of the areas to be prepared.

possible, thus decreasing the possibility during surgery of the entrance of bacteria into the wound from the skin surface.

Skin preparation usually is carried out during the afternoon or the evening before surgery. However, in some hospitals this procedure is carried out in the operating room suite just before surgery. Skin preparation may be done by nursing personnel from either the operating room or the ward.

A wide area of the skin is prepared, since this precaution further reduces the possibility of infection and eliminates the need for further skin preparation if the surgery must be somewhat more extensive than was planned originally. For instance, a patient who is to have excision of a small lump in her breast usually has the skin of the neck and the

thorax on that side prepared anteriorly and posteriorly, as well as the skin of the axilla and the upper arm. If later the tissue is found to be malignant, the removal of the entire breast and the surrounding lymph nodes can be carried out without further preparation of the skin. (In his explanation to this patient, the surgeon already will have included the possibility that the breast may have to be removed.) The patient's questions concerning the anticipated extent and the nature of the surgery should be referred to the surgeon. The nurse can assure the patient that it is customary to prepare a wide area of skin surrounding the incision.

Most hospitals have manuals describing specifically the areas of the skin to be prepared for certain types of surgery and the procedure to be used. Figure 15-2 shows areas of the body customarily prepared for common types of surgery. Before commencing any skin preparation, the nurse should look up the procedure and the area to be prepared in the hospital manual. If she is in doubt, she should consult the physician. It is very important to have the skin preparation meticulously complete before surgery, because last-minute additional preparation, along with the tension generated among the staff by the necessity for this procedure, is very upsetting to the patient and may shake his confidence in those caring for him.

Although the procedure for skin preparation varies in different hospitals, cleanliness of the skin and the removal of hair from its surface without injury to or irritation of the skin in the process are fundamental. The skin cannot be made completely sterile, but the number of microorganisms on it can be reduced substantially.

Plain soap and water are sometimes used for cleansing the skin. Bacteriocidal preparations that are particularly effective in decreasing the number of microorganisms on the skin are now very widely used. An iodophor or iodine is especially effective as a skin disinfectant when applied for a sufficient length of time (usually a ten-minute scrub). Plain water should be used and the skin dried. The umbilicus should be cleaned carefully with cotton swabs dipped in the soap or antiseptic solution.

Hair is shaved because microorganisms readily cling to it. Long hair, such as that on the head, the male chest, and the pubic-perineal area is shaved (when surgery is to be performed in these regions). This is necessary in order to prevent the presence of hair in the wound, which acts as a foreign body to prevent healing.

Shaving is made easier if long hair, such as that in the axilla and the pubic region, is first trimmed with scissors. A sterile disposable kit, or at least, a safety sterilized razor and new blade, is used for each patient.

Proper identification of the patient should be assured. A brief explanation of what is going to be done and why should be given before the procedure is begun. (Of course, this advice holds true for all preparations.)

The patient should be draped and screened to prevent unnecessary exposure. A good light should be ready for use, and the patient should be assisted into a comfortable position. The equipment should be arranged at a good working distance and the hair removed completely. The skin should be held taut and care should be taken to avoid cutting the patient; even a small cut can cause infection later in the operative area. Shaving the pubic hair can be very embarrassing for the patient. In most hospitals a male nurse or nursing assistant takes care of the skin preparation for male patients. Preparation for orthopedic surgery must be especially careful, because infections of bone are very difficult to cure.

**Elimination.** Before certain types of surgery it is particularly important that the bladder be empty. For example, in lower abdominal surgery, distention of the bladder can complicate the procedure and increase the possibility that the bladder may be traumatized during the operation. For this reason some surgeons ask that the patient be catheterized and that a catheter be left in place just before surgery on the lower abdomen. If the patient is not to be catheterized, care must be taken to see that he voids just before surgery. Even in operations far removed from the region of the bladder, such as surgery of the nose, the patient will be more comfortable and at ease if he has voided just before going to the operating room. Too often the patient is given the bedpan or the urinal hastily, with little attention to position or to privacy, when the stretcher arrives to take him to the operating room. Under these circumstances many patients become tense, are unable to void, or void in insufficient quantity. The patient's care must be planned in such a way that there is time for the important details of positioning and privacy, without obvious haste or impatience.

ENEMAS. Enemas are ordered often (but by no means always) before surgery. The reasons for their use are apparent—when the patient has surgery of his gastrointestinal tract, the tract must be as free of feces as possible. The act of straining to have a bowel movement is painful after any abdominal operation. If fecal matter is left in the bowel preoperatively, it may become hard and even impacted before the patient is able to bear down painlessly enough to evacuate.

Sometimes enemas are ordered for patients whose surgery involves distant organs. For instance, enemas often are ordered before eye surgery, so that the patient will be spared the strain and the exertion of moving his bowels in the immediate postoperative period; this exertion might cause hemorrhage in the operative area.

Having the bowel empty also prevents the possibility of involuntary bowel movement during or immediately after the operation, since general anesthesia produces muscular relaxation. The patient's comfort and peace of mind are enhanced if he has moved his bowels before going to the operating room.

Small-quantity commercially prepared enemas are being used with increasing frequency for preoperative preparation. Most patients find them more comfortable and less tiring than the large-quantity enemas, and they are usually quite effective.

The nurse should try not to develop a mechanical approach to preoperative care. Instead of saying to herself, "Enemas and catheterization are part of the preoperative routine," she should remember the principle that patients are not sent to the operating room with a full bladder or a full rectum.

The nurse should read the physician's preoperative orders carefully. Each patient's needs are different; each doctor has his own individual preferences concerning preoperative preparation. One patient may be given an enema the evening before surgery. Another patient's physician may order a bisacodyl (Dulcolax) suppository and no enema. When thorough preoperative cleansing of the bowel is essential, physicians often order "enemas till clear." This expression means that the enema is to be repeated until no more fecal matter is expelled with the solution.

**Food and Fluids.** It is essential that the patient have optimum intake of food and fluids during the days or the weeks preceding surgery. The patient whose diet and fluid intake have been consistently poor should be given supplementary nourishment and fluids. (The nurse's observation will be of value in detecting signs of malnutrition.) However, unless the surgery is to be a very minor procedure done under local anesthesia, the patient usually is allowed neither food nor fluids during the immediate preoperative period, in order to minimize the possibility of vomiting and aspiration of vomitus into the lungs.

The physician will leave specific directions concerning the length of time during which food and fluids are to be omitted preoperatively. Usually, midnight preceding surgery is specified as the time for terminating food and fluids. Before this time the patient should be encouraged to eat and drink in order to maintain fluid and electrolyte regulation and to provide nutrients necessary for wound healing. Protein and ascorbic acid (vitamin C) are especially important in promoting wound healing. Except in emergencies, patients whose nutrition is

poor usually have surgery deferred until deficiencies of food, fluids, or electrolytes can be corrected. Parenteral administration may be necessary if the patient is unable to take a sufficient amount of oral fluids.

The accidental feeding of patients who are fasting before surgery is a serious error, since usually it means that surgery must be delayed. Rescheduling the surgery is distressing to the patient, and it prolongs his hospitalization and expense. Careful instructions given to the patient and to all who care for him just before surgery are the most effective measures in avoiding this mistake. The nurse should not wait until midnight before surgery to explain this measure to the patient, nor assume that removing his water glass and pitcher is enough of a hint.

**Nails and Hair.** Details of personal grooming, such as trimming the nails and shaving, should be completed before surgery. Women are asked to remove bobby pins, because they might cause injury if the patient is restless during or immediately after surgery. Long hair should be braided to keep it neat and out of the way. The ends of the braids may be secured with elastic bands. Regardless of the length of a patient's hair, help him or her to arrange it so that it will be away from the face and mouth. Nothing is more distressing to the patient than to find that hair has become soiled with vomitus. Most hospitals provide turbans for patients to wear to the operating room. These serve the double purpose of preventing the straying of loose hair and of keeping the patient's hair clean and in place during the operation and the recovery from anesthesia.

**Attire.** Patients are given clean hospital gowns. If they ask permission to wear their own gowns or pajamas, explain that sometimes patients perspire a good deal and need to have their gowns changed while they are in the operating or recovery rooms. The patient's own clothing is harder to remove, and it might be put with the hospital laundry. For added warmth, patients in some hospitals are provided with long, white cotton stockings to wear to the operating room.

**Dentures and Prostheses.** In most hospitals the patient is asked to remove dentures, so that they will not become dislodged and cause respiratory obstruction during the administration of anesthesia. However, some anesthetists prefer that well-fitting dentures be left in to preserve the contours of the face. The nurse should acquaint herself with the policy at her hospital. If dentures are to be removed, she should tactfully ask the patient if he has any.

If he does, the nurse should give him an opaque denture jar; then, unless he needs help, leave him alone for a few minutes while he removes and cleans them and places them in the jar. In most hospitals the denture jar is left in the patient's bedside stand until he returns to the ward. Other prostheses, such as eyes or limbs, must be removed before surgery.

**Mouth Care.** All patients should have thorough mouth care before surgery; a clean mouth makes them more comfortable and prevents the aspiration of particles of food that may be left in the mouth. Needless to say, chewing gum is not permitted, since it, too, could be aspirated!

**Care of Valuables.** Attention is given to the care of valuables on admission. Sometimes, despite these measures, the nurse finds that the patient has valuable jewelry or documents with him on the morning of the operation. It is the policy in most hospitals that valuables be placed in the hospital safe before the patient goes to surgery. The nurse should always chart what has been done with valuables (such as depositing them in the safe). The nurse may not be working when the patient asks for them, but if she has written the information on the patient's chart, another nurse can locate them readily.

**Makeup and Jewelry.** Because the anesthetist carefully watches the color of face, lips, and nail-beds for cyanosis during surgery, patients are asked to remove their makeup. Jewelry should be removed for safekeeping; a valuable ring might slip off the finger of an unconscious patient and be lost. If the patient is reluctant to remove her wedding band, it may be tied to her wrist with a piece of gauze, by slipping the gauze under the ring, and then by looping the gauze around the finger and the wrist. Care should be taken not to tie it tightly enough to impair circulation.

Because operating-room attire further reduces the poise and self-assurance of the patient, the thoughtful nurse will explain the reasons for it. Many patients joke about their appearance, thus relieving some of their embarrassment. She should not be surprised if an occasional patient places great emphasis on one item of routine or appearance, because when people are anxious, they are likely to concentrate on some seemingly trivial detail.

Policies are designed for the safety of the patient and of his property. The nurse should try not to lose sight of this reason, or to enforce meaningless rules as assertion of authority or discipline. Sometimes exceptions can be made, even to valid rules, if in so doing the patient will be spared acute embarrassment.

## Transportation of the Patient to the Operating Room

When it is time for the patient to go to the operating room, he is placed on a stretcher and covered with cotton blankets. All necessary information should be recorded on the chart before the patient leaves the ward: medications, TPR (temperature, pulse, and respiration), voiding, disposition of valuables and dentures, and pertinent observations concerning the patient's condition. The blood pressure is taken and recorded by the nurse before the patient goes to the operating room; it is helpful to have a record of the patient's preoperative blood pressure so that it can be compared with blood pressure readings during surgery. The blood pressure should be taken before narcotics are administered, since they may lower the blood pressure. The chart and x-ray films are taken to the operating room with the patient.

The patient's identification bracelet and bed tag should always be checked before he is taken to the operating room to be sure the right patient is being taken for surgery.

It is important for the patient's nurse to help him onto the stretcher and to go with him to the operating room. Usually an orderly will assist in handling the stretcher. Before going to the operating room the nurse delegates to a member of the nonprofessional staff the task of making the patient's bed and preparing his unit for his return.

Measures to prevent spread of infection from the ward to the operating room during movement of personnel and patients are essential and should be worked out between the nursing staff of the ward and of the operating room suite. General considerations will be briefly discussed here. The stretcher used to transport the patient is specially cleansed and equipped in the operating room suite and is brought to the ward by an orderly from the operating room staff. Depending on the physical plan of the operating room suite, it may or may not be necessary for the nurse accompanying the patient to don a clean gown and a cap to cover her hair. When a separate area is available in the OR suite for nurse and patient to wait, it is not usually necessary for her to don a clean gown. If no such area is available, usually the nurse must wear a clean gown and cover her hair with an operating room cap. The nurse washes her hands thoroughly before leaving the ward with the patient, and she does not work with the patient if she has any infectious illness, such as a cold.

Accompanying the patient to the OR is of particular importance because undergoing surgery is a crisis situation for most patients, and they especially need the nurse's supportive presence at this time. Preoperative medication lessens, but does not eliminate, the patient's anxiety. In fact, some patients experience considerable confusion during their trip to the operating room, due to anxiety, the effects of preoperative medication, and the rapid changes in surroundings, such as going on the elevator and into the operating room suite. Confusion and apprehension can be lessened by a comment such as, "We are going on the elevator now."

It is important that the nurse remain with the patient until his care is taken over directly by the anesthetist or the operating room nurse. She should avoid "chatter," since it is important for the patient to relax and to drift into sleep, aided by her concerned presence and by the effect of preoperative medication. He should be placed so that bright light is not shining into his eyes as he lies on the stretcher. Sometimes the patient overhears remarks or observes events which seem inconsequential to a busy operating room staff who are accustomed to the environment of the operating room suite but which can frighten the patient. These should be explained and interpreted to the patient as necessary, so that he does not become unnecessarily apprehensive. A thoughtless remark by staff about the tightness of the schedule, or of some complication experienced by another patient, or some problem with equipment can raise anxiety to levels which greatly increase the physiologic and psychological hazards of surgery for the patient who is awaiting his operation. Such thoughtlessness occurs occasionally among the most dedicated of personnel due to the pressures and responsibilities of their work. One useful way of dealing with this problem is to have a nurse remain with the patient and focus her attention entirely on providing physical and psychological comfort during the waiting period (Fig. 15-3).

Some comment like "I'll be taking care of you this afternoon when you come back" is reassuring

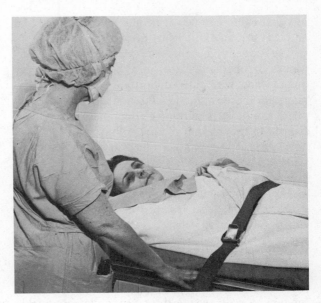

**Figure 15-3.** Emotional support prior to surgery helps alleviate the patient's anxiety. Here the operating room nurse reassures the patient as she waits for surgery. (Courtesy, Overlook Hospital, Summit, N.J.)

to the patient. It indicates that the nurse is expecting him back in the ward. If the patient is going to the recovery room before returning to the ward, he should be told, so that on awakening from anesthesia he will not be alarmed when he finds himself in a strange environment.

## ORGANIZING PREOPERATIVE CARE

Preoperative care involves many detailed observations and procedures that are carried out to protect the patient and his property and to enable him to arrive in the operating room in the best possible physical and psychological condition. Adequate preparation for surgery facilitates the patient's recovery from surgery and decreases the likelihood of postoperative complications. Because of the multitude of details, and the necessity of having the patient ready for the operating room at the scheduled time, it is especially important to organize the details of care and to carry them out in a way that avoids last-minute rush and confusion. Some details, such as having the patient void and giving the medications ordered for him, must be deferred until the time for surgery approaches. Other aspects of care, such as signing the operative permit, can be carried out well before the patient is scheduled to leave the ward. As the patient signs the permit, he needs to feel that calm, competent people are caring for him and that it is safe to entrust his welfare to them.

Occasionally, because the surgery is an emergency, preoperative care must be completed very quickly and with little opportunity for prior planning. In these situations the nurse should try to select the most important aspects of care. (For instance, if the patient's personal hygiene is good, the bath may be omitted; but skin preparation and signing the permission may not be omitted. The essentials must be completed.)

The patient's interests will not be served if, because of haste, the nurse forgets to give his preoperative medication! Instead of dissolving in confusion, when for any reason the stretcher arrives to take the patient to the operating room before his preparation is complete, the nurse can shield the patient from tension by asking the person who calls for him to wait outside the room while she quickly completes the essential care.

### CHECKLIST FOR PREOPERATIVE CARE

Some hospitals put a checklist or reminder sheet on the front of the chart of each preoperative patient. In any case, preoperative care should be organized in some way to provide an orderly approach to patient care. The following checklist covers the essential points in preoperative care:

A. General goals for the whole preoperative period
   1. Emotional support
   2. Instruction
   3. Spiritual needs; visit from clergyman
   4. Planning with family; teaching family
B. The afternoon before surgery
   1. Check preoperative orders carefully; note orders for enemas, catheterization, medications, and any other procedures that are to be carried out preoperatively
   2. Have patient sign consent
   3. Prepare skin of operative area
   4. Safeguard valuables
   5. Give sedative, if ordered, to promote sleep
   6. Withhold food and fluids as ordered (usually after midnight)
   7. Make certain that all specimens requested have been collected (urine, blood)
C. The morning of surgery
   1. Take and record TPR, BP
   2. Assist the patient with personal hygiene as necessary
   3. Help the patient to dress for the operating room

   4. Remove prostheses (including dentures, if it is hospital policy that they be removed)
   5. Administer preoperative narcotic, as ordered
   6. Have patient void
   7. Leave patient resting in bed, with call bell handy
   8. Make certain that all charting is complete

These measures cannot and should not be carried out always in this order. *The needs of each individual patient are more important than any routine.*

## REFERENCES AND BIBLIOGRAPHY

BAUDRY, F., and WEINER, A.: Preoperative preparation of the surgical patient, *Surgery* 63:885-889, June 1968.

BERKOWITZ, P., and BERKOWITZ, N.: The Jewish patient in the hospital, *Am. J. Nurs.* 67:2335, November 1967.

CALLISTA, SISTER RAY: Adaptation: a basis for nursing practice, *Nurs. Outlook* 19:254-257, April 1970.

DUMAS, R. G., and LEONARD, R. C.: The effect of nursing and the incidence of vomiting, *Nurs. Res.* 12:12, Winter 1963.

HADDON, W., SUCHMAN, E. A., and KLEIN, D.: *Accident Research,* New York, Harper and Row, 1964.

HEALY, K.: Does preoperative instruction make a difference? *Am. J. Nurs.* 68:62-67, January 1968.

KOLOUCH, F. T.: Indications for psychiatric evaluation of the surgical patient, *Lancet* 88:87-90, April 1968.

LEE, J. M.: Emotional reactions to trauma, *Nurs. Clin. N. Am.* 5:577-587, December 1970.

LEVINE, M.: *Introduction to Clinical Nursing,* ed. 2, Philadelphia, Davis, 1973.

MESERKO, V.: Preoperative classes for cardiac patients, *Am. J. Nurs.* 73:665, April 1973.

MESSICK, J. M.: Crisis intervention concepts: implications for nursing practice, *J. Psychiat. Nurs.* 10:3-5, September-October 1972.

MEZZANOTTE, E. J.: Group instruction for preoperative patients, *Am. J. Nurs.* 70:89, January 1970.

O'BRIEN, M. J.: The reaction of coronary patients to the sacrament of the sick, *Cath. Nurse* 16:36-43, June 1968.

OREM, D. E.: Nursing: concepts of practice, New York, McGraw-Hill, 1971.

QUIMBY, C. W., JR.: Preoperative prophylaxis of postoperative pain, *Med. Clin. N. Am.* 52:73, January 1968.

REEVES, R. B., JR.: What happens to the patient's religion? *Del. Med. J.* 45:40-43, February 1973.

RODMAN, M., and SMITH, D. W.: *Clinical Pharmacology in Nursing,* Philadelphia, Lippincott, 1974.

WAX, J. J.: The inner: a new dimension of rehabilitation, *J. Rehab.* 36:16-18, November-December 1972.

# The Postoperative Patient: Nursing Process

## CHAPTER 16

Postoperative nursing care involves intensive nursing designed to:

- **Assess the patient's condition, psychologically and physiologically, and to intervene effectively to promote recovery**
- **Prevent and detect complications**
- **Protect the patient from injury during his period of helplessness**
- **Relieve discomfort**
- **Help the patient to regain independence**

Factors such as the patient's age or nutritional status, or disease conditions requiring more intense therapy will affect the duration of the postoperative period. The kind of surgical intervention will have a bearing on how long the patient will require continuous observation beyond the immediate postanesthetic period.

During the immediate postoperative period, the patient is in the recovery room or in an intensive care unit. These are rooms specially designed for the care of the patient while he requires close observation and prompt care in the event of a sudden complication. Patients who go to the intensive care unit are sent there because the physician anticipates a more prolonged stay (over 24 hours), while patients in the recovery room usually stay just long enough to recover from the anesthetic. The intensive care unit may be equipped with electronic monitoring equipment which is used to carry on the continuous or intermittent monitoring of vital signs begun in surgery.

Nursing intervention during the postoperative period is based upon thorough knowledge of the patient, the physiology of the specific operative procedure, and an

231

understanding of the body undergoing stress. Continued assessment of the psychophysiologic measures indicating the patient's current status is used as the basis for nursing judgment and communication with the surgeon, anesthesiologist, and other staff members.

Using the data supplied from assessment and intervention provided in the earlier phases of the patient's illness, the nurse assesses the patient's current status in the light of the anesthetic agents and multiple drugs used, the medication ordered or required, and the surgical technique and its consequent care requirements. Of immediate concern are the intravenous fluids, dressings and drains, nausea or vomiting, the pain experienced, and the monitoring of vital signs. As the postoperative period progresses, careful attention to the patient's activity is necessary while the early signs of impending complications are noted. A more detailed analysis of these complications follows.

## POSSIBLE POSTOPERATIVE COMPLICATIONS

The first 24 hours after the surgery require alert attention to prevent or possibly detect the occurrence of four important complications of the immediate postoperative period: (1) hemorrhage, (2) shock, (3) hypoxia, and (4) vomiting. Because the patient may have been moved from the recovery room, each member of the nursing team must be alert to the signs of change that result from or point to these complications.

### Hemorrhage

Hemorrhage can be either external or internal. If it is internal, it is noted, not by visible bleeding, but by pallor, fall in blood pressure, rapid pulse, restlessness, and dehydration. For external bleeding, dressings must be inspected regularly for any sign of bleeding. Also the bedding and the dressing under the patient is inspected because blood may run under the patient's body and be more evident under him than on his dressing. (See Chapter 59 for a discussion of hematogenic shock.) In such an eventuality it may be necessary for the patient to be taken back to the operating room for ligation of bleeding vessels. Frequently, transfusions are ordered to replace the blood lost.

When reporting bleeding, the nurse should always note the color of the blood. Bright red blood signifies fresh bleeding. Dark, brownish blood indicates that the bleeding is not fresh. When the patient first is transferred to her care, the nurse should find out whether drains have been inserted and what type of drainage is expected. If she knows that a drain is in place, she will not be surprised when brownish-red drainage appears on a dressing. Dressings that become soiled may be reinforced, but they never should be changed except at the direction of the surgeon. If drainage is to be expected, the nurse should always explain to the patient that the drainage is a normal consequence of the surgery and does not indicate any complications.

The color and the amount of any drainage should be reported accurately on the patient's chart.

### Shock

The loss of fluids and electrolytes, trauma (both physical and psychological), anesthetics, and preoperative medications may all play a part in precipitating shock. The symptoms include pallor, fall in blood pressure, rapid, weak pulse, and cold, moist skin. Narcotics should never be administered to a patient in shock or to a patient in whom shock seems imminent. Narcotics given to a patient in shock may not be absorbed, due to the decreased volume of the circulating blood. Thus, as the patient recovers from shock, and the circulation improves, several doses of the narcotic may be absorbed at once, resulting in an overdose. Narcotics may precipitate shock in patients in whom this complication is imminent.

Patients in shock are placed with their heads lower than their feet. However, patients who have had brain surgery or spinal anesthesia should be kept flat; for these patients the foot of the bed should *not* be elevated. (The spinal anesthetic might travel upward and paralyze the diaphragm; placing the head lower than the rest of the body following brain surgery may increase cerebral edema.)

The treatment of shock includes the administration of whole blood, other parenteral fluids, such as plasma expanders, and drugs that help to raise blood pressure. Medications usually are administered intravenously to patients who are in shock. (See Chapter 59 for further discussion of shock.)

### Hypoxia

Hypoxia (oxygen deficiency) may complicate postoperative recovery. Sometimes anesthetics and preoperative medications depress respirations, thus interfering with oxygenation of the blood. Because mucus may block tracheal or bronchial passages and interfere with breathing, the amount of oxygen entering the lungs may be lowered. Oxygen and suction equipment always should be ready for emergency use, and the patient should be watched carefully for cyanosis and dyspnea. Remember that if breathing is obstructed (for example, by the tongue falling backward), the first thing to do is to relieve the obstruction (in this instance by bringing the tongue forward). Frequently, as illustrated in Figure 16-1, an oropharyngeal airway is used to maintain a clear passage for oxygen.

Other factors such as residual effect or overdose of drugs, pain, poor positioning causing pressure, or an obstructed airway also predispose to hypoxia. Signs of restlessness, tracheal tug, jerky and grunting respiratory efforts, perspiration, bounding pulse, and rising blood pressure all arouse suspicion of respiratory embarrassment. In view of arteriovenous shunting at the level of internal respiration, administration of oxygen should be used with some caution, and no time should be lost in securing supplemental information from blood gas analyses and determination of respiratory capacity through the use of the respirometer to develop an accurate diagnosis upon which specific therapy can proceed.

When indicated, positive pressure ventilation is applied by the use of a mechanical respirator. Any one of several types may be used. Many hospitals have the advantage of inhalation therapy services. Personnel in these services are specially trained to take care of the equipment and to assist with this important aspect of care.

As the patient gradually recovers, certain discomforts are manifest. Usually these can be relieved by careful medical and nursing techniques; therefore, they do not achieve the seriousness of complications. Sometimes they progress to the point of serious complications because the patient's response to surgery has been unusual or because preventive measures have not been sufficiently prompt and thorough.

## Vomiting

Vomiting is especially likely to occur after the administration of ether. In current practice other agents usually are used to commence anesthesia, even though ether may be added later. Some patients receive no ether at all but have a spinal anesthetic or some other type of anesthetic. Postoperative

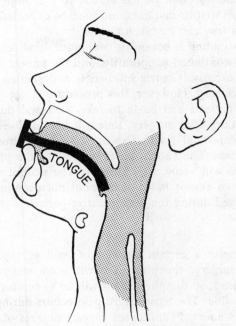

**Figure 16-1.** An oropharyngeal airway in place. Note how the airway prevents the tongue of the unconscious patient from blocking the air passages. As long as the airway is unobstructed and in place, there is a free route for air between the pharynx and the outside.

nausea and vomiting are not as severe now as they used to be, when more patients received ether.

Even today most patients do not feel like sitting up to dinner immediately after surgery. Although vomiting may not occur, most patients experience some nausea or some lack of appetite.

After the patient has vomited, he should be allowed to rest. Food should be avoided until he feels better. Then he may be offered a few sips of a liquid that he prefers or usually tolerates well. Many patients try water; others prefer a little tea or ginger ale. It should be suggested that the patient take only a sip or two and a little more later. Small amounts usually are tolerated better at first. Actions that precipitate vomiting should be avoided since this not only results in a loss of fluid and electrolytes but is distressing and discouraging for the patient. For instance, if the patient is nauseated at mealtime, no one should take a full tray of food to him. There is no surer way to make him turn away in disgust and insist that he cannot eat anything. Instead, the patient should be asked if he would like to try, for instance, a little jello or tea, and he should be taken only the dish that he has agreed to try. Sometimes he finds that he can eat more than he expected, and then a tray can be taken to him.

If vomiting is severe or prolonged, oral feedings are discontinued temporarily, and the patient is fed intravenously. Gastric intubation and suction may be necessary. However, this procedure is not usual. Most patients can begin to take food and fluids a few hours after surgery, unless it has involved the gastrointestinal tract. The nurse's own attitude is important. She should never suggest to the patient that he will vomit after surgery. The skillful nurse keeps an emesis basin nearby but not prominently displayed during the postoperative period.

## PAIN

Because a certain amount of pain is expected after surgery, the physician will leave orders for analgesics, so that the patient will be as comfortable as possible. The most severe pain occurs during the first 48 hours. Pain arouses varying degrees of anxiety in different people. Some take it in stride; others greatly fear it with the result that their tenseness and fear increase the pain.

The pain experienced as the patient recovers from anesthesia is usually rather severe and is often intensified by feelings of helplessness and of uneasiness at being in strange surroundings, as well as by the fact that administration of medication for relief of pain must often be delayed until vital signs become stabilized. Under such circumstances the supportive presence of the nurse is crucial, as are repeated calm explanations that medications for relief of pain will be given as soon as possible.

It is the responsibility of the nurse to evaluate the need of the patient for the narcotic. Usually the medication, such as morphine or meperidine hydrochloride (Demerol), can be repeated at four-hour intervals, if necessary. In no aspect of nursing is sound judgment more vital than in the administration of narcotics to postoperative patients. What at first appears a simple procedure (he has pain; you give the drug) is really a complex one. The following factors must be considered before administering the narcotic:

- Narcotics are not without side effects. For example, morphine may depress respiration or lead to constipation. Demerol often makes patients dizzy.
- Consider the timing of narcotics in relation to getting the patient out of bed. It is sometimes unwise to get a patient up shortly after he has had a narcotic, be-

cause he is more likely to feel dizzy and faint after receiving such medication. However, the timing of narcotics in relation to ambulation is a matter requiring astute judgment. Some patients require medication for the relief of pain before they can tolerate the additional discomfort entailed in getting up. In such instances it usually is wise to allow the patient to rest in bed for about an hour after administering the medicine to permit some relaxation, and then, when assisting him out of bed, perhaps to have the assistance of a second person in case the patient should become faint or dizzy.

- If narcotics are continued for prolonged periods, the danger of addiction arises. However, their use during the first two or three postoperative days does not cause addiction.
- Have nursing measures been tried to relieve the pain? Narcotics never should be administered as a substitute for nursing care. Sometimes helping the patient to turn, rubbing his back, and letting him express some of his worries about his condition are all that is required. Many a nurse who has left her patient to check on a narcotic order, after carrying out these measures, has returned to find him asleep.
- If the narcotic is required, it will have greater effect when the patient first has been made as comfortable as possible. A comfortable patient can rest undisturbed and receive the full benefit of the medication without being disturbed for ward routines.
- Never give a narcotic to a patient whose blood pressure is low and unstable without first consulting the physician. If shock is imminent, administration of a narcotic can precipitate it. This consideration is of particular importance during the immediate postoperative period, when the patient is in the recovery room.
- The purpose of the medication is to relieve pain, not to render the patient stuporous. Oversedation makes it impossible for the patient to practice such preventive measures as deep breathing and coughing.
- Morphine depresses respirations. Withhold it and consult the physician if the patient's respirations are less than 12 per minute.
- Narcotics and sedatives should be given with special caution to older people, because they have a tendency to become restless and disoriented as a result of the medication.
- When giving medicine for the relief of pain, take advantage of its psychological as well as its physiologic effect. All medicines convey some psychological meaning, along with their physiologic action. For example, do not rush in and give an intramuscular injection of Demerol, saying only, "Turn over." The patient may also be receiving penicillin or neostigmine (Prostigmin) as part of his therapy, and he may think that these are the medications being given and that nothing has been done to relieve his pain. Instead say, for example, "I'm going to give you some medicine to lessen the pain. In a few minutes you'll find it will be much less severe. Maybe you can doze off for a while."

- Give the medication promptly when it is required. Minutes seem like hours to patients who are in severe pain.
- Determine whether the pain is incisional pain, for which the narcotic is ordered, or whether it stems from another source. It is not enough to know that the patient has pain. Find out where the pain is. If he had abdominal surgery and the pain is in his chest, do not give the narcotic. Call the physician instead, so that he can discover the cause of the pain.
- Most patients do not require narcotics after the second or third postoperative day. If the patient continues to complain of pain and asks for medication, report this immediately. Perhaps a complication like wound infection is developing. Or perhaps the patient is beginning to rely on the drug to relieve worry and anxiety rather than pain. This tendency should be noted early, because it can lead to addiction.

Exercises in the early postoperative period also can increase the patient's pain. Assisting the postoperative patient to carry out measures to forestall complications and discomforts requires a great deal of tact, patience, and skill. It is all very well to say that the patient must turn, cough, and take deep breaths. Persuading him to do these things when they cause him considerable apprehension and pain is not so easy.

## EARLY POSTOPERATIVE CARE

### Intravenous Therapy

Intravenous fluids usually are given after major surgery to replace fluids and electrolytes. Transfusions may be necessary to replace blood loss. It is important to note whether the infusion is running, its rate of flow (it should run at about 60 drops per minute, unless otherwise ordered), and whether it is infiltrating (Fig. 16-2). The nurse should check the physician's order to see whether additional intravenous fluids are to follow or whether the treatment is to be discontinued after absorption of the present solution.

### State of Consciousness

The patient's state of consciousness must be noted. If general anesthesia has been given, he will be unconscious at first. Gradually he will become somewhat restless and then will open his eyes. Often the patient groans and moves a bit before he is fully conscious. The nurse should not be surprised if he seems not to hear her first few comments or explanations. As he begins to respond, she should talk with him quietly to reassure him that someone is with him and to help him realize that his surgery

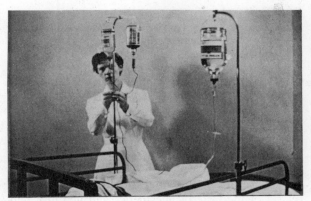

**Figure 16-2.** The recovery room nurse adjusts the rate of flow of the infusion. Note that the patient is protected by side rails.

is over and that he is in the recovery room. Because unconsciousness has been induced deliberately by anesthetics, the return of consciousness must await sufficient elimination of these drugs from his body.

Slapping an unconscious patient's face is not only useless but, if he is just beginning to be aware of his surroundings, physically and mentally traumatic. Shouting "Wake up, wake up!" also shows lack of understanding of the patient's needs and of his condition.

Taking hold of the patient's hand (particularly if he extends it, as though seeking to know if someone is there even before he can see her) is a reassuring gesture and seems to help many patients to feel more secure. Most patients who are recovering from anesthesia do not talk much or, contrary to a popular notion, tell secrets about their past lives. Most of what they say before they regain full consciousness is unintelligible, or it consists of brief comments or groans, showing that they are beginning to feel pain.

### Oral Fluids

Regardless of how much intravenous fluid the patient is receiving, nothing soothes his parched, dry mouth and throat like cool liquids that he can swallow. Patients usually ask for water almost as soon as they begin to complain of pain in the incision. However, several important points must be considered before giving the patient fluids by mouth:

- Check to make sure that the physician's order indicates that fluids may be given postoperatively.

    If the patient is not allowed oral fluids, rinsing his mouth and placing a cool, wet cloth or some ice chips against his lips will help to relieve the feeling of dryness.

- Make certain that the patient has recovered sufficiently from anesthesia to be able to swallow. Ask him to try swallowing without drinking anything. If he can, give him a small sip of water.
- Give only a few sips at a time. It will taste so good that the patient may gulp it, unless you instruct him to take only a few sips. Gulping the water will make him more likely to vomit it. Give fluids through a straw rather than directly from the glass, so that the patient does not have to sit up.

If the patient vomits, the nurse should assure him matter-of-factly that he will be able to retain fluids later. She should offer him mouthwash to help to get rid of the taste of anesthetics and vomitus, and make sure that he is kept dry and clean. She should try not to make him feel that the vomiting was a great calamity or that it is likely to continue for a long time.

However, emphasis on neatness and cleanliness should not obscure other essentials. For instance, if an unconscious or partly conscious patient starts to vomit, and an emesis basin is not handy (perhaps someone just went to empty it), the patient should not be left to look for a basin. The nurse should stay with him and turn his head to the side. Soiled bedding is more easily managed and less harmful than aspirated vomitus!

### Diet

The diet will be ordered by the physician in light of the patient's condition and special requirements. After surgery on the stomach the patient may be permitted nothing by mouth; later he may gradually be allowed small amounts of water. When the patient's condition permits, he is encouraged to resume a normal diet as soon as he can tolerate it. For instance, many patients who have appendectomies can eat a regular diet as soon as postoperative nausea has subsided. Many patients who formerly were permitted only clear liquids for one or two days after surgery now are permitted soft, easily digested foods as soon as nausea subsides.

### Urinary Retention

Patients who have had abdominal surgery, particularly if it has been in the lower abdominal and pelvic regions, often have difficulty voiding after surgery. Operative trauma in the region near the bladder may decrease temporarily the patient's sensation of needing to void. The fear of pain also causes tenseness and difficulty in voiding. The discomfort and the lack of privacy associated with using the bedpan may play a part. Position is very important. Many women cannot void lying down, but they can void if allowed to sit up. Men often have difficulty voiding when recumbent, but they can void normally if permitted to use the urinal while standing at the bedside.

Catheterization in the postoperative period formerly was used quite widely. However, because the procedure entails the risk of bladder infection, it should be avoided when simple nursing measures, plus a little patience, can result in adequate voiding.

The nurse should record the time and the amount of each voiding for one or two days after surgery (the length of time that this part of the record should be kept depends on how quickly normal function is resumed). She should follow any specific orders the physician may leave concerning the measuring of intake and output. However, notation of intake and output during the immediate postoperative period is a fundamental nursing responsibility.

If the surgeon anticipates that the patient will require catheterization, he sometimes inserts a retention catheter while the patient is in the operating room. The catheter may be left in until the patient can void normally. The catheter may be connected to a drainage bag by means of rubber tubing (straight drainage), or it may be clamped and released at intervals.

If the patient is unable to void, eight to twelve hours is the usual time that is allowed postoperatively before catheterization is considered. Overdistention of the bladder must be avoided. Not only does it make the patient restless and uncomfortable, but it can lead to infection of the urinary tract. The following signs indicate that the patient needs to void:

- Restlessness.
- Distention of the area just above the pubis. Palpation of this area causes discomfort and makes the patient feel that he has to void.
- Large intake of oral or parenteral fluid, with no unusual loss of fluid, such as that from prolonged vomiting or profuse sweating.

### Distention

Abdominal distention results from the accumulation of gas (flatus) in the intestines. It is caused by a failure of the intestines to propel gas through the intestinal tract by peristalsis, and it is aggravated by the tendency of some patients to swallow large quantities of air, especially when they are frightened or in pain. The handling of the intestines during surgery may cause postoperative distention, because the trauma of handling temporarily inhibits normal peristalsis. Contributing factors are immobility following surgery and interruption of the diet necessitated by surgery.

The patient's abdomen becomes swollen and painful. Often the pains are quite sharp. In fact, patients who have had severe distention say that their gas pains were worse than the pain from the incision. It is very important for the nurse to differentiate between the patient's complaint of pain around the incision, which can be relieved by narcotics, and pain that results from distention. If the latter is the cause, treatment must be given that helps the patient to expel the gas. The indiscriminate use of narcotics to relieve all complaints during the postoperative period represents very poor nursing. Too frequent use of narcotics can aggravate distention by further suppressing peristalsis and discouraging exercise.

Sometimes, if the symptoms are mild, they can be relieved by nursing measures. If the patient is permitted out of bed, help him to walk about and to go to the toilet. Sometimes the walking, plus some privacy in the bathroom, will help him to expel the gas. He should be encouraged to eat as normally as possible within the limits specified by the physician's orders.

Taking only fluids, particularly if these are always iced, often aggravates the problem. For instance, when the patient eats breakfast on the morning after surgery, suggest that he take a few bites of toast and cereal in addition to the liquids. Hot liquids, like tea and coffee, sometimes help to relieve distention.

If the patient's discomfort is severe, or if it is not relieved promptly by nursing measures, the physician should be notified. Usually he orders one or several of the following measures:

- Insertion of a rectal tube to dilate the anal sphincter and to release the gas that may have accumulated in the rectum. Insert the tube as though you were going to give an enema. Protect the bedding, in case some fecal matter should be expelled with the flatus, by covering the end of the tube with an absorbent disposable pad. The best results are achieved by leaving the rectal tube in place for about 20 minutes, removing and cleaning it, and then inserting it an hour or so later. The constant presence of the tube both day and night makes the patient uncomfortable and messy, and using the tube continuously can render it ineffective.

- Application of heat to the abdomen. A hot-water bottle or an electric heating pad usually is used. Be careful not to burn the patient. If available, a pad that makes possible accurate regulation of the temperature should be used. A device that permits the nurse to set the temperature and to maintain it constantly is preferable to devices that provide uneven amounts of heat.

- Use of neostigmine (Prostigmin) intramuscularly to stimulate peristalsis, thus helping the patient to expel gas. The usual dose is 1 ml. of a 1:1,000 or a 1:2,000 solution. Some physicians routinely order Prostigmin postoperatively to prevent distention.

### Paralytic Ileus and Acute Gastric Dilatation

A very serious condition called *paralytic ileus* sometimes occurs. The patient has paralysis of the intestines and thus absence of peristalsis.

Acute gastric dilatation, a condition in which the stomach becomes distended with fluids that do not pass normally through the gastrointestinal tract, is another complication similar to that of paralytic ileus. The patient frequently may regurgitate small amounts of liquid, his abdomen appears distended, and, as the condition progresses, he may develop symptoms of shock. Acute gastric dilatation is treated by passing a Levin tube to the patient's stomach, applying suction, and removing the gas and fluid. Some surgeons use suction of the gastrointestinal tract routinely to prevent paralytic ileus and acute gastric dilatation.

## COMPLICATIONS OF THE LATER POSTOPERATIVE PERIOD

### Constipation

Sometimes constipation results from interruption of the normal diet and the habits of elimination, as well as from the surgery itself, which may involve the handling of the intestines. Because the patient has not been eating normally, it is not expected that he will move his bowels for several days after surgery. If the patient knows that this is the expectation, he will be less likely to worry about bowel function. Of course, when surgery has involved only a minor procedure, the patient's normal bowel habits are affected little. Most postoperative patients have a normal bowel movement three or four days after surgery.

If the patient is troubled by constipation, often an enema or a suppository is ordered. While soapsuds enemas and oil-retention enemas are sometimes used, small, commercially prepared enemas like the Fleet or the Clyserol have been quite effective in stimulating defecation. The small amount of fluid required (usually 100 ml.) causes the patient little discomfort. Dulcolax suppositories, which stimulate peristalsis in the large intestine, are sometimes used in relieving constipation.

When a full diet is allowed, patients troubled by constipation should be encouraged to eat normal amounts of roughage, such as fruit, salad, and whole-grain bread and cereal. High fluid intake is helpful, as is the exercise of walking about on the ward. Of special importance are privacy, lack of hurry, and confidence (conveyed by the staff) that normal function will return.

Whether the difficulty is with voiding or defecating, the patient should be allowed to use the toilet rather than the bedpan, if he is able. The nurse should avoid going to the bathroom door with repeated questions of "How are you getting along?" Such behavior is likely to make the patient feel that you are hurrying him, and it is an intrusion on his privacy. Instead, she should give him a call light (or if there is none in the bathroom, a bell) and instruct him to call her when he needs her. If it is necessary for her to observe the results, she should ask the patient not to flush the toilet. She should suggest that he go to the bathroom at the same time each day (preferably the time that he is accustomed to at home).

### Parotitis

Patients who do not eat or drink for a period of time are likely to develop parotitis (inflammation of the parotid gland). The parotid glands, which produce saliva, are kept healthy by the normal stimulation of the saliva that occurs during eating. Patients who cannot eat or drink for considerable periods, whatever the cause, should have frequent mouth care. Symptoms of parotitis include the swelling of the parotid glands, pain, and fever. The treatment consists of antibiotics and, sometimes, incision and drainage. The patient is encouraged to chew gum or to suck hard candy to stimulate salivation. If parotitis as a postoperative complication is now rare, it is because conscientious practitioners provide good bedside nursing that includes oral hygiene for patients who cannot do this for themselves. Studies are being done to determine the best ingredients for hygienically sound methods of oral lavage. Gly-Oxide, among others, provides an effective disinfectant.

### Hiccups

Exactly why some people develop persistent hiccups after surgery is not understood clearly. However, gaseous distention seems to predispose to development of hiccups. If hiccups continue for hours, they may prevent sleep and strain the incision, thus causing pain.

Usually, simple methods of relief are tried first, like breathing in and out of a paper bag held tightly over the nose and the mouth. (The patient actually rebreathes his own exhaled carbon dioxide.) Carbon dioxide may be administered by a mask connected with a tank of 5 to 10 per cent carbon dioxide and 90 to 95 per cent oxygen. The nurse should always stay with a patient who is breathing a combination of carbon dioxide and oxygen. In a few minutes he will feel dizzy. Then the mask should be removed, because *continued administration could cause convulsions or coma.* Occasionally a small amount of sugar (one teaspoon) or salt taken without water may relieve the distress. Chlorpromazine (Thorazine), intravenously administered, sometimes relieves hiccups that are not relieved by carbon dioxide inhalations. If hiccups persist, the physician may inject a local anesthetic around the phrenic nerves in the neck, in order to stop the intermittent impulses that cause the diaphragm to contract.

Reassuring the patient that hiccups are usually a temporary phenomenon is also important.

### Pneumonia and Atelectasis

Pneumonia may result from failure to expand the lungs sufficiently, from accumulation of fluid in the lungs, which is favored by lying quietly in one position, and from failure to cough up mucus. Patients with chronic respiratory diseases, such as bronchitis, and elderly patients whose breathing has become more shallow are especially susceptible to postoperative pulmonary complications. Pneumonia of this type is sometimes called *hypostatic* or *postoperative pneumonia.* It occurs because the condition of the patient's lungs favors infection (any fluid which stagnates in the body tends to become a culture medium for bacteria) rather than because the patient has been exposed to virulent organisms, such as those which often cause pneumonia in healthy people. Because conditions in the patient's own respiratory system offer so little resistance to infection, it may be set up by organisms normally harbored in his mouth and throat, organisms that usually are not harmful. The symptoms of pneumonia include fever, cough, expectoration of purulent or blood-streaked sputum, dyspnea, and malaise. The treatment involves the use of antibiotics, such as penicillin. (See Chapter 29 for a further discussion of pneumonia.)

If a mucous plug should obstruct a bronchial passageway, causing the part of the lung served by that portion of the bronchial tree to fail to expand normally, this condition is called *atelectasis*. (Since unconsciousness and immobility are important predisposing factors, these complications can develop also in nonsurgical patients.)

The nurse should help the postoperative patient to maintain conditions in his respiratory tract that help to avoid pneumonia and atelectasis. Specifically, she can

- Suction mucus from his nose and mouth while the patient is unconscious.
- Have the patient rid his respiratory tract of mucus by taking deep breaths, coughing, and expectorating mucus.
- Help him to change his position frequently.

If the patient is unable to cough up secretions, the doctor may have to suction him through a bronchoscope (a long, hollow metal instrument that is passed down the trachea).

Now is the time for the nurse to have the patient do the exercises she taught him preoperatively. She cannot cough or take deep breaths for the patient; he must do these exercises himself. However, she can help by splinting the incision, i.e., placing her hands tightly over it to minimize the movement. Such splinting will lessen the pain in the incision when the patient coughs. As soon as he is a little stronger and more alert, the patient can learn to place his own hand over his incision when he coughs.

It is necessary for the patient to have tissues or a sputum cup in which to expectorate. Some fastidious people will require additional reassurance that it is "all right to spit it out." In polite society spitting is considered vulgar, but in postoperative treatment it is essential.

The nurse explains to the patient that it will be important for him to turn from side to side after his operation. Although frequency and specific ways of changing position must be adapted to the patient's particular condition and needs (for example, the patient who has had eye surgery often is permitted to turn only on one side and not on the

other), frequent change in position is important in the care of all postoperative patients.

Adaptations in methods and frequency in the change of position are discussed in later chapters. Patients whose condition does not require any unusual measure or consideration in turning usually are assisted to change their position every half hour, depending on the operative site and the patient's comfort. The patient may be positioned on either side, on his back, or on his abdomen.

### Thrombophlebitis

When patients lie still for long periods without moving their legs, particularly if there is pressure on their legs from a tight strap or a pillow roll under the knee, venous circulation may be impaired. Blood may flow sluggishly through the veins (venous stasis). This condition predisposes a patient to the development of inflammation, with consequent formation of clots within the veins, a condition called *thrombophlebitis*. There is another condition in which clots form, but in which inflammation is minimal or absent. This is called *phlebothrombosis*. These conditions occur most frequently in the legs. Inflammation helps the clots to adhere to the walls of the veins; therefore, thrombophlebitis is considered to be less dangerous than phlebothrombosis.

Clots that do not stick to the wall of the vein but travel in the bloodstream are called *emboli*. By lodging in a distant blood vessel they may obstruct circulation to a vital organ, such as a lung, and cause severe symptoms and even death. A patient with pulmonary embolism may have dyspnea, coughing, and cyanosis.

The symptoms, treatment, and nursing care of thrombophlebitis are discussed in Chapter 38.

**Preventive Measures.** The nurse may help to prevent thrombophlebitis by avoiding prolonged pressure on the patient's legs, which might impair circulation, and by encouraging him to exercise his legs. Although it is usually necessary to place a restraining strap across the patient's legs during surgery, the use of such straps during the recovery period is not a good practice and, except in unusual situations, is even unnecessary. If the patient is placed in a bed equipped with side rails rather than on a narrow stretcher during his recovery from anesthesia, he can move about without danger of falling. Moreover, on regaining consciousness he will be spared the uncomfortable feeling of finding that his movements are restrained. Often the pa-

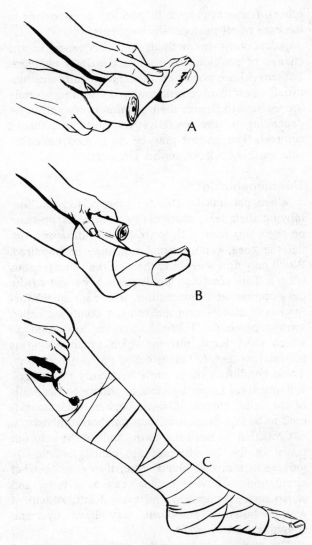

**Figure 16-3.** Steps in applying an elastic bandage. (A) Use four-inch bandages, starting as close to toes as possible to assure maximal venous return. (B) Anchor bandage around ankle, completely covering heel. (C) Overlap one-half to two-thirds of bandage. Continue wrapping to knee or thigh. Use additional bandages as needed. Secure with fasteners.

tient's arm must be restrained because of infusions. To restrain his legs as well will cause him to feel shackled and will increase his restless attempts to free himself.

In contrast with previous nursing practice, pressure on the legs resulting from the placing of pillows under the knees and elevating the knee gatch, and having the patient "dangle" (sit on the edge of his bed, with his legs hanging down over the side) now are avoided. Formerly, these measures were used

to relieve strain on the incision and to make the patient more comfortable. But in addition to causing pressure and possibly interfering with circulation, these practices discouraged movement and exercise of the legs.

SUPPORT STOCKINGS. Providing support for the veins by wrapping both legs with Ace bandages from the ankle to the midthigh also is considered helpful in preventing thrombophlebitis. A common method for the application of elastic bandages is shown in Figure 16-3. Support stockings which are commercially available are presently very commonly used and have the advantage of staying in place and providing firm, even support, without the frequent rewrapping required by elastic bandages.

EXERCISES. Unless the physician leaves orders to the contrary, postoperative patients should begin to move their legs as soon as consciousness returns. These exercises are not complicated and can be taught readily by the nurse during the preoperative period and then reviewed with the patient postoperatively. The patient should be instructed to move his toes and his feet, alternately flexing and extending them. Then he should flex and extend his legs by bending his knees and then straightening his legs. These exercises should be repeated regularly. It is much more effective to advise the patient, "Exercise each leg the way I have shown you ten times every hour," than to say, "Move your legs as much as you can." The nurse should remind the patient to exercise each time that she checks vital signs. If he is still sleepy from anesthesia, he cannot be expected to remember to do exercises.

### Wound Infection

The postoperative patient must be observed carefully for symptoms of wound infection. The first symptom may be increasing pain in the incision. (In normal recovery, pain in the incision decreases.) Other symptoms of wound infection include localized heat, redness, swelling, and purulent exudate. Systemic symptoms of infection include fever, chills, headache, and anorexia (loss of appetite).

The prevention of wound infection among surgical patients is an urgent problem, complicated by the evolution of many drug-resistant organisms. Staphylococcal infections are particularly widespread and especially difficult to treat because of their resistance to antibiotics. Prevention involves all the little unglamorous tasks often overlooked because they seem so trivial. In recent years too great reliance has been placed on the miraculous power of antibiotics to cure any and all infections, and vigilance in everyday routines designed to *prevent* infection has waned. The development of drug-resistant strains of bacteria is forcing us to reconsider some of the precautions that we had come to ignore as old-fashioned or unnecessary.

If a patient develops wound infection, every precaution must be taken to prevent the spread of the infection to others. The rational use of medical aseptic technique is essential in preventing the spread of infection.

The treatment of wound infections involves local and parenteral use of antibiotics, measures to drain pus, if any, and maintenance of the patient's resistance through rest and nutritious diet. Local applications of heat, such as hot compresses, sometimes are ordered to bring more blood to the part to help fight infection.

## Wound Disruption

*Dehiscence* means the separation of wound edges without the protrusion of organs. *Evisceration* means the separation of wound edges with the protrusion of organs. These complications are most likely to occur between the sixth and the eighth postoperative days, when the sutures hold the wound less firmly, and the wound itself may not yet be strong enough to hold the edges together. Predisposing factors include those which interfere with normal healing, such as malnutrition (particularly insufficient protein and vitamin C), defective suturing, or unusual strain on the wound from severe coughing, sneezing, retching, or hiccups.

The patient may say that he has a sensation of something "giving way." Pinkish drainage may appear suddenly on the dressing. If wound disruption is suspected, the patient should be placed at complete rest in a position that puts the least strain on the operative area. If evisceration has occurred, sterile dressings moistened with sterile normal saline should be placed over the protruding organs. The symptoms should be reported immediately. Emotional support and reassurance are as necessary as in any other emergency. The nurse might say, "Just lie there very quietly. I'm going to ask Dr. Jones to check your dressing. I'll be right back."

## EARLY AMBULATION

The term *early ambulation* is used widely to describe one aspect of postoperative treatment. *Ambulation* means walking. The patient is helped to walk about early in his postoperative period.

Since World War II the practice of early ambulation after surgery has helped patients to feel better sooner after their operations. As in every other treatment, achieving the desired results means that early ambulation must be carried out judiciously. When helping a patient out of bed for the first time, the nurse should remember that his body has suffered an insult that has emotional and physical repercussions. Pain at the site of his incision, which is to be expected, makes moving difficult at first.

The nurse should help the patient to a sitting position at the side of the bed. If dizziness is more than momentary, she should help him to lie down again. She should stand right at the bedside so that he will not fear tumbling to the floor. The nonadjustable hospital bed is much farther from the floor than the usual bed. If the height of the bed can be adjusted, it should be placed in the lowest position possible. If this type of bed is not available, a footstool should be used. While supporting the patient firmly with one hand under his axilla and the other on his forearm, the nurse should let him step to the floor and take one or two steps to the chair. He may be surprised to find that he can accomplish the walk within hours of having been on the operating table without having all his stitches pop open.

The exercise and the erect posture help the patient to breathe more deeply, and the change of position helps to prevent congestion of the lungs with fluid. Walking stimulates circulation in the lower extremities, thus lessening the problem of venous stasis. Erect posture and exercise also help to overcome problems of urinary retention, constipation, and distention. Early ambulation helps patients to regain their appetites, and greater activity during the day helps them to sleep better at night. Other important points to remember are:

- Early ambulation is a therapeutic measure. Its primary purpose is to prevent complications, not to solve nursing-service problems. Of course, early ambulation has affected the role of the nurse. Now more time is spent in teaching and encouraging the patient to move about, and less time is spent in bathing him. giving enemas, and doing catheterizations.
- Although early ambulation helps the patient to become self-sufficient more quickly, he continues to need attention and psychological support from the nurse in ways that do not interfere with his being up and about. In the days when patients were allowed barely to move after an operation, the nurse did practically everything for the patient. Now patients are out of bed a few days after surgery. Although the nurse no longer continues to give the patient a

complete bed bath day after day, she is still very much needed—to give skin care, backrubs, advice, attention to diet, and to help him to carry out gradually more of his own care and to plan periods of rest and activity.

- Ambulation means walking, not sitting. Frequently the treatment is misunderstood to mean just getting the patient out of bed in the morning, and assisting him to a chair, where he sits until evening! Prolonged sitting, by putting pressure on the legs, may predispose a patient to thrombophlebitis. The patient should sit for short periods, take frequent short walks, and alternate these with resting in bed.
- Walking soon after surgery often causes the patient pain and apprehension. He needs a great deal of explanation about the purpose of the treatment, so that he does not consider it merely a lack of attention or concern for his comfort.
- Special equipment, like catheters and infusion bottles, need not restrict the patient to bed. However, their management does require some ingenuity, so that the treatment may be continued safely and effectively while the patient is out of bed. Measures that are necessary for managing such equipment are discussed in later chapters. Whether the special equipment is a nasogastric tube or a Foley catheter, knowledge of the principles and the operation of the equipment will enable the nurse to adapt it for use when the patient is out of bed.
- Having plenty of assistance will add greatly to the patient's confidence, and will ensure his safety. The nurse should not hesitate to ask a male nursing assistant or another nurse to help, particularly if it is the patient's first time out of bed, or if he is elderly.

Early ambulation helps the patient to feel less helpless, and it tells him that he is recovering quickly

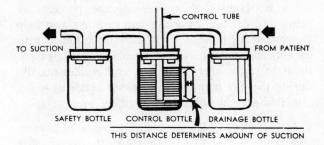

THIS DISTANCE DETERMINES AMOUNT OF SUCTION

**Figure 16-4.** Three-bottle suction. The air vent tube in the second bottle controls the degree of suction (negative pressure) by acting as a "break valve." This tube, usually called the *control tube,* is an alternate pathway for air to enter. The deeper the tube is submerged, the greater the water resistance that the incoming air must overcome. No matter how strong the suction exerted by the pump (example: 90 or 120 mm.), the suction of the patient will be only that which is determined by the *submerged* length of the control tube: (Jensen, J. T.: *Introduction to Medical Physics.* Philadelphia, Lippincott, 1960)

and satisfactorily from his operation. One of the dangers of early ambulation is this same confidence. Because patients look more self-sufficient, they themselves may be misled to walking down a hospital hall that is too long, returning to work too soon, resuming their full routine, or going on a camping trip before they have recuperated sufficiently.

## POSTOPERATIVE CARE OF CHEST-SURGERY PATIENTS

### Special Postoperative Nursing Measures

In addition to the general principles of postoperative care that apply to any patient who has had surgery, certain special postoperative nursing measures are necessary when the thoracic cavity has been opened. Preoperative care of this group of patients is similar to that of other preoperative patients. However, because of the specialized procedures that the patient experiences postoperatively, and because his participation is essential to the success of his postoperative regimen, giving careful instruction to the patient concerning what to expect postoperatively is especially important. The array of special equipment required for postoperative care can be very frightening if the patient does not understand its purpose or realize that its use after chest surgery is usual and does not indicate the development of complications.

The conditions for which chest surgery is performed are discussed elsewhere in the text. For example, surgery involving the lungs is discussed in relation to cancer of the lung. Heart surgery is considered in relation to treatment of heart disease. Chest surgery is considered as one treatment of esophageal hiatus hernia, cancer of the esophagus, and bronchiectasis.

Chest surgery is becoming increasingly common. Newer surgical techniques and anesthesia have made possible the surgical treatment of organs within the thoracic cavity. One particularly significant problem in relation to chest surgery is the interference with normal pressure relationships within the thoracic cavity. When the chest is opened, the air from the atmosphere rushes in, due to the negative pressure which normally exists in the thoracic cavity. The entrance of air under atmospheric pressure collapses the lung, causing serious impairment of respiratory function. By administering anesthesia and necessary oxygen through an endotracheal tube, collapse of the lung is prevented in spite of the opening of the chest. The lungs, inflated by the pressure of the vapors from the tube that passes through the mouth and the trachea, are able to function in spite of the interference with pressure relationships within the thoracic cavity.

## Chest Drainage

After chest surgery it is usually necessary to drain secretions and blood continuously from the thoracic cavity. Accumulation of blood and other fluids within the chest would prevent the necessary reexpansion of the lung. Drainage ordinarily must be carried out by the closed (underwater) method. An open drainage system would allow air to enter the thoracic cavity, for the air would be sucked in every time the rib cage expanded. The air entering from the atmosphere would collapse the lung further. Open drainage of the thoracic cavity, which permits

air to flow back into the chest, is used only when adhesions have formed that prevent the collapse of the lung.

Closed drainage of the thoracic cavity is accomplished by means of a catheter placed in the pleural space during surgery. Postoperatively it is allowed to drain under water into a bottle. Keeping the end of the drainage tube always under water prevents air from being drawn up through the catheter to the pleural space. A sterile drainage bottle, into which a measured amount (usually 500 ml.) of sterile water has been poured, is used for this purpose. In a three-bottle system, the drainage bottle is connected by rubber tubing with a control (trap) bottle, used to regulate the amount of suction being applied. The trap bottle is connected by rubber tubing with a suction device, such as a wall suction outlet (Fig. 16-4). The physician regulates the amount of suction being applied by adjusting the

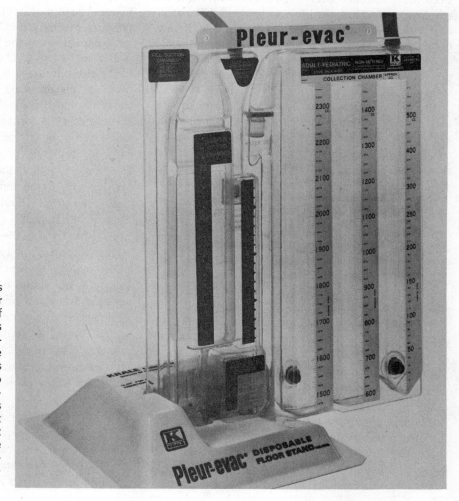

**Figure 16-5.** The Pleur-Evac is an effective disposable unit for underwater-seal drainage of the pleural cavity. Water is added to the left side to establish the water seal and regulate the amount of suction. This side is then connected to straight suction and the suction turned on until there is continuous bubbling. The right side is connected to the chest tube and provides an accurate measurement of chest drainage. (Krale, Division of Deknatel, Inc.)

position of a tube in the control (trap) bottle. The length that this tube is submerged under water in the trap bottle determines the amount of suction applied. The trap bottle is used because usually the amount of suction applied by the ordinary suction device is too great to be applied to the chest catheter. Therefore, the trap bottle lessens to the desired extent the degree of suction applied. The water in the trap bottle (in contrast with that in the chest drainage bottle) need not be sterile.

Any break in the system, either from the tubing becoming loose or from the bottles being broken, would present the hazard of air entering the tubing and being drawn up to the pleural space. All connections of stoppers and tubing are taped carefully to minimize the possibility, for instance, of having the end of a catheter slip off a glass connecting tip. Placing the drainage bottles in a holder is another precaution. The holder helps to protect the bottles from being knocked over and broken. More elaborate devices also are available to hold the bottles. A clamp always must be in readiness so that, if any break in the system occurs, the chest tube immediately can be clamped as close to the chest wall as possible. The clamp is placed where it can be easily seen.

Preventing fluids from flowing up through the catheter and entering the pleural space also is essential. While connected for drainage, the chest drainage bottle *never* is raised from floor level. Raising the bottle could result in a flow of fluid to the pleural space.

Often two chest catheters are used—one anteriorly and one posteriorly. In this instance two bottles are used into which the chest drainage flows, and each is labeled *anterior* or *posterior*. Two clamps are kept in readiness in case of any break in the drainage systems—one for each chest catheter. The amount and the character of the drainage in each bottle is noted and recorded separately.

The principles illustrated here are essentially the same even though the nurse may see different kinds of chest drainage apparatus. Commercial products are becoming available which are safer for the patient because they are designed to prevent backflow of air into the chest space (see Fig. 16-5).

The drainage tube must be patent to allow for the necessary escape of fluids from the pleural space. Clogging of the catheter, which may occur if a blood clot lodges in it, or if it becomes kinked, will cause the drainage to stop. This will prevent the lung from re-expanding normally, and it may cause the position of the heart and the great vessels to shift (mediastinal shift). In the first hours immediately after surgery the nurse is constantly alert to the functioning of the drainage system so that, if a malfunction should occur, precious minutes will not be lost in correcting it.

The fluid in the long glass tube in the drainage bottle will fluctuate with each respiration, and bubbling will occur in the drainage bottle if the system is working properly. Failure of the fluid to fluctuate in the long glass tube may mean that the catheter is clogged or that the lung has completely re-expanded. During the early postoperative period the former possibility is more likely. In some hospitals, milking the drainage tube from the patient toward the drainage bottle to remove an obstruction is considered a nursing responsibility. If drainage is not resumed by milking the tube, the physician should be notified at once. A roentgenogram (made by a portable machine) may be ordered to determine whether the failure of the fluid to fluctuate is due to re-expansion of the lung.

It is important to check the color and the amount of the chest drainage frequently and to note the condition of the dressings over the operative area. Although some bloody drainage is expected through the catheter postoperatively, it should not appear bright red or be copious. In some hospitals, measuring and emptying the drainage bottles is a nursing function; in others, the physician assumes this responsibility. If the nurse is to empty the drainage bottle, she first should clamp the chest catheter close to the patient's chest. The stopper then is removed from the bottle and the contents measured.

It is important to subtract from the total amount of drainage the amount of sterile water originally placed in the bottle. A sterile bottle to which sterile solution has been added to cover the end of the drainage tube is placed in position, the stopper inserted, and the clamp removed from the chest catheter. Drainage must be reinstituted promptly, so that the catheter does not become clogged or the necessary drainage delayed.

## Coughing and Deep Breathing

Coughing and deep breathing are additional measures which help to remove secretions, thus permitting the lung to re-expand. Although these measures are important in the care of any postoperative patient, they are especially so for a patient who has had chest surgery. The risk of developing complications, such as atelectasis, due to retained respiratory secretions, is particularly great in this patient. However, because the incision is in the patient's chest, the motion caused by coughing is extremely painful. The nurse can help by splinting the operative area with her hands when the patient coughs and, later, by teaching the patient to do this himself. The use of an expectorant, such as ammonium chloride, also helps the patient to raise secretions.

Abdominal distention, which pushes up the diaphragm, is a particular hazard after thoracic surgery, because it interferes with breathing. Sometimes, neostigmine (Prostigmin) is given to increase peristalsis and to help to expel flatus. Exercise in bed and early ambulation also help to decrease the problem of flatulence.

## Oxygen

Because the patient's respiratory processes are impaired temporarily, it is important for him to have supplementary oxygen for a time after his surgery. If this is ordered p.r.n., the nurse can determine the patient's continued need for it by his color, respirations, and pulse rate. Usually, oxygen is administered continuously during the immediate postoperative period, and then it is reduced and discontinued as the patient's condition warrants.

## Narcotics

It is important not to give the narcotic to the point at which it makes the patient so lethargic that he cannot move about, cough, and breathe deeply. Because of the particular danger of depressing respirations after chest surgery, drugs having this effect, such as morphine, must be used with caution. Observing respiratory rate and quality becomes more than a routine matter. On the other hand, for the patient to be able to carry out this strenuous postoperative regimen, the relief of pain provided by the use of narcotics must be sufficient. The use of narcotics is terminated gradually as the pain diminishes. The judicious use of narcotics is especially significant when the patient has had chest surgery. Because the incision is in the chest, coughing and deep breathing will be particularly painful, and yet they are particularly important, since there is greater likelihood of complications from retained secretions after chest surgery.

## Effect on the Patient

What does the patient see when he regains consciousness? Usually he sees a transfusion running, several drainage bottles beside his bed, suction equipment, and oxygen. He has a tube running into his nose (for oxygen), tubes running out of his chest, and a tube carrying fluids into a vein in his arm. Many other types of equipment also may be in use, such as monitoring devices which continuously record his ECG on a screen, hypothermia equipment, and a monitoring device which indicates his rectal temperature. (Use of hypothermia and of ECG monitoring are discussed in Chapter 61 in relation to heart surgery.)

Patients who have had chest surgery need nurses who are familiar with the equipment, have operated it enough to be at ease with it, and can center their attention on the patient, rather than on how to operate the machines. The nurse's manner of sureness and confidence as she performs necessary tasks can convey a feeling of confidence to the patient which no words, in the absence of such sureness of technical skill, can convey.

In addition, the patient needs nurses who are perceptive of his emotional as well as his physical reactions. He needs nurses who can detect a fleeting expression of fright on his face when, for example, he sees for the first time the bloody drainage that has come from his chest; nurses who, having seen his emotional reaction, can repeat quickly in a matter-of-fact yet compassionate way the explanation given preoperatively concerning the usualness and the purpose of the drainage.

Care of patients after chest surgery is an example of an aspect of nursing that makes heavy demands on the nurse's technical *and* interpersonal skills; such care illustrates vividly a type of situation in which both kinds of competence are required in high degree. The nurse whose perceptiveness of patients' reactions is so blunted that she views only the technical aspects of care, however competently, may by the second postoperative day have a patient who flatly refuses to cough—and who is accumulating a dangerous amount of respiratory secretions. The nurse who has undervalued the required technical competence may find that the patient has suddenly gone into critical condition because she did not notice that his chest tube was clogged and that necessary drainage from his chest has not been maintained. Small comfort, then, that her main concern had been helping him to understand his feelings in relation to the surgery!

**Posture and Arm Movements.** Particular attention must be given to the patient's posture and arm movements on the affected side, especially after certain types of chest surgery such as thoracoplasty, in which the surgery has had great effect on the muscles and the contour of the chest. In such instances a "ladder" is especially useful in helping the patient to exercise his arm on the affected side during the postoperative period. The ladder or rope, made of sturdy muslin, is placed at the foot of the bed on the affected side. By pulling on the ladder or rope the patient can raise himself to a sitting posture. In so doing he exercises his arm and shoulder on the affected side. Another way to encourage movement of the arm and shoulder is to move the patient's bedside stand to the affected side so that he is most likely to use the arm on the affected side to reach for his belongings. Patients whose surgery has had considerable effect on muscle strength and posture often are referred by the physician for physical therapy.

## VISITORS

The patient's relatives usually feel less worried when they are kept informed of the patient's condition and are given opportunities to express their interest and concern and to participate, when possible, in the patient's care.

Seeing the patient, if only for a few moments, often does a great deal to assure a relative that the patient really is all right—that he actually has come through the operation. Careful explanation of what to expect (that the patient is drowsy or confused, or that he is receiving intravenous fluids) is essential in lessening apprehension. A brief visit from a relative just after surgery often assures the patient that his family is there and that they are concerned about him.

Although visitors usually are not permitted in the recovery room, it is important to keep family members informed of the patient's condition and of the time when he returns to his own room. Some hospitals provide a visitors' lounge adjacent to the area of the operating room and the recovery room. Opportunities for contact with the staff are fostered by such an arrangement because of its convenience to all concerned. If the surgeons and the nurses know that the family are nearby, they can more easily stop to speak to them. The provision of such areas for the family conveys concern for them as well as for the patient. Such an arrangement is in marked contrast with the still prevalent practice of providing no particular place for the families of patients to wait during the surgery and recovery period. Especially in multiple-bed rooms the presence of the family over an extended period can be disturbing to the other patients. Wandering from lobby to coffee shop, family members frequently wonder uneasily how, if there were a need to communicate with them about the patient, they could be found. Often in such situations they are left on the periphery at a time when they are likely to be anxious and very much in need of reassuring contact with physicians and nurses. It is sometimes possible and desirable to allow a responsible member of the family to sit quietly beside the patient during the early postoperative period. Having a member of the family near is especially helpful if the patient is aged or extremely apprehensive or if he is unable to speak English.

## HELPING THE PATIENT TO REGAIN INDEPENDENCE

Helping a patient to regain comfort and independence after surgery is one of the privileges of nursing. Contrary to some opinions, modern surgical care requires not less nursing but different nursing measures. When the physician writes the order "out of bed," it is a treatment rather than an indication that the patient can take care of himself.

Measures that assist the patient to regain independence include:

- **Helping him to dress in his street clothes as soon as he is able.**
- **Assisting him to walk to a lounge and eat at a table with others.**
- **Encouraging him to bathe himself in the bathroom as soon as is feasible. This may be done at first by placing a chair in front of the sink where the patient can sit comfortably and bathe himself with running water. Later, he may be encouraged to use the shower.**
- **Assisting him to shampoo his hair. Many patients are accustomed to washing their hair frequently; thus their comfort and appearance benefit when the nurse helps with the first shampoo, which can be given at the sink with the patient sitting in a chair. A hand-held hair dryer can then be used.**

Of course, encouraging such measures depends on assessment of the patient's physical tolerance.

Although postoperative patients should be encouraged to assist with their own care, considerable physical help and a lot of encouragement are required. By providing patients with enough help and by staying with them when they attempt new activities, the nurse can show the patient that early ambulation and self-help are indeed treatment.

Persuading patients to do exercises that cause pain requires considerable tact, sensitivity, and assurance. The nurse must know that the measure is important and that it will not harm the patient. Her approach to the patient in encouraging activities ought to reflect this knowledge and assurance. The perceptive nurse who uses measures to relieve a patient's discomfort will minimize the patient's feeling that the staff does not understand how much pain he has and is pushing him to do what is beyond his endurance.

Allowing postoperative patients to help themselves more and to dress sooner in their own clothing is usually a point of encouragement for the patient. However, because a patient *looks* less sick two days after surgery, it is sometimes interpreted by the staff to mean that he is barely sick at all, and scarcely in need of any care. Some of these confusions are difficult to pinpoint; they affect the nonprofessional nursing staff, too. For instance, the patient in her own gown and robe, who had a cholecystectomy two days ago and has just finished coiffing her hair and applying lipstick, may find that her request to a nurse's aide for help in walking to the bathroom is met with surprise that such help should be needed. The professional nurse must examine carefully her own concepts of the nursing requirements of patients, and she must help auxiliary personnel to understand them also.

Regardless of how patient and tactful a nurse is, postoperative nursing care requires her to carry out procedures that the patient would not choose voluntarily. We cannot expect a patient who has pain to be delighted by the prospect of walking about and therefore suffering more pain. He will not say, "Oh, you're making me feel so much better!" Although some nursing procedures quickly and directly relieve discomfort and often prompt the patient to express gratitude, the reaction of most patients to early ambulation is one of skepticism. The nurse must be able to proceed gently and tactfully without expecting to hear the patient express approval and gratitude. Later, when the patient feels better and recognizes his progress, the nurse can feel the satisfaction of having helped him toward recovery.

## REFERENCES AND BIBLIOGRAPHY

AIKEN, L. H., et al.: Systemic relaxation as a nursing intervention technique with open heart surgery patients, *Nurs. Res.* 20:212-217, May-June 1971.

AYRES, S. M., and GIANELLI, S.: *Care of the Critically Ill,* New York, Appleton-Century-Crofts, 1967.

BRAINBRIDGE, M. V., and BRANTHWAITE, M.: *Postoperative Cardiac Intensive Care,* ed. 2, Philadelphia, Davis, 1972.

BENDIXEN, H., et al.: *Respiratory Care,* ed. 2, St. Louis, Mosby, 1972.

EISLER, J., et al.: Relationship between need for social approval and postoperative recovery and welfare, *Nurs. Res.* 21:520-525, November-December 1972.

HERSHEY, S. G.: Current concepts of shock, *Postgrad. Med.* 38:123, 1965.

LIPOWSKI, Z. J.: Physical illness, the individual and the coping process, *Psychiat. Med.* 1:91-102, April 1970.

McCAFFERY, M.: *Nursing Management of the Patient with Pain,* Philadelphia, Lippincott, 1972.

McCARTHY, R. T.: Vomiting, *Nurs. Forum* 3:49, 1964.

McLAUGHLIN, J. S., et al.: Clinical shock; a hemodynamic and metabolic assessment of treatment, *Amer. Surg.* 33:687, 1967.

MEDVEI, V. C., et al.: Understanding pain, *Lancet* 2:43, 3 July 1971.

MERSKEY, H.: Psychological aspects of pain, *Postgrad. Med.* 44:297-306, April 1968.

POWERS, M., and STORLIE, F.: The cardiac surgical patient—pathophysiologic considerations and nursing care, Toronto, Macmillan, 1969.

ROHWEDER, A. W.: Can love, compassion and involvement be scientific? *Nurs. Clin. N. Am.* 4:701-707, December 1969.

SCHMIDT, J.: Availability—a concept of nursing practice, *Am. J. Nurs.* 72:1086, June 1972.

SUTTON, A. L.: *Bedside Nursing Techniques in Medicine and Surgery,* ed. 2, Philadelphia, Saunders, 1969.

VILJOEN, J. F.: Postoperative respiratory adequacy affected by drugs, positioning, *Hosp. Top.* 46:95-96, May 1968.

# UNIT THREE

## Oncologic Nursing

# Care of the Oncologic Patient

## CHAPTER 17

## DEFINITION

Oncology is the study of neoplastic diseases generally grouped together under the term cancer.

For reasons that continue to confound scientists, certain body cells sometimes undergo changes in their structure and appearance; they begin to multiply and give rise to a colony of cancer cells. They may arise in any part of the body, at any time, and from any cell that can proliferate. They multiply rapidly, invading and destroying surrounding normal tissues by pressure and competing with normal cells for nutrients and oxygen. They can spread throughout the body by way of lymphatics or blood vessels (Fig. 17-1). Cancer cells, though changed in appearance, usually retain enough resemblance to the tissues from which they arose to be recognized, if found, in any other part of the body. For example, if a tumor from the neck shows malignant cells arising from breast tissues, it is recognized as having spread from the breast.

## HISTORICAL OVERVIEW

Cancer is as old as antiquity. Remains of the dinosaur and other long extinct animals and man gave evidence of bone cancer. The ancient Greeks called the disease *karkinos,* or crab, because of the clawlike extensions of some cancers. It was from this term that the word *carcinoma* was derived, as well as the Latin word *cancer* (Guthrie, 1946). The earliest medical records and the Bible also attest to the antiquity of cancer. The Ramayana, an old Indian epic of about

251

2,000 B.C., mentions the use of surgery and arsenicals in the treatment of cancer. The ancients often referred to cancer as "the stinking death." The Mosaic law suggested that extramenstrual bleeding

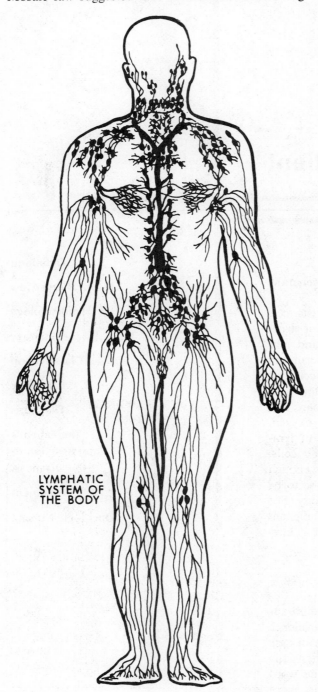

**LYMPHATIC SYSTEM OF THE BODY**

**Figure 17-1.** One route by which malignant cells can spread to other areas of the body is the lymphatic system. Cancer cells can also be carried by the blood.

be regarded as pathologic. Hippocrates gave accurate descriptions of many common types of cancer and described a "burning out" of a neck cancer (Guthrie). Other ancients, including Galen and Celsus, performed surgery for the removal of cancers. Galen probably gave us the first admonition that early diagnosis is necessary if cancer is to be cured. This was nearly 2,000 years ago (Guthrie).

Down through the ages many theories as to the cause of cancer have been propounded. Some of these include Galen's "melancholy" or "black bile" theory which persisted throughout the middle ages, Descartes' "sour lymph" theory, Boerhave's "inflammatory" theory, Sylvius' "chemical theory," and Hoffman, who not only combined the chemical and inflammatory theories, but also suggested an "hereditary" theory as well (Mettler, 1947).

Though many theories about cancer have been advanced throughout the ages, none has been accepted completely, and what progress in the diagnosis and treatment of cancer has been made, has come about as a result of such advances as the science of optics which led to the discovery of the microscope, Roentgen's accidental discovery of x-rays, the Curies' and Becquerel's discovery of natural radioactivity, and Morton's discovery of ether as an anesthetic agent.

There are now 1,500,000 Americans who have been "cured" of cancer with no evidence of disease five years after therapy. One of three patients is saved.

## EPIDEMIOLOGY

The number of deaths due to cancer is on the rise for three reasons:

1. The population is living to an older age as infectious diseases are controlled.
2. The population is increasing despite population control methods.
3. There is a true increase in cancer—in part due to environmental factors, but for the most part due to presently unknown factors (Fig. 17-2).

In addition to mortality, the morbidity associated with cancer demands early detection and knowledgeable medical and nursing care.

Cancer can occur at any age, but it is more common after the age of 40. Youth, however, is no guarantee against cancer. Cancer is now the second leading cause of death in children, second only to trauma. The longer life span is one reason for the increasing incidence of cancer in the United

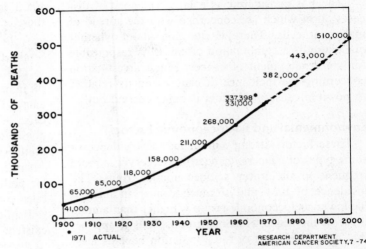

**Figure 17-2.** Forecast of cancer deaths if present trends continue. (The American Cancer Society.)

States. Having been spared death from such causes as poliomyelitis, diphtheria, and childbirth, more people are living long enough to develop cancer. Some forms of cancer are believed to be increasing in frequency to a degree not explained by the increased life span. For example, lung cancer has shown a rapid and relentless increase, while other types of cancers are decreasing or remaining at the same level. The rise in the rate of lung cancer seems clearly related to cigarette smoking (see Chap. 11). Both men and women are susceptible to cancer, but the incidence of cancer affecting different sites of the body varies considerably in the two sexes (Fig. 17-3).

## ETIOLOGY

So far the cause of cancer has eluded definite determination. Much stress is being placed on early detection, but not enough stress is being placed upon the prevention of cancer which in some instances is a preventable disease.

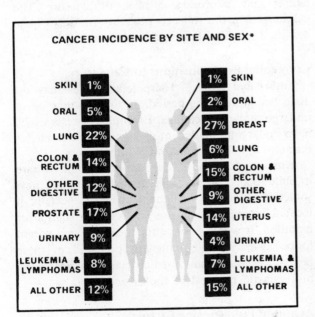

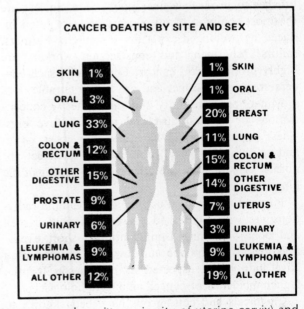

**Figure 17-3.** Cancer incidence (excluding superficial skin cancer and carcinoma in situ of uterine cervix) and cancer deaths by site and sex. (The American Cancer Society.)

Cancer is considered as a large category of diseases all of which are concerned with the spread of malignant cells. There is question about whether one cause or a combination of causes is responsible for the development of cancer. Much investigation concerning the incidence of cancer and its relation to possible causative factors is being carried out.

### Environmental and Socioeconomic Factors

These factors strongly influence the incidence of some types of cancers. Cancer of the cervix is more frequent in the lower socioeconomic group. The incidence of lung and stomach cancer in men in the lower socioeconomic group is higher than among those in the highest income group. Thus it appears that the largest part of the population benefits least from cancer control measures and that more effective programs are indicated.

Historically, the vocational environment has been discovered to be a cause of cancer. Sir Percivall Pott in 1775 observed that scrotal cancer was an occupational disease of chimney sweeps because of their constant exposure to soot, and he was the first to institute protective clothing and hygiene. These measures were successful in eliminating the cause of this type of cancer. Fatal bone cancers were observed in many workers in a New Jersey plant where women used radium salts to paint luminous dials on watches and often licked the brushes to produce a finer point. Skin cancers are the most common of all cancers and are often induced by prolonged exposure to sunlight. Farmers, sailors, fishermen, and construction workers are highly prone to skin cancer. Fortunately, such cancers are easy to detect and are highly curable.

Miners are constantly exposed to heavy concentrations of mineral dust and to radioactive ores. These workers should have periodic chest x-rays and sputum cytological examinations to detect abnormal cells that are the precursors to cancer of the lung.

Physical agents such as x-rays and gamma radiations are well-established causes of squamous cell and bone sarcomas. Long-continued short exposures to the fluoroscope and low levels of radiation have long been suspected as the reason for the higher incidence of cancer among radiologists.

Chemicals and cutting oils have been known to produce skin cancers in industrial workers. Protective clothing and good hygiene measures are instituted in most industries to prevent cancer from these causes.

### Social Customs and Cancer

The inhalation of cigarette smoke over a period of many years has been implicated as the major cause of lung, pharyngeal, oral, and laryngeal cancers. A large percentage of such cancer patients give a long history of smoking. Substances in cigarette smoke are known to produce cancer in experimental animals. It may be that other sources of air pollution such as exhaust fumes from automobiles contribute to the incidence of lung cancer.

Penile cancer is known to be practically nonexistent in Jewish men. This is thought to be due to the circumcision religious rite which is performed at the end of the first week after birth. In the United States penile cancer amounts to 0.33 per cent of all cancer; it conceivably could be eliminated with routine circumcision after birth.

In some Far Eastern countries such as Ceylon, India, Pakistan, and Burma there is a high incidence of oral and pharyngeal cancer which has been attributed to the national habit of chewing betel nuts and tobacco. In the southern part of the United States one encounters the term "snuff dippers' cancer." Powdered tobacco (snuff) is placed in the buccal cavity of the mouth (inside the lower lip) and is said to produce a sense of pleasure. The carcinogen in the tobacco probably produces local irritation which is followed by cancer.

### Congenital Predispositions to Cancer

**Embryonal Rests.** These fetal tissues may remain benign for long periods of time or may never undergo malignant change. Examples of rests which have undergone malignant change include medulloblastoma, glioblastoma, and Wilms' tumor.

**Moles and Nevi.** Malignant melanoma is rare in childhood. However, pigmented moles and nevi sometimes undergo malignant change especially if located in areas which are subjected to friction or irritation. It would be wise for the nurse and parent to be aware of the malignant potential of these benign lesions. Some pediatricians advocate the prophylactic removal of moles and nevi.

### Acquired Predisposing Factors

These lesions too may remain benign or undergo malignant change:

**Senile Keratosis.** Senile keratoses usually occur on the face, dorsum of hands, and so on.

**Leukoplakia.** Leukoplakia of the mouth or genitals are said to predispose to cancer and should be removed when feasible.

**Virus.** Extensive research is being conducted in an effort to determine whether cancer in human beings can be caused by viruses. No virus has yet been identified with the causation of human cancer, although viruses have caused cancer in animals. These include fowl leukosis, carcinoma of the skin of a rabbit (Rous, 1935), and breast carcinoma in mice (Bittner, 1942).

In 1958 the occurrence of a jaw tumor in Uganda drew much attention (Burkitt's tumor). The histology of the tumor was lymphoblastoma. Because the disease attacked children in a certain geographic location, it is believed that Burkitt's tumor is a vector-borne disease. The mosquito is being investigated as the probable vector. It is still too early to evaluate the significance of virus in the causation of human cancers. More research and data are needed.

**Parasites.** Parasites have been implicated in the development of cancer of the colon, bladder, and liver in the Near Eastern countries where schistosomiasis is endemic.

**Emotional Factors.** Some researchers believe that the development of cancer is related to emotional factors. It has been postulated that loss, particularly if the individual denies the loss and does not go through the normal grief process, can produce a physical effect which lessens the body's immunity to cancer, thereby increasing the likelihood that he will develop the disease.

It is considered likely that cancer occurs only when a certain combination of factors favors its development. These factors may include heredity, hormonal state, and exposure to carcinogens. In addition to efforts to find the cause(s) of cancer, attempts are being made to understand factors that affect host resistance in the hope that susceptibility to the development of cancer can be decreased.

## CLASSIFICATION

The objectives of classification are: (1) to aid clinicians cooperating in the care of the patient to plan treatment, (2) to give some prognostic indication, (3) to allow evaluation of different modalities of treatment, (4) to allow exchange of information by pooling similar patient information, (5) to aid in continuing investigation of cancer. The above statement is paraphrased from publications of the International Union against Cancer, one of the many international committees attempting to standardize nomenclature.

Descriptions sometimes used, such as "operable," "nonoperable," "resectable," "nonresectable," are subject to the individual criteria of the physician and refer only to surgical therapy. Anatomic and histologic criteria obtained by physical examination, nuclear medicine studies, and diagnostic x-rays, as well as operative and tissue findings, are essential.

Knowledge of the characteristics of the cancer and the extent of disease is useful in estimating the prognosis of the patient. One way of expressing extent of disease has been through the concept of staging, in which stages range from I through IV. A Stage I tumor would be limited to the site of origin whereas a Stage IV tumor would have widespread metastasis. Thus, in carcinoma of the cervix, Stage I indicates that the carcinoma is confined to the cervix. In Stage II, it has infiltrated the parametrium, but not the pelvic wall. In Stage III it has spread into the pelvic wall and may involve the lower third of the vagina, and in Stage IV it involves the bladder, or rectum, or has extended beyond the confines of the true pelvis. Staging, which is commonly clinical, is substantiated by histologic proof.

However, the definitions of staging for the types of neoplasms vary for each organ of the body. For this reason many oncologists favor a TNM (tumor, nodes, metastasis) staging to indicate extent of disease. This requires a statement for each of the following:

**a.** The primary tumor
  site
  size
  histology
**b.** The regional lymph nodes
  site
  size
  histology
**c.** Metastases
  absent
  present
    site
    size
    histology

A TNM staging can always be derived by the oncologist if the above-mentioned data are provided.

## PATHOLOGY

Tumors refer to new growths of tissue which persist and grow independently of their surrounding structures without normal body growth restraints, and which have no physiologic use.

Generally they are categorically divided into benign and malignant. For the sake of simplicity charts of differential characteristics such as Table 17-1 are helpful.

**Table 17-1.   Characteristics of Tumors**

| BENIGN | MALIGNANT |
|---|---|
| 1. Grow slowly. | 1. Grow rapidly. |
| 2. Often encapsulated. | 2. Rarely encapsulated. |
| 3. Do not infiltrate surrounding tissues. | 3. Infiltrate surrounding tissues. |
| 4. Remain localized. | 4. Metastasize via lymphatic or blood vessels. |
| 5. Usually no recurrence after surgical extirpation. | 5. May recur after surgical extirpation. |
| 6. Cells well differentiated in resembling those of parent tissues. | 6. Cells are not well differentiated and may be anaplastic. |
| 7. Produce minimal tissue destruction. | 7. Produce extensive tissue destruction generally. |
| 8. Do not cause death as a rule except when the size and position impair a vital function. | 8. May cause death unless treated aggressively and early. |
| 9. Do not produce cachexia. | 9. Produce typical cachexia. |

Specifically it may be difficult for the diagnostician to differentiate benign from malignant, and it is common practice to think of all tumors as belonging to a spectrum rather than a dichotomy, with a continuum from benign through potentially malignant to frankly malignant. Tumors at the malignant end of the spectrum are more or less malignant, depending not only on the cells themselves, but also on the host's (patient's) body defenses.

In order to name tumors some knowledge of embryology is necessary.

Malignant tumors may arise from any or all three embryonal tissues. When a tumor contains all three embryonal components it is referred to as a teratoma.

The embryonal tissues are as follows:

Ectoderm—outer layer of the embryo—which produces the skin and nervous system.

Mesoderm—middle layer of the embryo—which produces the bones, cartilage, muscle, fat, blood, and all other connective tissues.

Endoderm—inner layer of the embryo—which produces the linings of the gastrointestinal tract, respiratory system, spleen, liver, and so on.

Table 17-2 depicts a continuum of tissue behavior.

## SYMPTOMS

Cancer is an insidious disease that tends to develop slowly and with few or no early symptoms. Every effort must be made to discover it in its earliest stage, for early discovery facilitates complete extirpation and a good prognosis. It is now believed that cancer may develop even more slowly than was originally believed. Cancer cells may exist in the body (in situ) for many years without causing symptoms. According to one theory, if host resistance is good, these cells will not multiply and cause disease, but if conditions are favorable to malignant growth, the cells will multiply and cause symptoms. Two examples of this are the malignant cells present in the sputum of mine workers long before there is evidence of lung cancer and the malignant cells present in the cervix long before there is evidence of cancer.

Everyone should be familiar with the seven warning signals of cancer listed by the American Cancer Society.

- A sore that does not heal
- A lump or thickening in the breast or elsewhere
- Unusual bleeding or discharge
- Any change in a wart or mole
- Persistent indigestion or difficulty in swallowing
- Persistent hoarseness or cough
- Any change in normal bowel habits

If the disease progresses untreated, pain, weakness, weight loss, and anemia are characteristic. However, these symptoms frequently do not appear until late in the disease. Symptoms do not always progress from minimal to intense but often wax or wane, thereby giving the patient a false sense of security that they aren't important. Delay in seeking medical attention is still common. Attention must be directed to early diagnosis and treatment and emphasis placed on the prevention and avoidance of cancer. People must come to realize that cancer can arise from self-neglect.

As a tumor grows, it tends to press on adjacent tissues causing pain. Like cells anywhere in the body, malignant cells need nourishment. Because the tumor grows rapidly, the blood supply, normally adequate, becomes insufficient, and necrosis in the central portion of the tumor develops from lack of nutrients. Malignant tissues tend to bleed easily and to develop secondary infection. If the lesion is external or if there is drainage from it through a body orifice, an unpleasant odor may be noted. This

Table 17-2. A Continuum of Tissue Behavior

| TISSUE OF ORIGIN | LOCATION | BEHAVIOR | |
| --- | --- | --- | --- |
| | | BENIGN | MALIGNANT |
| Epithelial | surface | papilloma | carcinoma<br> basal cell carcinoma<br> squamous cell carcinoma<br> transitional cell sarcoma |
| | glandular | adenoma | adenocarcinoma |
| Connective | fibrous | fibroma | fibrosarcoma |
| | cartilage | chondroma | chondrosarcoma |
| | bone | osteoma | osteosarcoma |
| | fat | lipoma | liposarcoma |
| | blood vessels | hemangioma | hemangiosarcoma |
| | lymph vessels | lymphangioma | lymphangiosarcoma |
| | smooth muscle | leiomyoma | leiomyosarcoma |
| | striated muscle | rhabdomyoma | rhabdomyosarcoma |
| Hematopoietic (Reticuloendothelial) | lymphoid | | lymphoma<br> lymphocytic, well-<br>  differentiated<br> lymphocytic, poorly<br>  differentiated<br> lymphosarcoma<br> Hodgkin's disease<br> leukemia<br>  lymphocytic<br>  monocytic |
| | granulocytic | | myelocytic leukemia |
| | plasma cells | | multiple myeloma |
| Nervous | glia (supporting tissue of the brain) | | glioma (astrocytoma) |
| | meninges (covering of the brain) | meningioma | meningeal sarcoma |
| | nerve cells | ganglioneuroma | neuroblastoma |
| | retina of eye | | retinoblastoma |
| | adrenal gland | pheochromocytoma | |
| | nerve sheaths (covering) | neurolemmoma | neurolemmal sarcoma<br> (schwannoma) |
| Tumors of more than one tissue | multipotent cells | teratoma | malignant teratoma<br> (choriocarcinoma) |
| | breast | fibroadenoma | cystosarcoma phyllodes |
| | embryonic kidney | | nephroblastoma (Wilms') |
| Organ tumors which do not fit easily into one of the groups | testis | | seminoma<br>choriocarcinoma<br>carcinoma |
| | ovary | cystadenoma<br>(and others) | serous, mucous, or anaplastic<br>dysgerminoma<br>choriocarcinoma<br>malignant melanoma |
| | placenta | hydatidiform mole | |
| | melanoblast<br>  (is not of surface<br>  epithelium) | pigmented nevus | |

odor is not peculiar to cancer but can occur in any condition where there is necrosis, infection, and drainage. Patients whose cancers are contained within the body usually do not have an unpleasant odor.

The disease generally has a protracted course, but not always. The factors determining the severity and rapidity of progress of the disease are not fully understood. Some types of cancers have a more fulminating course than others. Host resistance is also believed in some way to play a part in the rate of progress of the disease. Cachexia is generally characteristic during the terminal stages of cancer (Fig. 17-4). Other symptoms relate to the disturbed function of the part of the body that is affected. Intestinal cancer may cause partial or complete obstruction; cancer of the larynx typically causes hoarseness. These symptoms are discussed more fully in later chapters dealing with the specific organs that are involved.

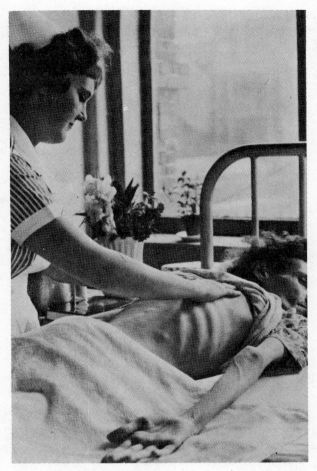

**Figure 17-4.** Appearance typical of cachectic patient.

## DIAGNOSIS OF CANCER

The diagnosis of cancer begins with the recognition that cancer may assume many forms and guises. Sometimes the symptoms are so typical that the patient proclaims the diagnosis himself. At other times a physician's or nurse's suspicion is aroused by an apparently minor condition that does not respond to therapy.

A complete regular physical examination is the first weapon in the struggle to discover cancer in its early stages. Every medical office, clinic, neighborhood health center, school, and industrial clinic should be a cancer detection center. With effective team work the physician, nurse, laboratory technicians, and others, can make the cancer detection examination a simple, routine, and sometimes, a life-saving procedure.

A pelvic examination should be a part of every woman's physical examination. In situ cancers can

be discovered early with the proper application of the "Pap" smears (see Chapter 52). Sputum examinations should be performed on all patients with a history of cough. Cytologic tests are performed to detect cancer cells that have been shed from malignant tissue. These tests are called "Pap" or Papanicolaou tests in recognition of the physician who developed this important technique. They are useful because in the normal scaling or "exfoliation" of epithelial cells, malignant cells may also be present in the secretions after they have been shed from a malignant lesion. Cytologic tests are now widely used, especially among groups where the risk of developing cancer is high. The patient at this time usually shows no symptoms of illness; thus it is possible to diagnose the disease in an earlier stage.

All tests permitting visualization of body structures are important in the diagnosis of cancer. Examination with simple instruments such as the nasal speculum, otoscope, ophthalmoscope, laryngeal mirror, tongue depressor, anoscope and vaginal speculum should be done as part of a routine physical assessment. Inspection of the patient from scalp to toes should be carried out. Skin cancer and precancerous lesions such as leukoplakia of the oral cavity, tongue, vulva, or penis can be observed. The observation of new growth on internal organs requires the use of such measures as proctoscopy, bronchoscopy, gastroscopy, and certain x-ray examinations or nuclear medicine studies. Proper preparation of the patient is necessary before these procedures are carried out.

The patient's history is very important. The physician can make a provisional diagnosis of cancer on the basis of the patient's history, symptoms, and appearance of the lesion. However, a definite diagnosis can be established only by histologic examination of specimens of tissue from the lesion. This technique is called biopsy. The ease with which a biopsy can be performed depends upon the location of the lesion. Biopsy of the skin can be performed readily. Biopsy of the cervix can be performed through a vaginal speculum; biopsy of the larynx through a laryngoscope. Specimens of lesions that are inaccessible must be obtained during surgical exploration.

In many communities several physicians form a "group" and share in the complete physical examination according to their area of expertise. In some large hospitals the patient is seen first by an internist for a complete medical evaluation before any treatment is carried out. If he has cancer, he is then assigned to a physician from the appropriate discipline for treatment. In many cancer centers the patient may remain under the care of a generalist (general practitioner interested in oncology) for day-to-day care, but treatment decisions are made by a group of oncologic specialists: surgical, medical (chemotherapist) and radiation (radiotherapist—nuclear medicine), with the consent of the patient. After his treatment for cancer is completed the patient returns to his primary physician, the internist, for continued follow-up care, i.e., periodic physical examination and interval history.

## THE PATIENT'S REACTION TO THE DIAGNOSIS

Illness other than cancer can cause death and disability. Most patients with heart disease know their diagnosis, and heart disease outranks cancer as a cause of death in our country. Why, then, does the question of knowing the true diagnosis loom so large in the care of the oncologic patient? Most people associate cancer with a lingering, painful death. This accounts for some of the widespread discussion over the advisability of telling cancer patients their diagnosis. Early diagnosis and modern treatment have altered this grim picture substantially. Today many patients with cancer can be cured. Others have had their lives extended and made more comfortable by advances in therapy. The new advances in therapy are changing the old attitudes toward the disease. The problem of "telling or not telling" reflects not only the nature of the disease, but individual attitudes toward it.

Some patients know their diagnosis and yet prefer to have it unconfirmed. Possibly such patients feel that a confirmation of the diagnosis by the physician would extinguish the last faint ray of hope that they do not have cancer. Usually, knowledge that they have the disease is not forced on patients who show that they do not wish or are not ready for such information. It is essential to keep one's antennae attuned to changes in the patient's response, and to modify the approach accordingly. Later the patient may seek more information than he did at first.

Some patients request their diagnosis. Some of those who learn their diagnosis possess or develop unusual strength and spiritual resources. Such patients command admiration and respect. They avail themselves of opportunities to talk with others—their clergyman, physician, nurse, and family—and obtain help. If the prognosis is unfavorable the knowledge of this gives the patient an opportunity to deal with his own response to imminent death, to set his affairs in order, and to plan realistically for the future needs of his family.

Some patients find the news too difficult to bear. They become depressed and apathetic. Occasionally they contemplate, and even commit, suicide. In any similar situation, when a person suddenly receives news that is shocking, it takes time for him to absorb it. This is true for both the patient and his family. At first there is shock and often disbelief (denial) and later, various degrees of acknowledgement that it has happened. Anger as well as fear is a frequent reaction to the diagnosis.

Some patients are told the truth, but not the whole truth. For example, they may be informed that a tumor was removed from the intestine. Whether the tumor is benign or malignant is often not disclosed unless the patient specifically requests this information. The patient has not been told a falsehood, and the door is left open for further discussion later without loss of the patient's confidence.

Some patients are aware of the diagnosis and so are their families, but each is unaware of the other's knowledge. In a futile attempt to "spare" each other, both are deprived of the opportunity for giving and receiving support in a family crisis, the so-called mutual pretense awareness context (see Chap. 12).

In certain circumstances some practitioners give a plausible explanation for the symptoms, because it is considered unlikely that the patient can accept the diagnosis. For example, the pain in the back and hip due to metastases may be ascribed to arthritis with the thought that the patient will be able to maintain optimism and hope for the future. (Oliver Wendell Holmes once cautioned a graduating class of young doctors, *"Be careful how you take away hope from a patient."*) Some patients might react to this approach by restlessly seeking a cure, or they may blame those who care for them for their lack of improvement, or they may insist that something is being kept from them.

In recent years there has been much emphasis on the doctrine of informed consent. Some practitioners operate on the principle that the patient is

259

the only one who has the right to say who should know his diagnosis, and that he must have factual information in order to give informed consent.

Probably there is no one best way of answering the question, "Should the patient be told?" Much also depends upon the patient's personality and his ability to cope with stress. Determining beforehand how the patient is likely to respond is the problem. Sometimes several people who know the patient well (e.g., his physician, pastor, and family) discuss the problem and decide. Sometimes the physician informs the family fully and leaves up to them the decision concerning what and how to tell the patient. In other situations the physician assumes entire responsibility for deciding what and how much to tell the patient. Often the decision is left to the patient himself, in the sense that he is given the information he specifically requests.

Whether or not the patient knows, a family member or responsible person is informed of the diagnosis and prognosis, so that he or she may help with realistic planning for future care. If the patient is unaware of his diagnosis, his family experiences a double burden—its own feelings and the need to keep the news from the patient. If the patient is aware of his diagnosis, the family has freedom to help him accept his illness. In either case the role of family members is crucial, and they need the continued support of the physician, the nurse, the pastor, and friends. In any event, the physician must also be cognizant of the fact that legally the patient must give informed consent for treatment.

How does this affect the nurse? She may or may not have a part in making the decision. If she is asked, she must suggest what she believes is best for that particular patient, whether or not this decision is what she would want done for her in like circumstances. Often nurses do not participate in making the decision. In such instances, they must accept the decision of others and be guided by it. Inconsistency and conflict among those who care for the patient are extremely upsetting to him. Whatever he has been told should be recorded in the nursing care plan so that all staff members will be aware of and consistent in the approach.

It is important for the nurse not only to know what decision has been made and to work within the limits of that decision, but also to assess the patient's reaction and discuss this with the physician so that the plan can be changed as necessary for the benefit of the patient.

## TREATMENT

Complete destruction or removal of malignant tissue is the only cure for cancer. There are several forms of therapy available for the patient with cancer: surgery, radiotherapy, immunotherapy, and chemotherapy.

### Surgery

Surgical treatment involves wide excision of the tumor and the node-bearing areas to which the disease might have spread. The need to remove all of the malignant tissue sometimes necessitates radical or disfiguring surgery or surgery that results in the alteration of body function, such as an opening of the colon on the abdomen (colostomy), or removal of the larynx (laryngectomy). In later chapters specific types of operations will be discussed in relation to the part of the body affected.

### Radiotherapy

Radiotherapy is used to destroy cancer tissue. Some forms of cancer are destroyed readily by radiation. The location of the tumor and its radiosensitivity help determine the usefulness of this form of treatment. Radiotherapy is given to cure, palliate, or control the spread of cancers. Some destruction of normal tissues around the tumor is inevitable if the tumor is to be completely treated by radiation.

It is known that increased oxygenation of poorly oxygenated malignant cells increases their susceptibility to radiotherapy. For this reason, some patients with cancer are being treated with a combination of radiotherapy and hyperbaric oxygen therapy. Hyperbaric oxygen therapy provides oxygen in an atmosphere at increased atmospheric pressure, resulting in an increased amount of oxygen being dissolved in body tissues and body fluids. This treatment is administered in a special pressure chamber which resembles an iron lung, and accommodates the patient. There are several different types of hyperbaric oxygen chambers. The principle of treatment, however, remains the same.

There is an increasing tendency toward the combined use of surgery and radiotherapy, and toward combining surgery and radiotherapy with chemotherapy. (See Chapter 18 for further discussion of radiotherapy.)

Palliative treatment of cancer is used to slow down the progress of the disease when possible and also to relieve distressing symptoms such as pain, and to clear up an open fungating tumor mass. For example, removal of an ulcerated tumor of the breast is desirable for esthetic reasons, even if it is not effective in curing the disease. Radiotherapy is useful in slowing down the progress of the disease even though the disease has progressed beyond the possibility of cure.

## Immunotherapy

Presently in the experimental stage, this form of therapy is aimed at involving or augmenting immune defenses as part of the systemic approach to the treatment of cancer. Immunotherapy is used as adjunctive therapy; that is, surgery, radiotherapy, or chemotherapy is used first to eliminate the bulk of the tumor (Silverstein and Morton, 1973).

## Chemotherapy

With the exception of many cures for choriocarcinoma with methotrexate and actinomycin D, no drugs have been discovered so far that can cure cancer (Shimkin, 1969). Some drugs can slow down the progress of the disease and provide relief. Patients with leukemia and lymphoma are living longer and more comfortably thanks to some of the newer chemotherapeutic drugs and better medical management. Chemotherapeutic drugs are toxic to normal cells, or they disturb the body's hormone balance. Much research is being done to discover drugs that destroy malignant cells without harming normal cells.

**Alkylating Agents and Antimetabolites.** There are several types of chemotherapeutic drugs. Alkylating agents, such as nitrogen mustard, are injurious to cells, particularly to the rapidly proliferating cancer cells. It is believed that this action results from reaction of the alkylating agent with the nucleic acids in the cells. Antimetabolites, of which folic acid antagonists are examples, interfere with cell growth and metabolism. Methotrexate and 6-mercaptopurine are examples of folic acid antagonists.

Both of these groups are potentially dangerous. Depression of the bone marrow, oral ulceration, nausea, vomiting, and diarrhea are some of the toxic effects encountered. The usefulness of these drugs lies in the greater susceptibility of malignant cells to their effects and their ability to exercise some control over the malignant process.

**Vincristine and Vinblastine.** Vincristine and vinblastine are derived from a species of the periwinkle plant. The mechanism of their action is to produce mitotic arrest and thus prevent new cancer cells from forming. Side effects from this group of drugs are bone marrow depression, areflexia, and muscular weakness.

Dosage of antineoplastic drugs is carefully adapted to the patient's particular form of disease and his response to the drug. Bone marrow depression resulting in decreased numbers of blood cells such as leukocytes is monitored by periodic blood counts. If the depression is marked, the chemotherapist may wish to modify the dosage or temporarily discontinue the drug, until the bone marrow recovers.

Many chemotherapeutic drugs are not effective until toxic levels have been reached. The dosage of the drug is in large part determined by the patient's weight in kilograms. It is important therefore to weigh the patient at the same time each day, for example before breakfast, using the same scale and having the patient wear the same attire.

**Steroid Compounds.** Certain hormones slow the growth of malignant cells by providing a less favorable environment for their growth. For example, men with disseminated prostatic cancer may have symptomatic improvement when the effects of male hormones are counteracted. This counteraction is achieved by the administration of estrogens to the male patient or by removal of the testes (bilateral orchiectomy).

Adrenal steroid hormones (adrenocorticotropic hormones [ACTH] and cortisone) are used in the palliation of cancer. By a mechanism not fully understood, they inhibit proliferation of malignant cells temporarily, providing symptomatic relief (see Table 17-3).

## Nursing Assessment and Intervention During Chemotherapy

Nursing responsibilities in care of the patient receiving chemotherapy for cancer include knowing the modes of action of drugs, toxic effects, and whether toxic effects are expected to have immediate or delayed manifestations and how these effects are to be monitored. These drugs are often equally toxic to normal cells such as red blood cells, white blood cells, and platelets. During the course of the treatment, the patient may require blood transfusions for anemia, special precautions relative to increased susceptibility to infection including care in

**Table 17-3.  Specific Agents Used In Cancer Chemotherapy**

| AGENTS | PRINCIPAL ROUTE OF ADMINIS-TRATION | USUAL DOSE | ACUTE TOXIC SIGNS | MAJOR TOXIC MANIFESTATIONS |
|---|---|---|---|---|
| *Steroid Compounds* | | | | |
| Androgen | | | | |
|    Testosterone propionate | IM | 50-100 mg. 3x weekly | None | Fluid retention, masculinization |
|    Fluoxymesterone (Halotestin) | Oral | 10-20 mg./day | | |
| Estrogen | | | | |
|    Diethylstilbestrol | Oral | Breast: 1-5 mg. 3/day | Occasional | Fluid retention, feminization |
| | | Prostate: 1 mg./day | | |
|    Ethinyl estradiol (Estinyl) | Oral | Breast: 0.1-1.0 mg. 3/day | N. & V.* | Uterine bleeding |
| | | Prostate: 0.1 mg./day | | |
| Progestin | | | | |
|    Hydroxyprogesterone caproate (Delalutin) | IM | 1 gm. 2x weekly | | |
|    6-Methylhydroxyprogesterone (Provera) | Oral | 100-200 mg./day | None | |
| | IM | 200-600 mg. 2x weekly | | |
| Adrenal Cortical Compounds | | | | |
|    Cortisone acetate | Oral | 20-100 mg./day | | |
|    Prednisone (Meticorten) | Oral | 15-100 mg./day | | |
|    Dexamethasone (Decadron) | Oral | 0.5-4.0 mg./day | | Fluid retention, hypertension, diabetes, increased susceptibility to infection |
|    Methylprednisolone sodium succinate (Solu-Medrol) | IM<br>IV | 10-125 mg./day | None | |
|    Hydrocortisone sodium succinate (Solu-Cortef) | IV | 100-500 mg./day | | |
| *Polyfunctional Alkylating Agents* | | | | |
| Methylbis ($\beta$ — Chloroethyl) Amine HCl (HN2, Mustargen) | IV | 0.4 mg./kg. Single or Divided Doses | N. & V. | Therapeutic doses moderately depress peripheral blood cell count; excessive doses cause severe bone marrow depression with leukopenia, thrombocyto-penia, and bleeding. Maximum toxicity may occur two or three weeks after last dose. Dosage, therefore, must be carefully con-trolled. Alopecia and hemor-rhagic cystitis occur occasionally with cyclophosphamide |
|    Chlorambucil (Leukeran) | Oral | 0.1-0.2 mg./kg./day 6-12 mg./day | None | |
|    Melphalan (Alkeran) | Oral | 0.1 mg./kg./day x 7 2-4 mg./day maintenance | None | |
|    Cyclophosphamide (Endoxan, Cytoxan) | IV<br><br><br>Oral | 3.5-5.0 mg./kg./day x 10 (40-60 mg./kg. Single Dose)<br>50-200 mg./day | N. & V. | |
| Triethylenethiophosphoramide (TSPA, Thio-TEPA) | IV | 0.8-1.0 mg./kg. or 0.2 mg./kg./day x 4-5 | None | |
| Busulfan (Myleran) | Oral | 2-6 mg./day | None | |
| *Antimetabolites* | | | | |
| Methotrexate (Methotrexate, A-methopterin) | Oral<br>IV | 2.5-5.0 mg./day<br>25-50 mg.<br>1-2x weekly | None | Oral and digestive tract ulcera-tions; bone marrow depression with leukopenia, thrombocyto-penia, and bleeding. Toxicity enhanced by impaired kidney function |
| 6-Mercaptopurine (6-MP, Purinethol) | Oral | 2.5 mg./kg./day | None | Therapeutic doses usually well tolerated; excessive doses cause bone marrow depression |
|    6-Thioquanine (6-TG, Thioguan) | Oral | 2.0 mg./kg./day | | |
| 5-Fluorouracil (5-FU, Fluorouracil) | IV | 12 mg./kg./day x 3 Smaller dose, 1-2 x weekly for maintenance | None | Stomatitis, nausea, GI injury, bone marrow depression |
| Arabinosylcytosine (Ara-C, Cytosar) | IV | 1.0-3.0 mg./kg./ day x 10-20 | N. & V. | Bone marrow depression, mega-loblastosis, leukopenia, throm-bocytopenia |

| AGENTS | PRINCIPAL ROUTE OF ADMINIS-TRATION | USUAL DOSE | ACUTE TOXIC SIGNS | MAJOR TOXIC MANIFESTATIONS |
|---|---|---|---|---|
| *Antibiotics* | | | | |
| Adriamycin | IV | 50-75 mg./m² in single or divided doses every 3 weeks | N. & V. | Stomatitis, GI disturbances, alopecia, bone marrow depression. Cardiac toxicity at cumulative doses over 600 mg./m² |
| Bleomycin | IV<br>SC | 0.25 mg./kg./day x 5-7<br>Maintenance: 1.0-2.0 mg./day | N. & V.<br>Chills<br>Fever | Mucocutaneous ulcerations, alopecia, pulmonary fibrosis in approximately 5% patients |
| Dactinomycin (Cosmegen) | IV | 0.01 mg./kg./day x 5 or 0.04 mg./kg. weekly | N. & V. | Stomatitis, GI disturbances, alopecia, bone marrow depression |
| Daunorubicin | IV | 0.8-1.0 mg./kg./day x 3-6<br>Total doses never to exceed 25 mg./kg. | N. & V.<br>Fever | Bone marrow depression with leukopenia and thrombocytopenia, alopecia, stomatitis; cardiac toxicity at cumulative doses over 25 mg./kg. |
| Mithramycin | IV | 25 micrograms every other day x 3-4 | N. & V. | Bone marrow depression particularly thrombocytopenia, bleeding, hypocalcemia, hepatic toxicity at large doses |
| *Miscellaneous Drugs* | | | | |
| L-Asparaginase | IV | 200-1,000 IU/kg. 3-7 x weekly for 28 days | N. & V.<br>Fever<br>Hyper-sensitivity reactions | Anorexia, weight loss. Somnolence, lethargy, confusion. Hypoproteinemia (including albumin and fibrinogen). Hypolipidemia and (?) hyperlipidemia, abnormal liver function tests, fatty metamorphosis of the liver. Pancreatitis (rare). Azotemia. Granulocytopenia, lymphopenia, and thrombocytopenia (usually mild and transient) |
| 1,3-bis (β-Chloroethyl)-1-nitrosourea (BCNU) | IV | 100 mg./m² every 6 weeks | N. & V. | Bone marrow depression with leukopenia and thrombocytopenia |
| o,p'-DDD | Oral | 2-10 gm./day | N. & V. | Skin eruptions, diarrhea, mental depression, muscle tremors |
| Hydroxyurea (Hydrea) | Oral | 20-40 mg./kg./day | None | Bone marrow depression |
| Procarbazine (Matulane) N-Methylhydrazine | Oral | 50-300 mg./day | N. & V. | Bone marrow depression, leukopenia and thrombocytopenia, mental depression |
| Quinacrine (Atabrine) | Intra-pleural | 100-200 mg./day x 5 | Local pain, Fever | |
| Vinblastine (Velban) | IV | 0.1-0.2 mg./kg. weekly | N. & V. | Alopecia, areflexia, bone marrow depression |
| Vincristine (Oncovin) | IV | 0.015-0.05 mg./kg. weekly | None | Areflexia, muscular weakness. peripheral neuritis, paralytic ileus, mild bone marrow depression |

* Nausea and Vomiting

Reprinted with permission from Krakoff, I. H., Cancer chemotherapeutic agents, Ca—A Cancer Journal for Clinicians 23:210, July/August 1973, The American Cancer Society.

an isolated environment, such as a life-island setting or laminar airflow unit, and early intervention to prevent hemorrhage.

Since with some drugs toxicity may be manifested before therapeutic effect can be obtained, the nurse should know the parameters of the therapeutic effect being assessed in each patient. For example, the therapeutic goal may be a change in the size of a tumor or lymph nodes, decrease in pain, or improvement in bone marrow or blood chemistry.

Additional aspects of nursing care include using nursing measures to lessen discomfort caused by drug therapy, explaining (within the framework already established by the physician) the purpose of the drugs and how the patient may participate to receive the best results possible, and supporting the patient emotionally during this treatment.

Just as chemotherapeutic response is on a highly individual basis, so also is the patient's emotional response to his situation. Some patients cope better when they are given as much factual data as is possible; others prefer minimal explanations and place their faith in the judgment of the oncologic team. Some patients understand that they will become sicker before starting to feel better. For example, the patient receiving fluorouracil may experience diarrhea as a result of taking this chemotherapeutic agent. The nurse's role involves noting and reporting the symptoms, recording intake and output, and using measures to promote cleanliness, relieve anal irritation, and provide ready access to bathroom or bedpan, as well as helping the patient to recognize that this unpleasant side effect is but a part of the drug's effects; that its use also involves helping him combat the illness. During such explanations it is essential to use terminology which has been agreed upon by all members of the health team, so that there is a coordinated approach to the patient. Sometimes the patient is told some of the truth; he may be told that the drug is being used to arrest his disease, but he may not be told that this effect of the drug probably will be only temporary (if this is the case). Such decisions must be based on the individual patient's situation and needs.

Because cure of cancer rests upon elimination of all malignant cells from the body, vigorous treatment is used when there seems to be any possibility of cure. Therapy may be continued despite the occurrence of distressing side effects, in the hope that cure, or at least considerable slowing of the disease process, may occur. The greater the likelihood of success with treatment, the more emphasis is placed upon continuing therapy despite associated discomfort. The skilled intervention of the nurse to lessen discomfort can make the difference between the patient's continuing with therapy, and abandoning it, thus possibly losing its beneficial effects.

**Emotional Support.** Patients who receive chemotherapy may be hospitalized for long periods of time or be treated as outpatients. This affords opportunity for the development of supportive nurse-patient relationships. The patient can be expected to have a wide range of emotional responses, such as denial, anger, depression, helplessness, and dependency. If the patient is to be helped through expression of thoughts and feelings, it should be recognized that nurses have feelings, too, and that they can benefit from nurse-specialist-led conferences or group sessions which help them to recognize their own responses so that they, in turn, can become more able to recognize and accept the emotional responses of patients.

An approach to the patient which is tolerant and understanding of his angry feelings, supportive of his denial when this is appropriate, yet which helps him face reality gradually and with sustained support and which promotes independence through encouragement of his participation in his care to the extent possible, are ways in which the nurse can help the patient cope. Ideally the staff and patient should be able to relate in an "open awareness" context, to the benefit of both (see Chap. 12).

Additional Supportive Therapy

Transfusions of whole blood, platelets, fluids, electrolytes, drugs for the relief of pain, and high protein and high vitamin diet are all important in the supportive therapy for the patient with cancer. Keeping a record of intake and output is important for monitoring fluid balance as well as the effect of certain chemotherapeutic drugs on kidney function. Diversional therapy for an individual patient or for groups of patients can do much to lighten their day. The nurse can promote the maintenance of the patient's emotional ties by preparing him for visiting hours and by establishing rapport with other sources of support, such as clergy, copatients, or social workers.

**Isolation Perfusion.** This is a technique whereby the blood supply to a section or organ of the body is separated from the systemic circulation and treated with a large dose of a chemotherapeutic drug. This technique makes it possible to administer larger doses of the drug directly to the tumor than would be possible through the general systemic circulation (Fig. 17-5). The part to be treated is cut off from the systemic circulation by the use of tourniquets, and the artery and vein serving the part are cannulated. Oxygenated blood to which the concentrated drug has been added is pumped into the artery, and from the artery it perfuses the tumor area. The blood is removed from the vein, reoxygenated, and recirculated. When the treatment is completed, the catheters are withdrawn from the blood vessels and the tourniquets are removed, allowing the systemic circulation to resume serving this part. The nursing responsibilities include assisting the physician with the procedure and observing the patient for possible side effects. For instance, an early side effect may include small ulcerations in the mouth. The patient may complain of burning after drinking fruit juice. Examination of the mouth with a flashlight will reveal the presence of small ulcerations. The entire mouth should be inspected. The physician administering the drug will place a protocol sheet on the patient's chart. This will tell the nurse and personnel from other disciplines everything known to date about the drug, including the side effects. The nurse must observe and report accurately all side effects of the drug. It must be remembered that many of these drugs are new, and

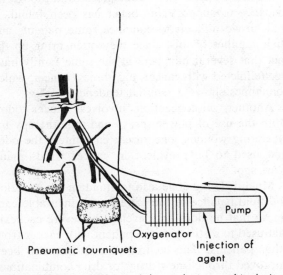

**Figure 17-5.** Diagram of the technique of isolation perfusion. The blood supply to one part of the body is separated from the systemic circulation, and the chemotherapeutic agent is introduced into the blood vessels servicing the part of the body affected by cancer.

an observant nurse may be quick to pick up a side effect that may not have been observed in the laboratory animal during the preclinical trials of the drug.

**Intra-arterial Infusion.** Chemotherapeutic drugs are sometimes administered by intra-arterial route to the tumor in special instances. This method involves the insertion of fine catheters into an artery for selective therapy to a tumor, for example, the external carotid artery is used to treat head and neck tumors. The internal carotid artery is used to treat brain tumors and branches of the celiac artery for liver tumors. With this technique the tumor itself receives the largest part of the drug. A simple pump (sigmamotor) is used to maintain a slow steady regulated flow of the drug to the tumor since gravity alone cannot overcome the arterial blood pressure. Fluorouracil is generally used to infuse liver tumors, methotrexate for head and neck tumors. Very close supervision of the patient and careful attention to details of the operation of the pump are important if this form of treatment is to be successful.

## ONCOLOGIC NURSING

### Prevention and Control of Cancer

**Educating the Public.** Information is important, but it is not enough. While much progress has been made in dealing with the cognitive domain through disseminating the facts about cancer, more work needs to be done in order to deal with the affective domain and to reach all segments of our society. People need to learn not only the facts, but also ways of protecting themselves. They must be helped to change attitudes of fear and despair about cancer, which unfortunately still persist. Cancer has been associated with disfigurement, pain, and death; attitudes will change slowly and only as a result of increased understanding of the disease, particularly of the possibility of cure when the disease is discovered early.

Public education has accomplished a great deal to encourage the awareness of warning signals and the willingness to seek diagnosis and treatment. Today more women are aware of the need to seek early treatment for breast tumor or abnormal vaginal bleeding. Some people have become so fearful of cancer that every symptom, however minor or transient, causes near panic. Such reactions do not indicate less need for public education.

On the contrary, they point to the extreme fear that people have of cancer and the need for continuing education in the ways by which cancer can be controlled and cured. These reactions emphasize also the importance of teaching in a manner that does not provoke needless alarm. People who are very frightened may react with apathy. Patients who refuse to go to physicians or nurse clinicians are not necessarily uninterested or even uninformed. Their fear of cancer may be so great that they are unable to face examination and the possible discovery that they have cancer.

**Aid by Groups.** The nurse works with groups such as the American Cancer Society, which is most active in public and professional education. Patient service is but one of their three basic programs. This organization provides professional consultation with registered nurses or social workers. Homemaker service is provided as needed to help keep the home well organized, clean, and pleasant. Licensed practical nurses may be provided for the patient who needs bedside care at home. In addition, such services as transportation to and from a clinic are provided, as well as drugs, prosthetic devices, sickroom equipment, dressings, speech therapy. The second basic program is education to keep the public alerted to the seven warning signals of cancer and the need for regular complete physical examinations, and to help the medical and nursing professions provide high quality care through such educational programs as workshops and seminars. The third basic program is support for cancer research, for without research, there can be no hope for the future conquest of cancer.

The American Cancer Society also sponsors or coordinates programs in which a patient with a diagnosis of cancer can be visited by a rehabilitated cancer patient with the same diagnosis. The Reach to Recovery program for postmastectomy patients and the International Association of Laryngectomees are examples.

In addition, intensive research is being carried out by the National Cancer Institute (NCI), which is a part of the National Institutes of Health (NIH). The assistance and guidance of members of the health professions and community groups, such as schools, churches, and clubs, also provide ample opportunity for public education.

As noted above the nurse collaborates in programs of cancer control and prevention. As a member of community groups and professional groups she is in an excellent position to teach and help bring the facts about cancer to the community. More active participation by the nurse is needed, however, if she is to be a health teacher in the true sense of the word.

Because of the nurse's specialized knowledge about health matters, neighbors, friends, and relatives often seek her advice. She can explain the need for early diagnosis, whatever the condition, without causing undue alarm. Nurses in industry, community health, and school, as well as hospital nurses are in an ideal position to detect certain skin cancers, neck lumps which may be Hodgkin's disease, lesions in the mouth, and other conditions which an observant nurse may see.

Besides teaching the seven warning signals of cancer and advising early diagnosis and treatment, nurses can encourage people to avoid practices believed to favor the development of cancer. Thus the school nurse has an important responsibility in preventing development of the smoking habit in schoolchildren, a habit easier to avoid entirely than to stop later. Nurses working with migrant laborers in many parts of the United States can encourage workers to minimize exposure of their skin to the sun to lessen their likelihood of developing skin cancer.

Nurses can also help people to correct misconceptions about cancer. For example, some people still believe cancer to be contagious even though no evidence to support this belief has been found. It may prove difficult to convince some patients and their families of this, since they often bring up the fact that several members in the same family have been afflicted with cancer, e.g., breast cancer, which sometimes shows a familial tendency.

Another misconception involves cancer odor. With the use of power sprays and radiotherapy for ulcerating wounds, one rarely encounters the odor that used to be prevalent in cancer wards many years ago.

Much is being done also to maintain the nutrition and fluid balance of the patient with incurable cancer so that he does not develop the severe cachexia that used to distinguish the patient with cancer from other patients. The control of pain has also been improved through new drugs or drug combinations, surgical procedures, and technological devices. Patients with cancer are no longer segregated or consigned to some back ward of the general hospital as they once were. This change has come about slowly as a result of public education and improved therapy.

## Nursing During the Illness

**Attitudes.** The nursing needs of the oncologic patient are varied and complex. They depend on his and his family's reaction to the diagnosis of cancer, the location and consequent impairment of body functions that may result from the disease or its treatment, the stage of the disease, and the prognosis. The quality of the care the patient receives depends not only on the scientific advances in drug therapy, surgery, radiotherapy, and on the availability of equipment, but also on the attitudes toward cancer of those who take care of him. Entering a health profession does not change attitudes magically. New knowledge can be acquired quickly, but emotional reactions toward cancer change slowly. This statement is no less true of professional personnel than it is of patients and their families. Feelings of fear and hopelessness, with consequent avoidance of the patient, sometimes interfere with the ability of the nurse to minister to the patient with cancer. Understanding her own feelings about the disease is important to a nurse as the first step in working with the patient. Most cancer patients are extremely sensitive. They can detect any insecurity and distaste on the part of the nurse as she works with them. If her attitude is calm, able, and understanding, the patient's confidence in her will help in his rehabilitation.

The attitude of the physician and others on the health care team toward the disease is also important as it affects not only the patient, but all those with whom he comes in contact. For example, if the physician is evasive in giving the patient necessary information concerning his illness, the patient may react by holding the nurse responsible for giving him this information. If the physician appears indifferent or hopeless toward the patient, the patient may become more anxious or hostile.

In similar vein, the nurse's attitude and care of the patient also affect the patient's view of the staff generally, and his responsiveness to therapy. Each staff member's actions and attitudes are important and affect the patient's response to others on the health care team.

**Communication.** A matter of particular concern involves communication among those who care for the patient. Evasion and subterfuge are common, lessening the patient's confidence in those who care for him. Two guidelines can help the oncologic nurse in communicating with the patient, and with colleagues.

- *Do not avoid the patient's questions and concerns.* He should be allowed to express them without being interrupted, or having the subject changed. When the nurse has heard a patient's question, she must decide whether it is one which she can, and should, answer. Because a patient asks a question, it does not follow that the nurse must answer it. But she can help him to find the answer, or refer him to the appropriate person with whom to discuss it. For instance, initial explanation of the diagnosis and plan of therapy is the responsibility of the physician. The knowledgeable nurse can clarify or reinforce the explanation or discuss with the physician those questions which are beyond her capability.

- *Have a clear understanding of about what others, particularly the physician, have explained to the patient.* Ideally such matters should be discussed regularly among all staff. If regular staff conferences are not yet established, it is essential for the oncologic nurse to take the initiative in establishing such communication. It is unwise to work with any patient without knowing the framework of explanation given to him by the physician. However, with the cancer patient it is especially necessary that communication be kept open among all who care for the patient. Sensitivity and judgment are required concerning what to tell the patient, in order to promote his comfort and well-being.

All who care for the patient must work together to foster the patient's trust in those who care for him and to help the patient to understand and to deal with his illness, in accordance with the patient's values and his emotional and spiritual resources.

**Supportive Care.** Although most of the problems that arise in nursing a patient with cancer are similar to those encountered in any other nursing situation, there is a tendency for many of these problems to occur simultaneously and to a severe degree. For instance, the patient may be plagued not only by incontinence, but also by severe pain or nausea, and by severe anxiety.

Helping the patient maintain dignity and equanimity is important. Perhaps in no other disease is there such a threat to "wholeness" as exists in cancer. The disease itself and the treatment are often destructive of tissue, and sometimes disfiguring. Some patients who know they have cancer state that they fear the pain or disfigurement or any other specific aspect of the illness not so much as they fear possible overall loss of self-control and dignity during the final stages of the illness. The oncologic nurse must not lose sight of this important concern of patients. The process of physical care is often demanding: tubes to keep patent, skin care, intravenous fluids, and many other tasks which can tax the resources of the nursing staff. Every effort should be directed toward helping the patient maintain his self-respect. Care in draping him during treatments, strict attention to cleanliness, allowing him to participate in planning his care as long as he is able to do so are all measures to help him maintain his dignity.

Nursing requirements have changed in response to changes in the total situation involving care of cancer patients. Many patients have their disease process slowed for considerable periods; many others experience cure, as a result of earlier diagnosis and vigorous use of newer methods of therapy. It is not unusual for a patient whose disease process is slowed and controlled to continue his usual activities for several years and to receive care and treatment on an ambulatory basis during this period. In years past, when there was less success with prompt diagnosis and with therapy, the diagnosis of cancer was often quickly followed by debility, cachexia, and death, and an aura of doom surrounded the patient and his family. It is essential for the nurse to assist the patient and his family to recognize that a diagnosis of cancer is not synonymous with death, to warn them if necessary about cancer quackery, to help them avail themselves of available treatment, and to establish a regimen which encourages as full a return to usual activities as possible. The patient who is physically able to continue working is encouraged to do so, as well as to continue his usual home life and recreation. Family members can assist the patient as they themselves are helped by professional staff to realize that the patient is likely to benefit (as will those in close association with him) if he is encouraged to live as full a life as possible. Often, in such situations, it is not known initially just what the patient's course and prognosis will be, and it is especially important, therefore, for the patient and his family not to draw dire conclusions and for the patient to become an invalid. Patients who have cancer and who nevertheless continue most of their usual activities have many realistic concerns. The oncologic nurse can help by listening, clarifying, and assisting the patient and family to find their own solutions. For example:

- To what extent should the patient discuss the diagnosis with others, such as friends and employer? Some patients find it preferable to discuss their con-

dition with only their closest family and friends, finding that they then are not burdened with reactions, such as pity or avoidance, which may occur among even the most well-meaning neighbors and business colleagues. Other patients find they feel more comfortable discussing the situation rather freely with others. Unfortunately, some employers are uninformed about improved cancer prognoses and may unreasonably terminate the employment of an employee with a diagnosis of cancer. The occupational or community health nurse's role includes promoting more positive employer attitudes.

- What constitutes the golden mean between effective self-care and excessive preoccupation with health, resulting in damage to relationships with others, as well as unnecessary narrowing of interests and life space? For instance, a patient who enjoys travel may decide to take the risk of requiring medical care while far from home, rather than give up plans for travel in order to be close to the facilities where he receives care. While it is important to assist the patient to view his situation realistically, in terms of the likelihood of his needing care, how effectively his requirements can be met away from home, and so forth, it is also necessary to recognize that the decision rests with the patient, to make according to his values.
- How much should the patient push himself? Some patients feel less anxious, and seem to manage best, when they continue their accustomed activities despite fatigue and discomfort, as long as they possibly can. Others, assessing their situation, decide they want and need more time for rest, reflection, and for the pursuits and relationships they most value and enjoy. (There is a difference between the latter decision and a premature recourse to invalidism in the belief that nothing else is possible.)
- How much protection and assistance should family members give? Overprotection can lead the patient to feel stifled, and lead to unnecessary dependence, or to resentment. But help *is* needed at various times, and particularly when the patient's strength diminishes. How can help be given in ways which preserve, as long as possible, the patient's independence, and which foster satisfying family relationships?

More patients are being cured of cancer, and these patients, too, require assistance of health professionals. Usually it is not certain, at the outset, whether or not the patient has been cured. A patient with cervical cancer may undergo hysterectomy. The physician explains to the patient that he believes all malignant tissue has been removed. Nevertheless, it is of the utmost importance that the patient return regularly for periodic medical examinations, so that any new evidence of the disease can be promptly detected and treated. Many patients, however, having been through the ordeal of facing the diagnosis of cancer and having surgery or radiation, or both, want nothing so much as to forget the experience. A visit to the clinic or physician not only reminds them of the experience, but brings with it suspense and dread concerning what may be found at follow-up examinations. Nurses, especially nurses in community health and industrial settings, can help by encouraging and supporting the patient, by showing understanding and acceptance of the patient's feelings, and also by stressing the necessity for, and the advantages to the patient, of follow-up care. As the years go by, and no new evidence of cancer is found, the patient usually relaxes more, as each favorable report brings greater feeling of security that he is, in fact, cured.

If the patient's disease becomes widespread, certain nursing considerations become especially important. The patient may conjure up dreaded fantasies of agonizing pain and mutilation. Too often his opening and sometimes fumbling comments and questions to express these concerns are met by avoidance or by an overly jolly approach which denies the seriousness of his situation. It is important to consider what the patient says, to patiently assist him in expressing his fears, and to discuss them with him. In so doing, some of the vague, enormous, and very threatening fears can be lessened and become more manageable. For instance, the patient who has opportunity to express the fear that the pain may later become unbearable can consider, with the nurse and physician, what is available to relieve his pain, and also important, can receive reassurance from them that they will not desert him—that they will be there and help him remain as comfortable as possible. It has been observed repeatedly that patients who receive emotional support from staff and who are in an atmosphere which fosters dignity, self-care to the extent possible, recreation, and companionship, experience less pain. Other fears, which patients often voice, and which also can become less paralyzing to the patient once he can speak of them, are fears of death, of separation from loved ones, loss of control, and mutilation.

During the spread stage of cancer it is especially important to observe the patient for complications. Bleeding or even serious hemorrhage may occur if a blood vessel is eroded by malignant tissue. Infection, manifested by such symptoms as fever and chills, may occur since the tissues undergoing malignant changes are vulnerable to infection. Pathologic fractures may result if the patient has metastases to bone. In addition, complications may occur as a result of physical inactivity: thrombophlebitis is an example. Vigilant nursing care is required to prevent complications when possible, and to detect their occurrence promptly.

For the patient who is not cured, the nurse must realize that the illness involves many stages, physically and emotionally, and plan care appropriate to each stage. It is important to assist the patient during each of these stages, not rushing him prematurely toward a phase which has not yet arrived, nor failing to recognize when a change in the patient's situation requires a change in his care.

For the patient whose resistance has been overcome by the disease, it is necessary to consider care required by the dying patient and by his family. In some areas there are specialized hospitals (hospices) for terminally ill cancer patients where nursing is the primary therapy. The openness of the staff's approach does much to assist patients to die with dignity (see Chap. 12).

## REFERENCES AND BIBLIOGRAPHY

AMERICAN CANCER SOCIETY: *A Cancer Source Book for Nurses,* New York, American Cancer Society, 1968.

———: *Cancer, a Manual for Practitioners,* ed. 4, Boston, American Cancer Society, 1968.

———: *Cancer Management,* Philadelphia, Lippincott, 1968.

———: *1974 Cancer Facts and Figures,* New York, American Cancer Society, 1974.

BARCKLEY, V.: A visiting nurse specializes in cancer nursing, *Am. J. Nurs.* 70:1680, August 1970.

BERGERON, J.: A patient's plea: tell me, I need to know, *Am. J. Nurs.* 71:1572, August 1971.

BOUCHARD, R.: *Nursing Care of the Cancer Patient,* St. Louis, Mosby, 1967.

CRATE, M.: Nursing functions in adaptation to chronic illness, *Am. J. Nurs.* 65:72, October 1965.

CRAYTOR, J. K.: Talking with persons who have cancer, *Am. J. Nurs.* 69:744, April 1969.

CRAYTOR, J. K., and FASS, M. L.: *The Nurse and the Cancer Patient,* Philadelphia, Lippincott, 1970.

DAVIS, M.: Cancer dwells here, *Nurs. Forum* 6:379, 1967.

DONALDSON, S., and FLETCHER, W.: The treatment of cancer by isolation perfusion, *Am. J. Nurs.* 64:81, August 1964.

ENGEL, G. L.: Grief and grieving, *Am. J. Nurs.* 64:93, September 1964.

EVANS, R. B., et al.: Some psychological characteristics of men with cancer, *Cancer* 17:307, 1964.

EVERSON, T. C., and COLE, W. H.: *Spontaneous Regression of Cancer,* Philadelphia, Saunders, 1966.

FEIFEL, H. (ed.): *The Meaning of Death,* New York, McGraw-Hill, 1959.

FOX, J. E.: Reflections on cancer nursing, *Am. J. Nurs.* 66:1317, June 1966.

FRANCIS, G. M.: Cancer: the emotional component, *Am. J. Nurs.* 69:1677, August 1969.

GARNER, H. H.: *Psychosomatic Management of the Patient with Malignancy,* Springfield, Ill., Thomas, 1966.

GEORGE, M. M.: Long term care of the patient with cancer, *Nurs. Clin. N. Am.* 8:623, December 1973.

GRANT, R.: Nursing the cancer patient, *Nurs. Forum* 4:57, 1965.

GUTHRIE, D.: A *History of Medicine,* Philadelphia, Lippincott, 1946.

HOFFMAN, E.: "Don't give up on me," *Am. J. Nurs.* 71:60, January 1971.

KISSEN, D. M., and LeSHAN, L. L. (eds.): *Psychosomatic Aspects of Neoplastic Disease,* Philadelphia, Lippincott, 1964.

KLAGSBRUN, S. C.: Cancer, emotions, and nurses, *Am. J. Psychiat.* 126:1237, March 1970.

————: Communications in the treatment of cancer, *Am. J. Nurs.* 71:944, May 1971.

KRAKOFF, I. H.: Cancer chemotherapeutic agents, *Ca— A Cancer Journal for Clinicians,* 23:208, 1973.

LeSHAN, L. L., and GASSMAN, M. L.: Some observations on psychotherapy with patients suffering from neoplastic disease, *Am. J. Psychotherap.* 12:723, 1958.

LUNCEFORD, J. L., et al.: Nursing Care of Patients in the Laminar Air Flow Room, USDHEW Publ. No. (NIH 72-93), Nursing Clinical Conferences, 1-16, December 1971.

MANGAN, H.: Care, coordination and communication in the life island setting, *Nurs. Outlook* 17:40, January 1969.

MEINHART, N.: The cancer patient: living in the here and now, *Nurs. Outlook,* 16:64, May 1968.

METTLER, C. C.: *History of Medicine,* Philadelphia, Blakiston, 1947.

NEALON, T. F. (ed.): *Management of the Patient with Cancer,* Philadelphia, Saunders, 1965.

NEELON, V. J.: Hyperbaric oxygenation, *Am. J. Nurs.* 64:73, October 1964.

NOWAK, P. A.: Nursing care in isolation perfusion, *Am. J. Nurs.* 64:85, August 1964.

*Nursing and the Cancer Patient,* Contemporary Nursing Series, Browning, M., and Lewis, E., comps., New York, The American Journal of Nursing Company, 1973.

PAYNE, E., and KRANT, M. J.: The psychosocial aspects of advanced cancer, *JAMA* 210:1238, 1969.

PRENSCHKE, D.: Guardedness or openness on the cancer unit, *Nurs. Res.* 22:484, November–December 1973.

ROSENFELD, L., and CALLAWAY, J.: Snuff dippers' cancer, *Am. J. Surg.* 106:840-844, 1963.

RUBIN, R. (ed.): *Clinical Oncology for Medical Students and Physicians: A Multidisciplinary Approach,* ed. 3, New York, The University of Rochester and the American Cancer Society, 1970-71.

SHIMKIN, M. B.: *Science and Cancer,* Washington, D.C., U.S. Department of Health, Education and Welfare, 1969.

SILVERSTEIN, M. J., and MORTON, D.: Cancer immunotherapy (pictorial), *Am. J. Nurs.* 73:1178, July 1973.

WOLF, E. S.: Where hope comes first, *Nurs. Outlook* 12:52, April 1964.

# Nursing Management in Radiotherapy

## CHAPTER 18

The term "radiotherapy" refers to the therapeutic application of ionizing radiation from x-ray machines or from radioactive materials. Radiotherapy deals mainly, but not exclusively, with the treatment of cancer. For this reason the medical specialist who practices radiotherapy prefers to be called a *radiation oncologist* or *radiotherapist*.

The aim of radiotherapy is an orderly destruction of malignant, rapidly dividing cells, while leaving the rest of the body well or able to recover and capable of eliminating the killed cancer cells. This destruction is accomplished by x-rays or radioactive materials.

When the malignancy is far advanced, radiotherapy is used palliatively to cause a remission of symptoms so that the patient will be more comfortable. Radioactive isotopes are used for both diagnostic and therapeutic procedures.* Radiotherapy is used to heal lytic lesions in the bones. As the lytic lesions heal, pain diminishes. Radiotherapy is both palliative and curative in late-stage malignancy.

An adequate knowledge of radiation is necessary not only for the safety and protection of personnel, but also for countering the superstition, misconception, and fear brought about by the atom bomb. A more realistic attitude concerning clinical uses of radiation is necessary if the health care team is to be truly successful in the management of patients receiving radiotherapy. Uncertainty or confusion on the part of hospital personnel will only increase the patient's fears and damage his morale. That radiation is invisible and inaudible

---

* The diagnostic uses of radiation are discussed in the various clinical chapters where appropriate.

271

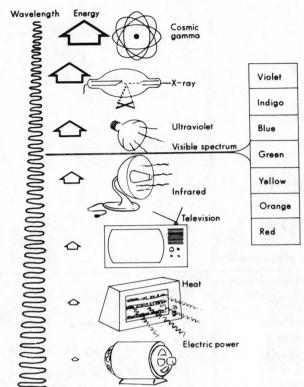

Wavelength   Energy

Cosmic gamma

X-ray

Ultraviolet

Visible spectrum

| Violet |
| Indigo |
| Blue |
| Green |
| Yellow |
| Orange |
| Red |

Infrared

Television

Heat

Electric power

**Figure 18-1.** The electromagnetic spectrum. (Early, P. J., Rozzati, M. A., and Sodee, D. B.: *Textbook of Nuclear Medicine and Technology,* St. Louis, Mosby)

makes it seem menacing and difficult for some patients to understand. Diagnostic tests and treatments often involve the use of large machines that are, for the patient, strange to behold. Because radiotherapy is used for the treatment of cancer more often than for any other condition, and because most patients know this, radiotherapy itself suggests a serious condition. The nurse whose practice is based on an understanding of the physical laws that govern radiation will be able to protect herself from possible damage that can be produced by radiation. Her skill in applying the principles underlying nursing care is necessary for the safe and effective use of radiotherapy.

Radiation deserves the same respect given to other modalities of therapy for cancer. As noted in Chapter 17, radiotherapy is one of four accepted forms of treatment for cancer and allied diseases. These methods are used singly or in combination. The choice is left to the judgment of the physician. It must always be remembered that it is the patient rather than the cancer which is being treated. All available means must be used to support the patient while he is receiving radiotherapy for his disease.

## WHAT IS RADIOACTIVITY?

Light waves, radiowaves, ultraviolet waves, and so on, are energy waves, or rays of electric and magnetic influence. In the electromagnetic spectrum, radiations are grouped according to wave lengths (Fig. 18-1). These waves act as packets of energy called "quanta" or "photons" (Tievsky, 1962). They contain a precise amount of energy depending upon the wave length. The energy of the quantum is proportional to the frequency of the radiation. The shorter, more energetic waves are located in the upper part of the spectrum, while the longer, less energetic waves are located in the lower part. The laser beam is the most recent addition to the spectrum (1959). Nearly all parts of the electromagnetic spectrum can now be used for the diagnosis or treatment of disease.

### Natural Radioactivity

Radioactive atoms such as radium or uranium occur in nature and are said to be naturally radioactive. Natural radioactivity also exists in minute amounts in soil, air, water, and building materials, as well as in our own bodies. Cosmic radiation is present everywhere, but slightly more is found at higher altitudes. For example, a person living in Denver, Colorado, gets more background radiation than a person living in New York City. This natural background radiation is a normal part of the environment.

Radioactive elements fall toward the heavy end of the Periodic Table of elements, have a high atomic number and mass, and are unstable. The lighter elements have approximately the same numbers of protons and neutrons and are stable. With heavier elements the atomic nuclei are larger and inherently unstable. It becomes increasingly difficult for the nucleus to remain intact regardless of the numbers of neutrons it has. Radioactivity is instability of radioactive atoms, which results in spontaneous disintegration of the atom. In an attempt to reach stability, the nuclei of unstable atoms give up energy in the form of particles or waves, called alpha and beta particles, and gamma waves.

**Alpha Particles.** Alpha particles are positively charged; they can penetrate tissues only a fraction of a millimeter and their energies are quickly dissipated because of their low penetrating power and short range. If an isotope whose disintegration gives off alpha particles is accidentally ingested or enters the body through a wound, alpha particles will become dangerous, and perhaps even lethal, because they will ionize tissues. Internal ionization from isotopes is more harmful than ionization by external beam therapy.

**Beta Particles.** Beta particles are negatively charged. They are streams of fast-moving electrons produced by nuclear disintegration or x-ray machines. Their ability to penetrate tissues is much greater than that of alpha particles, usually 1 to 4 mm., and the energies produced are dissipated more slowly than are the energies produced by alpha particles. Beta particles, or electrons, produce useful therapeutic results in the vicinity of their release. When radioactive pharmaceuticals which are beta emitters are injected or ingested for therapy, the patient's own body will serve as an effective shield, so that other persons are not affected by radiation.

**Gamma Waves.** Gamma waves (photons) produced by radioisotopes or x-ray machines are highly energetic, travel with the speed of light ($3 \times 3^{10}$ cm. per sec.), and can penetrate deeply into body tissues. When used internally, they can pass directly through the body, and present the greatest external hazard.

For comparison of their ability to penetrate: a sheet of paper can stop alpha particles, a block of wood, or 1 to 4 mm. of tissue can stop beta particles, and a thick concrete wall can stop gamma waves (Fig. 18-2).

## Artificial Radioactivity

The credit for discovering artificial radioactivity (1934) belongs to Irene and Frederic Joliot-Curie. While bombarding aluminum with alpha particles

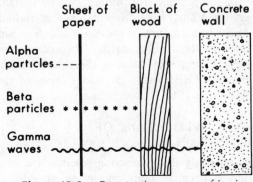

**Figure 18-2.** Penetrating power of ionizing radiations.

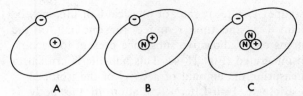

**Figure 18-3.** Hydrogen, the lightest and simplest element, has three varieties: (A) Hydrogen ($H^1$, stable); (B) Deuterium ($H^2$, sea water, heavy water, heavy hydrogen); (C) Tritium ($H^3$, unstable).

from polonium, the aluminum continued to give off electrons, even after the removal of the polonium. The short-lived phosphorus thus obtained was shown to be radioactive. Since then many artificial isotopes have been produced by using various particle accelerators and reactors (Fig. 18-3). Like natural radioactivity, artificial radioactivity will also produce alpha and beta particles and gamma waves. Man-made isotopes are valuable in therapy because they are relatively inexpensive and readily obtainable. An isotope chart, known as the Seaborg chart, is convenient for the radiotherapist and nuclear chemist. It shows the important characteristics of each radioactive element, e.g., the atomic number, mass, half-life and type(s) of radiation emitted. Many artificially produced isotopes have short half-lives and little material is needed to get a sufficient number of disintegrations; by the time ten half-lives have elapsed, the amount of radioactivity is negligible (1/100 of the original amount).

There are now many radioisotopes used in the medical, biological, and industrial fields, and their numbers are increasing. As newer isotopes become available for diagnosis and therapy, it becomes an important responsibility for the nurse to find out all she can about them, just as she would for a new drug. When caring for a patient receiving radiotherapy, she should know (or refresh her memory through consultation with a specialist who knows) the rays and particles emitted, the half-life, and how the isotope is eliminated from the body so that nursing precautions, if indicated, can be observed and nursing care plans instituted.

## Radioactive Disintegration (Physical Half-Life)

All radioactive isotopes are continuously undergoing spontaneous disintegration until stability is reached. This decay is constant and cannot be speeded up or slowed down. The decay rate is different for each isotope and is a characteristic of the isotope. The decay rate, or physical half-life, may be defined as the time required for one-half of the atoms of a radioactive substance present to become disintegrated (Fig. 18-4). This half-life is critical in measuring the amount of activity of the isotope.

**Biologic Half-Life.** Radiation in the body is disposed of by metabolic processes as well as by the physical half-life. The term "biologic half-life" refers to the time it takes for one-half of the radioactive atoms to be eliminated from the body as a result of natural biologic processes.

**Effective Half-Life.** This term is used to refer to the time required for a certain amount of radioactive material in the body to lose one-half of its original activity as a result of both natural biologic elimination and radioactive decay processes. For example, the physical half-life of radioactive iodine ($^{131}$I) is 8.1 days, and the biologic half-life is about 18 to 24 days. With internal radiation it is important to know the body's pattern of distribution, the metabolism, and the excretion of each isotope. An isotope which is dispersed throughout the body is less hazardous than one which confines itself to an organ, e.g., $^{131}$I which concentrates in the thyroid. Also, an isotope which is excreted rapidly or has a short half-life is less hazardous than one which remains in the body for a long period of time.

## MEASURING RADIOACTIVITY

Measures of ionizing radiation often appear in medical and nursing publications; therefore, a knowledge of the more common terms is essential for nurses. Radioactivity is measured as units of source strength and as units of dose.

**Units of Source Strength.** The source strength is a measure of the number of radioactive disintegrations per second. The curie, so named to honor Madame Curie, is equal to the radiation power of 1 Gm. of radium or, the quantity of radioactive material in which 37 billion disintegrations occur per second ($3.7 \times 10^{10}$). The curie for practical purposes of therapy is too large. The following terms are used in nuclear medicine to measure amounts of radioactivity:

1 curie (c.)       = $3.7 \times 10^{10}$ disintegrations per second
1 millicurie (mc.)   = $3.7 \times 10^{7}$ disintegrations per second
1 microcurie ($\mu$c.) = $3.7 \times 10^{4}$ disintegrations per second
1 picocurie (pc.)   = $3.7 \times 10^{1}$ (or 37) disintegrations
           per second

The amounts of radioisotopes given to patients can be classified as follows:

Small amounts . . . . . . . . less than 200 microcuries
Moderate amounts . . . . 200 microcuries to 5 millicuries
Large amounts . . . . . . . over 5 millicuries

**Units of Dose.** The primary unit of dose is the roentgen, so called to honor Wilhelm Roentgen, discoverer of x-rays. The roentgen, or "R," is the measure or quantity of exposure to x-rays or gamma radiation. It is defined as the amount of ionization produced in 1 ml. of air under specified conditions (Tievsky, 1962). The therapeutic dose is measured in terms of roentgens or milliroentgens (1/1000 of a roentgen), and abbreviated as mr. Dose units are used for calculating the dosage of radioactive material before internal administration, for describing effects of radiation on tissues, and to ensure the safe handling of radioactive materials.

The term rad (radiation absorbed dose) is another unit of dose. It refers to the amount of radiation absorbed by the tissues.

The term rem (roentgen equivalent—man) is used to compensate for differences in ionization and energy transfer of different types of radiation. The rem is the amount of radiation which produces the same biologic effect as the absorption of one roentgen, taking into account the relative biologic effectiveness (RBE) of the various types of radiation (Tievsky, 1962).

## CLINICAL APPLICATION OF RADIOTHERAPY

Radiotherapy is an exacting science. Its administration is as meticulous and often as tedious as that of surgery or chemotherapy. The application

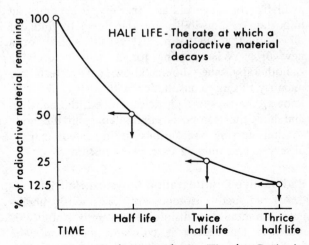

**Figure 18-4.** Radioactive decay. (Tievsky, G.: *Ionizing Radiation*, Springfield, Ill., Thomas)

can be as extensive as that of an operative procedure. Major and minor procedures are often performed concomitantly for the express purpose of treatment with radioisotopes, e.g., a thoracotomy with an implant of either radon or iodine seeds into an unresectable lung tumor. Radiotherapy is not an easy way out in the management of cancer. Like surgery, it can result in painful and unpleasant complications.

## Planning for Radiotherapy

Many factors must be taken into account before radiotherapy can be initiated. Of importance are the following: (1) the location and extent of the tumor, (2) the histology of the tumor, (3) the presence and sites of metastases, (4) the radiosensitivity of the tumor, (5) the age and physical and psychological condition of the patient, and (6) the efficacy of radiotherapy in terms of cure rate, palliation, and so on, as compared with such other modalities of therapy as surgery or chemotherapy.

In addition to a thorough history and physical examination, all recent laboratory data must be reviewed and studied. Consultation with the radiotherapist is requested. In many large centers, the patient is presented at a conference of medical (chemotherapy, immunotherapy), surgical, and radiation oncologists to determine the particular type of therapy best suited to the patient's malignancy. A biopsy is necessary to establish the histology of the tumor. The patient is examined by several radiotherapists, and after consultation he is then told how he will benefit and what to expect from the various forms of treatment. Radiotherapy and its effects are best explained by the radiotherapist. Informed consent is then obtained.

In some radiation centers the patient is taken to an area of the hospital containing an x-ray simulator (a machine used to demonstrate, but not to administer, radiotherapy), where he is placed on a treatment table and special films outlining the tumor area are taken. Skin markings are applied to the areas to be treated. Carbol fuchsin or other appropriate skin markers are used. Operational factors such as timing, distance, and port size are determined by the radiation oncologist and members of the planning team, including the physicist. The patient is encouraged to ask questions while the therapist explains the treatment routines and the part the patient is expected to play. With this un-

hurried approach an effort is made to establish a supportive relationship with the patient and to reduce his fears in order to help him accept radiotherapy with confidence and hope.

## Nursing Support

The nurse's role at this time is largely supportive. Some patients feel "doomed" to die if surgery cannot be performed. They must be reassured that radiotherapy, like surgery, is another form of treatment for tumors and that excellent results are frequently obtained. Repeated explanation and reassurance are often necessary to help the patient adjust to radiotherapy. The patient must know why he is left alone during actual therapy, and the intercom system and television monitor should have been explained in advance of therapy. The patient's basic needs for information must be met. Silence or vague answers can be more disturbing to him than the truth.

It is well to remember and use the exact terms the therapist has used to explain the effects of treatment ("melting" or "shrinking" of the tumor). This should be noted on the nursing care plan. Lay terminology is best understood by most patients. Technical terms may add to the patient's fears. Most patients tolerate therapy and bear some discomfort if they are given simple explanations.

Discussion of the side effects of therapy should be minimized until they are imminent or actually occur. Psychological effects include depression, apprehension, overreaction, and belief in "old wives' tales" which seem to persist. Frequent reassurance and consistency of explanation by members of the health care team are important in dispelling doubts and maintaining morale.

It is particularly important to help the patient work out a regimen of nutritious and appetizing meals, pleasant diversion, rest, and companionship during the period of radiotherapy. Most patients receiving therapy are able to live at home and come to the hospital for their treatments.

When preparing the patient for radiotherapy and assisting him during the period of therapy, it is important for the oncologic nurse not only to clarify or reinforce the explanation of the treatment to him, but also to listen to his views, doubts, and concerns about the treatment. Too often this is overlooked, and the patient, though exposed to a good deal of instruction, continues to harbor doubts, fears, and fantasies concerning the effects of radiation which are not discussed with the professional staff who could help him to deal with them, and thus assist him to channel his energies from worry to constructive action as a participant in his program of therapy. The generalist nurse should confer with other team members such as the radiotherapist, physicist, or oncologic nursing specialist, when she is unable to answer the patient's questions or when the answers are not in her domain.

### Sensitivity of Tissues to Radiation

Rapidly dividing cells are more sensitive to radiation than those which divide slowly. This generalization was made by Bergonie and Tribondeau (1906) who stated that "cells are sensitive to radiation in proportion to their proliferative activity."

The following is an outline of cells arranged according to their sensitivity to radiation, with the most sensitive cells listed first:

1. Lymphocytes
2. Erythroblasts
3. Myeloblasts
4. Epithelial cells
   a. Basal cells of testes
   b. Basal cells of intestinal crypts
   c. Basal cells of the ovaries
   d. Basal cells of the skin
   e. Basal cells of secretory glands
   f. Alveolar cells of the lungs and bile ducts
5. Endothelial cells
6. Connective tissue cells
7. Tubular cells of the kidneys
8. Bone cells
9. Nerve cells
10. Brain cells
11. Muscle cells

This summary is now called the law of Bergonie and Tribondeau (Behrens el al., 1969).

Radiosensitivity does not imply curability of cancer. For example, the lymph nodes in some lymphoma or in the leukemias are quite radiosensitive, and radiotherapy may be the treatment of choice, but some types of lymphoma and leukemias are progressive.

### EXTERNAL BEAM THERAPY

X-rays, or roentgen rays (waves), vary in wave length and in penetrating power. They are high frequency waves having short wave lengths (Fig. 18-1). X-rays are produced in a vacuum tube (Fig. 18-5).

At one end of the tube is the cathode or negative pole; at the opposite end is the anode or positive pole. A wire attached to each pole leads to a high voltage source. When the cathode is heated by means of a filament, free electrons are boiled off and driven by the difference in electrical potential. These electrons, flowing at tremendous speed, strike the target, producing x-rays. The rate at which these electrons flow can be altered by increasing or decreasing the voltage supplying the tube. Since x-rays vary in wave length and penetrating power, it is this principle which is used to determine the kind of x-ray apparatus to be used in the treatment of the various kinds of tumors. Soft x-rays (longer wave lengths) are generally used for treating superficial cancers and for diagnosis. Hard x-rays (shorter wave lengths), are generally used for treatment of deep-seated tumors. X-ray machines in general use are in the 30 to 120 kilovolt range. More powerful are the linear accelerators (Fig. 18-6) that deliver up to 33 million electron volts and the betatrons that will deliver up to 35 million electron volts. Cobalt teletherapy units (Fig. 18-7) use radioactive cobalt ($^{60}$Co) as a source of radiation.

**Timing (Fractionation).** In external beam therapy, doses are not given in a single application, but in daily or less frequent fractions distributed over a total treatment period of several weeks. Fractionation is said to increase the effect of radiation on the tumor, while allowing normal cells to recover. Each daily fraction of the dose permits progressive biologic damage to the tumor cells. This division of dose kills tumor cells in the premitotic stage, and since mitosis is a continuing

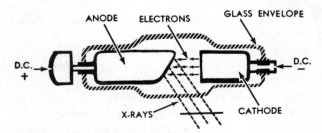

**Figure 18-5.** Simplified diagram of an x-ray tube. Although in this diagram the x-rays appear to be concentrated in one area, actually radiation danger exists anywhere in the presence of the machine, and precautions should be taken accordingly. (Jensen, J. T.: *Introduction to Medical Physics,* Philadelphia, Lippincott, 1964)

process, the tumor cells are radiated many times instead of just once. Fractions may vary; often five fractions per week are used.

**Rotational Therapy.** In some treatment situations rotational therapy, which can be accomplished with many of the newer supervoltage machines, is employed. Anterior, posterior, and lateral fields can be used and the x-ray beam can be directed at the tumor from several angles, not just one. With this technique, normal tissues are spared to a large degree, and sensitive tissues in front or in back of the tumor are avoided. Also with supervoltage and rotational therapy there is a "skin sparing effect" with the maximum buildup of energy directed to the tumor (Nealon, 1965). Bone structures are also spared, avoiding bone necrosis, and better depth dosage is achieved. Special shields are used also to protect normal structures near the tumor, thus avoiding the complications such as lung fibrosis, radiation nephritis, and bone marrow damage. Orthovoltage therapy (deep therapy) has largely been replaced by supervoltage therapy. Patients appear to tolerate supervoltage therapy better than orthovoltage therapy.

**Individual Reactions.** Individual differences may alter the patient's response to therapy. Infection or ischemia may decrease the radiosensitivity, and poor response is evident more often among the cachectic than in well-nourished patients. On entering tissues, radiation produces ionization of atoms with chemical alteration of tissue proteins. Ionization is facilitated by the large amounts of water and oxygen present in the tissues. The maintenance of good hydration of the patient receiving radiotherapy is an important nursing responsibility. When the oxygen carrying ability of the blood is impaired as a result of anemia, there is a reduced response to radiotherapy. It is important therefore that the patient's hemoglobin be maintained at near normal levels. Hypoxic cells within a tumor are protected to some extent from radiation destruction. Based on this concept, clinical trials have been undertaken in administering radiotherapy while the patient breathes in oxygen under increased barometric pressure. This involves the use of the hyperbaric chamber. There is great complexity in the relationship of factors such as oxygen tension, dose rate, and fractionation in the many types of radiation of differing energies. Hyperbaric radiotherapy is still in the clinical trial stage and more experi-

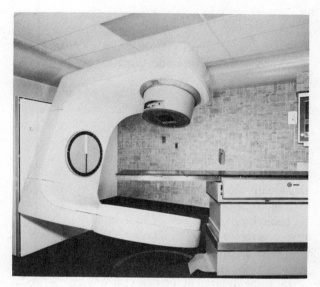

**Figure 18-6.** Clinical linear accelerator (Cliniac). (Varian Associates—Radiation Division, Palo Alto, Calif.)

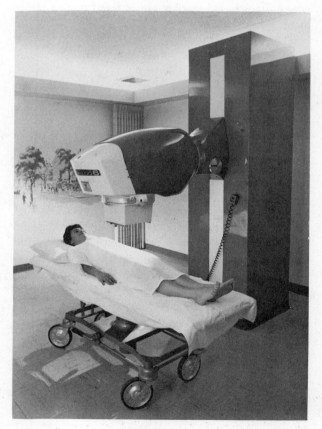

**Figure 18-7.** A vertical teletherapy unit. The radioactive source is Cobalt[60]. (Atomic Energy of Canada, Ottawa, Canada)

ence is needed to make definite statements about its value.

Radiation reactions may be acute or chronic depending upon the dose and time; thus the fractionated dose plan may require some adjustment to the pathology and tolerance of individual patients.

### Nursing Care

#### Patient Education

Most patients know that they are receiving x-ray therapy for cancer. The physician discusses the diagnosis with the patient and his family and is guided by the legal principle of informed consent as well as behavioral principles of individual variations in response to seemingly similar situations. It is important that all members of the health care team be aware of the explanation given the patient and family.

In some treatment centers the patient is given a booklet which presents basic information about radiotherapy, including how to care for the skin after treatment, why soap and water are not used, why certain blood studies are ordered during treatment.

The nurse encourages the patient to take plenty of fluids and to have a well-balanced diet, sometimes with protein supplements.

The nurse is perhaps of greatest help when she listens and allows the patient to express his feelings. By her quiet acceptance of his emotional state, she can help him accept therapy and come to terms with his illness. Many social and psychological problems can be resolved once the diagnosis and its implications are openly or tacitly accepted. If the patient's disease is curable, this fact should be stressed to the patient and his family. The discomforts of therapy can be tolerated better, if the patient knows that a cure is imminent. For the patient with incurable disease, the palliation achieved may permit normal or near normal activities for a long period of time. If radiation reactions should become severe, the therapist may halt treatments to give the body a chance to recover. The reason for this should be explained to the patient and his family to avoid misunderstandings, feelings of discouragement and setback. It should be explained that deviations from the original plan of therapy are not unusual.

#### Helping with Administration

When external beam therapy is used, the patient must be reminded not to remove the skin markings. Markings are reinforced as necessary when the patient returns for therapy. Perspiration may cause the markings to fade. Sandbags or individually constructed molds made of laminated plaster of paris or an acrylic resin or a clear plastic are sometimes used to immobilize the part to be treated. Molds are especially helpful in treating head and neck tumors where a precise beam to a small area is to be used. Special precautions must be taken to shield the eyes or other critical tissues from possible stray radiation. It is especially important to protect the lens of the eye, the gonads, and the hematopoietic system; these have been termed the "critical tissues" (Tievsky, 1962).

#### Patient Activities

Normal activities are encouraged as much as possible. Rest periods should be provided after therapy as some patients tire easily. Most patients are ambulatory, however, and continue radiotherapy on an outpatient basis. Some find they eat better before the treatment and a highly nutritious breakfast should be provided if treatment is later in the day.

#### Radiation Reactions

**The Skin.** Certain radiation reactions are anticipated, and appropriate supportive measures are instituted. With better radiation techniques and patient management, many side effects have been reduced or nearly eliminated. It is unwise to burden the patient by telling him of side effects which may or may not occur. However, he should be advised to report any discomforts he experiences to the staff. When the patient reports symptoms, such as itching or burning, it is essential to take his statements seriously and to see that the appropriate member of the health care team receives the information about the patient's symptoms. The patient should know that the skin in the treated area may become reddened, and that this is a normal reaction to therapy. The term "burn" should never be used as it may connote overtreatment or carelessness.

The patient is instructed to keep the radiated skin clean by patting with a soft cloth wet with warm water and then by patting it dry; and specifically not to scrub it with soap and water, and to avoid unprescribed ointments, creams, or powders. Cornstarch may be used two or three times a day for a mild "blushing" of the skin. The radiated skin should be protected against extremes of heat or cold, and a shower spray should not be directed on it. Heat pads, ultraviolet light, diathermy, whirlpool, sauna or steam baths, and direct sunlight must be avoided. No adhesive tape or other tape should be used. Constricting garments such as girdles or collars can irritate the skin. Loose clothing is advised to avoid irritation. Nylon clothing is not porous and tends to keep the skin moist which encourages breakdown.

Intense itching, especially in patients with Hodgkin's disease, is sometimes experienced. A steroid type cream or aerosol spray is sometimes prescribed for relief. Cornstarch may be used on radiated areas where two skin surfaces are in contact, e.g., axillary and groin areas, and areas under the breasts, provided there is no breakdown of the skin. When therapy is completed, talcum or zinc stearate powder may afford some relief from itching.

**The Hair.** If the scalp is being irradiated, shampoos, tinting, and permanent waving should be avoided. Upon completion of therapy, the therapist may recommend a mild baby shampoo. Partial hair loss is seen. This epilation is temporary, regrowth occurring in from four to six months, and the patient should be reassured that this condition is temporary. A wig is recommended to restore appearance and morale.

**The Bone Marrow.** Patients receiving radiotherapy may develop varying degrees of bone marrow depression. The need for periodic blood counts and occasional, small whole blood, packed cells, or platelet transfusions to tide over the patient until his therapy course is completed must be explained to the patient. The lowered leukocyte count makes the patient easy prey to infection. Visitors and hospital personnel with colds or other infections should not be in close contact with radiotherapy patients. If the leukopenia is severe, the therapist may temporarily halt treatments and perhaps put the patient on reverse isolation precautions.

**Fluids and Diet.** Most patients tolerate a well-balanced diet. Because large amounts of tumor are being lysed during therapy, it is important to maintain effective kidney function to avoid uric acid crystalluria and possible kidney shutdown. Good hydration and maintenance of dilute urine are measures used to prevent this rare complication. The patient should take up to 3,000 ml. of fluid daily. If the fluid intake is inadequate, the therapist may wish to order a supplementary intravenous infusion to make up the deficit. Accurate intake and output records are essential. Most patients who are able like to do this themselves once they have been taught. Unless the patient has been on a special diet for some medical reason, a regular diet is usually recommended. Allopurinol is sometimes prescribed when the uric acid level in the blood is high.

### Follow-up Care

Most patients receive radiotherapy on an outpatient basis; hospitalization is avoided as much as possible. Outpatients are often able to carry out their usual activities during the period when they are receiving radiotherapy. It is important to consider the patient's family as well as the patient when planning for continuing care. Patients' families often have questions and misgivings, and it is essential for them to have an opportunity to talk with members of the staff so that they can be more comfortable about the situation themselves and, therefore, better able to offer assistance and support to the patient.

On each visit, the patient may be given a slip for his next appointment with the radiotherapy department. He may also be given the name and telephone number of the therapist on duty in case of emergency. He is advised to keep his follow-up appointments. The patient is referred to the social worker for assistance with such matters as temporary housing, transportation, and family problems. In some instances homemaker or housekeeping services may also be necessary. It is important for the nurse in all clinical settings to be alert to the need for continuity of care and to initiate referral to other nurses when necessary. For example, if the patient is treated initially in the hospital and subsequently as an outpatient, referral to a community health nurse may be indicated. Side effects from therapy can occur after the course of treatment has terminated. The therapist will therefore prepare the patient for this possibility and stress the importance of returning to the clinic if he experiences any discomfort, so that medication and treatment can be prescribed if necessary.

### The Management of Radiation Reactions

A systemic effect known as radiation sickness is sometimes experienced by patients undergoing extensive radiotherapy. The amount of radiation sickness depends upon the site, dose, and volume treated; for example, a patient undergoing therapy for a small basal cell cancer of the face will not be expected to experience radiation sickness. Patients who have large areas of the body treated may experience radiation sickness. The symptoms may include weakness, nausea, vomiting, diaphoresis, and sometimes chills. The symptoms are handled prophylactically and symptomatically.

**Prophylactic Management.** Symptoms associated with radiotherapy are often influenced by the emotional state of the patient. He should be reassured that side effects are not frequently encountered today. Care of the patient should emphasize support, explanation, and a program of rest and diversion in pleasant surroundings. It is possible for most patients to remain at home among familiar surroundings, and to continue accustomed activities.

To avoid nausea and vomiting, the nurse and dietitian should plan the patient's meals to be served so that food is avoided at least one hour before and after therapy. Some therapists may decide to order an antiemetic to be given one half hour before therapy. Rushing the patient should also be avoided, and diagnostic tests should not be scheduled immediately before or following therapy. Emphasis upon emotional support and a program including necessary rest and pleasant diversion often obviate the problem of nausea.

**Leukopenia.** If a large area is being treated, the patient will need regular blood counts. If the white blood count falls below 2,000, daily blood counts are ordered and therapy halted temporarily, or the therapist may decide to continue treatments if there is a reason for continuance, e.g., the treatment series is almost completed. The patient usually recovers from leukopenia in from two to four weeks.

**Anemia.** Successful radiotherapy does not produce anemia. Usually anemia due to cancer improves during therapy. Persistent anemia is not common, but when present it may make radiotherapy inadvisable.

**Skin Care.** As stated previously, with the skin-sparing effects provided by modern supervoltage machines, reactions are usually minimal. Mild or "dry" erythema can occur in from 10 to 14 days following therapy. Itching or burning may or may not accompany erythema. The best treatment is to keep the area dry and exposed to the air as much as possible. Cornstarch may be used.

Moist erythema sometimes occurs with vesication or denudation of the epidermis. Healing will occur within the lesion and its borders. The dry method of skin care is preferred by most therapists. Medications such as 2 per cent gentian violet spray may be prescribed to assist drying and healing. Creams such as lanolin are sometimes prescribed. It is essential to seek the recommendation of the radiotherapist concerning any application to the patient's skin. No perfumed soaps or lotions should be used.

**Infection.** If infection is present, a culture is taken and the appropriate antibiotic or antiseptic is prescribed, usually topical applications that are absorbed and not those which tend to keep the skin moist and away from air. Meticulous aseptic technique must be observed once the skin is opened. Sterile dressings should be held in place with hypoallergenic tape to avoid further irritation. Radiation ulcers, rarely seen anymore, involving large areas of skin may necessitate surgical intervention such as debridement or skin graft (Nealon, 1965).

**Telangiectasis.** Varying degrees of telangiectasis are sometimes seen as a late residual reaction. There is a slight darkening of the radiated skin with reddish or purplish weblike markings which are caused by capillary dilatation. Some fading does occur with time. This reaction seems to develop more in patients who have received low energy radiation (orthovoltage), and it is rare with supervoltage. With the therapist's approval, a covermark type of cosmetic may be used to camouflage the area if it is on the face or other exposed part of the body. A good waterproof cosmetic will blend with the patient's own skin coloring and will do much toward restoring the patient's appearance and morale. The makeup is removed at night with an albolene type cream.

**Conjunctivitis.** Stray radiation to the eye is largely avoided by more precise beam direction and specially constructed shields and molds. In treating lesions near the orbit, a conjunctival reaction may occur. These are usually mild and clear up with simple treatment. An eye bath with normal saline or other solution is sometimes ordered. If the eye is painful, an anesthetic analgesic type of eye drops is sometimes prescribed, e.g., butyn sulfate 2 per cent with metaphen. When there is painful sticking of the eyelids the therapist may prescribe sterile castor oil drops to be instilled at the hour of sleep. Temporary or permanent epilation of the eyebrow or eyelids may occur. If infection is present, a culture should be taken and an ophthalmologist should be consulted. Cosmetics can camouflage this disfigurement.

**Mucosal Reactions in the Head and Neck.** Mucous membrane reactions precede skin reactions. After about the tenth day of therapy the mucous membranes may become red. This is followed in a few days by a white fibrinous membrane which may become adherent. The patient experiences cough, hoarseness, sore throat, dryness, and dysphagia. Mild antiseptic mouthwashes may alleviate the discomfort. Moderate pain may be relieved by sucking on anesthetic type lozenges. Dysphagia is sometimes treated with viscous lidocaine which is swallowed and which coats and soothes the painful mucous membranes, allowing the patient to swallow liquids and take soft foods. If the severity of the reaction greatly impedes nutrition, the therapist may halt therapy for one to two weeks and then resume treatment. Adequate hydration and nutrition must be maintained.

Following therapy to the mouth or salivary gland, dryness and a "metallic" taste is experienced by some patients. This may be somewhat ameliorated by carbonated soda or hard lemon candy.

**Laryngeal Edema and Atrophy of Nasal Mucous Membrane.** Laryngeal edema is rarely seen. If the edema is severe, a tracheostomy may be performed as an emergency measure. Atrophy of the mucous membrane of the nose after therapy to the nose is an irreversible complication. Some relief may be obtained by prescribed nose drops.

**Respiratory System.** Cough can be produced by radiotherapy to the trachea, bronchi, or lung. Relief is sometimes obtained by prescribed cough medication. Steam inhalations without medication also provide some relief. Radiation pneumonitis is the acute phase of radiation reaction seen when treating lung or breast cancer, and radiation fibrosis is the late stage of the same process. This is not common, but does occur, especially when larger volumes of tissues have been treated, or the patient has underlying chronic lung disease.

**Pelvic Sites.** Patients receiving therapy to either the abdominal or pelvic organs may develop varying degrees of nausea, vomiting, or diarrhea. Several medications are available for the relief of these unpleasant side effects. The patient should understand that these symptoms are temporary and will subside upon completion of treatment. The maintenance of adequate nutrition is important. Diarrhea may be controlled with prescribed doses of medications such as paregoric, kaopectate, or diphenoxylate (Lomotil). The appearance of blood and/or mucus in the stool should be reported at once. The patient's vital signs should be checked and a stool specimen should be saved for the physician's inspection and laboratory examination. Cessation of therapy may be indicated.

Tenesmus, a painful and ineffectual effort to evacuate the bowels or bladder, is sometimes experienced during radiotherapy to the pelvic area. Rectal instillations of warm olive oil or sodium bicarbonate solution are sometimes helpful. Medications such as dibucaine (Nupercainal) or belladonna and opium suppository may also afford relief.

Pyridium, a urinary analgesic, is sometimes prescribed for its soothing effect on the urogenital mucosa. Perforations causing fistulae are rare complications and may require correction by surgery.

**Hemorrhage.** Invasive tumors anywhere in the body may invade blood vessels and cause sudden hemorrhage. This emergency is not directly related to radiotherapy but is a surgical emergency which may occur in a patient receiving radiotherapy. When bleeding is severe, or when it is internal and therefore not quickly detected, treatment in time may not be possible. Hemorrhage is sometimes seen in patients with recurrent disease in the head, neck, or groin areas. Prevention of carotid hemorrhage (carotid blowout) may be possible when the physician suspects that the artery will rupture and does a prophylactic ligation. If ligation is not done and the vessel perforates, firm pressure should be applied and not released while a call is put in for the emergency team. The patient will then probably be taken to the operating room for a ligation of the artery. In some instances a small tumor will invade a large vessel causing massive bleeding. When hemorrhage is a possibility the patient should be placed on hemorrhage precautions. He should be kept close to the nurses' station for frequent observation. He should have two units of blood available for him in reserve in the blood bank. This will mean that he must be retyped every five days, depending upon institutional policies. Sometimes such a patient is put on the critical list.

### Emergencies Responding to Radiotherapy

**Superior Vena Cava Obstruction.** This condition, found for example in association with enlargement of mediastinal nodes in lymphoma or anaplastic carcinomas, is considered to be a medical neoplasia emergency. Patients are admitted for treatment as soon as the diagnosis is suspected. In addition to emergency radiotherapy and/or chemotherapy, oxygen, diuretics, bed rest in Fowler's position, and digitalization if congestive heart failure is present are accessory treatment measures.

**Impending Cord Compression.** This is sometimes seen in patients with metastases from many sources, but especially in lymphomatous disease. This serious complication must be recognized early so that steps may be taken to prevent paraplegia. This is considered an emergency situation and radiotherapy should be started within 24 hours (Millburn, 1968).

## RADIATION PROTECTION

All persons involved in the care of patients receiving radioisotopes must recognize the necessity for limitations to radiation exposure. The degree of possible hazard depends upon the type and amount of radioactive material used for treatment.

Generally, no special precautions are required when patients receive small amounts of radioactive material for diagnostic studies (less than 200 microcuries). If any precautions are necessary, they are specified by the radiologist. There is usually no

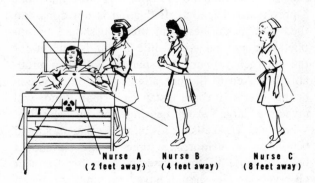

**Figure 18-8.** Examples of distance. Nurse B four feet away) receives approximately 25 per cent of the radiation received by Nurse A two feet away), and Nurse C (eight feet away) receives approximately 25 per cent of the radiation received by Nurse B.

hazard to personnel or visitors. Patients receiving moderate or large amounts (200 microcuries to over 5 millicuries) may present a hazard unless simple precautions written by the radiation safety officer are carried out.

The safety principles of time, distance, and shielding (where applicable) should always be borne in mind.

**Time.** This refers to the length of exposure. The less time spent in the vicinity of a radioactive substance the less the radiation received. Nurses should plan carefully so that less time will actually be spent at the bedside. The nurse must learn to work quickly and efficiently. Careful psychological preparation helps the patient to accept the limited amount of nursing time.

**Distance.** This refers to the distance from the radioactive source. The patient's bed assignment and degree of isolation are determined by the radiation safety officer after monitoring the patient. The inverse square law applies to radiation exposure. The rate of exposure varies inversely as the square of the distance from the source (patient). A nurse standing four feet away from the source of radiation receives 25 per cent as much radiation as she would if she were standing two feet away from the source (patient). (Fig. 18-8.)

**Shielding.** This refers to the use of any type of material to attenuate radiation. The material usually used is lead, but other materials have the capability of shielding. Examples include the concrete walls usually found in radiation therapy and diagnostic radiology departments. Lead-lined gloves, leaded aprons and drapes are also examples of shielding.

The term HVL (half value layer) may be defined as the thickness of a material needed to reduce the dose rate by one half. When discussing HVL, the type of shielding material and the energy of the radiation should be stated. Each successive HVL decreases the previous dose rate by one half. In the recovery ward where there may be several patients who have received permanent implants, a movable shield may be used to reduce exposure to radiation. Many nursing functions such as monitoring of vital signs, performing a treatment, and so on, may be done from behind such a shield (Fig. 18-9).

**Other Control Procedures.** Since radiation produces no immediate symptoms, one can receive radiation injury without being aware of it. The National Committee on Radiation Protection publishes guides for radiation safety for all hospitals, clinics, and laboratories engaged in the handling of x-rays and radioactive materials. Many of the early radiation pioneers were not afforded the benefits of radiation safety rules and regulations, and many received radiation damage as a result of prolonged and unnecessary exposures. The effects of long and short exposures must be taken into account. The latent period between the exposure and the accumulated biologic effect is often long. Today, great care is taken to protect occupationally exposed workers from radiation injury which can accumulate over the years. In many hospitals, afterloading techniques have cut down on amounts of exposure to personnel involved in radiotherapy with isotopes. The control of x-ray machines is precise and they are operated by remote control, often with fail safe devices in case of emergency or accident. Radium is stored in lead safes. The central isotope laboratory and cyclotron are off limits to all except radiation personnel. Radioisotopes are stored in lead containers.

However, absolute protection for all personnel is not possible and those who work in this field must deal with the small risk involved. Radiation risks are very small, and scientists have come a long way in reducing radiation exposure to the barest minimum. However, all women who are pregnant (whether staff or visitors) should avoid any exposure to radiotherapy.

**Delayed Effects of Radiation.** These may include radiation dermatitis especially on the exposed portions of the body due to beta and gamma exposures. The hematopoietic system may show changes in the blood-forming organs and blood cells from exposure to radioisotopes or x-ray machines. Damage to the lens of the eye causing cataract may result from low dose exposures. Genetic mutations may occur, as well as cancer which can be induced from whole body exposures. Radiation of the gonads can sometimes produce gene mutations of the reproductive cells. There is also the possibility of these mutations being passed on to the children of the parent who received radiotherapy. Generally, the greater the exposure, the greater the likelihood of producing gene mutations. On the other hand, some genetic changes may occur spontaneously without exposure to radiation.

**Radiation Safety Officer.** In many large centers

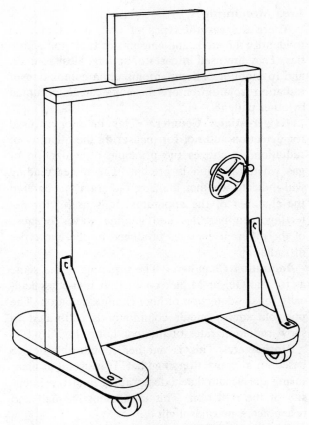

**Figure 18-9.** An example of shielding. The wheel on the right of the shield can raise or lower the breast plate. The shield is made up of two pieces of Bakelite with a one-inch thickness of lead sheeting sandwiched between.

a radiation safety officer or health physics officer is employed. This person is a qualified medical physicist, not necessarily a physician. In smaller hospitals or clinics, the chief radiotherapist may assume this role. It is his responsibility to see that all hospital personnel abide by the safety rules and regulations recommended by the National Committee on Radiation Protection (NCRP). He is responsible for the measurement and control of radiation within the hospital, e.g., patient and personnel monitoring, and checking radiation machines for possible safety hazards. It is essential for representatives of the nursing department to meet periodically with the radiation safety officer to review and to revise as necessary the procedures in use for protection of personnel and visitors, as well as to consider any problems in carrying out the procedures which have been developed.

## Area Monitoring

There are several types of area monitors used to identify the kinds and amounts of radiation activities. They are used in cases of spillage, lost sources, and to monitor patients' rooms upon completion of radiation isolation before the units can be occupied by other patients.

**Geiger-Müller Counter.** This monitor is used for detection and not for measuring the quantity of radiation. It utilizes the principle of ionization of gas when radiation is present. The meter reading will indicate whether ionizing radiation has entered the chamber of the apparatus. It is useful for detecting beta particles and gamma waves because of the different energies produced by the two types of radiations.

**Ionization Chamber.** The principle is the same as for the Geiger-Müller counter. It is used specifically for the detection of high gamma radiation. The portable survey meter commonly is calibrated to show radiation rates of mr. per hour (Fig. 18-10).

**Dosimeter.** This is another monitoring device based on an ionization chamber. It is useful in measuring the accumulated dose rather than the intensity of the radiation. This instrument is small and resembles a pen flashlight.

**Scintillation Counter.** This monitoring device contains crystals that fluoresce when exposed to radiation. The faint light is converted by large image amplifiers into electrical impulses which are then amplified by a photomultiplier tube. This apparatus is used primarily in the radioiodine laboratory for monitoring laboratory samples from the patient.

**Film Badge.** A film badge is usually worn over the employee's breast pocket and is used to measure the amount of radiation exposure of the employee (Fig. 18-10). The films inside the badge are darkened by exposures to ionizing radiation. They are read by the radiation safety officer every month and exchanged for a fresh badge. Overexposures are investigated by the radiation safety officer to determine and correct the cause. A record of the employee's exposure is kept on file in the health physics department.

**Maximum Permissible Dose.** The maximum permissible dose (MPD) for workers in the radiation department (radiologists, therapists, technicians) is set at 100 mr. per 40-hour week, or 5 rads per year. Nonworkers (general population, nurses, and so on) should not receive over 1/10 the MPD of workers in the radiation field. The MPD for nursing personnel is set at 500 mr. a year and is well below the standard set for workers in radiation. Overexposures among nursing personnel are rare, and if they should occur, steps are taken to determine and correct the cause. If a nurse receives over 100 mr. in one month, she is informed of this fact as well as the previous accumulated amount since the beginning of the year.

### Safety in the Hospital

The hospital has a responsibility to provide a safe controlled environment for its employees. Written policies must be available on nursing units

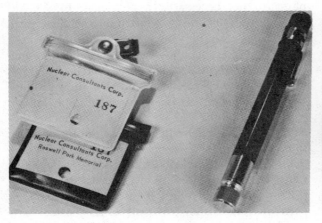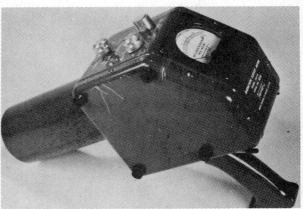

**Figure 18-10.** Monitoring devices. (*Left*) Film badges and dosimeter, used for personnel monitoring. (*Right*) Survey meter, used for area monitoring ("Cutie-Pie").

where radioactive sources are being used. Radiation safety courses should be available to help nursing personnel function effectively and intelligently, and immediate expert consultation must be available for problem solving or answering the nurse's questions. The nurse who works with radiotherapy patients has a responsibility to herself and the hospital to keep abreast of the newer developments in radiotherapy, and to work with the radiation safety officer in reviewing, implementing, and revising procedures.

For the Protection of Yourself and Others:

1. Be sure you know what radiation is emitted by specific isotopes and how the isotope is eliminated from the body.
2. Do not remain in the room while a patient is being x-rayed or fluoroscoped.
3. Do not hold children for x-rays. Suitable molds and restraints are available and should be used for restraint if necessary.
4. Know the procedures set up for the protection of yourself, other patients, and personnel.
5. Know how the isotope is stored when not in use.
6. Know the procedure to follow for lost sources or accidental spillage of a radioactive liquid such as $^{32}P$, $^{131}I$, or $^{198}Au$.
7. Know how radioactive excreta are handled.
8. Know what should be done in the event a radioactive patient is to be discharged from the hospital.
9. Know what should be done in the event of sudden death of a radioactive patient.
10. Know how contaminated linen or other material is disposed of in the hospital.
11. Be sure the patient and his family are informed about the radioactivity, the protecting barriers, and the reasons for the precautions that are taken.

Detailed information concerning all these matters should be sought from the radiation safety officer.

## RADIOISOTOPES

In certain instances it may be more advantageous to use radioactive sources within the tumor itself (interstitial), as opposed to using a distant source (external beam therapy) (Table 18-1). This method has the advantage of delivering the highest dose within the tumor, with a rapid fall-off of dose in the surrounding tissues. Radioisotopes also may be administered orally or intravenously for systemic effect, into body cavities for local effect, and applied topically for local lesions using various kinds of applicators. Radioisotopes are used for diagnosis, employing small doses in the microcurie range, and for internal therapy, usually in the millicurie dose range. Many patients receive radioisotope therapy on an outpatient basis. However, patients who have received more than 30 millicuries of a radioactive substance must be hospitalized. This is the ruling of the National Committee on Radiation Protection (NCRP) and the Atomic Energy Commission (AEC).

## RADIATION SOURCES FOR THERAPEUTIC USE

### Radium Therapy

Radium is a naturally occurring radioactive metal obtained from pitchblende ore. It has an unstable nucleus which decays at a fixed rate emitting alpha and beta particles and gamma rays. $^{226}$Radium is a most widely used radioactive material. The half-life is 1620 years. Radium, usually in the form of radium chloride, is used in platinum capsules to filter out the alpha and beta particles and some of the softer gamma emissions. For implantation, the radium is in a needle applicator with an eyelet and a trochar point. For intracavitary or mold use, the container may be in tube form. The type and number of applicators used in treating specific tumors depends largely upon the location, size of the lesion and the amount of radiation to be given (Fig. 18-11).

Some commonly employed radiation sources include: radium needles, tubes, capsules, applicators, and molds; cobalt needles, tantalum wires, radon seeds, or iodine seeds.

**Radium Needles, Tubes, and Capsules.** Radium needles may be used exclusively for delivering large doses of radiation to a localized tumor such as the tongue, floor of the mouth, or neck nodes. This type of therapy is sometimes used in combination with external beam therapy. Radium needles are implanted interstitially and remain in place for a prescribed period of time depending upon the dose desired. Radium tubes or capsules are used for treating vaginal or uterine cancers. Radium applicators may be used for treating tumors or recurrent disease in the nasopharynx, nasal cavity, or maxillary sinus.

Radium substitutes such as cesium are rapidly replacing radium.

**Radium Molds.** These applicators are tailor made according to the area to be treated. Molds

## Table 18-1. Radioactive Isotopes Used Therapeutically

### UNSEALED SOURCES

| ISOTOPE | HALF LIFE | RADIATION | CHARACTERISTICS | CLINICAL APPLICATION | NURSING PRECAUTIONS AND COMMENTS |
|---|---|---|---|---|---|
| Iodine $^{131}$I | 8.1 days | Beta Gamma | Colorless, odorless, tasteless clear liquid | Hyperthyroidism, cancer of thyroid and thyroid metastases | Maximum precautions—room isolation, special handling of urine and wetted linen |
| Gold $^{198}$Au | 2.69 days | Beta Gamma | Beet red solution | Malignant effusions | Maximum precautions—room isolation, special handling of wetted linen. Rotate patient every 15 min. for 2 hours |
| Phosphorus $^{32}$P | 14.3 days | Beta | Blue liquid | Malignant effusions, leukemia and polycythemia vera | Special handling of contaminated linens. Isolation unnecessary. Rotate patient every 15 min. for 2 hours |

### SEALED SOURCES

| ISOTOPE | HALF LIFE | RADIATION | CHARACTERISTICS | CLINICAL APPLICATION | NURSING PRECAUTIONS AND COMMENTS |
|---|---|---|---|---|---|
| Radium $^{226}$Ra | 1620 years | Alpha Beta Gamma | White solid in applicators | Uterine, cervical, nasopharyngeal cancer | Maximum precautions—room isolation |
| Radon $^{222}$Rn | 3.83 days | Alpha Beta Gamma | Gas in seeds or tubes | As implant in inoperable tumors | Maximum precautions—room isolation |
| Cobalt $^{60}$Co | 5.27 years | Beta Gamma | White solid in seeds or applicators | Same as for radium, radon | Maximum precautions—room isolation |
| | | | Pellet form in teletherapy machine | Deep tumors | No hazard in teletherapy |
| Cesium $^{137}$Cs | 30 years | Beta Gamma | Alkali metal in seeds or applicators | Same as for radium | Maximum precautions—room isolation |
| Iodine $^{125}$I | 60 days | Beta Soft Gamma | White solid in seeds | Permanent seed implant for inoperable tumors | No isolation necessary (soft gamma emitter) |
| Iridium $^{192}$Ir | 74.4 days | Beta Gamma | Platinumlike metal in applicators | Temporary implants | Maximum precautions—room isolation |
| Cesium $^{131}$Cs | 9.7 days | Gamma | Alkali metal in seeds or applicators | Permanent implants | Maximum precautions |

(moulages) are used in certain cases of cancer of the skin, penis, vulva, some tumors of the buccal mucosa, or palate. The molds are made by specially trained mold technicians. The mold containing the radioactive source is left in place depending upon the dose-time relationship specified by the radiotherapist. This may vary from a few hours a day for several days (intermittent therapy), to many consecutive hours.

**Radon Seeds ($^{222}$Rn).** Radon is a gas which is obtained from the gradual disintegration of radium. The gas is collected and purified in a special apparatus known as a radon plant. The gas is collected in long thin gold tubes which are cut after being pinched off and sealed in small segments. Radon seeds are generally used in the treatment of inoperable or recurrent tumors. The implant is permanent when seeds are injected directly into the tumor, or can be temporary when administered in applicator form when it is desirable to deliver a high dose. Radon emits beta particles and gamma rays. Temporary isolation of the patient is necessary and radiation precautions must be observed. The seeds may be considered inert at the end of a month.

**Iodine Seeds ($^{125}$I).** These seeds are said to be as effective as radon seeds. $^{125}$I is a soft gamma emitter with a half-life of 60 days. There is no external hazard, since the patient's body acts as an effective shield, and temporary isolation is not necessary.

### Nursing Care of Patients with Radionuclide Application or Implantation

The highly radioactive qualities of radium make it dangerous to handle because of its destructive effects on normal tissues. Therefore, extreme caution must be exercised in the use, storage, and

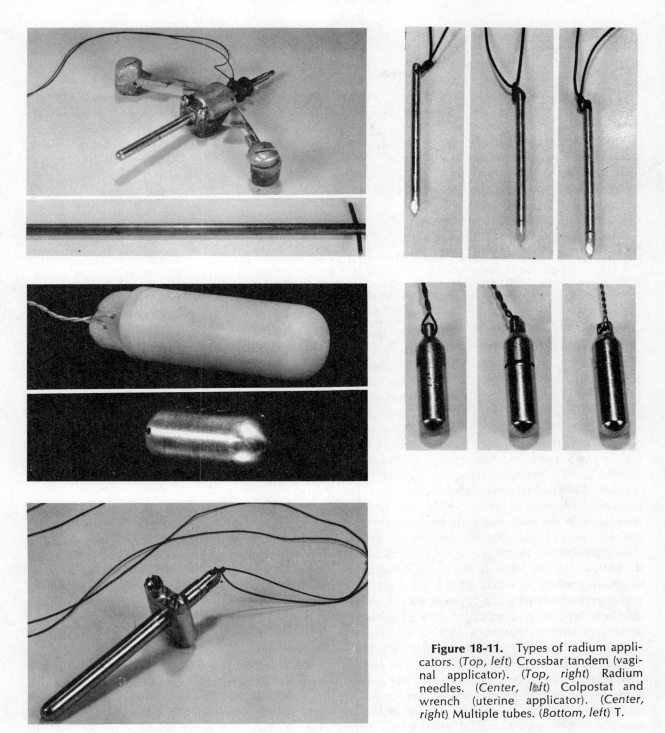

**Figure 18-11.** Types of radium applicators. (*Top, left*) Crossbar tandem (vaginal applicator). (*Top, right*) Radium needles. (*Center, left*) Colpostat and wrench (uterine applicator). (*Center, right*) Multiple tubes. (*Bottom, left*) T.

transportation of radium and cobalt. Since its discovery, radium has been used extensively for practically every form of cancer. Today, its advantages and disadvantages are better understood. Radium continues to have a definite place in the treatment of cancer in specially selected sites such as the cervix, uterus, tongue, nasopharynx, and other sites which may lend themselves to the use of applicators. In many European countries radium is used more extensively than in the United States.

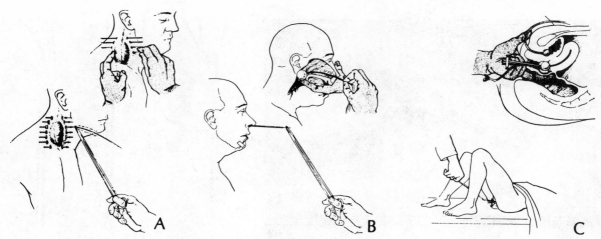

**Figure 18-12.** Afterloading techniques. (A) Afterloading for removable radioactive implants: (*top*) insertion of unloaded nylon tubes in and around the tumor; (*bottom*) afterloading with radioactive seeds in nylon ribbons. (B) Afterloading for nasopharynx applicator: (*top*) insertion of unloaded applicator; (*bottom*) afterloading with radioactive sources. (C) Afterloading for uterus applicator: (*top*) insertion of the unloaded applicator; (*bottom*) afterloading with the radioactive source. (Henschke, U. K., Hilaris, B. S., and Mahan, G. D.: Afterloading in interstitial and intracavitary radiation therapy, *Am. J. Roentgenol.* 90:386-95)

**Afterloading Techniques.** These are relatively new techniques devised to reduce radiation hazard to a minimum (Fig. 18-12). These techniques utilize polyethylene or Nylon tubes or metal applicators which receive the radioactive source. This technique is usually reserved for treating patients with high gamma radiation. The empty applicator is inserted into the patient in the operating room or a specially equipped treatment room, under local or general anesthesia, depending upon the circumstances. This method makes it possible for the surgeon and radiotherapist to make better use of their digital skills. Depending upon circumstances, the patient may be taken to the x-ray department to assure correct placement of the applicator. In some hospitals and clinics, x-ray equipment is available in the operating room. After correct placement of the applicator, the patient is taken to the recovery room to react from the anesthesia. When he is fully reacted and his vital signs are stabilized, he is discharged to a single room on the ward. The radioactive source is then inserted into the applicator by the radiotherapist for a specified number of hours. In some instances the patient is "afterloaded" daily for short treatment periods. Upon completion of treatment the applicator and source are removed.

**Preparing the Patient.** Both physical and psychological preparation of the patient are important.

As with all radiotherapy procedures, the radiotherapist is responsible for explaining the procedure and for obtaining the patient's consent. The nurse reinforces the physician's explanations and supports the patient as he goes through the preparation and the treatment. The need for enforced bed rest when indicated, as well as limited activity and temporary isolation, must be explained to the patient and his family.

Before a cervical, uterine, or bladder applicator is inserted, the patient will need a cleasing enema and insertion of a Foley catheter. This is done to avoid possible displacement of the applicator. Laxatives are discontinued and the patient is placed on a constipating diet. Some therapists recommend mild immobilization of the thighs and hips using a binder or other appropriate material. The patient may "log roll" from side to side and may also lie on his back. Some therapists believe the bed must not be gatched, but others permit the semi-Fowler's position or the use of one pillow under the head. Detailed personal care such as shampoo, manicure, and complete bath should be carried out the day before therapy. Careful attention to these details will help the patient and his family accept and cope with the temporary enforced isolation. Necessary nursing care should be given without rushing the patient.

**Safety Precautions.** The radiation safety officer will specify safety precautions such as the time and distance required for safe visiting. A narrow strip of adhesive is used on the floor of the patient's room in some centers to designate safe distance for visiting. A wristlet (Fig. 18-13) reading RADIATION PRECAUTIONS is placed on the patient's wrist. This must remain until removed by the radiation safety officer. This precaution is applied to all patients treated with internal sources of radiation. The bed, door, and patient's chart are also appropriately identified with radiation tags and adhere type labels (Fig. 18-13). The radiation principles of time, distance, and shielding (when applicable) are observed. Film badges must be worn by all personnel involved in direct care of the patient, and rotation of nursing assignment, if recommended, is carried out.

The nurse must be aware of the number and types of applicators used, the time the applicator(s) was inserted, and the time the applicator(s) is to be removed. The applicator(s) must be checked periodically to avoid displacement or loss. The removal of the applicator(s) must be done at the specified time, and the therapist should be notified

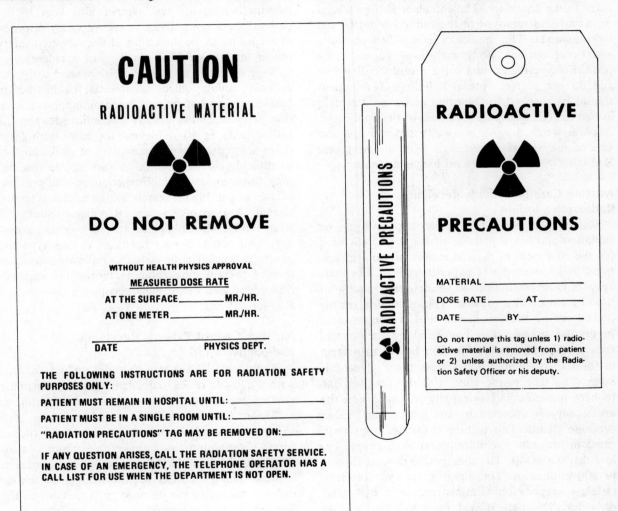

**Figure 18-13.** *(Left)* Radiation placard for door of patient's room and for front of patient's chart; also used on the record of patient's chart. *(Center)* Patient's wristlet. This may be removed only by the radiotherapist. *(Right)* Radiation tag for patient's bed. Three radiation tags are also used on the body of the radioactive patient: one on the wrist, one on the outside of the shroud, and one on refrigerator door in morgue.

if necessary. If an applicator should fall out, it should be picked up carefully, using long-handled tongs, and placed in the lead container (pig) which is usually kept in the patient's bathroom. This is a rare occurrence, but occasionally does happen with cervical or intraoral applicators. With cervical or uterine applicators, the Foley catheter is removed just prior to removal of the applicator. The radiotherapist will remove the applicator. An assistant, wearing disposable gloves and using long-handled tongs and brush, will wash the applicator in a basin of soapy water before returning the applicator to the container. The container is then placed on a cart and removed to the radium room by the radiotherapist. The applicator is handled carefully and never opened. Body excretions, vaginal tampons, Foley catheter, and urine are not radioactive and do not require special handling. The patient should be checked for bleeding and should remain in bed for one hour after removal of the applicator. A plain water douche is usually ordered and the patient may be transferred to a multi-bed room. Radiation precautions are no longer necessary.

### Nursing Care of Patients Receiving Radioactive Iodine

Radioactive iodine ($^{131}$I) emits beta and gamma radiation and has a half-life of 8.1 days. It is used for the treatment of thyroid cancer, thyroid metastases, and some types of hyperthyroidism. For therapy, radioactive iodine is administered orally in liquid form or in a capsule. This isotope is readily picked up by the circulation and is concentrated in thyroid tissues. It is converted by the thyroid cells to thyroxine, which is then bound to protein to form thyroglobulin and stored in the gland follicles. The therapeutic effect (90 per cent) is due to beta particles. $^{131}$I is rapidly absorbed and the excess rapidly excreted by the kidneys and other exocrine glands. This isotope is usually contraindicated in pregnancy, children, and most people below the age of 40. The therapeutic dose is from 1 to 100 millicuries. The liquid is a clear, colorless, tasteless preparation administered in a half glass of water. The patient will need to fast, because food delays the absorption of the isotope. The precautions set forth by the radiation safety officer must be strictly observed. In some clinics visitors are not permitted for 40 to 72 hours, or the period of greatest radioactivity. In some institutions visitors may visit for a brief period (10 min.) provided they sit near the entrance of the room. The radiation safety precautions of time and distance are thus observed. Contamination from perspiration, vomitus, or diarrhea will present the greatest hazard within the first 24 hours. Unnecessary or sustained contact must be avoided and only essential nursing care is performed. If close contact becomes necessary, an isolation gown and disposable gloves should be worn. Urine is collected carefully by the patient and put into gallon jugs which are contained in a lead-lined box kept in the patient's bathroom. Linen which is wet is placed in a plastic laundry bag in a linen hamper also kept in the patient's bathroom. These items are safely disposed of according to the directions of the radiation safety officer after monitoring. In case of accident, e.g., spillage of urine, all activity is suspended while the radiation safety officer is notified for instruction and supervision of proper decontamination. Radiation precautions are usually discontinued when the radioactivity is 30 millicuries or less. With large doses some patients may complain of neck soreness or difficulty in swallowing. A rare severe reaction may threaten tracheal obstruction or compression of the larger blood vessels if the gland is retrosternal. A rare severe general collapse related to acute endocrine imbalance (thyroid crisis, storm) may also occur. Severe reactions of this type are generally treated with steroids. Following completion of therapy, the room is thoroughly cleaned, then monitored before new occupancy (Benna and Rawson, 1965).

### Nursing Care of Patients Receiving Radioactive Gold

Radiogold ($^{198}$Au) is a beet red colloid solution with a half-life of 2.7 days. It is a beta and gamma emitter and is used to retard the accumulation of malignant effusions in body cavities. Also, this isotope is sometimes injected interstitially (liquid form) directly into an unresectable tumor, or interstitially in stainless steel seeds as a permanent implant. Small amounts of this isotope are eliminated in the urine, while most of it remains in the injected area. Contamination may easily be seen by the appearance of a pink or red stain on the dressing, gown, or bedding.

With intracavitary use, radiogold produces irradiation of the lining of the cavity. It will reduce or suspend tumor activity and will deliver a lethal dose to tumor cells. The radiotherapist will use and remove his own equipment, usually sterile disposable paracentesis or thoracentesis sets. When the isotope is used in body cavities, the position of the patient must be rotated every 15 minutes for at least two hours. This will assure equal distribution of the isotope throughout the cavity. Sometimes the polyethylene tubes used for administering the isotopes are clamped and left in place to facilitate further treatment at a later date.

### Nursing Care of Patients Receiving Radioactive Phosphorus

This isotope ($^{32}$P) is a tasteless, odorless, blue colored liquid with a half-life of 14.3 days, and is a beta emitter. The indications for use are about the same as for radiogold. This isotope concentrates in the nuclei of cells where it forms an important constituent of their chemical structure, nucleic acid. The nuclei of rapidly proliferating cells tend to have more nuclear material than normal cells, so they concentrate the radiophosphorus. Temporary isolation is not necessary because the patient's own body serves as an effective shield. Contamination can easily be seen by the appearance of a blue stain on the dressing, gown, or bed linen. Contaminated items must be handled carefully; disposable gloves should be worn and waterproof containers used. Contaminated items are removed for proper disposition by radiation safety personnel after monitoring. Radiophosphorus may be administered orally or intravenously for the treatment of chronic leukemia or polycythemia vera. The isotope tends to deposit in bones and in the cells of the reticuloendothelial system. Some of the isotope is excreted in the urine and stool in the first few days. The patient should flush the toilet three times and should wash his hands thoroughly. As with radiogold and all radioisotopes the patient's chart should contain the appropriate labels. The patient's bed should have a radiation tag as a reminder that a possible hazard can exist if there is contamination. The patient should also wear a wristlet reading RADIOACTIVE PRECAUTIONS. The radiation safety officer should always be consulted for problems.

### Nursing Care of Patients Receiving Cobalt Therapy

This isotope ($^{60}$Co) is a white solid and has a half-life of 5.3 years. It is a beta and gamma emitter and is never used as a permanent implant.

It has many applications in the treatment of tumors. The nursing considerations are the same as for radium and radon when the isotope is used in applicator form. No contamination problems occur because the isotope is in a sealed container. The patient will need to be isolated while the radioactive source is in place. He is assigned to a single room and maximum precautions are observed.

Cobalt teletherapy is external beam therapy. The isotope is used as a distant source for treatment. The radioactive cobalt pellet is located in the loading head of the tungsten housing of the installation. The beta particles are screened out by a thin filter and only gamma radiation is used for treatment. This form of therapy is generally used to treat deep-seated tumors. There is no hazard except in the treatment room when the shutter on the installation is open during actual treatment. The patient does not become a radioactive source.

## GLOSSARY

**AEC.** Atomic Energy Commission.

**Alpha particle.** Positively charged subatomic particle emitted by radioactive substances in their change from one element to another. They are identical to the nuclei of helium atoms.

**Background radiation.** Term used to describe the natural radiation of the earth, its atmosphere, and cosmic radiation from outer space.

**Bergonie Tribondeau law.** The radiosensitivity of cells varies directly with their proliferative activity and inversely with their degree of differentiation.

**Beta particle.** The name given to electrons emitted from radioactive nuclei. Also called beta radiation.

**Biological half-life.** The time required for radioactivity to diminish by one half by the combined processes of excretion and radioactive decay.

**Cathode ray tube.** A high-voltage discharge tube so constructed that the cathode stream can emerge from the tube.

**60 Cobalt.** A radioisotope of cobalt frequently used both internally and externally in the treatment of cancer.

**Contamination.** As applied to radioactive substances it is the result of mixing a radioactive material with part of one's environment; i.e., equipment, skin, clothing, etc.

**Cosmic radiation.** High energy particles that enter the earth's atmosphere from outer space at speeds approaching the speed of light.

**Critical tissues.** Tissues which are most sensitive to radiation. These include the lens of the eye, the gonads, hematopoietic system, and the skin.

**Curie.** A quantity of radioactive material the atoms of which decay at a rate of 37 billion disintegrations per second. It is the amount of radioactivity associated with one gram of radium.

**Daughter product.** An atomic species that is the immediate product of the radioactive decay of a given element, e.g., radon gas is the first daughter product of radium. In many instances, such as with radon, the daughter product is also radioactive.

**Decay.** Disintegration of a radioactive substance.

**Desquamation.** The scaly peeling off of the outer layer of skin as a result of radiation therapy, not unlike a first degree sunburn when the redness has subsided.

**Electromagnetic spectrum.** The entire range of wave lengths or frequencies of electromagnetic radiation extending from gamma rays to the longest radio rays (waves), and including visible light.

**Electromagnetic waves.** Waves propagated by the simultaneous periodic variations of electric and magnetic field intensity.

**Electron.** A fundamental, elementary particle with a negative charge.

**Emitter.** Throws off or gives out particles or waves, e.g., alpha and beta emitters and gamma wave emitters.

**Epilation.** Temporary hair loss sometimes seen after x-ray therapy to a part of the anatomy which normally produces hair, e.g., axilla, chest, head, etc.

**Epithelitis.** Skin changes secondary to radiation.

**Erythema.** Reddening of the skin due to capillary distention with blood normally seen after external beam therapy. This should not be mistaken for a burn.

**Fall-out.** Radioactive debris following detonation of atomic weapons.

**Film badge.** A photographic film packet which is sensitive to ionizing radiation. It is used to estimate the amount of radiation exposure of personnel working with radioactive substances or x-rays.

**Filter.** A metallic plate made of copper or aluminum at the opening of the x-ray tube through which x-rays must pass before reaching the part to be photographed or treated.

**Fission.** The splitting of an atomic nucleus resulting in the release of large amounts of energy.

**Fluorescence.** The property of a substance to emit radiation in the visible portion of the electromagnetic spectrum after exposure to x-rays.

**Fractionation.** Separation into different portions. X-ray therapy, for example, is not given as a single dose but in fractionated doses.

**Fusion.** Opposite of fission. The union of atomic nuclei to form heavier nuclei resulting in the release of enormous quantities of energy.

**Gamma rays.** Electromagnetic radiations emitted during radioactive decay. They are more penetrating than alpha or beta particles.

**Half-life.** The time required for half of the atoms of a radioactive substance to disintegrate.

**Hard radiation.** The term usually applied to radiation having short wave length, high energy, and deep penetrating ability.

**Health physics.** The department of occupational health dealing with the protection of personnel engaged in the handling of x-rays and radioactive materials.

**Hematopoietic system.** The tissues which are responsible for the formation of blood cells. These specialized tissues are located in the bone marrow, lymphatics, and spleen.

**ICRP.** International Committee on Radiation Protection. This international group of experts is charged with recommending safety standards for the protection of workers in the field of radiation.

**Implant.** To insert into a living site.

**Interstitial.** Situated in the interspaces of the tissues.

**Intracavitary.** To introduce into a body cavity.

**Inverse square law.** The intensity of the x-radiation is inversely proportional to the square of the distance from its source.

**Ionization.** The process whereby one or more orbital electrons are removed from a neutral atom.

**Ionizing radiation.** Refers to x-rays and radiation from radioactive substances because of their strongly ionizing effect on matter.

**Isotope.** Any of two or more species of atoms of a chemical element with the same atomic number and position in the periodic table. They are nearly identical in chemical behavior but differ in atomic mass and show different behavior in mass spectrograph, in radioactive transformation, and in physical properties.

**Kilo (K).** Thousand.

**Kilovolt (KV).** Thousand volts.

**Leukopenia.** A condition in which the number of white blood cells in the circulating blood is abnormally low.

**Maximum permissible dose (MPD).** This is the rule established by the NCRP. The MPD for workers in the field of radiation (radiologists, therapists, etc.) has been set at 100 mr. per 40-hour week or 5 rads per year. Nonworkers should not receive over 1/10 of the MPD set for workers in the radiation field.

**MEV.** Million electron volts.

**Microcurie.** One millionth of a curie.

**Millicurie (mc).** One thousandth of a curie.

**Milliroentgen (mr.).** One thousandth of a roentgen.

**Monitor.** To test for intensity of radiation, especially if due to radioactivity.

**Moulage (mold).** An impression or cast used to contain a radioactive substance to a certain part of the body.

**National Committee on Radiation Protection (NCRP).** The national committee which developed standards of protection for personnel engaged in the field of radiation (1928).

**Neutron.** An uncharged elementary particle that has a mass nearly equal to that of the proton and is present in all known atomic nuclei except the hydrogen nucleus.

**Nucleic acid.** A component of the cell nucleus, comprising a union between phosphoric acid, ribose or desoxyribose, and the four bases: adenine, guanine, cytosine, and tyrosine.

**Nucleus (atom).** The positively charged central portion of the atom that comprises nearly all of the atomic mass and consists of protons and neutrons, except in the hydrogen atom, which consists of one proton only.

**Nucleus (cell).** A portion of the cell protoplasm held to be essential to vital phenomena and heredity.

**Photon.** A quantum (packet) of radiant energy. It has no charge and is characterized by its wave length or frequency.

**Positron.** A positively charged particle having the same mass and magnitude of charge as the electron.

**Proton.** An elementary particle that is identical with the nucleus of the hydrogen atom. Along with neutrons, it is a constituent of all other atomic nuclei, and carries a positive charge.

**Radiation sickness (syndrome).** A systemic effect sometimes experienced by patients receiving radiotherapy to large areas of the body. The symptoms encountered may include weakness, nausea, vomiting, diaphoresis, and perhaps chills.

**Radioactivity.** The phenomenon whereby atoms disintegrate and emit radiation.

**Radioiodine ($^{131}$I).** A radioisotope of iodine having a half-life of 8.1 days.

**Radioisotope.** An isotope which is naturally or artificially radioactive.

**Radiologist.** A physician with specialized training in the diagnosis and treatment of disease by the use of ionizing energy; certified by the Board of Radiology.

**Radioresistant.** Opposition offered by the body to radiation.

**Radiosensitive.** Susceptibility of tissues to radiation.

**Radiotherapy.** Treatment of human ailments with the application of ionizing radiation.

**Radium (Ra).** A natural radioactive element obtained from pitchblende ore. It emits alpha, beta, and gamma radiations and has a half-life of 1,620 years.

**Radon ($^{222}$Rn).** A heavy radioactive gaseous element formed by the disintegration of radium, with a half-life of 3.83 days.

**Roentgen (r).** The primary unit of dosage of x-rays.

**Roentgen (Wilhelm Conrad).** Discoverer of x-rays (1895).

**Scattered radiation.** Refers to a change in direction of the x-ray photon as a result of collision of matter.

**Soft radiation.** Long wave length x-rays of low penetration.

**Strontium ($^{90}$Sr).** A radioisotope which emits beta particles and has a half-life of 28 years.

**Telangiectasis.** An abnormal dilatation of capillary vessels and arterioles that is sometimes seen on the skin as a late reaction to radiation therapy.

**Teletherapy.** The radiation treatment given by a radioactive substance external to the body. The treatment is similar to that given by high energy x-ray machines.

**Transmutation.** The conversion of one element or nuclide into another either naturally or artificially.

**Tungsten.** A gray-white, heavy, high-melting, ductile, hard metal used especially for electrical purposes and in hardening alloys. It is used in radiotherapy to house cobalt ($^{60}$Co).

**Uranium.** A silvery heavy radioactive metal found in pitchblende ore.

**X-ray.** Electromagnetic radiations discovered by Roentgen in 1895. X-rays have the ability to penetrate opaque materials and affect a photographic film.

## REFERENCES AND BIBLIOGRAPHY

ADELSTEIN, S. J.: The risk:benefit ratio in nuclear medicine, *Hosp. Pract.* 8:141, January 1973.

AMERICAN CANCER SOCIETY: *Cancer Management—A Special Graduate Course on Cancer,* Philadelphia, Lippincott, 1968.

ARENA, V.: Radiation accidents: What you need to know about them, *RN* 36:42, September 1973.

BARNES, P., and REES, D.: *Textbook of Radiotherapy,* Philadelphia, Lippincott, 1972.

BEHRENS, C. F., KING, E. R., and CARPENDER, J. W.: *Atomic Medicine,* p. 135, Baltimore, Williams & Wilkins, 1969.

BENNA, R., and RAWSON, R.: Treatment of thyroid cancer with radioactive iodine, *in* BLAHD, W. H. (ed.): *Nuclear Medicine,* pp. 643-644, New York, McGraw-Hill, 1965.

BOEKER, E.: Radiation safety, *Am. J. Nurs.* 65:111, April 1965.

————: Radiation uses and hazards, *Nurs. Clin. N. Am.* 2:32, March 1967.

BOUCHARD, R.: *Nursing Care of the Cancer Patient,* St. Louis, Mosby, 1967.

BUSCHKE, F., and PARKER, R.: *Radiation Therapy in Cancer Management,* New York, Grune and Stratton, 1972.

COREY, P., and BENNA, R.: Progress in radioactive isotope scanning, *Med. Clin. N. Am.* 50:689-700, May 1966.

CURIE, M.: *Radioactive Substances,* New York, Philosophical Library, 1961.

DUGAN, J.: No ashes for the phoenix (poem), *Nurs. '74* 4:66, January 1974.

DUNN, E.: Diagnostic radioisotopes, *Hosp. Med.* 1:30, February 1965.

EARLY, P. J., RAZZAK, M. A., and SODEE, D. B.: *Nuclear Medicine and Technology,* St. Louis, Mosby, 1969.

EBERT, R. V.: Radiation pneumonitis, *in* BEESON, P., and McDERMOTT, W. (eds.): *Cecil-Loeb Textbook of Medicine,* ed. 12, p. 516, Philadelphia, Saunders, 1967.

GREENBERG, E., et al.: Bone scanning for metastatic cancer with radioisotopes, *Med. Clin. N. Am.* 50: 701, May 1966.

HENSCHKE, U. K., HILARIS, B. S., and MAHAN, G. D.: Afterloading in interstitial and intracavitary radiation therapy, *Am. J. Roentgenol.* 90:386, August 1963.

HILKEMEYER, R.: Nursing care in radium therapy, *Nurs. Clin. N. Am.* 2:83, March 1967.

KAUTZ, H. D., STOREY, R. H., and ZIMMERMANN, A. J.: Radioactive drugs, *Am. J. Nurs.* 64:124, January 1964.

MILLBURN, I., et al.: Treatment of spinal cord compression from metastatic carcinoma, *Cancer* 21:447, March 1968.

MILLER, A.: The nurse on the radiological team, *Am. J. Nurs.* 64:128, July 1964.

NEALON, T. F., JR. (ed.): *Management of the Patient with Cancer,* p. 784, Philadelphia, Saunders, 1965.

The patient in radiation therapy, Chapter 6, *in* CRAYTOR, J., and FASS, M.: *The Nurse and the Cancer Patient: A Programmed Textbook,* Philadelphia, Lippincott, 1972.

Radiation Therapy—a treatment modality for cancer, *in* BEHNKE, H. (ed.): *Guidelines for Comprehensive Nursing Care in Cancer,* New York, Springer, 1973.

RUMMERFIELD, P. S., and RUMMERFIELD, M. J.: What you should know about radiation hazards, *Am. J. Nurs.* 70:780, April 1970.

SELBY, B.: Proper preparation of a patient for x-rays, *Hosp. Med.* 1:17, October 1964.

TIEVSKY, G.: *Ionizing Radiation,* pp. 20, 48-57, 138, 141, 147, Springfield, Ill., Thomas, 1962.

# UNIT FOUR

## Disturbances of Body Supportive Structures and Locomotion

# The Patient with a Fracture

## TYPES OF FRACTURES

A fracture is a break in the continuity of a bone and may be classified as follows:

- *Open* (compound). The bone breaks through the skin. Because there is an open wound, the danger of infection is increased greatly.
- *Closed* (simple). Any fracture that is not open is a closed fracture.
- *Displaced*. The bone ends are separated.
- *Greenstick*. The bone bends and splits, but it does not break clear through. This kind of fracture occurs primarily in children.
- *Complete*. The fracture line goes all the way through the bone.
- *Comminuted*. The bone is broken in several places.
- *Impacted*. One portion of the bone is driven into another.
- *Complicated*. A fracture with injury to the surrounding tissues, such as blood vessels, nerves, joints, or internal organs.
- *Pathologic* (spontaneous). The bone breaks without sufficient trauma to crack a normal bone. This kind of fracture occurs in such conditions as osteoporosis (porous bones), cancer, certain instances of malnutrition, and Cushing's syndrome, and as a complication of cortisone and ACTH therapy.

## THE PATHOLOGY OF FRACTURE AND THE PHYSIOLOGY OF BONE REPAIR

For ten to forty minutes after the fracture, the muscles surrounding the bone are flaccid. Then they go into spasm, and when they do, they cause increased deformity and additional interference with the vascular and lymphatic circulations. Traction at this later stage is

297

accomplished only with difficulty. The application and maintenance of traction immediately after a fracture avoids the later complication of spastic muscles.

When there are bone fragments as a result of fracture, the local periosteum and surrounding blood vessels are torn. The tissue surrounding the fracture shows an aseptic inflammation (unless the skin is broken), with swelling due to hemorrhage, inflammatory exudate, and edema. The blood in the area clots, and fibrin network forms between the bone ends. This changes into granulation tissue. The osteoblasts, proliferating in the clot, increase the secretion of an enzyme that restores the alkaline pH. The result is the deposition of calcium in the callus and the formation of true bone. At the stage of the consolidation of the clot (six to ten days after the injury) the healing mass is called a *callus*. The callus holds the ends of the bone together, but it cannot endure strain.

Interference with the removal of the debris will interfere with the healing process. Nonunion of the fracture (a permanent break in the continuity of the bone) may result. Nursing measures that promote adequate circulation in the affected part foster deposition of calcium and healing of the bone. This is one reason that elevation of the affected limb, which helps to reduce edema, is so important. Because early mobilization of the patient encourages favorable nitrogen balance and counters sluggish circulation, many patients with a fractured hip are treated with pin fixation instead of traction.

Consolidation of bone takes about half as long in a 6-year-old as in a 60-year-old; but, interestingly enough, once a person becomes an adult, age does not affect healing. Nor do most systemic diseases, including osteoporosis, influence the time it takes for a fracture to heal, although the older or debilitated patient is in greater danger of not surviving the injury because of complications. Bone repair is a highly local process. About one year of healing must take place before bone regains its former structural strength, becoming well consolidated, remolded, and possessing fat and marrow cells.

## FREQUENCY

Most accidents occur in the home and on the highways. Slippery, wet tubs, scatter rugs, highly polished floors, roller skates on a dark stairway, and activities involving a precarious balance, such as standing on a rickety chair to hang a curtain can all be hazardous. The frequency of fractures is greater among persons who have predisposing conditions, such as osteoporosis and cancer, which affect bone. Poor coordination, diminished vision and hearing, the frequency of dizziness and faintness, and general feebleness make falls and resultant fractures a common problem among the elderly. Other high-risk groups include patients with diseases affecting locomotion, such as arthritis, Parkinson's disease, and multiple sclerosis. The fact that bone breakage in older persons is more frequent across the neck of the femur is attributed partially to atrophy of bone. Up to the age of 45, men suffer more fractures than women. After that age the frequency is higher in women.

## SYMPTOMS

- *Pain.* One of the most consistent symptoms of a broken bone is pain. It may be severe, and it is increased by attempts to move the part and by pressure over the fracture.
- *Loss of function.* Skeletal muscular function is dependent on an intact bone.
- *Deformity.* A break may cause an extremity to bend backwards or to assume another unusual shape.
- *False motion.* Unnatural motion occurs at the site of the fracture.
- *Edema.* Swelling usually is greatest directly over the fracture.
- *Spasm.* Muscles near fractures contract involuntarily. Spasm, which accounts for some of the pain, may result in the shortening of a limb when a long bone is involved.
- *Discoloration and paralysis.* If the sharp bone fragments tear through sufficient surrounding soft tissue, there will be bleeding and black and blue discoloration of the area. If a nerve is damaged, there may be paralysis.

## FIRST AID

**Bleeding.** If the nurse is present at the accident, she first should notice if there is any bleeding and take measures to stop it and to combat shock. The average amount of blood lost to the general circulation in a closed fracture of the femur is 800 to 1,200 ml. Of course, there may be a great deal more bleeding in an open fracture.

**Evaluation.** It is safe to assume that a fracture has occurred if the limb is misshapen, if the patient states that he has heard the bone snap, or if there is a loss of function. Overcaution is never misplaced. It is better to splint a sprain than not to splint a fracture.

**Getting the Right Kind of Help from Others.** The patient with a possible fracture needs protection against well-meaning but untrained passersby who try to sit him up or to move him immediately. Such interference usually can be stopped by the self-assured presence of the nurse who identifies herself. Although she may feel neither calm nor self-assured, others will listen if she can convince them that she knows what she is doing. Immediately taking the patient's pulse gives her valuable information about his condition. Also, this professional gesture often will convince even a stubborn lay bystander that one more competent than he has taken charge. Taking the patient's pulse has the added advantage of giving the nurse a full minute to collect her thoughts and to plan what to do next. If the patient is lying in a busy street, someone should redirect traffic around him until the ambulance comes. The patient should be covered, and the crowd kept away. Perhaps one bystander can take the responsibility of keeping people back, another can call for the police or an ambulance, and a third can direct traffic to protect the patient and those ministering to him from being struck by oncoming cars.

**Splinting.** *Splint them where they lie* is the motto. The ragged edge of a broken bone can do great damage to the soft tissues around it. Fragments of bone can cut through periosteum, fascia, muscle, nerves, blood-vessel walls, and even skin. The protrusion of a fragment of bone through skin is very dangerous, since dirt or perhaps bits of clothing may be introduced into an otherwise clean wound. Frantic efforts to remove the patient to a hospital in all haste are perilous. Pulling a patient to the side of the road and lifting him into a car without supporting the fracture can create an open fracture from a closed one. It is far better to stop hemorrhage, treat shock, and immobilize the fracture before moving the patient from the place where he fell. Patients with fractured ribs should be transported in a sitting position.

To splint an arm or a leg, use padded wood, a folded telephone book, or anything that is stiff. If such items are not available, a broken leg can be splinted to the intact leg. If possible, apply the splint so that it includes the joints above and below the fracture site. For example, if the tibia is broken, include both the ankle and the knee in the splint. Be sure to pad the appliance, so that the soft tissues are protected uniformly. Remember that the arm and the leg bones are especially close to the skin, and that extreme gentleness is needed in handling a fractured limb to prevent a simple fracture from tearing the skin and becoming a compound fracture. Tie the splint in place securely but not so tightly that circulation is impaired. For further details see first-aid manuals, such as that published by the American Red Cross.

**Traction.** As the ends of broken bones in the arms and the legs tend to override, traction should be applied before splinting, except in open fractures. Traction holds the broken edges of the bone still, thus preventing further damage to soft tissues and reducing pain and shock. Traction is accomplished by steady pulling of an intact part that is distal to the fracture, such as the wrist, the head, or the ankle. Be sure that the pull is steady. A jerky movement can cause more damage to muscles, nerves, and blood vessels. The amount of traction should be just enough to support the extremity in such a way that motion of the fracture area is minimized. Traction is not necessary in every fracture, but it should be applied to fractures that are unstable or those that cannot be externally splinted.

Pull in line with the part proximal to the fracture. Traction should be applied at a more distal point: in a fracture of the wrist, at the fingers; in a fracture of the ankle, at the foot. In a fracture of a long bone the application of a traction splint, such as the Thomas type (Fig. 19-1), should be applied before the patient is transported. These splints are carried regularly by ambulances. After traction has been started, it must not be released until a splint that can maintain the pull is applied. It is absolutely necessary to transport the patient without a traction splint, an improvised appliance should be made or manual traction on the otherwise splinted limb should be maintained continuously until the patient reaches the hospital, and the physician takes over.

**Open Fracture.** In first-aid treatment of an open fracture, cover the open wound with a sterile dressing. If none is available, keep dirt away from the wound by other means, such as placing the inside fold of a clean handkerchief over the wound. If the bone disappears into the wound, it most likely has carried some dirt back with it. Write a note that the bone has broken through the skin, and pin the note to the clothing of the patient. When he gets to the hospital, the physicians then will know that deep, thorough cleansing will be necessary. Do not apply traction if the bone protrudes through the open wound; however, immobilize the area by splinting. Try to prevent the contaminated end of the bone from slipping into the wound.

**Complications.** INFECTION. Infection is a prime concern in an open fracture. For this reason early debridement of the wound in the operating room is considered essential. Excision of necrotic and severely traumatized tissue, plus careful cleansing and flushing out of the wound, helps to remove the contaminated foreign materials, thus decreasing the likelihood of infection. Osteomyelitis (infection of bone) can be a catastrophic complication of open

fractures. In compound fractures the incidence of delayed union and nonunion tends to be increased, especially if infection occurs.

DANGERS OF TOURNIQUETS AND ANTISEPTICS. Although authorities are not in complete agreement, the prevailing current opinion is that the emergency use of tourniquets and antiseptics is dangerous. A tourniquet may control venous flow while the patient bleeds to death from an artery; or if the tourniquet occludes the artery, the resulting ischemia may cause gangrene, nerve compression, or further soft-tissue damage. Instead of applying a tourniquet, elevate the injured part and use direct pressure over the bleeding. Compress pressure points. Use a tourniquet only if bleeding cannot be stopped by these other methods. After a tourniquet has been applied, it should remain in place until the patient is seen by the physician.

Antiseptics may traumatize the tissue further, without truly disinfecting the wound. Thus they should not be used. The physician will order a cleansing procedure once the patient is in his care.

**Fractures of the Spine.** See Chapter 24 for first-aid measures.

## HOSPITAL TREATMENT OF FRACTURES

When the patient arrives at the hospital, traction is maintained if it has been started earlier. If the patient arrives with a splint, it should not be removed. X-ray films are taken before any treatment is given. If the fracture was not splinted outside the hospital, a splint is applied to immobilize the part while the patient goes to the x-ray department and waits for the x-ray films to be developed and read. Immobilization helps to reduce pain. In addition, the physician usually orders medication for pain. The patient should travel in a wheelchair or on a stretcher, and the injured part should be kept elevated to minimize edema.

In removing clothing, help the patient to keep the injured part as motionless as possible. To remove a jacket when the left arm is broken, have the patient remove his arm from the right sleeve first, freeing the jacket, so that it can be slipped off his left arm without moving that arm. On occasion it may be necessary to cut clothing away. When it is possible, cut along the seam, making sure that no threads fall into any open wound.

When a patient is admitted to the hospital with multiple injuries, a decision is made as to which

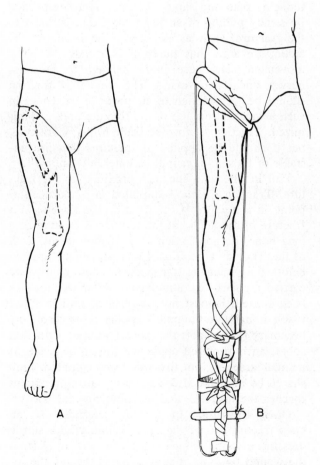

**Figure 19-1.** (A) Diagram of a fractured femur, showing the bone fragments pulled out of alignment by muscle spasm. (B) Application of Thomas splint at the scene of the accident. Traction maintains the alignment of the bone fragments and prevents their injuring nearby tissues.

problems are to be given priority. Bleeding and shock will be first on the list. The nurse and the physician work as a team, the nurse supplying the physician with materials as he needs them, such as intravenous setup, fluids, and bandages. She observes the patient, checking vital signs, color, urinary output, and so on, and she helps to make him as comfortable as possible by such measures as providing an emesis basin, covering him with a blanket, and promptly giving him the medications ordered.

The aim of treatment is the support of the physiologic process of bone healing. One aspect of treatment does pose a dilemma: the fragments will not heal unless they are immobilized absolutely; at the same time, it is necessary to treat the limb in such a fashion that circulation is maintained and muscles will not atrophy. Early, active use of nearby muscle groups is one of the most effective ways to encourage adequate circulation. The solution to this problem is active use of the injured part without disturbance of the injured bone.

## Types of Reduction

The method of treatment which the physician selects for a fracture depends on many factors: the first aid given, the location and the severity of the break, and the age and the overall physical condition of the patient. First, the physician *reduces the fracture* (replaces the parts in their normal position) by manipulation of the fragments. He takes the broken limb in his hand and, by gentle manipulation, redirects it to its normal position. Then he immobilizies the part by bandage, cast, traction, or internal fixation. This kind of reduction is a *closed reduction.*

In an *open reduction,* which is performed in the operating room, the bone is exposed and realigned under the direct vision of the orthopedist. The operation usually is performed under general or spinal anesthesia. A cast is applied, and roentgenograms are taken while the patient is still anesthetized so that any needed correction can be made without giving him more anesthesia. This method is used most frequently for dealing with soft tissue, such as nerves or blood vessels, caught between the ends of the broken pieces of bone; for wide separation of the fragment; for comminuted fractures; for fractures of the patella and other joints; for open fractures when debridement of the wound is necessary; and for internal fixation of fractures.

Thanks to the availability of more reliable and less reactive metals, internal fixation is possible in many cases in which it was previously ruled out. This procedure may at times become the more conservative form of treatment. However, open reduction and internal fixation are usually reserved for only those cases that cannot be adequately handled by closed methods.

**Skin Preparation for Open Reduction.** Because osteomyelitis is extraordinarily difficult to cure and may result in the patient's being permanently crippled, careful attention is paid to the preparation of the skin before any orthopedic surgery. In an emergency, shaving and cleaning the skin may be done in the operating room. When there is time, preparation usually begins the day before the surgery. The skin is shaved and scrubbed with providone-iodine (Betadine) and similar preparations, after which an antiseptic is applied. The area then may be wrapped in a sterile covering, which is removed the next day, when another scrubbing with Betadine and application of an antiseptic are repeated. A new sterile covering may be put on and left in place until the operation. In some hospitals the scrubbed area is left open.

The aseptic technique carried out in the operating room is even more important. Scrupulous attention to every detail of the technique is essential. Because the orthopedists are handling bones that are both hard and sharp, it is common for rubber gloves to tear, exposing unsterile skin to the operating field. For this reason many orthopedists now use two pairs of gloves.

## THE PATIENT IN A CAST

### Cast Application

Patients with fractures being treated by closed methods will usually be immobilized in casts. Casts hold the bone in place while it heals and often permit early ambulation, even when a leg is broken. The patient may be given a narcotic before the cast is applied, or general anesthesia may be used. Sometimes a local block is performed, such as infiltrating the brachial plexus with procaine hydrochloride, when reduction of a fracture of the arm is to be undertaken.

The orthopedist determines how he wishes to immobilize the parts and positions the patient accordingly. An assistant holds the arm or leg exactly in

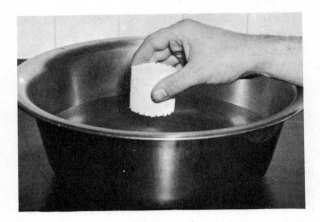

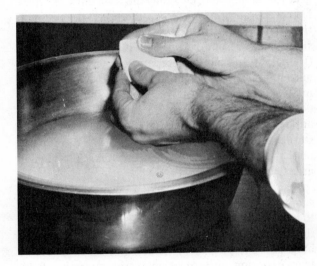

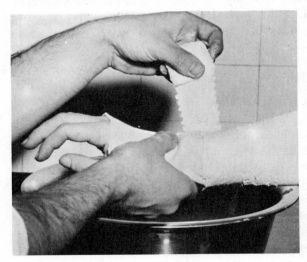

**Figure 19-2.** Applying a cast. (*Top*) The roll is soaked in an upright position. (*Center*) The water is pressed out evenly and gently. (*Bottom*) The part is supported in the proper position during the bandaging.

place. Casts that include joints usually are applied with the joints flexed to lessen stiffness later.

A technician prepares the rolls of plaster (Fig. 19-2). He places two rolls of plaster bandage in a bucket of tepid water. Each roll is stood on its end. He watches until the bubbles stop, at which point he immediately removes the first, lays it on its side on his hand, and with the other hand very gently presses the extra water out of it. He unrolls three or four inches of plaster bandage, hands the roll to the orthopedist, puts a fresh third roll in the water, and removes the second roll.

Each motion that the technician makes with the plaster of Paris bandage has its reason. The roll is placed in the bucket on end instead of on its side so that air can escape, and water can penetrate all the folds with a minimum loss of plaster in the surrounding fluid. The roll is removed from the bath as quickly as the last bubble leaves it, because air then has been replaced by water. The longer the roll stays in the water, the more plaster it loses. If the roll is left in too long, all that remains is limp, wet gauze. The roll is grasped at either end and is gently squeezed to express excess water and to push the plaster centrally into the roll. This also prevents the roll from twisting as it is applied.

Some orthopedists use a stockinette or padding under the cast as a lining to protect the skin, especially over bony prominences; others feel that padding defeats the purpose of the cast. If a stockinette or padding is used it should be ready when needed and should be kept from wrinkling.

During the application of the cast the technician, or sometimes the nurse, stays in the operating room, handing the orthopedist the equipment he needs, perhaps manually supporting the patient's arm or leg while the orthopedist's hands are busy, and giving verbal support to the patient. The orthopedist may be concentrating too hard to talk to the patient. A quietly spoken word from the nurse reminds the patient that he is not forgotten.

After the fragments of bone have been manipulated into place, and the cast has been applied, a second x-ray film is taken, so that the physician can see that the alignment is proper. Subsequent x-rays are taken as the physician deems necessary.

When the treatment room is cleaned the contents of the bucket can be drained into the sink if there is a trap on the sink outlet. Otherwise, the bucket should be emptied into the garbage to prevent the plumbing from becoming clogged.

## Drying and Finishing the Cast

Although plaster of Paris becomes hard in only a few minutes, it takes 24 to 48 hours for a cast to dry completely. During this time it needs protection. Something as simple as a thumbprint on the cast can leave an indentation that may cause a pressure sore on the patient's skin. To avoid this, support the cast with the palm of the hand rather than the fingertips. Protecting the patient from extremes of temperature is also important. Since the damp cast may feel cold, a warm blanket over the rest of the patient may be appreciated. If it is a hot day (on a hot day the inside of a cast feels like an oven) or if the patient is very anxious, a cool bath or the use of fans for good ventilation may help. However, no draft ever should be allowed to fall directly on a patient in a wet cast. Many patients become disturbed because of the heat generated by the chemical reaction of the plaster of Paris as it sets. They should be reassured that the heat level is within safe limits and will be of short duration.

The cast itself must be left uncovered so that water can evaporate from it. Many physicians prefer natural evaporation, but some ask the nurse to use cast dryers to speed the drying. Never use intense heat. Not only is there danger of burning the patient, but the heat will dry the outside of the cast and leave the inside wet, so that later, it may become moldy. Intense heat can crack the plaster.

The damp cast never should be placed on a hard bed, where it automatically will flatten over bony prominences, later causing damage to the soft tissue between the cast and the bone. Instead, the cast should be placed on a pillow or a series of pillows, covered with oiled silk, rubber, or plastic to protect the pillow from the dampness of the cast. The pillow prevents flattening of the cast and elevates the part.

A spica (body cast) is supported on pillows until it is dry along its entire length (Fig. 19-3). After several hours, turn the patient as directed by the physician to allow the undersurface of the cast to dry. Handle the damp cast with a flat hand, keeping your fingertips away to avoid indenting it. Never lift a spica cast by the foot or the ankle; rather, slip your hand under the buttocks of the patient.

After 48 hours, when the cast is thoroughly dry, it can lie on a hard surface. Although casts are durable, like bones, they do break. A particularly active patient may need to be told of this possibility.

**Edges.** After a cast is dry, the nurse can finish the edges. The roughened edges of plaster crumble, and cast crumbs can find their way up under the cast and cause decubitus ulcers wherever they settle. If the cast is lined with a stockinette, the nurse should pull it over the edge and tape it to the cast. Some physicians secure the stockinette over the edge of the cast with plaster (Fig. 19-4). If there is no stockinette, the nurse can line the edge with adhesive tape.

## Types of Casts

**Spica Casts.** In a spica cast special attention needs to be given to finishing the area near the buttocks. If there is not enough room for defecation, the nurse should tell the physician, so that he can enlarge the space. To protect the cast from getting wet and soiled, the nurse can fit some waterproof material—oilskin or plastic—around the edge and tape it to the cast. She may prefer to shellac or varnish the section of the cast that is in danger of becoming wet. A consistently damp cast will become moldy and very malodorous.

Whenever the patient is turned, inspect the buttocks and brush away any cast crumbs that may have accumulated. Note that the buttocks are creased where the cast has pressed against the skin; these creases are lines of potential skin breakdown. Consult the physician about any local medication that may be applied. He may recommend rubbing the involved areas with skin cream or oil, or painting them with tincture of benzoin.

**Light Cast II.*** This is a fiber-glass cast which hardens rapidly on exposure to ultraviolet type of light. Once the cast is applied, it is held under a cradle containing the light and hardens in a few minutes. The cast is lightweight, strong, porous, and durable. It is particularly useful for treatment of elderly persons where the weight of a conventional cast may pose particular problems. This type of cast will probably find its greatest use in immobilizing undisplaced fractures and in second casts (cast applied following initial treatment with a conventional cast).

**Bivalve Cast.** If a cast is put on an extremity before edema has developed fully, compression of the tissues will result, because there will be no room for expansion inside the cast. To avoid this

___
* Trade name

possibility, the physician may apply the cast, and as soon as it is dry, split it along both sides. The sides are then refitted on the patient's limb and bandaged in place. This kind of cast is called a bivalve cast. It may be used when a patient is being weaned from a cast, when a very sharp x-ray film is needed, or in the treatment of such conditions as arthritis, in which the method is a convenient one for splinting the part intermittently.

A bivalve cast should be removed daily, unless the physician indicates otherwise. Note any pressure areas on the skin. While the patient is out of the cast, bathe the part, apply an emollient lotion, and assist the patient with any prescribed exercises.

### Assessing the Patient in a Cast

- **Assess the part, especially when the cast has been newly applied, for any swelling, pressure or irritation.**

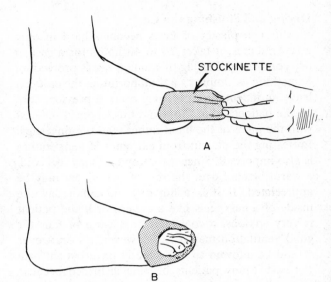

**Figure 19-4.** The edges of this cast are made smooth by pulling out the stockinette (A) and fastening it to the outside of the cast (B).

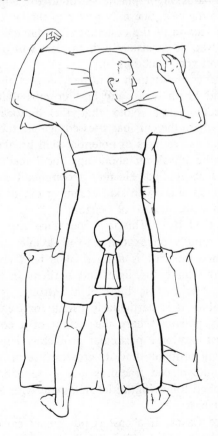

**Figure 19-3.** The wet spica cast is supported on pillows until it dries. When the patient lies on his abdomen, his feet are positioned over the edges of the pillows, which are so placed that they support the patient in good body alignment.

To lessen edema, keep the part elevated, using pillows with plastic protective covers if available.

- **Note also the color and temperature of the skin of the extremity. Blanching, cyanosis, mottling, and coldness are indicative of circulatory impairment and should be reported at once. Prompt cutting of the cast by the physician is essential if circulatory impairment occurs.**
- **Note any odor coming from the cast. A fetid, unpleasant odor may indicate the presence of a decubitus ulcer or infection under the cast.**
- **Pay careful attention to the patient's complaints, such as of numbness, tingling, pressure, or pain, and bring them to the physician's attention. A cast window may be cut over the area of discomfort to permit visualization of the skin.**
- **Observe the cast for any discoloration, such as from bleeding or drainage from a wound. Circle the area on the cast with a pencil, report the symptoms, and note whether the discolored area spreads beyond the original pencil marking.**
- **Make sure that very old or very young patients do not push various objects, such as coins, spoons, and toothbrushes under the cast, they may do so in an attempt to alleviate itching. If an object does become lodged under the cast, pain may occur at first, due to pressure, but then may disappear in a few days as the wound becomes anesthetized. However, a hot spot may appear or drainage may be evident on the cast over the affected area. Observe such patients carefully and avoid leaving them with a variety of small objects. If itching occurs under a body cast, threading a long turkish towel through the cast and pulling it back and forth can scratch an itchy back.**

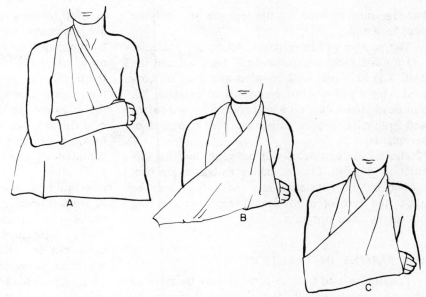

**Figure 19-5.** (A) The arm is positioned with the fingers higher than the elbow. (B) The entire arm is enclosed in the sling. (C) The flap is fitted snugly around the elbow.

● **Use a sling when needed. If the patient has a fractured arm, he must still keep it elevated when he gets out of bed. A sling is used to support the entire arm, including the wrist. Adjustable slings, which are now available, eliminate the need for safety pins and a knot at the neck (Fig. 19-5). To prevent edema of the fingers, adjust the sling so that the fingers are higher than the elbow.**

## Moving the Patient

The patient in a body cast requires special care when being turned. Because of his helplessness, turning is at first a frightening experience for him. Explain the procedure before beginning, and make certain to have plenty of help available. Remove the head pillow and raise the side rail on one side of the bed. Have the patient move to that side of the bed, while you go to the opposite side. The affected leg is the one which swings up and over. Before turning, the patient should put the arm on the unaffected side over his head, to get it out of the way. If the patient can be turned alone, place one hand on the patient's shoulder and the other on his hip, and turn him toward you. If the patient is heavy or is inexperienced in turning, it is important to have two people to assist with turning. Never pull on the abduction bar to turn the patient.

When the patient is in prone position, make certain that his toes do not dig into the mattress. Position him so that his toes hang free over the edge of the mattress, or elevate the lower portion of the cast on a pillow, leaving the toes hanging free over

the end of the pillow. Inspect the exposed skin carefully each time the patient is turned.

## Removal of Cast

Casts are removed by a mechanical cast cutter. Although cast cutters are noisy and frightening, the patient should be assured that the machine will not cut him. When the cast has been removed, continued support to the limb is necessary. An Ace

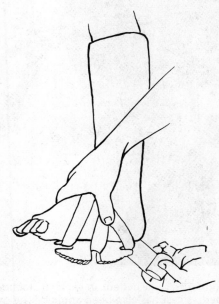

**Figure 19-6.** Rubber walking heel being applied to cast. (Richards Manufacturing Co., Memphis, Tenn.)

bandage may be used for the leg; the arm may be kept in a sling.

The patient will have pains, aches, and stiffness, and the limb will feel surprisingly light without the cast. The skin will look mottled and may be covered with a yellow crust composed of exudate, oil, and dead skin. Olive oil and warm baths will soften and gradually remove this crust over a period of several days.

The patient's muscles will be weak, and his circulation sluggish. Graded active exercises are prescribed by the physician, and the patient may be under the care of a physical therapist in carrying out his exercise program.

## THE PATIENT IN TRACTION

Traction is used both as a temporary measure to disengage the fragments and as a continuous measure to maintain the alignment of the bones. Sus-

pension traction (in which weights and pulleys are used) is commonly used in oblique and comminuted fractures of long bones, especially those of the legs, on which the muscle pull is strong. The pull of the traction is just enough to correct the overriding of the fragments caused by muscle spasm and to place the fragments in the position in which they should heal. Eight to ten pounds of pull is the usual weight for the leg of an adult. Traction must be maintained continuously and smoothly.

Traction can be applied by means of adhesive or moleskin tape attached to the skin (Buck's extension or Russell traction), or it can be applied directly to the skeletal system (skeletal traction) by inserting a pin or a wire through the bone (Fig. 19-7). A Steinmann pin or a Kirshner wire is threaded through the bone in leg fractures. As illustrated in Figure 19-8, Crutchfield or Vince tongs are attached to the skull, when traction is used in the treatment of fractured cervical vertebrae.

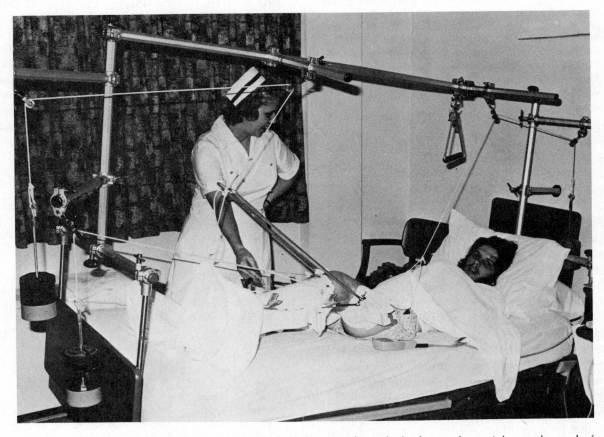

**Figure 19-7.** A patient in skeletal traction. Note the pin through the bone, the weights at the end of the bed. A cast has also been applied. The overhead trapeze assists the patient to move in bed. Call bell is within patient's reach. (Reprinted with permission from the July 1973 issue of *Nurs. '73,* Copyright © 1973 by Intermed Communications, Inc., Jenkintown, Pa. 19046).

**Traction Cart.** In some hospitals a traction cart is used. It is stocked with such equipment as adhesive tape, felt, stockinette rolls, bandage, scissors, screwdriver, tincture of benzoin, acetone, adhesive remover or ether, razor and blades, pulleys, weights, carriers, rope, sandbags, shock blocks, pelvic girdles, skin halters, trapezes, and lengths of pipe. Keeping the equipment on the cart is a convenience, since all needed articles can be rolled to the bedside.

### Pretraction Preparation

Before the orthopedist places the patient in traction it is important to check to see that the mattress is firm and level. A bed board is often used under the mattress to provide additional firm support. If skin traction is to be applied, the limb is shaved carefully. Careless shaving may remove epithelium which would invite infection under the tape. Some physicians prefer that the limb remain unshaved. To toughen the skin, tincture of benzoin is swabbed on the area that will receive the adhesive. The orthopedist applies the tape, sets up the pulleys and weights, and positions the part in traction.

### Types of Traction

**Russell Traction.** Russell traction permits the patient relative freedom to move about in bed. The knee should be bent, not kept straight. The traction cord passes first through the overhead pulley, attaches to the Balkan frame, then goes to the foot of the bed, then back to the pulley on the spreader at the patient's foot, then to the second pulley at the foot of the bed, and finally to the weights. The resulting pull on the leg is in a forward, upward direction. To keep the patient from slipping down in the bed, the foot of the bed may be elevated to provide a countertraction force. Gravity then will help to pull the patient's body toward the head of the bed.

**Buck's Extension.** Buck's extension is a simpler traction (Fig. 19-9). It may be used to align bone fragments temporarily while the patient awaits internal fixation. Foam-rubber strips, moleskin tape, and then an elastic bandage are applied to the skin of the leg; traction is accomplished with a single pulley.

### Physical Assessment and Nursing Care for the Patient in Traction

Assessment and related nursing intervention should include the following considerations.

**Position of the Limb.** Assess the position of the limb in relation to the maintenance of traction. If the patient slides down in bed, and the footpiece touches the pulleys at the foot of the bed, traction is disrupted. If suspension traction is used and is working properly, the patient's leg will rise when he lifts his hips. If his leg does not rise, check to be sure that the traction rope is in the grooves of the pulley and that the weights are hanging free. If the leg still does not rise, inform the physician.

The affected leg should be in alignment with the patient's body and with the traction apparatus. Firm pillows are sometimes placed under the leg, when the orthopedist recommends their use. When they are used, pillows support the thigh and the calf along their entire length. The covering on the pillows should be slippery (powdered plastic material may be used) to decrease friction, which impedes traction. The patient's heel should be placed beyond the edge of the pillow, to avoid pressure on the heel.

**Condition of the Affected Limb.** Assess the color and temperature of the limb. The foot should be warm and the same color as its healthy opposite member. Sensation should be normal when the foot or the hand is touched; there should be no numbness or tingling. Coldness, blanching, cyanosis, and disturbances of sensation indicate diminished circulation to the part and should be called immediately

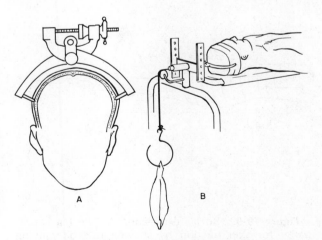

**Figure 19-8.** Crutchfield tongs. (A) The prongs are inserted into the skull and securely clamped in place. Note that there is ample bone between the tongs and the brain. (B) The patient is on a Stryker or a Foster frame, which allows turning of the patient while constant traction is maintained.

to the physician's attention. Adhesive tape on the patient's skin should be smooth, so that it does not irritate and denude the skin. If the patient is in Russell traction, be sure that the skin under the popliteal space, where the pull of the hammock is exerted, is protected with foam rubber. The extremity in traction should not be covered by a blanket, because this would hamper the movement of the cord. If the patient wishes, place a towel over his foot, but not touching the cords, to keep the foot warm.

Inspect the skin of the affected limb carefully and frequently for redness, irritation, and early signs of decubitus ulcers.

**Equipment.** Check the equipment carefully. All ropes should be in their grooves. If a cord is frayed, it should be replaced before it breaks. Manual traction is applied to the extremity while the cord is being changed. Knots should be tied tightly, and their ends taped together. The weights should swing free. A visitor may inadvertently push a chair against them, or they may get caught on the bed. Pulleys should not squeak. A drop or two of oil applied to the pulley can eliminate squeaking. Never

remove weights unless the physician specifies that this be done.

**Positioning.** Note the patient's position in bed. Avoid allowing him to slump down, as this interferes with deep breathing. Note the skin of the patient's elbows and unaffected heel. Sometimes the skin becomes dry and red from friction, as the patient presses down on the mattress with his elbows and unaffected heal in order to raise himself in bed. Teach the patient to use the overhead trapeze, thus sparing his elbows. Apply lanolin to reddened areas. A long-sleeved gown may help to lessen irritation of elbows.

When positioning the patient for use of the bedpan, use pillows behind the bedpan to raise the patient and prevent excreta from running down his back. A flat "fracture" bedpan is particularly useful for these patients.

**Skin Care.** Encourage the patient to carry out as much of his bath as possible, since this provides exercise and fosters independence. When washing the buttocks, massaging the lower back, or placing the patient on the bedpan, ask him to raise himself with the trapeze. When he is tired, provide a respite and then resume the care with the patient again raising his buttocks off the bed. It is important, when giving back care, to bend down and look at the skin to detect redness and breaks in the skin.

**Exercise.** All unaffected parts of the body should be exercised regularly. Teach the patient simple exercises to carry out with his arms, unaffected leg, shoulders, and his abdominal muscles, to counteract the muscle weakness which is caused by bed rest. Exercise must be gradual and appropriate to the age and condition of the patient.

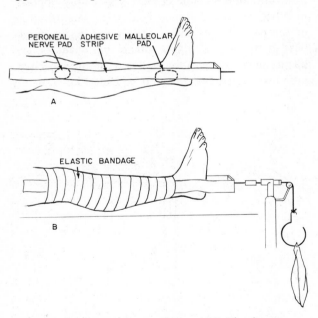

**Figure 19-9.** Buck's extension. (A) The leg is prepared for skin traction by shaving it and applying tincture of benzoin. It is padded, and adhesive strips and an elastic bandage are applied by the physician. (B) Leg in Buck's extension. The patient should be cautioned to keep himself high enough in bed so that the footplate does not rest against the bedpost.

## Removal from Traction

When a patient is removed from traction, first soak the adhesive tape, to help loosen it before removing it from the skin. Wash the limb and apply an emollient. Find out from the physician when movement is permitted and explain this to the patient. The limb will at first feel stiff, and, if it was in traction for a considerable time, the muscles will have undergone some atrophy, and the limb will look thinner than its opposite member. Explain to the patient that the stiffness will eventually disappear and that his muscles will grow strong again as he keeps using his leg.

## NURSING ASSESSMENT AND INTERVENTION FOR THE PATIENT IN A CAST OR IN TRACTION

### Explanation

Most fracture patients come to the hospital on an emergency basis and are highly anxious about the injury they have sustained as well as the emergency treatment. Explanation of the patient's condition and treatment is very important. Give only brief, simple explanations at first. When the patient becomes less anxious and more oriented to his situation, detailed explanations of his condition and treatment can begin. Such simple, direct explanations are essential, since the array of bars, ropes, and pulleys may further frighten the patient. Tell him that he will be cared for. Show him the call light, and explain its use. Indicate the things that he *can* do for himself, since this can diminish feelings of helplessness. Place such articles as the urinal, drinking water, and tissues within his reach.

Sometimes, particularly with elderly and with very anxious patients, perceptual distortion and confusion occur. For example, a patient may become agitated during the night and ask, as he looks at the bars of the frame over his bed, why he is caged. If this should occur, turn on the light and slowly and calmly explain what the apparatus is, where the patient is, and what happened which led to hospitalization.

Family and friends can also help the patient understand what has happened. Help the patient to get in touch with them.

**Motor Ability.** Motor ability of all accessible parts of the body should be assessed since limited mobility caused by such treatments as a spica cast can lead to muscle weakness. Special attention should be given to the mobility of the affected part. (Thus, it is important for the patient to move the wrist and fingers, and the elbow, even though a cast is on the forearm.)

**Respiratory Function.** Shallow breathing is a problem among patients with decreased mobility. Pulmonary congestion is also likely to occur, particularly among smokers and individuals with pre-existing lung disease, such as emphysema. It is essential to encourage the patient to breathe deeply at regular intervals and to cough up secretions. Change of position is beneficial, whenever possible.

Thus, the patient in a spica cast is turned so that he alternately lies in a supine or a prone position.

**Circulatory Function.** Special attention should be given to the circulation of the affected part. The toes of the patient in a leg cast or in traction should be inspected regularly for edema, coldness, blanching, and cyanosis. The nurse should be alert to any complaint of numbness or tingling in the part. The injured limb is kept elevated to prevent edema. Regular exercise of the part also aids in maintaining circulation.

Observation for thrombophlebitis is important, especially when prolonged bed rest is required. Any redness, induration, pain over the course of a vein, and any mottling of the skin of the part should be noted. Although regular exercise can help to prevent thrombophlebitis, if any symptoms of the condition appear the part should be kept at rest until a medical evaluation is made.

**Nutrition.** The patient who is inactive is likely to gain weight. Sometimes it is quite feasible for the patient to get on the scale (such as when he has a leg cast). Of course, the weight of the cast must be taken into consideration. When weighing the patient regularly, it is possible for the nurse to note fluctuations in body weight, with the weight of the cast remaining constant. If the patient must remain in bed, it is important for the nurse to note weight gain by observing the patient and checking the tightness of the cast. It may be necessary to place the patient on a low calorie diet if weight gain occurs. On the other hand, depression (so often a problem in these patients) and inactivity can lead to anorexia, so that it may be necessary to encourage food intake by between-meal snacks.

Fluid intake should be encouraged unless it is contraindicated. Prolonged immobility predisposes the patient to urinary calculi, infections, and difficulties in effective emptying of the bladder. Generous fluid intake can help to prevent and to alleviate these problems.

**Elimination.** As noted above, it is important to assess the adequacy of urinary output. Positioning the patient in the most natural position possible when a bedpan or urinal is used, is important. Constipation is frequently a problem among patients whose activity is restricted. Frequency of bowel movements and whether the stool is hard and difficult to expel should be noted. In addition to encouraging fluids and providing bulk-producing foods in the diet, suppositories, stool softners, laxatives and enemas may be necessary.

**Skin.** The skin should be observed—especially over bony prominences, over the back, and at any points where there is pressure from such devices as casts and traction. Any redness or possible broken areas should be noted. Prompt relief of pressure whenever possible and massage of the part, using an emollient lotion are essential. Sponge rubber, and cotton pads can be used to relieve pressure and irritation from the edge of a cast or from traction equipment. An alternating pressure pad, placed over the mattress, is helpful and should be used whenever the patient is especially vulnerable to decubitus ulcers (such as in the case of an elderly person who must lie on his back.) Since the skin tends to become dry and scaly, regular exercise (noted above) and the use of emollient lotions after bathing are important.

Aesthetic considerations are also important. The patient in a large cast or traction, who cannot use tub or shower, may feel unclean despite sponge baths. He should be helped with the niceties of care so that he can feel more acceptable. For example, he should be encouraged to use deodorants, powder, and toilet water.

Regular hair shampoos are also important. Many patients are accustomed to shampooing their hair several times a week and are greatly distressed by the frequent inattention to this aspect of personal hygiene in hospitals. Often it is possible to place the patient on a stretcher and take him to the sink, where his hair can be thoroughly washed and rinsed. Small hand hair driers, provided by the family or hospital, can then be used to promptly dry the hair.

## COMPLICATIONS FROM CASTS AND TRACTION

### Hypostatic Pneumonia

Hypostatic pneumonia is a frequent secondary cause of death in the older patient who breaks his hip and is put in traction. This dread complication is a danger for any patient who remains long in one position. For this reason the patient should engage in deep-breathing exercises every three to four hours through such activities as blowing bubbles into a glass of water with a straw or blowing up balloons. Lifting exercise weights is also good practice for those using a trapeze.

### Footdrop

Footdrop is a paralytic deformity that results in an inability to hold the foot in normal position. The foot in traction should be in a natural walking position. The other foot must not be allowed to grow weak from disuse. It must be exercised, and when it is at rest, it should not be pushed down with covers. A small splintlike footboard is used with traction. A footboard not only keeps the covers off the patient's toes, but also helps to prevent him from slipping down in bed. Walking is a precious ability; thus every effort should be made to prevent this deformity since patients cannot walk if they develop footdrop.

The most dangerous position for the unaffected leg—and this statement applies to all bed patients—is outward rotation. Although it may feel comfortable for the patient in bed, it leads easily to contractures of the strong abductor muscle groups. All bed patients should be taught to "toe in" while they are resting on their backs. If necessary, sandbags are used for support, although they are a poor substitute for muscular control. Care should be taken to see that the patient does not become confined in one position for many hours.

### Pressure Sores

Since patients in traction are often unable to move about they are more prone to develop pressure sores. In addition the mechanical devices used for immobilization can cause pressure and lead to skin abrasions. However, many measures are available for coping with this problem. For example, silicone cushions are available for use with Stryker frames.

### Delayed Union or Nonunion of the Bone Ends

In some instances, delayed union or nonunion results. *Delayed union* means that the bony union is slower than usual. For example, a fracture of the tibia might be considered as showing delayed union if there is little, if any, x-ray or clinical evidence of union by four months. *Nonunion*—a permanent break in the continuity of the bone—would be considered if there are no signs of union clinically or by x-ray some months later. It is to be stressed that these are arbitrary periods of time and will vary with the individual case and the attending physician.

Either of these conditions can be caused by (1) inadequate immobilization of the part, (2) distraction (bone fragments are held apart, as in those cases in which traction is excessive), (3) infection, or (4) poor circulation. The location of the fracture and the extent of the injury also may be factors that delay or prevent bone healing.

## Kidney Stones

The combination of local decalcification and a decrease in body activity increases the amount of calcium salts excreted by the kidneys. Some of this increased load of calcium salts may precipitate from the urine, forming calculi. Increased fluid intake and regular exercise for those parts that do not need to be immobilized may prevent this particular complication.

## Thrombophlebitis, Phlebothrombosis, and Emboli

These dangers can result from trauma and from immobilization of an injured leg. This is one reason that elevation of the affected limb, which helps to reduce edema and improve circulation is so important. In addition, it is necessary to encourage *active* motion of the fingers and toes not just weak wiggling. Joints not immobilized should be activated early—as soon as pain permits—and isometric exercises of the immobilized parts should be started early. All of these measures are of great help in improving circulation to the part.

One of the major complications of trauma to the lower extremities or of prolonged bed rest is thrombophlebitis and thromboembolism. Muscle and joint activity carried out early can reduce the incidence appreciably. Preventive measures are far better for the patient than treatment of phlebitis or pulmonary embolism.

**Symptoms.** Symptoms of thrombophlebitis of the leg are pain in the calf, swelling, local heat, and redness. Phlebothrombosis is a particularly serious problem since it may result in pulmonary embolism. Pulmonary embolus, if it occurs, may happen any time from a few days to several months after the injury.

## Fat Embolism

Fat embolism develops most often in patients with multiple fractures of long bones or with ex-

tensive damage to soft tissue. Symptoms of fat embolism usually develop 24 to 48 hours after trauma. Two hypotheses explain the formation of fat embolism: (1) Trauma causes fat to be released from the marrow of the bones into the circulation, where the fat globules become emboli which can travel to the lungs, brain, and other organs. (2) The body's physiologic response to trauma alters the natural emulsion of fats in the blood. Fat is not broken down as rapidly and accumulates, forming emboli (Law, 1973). Symptoms of fat embolism include various indications of damage to the affected organs. For example, the patient with cerebral embolism may become irritable and restless and then lapse into coma. The patient with pulmonary embolism may experience dyspnea, cyanosis, cough. Fat globules may be demonstrated in the urine in some cases. Prompt immobilization of the fracture helps prevent fat embolism by minimizing the release of fat from bone marrow into the circulation.

## Constipation

This is a frequent complaint of patients in traction or a cast. Abdominal distention and retention of waste products can make the patient very uncomfortable. The causes are many. It may result from a lack of exercise, or it may be that some people find it difficult to change eating habits to fit a hospital schedule. In extreme cases in which people can not make this adjustment, a long hospitalization may result in malnutrition. In the case of elderly people the problem may be caused by a lack of teeth. If this is so, the dietitian should be alerted that the patient has a problem with chewing, so that she can prepare dishes that the patient can eat. To prevent or treat constipation quickly, the nurse should note whether or not the patient has a bowel movement. She should encourage fluids and roughage in the diet, and give the patient a bedpan regularly, perhaps every day after breakfast. She should report constipation to the physician promptly. It is easier to deal with this problem if measures are taken promptly to relieve it, such as use of bisacodyl (Dulcolax) suppositories or small, commercially prepared enemas, such as Fleet's.

## Retention of Urine

The causes of urine retention may be the inactivity of the patient and a decrease in fluid intake. The absence of urine is an observation of vital importance for the nurse to make. On a busy ward it is all too easy to fail to notice the retention of urine. Urinary incontinence calls attention to itself, but retention is less obvious. If retention occurs, the patient may need to be catheterized. However, other measures are tried first, such as proper positioning of the patient and attention to privacy. Because catheterization carries some risk of infection, it is avoided when possible.

## Infection

Wound infection slows or prevents bone healing, and if the bone itself becomes infected, the patient may be crippled the rest of his life. In compound fractures, because the wound is deep, there is the possibility of infection with the gas-gangrene bacillus, *Clostridium welchii* (*Clostridium perfringens*). The anaerobic organism is so contagious and so deadly that its presence may demand that the ward be closed to any new patients.

Symptoms of *gas gangrene* are sudden local puffiness (with discoloration), pain, thin, watery exudate, which is very foul smelling, fever, and an expression of severe illness. The crepitation that may be felt under the skin is caused by gas bubbles in subcutaneous tissue and the muscles. Therapy in a hyperbaric oxygen chamber has recently proved effective.

*Tetanus* is another danger. Both infections are treated by opening the wound widely, so that air can enter and by administering antibiotics and providing continuous drip irrigations of hydrogen peroxide or Dakin's solution. Tetanus prophylaxis is important as a preventive measure and should be started promptly after the patient's injury has occurred. The trend now is toward use of an immunizing preparation (tetanus immune globulin) made from human serum rather than from horse serum. Tetanus toxoid is usually administered at the same time as the tetanus immune globulin, made from human serum.

## PATIENT EDUCATION

The patient's understanding of the type of fracture he has and the therapy entailed can assist him to avoid complications. While the actual healing process in the bone cannot be hurried, it is most important that the patient trust that the staff will insure skillful care in reducing and immobilizing the fracture site and in avoiding any interference with reparative processes (such as further injury to the site). Such a situation is difficult for some patients to accept, particularly if they rely greatly upon their ability to control the events affecting their lives.

The patient's challenge is to cooperate with the healing and treatment process, by not interfering with it and by promptly reporting any indications that the healing is not progressing satisfactorily, or that measures to provide immobilization are either not effective or are interfering with other body processes, such as circulation.

For many patients with fractures the treatment includes reduction of the fracture and application of a cast, after which the patient is sent home. For this reason, he should be given explicit instructions and assured that he may come to the emergency room at any hour, if he needs care or if he requires the reassurance of professional evaluation of his condition. The hospitalized patient, too, requires the same teaching, so that he will understand the purpose of the observations being made by the staff and the need to promptly call to the attention of the staff any symptoms requiring their intervention.

In this vein, the patient should be instructed to:

- **Note the color of the extremity which extends beyond the cast (e.g., the toes or fingers), and to report any discoloration, such as blanching or cyanosis.**
- **Note the temperature of the extremity: If they are cold, he should report this immediately.**
- **Observe the cast for any discoloration, which would indicate that drainage is occurring inside the cast, and to report such drainage.**
- **Assess pain. If pain continues unabated or begins to grow worse, the patient should seek care.**
- **Observe the extremity for swelling and for a feeling of increased tightness of the cast. He should seek immediate professional care for these symptoms.**
- **Elevate the extremity as directed, to lessen the swelling and pain. The physician will indicate the amount of elevation needed.**
- **Elevate the part when out of bed, by use of a sling (for the arm) or a hassock (for a leg).**
- **Allow the cast to dry evenly on all sides, realizing that the inner layers of the cast are still damp when the outside is dry. The cast is fragile when it is damp. Care must be taken not to bump it or to cause a depression in it by pressing on it. Never get the cast wet, once it has dried. The cast may be cleaned by using a small amount of cleansing powder and a slightly damp cloth and by working quickly.**
- **Never place anything inside the cast. If the stockinette has not been pulled over the edge of the cast, the patient should be taught how to make a smooth edge for the cast by "petaling" it with adhesive tape.**

If the patient is hospitalized, the nurse makes these observations and carries out whatever aspects of care the patient is unable to perform himself.

## FACTORS AFFECTING RECOVERY

**Emotional Aspects.** Anger, resentment, and feelings of extreme helplessness are common among patients whose mobility is seriously curtailed by a cast or traction. Because of their dependence upon others to care for them, it is especially difficult for these patients to express their feelings for fear that they will be labeled uncooperative and receive less care. Too often such expressions of anger are discouraged or viewed as evidence of ingratitude.

Thus it is important for the nurse to help the patient to channel expressions of his anger, either directly, by talking about how furious he is that this happened and about how much it hurt; or indirectly, by engaging in the exercise permitted which not only aids circulation and respiration, but also dissipates the energy and tension generated by anger. Competitive games, such as checkers and chess, may also serve as a safety valve for angry feelings.

Long-term patients, particularly, should be encouraged to participate in group activities, such as singing and games, which can lessen feelings of helplessness and isolation. Singing also has the advantage of promoting deep breathing and helping to prevent hypostatic pneumonia.

It is important to distinguish between feelings of helplessness and actual helplessness. A patient with a broken arm may be more distressed by feeling helpless than a patient in a body cast. It is essential to deal with the individual patient in relation to his response.

Feelings of helplessness are a pervasive problem and are expressed in various ways and with varied degrees of intensity. The patient may engage in outbursts of anger or may withdraw, behaving submissively, and resisting self-care and other activities. Helping this patient to talk about his experience will enable him to express some of his feelings of powerlessness so that he may become more able to express anger and, begin to participate more in his own care.

A consistent show of interest in the patient's welfare and recovery can in turn kindle his own efforts. Arranging the environment to foster self-help and encouraging groups of patients to assist one another are also important. It is particularly important that a patient who is confined to bed in a large cast or in traction have his belongings handy so that he can be as self-sufficient as possible. Placing a shoe bag, with its multiple compartments, at the head of the bed is one useful way of keeping writing paper, pens, and toilet articles within reach. In addition, the food tray can be placed in a position which enables the patient to feed himself. The nurse can provide assistance, if needed, with such activities as cutting meat or pouring hot coffee.

The patient will also feel less helpless if he knows what injury he has sustained, what treatment is necessary, approximately how long it is expected to take, and how he can participate in his recovery. The nurse and physician provide this information, and can assist the patient to be aware of his own progress by allowing him to look at his x-rays.

It is also important to include the patient's family or close friends in explanations and discussions to lessen their apprehension and to facilitate their helping the patient make realistic plans. While some patients chafe at the restrictions and eagerly accept opportunities for more independence as soon as they are able, others become timid and require a great deal of support and encouragement in availing themselves of opportunities for more activity.

**Age.** Fractures present a special hazard to the elderly. Problems with vision, hearing, position sense, and agility make the elderly more prone to falls and to accidents, resulting in numerous types of fractures, especially fractures of the hip.

Assessment of the elderly patient with a fracture should emphasize such considerations as: his ability to perform self-care activities within the limits imposed by his treatment; his sensory abilities and the need for devices such as glasses and hearing aids; his orientation, alertness, and responsiveness to activities and people around him; and any early symptoms of complications. Newer methods of treatment (such as hip pinning) emphasize early mobilization of the patient, thus reducing bed-rest time and lessening the likelihood of hypostatic pneumonia and decubitus ulcers which occur readily in elderly patients on extended bed rest.

Nevertheless, the elderly person with a fracture, even when treated with the most up-to-date methods, presents a challenge to the nurse to devise ways to exercise unaffected parts and to lessen the negative physical and emotional consequences of prolonged inactivity. Maintenance of fluid intake, observation for adequate voiding, prevention and early detection of constipation, skin care, deep breathing, opportunities for diversion and for social contacts, are all examples of important aspects of care. Prompt assistance in maintaining and regaining independence in self-care is essential. Unfortunately, some elderly people, through neglect and their own discouragement, unnecessarily become semi-invalids following a fracture. Effort is required to help the patient return to his own home and to his accustomed activities, whenever this is feasible.

For the young adult and the person during middle life, the experience of a fracture often is especially disturbing due to interruption of work, education, and family responsibilities. The younger person, thanks to greater muscular strength, agility, and coordination, typically copes more effectively than the elderly with such tasks as learning to use crutches.

**Socioeconomic Factors.** For all patients, regardless of age, a fracture may present serious social and economic problems. Economically, equipment, such as walkers, crutches, and wheelchairs, is costly. If the need for it is temporary, it is important for the patient to realize that he can rent (or sometimes borrow) such items rather than purchase them. Prolonged treatment, particularly when in a hospital or in an extended care facility, is expensive, and such costs present particular hardships for the elderly. Isolation from work, family, and friends

due to hospitalization presents difficulties for most patients and is especially problematic for individuals who lack close family ties and secure employment, or those who rely heavily upon work, social contacts, and physical activity to lessen anxiety and to give purpose and meaning to their lives.

Group experiences are especially important for fracture patients who are confined to hospitals for more than a few days. Anxiety over disability is usually severe, and threats to the patient's body image and view of himself as an active, capable person are very real. Group discussions with a nurse can assist patients to express some of their feelings as well as lessen their loneliness.

## SPECIFIC FRACTURES

### Fracture of the Hip

Fracture of the hip occurs in one of three places in the femur: the head of the femur, the neck of the femur (both are intracapsular), or the intertrochanteric region (extracapsular) (Fig. 19-10). Treatment and nursing care depend not only on the age and the general condition of the patient, but also on the location of the fracture, because treatment of fractures in each region presents characteristic problems.

Fractures in the intertrochanteric area usually result from a direct fall on the hip and occur in people who are slightly older than those with hip fractures in the other regions. Eighty per cent are over 60 years of age. Although there is a high early mortality (17 per cent), late complications are rare. Hemorrhage and shock are seen more frequently in patients with an extracapsular fracture than in patients with an intracapsular fracture. Late complications include nonunion, malposition of the femur, migration of the nail, and fracture of the metal used in treatment.

### Treatment

**Internal Fixation.** Because the patients usually are elderly, prolonged traction, which requires prolonged, debilitating bed rest, is avoided when possible. Early mobilization is desirable and possible with the use of the Jewett, the Neufeld, and the Austin Moore pins, the Smith-Petersen nail (Fig. 19-11) and the Thornton plate, the Pugh and the Ken nails, the Massie nail and plate, screws, and bands. Other types of devices for internal fixation of fractured hips include the Modny apparatus,

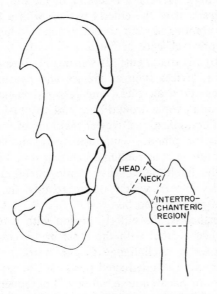

**Figure 19-10.** Areas in which hip fractures are most common.

Deyerle pins, and modifications of both. These appliances are made of nonelectrolytic metals, such as Vitallium and stainless steel. The bone heals around the metallic device, which in the meantime holds the bone together. Thus the bone is immobilized immediately, and patients can be mobilized much earlier than they can with treatment by traction. Plates, bands, screws, and pins are removed only after the bone has healed, and only if they become loose or otherwise troublesome to the patient.

Another device to produce internal fixation is the intramedullary rod, which is inserted in long bones. It may be used to stabilize a fracture of a long bone which is not significantly comminuted, or in some cases of fracture or threatened fracture of long bones. This may permit early ambulation. The patient usually is placed in traction after this procedure and may bear weight in about three weeks.

**Bone Grafts.** Sometimes cancellous bone (the reticular tissue of bone) is packed around the fracture line to stimulate bone growth. Heterogenous bone (bone from another species), homogenous bone (bone from the same species but another person), or autogenous bone (bone from the body of the patient) may be used. Autogenous bone, which may be taken from the tibia or the iliac bone, seems to be accepted best by the body. Bone grafts in general do not stimulate as profound an antigen-antibody response as do grafts of other tissues. The grafted bone eventually is replaced by the growth of new bone.

**Complications.** Intracapsular fractures in general are caused by far less trauma than extracapsular fractures. Sometimes, the patient twists his body while his foot is in a fixed position, and the neck of the femur cracks. The mortality rate is less in intracapsular fractures than in extracapsular fractures, but there is a high incidence of complications. Blood vessels run close to the neck of the femur. When the bone fragments produced by the fracture divide these vessels, the neck and the head of the femur suffer a loss of blood supply, which may cause avascular necrosis (called also aseptic necrosis). The problem is not always obvious since dead bone may initially look like live bone on an x-ray film. Dead bone will unite with the live part of the femur and may even support the weight of the patient for some months following an internal fixation, but then it collapses. Approximately 30 per cent of intracapsular fractures have this unfortunate outcome.

Methods are being investigated to discover whether the femoral head is viable or not. Still experimental are the use of radioactive phosphorus, staining the bone, and testing the oxygen tension of the blood. Subcapital fractures and some other fractures of the neck of the femur present problems in relation to solid internal fixation, with a high incidence of nonunion and aseptic necrosis.

The frequency of nonunion varies in different reported series, but may be in the neighborhood of 14 per cent. Some degree of aseptic necrosis and secondary arthritic changes in the joint occur in 45 to 50 per cent of patients.

When there is necrosis of the femoral head after a fracture, the patient may have pain and muscle spasm and develop a limp. Depending on the patient's age, his condition and the degree of disability, re-operation for insertion of a femoral head prosthesis may be considered. A "total hip" prosthesis is now sometimes used (see below).

After the insertion of a prosthesis, the position of the patient is determined by the line of the incision in the capsule (Fig. 19-12). The objective is to prevent strain on the incision that would result in pushing the prosthesis through it. When the surgical approach has been posterior, the patient is kept relatively flat in bed, with the operative leg somewhat abducted and in external rotation (here is an exception to the rule). When the incision is anterior, the leg is kept in internal rotation, and the patient may sit up. He is helped out of bed on the first postoperative day and is encouraged to walk

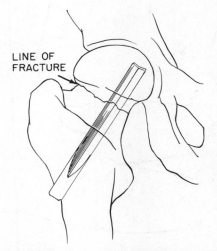

LINE OF FRACTURE

**Figure 19-11.** A Smith-Petersen nail through the fractured neck of a femur.

with weight bearing as soon as the soft tissues have healed. X-ray films are taken about every three months the first year.

### Postoperative Nursing Care

Because these patients usually are elderly and have suffered two major physical insults (the trauma of the fracture and the surgery), alert, supportive nursing care and careful judgment are especially important to the life and the comfort of the patient. Hemorrhage is an immediate postoperative concern. So is postoperative pain, which may be severe. Narcotics should be administered judiciously and with consideration of the dangers of disorientation and depression of respiration.

Postoperative exercises of deep breathing and the

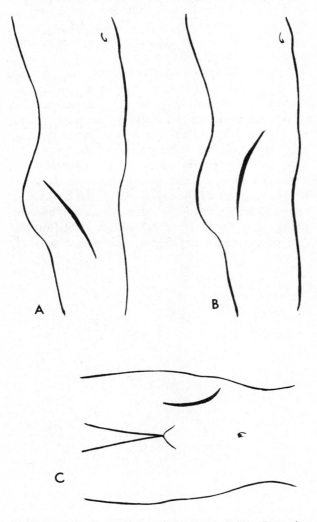

**Figure 19-12.** Lines of incisions. (A) Posterior approach. (B) and (C), anterior approaches.

use of intermittent positive pressure breathing (IPPB) help minimize the pulmonary complications so common in elderly people. Combined with active motion of the extremities these measures can minimize the dangers of vascular complications. This is important from the standpoint of mobilizing the patient, but more important with respect to reducing the morbidity or mortality associated with pulmonary emboli.

When there is a surgical wound in which a large skin flap covers a dead space, the patient may come from the operating room with a drain that may be connected to a low suction drainage device, such as the Hemovac (Fig. 19-13). The drain may be left in place for one or two days to prevent the collection of fluid in the space.

When a fractured hip is nailed there is seldom the need for a cast.

**Positioning.** Postoperatively, the physician will order to which side the patient may be turned. If it is toward the affected leg, the bed provides a comfortable splint and reduces the pain of movement. A pillow should be placed lengthwise between the patient's legs before he is turned. He should be turned all at once, with the fractured leg kept in a straight line with the trunk. If the patient may be turned to his unaffected side, one pillow should be used lengthwise under his upper leg and another behind his back.

**Exercise.** Depending on the condition of the patient, exercises prescribed by the physician are started by the physical therapist, possibly on the day after the operation. The role of the nurse is to encourage the patient to do the prescribed exercises and to make the exercises as pleasant as possible. Again, the nurse reminds the patient to avoid external rotation while he is in bed by "toeing in."

After pinning for internal fixation some patients are placed in traction for one or two days to help to relieve muscle spasm. Then they are helped out of bed, sometimes to ambulate without weight bearing on the affected leg and sometimes just to use a wheelchair. Weight bearing on the operative side is avoided until evidence of healing is seen on x-ray film.

## THE PATIENT WITH TOTAL HIP AND TOTAL KNEE REPLACEMENT

When a joint is badly damaged by injury or disease (commonly severe arthritis) total replacement of the joint with a prosthesis may be performed.

This type of surgery is usually undertaken in treating older people with severe joint pathology who do not respond to more conservative therapy. The joints most commonly replaced are the hip and the knee.

**Preoperative Preparation.** Careful preoperative instruction is essential, particularly in light of the newness of this surgical procedure. The patient is taught exercises, such as quadriceps setting, how to get on and off the bedpan using the trapeze, how it feels to keep his legs in abduction and how the splint for maintaining this position is applied. He is also instructed as to the procedures for preventing pulmonary complications, such as coughing, deep breathing, and use of blow bottles and (if prescribed) IPPB. It is essential that this preoperative instruction be given carefully and slowly, with opportunities for the patient to practice the skills and to ask questions.

### Hip Replacement

#### Postoperative Nursing Care

**Position.** Following total hip replacement, the patient's legs are placed in abduction by means of a splint which is applied to both legs. This position is maintained to prevent dislocation of the prosthesis. (In this operation, both the acetabulum and the head of the femur are replaced with prostheses and are held in position with cement.) Procedures vary for postoperative care, depending upon the experience and preference of the surgeon. In some instances the patient's affected leg is placed in Russell traction, and Ace bandages are applied to both legs to prevent thrombophlebitis. In other situations, only the abduction splint is applied, and surgical elastic stockings are applied to both legs to prevent thrombophlebitis. The length of time that the patient is required to wear the splint varies, as does the time when he is allowed to begin to walk. Bed rest with splinting in the position of abduction may, for example, be maintained for a week, with gradual resumption of activity beginning during the second week postoperatively. Even after the splint has been removed the patient is instructed to maintain the position of abduction as fully as possible.

**Assessment.** When working with the patient, assess the position of the legs: both should be abducted. Note any drainage from the operative site, and whether the patient is in pain. Pain is often severe for the first two to three days, and analgesics are important to provide relief. Observe whether

the splint is causing redness or irritation of the skin. Note the circulation of the affected leg (warmth, color, pulses). Observe also any complaints which may indicate nerve damage, such as sensations of numbness or tingling, a burning sensation in the leg, or changes in reaction to pin pricks over the dorsum of the foot. Be alert for symptoms of dislocation of the prosthesis: severe pain, a palpable lump over the head of the femur, and changes in circulation and in nerve functioning.

**Daily Care.** Following total hip replacement, the patient is not permitted to turn on either side. Usually two people are needed to help him move. When back care is given one person helps the patient to raise himself off the bed with the aid of an overhead trapeze while the other administers back care. The patient uses this maneuver also for getting on and off the bedpan and when his bed linen is being changed. The bed is made from top to bottom, by two nurses working together, sliding the soiled sheets out from the top of the bed downward, as the patient raises himself with the trapeze and with the assistance of the nurses. A small flat bedpan is preferable for these patients, since it can be slipped under them more easily and with less exertion for the patient. Only liquids and a very light

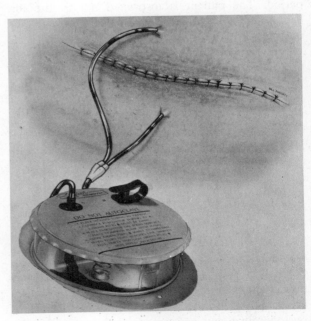

**Figure 19-13.** The Snyder Hemovac. This is one type of low pressure suction device which is used to drain blood and other exudates from wounds, thus facilitating healing. (Zimmer Company, Warsaw, Ind.)

diet are allowed for the first three postoperative days, in order to keep the patient from having a bowel movement. At the end of three days the diet is increased, and an enema may be prescribed to aid defecation.

**Exercises.** The patient is encouraged to exercise his upper extremities and to breathe deeply. Sometimes IPPB is prescribed. Blow bottles are also helpful. The patient is taught quadriceps-setting exercises, which he practices in the postoperative period, contracting and relaxing his quadriceps muscles approximately ten times every hour to strengthen his muscles in preparation for walking. Gentle, frequent movement of both feet and ankles is recommended, particularly while the patient's legs are in the splint. The bed is placed in a flat position several times daily in order to extend the hip fully.

During the second postoperative week, the patient begins to ambulate: at first with a walker, then with crutches or a cane, and finally, with no assistance. Sometimes only partial weight bearing is permitted at first; in other instances, the patient is allowed full weight bearing. The speed of this progression depends greatly upon the patient's condition. A very debilitated elderly patient may continue to use the walker for a considerable period. The patient is instructed not to use low chairs, but to sit in firm straight backed chairs and to use a raised toilet seat—these measures help to prevent dislocation of the prosthesis. Both the use of the raised toilet seat and the firm chairs are begun in the hospital and continued in the patient's home. Regular exercise such as walking is important when the patient returns home. The patient's response is often dramatic, as he discovers that after years of pain and disability he is able to walk comfortably.

### Knee Replacement

Following total knee replacement a Zimmer splint is applied to the affected leg. It is important to check the circulation to the leg while it is in the splint. Surgical stockings to help prevent thrombophlebitis are usually worn while the patient's movement is restricted. Range-of-motion exercises are usually prescribed beginning at about the third postoperative day and are carried out at first by the physical therapist. The patient is usually confined to bed for five or six days. Afterward he gradually ambulates with the aid of a walker and crutches and then is usually able to walk without either of these aids.

## CRUTCH WALKING

The physical therapist measures the patient for crutches. It is important that they be the proper height, so that as the patient learns to walk he can hold himself erect and experience as little strain as possible. A principle of any rehabilitative measure is that it should produce the most natural situation possible. Crutches that fit properly allow the patient to walk more naturally than do ill-fitting ones.

The patient has time to think about crutch walking. It can become a goal. Warn him that progress will be slow, but mark each hard-won advance with the praise that it certainly deserves.

### Preparation

In preparation for walking with the aid of crutches, the patient may be taught the following exercises to strengthen his arm and his shoulder muscles: to lie on his abdomen and do pushups, to lift sandbags while he is lying on his back, and to sit up with both palms on the mattress and to push up until his buttocks clear the bed. Sawed-off crutches may be given to him for practicing straight elbow pushups. At this stage he learns not to hunch his shoulders and not to lean on his crutches. In crutch walking the weight is carried on the hands, not the axillae. Branches of the brachial plexus run through the axilla; the patient who leans on his crutches may damage these nerves, so that paralysis of his arm results. This condition, known as *crutch palsy*, has been known to develop after only four hours of leaning on crutches without the use of handgrips.

For a day or two the patient stands before he walks. Parallel bars may be used before he tries his crutches. Standing gives him the feel of being upright with crutches. He is taught the tripod position, with the crutches ahead of him and to the side. He leans forward slightly from the ankles —not from the neck, the waist, or the hips. A mirror helps the patient to obtain and to maintain good position. The patient with a pinned hip may be advised not to touch the foot of the affected side to the floor.

Shoes should fit well and have nonslip soles and heels. Women should not wear high heels.

## Types of Gaits

The patient is taught by diagram and demonstration before he actually tries his crutches. The following are frequently used types of gaits:

- *Swing-through.* The two crutches are advanced simultaneously. The patient swings through, landing beyond the crutches (Fig. 19-14). This system is used where there is complete paralysis of the hips and legs. Otherwise, it is an undesirable method, since it leads to atrophy of the legs and the hips. However, this gait is the fastest of all, and it is permissible for a patient to resort to it when he is in a hurry, such as when he is crossing a street.
- *Two-point.* The left foot and the right crutch are advanced simultaneously, and then the right foot and the left crutch are advanced. This gait is the most natural of the gaits, and it is faster than the four-point.
- *Three-point.* When the patient is allowed little or no weight bearing on one extremity, as in a hip nailing, or when there is no extremity, three-point walking is done. Advance both crutches, using the strong leg to stand on, then swing the strong leg through the crutches. The involved limb can go with the crutches or it can stay in line with the strong leg.
- *Four-point.* One at a time, the right crutch, the left foot, the left crutch, and the right foot are placed down.

The two- and the four-point gaits are used especially for polio, arthritis, and cerebral palsy. They allow equal but partial weight bearing on each limb. If a single crutch is used, it is placed on the unaffected side. Also, a disabled person should be helped to get in and out of bed, up and down stairs, or simply to walk, by support on his unaffected side. This position may seem contrary to logic, but it works much better, because it supports and augments the patient's own strength of the unaffected parts.

## Teaching Crutch Walking

Try these different gaits yourself with a pair of crutches. You will find yourself making some of the common errors of beginners, such as trying to lift a crutch while your weight still is on it. Beginners also have a tendency to take a longer step with the weaker leg. Skilled crutch walkers take a short step of equal length with each foot. You can teach better if you know how it feels to use crutches. You will discover problems that may surprise you.

Ordinarily, the physical therapist teaches crutch walking. (If there is no physical therapist, the nurse carries out the teaching.) She should work with the physical therapist and know what he has taught the patient. When the patient practices crutch walking in his room, on the ward or in the hall, the nurse should tell him what accords with the teaching of the physical therapist. Besides teaching exercises and crutch walking, the physical

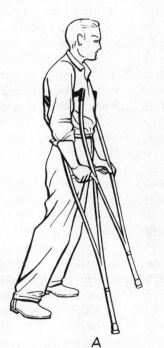
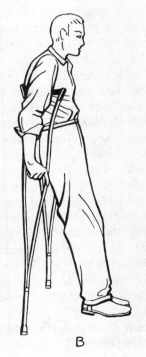
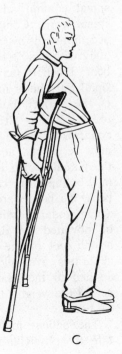

**Figure 19-14.** A man with paraplegia using the swing-through gait. (A) He puts the crutches well in front of him. (B) The swing through. (C) The position in which he lands. He next puts the crutches in position (A).

therapist also may use heat—by hot pack, with a cradle and a light bulb, or deep heat with a diathermy machine. Whirlpool baths, massage and electric stimulation may be used to improve muscle tone.

It is a tragedy if the patient falls down in the early stage of ambulation. He may be hurt or suffer a severe blow to his self-confidence. Therefore, take all possible precautions. Inspect the crutch tips for wear, and teach the patient to do likewise. If the rubber shows signs of wear, discard the tip and use a new one. When the patient first starts to walk, one person stands behind him, and one stands in front. Physical therapy workers often stand behind the patient and hold him by his belt. Watch that the way is clear for the patient, and teach him to do the same. There must not be a wet or oily spot on the floor, no dropped piece of gauze, no footstool, or anything else on which he can slip or trip. After looking down to see that the way is clear, he then can walk with head erect and eyes up.

## OTHER FRACTURES

### Fracture of the Spine

The patient with a fracture of the spine usually is placed in a position of hyperextension, a position that best reestablishes the normal position of the spinal column and exerts least pressure on the spinal cord. Continuous hyperextension may be accomplished by a cast or by immobilizing the body with head traction and sandbags over a gatch bed. Traction may be accomplished by making small burr holes in the skull into the outer layers of the parietal bones on each side and inserting tongs, such as Crutchfield tongs, which then are connected with a pulley and weights. Sandbags may be placed at the shoulders to help to keep the patient down in bed, or the head of the bed may be raised for countertraction. In many hospital beds, the headboard is a solid piece and does not accommodate cervical traction. Sometimes this can be obviated by placing the head of the patient at the foot of the bed. There are also pieces of apparatus available commercially which can be applied to the head portion of the frame which permit the weights to be suspended over the side of the bed.

The patient may turn from side to side only with the physician's permission. The patient must be turned without bending his spine. If the patient may be turned, a Stryker or a Foster frame facilitates care.

If, as rarely may be the case, the patient is not allowed to turn, his body may be held still by sandbags at his sides, or a drawsheet may be placed over his abdomen. As the patient may have to lie still in the same position for as long as six weeks, the care of the skin is of the utmost importance. Back care is given by compressing the mattress with one hand and slipping the other hand under the back of the patient. All of the back cannot be washed and rubbed at one time, but no area should be neglected. Beware of the development of decubitus ulcers at the back of the head. The patient is not allowed to have a pillow, but a thin piece of foam rubber under his head may help to prevent a pressure sore. Because the traction relieves pain, patients often are more comfortable in tongs than they appear to be. However, the family may need to be assured that the tongs grip only the bones of the head and that there is no danger of puncturing the brain of the patient. Watch for signs of infection around the burr holes.

Sometimes traction is accomplished by leather or webbed straps on the head and under the chin. These can cause considerable skin irritation. Thin strips of foam rubber between the skin and the leather may help. Traction may be released momentarily for skin care only if the head is supported in the same position with the other hand, and only if the physician allows it. Use alcohol and powder. A physician's order is required for release from traction long enough for a barber to shave a male patient. Be especially careful that there is no jerk when traction is reapplied.

Patients in the position of hyperextension may have difficulty swallowing. Feed the patient slowly. Have a suction machine nearby in case he needs it. The position is a tiresome one. There is little for the patient to look at, and his body grows weary from lying so still. A radio, a mirror, and visits from family and friends may help his morale. Prism glasses enable him to read.

Massage the parts of his body on which he lies and institute range-of-motion exercises for his limbs to help maintain muscle tone. Patients who are in casts and traction are particularly susceptible to hypostatic pneumonia. Deep-breathing exercises, blowing into a bottle of water through a straw, or singing should be carried out five or six times a day.

If a patient has a fracture of a cervical vertebra, he may graduate to a neck brace. Since he cannot look down with this brace on, he has to be careful when he walks.

## Fracture of the Mandible

Fractures of the mandible are treated frequently with wires that splint the lower jaw to the upper jaw. The nurse should be familiar with the wire loops that can be unhooked, and she should keep a pair of scissors strapped to the head of the bed for use in case the patient vomits. Because the patient cannot chew, he is given a liquid or, at best, a semi-liquid diet and may be fed through a straw. The patient's mouth should be cleansed thoroughly after each meal and every two hours. Retract the cheeks with a tongue depressor, and use a flashlight to see into the mouth. These fractures usually are compound. Complications include primary hemorrhage, asphyxia, and infection, which may lead to osteomyelitis.

## Fracture of the Clavicle

A fractured clavicle may be immobilized by a figure-of-8 bandage. When a fractured clavicle is immobilized with plaster, the cast usually is placed over padding applied in a figure-of-8 design. Felt is placed in the axilla to protect the axillary vessels and nerves. Initially, the patient may be uncomfortable. Pressure against the axilla can be relieved by abducting the arm or resting the elbows on the arms of a chair or a table. Encourage the patient to use his arms as naturally as possible. Motion will help to prevent "frozen shoulder."

## Fractured Ribs

Broken ribs are uncomfortable, since they must move when a person breathes. Often they are strapped for support, and usually they heal without trouble. They are treated with adhesive strapping, which crosses the midline to the unaffected side, front, and back, and is applied as the patient exhales. Shave the skin first to facilitate the removal of the tape. Pad the nipple area.

# DISLOCATIONS AND SPRAINS

*Dislocations* occur when the articular surfaces of a joint are no longer in contact. In adults they are caused by trauma or, less frequently, by disease of the joint. The symptoms are pain, malposition, leading to an abnormal axis of the dependent bone, and loss of the function of the joint. Treatment consists of manipulation of the joint until the parts are again in normal position, followed by immobilization by Ace bandage, cast or splint for several weeks to allow the joint capsule and surrounding ligaments to heal.

Manipulation never should be attempted by anyone except a physician, who usually makes an x-ray examination first and may anesthetize the patient for the procedure. Amateur attempts at reduction may injure further the capsule of the joint and surrounding structures and sometimes cause fractures or hemorrhage.

If the patient must be transported to the doctor, the affected joint should be splinted. After the reduction of the dislocation the nurse watches for compression resulting from tight bandages or a tight cast.

*Sprains* are injuries to the ligaments surrounding a joint. They are accompanied by pain, swelling, and loss of motion. They may become ecchymotic because of the rupture of the nearby blood vessels. An x-ray film may be taken to differentiate a sprain from a fracture. Treatment consists of elevation of the part and application of an elastic bandage. Buccal Varidase may be used early to minimize swelling. An injection of hydrocortisone and lidocaine at the point of maximum tenderness helps to relieve pain. There is a tendency now to treat sprains by having the patient continue to use the affected part after providing support with elastic bandage. An ankle, for example, may be strapped, after which the patient is allowed to walk.

## REFERENCES AND BIBLIOGRAPHY

ANDERSON, N.: Rehabilitative nursing practice, *Nurs. Clin. N. Am.* 6:303, June 1971.

BAILEY, J. A.: Tractions, suspensions, and a ringless splint, *Am. J. Nurs.* 70:1724, August 1970.

BENNAGE, B. A., and CUMMINGS, M. E.: Nursing the patient undergoing total hip arthroplasty, *Nurs. Clin. N. Am.* 8:107, March 1973.

BETTS, G. A.: An adjustable plastozote splint for the hand or arm, *Nurs. Times* 66:1556, December 1970.

BLAKE, F.: Immobilized youth—a rationale for supportive nursing intervention, *Am. J. Nurs.* 69:2364, November 1969.

BRADLEY, D.: Fractures of the pelvis, *Nurs. Times* 68:376, March 1972.

————: Fractures of the upper end of the femur: Clinical features, *Nurs. Times* 66:1523, November 1970.

————: Fractures of the upper end of the femur: Treatment, *Nurs. Times* 66:1552, December 1970.

BRUNNER, N. A.: *Orthopedic Nursing: A Programmed Approach,* St. Louis, Mosby, 1970.

CLISSOLD, G. K.: *The Body's Response To Trauma: Fractures,* New York, Springer, 1973.

CONWELL, H. E.: Injuries to the wrist, *Ciba Clin. Symp.* 22:1,3, 1970.

CORBEIL, M.: Nursing process for a patient with a body image disturbance, *Nurs. Clin. N. Am.* 6:155, March 1971.

DAVIS, L.: *Christopher's Textbook of Surgery,* ed. 9, Philadelphia, Saunders, 1968.

EATON, P., and HELLER, F.: Therapeutic nursing care of orthopedic patients, *Nurs. Clin. N. Am.* 2:429, September 1967.

ESAH, M.: Fractures of the tibia and fibula, *Nurs. Times* 68:258, March 1972.

EYRE, M. K.: Total hip replacement, *Am. J. Nurs.* 71:1384, July 1971.

GARTLAND, J. J.: *Practical Orthopedics,* ed. 2, Philadelphia, Saunders, 1972.

GRAVES, S., and VINCENT, S.: Total hip replacement is a family affair, *RN* 34:35, June 1971.

GRIFFIN, W., et al.: Group exercise for patients with limited motion, *Am. J. Nurs.* 71:1742, September 1971.

LARSON, C., and GOULD, M.: *Orthopedic Nursing,* ed. 8, St. Louis, Mosby, 1974.

LAW, J.: The fat embolism syndrome, *Nurs. Clin. N. Am.* 8:191, March 1973.

ROBERTS, J. M.: New developments in orthopedic surgery, *Nurs. Clin. N. Am.* 2:386, September 1967.

SMITH, A. P.: A day in my double life, *Am. J. Nurs.* 71:84, January 1971.

WILMOT, A.: Total knee joint replacement, *Nurs. Times* 69:626, May 1973.

# Patients with Diseases of the Bones and Joints

## CHAPTER 20

## ARTHRITIS

Numerous terms are used to describe the presence of pain in skeletal tissue.

*Rheumatism* refers to pain in the joints and other supporting tissues of the body, such as muscles, tendons, and bones. Pain in the joints alone is known as *arthralgia*. When arthralgia is associated with inflammation, the term *arthritis* is used.

Arthritis is not confined to man and may, in fact, afflict all higher animals, especially those whose capsular joints are lined with thin synovial membrane. Nor is it a modern phenomenon. Evidence of arthritis has been found in dinosaurs and other prehistoric animals and in the early remains of man, such as Egyptian mummies. Descriptions of arthritis are found in the earliest medical writings, including those of Hippocrates. The contemporary description of inflammation, as pain, swelling, localized redness, heat, and alteration of function goes back to Galen.

There are many forms of arthritis. The term is usually applied to diseases in which the major symptom involves joints. For most forms of arthritis, the cause remains unknown, and the various theories of causation are still subject to controversy. Rheumatoid arthritis, potentially the most crippling disease in this category because of its progressive nature and widespread involvement, has been included among the connective tissue disorders. This grouping, also called *collagen diseases,* suggests an underlying involvement of the connective tissues of the body and includes systemic lupus erythematosus, polyarteritis nodosa, progressive sys-

323

temic sclerosis, dermatomyositis, as well as rheumatoid arthritis and perhaps rheumatic fever. While the cause (or causes) of rheumatoid arthritis remains unknown, it can be fairly well-defined clinically in terms of its manifestations, Rheumatoid arthritis and many conditions similar to it will be discussed in this chapter; discussion of other diseases, seemingly closely related, will be found in other chapters.

### Incidence

Arthritis and the rheumatic diseases in general rank first among the causes of physical disability in the United States. Between 15 and 16 million people have arthritis of sufficient severity to interfere with the way they live their lives and the degree to which they are able to perform work. Perhaps half a million people are totally disabled by arthritis. However, some evidence of arthritis may exist in almost everyone over the age of 55, and it has been estimated that 30 to 50 million Americans may be afflicted, even if in the majority, few if any symptoms are present (other than some feelings of creakiness, temporary stiffness of joints, and minor aches in association with weather changes and excessive exercise). In adults the two major causes of disability due to arthritis are rheumatoid arthritis and degenerative joint disease.

### Types of Arthritis

A partial classification of the complex disease entities usually included in the term *arthritis* follows:

- Infectious arthritis
- Traumatic arthritis
- Polyarthritis of unknown etiology (example, rheumatoid arthritis)
- Degenerative joint disease (example, osteoarthritis)
- Arthritis associated with biochemical or endocrine abnormalities (example, gout)
- Tumor
- Allergy and drug reaction

## INFECTIOUS ARTHRITIS

Infectious arthritis may be caused by one of several specific microorganisms. With the current rise in the prevalence of venereal disease, increasing numbers of cases of gonococcal arthritis are being diagnosed. Staphylococci and streptococci also may cause arthritis, often in patients debilitated by other diseases, including rheumatoid arthritis, or those treated with corticosteroids. In both types of pa-

tients, the natural resistance to infections is lowered. While these three microorganisms all produce acute arthritis chiefly in adults, other bacteria may produce arthritis in children. A more chronic form of arthritis may result from invasion of joints by tubercle bacilli in untreated tuberculosis, and as part of fungal diseases, such as histoplasmosis or coccidioidomycosis, especially in parts of the country where these diseases are prevalent. Usually, only one joint is involved, with severe inflammation and associated adjacent muscle wasting in the cases of acute infections and more subtle signs in chronic infection.

The invasion by microorganisms produces an outpouring of synovial fluid, resulting in swelling because of *effusion*. The effusion contains innumerable white cells attempting to combat the infection, and in the process of ingesting the microorganisms, these cells release enzymes that may be destructive to protein complexes in the joint fluid and to the structure of the joint itself. While normal synovial fluid is clear, acellular, and viscous, infected fluid tends to be thin and cloudy, often purulent. Effusion results in swelling and pain.

If the fluid is removed from the joint, usually by aspiration into a syringe, it can be examined and cultured to identify the responsible microorganism. The appropriate antibiotic to eradicate the infection is usually administered systemically but sometimes is injected directly into the joint as well. Early diagnosis usually results in cure, although tuberculous arthritis and the arthritis resulting from untreated syphilis may require surgical correction.

## TRAUMATIC ARTHRITIS

Direct blows to the joint, such as those suffered by football players and other athletes, or a multitude of small insults to the joints, as in joggers and ballet dancers, may produce traumatic arthritis.

## RHEUMATOID ARTHRITIS

Rheumatoid arthritis is an inflammatory disease of connective tissue, characterized by chronicity, remissions, and exacerbations. Constitutional symptoms and joint changes, which may become permanent deformities, are part of the disease.

### Incidence

Rheumatoid arthritis is found throughout the world, although some believe that it is more common in temperate than in torrid climates. In the United States, 6 million people are estimated to have this form of arthritis; half of these are under the age of 45. This crippling disease strikes during the most productive years of adulthood. The majority of new cases begin between the ages of 25 and 50, but no age is spared, as rheumatoid arthritis may afflict infants or even the very old. An oddity is that while women barely outnumber men in the propensity to develop the disease, three times as many women as men develop sufficiently severe disease to need medical attention.

## Pathology

Rheumatoid arthritis is a systemic disorder; its nature is not fully understood, and its etiology is as yet unknown. However, the local effect in the joint can be described (Fig. 20-1). Some of this effect is due to the disease itself and some to the body's reactions against it. For example, the replacement of damaged tissue by fibrosis is a defense mechanism of the body. However, scars due to fibrosis can lead to crippling contractures.

Synovitis, the earliest pathologic change, causes congestion and edema. Fibroblasts, leukocytes, lymphocytes, plasma cells, and other materials proliferate from the synovial membrane, forming a tissue called a *pannus,* which soon invades the articular cartilage, slowly causing its lysis (breakdown)

and replacing it with tough fibrous tissue. When this tissue adheres also to the opposite joint surface, motion is inhibited. This is the stage of *fibrosis ankylosis* (abnormal immobility of a joint).

When the restricting band of tissue becomes calcified, as it may, the stage of *osseous ankylosis* has arrived, and the joint no longer exists. This process from nonspecific synovitis to complete ossification of the joint may take years, and it may proceed at different rates in different joints in the same patient.

On the other hand, the opposite phenomenon may occur. Rather than fusing the joint through ankylosis, rheumatoid arthritis may cause such severe destruction of the bone ends that the joint ceases to exist as a functional entity. Such mutilating arthritis may also take a long time to develop and is characteristically seen in some patients who have a disease resembling rheumatoid arthritis in association with a skin disorder known as psoriasis.

Nodules in the subcutaneous tissue develop in approximately 15 per cent of patients, especially those with the more severe forms of rheumatoid arthritis. They usually appear over pressure points, such as the elbows, extensor surfaces of the forearms, base of the spine, and back of the scalp and at the Achilles tendons of both the heels. They may be lodged in the subcutaneous tissues or bound to the underlying bone. They generally become painful only if continuous pressure is applied to them,

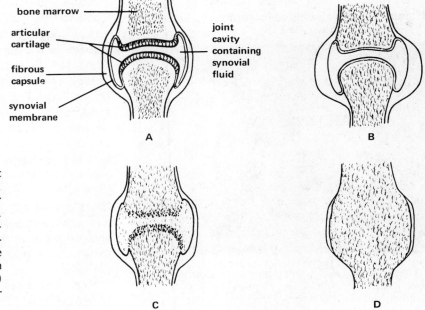

**Figure 20-1.** Pathologic changes in rheumatoid arthritis. (A) Normal joint, as in knee or between digits of fingers or toes. (B) Same joint, showing progression of pannus formation, destruction of cartilage and acute inflammation. (C) Inflammation subsided; fibrous ankylosis. (D) Bony ankylosis; the joint is immobile.

bone marrow

articular cartilage

fibrous capsule

synovial membrane

joint cavity containing synovial fluid

A

B

C

D

in which case they may cause a breakdown of overlying skin with resultant ulcers.

Muscles become weak and atrophy, partially from disuse. Because of connective-tissue changes and neurovascular changes, the extremities often have a smooth, glossy appearance and may be cold and clammy.

### Etiology

Although the causative factors of rheumatoid arthritis have not yet been discovered, some previously suspected theories have been ruled out. This disease is not caused by faulty diet, lack of vitamins, overdose of vitamins, or cold and damp weather. It is probable that arthritis is not caused by a single factor, but that one or more factors trigger the onset. Theories of etiology include the following.

**Infection and Immunity.** Although many types of organisms have been implicated as etiologic agents in rheumatoid arthritis over the past 50 years, none has withstood the test of close scrutiny. In spite of this there is a strong feeling that a viable agent (probably viruslike), will be found as research techniques improve. The organism itself may be the cause of the abnormal "autoimmune" reaction which causes the body to produce antibodies against its own tissues. These "autoantibodies" are of both diagnostic and pathologic significance.

**Faulty Adaptation to Physical or Psychic Stress.** Psychic stress as a cause of rheumatoid arthritis is associated more often with degenerative joint diseases. Studies, such as that conducted by Dr. Thomas Holmes and his colleagues at the University of Washington, have shown that illness is more likely to occur when an individual experiences stress. Thus, although a cause-and-effect relationship between illness and stress is often a matter of conjecture in an individual patient, data implicating psychological stress as a causative factor in the onset of many illnesses among groups of people studied indicates the need for concerned attention to the patient's history and present life circumstances when illness strikes.

**Inherited Factors.** Children of arthritic parents have a greater tendency to develop the disease than those whose ancestors have no such history. Heredity may be a factor, but the evidence pointing to this theory could be explained also by environmental factors. Perhaps a latent virus infection was passed from the mother to the child.

### Symptoms

In 75 to 80 per cent of the patients the onset is insidious. Over a period of time patients notice that a joint or two is stiff when they wake up in the morning. There are twinges of momentary discomfort in a finger or two. Slowly some joints, usually the fingers, become moderately sore, red, and swollen (Fig. 20-2). Over a period of weeks other joints become involved. Swelling and pain come and go. In the meantime the patients find that they tire easily. They lose weight and may develop a fever and a feeling of malaise. Tolerance for any kind of stress is lessened. Even temperature changes are tolerated poorly. Although the diet may be adequate in iron, patients characteristically have a persistent anemia because of the effect of this chronic disease on the blood-forming organs.

As the disease progresses, the muscle wasting around affected joints accentuates the appearance of swelling. The proximal finger joints swell the most, and as deformity develops, the fingers deviate toward the ulnar aspect of the hand. Extremities become cold, moist, and mauve-colored. Patients in this stage of the disease have considerable pain even at rest and especially on motion. Although the supporting muscles are in spasm, the ligaments are lax. Consequently, the affected joints are unstable and move in unnatural directions. They easily become dislocated; each time a dislocation occurs, there is some further damage to the supports and the joint surfaces.

Rheumatoid arthritis is a capricious disease. The symptoms may vanish suddenly for reasons appar-

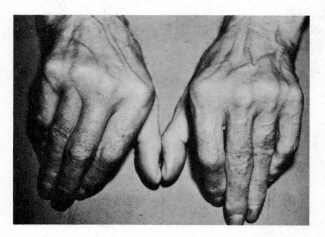

**Figure 20-2.** Appearance typical of arthritic hands. The joints become sore, swollen and deformed. (Medichrome—Clay-Adams, Inc., New York, N.Y.)

ent to neither the physician nor the patient. Inflammation leaves the joints that were sore and red; the patient is not stiff, he has no fever, and his pain is gone. However, the symptoms almost invariably return after the patient has had a symptom-free period. Inflammation causes more joint damage, and then there is another remission. The pattern of remissions and exacerbations continues over the years.

Without treatment—and sometimes with it—the joint may be destroyed totally. As the synovial space is replaced with bony growth, motion is lost. When the joint becomes immobile, the pain of the inflammation is lessened, but there is still discomfort because of contractures and immobility. One of the aims of treatment is to decrease the inflammation of the joint before it has become one bone.

## Treatment

Although the cause of rheumatoid arthritis is still a mystery, and the disease cannot be cured, much can be done to lessen its damage. Early treatment before the onset of fibrous or bony ankylosis gives the best results. Treatment is designed to make the patient more comfortable, to prevent or to correct deformities, and to maintain or restore function of the affected parts of the musculoskeletal system.

Optimal health conditions should be maintained, since supporting the resistance of the body to the inflammation is one of the few truly therapeutic steps that medicine has to offer. Rest, both systemic and local, is balanced carefully with exercise. Even during an acute phase of the illness some movement of the affected parts usually is prescribed to help lessen the possibility of bony ankylosis, muscle wasting, osteoporosis, and the debilitating effects of prolonged rest. Deep breathing and prescribed exercises, graded to the condition of the patient, strengthen general body tone and keep specific muscle groups from atrophying. The patient should be encouraged to eat an optimum diet, even though he may have little appetite. Unless there are other medical complications such as diabetes or hypertension, this diet need not be modified from that of a normal individual.

### Drug Therapy

Drug therapy in rheumatoid arthritis is not curative, but it helps the patient to feel less pain, and in some instances it depresses the inflammatory process (antiphlogistic action). Because of the long-term nature of this disease, the relief of pain by the use of narcotics is avoided.

**The Salicylates.** Aspirin (acetylsalicylic acid) is the major drug in this group. In early rheumatoid arthritis, it seems to reduce inflammation and to afford specific relief of joint pain and stiffness. In chronic rheumatoid arthritis the relief appears less dramatic, but it still is present, and probably it is more related to the general analgesic properties of aspirin than to any specific action. The manner in which this common drug works still is not fully understood.

The usual dose in rheumatoid arthritis is two to four (0.3 Gm.) tablets two to six times a day. Some physicians give the drug until the serum level of salicylates reaches 25 mg. per 100 ml.

SIDE EFFECTS. Some people have an allergy to aspirin, which briefly manifests itself as a skin rash or as asthma. Large doses of aspirin, which may help the inflammatory process to subside, also may give rise to the side effects of salicylism: nausea, vomiting, tinnitus, deafness, drowsiness, hyperpnea (rapid respiration), slow pulse, and peripheral vasodilation.

Hyperpnea, rare in adults, may lead to alkalosis through the excessive loss of carbon dioxide. These effects are reversible by stopping the medication.

Dehydration should be prevented since it can lead to serious salicylate toxicity (particularly in children), during hot summer months.

Another serious problem is that aspirin may erode the mucosa of the stomach, leading to multiple small spots of bleeding. Patients on high doses of aspirin should be instructed to watch their stools for evidence of gastrointestinal bleeding (black, tarry stool). Rarely, there may be interference with kidney function or blood clotting.

Milk and crackers taken before the drug may help to prevent gastric distress. Buffered or enteric-coated aspirin sometimes is ordered. If the patient experiences distress that seems to be related to his aspirin intake, the physician should be notified. Some patients decrease the dose or omit the tablets entirely without consulting the physician, and yet control of the symptoms depends on a high, sustained blood level of the drug. If the patient is experiencing toxic side effects, the physician should be informed.

**Phenylbutazone (Butazolidin).** This drug has been found to be effective as an analgesic and antiphlogistic in about 50 per cent of the patients with rheumatoid arthritis. If phenylbutazone is not effective within one to two weeks, it is discontinued. It is given by mouth in doses of 100 to 400 mg. a day.

SIDE EFFECTS. Side effects include nausea, abdominal pain, skin rash, visual disturbances, dizziness, lethargy, fever, anemia, and edema from sodium retention, especially in patients with cardiac problems. Serious toxic reactions may occur, such as the reactivation of a peptic ulcer with gastric bleeding, agranulocytosis, leukopenia, thrombocytopenic purpura, exfoliative dermatitis, psychosis, hypertension, and toxic hepatitis. Many patients receiving this drug have adverse effects. Patients maintained on phenylbutazone need periodic blood counts.

*Oxyphenbutazone* (Tandearil) is a related compound with much the same effects and dosage.

**Indomethacin (Indocin).** This drug is an unrelated anti-inflammatory drug which also has been found useful in about 50 per cent of patients. Unfortunately, it is not yet predictable which patients will respond well to it. The dosage is usually 25 mg. given three or four times daily *with meals.*

SIDE EFFECTS. Gastrointestinal intolerance, mental changes, dizziness, visual problems, and, rarely, effects upon blood-forming tissues may complicate prolonged therapy.

**Other Anti-inflammatory Drugs.** Many other anti-inflammatory agents are currently in various stages of development and testing. No others have as yet been released for prescription use in the United States, but many are available in foreign markets. Some are chemically similar to agents already discussed, and others are entirely new formulas. Effort is underway to develop anti-inflammatory agents that may prove to be more effective than existing ones, require less frequent administration, help a greater proportion of patients, or produce fewer undesirable toxic effects. Tests thus far have suggested several of the newer compounds may well qualify on more than one count. In the near future, one or more may well be approved by the federal Food and Drug Administration.

**Immunosuppressives.** Chief among a number of experimental drugs are the so-called immunosuppressive agents, notably cyclophosphamide (Cytoxan) and azathioprine (Imuran) which were developed as anticancer drugs. They are utilized only in advanced active disease and result in depression of the lymphoid cells which are immunologically active. It is not known whether this is the reason for their effect on rheumatoid arthritis and other collagen diseases.

**Antimalarials.** Antimalarials include quinacrine hydrochloride (Atabrine), chloroquine (Aralen), and hydroxychloroquine (Plaquenil). These drugs show an affinity for connective tissue and so are used sometimes to help to control the inflammation of arthritis. They usually require some time to show their effects (three to six weeks). Quinacrine hydrochloride is used rarely, because it turns the skin yellow.

SIDE EFFECTS. Toxic effects may include anemia, such eye symptoms as blurred vision, halo around lights, and difficulty in adjusting to glare, and gastrointestinal symptoms. Chloroquine and hydroxychloroquine may deposit in the retina of the eye, and if the damage they produce is not detected in time, it may result in blindness. For this reason, chloroquine is no longer recommended for use in rheumatoid arthritis. Hydroxychloroquine, however, is more likely to be used in life-threatening diseases related to rheumatoid arthritis.

**Soluble Gold Salts.** Soluble gold salts are gold sodium thiomalate (Myochrysine) and gold thioglucose (Solganal). Recent studies seem to have confirmed what rheumatologists have long suspected on the basis of clinical observations: administration of gold salts seems to be the most effective therapeutic approach for inducing suppression of ongoing rheumatoid arthritis. The reason for the effectiveness of gold salts remains obscure; however, prolonged administration can offer a sizable proportion of patients considerable relief and may prevent destructive changes in the joints in a majority. A minority of patients develop toxic symptoms of sufficient severity to require discontinuation of the drug, but many of these patients simultaneously develop remission of their symptoms. Only a small minority of patients fail to respond. From the initiation of gold salt administration, also known as *chrysotherapy,* there is usually a two or three month lag before efficacy becomes apparent. During this time, control of symptoms must be achieved with anti-inflammatory or other medication.

Administration of gold salts should always be intramuscular, preferably into the outer upper gluteal quadrant. Gold sodium thiomalate, being a solution, is easier to administer. Gold thioglucose is a suspension and must be shaken very well before being drawn into the syringe, and usually requires a 20-gauge needle for administration.

SIDE EFFECTS. Toxic reactions of minor degree may occur in about one-third of the patients; these include itching of the skin, mild albuminuria, or mouth sores. These may be regarded as danger signs and if they occur, gold salts are either reduced in dosage or discontinued. More severe reactions include exfoliative dermatitis, nephritis, hematuria, and suppression of platelets, white blood cells, or red blood cells, sometimes to an alarming degree. Most toxic reactions are reversible, usually some time after discontinuation of the drug. In some instances they require antidotes in the form of corticosteroids or BAL. As the antidotes themselves may cause serious unwanted reactions, they are employed only in life-threatening situations.

Some patients may develop nitritoid crises immediately after administration of gold salts; the symptoms include a flushing feeling, light headedness, and pounding headache. They represent an allergy to the solvent, not to the gold salt itself, and last only a few minutes. An occasional patient will develop an exacerbation of joint pain within a day or so after each injection of gold salts. Other toxic manifestations, such as jaundice, hepatitis, and severe gastrointestinal upsets have been claimed to result from gold salts, but the evidence is not conclusive.

Many patients receive a test dose of 10 mg. intramuscularly, followed by a 25-mg. dose a week later, and then, if no signs of intolerance have appeared, 50 mg. weekly, or less, depending upon the judgment of the physician. When the total dose approaches 1 Gm., a maintenance regimen is introduced, with the interval between injections gradually increasing to approximately one month. Patients who show positive response and fail to develop signs of toxicity may well receive gold salts for long periods, perhaps for life.

**Corticosteroids.** Synthetic hormones designed to duplicate the action of adrenocortical steroid hormones are widely used because they give fairly prompt relief from pain and stiffness. Physical and mental well-being are improved, and patients are able to remain active at work and in their daily activities. However, the progression of rheumatoid arthritis is not halted, so that the ultimate outlook is not improved. Moreover, the long-term use of corticosteroids may result in untoward effects that may be more disabling and ultimately life threatening than the disease being treated. Ideally, the lowest dose possible to achieve partial suppression for the shortest period of time should be given. Unfortunately, it is difficult to discontinue corticosteroids once they have been started, so that great care must be used in selecting the patients who receive these drugs. Continued close supervision by a physician is imperative.

Prednisone, prednisolone, methylprednisolone, betamethasone, dexamethasone, and triamcinolone are the most commonly used synthetic corticosteroids. Their relative potency varies, but as a rule of thumb, one standard-sized tablet of any of these is approximately equivalent to any other. The standard of measure is prednisone, and most patients will respond to doses of 2.5 to 5.0 mg. daily. Only a rare patient receives more than 15 mg. a day.

Hydrocortisone (cortisone) is another of the corticosteroids used. Among the functions of hydrocortisone are the regulation of carbohydrate metabolism and ionic balance and the ability to stand stress. It is administered orally in 10-mg. dosages, four times daily.

CORTICOTROPIN (ACTH, ACTHAR). This drug is derived from the pituitary gland and acts to stimulate the adrenal cortex. It is given to patients to stimulate their own production of hydrocortisone. When ACTH is given to a patient, his natural anterior pituitary gland production is reduced, and his adrenal cortices hypertrophy as they are stimulated to do increased work.

Because ACTH is destroyed in the gastrointestinal tract, it is given intramuscularly or intravenously rather than orally. A usual dose is 10 U. o.d. IM of corticotropin gel.

ADMINISTERING CORTICOSTEROIDS. In addition to oral doses and intramuscular and intravenous injections, corticosteroids can be administered directly into the joint. Hydrocortisone derivatives are used. The dose usually depends on the size of the joint. There are a variety of techniques; some physicians merely inject the corticosteroid, others first aspirate fluid for analysis. Some physicians inject the joint after careful cleansing of the skin alone, while others use surgical drapes and gloves. Aspiration of fluid tends to relieve some of the pressure within the joint and results in transient pain relief. The injection of corticosteroids can prolong pain relief and diminish signs of inflammation. A tray for this purpose usually includes ethyl chloride spray, various-sized syringes and needles, antiseptic solutions (preferably iodine-containing), lidocaine for skin infiltration when desired, and vials of corticosteroid designed for intralesional or intra-articular use.

Most patients who have rheumatoid arthritis can expect about three weeks of relief of inflammation in the injected joints, and some may even show transient general well-being suggesting absorption of corticosteroid from the joint. The injections are not without hazard; a rare infection may be introduced during injection, and repeated injections of a given joint may promote breakdown of the joint, probably as a result of overuse of a diseased joint that feels well. Nevertheless, corticosteroid injections represent valuable adjunctive therapy for control of acute symptoms that punctuate the chronic disease, and aspiration of joints yields valuable diagnostic clues.

SUPPLEMENTS. Since therapy with corticosteroids results in a negative nitrogen balance in the body, supplementary gonadal hormones, because of their anticatabolic action, also are prescribed by some physicians, especially for elderly and postmenopausal patients. Unexpected vaginal bleeding should be reported to the physician, and the female patient should have regular pelvic examinations.

Since the various preparations of cortisone depress natural adrenocortical activity, and ACTH depresses natural anterior pituitary activity, the sudden withdrawal of the drugs causes severe symptoms. When cortisone is discontinued abruptly, the patient has headache, nausea, retching, severe anorexia, weight loss, malaise, aches and pains, restlessness, insomnia and fatigue. To allow the body to resume its own production of hormones, both cortisone and ACTH are tapered off slowly; each day a little less is given.

SIDE EFFECTS. Side effects of both the corticosteroids and ACTH are frequent, as patients usually are kept on these drugs for long periods of time. The lower the dose, the less is the chance of developing serious side effects.

One of the most dangerous effects, the suppression of inflammation, is what makes the arthritic patient feel better; but this advantage carries with it a penalty. Inflammation is a body defense that serves the dual purpose of fighting infections and, by pain and swelling, calling attention to the troubled part of the body. A patient on steroids loses along with the pain of inflammation much of his ability to fight infection. Symptoms are suppressed, and because they can go unnoticed, they can go untreated. An arthritic patient on high dosages of steroids may have an infected tooth or appendicitis and never know it because the symptoms are masked. The unchallenged infection can proceed to septicemia or a ruptured appendix, as the steroids depress the symptoms of inflammation without curing the infection. One of the most important points in the nursing care of the patient on steroid therapy is observation for the slightest sign of trouble anywhere in the body. The smallest rise in temperature or the slightest discomfort in a new area is reported immediately to the doctor.

Another common side effect is weight gain due both to an accumulation of fat and to a redistribution of ions in the fluid compartments of the body. Sodium is retained, and potassium is lost. The patient frequently becomes edematous; he acquires a moonface and perhaps a buffalo hump. These changes are not usually considered an indication to discontinue the drug. A low sodium diet may be ordered. Because of the possibility of developing edema, the patient's weight is observed carefully both in the hospital and at home. The patient should be instructed to keep a record of his weight, weighing himself at intervals as recommended by his physician.

Steroids can give rise to peptic ulcers. Complaints of gastric distress should be noted, and reported promptly to the physician. Acne may appear in a patient who believed that he was far enough beyond adolescence never again to be troubled with it. There also may be increased pigmentation of skin, hirsutism (hairiness), easy bruising, amenorrhea (cessation of menstruation), osteoporosis, weakness, and mental depression.

Posterior subcapsular cataracts frequently develop during long-term corticosteroid therapy. These do not always interfere with vision but sometimes require surgical removal. Severe skin ulcers, which heal slowly at best, may develop and cannot readily be corrected by grafts. Peripheral neuritis is a danger symptom, usually indicating the onset of vasculitis. This condition, an inflammation around small blood vessels, mimics the potentially fatal disease, polyarteritis nodosa and is seen predominantly in rheumatoid arthritis patients receiving corticosteroids, so that the inference has been drawn that the corticosteroids may well be responsible. Indeed, reduction of corticosteroid dosage can result in amelioration of vasculitis, but so can increase of corticosteroid dosage. Destructive changes of the femoral and to a lesser extent the humeral leads because of aseptic necrosis is also thought to be a result of prolonged corticosteroid administration.

Some studies have indicated a considerable increase in mortality in patients receiving these powerful hormones. In part, this may be the result of reduced ability to withstand stress, such as surgery, accidents, and other trying situations because of relative adrenal suppression. During periods of stress, such patients must receive larger doses of corticosteroids, and up to a year or more after discontinuation of corticosteroid administration, patients undergoing surgery should be "covered" with adequate corticosteroid dosage preoperatively and postoperatively.

Many patients are naturally concerned about the changes in their appearance resulting from corticosteroids. Generally, these changes are minimized by low dosage and may ultimately disappear almost completely when corticosteroids are stopped. However, corticosteroid reduction is a slow and agonizing process, often giving rise to new symptoms of diffuse pains, depression, lassitude, loss of appetite, weight loss, and stiffness for longer periods of time. These do not necessarily mean that the disease being treated is coming back, and if patients are willing to persevere, these symptoms may abate.

## Other Therapeutic Modalities

**Heat.** Heat is more of a comfort than a curative measure. Because it improves circulation and relieves muscle spasm and pain, it allows the part better rest and easier exercise. Heat can be applied dry or wet. Dry heat sometimes is applied by a heating pad (on low—to prevent burns), a paraffin bath, an infrared bulb, a hot-water bag or an appliance such as the Aquamatic pad which maintains a constant degree of heat. The ordinary heating pad is not as effective as other measures. Infrared heat penetrates deeper than the level of the skin. Even superficial heat affects deeper-level blood vessels by reflex action. Diathermy and ultrasonic therapy do not seem to have a special advantage in rheumatoid arthritis (Beeson and McDermott, 1971).

Many arthritic patients prefer wet heat, claiming that it penetrates better. Wet heat can be applied in the form of baths, either local or tub (Fig. 20-3). Patients who have advanced disease may find getting in and out of a tub too much of a struggle; in such cases, towels dipped in water at 116 degrees F., wrung out and applied are effective. Heat in any form should be applied for 20 to 30 minutes.

The application of pure lanolin or other lotions may help to counter the drying effects of this treatment.

There has been an increasing interest on the part of physicians and physical therapists in the use of cold rather than heat for relief of pain and spasm. There are strong advocates for both modalities. Patients frequently find much greater relief with one modality over the other.

Massage improves the flow of both blood and lymph, but it is not used on a joint that is actively inflamed, as it may aggravate the disease.

**Splinting.** An extended rheumatoid arthritic joint is under greater pressure than a flexed one, accounting for the tendency of patients to keep their joints bent. While these measures help, they may not be enforceable because of discomfort. In such cases, splinting may be a valuable adjunct.

*Braces, bivalve casts, or splints* applied to joints that are painful and in spasm help to prevent dislocations and deformity and to keep the rest of the joints mobile. Splints have three basic functions:

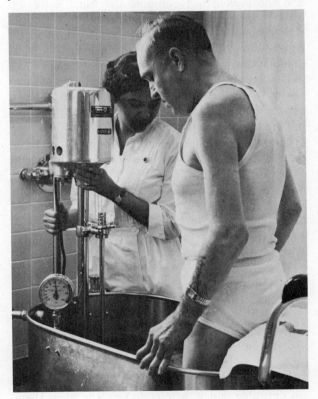

**Figure 20-3.** The warmth (the water temperature is 104 degrees F.) and the swirling action of the whirlpool, here administered by the physical therapist, is beneficial to inflamed arthritic joints. Note the deformity of the patient's hands.

(1) to immobilize the part for local rest during an active phase of the disease; (2) to correct deformities, such as provided by a long brace with a turnbuckle across the back of the knee to help place that joint in extension; and (3) to help overcome weakness.

Resting splints can be fabricated of plaster of Paris, or commercially available lightweight plastic splints may be used. A splinted joint tends to hurt less or to lose all its pain, so that the splint will find ready acceptance. Long leg splints to keep the knee straight are the most common resting splints, and many therapists also use resting splints for the hand to keep wrists and fingers straight. Rest can also be achieved during activity by use of a functional splint, which supports some joints while leaving others free to act.

The most commonly used of these are functional splints for the wrists which support the wrist and hand while leaving the thumb and fingers completely free. As a result, grip strength is enhanced, and the patient can continue the usual activities. This splint is applied in a position of function, which means very slight extension of the dominant hand (for power) and very slight flexion of the nondominant hand (for toilet activities) (Ehrlich, 1972).

Braces attached to shoes to support unstable ankles or similar braces for the knees also serve to assure some stability and decrease pain while permitting the patient to function.

If poor posture is imposing an abnormal strain on weight-bearing joints, the patient may be fitted with a corset that improves posture. The splint or brace must fit well, be neither constricting nor loose, be lightweight, and must maintain the joint in a good functional position. Observe for friction on the skin. Adequate padding and good skin care protect the skin. Check for rough edges that might tear the skin of the patient. Once a week the leather parts should be saddle-soaped, and the metal joints oiled.

**Stretch Gloves.** Sometimes the overnight wearing of two-way stretch gloves (such as those made of nylon and spandex that are readily available at department store glove counters) will help relieve some of the stiffness and discomfort in arthritic hands. These gloves are strictly adjunctive, but they are desirable and well tolerated except when rheumatoid arthritis or osteoarthritis is accompanied by severe local inflammation, in which case the pressure they exert may not be tolerated well (Ehrlich, 1973).

**Surgery.** The use of surgery to overcome or prevent deformity is becoming an increasingly important aspect of early treatment. Previously surgery was resorted to only late in the disease after extensive damage had been wrought. Synovectomy (removal of the diseased lining) performed early is being extensively investigated as a means of preventing destructive changes in affected joints, particularly those of the hands, feet, and knees. When muscle spasm is causing progressive deformity, tendons may be transplanted to change the direction of pull to a corrected one. An artificial angling of the bone through surgical fracture (osteotomy) may improve the utility of a deformed limb.

ARTHROPLASTY. Arthroplasty, the fashioning of a new joint with artificial material, may be resorted to.

Initially, only parts of joints were replaced, such as the Vitallium cup for the acetabulum, or new heads of bones. Now, many of the operations are total arthroplasties, in which both components of the joint are replaced. Two different materials are usually used—steel and some form of plastic. Thus, hips, knees, elbows, shoulders, and carpal bones have been replaced. For the fingers and knuckles, the ends of the bone are removed, and silicone-plastic spaces are introduced to keep the joint open, stable, and mobile. Many of these operations employ surgical cement (methylcrylate) for fixation. This cement hardens very quickly in the operating room, and patients can often use their new joints within a week of surgery. The length of postsurgical convalescence has thus greatly been decreased. So successful has this approach been, that the arthrodesis (fusion of the joint surfaces) which was formerly advocated for severely painful and unstable joints has been all but abandoned (Ehrlich, 1973).

It is especially important that postoperative exercises be applied when and as prescribed by the surgeon. For example, following synovectomy and arthroplasty of the fingers there may be lateral instability, and exercises requiring wide spreading of the fingers with abduction and adduction motions must be avoided.

## NURSING ASSESSMENT AND INTERVENTION

### Cognitive and Affective Factors

Arthritis is usually a long-term condition, and, except during periods of acute exacerbation, the patient's care is carried out at home with periodic visits to the physician or clinic. Family health practitioners and nurses in independent practice may carry considerable responsibility for the patient's health care over extended periods, assessing the condition of the patient's joints and his response to medication, exercise, and other treatment. Such practice requires a high degree of collaboration between nurse and physician, so that each contributes maximally to the patient's care and rehabilitation. Assessment of the patient's understanding of his illness and of his ability to care for himself is of primary importance.

**Patient Education.** Arthritis is a well-known cause of pain, crippling, and deformity. Often the patient makes the diagnosis himself on the basis of his symptoms. The physician's confirmation of the diagnosis can spark fears of incapacity, even though the disease may at the time cause only moderate pain and stiffness in a few joints. The patient with rheumatoid arthritis is faced with a disease whose course is typically unpredictable. Intelligent management of his symptoms by such measures as heat, analgesics, exercise, and rest often are effective in helping the patient continue his usual activities.

It is essential for the patient to learn that rheumatoid arthritis has spontaneous remissions. This tendency toward an uneven course of remissions and exacerbations promotes quackery, because remission may coincide with the use of some "miraculous" cure. The well-informed patient who is helped to accept the fluctuations in his symptoms is less likely to fall prey to worthless and misleading treatment and remedies, such as vibrating pillows ($12 to $50), copper ankle disks and bracelets ($30 to $300), vibrating chairs ($600), "radioactive earth" ($10), and uranium mine visits (four for $100).

There are various remedies which do help patients, although their effectiveness may sometimes seem overstated. Local applications such as oil of wintergreen, which contains methylsalicylate, may be helpful. By causing vasodilation, it can promote feelings of warmth and relaxation of the part. The warm whirlpool bath of a nearby health spa may ease stiffness and pain. For patients who can afford it, a vacation at a residential spa may ease symptoms by providing release from a tense environment at home or work. Climate is neither causative nor curative. However, if the patient enjoys warmer weather, and if his spirits improve and he is able to relax and exercise more comfortably, such a change may be beneficial.

**Emotional Factors.** Disease processes often make their appearance when an individual is under stress, and the anxiety over illness becomes an additional emotional, as well as physical, burden. The nurse who is sensitive to the patient and who recognizes his emotional and physical responses can assist him to break the vicious circle. Expressing such feelings as anger, frustration, or a sense of immobilization in a disturbing life situation can assist the patient to deal more effectively with his physical ills and may lessen the severity of his symptoms. Relief of anxiety is particularly important among patients with arthritis, since increased muscle spasm, with resultant intensification of pain, may occur when the patient is anxious.

Arthritis requires considerable self-care. For some patients, willingness to spend time in such activities as using warm applications or baths and making an effort to work out a daily schedule providing for alternating periods of rest and activity may conflict with ideals of caring for the needs of others. In any illness requiring considerable self-care, it is essential to assess the patient's willingness to carry out the care and to assist him to understand his own values and attitudes toward the necessary treatment. Often the nurse can serve as a "sounding board" to whom the patient may reveal problems or anxieties kept from the physician, either because the patient was too shy to talk of them or because the physician seemed too busy.

An important area is the patient's sexual adjustment, which usually suffers because of the physical derangements or emotional problems induced by arthritis. The nurse can help the patient through discussion and consideration of the problems, and can collaborate with the physician on measures recommended that can solve the problems. This important area of human functioning need not be compromised by arthritis (Ehrlich, 1973).

## Age and Developmental Level

Assessment of the patient in relation to age, developmental level, and socioeconomic factors is essential, so that care can be planned to assist him in furthering his own goals despite the illness.

Frequently rheumatoid arthritis has its onset in early adulthood, when responsibilities to a developing career and family are heavy. Curtailment of the patient's physical abilities may result in irreparable loss of opportunities for further education, occupational advancement and increased income, and personally enjoyable activities such as hobbies, travel, or sports. Early and persistent efforts to treat the disease may lessen these destructive results. The focus of nursing should be creative, in helping the patient to fulfill his life, as contrasted with custodial care which is concerned with maintaining the status quo.

The adult who experiences the long-term effects of rheumatoid arthritis or the onset of osteoarthritis needs help to avoid acquiescence to premature withdrawal from his vocational and leisure-time activities. If he allows himself to be discouraged by the stiffness and pain and willingly accepts the view that nothing can be done for such symptoms in later life he will forfeit numerous opportunities and enjoyments.

For the elderly, the problems are multiple. Aching, stiff joints may lead the patient to stay at home, since public transportation is too arduous, and taxi fare is beyond his means. Gnarled fingers may make food preparation difficult, opening the safety caps on medicine bottles may also pose a problem. Shopping, with the necessity for handling bags of groceries, may present serious difficulties, and the patient's nutrition may suffer. Shopping services for such patients, and such community programs as "Meals on Wheels," providing one hot meal per day delivered to the patient's home, can greatly improve nutrition and help the patient to continue to care for himself in his own home.

Costs of health care loom large, presenting a particular hardship for those of moderate and low income who may find that opportunities for economic advancement are wiped out by the continued financial drain of long-term treatment and the curtailment of earning power which may result from the condition. It is essential for the nurse to assist the patient to seek the financial assistance for which he is eligible, through such programs as veterans benefits and insurance plans.

### Physical Factors

**General Assessment.** Physical assessment of the patient with arthritis involves such factors as inspection of joints, consideration of the subjective symptoms reported by the patient, and assessment of overall health.

Observe the joints for heat, redness, swelling, deformity, and limitation of motion. Note whether subcutaneous nodules are present over such areas as the elbows, heels, and the base of the spine. The patient's skin over the affected joints is usually smooth, shiny, thin, and fragile.

Ask the patient about the presence of pain and stiffness, and the circumstances under which these symptoms are aggravated and relieved. Evaluate with him his ability to perform various activities. If his condition is acute, most of this evaluation will be verbal. If his condition is less acute, ask him to demonstrate range of joint motion and to describe recent losses or gains in function.

It is particularly essential with the rheumatoid arthritis patient to note changes in symptoms at frequent intervals, since symptoms tend to fluctuate. Because of lessened activity, muscle strength is often appreciably diminished. Thus in the acutely ill patient breathing may be shallow, and tachycardia may result from even mild exertion.

For the patient with acute rheumatoid arthritis, the following aspects of assessment are also especially important: body temperature, diaphoresis, weight (particularly weight loss), appetite, and bowel function (because of limited exercise, constipation may present a problem). Particularly in the acutely ill patient who has fever and whose discomfort has led him to neglect fluid intake, the urine may be concentrated and scanty.

The physical aspects of nursing intervention involve rest, exercise, positioning, and alleviating such symptoms as undernourishment, dehydration, constipation, fatigue, and the pain and stiffness of joints.

**Rest.** The acutely ill patient particularly requires rest. A bed cradle can provide comfort by keeping bedclothes off inflamed joints. Because joints limited in motion tend to take the form of flexion, which leads to contractures, the resting position of the joints should be the position of greatest possible extension without actual pain. Splinting, if ordered by the physician, can alleviate pain and lessen the possibility of deformity. The *bed* should be flat and firm with only one small pillow. A bed board that fits should be placed under the mattress and firmly attached, so that when the patient moves near the edge, he is not in danger of tipping the bed board over. The height of the bed should be level with that of the wheelchair, if the patient moves back and forth between the two. The bed should not be so low that it causes the person who cares for the patient to develop backache. A bed adjustable in height is desirable, not only to facilitate care while the patient is in bed, but also to make it easier for him to get out of bed. If such a bed is not available, and the bed is too low, it can be elevated on cinder or wood blocks. If a conventional footboard is not available, one can be made from a wooden box.

*A good chair* for an arthritic patient, be it mobile or stationary, should be 3 to 4 inches higher than the usual chair to prevent excessive bending at the hips. The patient's feet should be firmly planted, and the body should be firmly supported throughout and kept in good alignment. Pillows are not as comfortable as their softness implies, because they tend to cause the patient to hunch over, and they lead to fatigue. Since a wheelchair may seem cumbersome in a small apartment or a house and may not pass through the doorway, a straight-backed kitchen chair with arms can be fitted with four casters.

**Nourishment and Elimination.**  Small, tempting, easily digested meals with between-meal snacks can encourage the patient to eat. Fluid intake should be encouraged, unless the physician indicates that this measure is contraindicated. Stool softeners, suppositories, or Fleet's enemas may be ordered to alleviate constipation.

**Pain Relief.**  Sedatives or tranquilizers may be ordered to lessen anxiety and promote rest. Medications (previously discussed) are prescribed by the physician to relieve distressing symptoms of painful, stiff joints. Observation of the patient's response to any drug prescribed, particularly if corticosteroids are prescribed, is essential and must include awareness of side effects as well as therapeutic response. Drug interactions also must be considered. These patients are advised against taking both aspirin and warfarin (Coumadin).

**Exercise.**  Appropriate exercise can often preserve or increase the function of the joint by preventing ankylosis, maintaining muscle tone, and improving strength and coordination. Only gentle stretching is permissible. Excessive exercise can lead to pain or fatigue, while vigorous exercise of an inflamed joint or movement that increases joint instability and abnormal deviation and dislocation can cause further damage. The type and amount of exercise are prescribed by the physician. The physical therapist has a primary responsibility for carrying out this aspect of the treatment when the patient is under his care.

The nurse has an important role in carrying out the objectives concerning positioning and exercise during the patient's daily care and in teaching the patient to implement these objectives himself.

Whenever possible (in relation to severity of the joint involvement) each joint should go through its full range of motion at least once daily. Active exercise is preferable to passive exercise. As the patient's condition improves and his tolerance increases, the amount of exercise is gradually increased.

Teach the patient to:

- **Exercise affected joints several times a day, carefully following the physician's recommendations concerning which joints to exercise and what exercises to use.**
- **Expect some discomfort but avoid exercising to the point of pain and fatigue.**
- **Use several short periods of exercise daily, rather than fewer longer periods. For example several periods of 5 to 10 minutes are usually better tolerated than one 30-minute period.**
- **Maintain a balance between rest and activity. Rest stops on long drives can prevent stiffness, as can walking about at intervals while watching television.**
- **Consult the physician about whether the patient may take aspirin before he exercises. Some patients find that taking analgesics and applying heat before and after exercise alleviates pain and stiffness.**

**Equipment.**  Various mechanical aids have been devised to help the disabled in the performance of day-to-day tasks (Fig. 20-4). Rare is the arthritic for whom a mechanism cannot be fashioned that helps him to feed himself, comb his own hair, select his own programs on the television set, and cope with more complex and specialized problems. Some mechanical aids are currently on the market; others can be custom-built, very often of improvised materials, if a little ingenuity is employed. A device should be lightweight and as simple as possible. If the patient finds it inconvenient or does not like it for any reason, he will not use it.

Not every action of the arthritic should be governed by a gadget. Indeed, his life will be simpler if he has to take care of only a few appliances, but if a device can give the patient the necessary independence, encourage him to use it.

## Other Considerations for the Arthritic Patient

Because most types of arthritis, once acquired, will stay with the patient the rest of his life, and because at least some of the course that the disease takes will depend on how he handles himself, nursing attention must turn also to the long-term status of the patient's mind, body, and emotions.

Any chronic disease tends to make a person think more about his body than he would ordinarily. This tendency is especially true in arthritis. What the patient does for and to himself can make a difference in the progress of his disease: the patient with gout who resists a sweetbreads dinner, the patient with osteoarthritis who improves his posture when he loses weight, the patient with rheumatoid arthritis who follows his prescribed regimen of exercise and rest. Yet too much concentration on self can warp a personality. Activities that truly interest the patient, especially those that bring some income, help to divert the patient from unhealthy preoccupation with himself. With a regimen of rest, exercise, medication, good diet, and physical therapy, some patients avoid becoming crippled.

## Home Care

Many arthritic patients are confined to the home. Nursing attention then broadens to include the patient's total environment. A nurse going into the patient's home might ask herself questions such as these: What is the physical setup? How can it be arranged to allow the patient to be as active as he can be? How can it be arranged for maximum privacy for both the patient and others in the family? Does the patient have his own room? Can he get in and out of his room without help? What work can the patient do? Can the ironing board or the sink be arranged so that the patient can reach them?

Some arthritic patients have deformities that are far advanced, and the nurse finds them seemingly beyond rehabilitation. Sometimes the disease is overpowering; treatment was not begun in time, or it was inadequate.

Whatever the condition of the patient, the nurse should concentrate on making the most of his re-

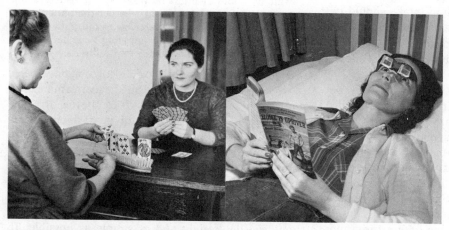
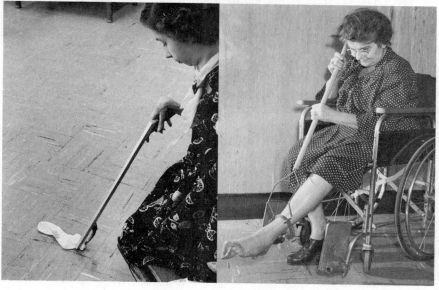

**Figure 20-4.** (*Top, left*) An ordinary scrubbing brush holds the cards for this patient, whose hands are deformed. (*Top, right*) Prism glasses permit reading while the patient is lying flat in bed. (*Bottom, left*) This patient uses reaching tongs to retrieve her sock. (*Bottom, right*) No help needed in putting stockings on. (Institute of Physical Medicine and Rehabilitation, New York University Medical Center, New York, N.Y.)

maining capabilities (Fig. 20-5). The best way to begin is to look for little things that hold promise of improving the situation. For example: What activity has the patient not yet tried that seems likely to succeed? Dusting? Doing dishes? Cooking? Can the nurse devise a way for him to do it? Remember it is the patient's goals that are important. The nurse's job is to help him to reach his own objective.

**Family Considerations.** The patient is not the only one to be considered. How do the other members of the family feel? However devoted the family may be, the progressive helplessness of the arthritic is a 24-hour burden that invariably leads to tensions. Arthritis can make other existing problems worse. Children, especially, who begin by resenting the disease, slowly and without realizing it often end by resenting the person with the disease. The nurse should talk with them without prying. They may be unable to say in front of the patient how guilty they feel (if they do) at not doing more, and how angry, impatient, and resentful they become at times.

**Volunteer Help.** What other people could be of help? Perhaps a volunteer of some medical or social group could take the patient for a ride occasionally. Are there women in the church who could wheel the patient out in the air once a week? Talk to the physician and the social worker. Remember that one person's interest can spark the interest and the enthusiasm of others. It is easier to tackle a hard problem with someone else than to face it alone. Sometimes the nurse is the catalyst; sometimes it is the physician or the social worker or a family member.

The Arthritis Foundation, 1212 Avenue of the Americas, New York, N.Y. 10036, distributes a number of excellent pamphlets and other teaching aids which are available to nurse and patient. The Foundation can also provide sources of local information and assistance which would be more directly available to the patient. The State Division of Vocational Rehabilitation can also be a source of help.

To care for a patient with as severe a disability as advanced arthritis calls for persistence, creativity, and realistic appraisal of one's own feelings. If the nurse feels defeated, she may do a minimum for her patient and let everything continue as it is. If the patient has not been out of the house for five years, no one—not the physician, the supervisor,

the social worker, the patient himself—will criticize a new nurse for not finding a way to change this situation. If the nurse asks it of herself, though, perhaps a way can be found.

## ANKYLOSING SPONDYLITIS (RHEUMATOID SPONDYLITIS)

Ankylosing spondylitis is a chronic inflammatory disease of the joints of the spinal column that is characterized by progressive stiffening and pain. It was formerly believed that this disease was a manifestation of rheumatoid arthritis, hence the name rheumatoid spondylitis. It is now generally felt, however, that while related, the two diseases are distinct entities.

### Incidence

A disease mainly afflicting young men, its onset is almost always before the age of 50. It is seen in men ten times more frequently than in women.

### Pathology

The synovitis of the spinal joints starts usually in the sacroiliac region and moves upward. Ossification gradually occurs, eventually fusing the spinal column into a rigid unit.

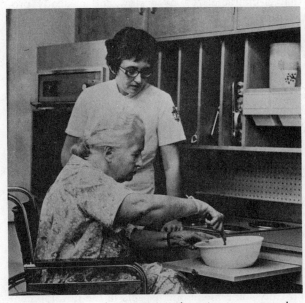

**Figure 20-5.** This woman is learning to resume her usual tasks with the assistance of the occupational therapist. The bowl she is using is held steady by the hole in the board. (Overlook Hospital, Summit, N.J.)

## Symptoms

In 85 per cent of the patients the onset is gradual, starting with aches and pains and frequent remissions. As the costotransverse and the costovertebral articulations are involved, there is limitation of chest expansion, subjecting the patient to the possibility of pulmonary complications. As the spine stiffens, the normal lumbar curve is lost, and there may be kyphosis (humpback curvature) of the thoracic spine. As the neck and the head become immobilized, the patient must rotate from the hips to see from side to side.

Although the overall health of the patient may remain robust, he has considerable joint pain and muscle spasm.

## Treatment

Salicylates relieve the pain, while moist heat relieves muscle spasm. Phenylbutazone or indomethamin may be given. Properly graded exercises are planned to keep the spine mobile and especially to preserve chest expansion. Exercises are important to maintain the spine in a position of function, even though ankylosis occurs frequently.

## DEGENERATIVE JOINT DISEASE (OSTEOARTHRITIS)

This type of arthritis is a disease of the joints that is characterized by a slow and a steady progression of destructive changes. Unlike rheumatoid arthritis, degenerative joint disease has no remissions and no systemic symptoms, such as malaise and fever.

## Incidence and Etiology

This is a wear-and-tear disease that may start as early as the middle 30's, but it is mainly an affliction of later middle life and old age. Repeated trauma may lead to degenerative changes. Obese people, whose joints must bear heavy weight, are more likely to develop early symptoms than lean people. It has been suggested that osteoarthritis is more common in people who use muscular effort as a way of coping with anxiety and aggression. Men and women are affected equally.

Recent studies and experiments in animals indicate that probably there is a hereditary factor and possibly some metabolic aspects in the development of osteoarthritis. This disease certainly occurs in some kinds of individuals more than in others and in certain animal strains more than in others.

## Pathology

Osteoarthritis is a reflection of generalized aging. The cartilage that covers the bone edge becomes thin and ragged, and it no longer springs back into shape after normal use. Finally, the bone end becomes bare. There is breakdown in the fibrillar components of the joint, but collagen is retained. The synovial membrane, which at first is normal, becomes thickened. The fibrous tissue around the joint ossifies. These changes, which occur slowly, give the patient pain and limited motion of the joint. Ankylosis does not occur.

## Symptoms

Degenerative joint disease starts slowly with morning stiffness, especially in damp weather or after a period of heavy activity. General health is not affected. Slowly the involved joints, which may be any in the body, are uncomfortable, and finally they are painful when they are exercised. The joints most commonly affected are hips, knees, and spine. There is little or no swelling, and no regional loss of muscle bulk. The discomfort yields to rest, aspirin, and warmth, only to reappear with activity. Over the years there is limitation of motion.

## Inflammatory Osteoarthritis

Asymmetrical arthritis that resembles rheumatoid arthritis has recently received considerable attention. It usually begins with pain, swelling, and redness—the symptoms of inflammation—at the distal or proximal joints of the fingers and the interphalangeal joint of the thumb. The predominant victims are women, chiefly at the time of menopause or later. A strong family history usually exists. The early inflammatory changes ultimately resolve to leave gnarled bumpy fingers. However, while deformity is common, crippling is rare (Ehrlich, 1972.) The x-ray changes late in the disease show signs of bony proliferation at the joint margins and cystic erosions adjacent to the joints. Hand function is weakened but not lost. Often, the most distressing symptom occurs at the base of the thumb, where the joint between the carpal bones and the metacarpal bone of the thumb is deranged, becomes unstable and swollen. In association with the changes in the hand, there may be osteoarthritic changes in the cervical spine, hips, and knees. Bunions are common. After a period of time, lasting up to several years, the acute symptoms generally subside leaving behind some deformities. Some of these patients, at least, seem predisposed later to develop a disease indistinguishable from rheumatoid arthritis but generally milder and affecting the upper extremities more than the lower. Of course, similar bumpy changes in the fingers, called Heberden's nodes, may develop benignly and without symptoms in women of middle age, and are not necessarily associated with degenerative changes elsewhere. These patients seem to respond well to the overnight wearing of stretch gloves, previously cited in the discussion of treatment of rheumatoid arthritis (Ehrlich, 1972).

## Treatment

Proper local rest of the affected joints is more important than total body rest. Short periods of moderate exercise are helpful. Exercises never should be a strain to the patient. Normally repeated five to six times a day, they should be regulated by the feeling of the joint. Postural defects that add to the strain on a joint theoretically should be corrected; but since posture is the result of the habit of a lifetime, it probably will not be changed after middle age. Heat to the part is a comfort to the patient. If massage is used, it must be done gently to avoid further damage. Obese patients should lose weight. Anything that helps to relieve strain on the sore joints helps the patient. Support may be given with strapping, belts, braces, canes, or crutches. In some instances the patient may gain relief while he is in traction.

Aspirin affords relief from pain. However, narcotics are to be avoided. Corticosteroids may be injected into areas of inflammation during an acute stage. Daily traction and swimming may be prescribed.

Because both osteoarthritis and rheumatoid arthritis are called "arthritis," and patients may know that rheumatoid arthritis causes deformity, those with osteoarthritis may worry that their disease also will result in deformity. This worry can be relieved because this disease does not have the crippling effect of rheumatoid arthritis.

## GOUT

Gout is a metabolic disease, a familial arthritis that may attack any joint, but often it settles in the big toe, the ankle, the knee, or the instep. There are periodic acute episodes of swelling and pain, which can be excruciating, with eventual limitations of motion. According to the Committee of the American Rheumatism Association, 90 to 95 per cent of the patients are men, and the disease is rare in women before the menopause.

## Pathology

The basic disorder in gout seems to be an inability to metabolize purines, which are products of the digestion of certain proteins. This inability results in an accumulation of uric acid in the bloodstream. Deposits of sodium urate crystals (tophi) occur in the margins of the joints, in the cartilage of the ear, in the kidneys, on the skin, and, rarely, in the heart and other organs (Fig. 20-6). Fibrous or bony ankylosis of the joint may develop.

It is possible to have hyperuricemia without having gout. This occurs frequently in the siblings of gouty patients. Primary gout is the hereditary defect in the ability to metabolize purines. However, secondary gout can arise as a result of increased purine metabolism resulting from some blood dyscrasias, such as polycythemia and certain leukemias.

## Laboratory Findings

The most important diagnostic test for the presence of gout is the demonstration of monosodium urate crystals in freshly aspirated joint fluid. When

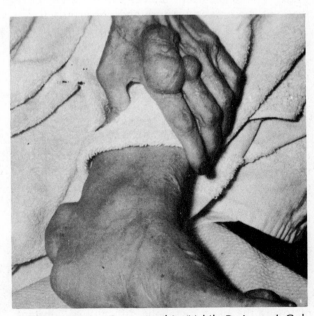

**Figure 20-6.** Gouty tophi. (Vakil, R. J., and Golwalla, A.: *Clinical Diagnosis*, Bombay, Asia Pub. House)

the physician removes such fluid for testing, it is imperative that the laboratory receive it immediately so that the demonstration of the crystals within scavenger white cells under polarized light can be accomplished. Of lesser importance is the demonstration of elevation of uric acid in the blood. Levels above 7 mg. per 100 ml. in men and 6 mg. per 100 ml. in women are usually associated with gout, although elevated uric acid levels are far more common than is gout, and perversely, gout may occur even in the presence of normal uric acid levels.

### Symptoms

An attack of gout begins usually with sudden, agonizing pain. The skin turns red, and the part swells. The attack lasts three days to several weeks and then disappears, to return in a month or perhaps a year later. The joint recovers completely after the early attacks.

During an attack the pain usually is so severe that the weight of the bedclothes or even the touch of a passing draft is intolerable. Movement of the joint is out of the question. Spontaneously, in about two weeks—or sooner with treatment—swelling, redness, and pain are gone, and the joint appears to be as good as ever. However, after years of attacks the permanent damage to the joint becomes evident. With recurrent attacks the involvement of the joints becomes migratory and polyarthritic.

The tophi that form in joints can eventually result in a chronic inflammatory reaction that causes structural damage and deformity. Sodium urate deposits in the kidney can endanger the life of the patient. The occurrence and the size of tophi are not necessarily related to the frequency of acute episodes.

Attacks become more and more frequent over the years. An attack may be triggered by surgery, trauma, infection elsewhere in the body, allergy, excessive alcohol, weight gain, a weight-reducing diet, emotional upset, and such drugs as liver extract, vitamin B, antibiotics, ergotamine tartrate, and diuretics. Even environmental changes may cause an attack.

### Treatment

Although gout cannot be cured in the sense of removing the basic metabolic difficulty of constant or recurrent hyperuricemia, the attacks usually can be controlled to the point that they no longer occur.

The regimen must be individualized for each patient and changed from time to time in response to the changes in the course of the disease. Understanding the nature of gout, practicing self-discipline, and conscientiously maintaining contact with his physician are all necessary for success.

When attacks become prolonged or tophi develop, attempts are made to reduce the uric acid level in the blood. This can be accomplished either by promoting the excretion of urates by the kidney through inhibition of tubular reabsorption of urates or by preventing the breakdown of purines to uric acid by inhibiting the metabolic cycle.

**Diet.** The excess uric acid in the body of a patient with gout is derived from a process of internal biosynthesis; consequently, except for severe tophaceous gout, there is less emphasis on strict diet restriction. Dietary management was formerly regarded as most important in gout control, and rigidly prescribed. However, since the effect of dietary control upon urate levels is relatively small, a much more lenient attitude has lately been taken. The most important feature of dietary management is moderation, and patients should probably be counselled to avoid not only dietary excesses, but excesses of all kinds in their daily lives. While the majority of patients are not placed on a rigid diet, they are instructed not to take high-purine foods. The reaction to food and alcoholic drinks is extremely individual.

*The prescribed diet* is adequate in proteins—with concentration on low-purine proteins—low in fat and rich in carbohydrates. Large fluid intake and moderate alcoholic restriction usually are recommended. High-purine foods, to be avoided, include liver, kidneys, brains, anchovies, sardines, herring, smelts, bacon, goose, haddock, mackerel, mutton, salmon, turkey and veal, yeast, beer, meat broth, and leguminous vegetables, such as beans.

Low-purine or purine-free foods, usually allowed, include chocolate, coffee, tea, fruit juices, fruits, breads, cereal and spaghetti, eggs, gelatine, milk, nuts, pies (except mincemeat), sugar, and other than leguminous vegetables.

**Drugs.** Because of the urgent nature of the pain, narcotics may be justified. However, they are rarely used, because more specific drugs are known.

*Colchicine* is a blessing to the patient with gout. Although this drug has been known to mankind for many centuries, in spite of intensive research and many theories nobody knows to this day how it works. It relieves the symptoms of an acute attack, even though, strangely enough, it is not analgesic or antiphlogistic in any other type of joint pain. Nor does it affect uric acid metabolism. If it is given promptly enough, colchicine gives relief within 12 to 24 hours. It is given by mouth in tablets of 0.5 to 0.6 mg. every hour until either the joint symptoms are relieved or nausea, vomiting or diarrhea appear, but no more than 16 tablets of colchicine should be given within a 24-hour period. More than this number of tablets may produce severe toxic gastrointestinal reactions with shock or acute renal failure, leading even to death. Intravenous therapy may be used, but intramuscular and subcutaneous injections never are used, because colchicine is very irritating to tissues. A positive response to colchicine can be considered a diagnostic test for gout, since this is the only rheumatic disease that readily responds to this agent.

Patients with gout should always have colchicine tablets handy. The earlier the pills are taken in an attack, the quicker the attack will be over. If the drug is not taken early, more of it may be needed for relief, which then may not be accomplished before nausea, vomiting, or diarrhea start. Regular, small amounts may be prescribed to prevent attacks.

*Phenylbutazone,* used for stubborn attacks, is given in the dose of 100 mg. to 200 mg. by mouth four times daily for two to three days. The patient taking this drug, should be watched for edema, nausea, epigastric pain, vertigo, stomatitis, and a rash. Toxic reactions can be serious. Phenylbutazone is considered by many physicians to be the drug of choice in treating the acute attack of this disease. Usually it needs to be taken for such a short period of time that toxic effects do not appear. This drug is uricosuric.

Indomethacin is also effective in treating attacks of gout.

*Probenecid* (*Benemid*) also increases the excretion of uric acid. It is given in doses of 0.5 to 2.0 Gm. daily. A newer unicosuric agent is sulfinpyrazone (*Anturane*). Constipation, nausea, anorexia, and rash are toxic reactions. When patients are treated with one of these drugs, encourage the intake of fluids, at least 3,000 ml. a day, to prevent kidney stones. Salicylates interfere with the action of probenecid, and so the patient should be instructed not to take the two drugs together.

*Allopurinol* (*Zyloprin*) inhibits the enzymes leading to the formation of uric acid. This leads to more effective renal excretion and diminution of body stores. It is of particular value where kidney disease is present.

The initial dose of 100 mg. daily is gradually increased to the level necessary to maintain normal uric acid levels. That may require 400 to 600 mg. a day. During the first few months of therapy, however, patients may sometimes experience an increased frequency of gouty attacks. The uricosuric agents and allopurinol do not treat the acute symptoms of gout, and are therefore not a substitute for colchicine or anti-inflammatory medications.

**Other Treatment.** Other treatment of advanced gout includes hemodialysis when there is renal involvement, and surgery to remove large tophaceous masses. Surgery may be employed also in an attempt to correct crippling deformities that may result when treatment is delayed and to fuse unstable joints to increase their function.

During an attack a bed cradle is placed over the affected joint to protect it from bedclothes, breezes, and bumps. A sign "Don't Bump the Bed" may remind auxiliary personnel and visitors to be careful. Either warm or cold compresses may be ordered and applied very gently. Elevation of the joint may make the patient more comfortable. Only after the pain and the redness have disappeared is the joint to be exercised. Then early ambulation is a necessity to ensure good joint function.

## LOW BACK PAIN

Pain in the lumbosacral region is a very common symptom and an important cause of loss of work time in industry. Because the symptom may be caused by a multitude of disorders, and because neuromusculoskeletal mechanisms of the back are complex, a thorough diagnostic examination is required when the patient has low backaches. In women the cause may be gynecologic, and in both sexes it may be urologic, metabolic, orthopedic, or psychosomatic in origin. The four most likely orthopedic causes of low back pain are:

1. Acute lumbosacral strain, which is treated with bed rest, muscle relaxants, analgesics, and local heat to relieve musle spasm.
2. Unstable lumbosacral mechanism, which is treated with measures to relieve muscle spasm and exercises designed to increase the strength of the paravertebral muscles. Sometimes a lumbosacral belt or brace is prescribed, and occasionally a spinal fusion is done.

3. Osteoarthritis.

4. Herniated intervertebral disk.

Since disuse of muscles and joints leads to stiffness and weakness, those patients who are given the external support of a brace probably will have exercises prescribed also. Patients with low back pain should be taught body mechanics that minimize back strain, such as how to lift heavy objects from the floor. The industrial nurse especially is in a position to prevent disorders of the back by teaching good body mechanics to the men and the women of her industrial population. She may post signs showing ways of moving that lessen strain, visit the workers on the job, and give demonstrations.

## BONE TUMORS

There are two kinds of bone tumors: (1) primary, those that originate in bone, and (2) secondary, those that are metastatic, starting somewhere else in the body and traveling to bone. The older the patient, the more likely it will be that the bone tumor is malignant. Many tumors never invade bone, but uncontrolled cancer of the breast, the prostate, the kidney, the lungs, and the thyroid do have a tendency to settle in bone as a secondary site of involvement.

Pain and swelling are the principal symptoms of a bone tumor. Biopsy of marrow tissue may be taken to establish the type of tumor. Treatment may consist of excision of a primary tumor (if it is caught before it spreads) and roentgen therapy, which all too often is unsuccessful. Sometimes the affected section of bone is removed, and the defect is filled with bone graft chips. In other instances there is amputation of an entire part of the body, and the surgery may be extensive. For example, in a hemipelvectomy, half of the pelvic bone with its entire adjacent limb is removed. Chemotherapy temporarily may suppress the progress of malignancy. The aim of the palliative treatment is to help the patient to remain as comfortable as possible. The ingenuity of the nurse is called on to keep the patient from suffering unnecessarily.

Some bone and joint cancers, while quite uncommon, sometimes develop in children. While the prognosis in these is guarded, the youngsters may undergo amputations and prolonged courses of drug treatment and radiotherapy which will require considerable emotional support for the patient and the family members.

## OSTEOMYELITIS

Osteomyelitis, infection of bone, can result from a compound fracture in which the bone is exposed to the bacteria of the outside world, or it may occur if a nearby infection erodes into bone. However, the infection is more often blood-borne, starting at a parent focus of infection somewhere else in the body, perhaps a boil or a squeezed pimple. Staphylococcus is the most common offending organism, and streptococcus is the second. Penetrating wounds that extend to bone are a good breeding ground for anaerobic bacteria. Streptococcal infections start with more violent symptoms than those caused by staphylococcus, but they have less tendency to become chronic.

### Symptoms

No matter what the organism, the onset of the illness usually is stormy, and the danger of chronicity is ever present. The patient has a fever and feels severe pain, perhaps a headache or nausea. His leukocyte count is increased. There is local swelling.

### Pathology

The pain of osteomyelitis is caused by pressure due to pus formation and also to the destruction of bone. The infection spreads within the shaft of the bone, and the resultant pus gathers beneath the bone itself causes necrosis. Dead bone, called *sequestrum,* becomes detached and must be removed. The periosteum begins the formation of new bone, called *involucrum.* Thus a chronic process of bone destruction and regeneration may occur.

### Treatment

There are three weapons to combat osteomyelitis: (1) the patient's own defenses, aided by rest and good nutrition; (2) antibiotics; and (3) surgical drainage of the pus that forms. In the early stage of treatment the antibiotic may be given by continuous drip infusion. Some physicians make a series of drill holes in the bone to evacuate pus and to relieve the pressure. Antibiotics are put directly into the wound, and a catheter may be left in place for periodic irrigation or continuous drip of antibiotic solution. The wound is kept open for drainage, and the extremity positioned so that the mouth of the wound is down, utilizing the help of gravity in draining the pus. Sometimes a closed irrigation and drainage system is used, with a low-pressure pump providing intermittent suction that allows the wound to fill periodically. The affected part may be immobilized with plaster, such as a half cast.

## Nursing Care

The nurse caring for a patient with osteomyelitis must be especially mindful of the patient's pain. Movement causes great distress to the patient; yet he cannot lie continuously in one position. When she turns the patient, the nurse's hands should be extremely smooth, careful, and unhurried. The limb should be well supported over its entire length, perhaps splinted with a pillow, and never allowed to lag behind. A firm pillow supports it, and sandbags hold it still. Immobilization of the part, which is a comfort to the patient while slightest movement is agony, can be accomplished by a cast, a brace, or the judicious placement of sandbags. The nurse should take extra care to see that the patient's bed is placed where it is least likely to be jarred. She should avoid bumping into it, and warn visitors, cleaning maids, and others to be careful.

Whenever it is possible, the patient should be given foods that he enjoys. He needs a nutritious diet. The physician may order a high caloric diet. Fluids are encouraged.

The nurse, aware that the infection can spread to other bones, is quick to tell the physician of any swelling, redness or pain elsewhere over a bone. She knows also that pathologic fractures (fractures that occur without severe trauma) may occur. These are singularly difficult to recognize, because the pain of osteomyelitis is so great that the pain of the fracture is masked.

## Complications

The diseased bone may lengthen as bone growth is stimulated, or it may shorten because of the destruction of the epiphysial plate. Another complication of osteomyelitis may be the result of negligence on the part of the nurse. If dressings become too routine over a period of months, she may become careless with her aseptic technique, and fresh organisms may be introduced into the wound.

Perhaps the most discouraging complication of all is the tendency of osteomyelitis to become chronic. The sinus from the bone to the outside may drain for years. The inactivity of the part, the muscle spasm, and the despair of the patient take their toll. The patient with chronic osteomyelitis frequently is wasted, weak, and burdened with a deformed extremity. Sometimes amputation is necessary. Fortunately, antibiotic therapy has lessened the incidence of chronicity and heightened the chances of recovery.

## REFERENCES AND BIBLIOGRAPHY

THE ARTHRITIS FOUNDATION: *Arthritis and Related Disorders,* New York, (n.d.).
———: *Arthritis Manual for Allied Health Professionals,* New York, 1973.
———: *Arthritis Quackery Today,* New York, (n.d.).
———: *Home Care in Arthritis,* New York, 1966.
———: *Primer on the Rheumatic Diseases,* New York, 1973.
BEESON, P. B., and MCDERMOTT, W. (eds.): *Cecil-Loeb Textbook of Medicine,* ed. 13, Philadelphia, Saunders, 1971.
BRASSELL, M., et al.: Helping patients adjust to rheumatoid arthritis, *Nurs. '72* 2:11, October 1972.
BRUNNER, N. A.: *Orthopedic Nursing: A Programmed Approach,* St. Louis, Mosby, 1970.
CALABRO, J. J.: Rheumatoid arthritis, *Ciba, Clin. Symp.* 23,1:2, 71.
CIUCA, R., et al.: Range of motion exercises, active and passive: A handbook, *Nurs. '73* 73:25, December 1973.
CORBEIL, M.: Nursing process for a patient with body image disturbance, *Nurs. Clin. N. Am.* 6:155, March 1971.
DI PALMA, J. R.: Drug therapy today. Recent developments in bone-disease treatment, *RN* 36:63, January 1973.
DITUNNO, J., and EHRLICH, G. E.: Care and training of elderly patients with rheumatoid arthritis, *Geriat.* 25:165, 1970.
DUTHIE, J. J. R., et al.: Course and prognosis in rheumatoid arthritis, *Ann. Rheum. Dis.* 23:193, 1964.
EDWARDS, M. H., CALABRO, J. J., and WIED, M. E.: Patient's attitudes and knowledge concerning arthritis, *Arth. Rheum.* 7:425, 1964.
EHRLICH, G. E.: Inflammatory osteoarthritis. I. The clinical syndrome, *J. Chron. Dis.* 25:317, 1972.
———: Inflammatory osteoarthritis. II. Superimposition of rheumatoid arthritis, *J. Chron. Dis.* 25:635, 1972.
———, (ed.): *Total Management of the Arthritic Patient,* Philadelphia, Lippincott, 1973.
EHRLICH, G. E., KATZ, W. A., and COHEN, S. H.: Rheumatoid arthritis in the aged, *Geriat.* 25:103, 1970.
FRANKS, A.: Please don't turn me off! *RN* 32:52, October, 1969.
GIFFORD, R. H.: Corticosteroid therapy for rheumatoid arthritis, *Med. Clin. N. Am.* 57:1179, September 1972.
GRAHAME, R.: Caring for patients with rheumatoid disease, *Nurs. Times* 67:701, June 1971.

————: Rheumatoid disease and clinical aspects, *Nurs. Times* 67:664, June 1971.

HARTUNG, E. F.: Treatment of degenerative arthritis, *Mod. Treat.* 1:1187, 1964.

————: The nonspecific management of rheumatoid arthritis, *Bull. Rheum. Dis.* 15:366-369, 1965.

HERMANN, I. F., and SMITH, R. T.: Gout and gouty arthritis, *Am. J. Nurs.* 64:111, December 1964.

HOLLANDER, J. L., and McCARTY, D. S.: *Arthritis and Allied Conditions,* ed. 8, Philadelphia, Lea and Febiger, 1972.

KELLGREN, J. H.: The epidemiology of rheumatoid diseases, *Ann. Rheum. Dis.* 23:109, 1964.

KERR, A.: *Orthopedic Nursing Procedures,* New York, Springer, 1969.

LAMONT-HAVERS, R. W.: Personal communication.

————: Arthritis quackery, *Am. J. Nurs.* 63:92, March 1963.

LARSON, C. B., and GOULD, M.: *Calderwood's Orthopedic Nursing,* ed. 7, St. Louis, Mosby, 1970.

LOWMAN, E., and KLINGER, J.: *Aids to Independent Living,* New York, McGraw-Hill, 1969.

LOXLEY, A. K.: The emotional toll of crippling deformity, *Am. J. Nurs.* 72:1839, October 1972.

MAGGINNISS, O.: Rheumatoid arthritis—my tutor, *Am. J. Nurs.* 68:1699, August 1968.

OSTROW, E. K.: *The Effects of Arthritis on the Life Adjustment of a Group of Arthritis Clinic Patients,* New York, Arthritis and Rheumatism Foundation, (n.d.).

REYNOLDS, F., and BARSAM, P.: *Adult Health: Services for the Chronically Ill and Aged,* New York, Macmillan, 1967.

RODNAM, G. P.: Gout, *Mod. Treat.* 1:1203, 1964.

THOMAS, B. J.: Nursing care of patients with cancer of the bone, *Nurs. Clin. N. Am.* 2:459, September 1967.

WALIKE, B., et al.: Rheumatoid arthritis, *Am. J. Nurs.* 67:1420, July 1967.

# The Amputee:
## Nursing Considerations

## CHAPTER 21

## PSYCHOSOCIAL IMPLICATIONS

Usually, the loss of a limb is psychologically damaging. An amputation can make a patient feel that he is less acceptable than others, can lessen his self-esteem, and can affect his self-image. The patient can be expected to experience grief over his loss and, depending on his adjustment, work through the various stages of the grieving process. The nurse helps by assessing the stage of grief the patient is in and providing appropriate support. (See Chapter 6 for the nursing needs of patients experiencing grief and change in body image.)

Not only does the loss of a limb mean that the person may consider himself to be no longer whole, but it may also create some difficult practical problems. According to his situation, the patient will face the possibility of loss of locomotion, lifelong invalidism, a change in homemaking practices, and perhaps the loss of a job.

Even if the mechanics of rehabilitation can be accomplished perfectly, the loss of a limb may cause such anxiety and grief that the patient is unable to use a prosthesis. A young healthy person who loses a leg in an automobile accident often is able to make the necessary physical adjustments, so that after only a relatively short time he can continue a full, active, and productive life. On the other hand, the young college athlete or cheerleader who has an amputation due to cancer of the bone has overwhelming adjustments to make. Yet these people need rehabilitation also. Persons who undergo amputation for metastatic disease survive for an average of 3.5 years and occasionally for five to ten years (Dietz, 1969). The young war amputee has his own problems to cope with and these will be different from the young patient with bone cancer (Anders et al., 1972).

While the entire response to amputation is highly individual, it is affected by such factors as age, prognosis regarding underlying condition, and the patient's emotional state and developmental level.

At best, the psychological adjustment to the loss of a limb is far from easy, and the suddenness of an amputation resulting from an accident gives the patient no time to build up defenses. An amputation is irrevocable, carrying a deep sense of loss, even for the patient who has had severe pain in the leg. The patient who awakens from anesthesia to find a limb amputated needs people around him who can help to cushion the emotional impact by their acceptance of his feelings and their faith in his ability eventually to cope with the problems.

**The Older Amputee.** An older patient who loses a limb because of peripheral vascular disease may find the multiple adjustment overwhelming and may not be able to profit from rehabilitation facilities. Realistic goals for this patient might be limited to transfer activities and wheelchair independence.

The older person requiring an amputation has a greater likelihood than the younger person of having widespread concomitant disease that may be disabling in itself. There may be generalized weakness, poor vision, or the aftermath of a cerebral vascular accident.

In the elderly, amputation arouses fears of death, incapacitation, abandonment, pain, helplessness, and disturbance or loss of previously established interpersonal relationships. The elderly amputee who jokes that he has "one foot in the grave" may be using a cliché to seek out someone to listen to his feelings about dying, since loss of a body part symbolizes the approach of his total death (Leonard, 1972).

It is possible that the older person especially may fear abandonment so much that he assumes a state of helplessness as a way of control over people and environment. But passivity impedes progress toward optimum health. The patient should be encouraged to do as much as possible for himself with the support of the nurse's presence and direction.

Changing lifelong habits requires stamina, courage, patience, help, and a certain degree of health. Yet some elderly patients, especially those who are supported emotionally by loved ones, do very well in adjusting to great changes in their lives.

**The Family.** The physician may decide that it is better for the family to learn of an impending amputation before the patient does, so that they will have time to adjust to the idea and can help the patient when he learns about it.

While the family may be of great assistance to the patient in helping him to reintegrate his body image, the nurse must realize that family members react to amputation in as individual a way as does any patient. Some may react with panic or with guilt because of ambivalent feelings toward the patient. Some may be angry because, in their perception, amputation could have been avoided if the patient adhered to his medical plan. Some may be afraid to look at or touch a stump. (The nurse may share some of these feelings herself.)

The nurse supports the family by listening to their expression of feelings about the body image change, preparing them for each stage of care, helping the patient and family to set realistic goals, and recognizing assets as well as limitations. Some patients and families who have difficulty coping may require psychotherapy.

## INCIDENCE

Amputation is a medical entity of a special nature because the disability results not from a form of pathology, but from a form of treatment which has eliminated the pathology. It is particularly unfortunate when acute trauma necessitates the amputation of a formerly healthy limb. It is estimated that one out of every 250 to 300 people in the United States has a major amputation and that each year there are more than 30,000 new amputees as a result of congenital defects or surgery, with a ratio of three in the upper extremity to every ten in the lower extremity. During and following World War II there was a considerable surge of interest in research in amputees and amputations because of the 21,000 amputee casualties in that war. In the same four-year period, however, there were more than five times that many amputations in the United States for other than war injuries, a situation not recognized as a national medical problem. Almost every nurse, regardless of the type of institution or agency she works in, will encounter amputees during her professional career.

## ETIOLOGY

The causes of amputation are: (1) accidental and extensive violence to extremities, (2) death of tissues from peripheral vascular insufficiency of arteriosclerosis or diabetes, (3) death of tissues due to peripheral vasospastic diseases, such as Buerger's disease and Raynaud's disease, (4) malignant tumors, (5) long-standing infections of bone and other tissues which leave no chance of restoration of function, (6) thermal injuries, due to both heat and cold, (7) a useless deformed limb which is objectionable to the patient, and (8) other conditions which may endanger the life of the patient, such as vascular accidents, snake bites, and gas bacillus infections.

## MANAGEMENT

Amputee management is viewed as a team effort. Optimally, the team includes the patient, the family, physicians, nurses and their assistants, occupational and physical therapists, the physiatrist, the prosthetist, the social worker, the psychologist, and the vocational counselor.

Although amputation involves loss of a significant body part and all that it entails for the patient, it can also be viewed as reconstructive surgery. A functioning organ, the amputation stump, is left, providing an opportunity to use one of the modern designs of prostheses from which the patient can gain the greatest degree of functional performance. In line with the modern concept of management, the potential amputee passes through a number of phases toward his functional restoration: (1) investigation and beginning assessment for rehabilitation, (2) preoperative, (3) surgical, (4) postoperative care, (5) caring for the stump, (6) fitting with a prosthesis, and (7) training with a prosthesis.

### Investigation and Beginning Assessment for Rehabilitation

Whenever trauma, infection, vascular insufficiency, or ulceration threaten the viability of a limb, an all-out attempt is made to save it. In recent years improved traumatic and orthopedic procedures and surgical control of infection and even resuture of amputated parts have saved many limbs. When this is not possible, the patient requires amputation. Vascular surgery, such as bypassing obstructed vessels and endarterectomy and sympathectomy are having increasing success. The use of hyperbaric oxygen has also been of value for indolent ulceration and threatened gangrene. If treatment is carried out in a chamber with oxygen under pressure, the nurse must be prepared to go through the prescribed procedures when entering the chamber. These are the same as those for deep sea divers working under pressure, requiring decompression when leaving the chamber (Zilm, 1969).

Treatment for control of diabetes, nutritional deficiency, peripheral circulatory insufficiency, systemic infections, and tissue metabolism can save some limbs. It is important for the nurse to give accurate dosages of insulin and other medications on time and to dress open lesions meticulously to help bring threatening disorders under control and to save the limbs.

### Preoperative Phase

#### Psychological Preparation

When amputation is inevitable, the physician discusses with the patient and family the extent of physical disability and the psychological, esthetic, social, and vocational implications, as well as the realistic possibilities for prosthetic restoration. He promptly attempts to reduce anxieties and misunderstandings because radical surgery constitutes a severe threat to most people. Nevertheless, the patient is still faced with a crisis. However, this approach establishes the groundwork for assisting the patient to accept and to adjust to the realities of the situation. Not all amputees can benefit from a prosthesis and the surgeon is careful not to make casual promises to soothe a patient prior to surgery.

Patients vary in their reaction to the impending loss of a limb. These reactions are based upon such variables as the patient's age, his educational, intellectual, economic, and emotional status, what the loss of the part means to him, and how he has dealt with previous losses. In general, a gradual state of depression and a degree of hopelessness are most common. Those with diabetes, for example, may be angry because in spite of the extra care they gave their legs and their dietary deprivation, they must lose their limb, after all.

The nurse can help the patient and family by accepting their reaction of shock and grief at the news and by letting the patient and his family talk about their feelings. Before the operation, she can help them to learn how others have managed with one arm or one leg, how the patient can help himself (by diet and exercises), and what to expect during the postoperative period. She can resist the temptation to make preoperative promises that cannot come true when attempting to aid the patient to accept the thought of an amputation.

Although it has been stated frequently that nurses should encourage patients by showing enthusiasm and optimism themselves, this does not necessarily result in the patient sharing this attitude. Sometimes, it results in the patient perceiving the subtle message that he is expected to smile bravely and undertake his rehabilitation exercises with enthusiasm. This he may do as a facade to smooth relationships with the staff. He meets their need for an eager, smiling patient, rather than his own needs. Although it is important for the nurse to feel and show confidence in the patient's ability, a forced cheeriness may not be the best way to do this. It is usually preferable to listen while the patient discusses his concers, realizing that he is likely to express grief and anger. If it is possible, the nurse can have an amputee who has coped successfully with his handicap visit the patient.

Many of the serious psychological problems at the thought of amputation are lessened by recently improved surgical procedures, making it possible for amputees to ambulate almost immediately after surgery. But despite immediate postsurgical fitting and early amputation, the patient cannot be hurried through his stages of grieving, and each patient needs support to proceed at his own pace to fully integrate the experience.

Most physicians assure a patient who will lose one limb and still have three remaining normally functional limbs that he will derive practical function from the use of a prosthesis. This applies to almost all lower extremity amputees and most upper extremity amputees, regardless of age. The great majority of amputations in the lower extremity are performed on patients over the age of 60. Unfortunately, it is this older age group which has coexisting debilitating and degenerative diseases, many of which are disabling in themselves. The nurse must be careful not to become overenthusiastic about how much function will be regained after the amputation, since in the older age group the quality of performance with protheses falls far short of the normal, both for upper extremity and lower extremity amputations.

Some patients are unable to accept the amputation. Many of these, unfortunately, do not receive the help which is sufficient for their emotional requirements. One task of the nurse is to continually support those patients who initially cannot accept it. At a later time they may begin to progress toward acceptance, especially if they have family and friends as well as nurses and physicians who don't give up on them.

**Phantom Limb.** The surgeon also informs the patient of the phenomenon of phantom-limb sensation (not phantom-limb pain). This is the patient's sensation of the presence of the amputated limb. It is a normal, frequently occurring physiologic response following amputation surgery. If the phantom is painful, however, it can be an extremely serious problem with regard to the emotional status of the patient and his ability to use a prosthesis. The sensation of a phantom limb should be explained to the patient as a normal phenomenon so that he will not be disturbed by his awareness of the amputated part. After a patient learns to use a prosthesis for practical purposes, although he still is aware of the phantom, he usually learns to ignore its presence. The patient may merely feel that the foot or the hand is still there. He should be encouraged to talk about the sensation. He may be embarrassed, or he may fear that he is losing his mind or that the staff will think that he is emotionally disturbed.

The experience of phantom limb as a usual occurrence after amputation consists of somesthetic and kinesthetic sensations which feel as real as those in the opposite limb or as in the phantom limb before amputation. Amputation phantoms can persist for months or decades, or can come and go.

Psychological explanations for painful phantom limbs are varied and inconclusive. Various studies suggest that the patient's pain is an expression of anger turned toward himself, a denial of the loss and associated grief, a way of satisfying unacceptable dependency needs, or an expression of anxiety related to disposal of the amputated part. It is also suggested that underlying all these motives is depression and that relief of the depression by psychotherapy, electroshock therapy, or other antidepressant methods may be expected to relieve the pain. Another successful mode of therapy is nonpsychiatric in nature and involves intensive concentration on several sensorimotor tasks. Concentration, ignoring distractions, and habituation to rhythmic stimuli over a period of weeks effect a reorganization of central sensory processes.

Aldrich (1966) suggests that the incidence of painful phantom limb is less likely if the patient's physician helps him to express his feelings about the amputation, both pre- and postoperatively. The nurse, by her supportive listening presence, helps the patient to accept and deal with the loss. The reactions of patients who lose limbs resemble reactions of grief at the loss of a friend or relative. The patient's failure to communicate or even to recognize his reactions may result in later emotional problems. For example, the physician may say, "The operation is safe and necessary," but the patient may hear, "You will feel better after it." When during the postoperative period the patient is not better, he feels deceived and angry at the surgeon.

The amount of grief is thought to be proportional to the symbolic significance of the part and the resultant degree of disability and deformity. It is recommended that the physician in his preoperative explanation emphasize the necessity for the amputation without criticizing the patient for his reservations and recognize the anger the patient may feel about the threat to his body integrity. This helps clear the way for the expression of grief as well as the patient's concern about the disposition of the amputated part. The patient usually wants the separated part of himself treated with respect, which includes decent burial of the part. The nurse discusses with the physician what was told to the patient and how the patient has responded. She also gives the patient the opportunity to further express his thoughts and feelings.

## Physical Preparation

If the operation is not an emergency, there is time to prepare the patient for some of the things he will be required to do after amputation. A good diet, including plenty of fluids, helps the patient to withstand the shock of the operation. If the patient's condition permits it, he is prepared for postoperative exercises by starting them preoperatively. The patient can do pushups while he is lying prone. In anticipation of crutch walking, he can push down on the bed with his hands while he is in the sitting position. The patient practices until he can lift his buttocks off the bed. The three unaffected limbs are put through the normal range of motion. If the patient is old, ill, or weak, care is taken not to tire him. An exercise done two or three times a day is

better than one done ten times all at once. An overhead bar and trapeze should be put on the bed.

**Vascular Integrity.** Preoperatively, an arteriogram (see Chap. 34) may be done on the leg, especially when no popliteal pulsations can be felt, to help identify those patients whose legs can be saved by such vascular surgery as endarterectomy and bypass grafting. These surgical procedures are helpful when there is occlusion of a segment of an artery. However, they are not applicable when there is generalized arteriosclerosis in the limb that is being considered for amputation. Palpation of the popliteal artery and an arteriogram also may be done to help determine whether there is sufficient circulation intact in the lower part of the leg so that a BK (below-knee) amputation will be successful, or whether an AK (above-knee) is necessary. If there is necrosis, surgery may be delayed until there is a clear demarcation between healthy and unhealthy tissue.

In some hospitals, when it is believed that the patient cannot tolerate general anesthesia, dry ice refrigeration anesthesia of the limb may be used. The limb, kept at 45 degrees to 74 degrees F., becomes numb, but it does not actually freeze. Refrigeration decreases the metabolic rate in the limb, lessens the blood loss, and inhibits the growth of microorganisms (Gorman and Rosenberg, 1967).

Just before the operation the refrigerated limb may be elevated to drain venous blood out of it; then a pressure dressing and a tourniquet may be applied. An infusion usually is started, and blood is made available in case of need.

## Surgical Phase

**Level of Amputation.** Amputation can be performed at any level in the lower extremity. There are preferred levels of choice above and below the knee to facilitate fitting with available prostheses. A stump too long or too short creates fitting problems and discomfort. Over 90 per cent of amputations in the lower extremity are at the standard above- or below-knee levels. The ideal level above the knee is in the middle third of the thigh, the longest preferred stump being to within four inches of the knee. The standard below-knee level of choice is in the middle third of the leg, but not lower than the musculocutaneous junction of the calf muscles. Hemipelvectomy and hip disarticulations are relatively infrequent and are performed almost exclusively for malignant tumors. Knee disarticulations, ankle disarticulations (Syme's amputation), and partial foot amputations are occasionally performed, but these are rare.

When the surgeon decides that amputation is inevitable, the first decision he makes is the level of amputation. Although he has a number of tests available, including arteriography, the final decision can be made only by observing the vascularity of the tissues on the operating table.

In the upper extremity the principle followed is to have all possible length and tissue with the exception of partial hand amputations. An amputation through any part of the hand that does not leave functioning elements is obstructive to the use of a prosthesis. In such cases, amputation is generally by disarticulation through the wrist or just proximal to the wrist.

In the lower extremity, unless there is unequivocal evidence that the knee cannot be saved, an attempt is made to amputate below the knee. Amputation above the knee is considerably disabling. Since function is achieved in relationship to agility, older people do not do as well with an amputation above the knee, although the majority of them can be fitted with a prosthesis.

With modern techniques and the use of a rigid plaster dressing applied at the time of surgery, a good many patients who were considered to be candidates for above-knee amputation, particularly diabetics with gangrene of the toes, can survive with below-knee amputations in greater proportion than was previously recognized.

NORMAL PHYSIOLOGY OF WALKING. In order to understand what the surgeon will do, it is necessary to review what happens when an amputation takes place. The normal individual when walking is not aware of the physiologic activity created by and controlled by the muscles. Normal physiologic muscular activity is not limited to contraction, relaxation, movement of the joints. It is intimately related to the central and autonomic nervous systems, bringing about muscle balance, synergy, and reciprocation, either directly or reflexly. It also affects local circulation and builds up afferent input and feedback information relating to skill and coordination through the spinal tracts. In the brain the end result of this cerebrospinal complex is awareness. From this highly complicated mechanism the patient derives his sense of balance, proprioception, and kinesthetic sense. These in turn, combined with the emotional pattern of the individual, relate to his sense of security, confidence, comfort, cooperation, and motivation. Amputation seriously disturbs this chain of events from the level of the sectioned muscles to the neurologic silence below it. In an effort to compensate for these losses, the patient derives false information from the phantom—each interpreting it in his own way. The surgeon will attempt to restore the physiologic losses by the technique of his amputation.

**Myoplastic Amputation.** The myoplastic form of amputation consists of sewing opposing muscles to each other and down to the bone from which they originate. This allows the muscles to contract isometrically so that even though the muscle is sectioned, it is giving information to the patient as to the degree of tension, the position of the limb, and the amount of force exerted upon it. If the muscles are simply severed and allowed to retract as they are in a guillotine type of *open* amputation, these muscles do not reattach to bone and do not contract isometrically in the phase of gait in which they normally contract. Thus, they do not provide the feedback information which the patient needs to have a sense of balance and position of the limb. When myoplastic amputation is performed in the manner described, phantom limb pain is seldom a problem.

When the surgeon performs a myoplastic amputation and sutures the muscles under a slight degree of tension, he creates a functioning organ which is adaptable to the total contact method of fitting a prosthetic socket. The uniform surface contact, including the end of the amputation stump, provides feedback information to the patient which improves his proprioception and gives him confidence and skill in the use of a prosthesis.

Immediate Postoperative Stump Dressing

The former conventional manner of dressing the amputation stump upon completion of the procedure was to apply a fluffy dressing supported by an Ace bandage for slight compression. In recent years the rigid dressing has been considered to be far superior to the elastic compressive dressing. This consists of applying very few layers of gauze contoured to the end of the amputation stump, protecting the patella and other subcutaneous bony points with felt pads, and applying a sterile stump sock and a cast of elastic plaster of Paris. The cast extends above the knee in the below-knee amputation and as high as possible in above-knee amputations, and is retained by a suspension mechanism —either by a broad belt or by straps and waistbelts. The elastic plaster of Paris is highly compressive when it is applied, but when the plaster sets, it is firm and accurately fitted to the amputation stump. This prevents swelling and bleeding and in the encased rigid dressing the phantom remains quiescent. A coupling device can be attached to this rigid dressing and a temporary prosthesis created at the time of surgery by adding a tube and a foot (a walking pylon or "peg leg"). There are commercial devices for making such temporary limbs (Fig. 21-1).

The generally accepted technique of amputation above and below the knee involving the use of equal flaps can be adapted for satisfactory use of modern prostheses. In below-knee amputation, however, there is a tendency to make no anterior flap and to make one long posterior flap. The reason is that the circulation in the posterior flap is better than it is in the anterior flap, placing the scar anteriorly and making it possible to use a total contact socket early after amputation without placing stresses upon the scar of surgery.

If the rigid dressing is not used at the time of surgery, the amputation stump must be shaped and conditioned by bandaging with elastic bandages or the use of elastic stump-shrinking socks or both (Fig. 21-2). With the use of the rigid dressing and immediate or early ambulation, the entire preprosthetic management period is altered since the most efficient way of conditioning, shrinking, and

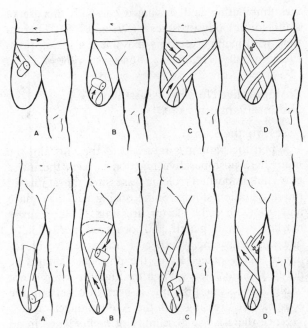

**Figure 21-2.** In bandaging a stump of the upper leg, the bandage is anchored at the waist. The bandage is applied while the patient is standing on his unaffected leg. A crisscross (rather than a circular) pattern is followed around the leg, starting at the stump end. Each loop overlaps the previous one by at least half its width. The same principles apply to bandaging a stump of the lower leg. Anchoring is accomplished without a circular turn around the leg.

shaping the amputation stump is by using it. Even when immediate ambulation is not anticipated, the use of the cast considerably lessens the former lengthy period of stump conditioning for prosthesis fitting.

### Other Amputations

Hemipelvectomy, interscapulothoracic amputation, and translumbar amputation (hemicorporectomy) are radical procedures used in specialized centers when the patient has a bone or soft tissue malignancy. The nursing care is complex depending upon the patient's disturbance in self-image, loss of function, and involvement of other organ systems. Special prostheses are required for some return of function. In one report a 49-year-old male underwent total amputation of the lower body at the level of L4 to L5 for cancer of the bladder and intractable pain. Four and one-half years later he

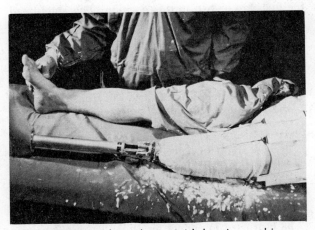

**Figure 21-1.** Above-knee rigid dressing and immediate fitting in the operating room. (Institute of Rehabilitation Medicine, New York University Medical Center, New York, N.Y.)

was ambulating and driving a car with the use of a full lower body prosthesis (Dietz, 1969). The patient with hemipelvectomy may have a sitting prosthesis initially (Hampton, 1964).

### Postoperative Nursing Assessment and Intervention

#### Assessing the Stump

When the patient is returned to the unit and the immediate postoperative reaction is past, the nurse plays an important role in assessing the status of the amputation stump. Some oozing will take place and stain the rigid plaster dressing. If the stain is marked with a pencil and observed periodically, one can determine whether or not excessive bleeding is taking place. If so, the physician should be notified immediately. When the rigid dressing is not applied, the same principle is used in observing the compressive dressing with the Ace bandages.

Since there is the possibility of *hemorrhage* in an amputation stump when a rigid dressing is not applied, the nurse observes the degree of bleeding carefully. A tourniquet should be in view, tied to the bed in the event that massive bleeding is evident. With the use of the rigid dressing, however, hemorrhage is not possible.

Most of the amputations that are done on an elective basis are completely *closed* without the use of a drain. It is usually not necessary to drain a stump which is encased in a rigid dressing since it cannot bleed and cannot swell. If there is any possibility of infection, the rigid dressing is not applied and a closed amputation is not performed. When a drain is used it is removed through a cast window on the first or second postoperative day.

*Open* amputations (guillotine operation) are often performed in the presence of *infection*. These are left open and the skin placed in traction so that a secondary closure may be accomplished at a later date. Close observation by the nurse is necessary to observe the degree of oozing from the amputation stump. The nurse should be alert for the odor which is characteristic of infection and notify the physician with regard to both bleeding and the development of an odor from the amputation stump.

If the wound is infected, reoperation or perhaps amputation at a higher level may be performed after the infection is cleared and the patient's condition is improved. Sometimes the stump is allowed to heal without revision (reamputation). Sometimes revision is done. For instance, a guillotine operation may be revised later to provide a stump suitable for the prosthesis.

Another important consideration in an open amputation is maintenance of skin *traction* which is used to prevent the skin and muscles from retracting. In such a situation, the traction must be continuous. The surgeon may arrange the traction so that the patient can turn over in bed and even get up in a wheelchair with a specially designed traction board without interrupting the pull of the weights.

#### Preventing Contractures

When a flap operation (closed amputation) has been performed and a rigid plaster dressing is not used, the patient returns to the ward with a pressure dressing and perhaps a splint. The splint may be applied to prevent contractures at the knee or the elbow. The splint should be padded well to prevent skin irritation and the breakdown that may be caused by the pull of muscle spasm against the splint.

Bed positioning of the patient must be considered. With the rigid dressing there is no danger of the development of flexion contractures of the stump. When the rigid dressing is not used, bed positioning to prevent contractures is quite important. The patient can be made comfortable by placing a pillow under the thigh or under the knee if he has a great deal of pain. No harm is done in the first day or two in this position. The amputated limb, however, should be kept in extension alignment with the body thereafter at all times. The nurse may assist in the prevention of contractures by carrying out the following directives:

- **Assist and teach the patient to roll from side to side and to assume a face-lying position (prone) in order to create extension for the amputation stump. Know what the physician and physical therapist permit. Because the patient may experience a great deal of pain in the immediate postoperative period, a good time for placing him prone is about one half-hour after he has received medication for pain. Then he will be more comfortable and better able to move.**

  **While he is lying on his abdomen, the patient may be instructed to adduct the stump so that it presses against his other leg. His toes should extend over the end of the mattress so that they are not pressed down**

into the mattress. When the patient lies on his un-affected side, he may be taught to flex gently and to extend his stump. When a patient with a below-knee amputation is in the supine position, and a pillow has been placed momentarily under his knee on the oper-ative side, he can flex gently and extend his knee. He is taught to pull himself up in bed by using his arms and the overhead trapeze rather than to push with his heel, which may become sore.

- **The patient's mattress must be firm. A sagging mat-tress can cause a flexion contracture.**

- **The foot of the bed is elevated on blocks, if this is permitted, instead of using a pillow. The foot gatch should not be raised as this would have the same effect as using a pillow.**

- **Work with the physical therapist so that a program of exercises to prevent contractures is implemented for the patient who progresses to the point where he is up in a wheelchair most of the day. For example, to prevent hip flexion contracture, the patient can be taught to suspend his stump over the edge of the bed and go through the full range of joint motion before he gets up and when he returns to bed. Attention is paid to the remaining limb as well as to the stump. Good muscle tone is maintained by range-of-motion exercises, with the patient doing the work. Footdrop is avoided by ankle exercises and the use of a foot-board.**

Amputation is major surgery and a great strain even for the young and the robust. The patient, especially the older one who may be in poorer physical condition should not be permitted to over-strain himself and become fatigued.

### Temporary Prosthesis

When immediate fitting of a temporary prosthesis is performed in the operating room, it is intended to get the patient up as soon as possible. Thus, the patient with a rigid dressing may be allowed to sit on the edge of the bed and dangle his unaffected leg on the day of surgery. If he has the stamina the next day or the second postoperative day, he may be permitted to stand and regain his sense of bal-ance. Touching down on the floor with the impro-vised prosthesis and weight bearing of about 10 per cent of body weight is permitted.

The pylon which serves as a temporary pros-thesis is detached when the patient is in bed but must be attached at all times when he is out of bed to prevent the stump from being pulled out of the cast (rigid dressing) by the effect of gravity or the weight of the cast. The nurse checks the suspension straps and notifies the appropriate team member if a suspension strap is loose and cannot be tightened. If the cast comes off accidentally the nurse should immediately bandage the stump with an elastic bandage to prevent swelling and edema, then notify the physician.

If the rigid dressing is applied properly, the pa-tient can progress to walk with crutches or a walk-erette or in parallel bars one, two, or three days after the amputation with a high degree of safety. He is not permitted to put full weight on the am-putation stump until six weeks after amputation. The reason is that the skin may heal in two weeks, but the deep tissues take at least six weeks for the scars to mature to the point where the tissues can withstand the forces of full weight bearing. If a walking pylon has been applied, the patient will be ambulating under the supervision of the physical therapist. He will also participate in activities in the physical therapy department. The nurse works with the physical therapist by positioning the pa-tient properly in bed, by encouraging exercises, and by supervising him as he attempts to stand, transfer weight and maintain balance in his room. Thus, it is important that the nurse keep in touch with the physical therapist to know what exercises are to be continued on the ward.

Whenever the patient returns from the physical therapy department, the nurse should question him with regard to shortness of breath, the presence of pain, his response to exertion, and the condition of the phantom. She should also encourage the patient to continue his program so that he may make progress. Two or three weeks after ampu-tation, the cast is removed so that the skin sutures can be removed.

After the sutures are removed, the patient is fitted with a temporary prosthesis (Fig. 21-3) with which he walks until his stump is in condition to tolerate a permanent prosthesis. Under these con-ditions it is possible for the patient to be ambula-tory on two legs when he leaves the hospital about a month after surgery, provided the scar is healed and all other conditions are satisfactory. This is far better than the previous standard technique of dis-charging a patient and having him wait for several months before his amputation stump is ready to be fitted with a prosthesis. In this waiting period there is a great deal of time lost. Depression and atrophic phenomena may develop because he often has no means of maintaining himself in satisfactory physical condition.

In some centers, upon removal of the initial cast socket as a rigid dressing, the patient is fitted with a removable plastic socket (Fig. 21-3). Under these conditions, the amputation stump will have a tendency to swell and the nurse may be required to bandage it or apply an elastic stump-shrinking sock so that the patient may sleep in it. This prevents excessive swelling so that the prosthesis will fit in the morning when he is ready to use it. The amputation stump will have a tendency to swell for about three weeks. This is why in most centers where immediate or early ambulation is carried out, the initial cast is left on for about 21 days, so that a removable prosthesis can be applied, avoiding the need to fit another socket.

The whole process of postoperative management has changed in recent years since it is known that even if a standard amputation is performed and the stump heals in a reasonable length of time, the pa-

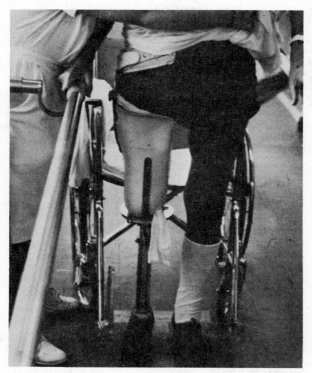

**Figure 21-3.** Temporary, removable above-knee socket and walking pylon. (Institute of Rehabilitation Medicine, New York University Medical Center, New York, N.Y.)

tient can be fitted with a prosthesis three or four weeks after amputation. If he is using a walking pylon, the concept of doing exercises and strengthening muscles is less important since the patient is active rather than passive during the postoperative period, and the activities in which he is engaged are precisely the ones which he needs to keep his muscles strong and functioning without additional exercise.

### Caring for the Stump

The type of surgery performed influences the length of time for stump conditioning, shrinking, and shaping. However, there are some general principles to be observed.

**Bandaging.** To help the stump shrink and shape properly for the wearing of a prosthesis, two or three elastic bandages may be sewn together and applied to the stump. The physician generally determines the method for applying the bandage. The stump usually is bandaged first with an over-and-under motion and then with a spiral motion (Fig. 21-2). All parts of the wrapped limb should be equally compressed. If the proximal part of the stump is compressed more tightly than the rest of the limb, edema will result in the end of the stump (bulbous edema). When a bandage is applied to an above-knee amputation, the spirals are continued as high as possible to avoid a roll of flesh above the bandage. The bandage is changed at least twice during the day and before the patient retires for the night, at which time the underlying skin is inspected. In the summer especially, when the patient perspires profusely, the stump should be washed each time that the bandage is changed, and talc applied. If the skin is dry, a little petrolatum or cold cream may be used.

If the patient will have to bandage his stump at home, he and a member of his family should be taught how to apply the bandage and how to care for the stump. He should also be taught to wash the bandages between wearings, to rinse them well, and to lay them flat to dry, since hanging tends to decrease the elasticity. When the bandages are dry, they should be rolled without stretching. It is safer to use safety pins instead of clasps to secure the end of the bandage. If the patient uses a leather shrinker, he should be cautioned to use it with the same precautions that he would use with elastic bandages, giving special attention to cleanliness, frequent changes, prevention of tightness on the top, and skin irritation.

The nurse should check to make sure that the patient is applying the elastic bandage or any other device for shrinkage with even pressure from the tip of the stump on up the limb. The patient and the nurse should look for shrinkage without pockets of flabbiness. The patient should return to his physician if the stump becomes uneven.

**Protecting the Stump.** Successful ambulation depends on maintaining both the stump and the prosthesis in good condition. The patient should learn to protect both. Trauma to the stump may necessitate a return to the wheelchair or even to surgery, and repair of the prosthesis is an added expense. The stump is protected also by good daily care. It should be inspected for skin irritation and should be bathed, aired, and powdered twice a day. Stump socks should be washed every day. When they tear or stretch, they should be discarded; the roughness of a darn or the crease of a stretched sock may cause a decubitus ulcer.

## Upper Extremity

A similar approach is used in amputations of the upper extremity. The surgical objective here is to create a gently tapering stump with muscular padding over the end. The upper extremity amputation stump moves within the socket more and is subject to more variations in friction than the lower extremity stump. For this reason the myoplastic closure and loose approximation of the skin flaps are essential. Tight skin across a subcutaneous cut bone end is the primary cause of the pain in an upper extremity amputation at any level.

**Postoperative Dressing.** The application of a rigid dressing can simplify the postoperative care of the upper extremity amputee, but it is seldom used. The reason is that most upper extremity amputations are performed following extensive trauma or infection. In addition the greatest length is preserved. In emergency circumstances, the application of a rigid dressing adds to the risk of complications since the necessary, frequent inspection of the part would not be possible.

The dressing of an upper extremity stump usually consists of a thin strip of nonadherent material such as Telfa, silk, or petrolatum gauze, covered with fluffy gauze and kept in place with a gently compressive bandage. This bandage is not designed for shrinkage, but simply for external support to hold the dressing on and to some extent control posttraumatic and surgical edema.

**Exercise.** During the healing period the patient may become ambulatory and is made aware of the importance of good posture. In amputations above the elbow and higher, there is a tendency for the trunk to tilt away from the side of the amputation and for the head to tilt toward it. Eventual foreshortening of the shoulder girdle results in scoliosis. This is of greater importance, of course, in growing children. For this reason, deep breathing, bilateral adduction and abduction exercises for the scapulae, and shoulder shrugging should be practiced several times daily.

Most patients with upper extremity amputations can be measured for a prosthesis shortly after the surgical scar has healed. It is necessary to maintain full range of motion in the remaining joints and build up strength in the muscles by the time the prosthesis is finally delivered. This is accomplished by carrying out passive exercises and by encouraging the patient to perform active exercises within his tolerance. The nurse gives the patient support and supervision as necessary and is guided by the physical therapist.

**Bandaging.** Only when there is no longer the possibility of infection and the scar is well on the way to healing is shrinking bandaging done. The elastic bandage is applied in the same manner as for lower extremity stumps. Compression proximally is achieved by spirals and doubling back the bandage to avoid circular constriction. Upper extremity stumps do not need massive shrinkage over a long period as do those of the lower extremity. They will not be subjected to the great forces of body weight support even while using a prosthesis, and usually stabilize in about six months.

**Other Considerations.** A person who loses his dominant hand has the choice of learning to do everything (write, light a match, count change, eat, and so on) with his other hand or of learning to use a prosthesis. There are many things a one-handed person cannot do for himself. For example, he cannot wash his hand. Since the loss of a hand is a devastating disability, one that makes a difference to the patient almost every minute of the day, early restoration of the sense of purposeful use is important and can be accomplished by placing a temporary cuff over the stump and fitting it with a clip or clamp which can hold a pencil, a piece of chalk, or a spoon. The patient can then have the satisfaction of practicing writing on paper or a blackboard and attempting to feed himself as training procedures.

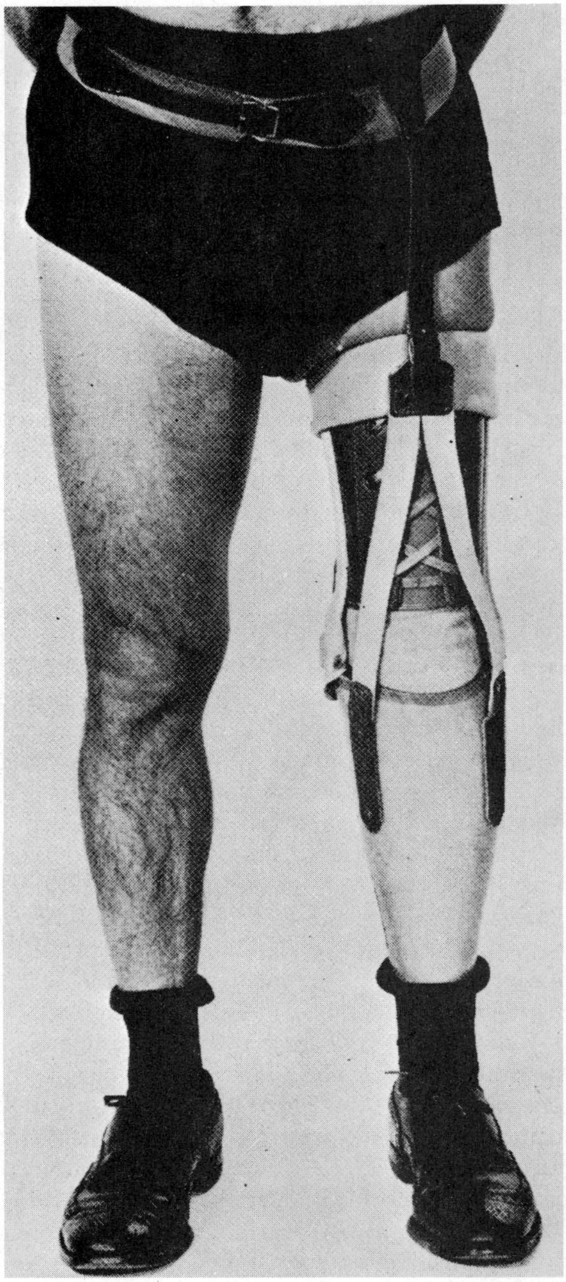

The upper extremity phantom is more active and liable to be more painful than the phantom of the lower extremity. The more violent the injury or the more painful the condition for which the amputation was performed, the more troublesome will the phantom tend to be. Many patients feel that the absent hand is bleeding, or is in a cramped position. A common complaint is that the thumb is dug into the palm of the hand. Exercising the muscles of the stump as if the limb were still there should be part of the daily routine. For example, the patient closes his eyes and moves the stump as if he were putting the limb through full range of motion. Bilateral opening and closing of the hands, movements of the individual fingers and shaking of the wrists are part of the phantom exercise routine. The nurse can play a very important part of this preprosthetic training program in association with the occupational therapist. With persistence and support, the painful phantom is eliminated by purposeful use of a functional prosthesis, whether the upper or the lower extremity is involved.

Complications that may occur late in the postoperative course include chronic osteomyelitis (following persistent infection) and, rarely, a burning pain (causalgia), the etiology of which is not known. Pain may also be caused by a stump neuroma, which is formed when the cut ends of nerves become entangled in the healing scar. A neuroma may be treated with injections of procaine, or reamputation may be necessary.

## Fitting with a Prosthesis

With few exceptions artificial limbs are made by commercial prosthetists working closely with physicians. Prostheses are not made by type, but are assembled from components prescribed by a physician. Components are individually prescribed for the special requirements of each patient. The basic components of a prosthesis are:

| LOWER EXTREMITY (FIGS. 21-4 to 21-6) | UPPER EXTREMITY (FIG. 21-7) |
|---|---|
| Socket | Socket |
| Suspension | Harness |
| Joints (hip, knee) | Joints (elbow, wrist) |
| Foot and ankle | Terminal devices |

Each component allows the physician a choice to suit the individual. Lower extremity sockets are usually made of laminated plastic of open, closed, or total contact design. Plastic sockets are made

**Figure 21-4.** Conventional below-knee wood socket with knee joints and laced thigh corset. (Institute of Rehabilitation Medicine, New York University Medical Center, New York, N.Y.)

from a modified plaster cast of the stump. Willow wood or extra light wood sockets are made from measurements and shaped anatomically to support weight on predetermined landmarks.

The socket is suspended or kept on by suction, waist belts, hip joint and pelvic bands, shoulder straps, laced leather thigh corset or supracondylar strap, depending on the level of amputation and the characteristics of the amputation stump. Suction is created in a closed socket with a valve which allows air to be expelled from it, but not to get into the socket.

**Knee Joints.** Knee joints may be of single axis type, polycentric, positive friction, locking (safety) or hydraulic. The physician may choose to order a manual lock which keeps the knee stiff on weight bearing, but which the patient can unlock when he sits. The ankle and foot may be of the single axis type with an articulated foot or Sach (solid ankle, cushion heel), which is one piece with a compressible rubber heel wedge.

**Upper Extremity Sockets.** Upper extremity

sockets are made of laminated plastic and are suspended by a harness. The harness is usually the figure-of-8 type with a closed loop over the unin-

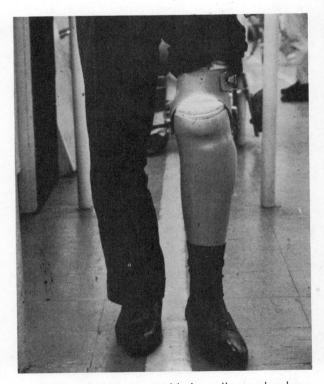

**Figure 21-5.** Plastic, molded patellar tendon-bearing below-knee socket suspended by a supracondylar strap. (Institute of Rehabilitation Medicine, New York University Medical Center, New York, N.Y.)

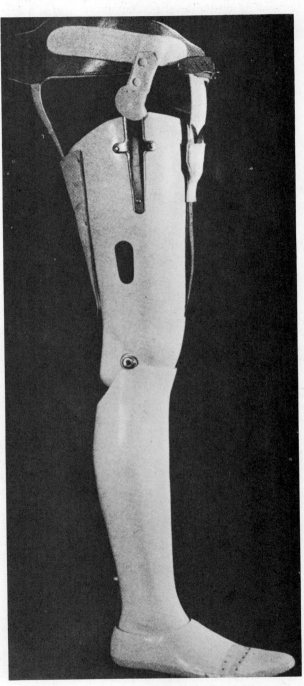

**Figure 21-6.** Conventional above-knee wood socket with hip joint and pelvic band; single axis knee and ankle. (Institute of Rehabilitation Medicine, New York University Medical Center, New York, N.Y.)

volved shoulder. The other loop is split so that one strap holds the limb on and the other is attached to a cable which operates the terminal device (Fig. 21-8). Many variations of harnessing are available depending on the level of amputation and the special requirements of the individual (Fig. 21-9). The elbow may be of the automatic alternating locking type for above-elbow or the rigid, flexible or polycentric for below-elbow amputations. Wrist units are of manual friction, quick disconnect type for changing terminal devices, or with flexion unit, all of which are round. For amputations near the wrist, the unit is oval, corresponding to the shape of the wrist. The terminal devices consist of steel and aluminum split hooks, with or without rubber inserts in the "fingers," or voluntary opening and

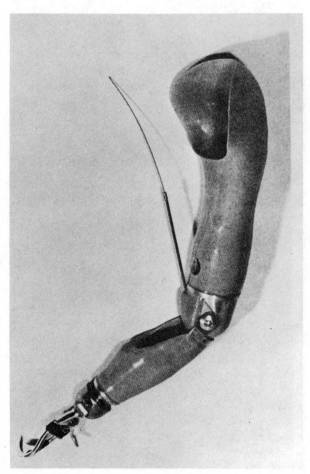

**Figure 21-7.** Standard above-elbow prosthesis with wrist flexion unit, voluntary opening hook. (Institute of Rehabilitation Medicine, New York University Medical Center, New York, N.Y.)

voluntary closing hands (Fig. 21-10). The hooks and hands all provide one function—pinch. The pinch or prehension of the hand consists of the index and middle fingers approximating the thumb. On the split hooks, one prong or finger is stationary while the other, or thumb, moves. The fingers are held in approximation by rubber bands and are separated by a pull on the cable.

**Fitting the Prosthesis.** The prosthetic prescription utilizes the proper combination of these components and obviously should be written by a knowledgeable physician. Prostheses should be made by a certified prosthetist—one who has a certificate of professional competence from the American Board for Certification of Prosthetists, by examination. Fitting and fabrication of a prosthesis is a skillful process. With an ill-fitting prosthesis or one with the wrong components or poorly aligned, the amputee has no chance to reach his best potential.

### Training with a Prosthesis

A prosthesis is not designed to replace the lost part, its functions, or its appearance. Therefore the function achieved should not be compared to normal function but is to be evaluated against the patient's best potential. The amputee's potential depends upon such variables as his age, the type of amputation, condition of the amputation stump, physical status, condition of the remaining limbs, concurrent debilitating illness, visual motor coordination, motivation, acceptance, cooperation, and insight. Patients vary greatly in their capability of deriving function and in their learning capacity with their prosthesis; the period allotted for their training varies and is affected by such factors as the speed with which the patient learns and his potential for rehabilitation.

For some patients a prosthesis signifies tragedy; to them it is a constant reminder of inadequacy. For others a prosthesis is an expensive, sometimes troublesome piece of machinery that nevertheless is of great help. Al Capp, the cartoonist, who lost a leg at the age of nine, said:

> . . . I had learned how to live without resentment or embarrassment in a world in which I was different from everyone else. The secret, I found, was to be indifferent to that difference. . . . As you sway through life on a wooden leg, an odd and blessed thing happens. The rest of the world be-

comes accustomed, and then forgets that you have one, just as it becomes accustomed to, and then forgets the color of your eyes or whether you wear a vest. And you become accustomed to the limitations of one-legged life, such as not being able to pole-vault or drive a shift car, or being limited to half as much athlete's foot as other people have (Capp, 1960).

A prosthesis is expensive. If mental depression prevents its use, it is of equal importance to relieve the depression as well as concentrate on ambulation or dexterity. For some patients, alleviation of despair is a more important consideration than the mode of getting from one place to another.

## Lower Extremity Prosthesis

The purpose of a lower extremity prosthesis is to provide weight support and comfort as well as the capacity to ambulate with safety, with or without mechanical aids. The process is begun by teaching the patient to apply the prosthesis properly without assistance. His training starts with standing and weight shifting to get the feel of weight support and balance, between parallel bars. He is then taught heel and toe balance and rocking and hip hiking to get the prosthesis off the ground. Early steps begin by advancing the prosthesis first and bringing up the other leg to the standing position. With practice, alternate steps and increasing weight bearing are progressively accomplished. Initially crutches, the walkerette, or canes are used until the patient has sufficient confidence and stability to discard them. It takes about two weeks of daily training to determine what any individual patient's best function will be. Daily practice for about two months thereafter usually permits the patient to achieve a satisfactory level of function. During this time and for about two years, the use of the prosthesis will cause the stump to shrink in volume, making the socket loose. The sign of shrinking is sinking of the stump too far into the socket, causing pressure in the groin or over the patella. Additional stump socks take up this volume, or placing a leather liner in the socket will improve the fit and comfort. After a first fitting, the prosthetist should check the fit every month for six months and make the necessary adjustments in fit and alignment. Painful stumps are basically medical problems and cannot be solved by changes in the prosthesis. Any discomfort caused by the prosthesis itself should be corrected as soon as possible. The nurse is in a position to discuss the progress with the patient and to examine the stump. Any observations relating to fit, comfort, or general physical stress should be reported to the physician, the physical therapist, or the prosthetist.

Learning to walk correctly takes time and practice. The patient may learn this skill in a physician's office, a rehabilitation center, or a hospital clinic.

As with any physical skill, learning good technique right from the beginning will lead eventually to a more polished performance. If the patient develops poor habits, such as taking a longer step with the prosthetic foot or hiking the hip and shoulder on the amputated side with each step, or walking with the feet too far apart, his walk will be less normal. Handicapped by such habits, it will be more difficult later for him to attain normal speed. It is much harder to correct a well-established fault in any physical skill, be it playing tennis or walking with a prosthesis, than to learn correct technique in the first place. The nurse should work closely with the physical therapist and help the patient early to overcome defects in gait, so that eventually his walk will be as smooth as possible.

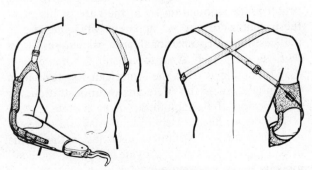

**Figure 21-8.** Below-elbow figure-of-8 harness. (Institute of Rehabilitation Medicine, New York University Medical Center, New York, N.Y.)

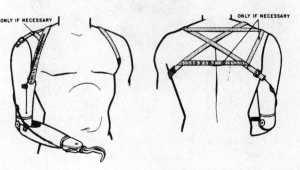

**Figure 21-9.** Above-elbow figure-of-8 harness. (Institute of Rehabilitation Medicine, New York University Medical Center, New York, N.Y.)

## Upper Extremity Prosthesis

Upper extremity amputees are trained by occupational therapists and assisted by the nurse. The training consists of teaching the patient to apply and operate the prosthesis. He is taught procedures to bend and lock the elbow and proper methods for using the harness. He is given very small increasingly difficult operations to perform with the terminal device, whether it is the hook or the hand. The prosthesis is not operated by the opposite shoulder. The loop over the uninvolved shoulder is for anchorage. The reaction point is at the cross over between the figure-of-8 loops. All of the operations of the elbow and terminal devices are controlled by the shoulder on the amputated side. The cable is pulled by protraction of the scapula on the amputated side. This increases the distance between the reaction point and the attachment of the cable to the thumb of the hook or hand, causing it to open. With practice, the amputee can operate the prosthesis with almost imperceptible motions.

## Recent Advances

Within the last decade or so great advances have been made in the operative concepts and the design and function of prostheses. They can be made exceptionally light in order to make it possible for a patient to function, even at a low level, with a de-

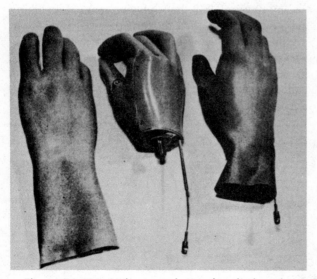

**Figure 21-10.** Voluntary closing hand plus glove. (Institute of Rehabilitation Medicine, New York University Medical Center, New York, N.Y.)

gree of comfort which makes ambulation practical. Heavy plastic and steel are usual components of prostheses, but light woods, including treated balsa wood, aluminum, and light plastics can be substituted and be made functional.

**Teamwork.** One of the most important advances is the concept of the teamwork approach in the rehabilitation of the amputee. The nurse has more personal contact with the amputee than any other member of the team. In this role she is in a position to encourage and to help him become motivated, to promote wound healing and gain his confidence and participation. Rehabilitation is not an all-or-nothing proposition. It does mean assessing strengths and liabilities and helping the patient to make the most of what he has. It is equally vital that the physician, the nurse, the physical therapist, the family, the patient, and other team members be realistic about what is expected. They should help the patient to set goals that are possible for him. A 71-year-old man with generalized arteriosclerosis and diabetes may never be able to walk without a cane for extra support. That he can ambulate at all is an important consideration.

The nurse can help the patient to realize that he has assets as well as problems. When people are discouraged, they sometimes fail to see that they have strengths with which to work. The nurse who can help her patient to see both sides of the ledger will be better able to help him to become self-directing. She herself must not give in to hopelessness, nor must she expect her efforts to yield spectacular results. Effective action—even, at times, unexpected success—will lie somewhere between these extremes.

Long-term medical and nursing supervision usually is desirable. A community health nurse who visits the home may help the patient to solve some problems in ambulation or in the care of his prosthesis that were not yet apparent when he was in the hospital. Organizational and printed resources that the nurse may wish to consult for her patient may be obtained from the American Rehabilitation Committee, Inc., the Veterans Administration, or the Division of Rehabilitation of each state.

The local health department may be able to give the names of volunteer agencies in the locale of the patient that may provide financial, medical, job placement or counseling facilities.

"My Well-balanced Life on a Wooden Leg" was written by Al Capp in *Life* magazine, May 23,

1960. If you can obtain a copy of this article for your patients to read, do so. They probably will find Mr. Capp's account of his experiences not only humorous but a real morale-builder.

## REFERENCES AND BIBLIOGRAPHY

ALDRICH, C.: *An Introduction to Dynamic Psychiatry,* New York, McGraw-Hill, 1966.

ANDERS, R. L., et al.: Amputee discussion program, *J. Psychiat. Nurs.* 10:21, July-August 1972.

ARNOLD, H. M.: Elderly diabetic amputees, *Am. J. Nurs.* 69:2646, December 1969.

BLISS, R.: Covert behaviors: Recognition and intervention, *ANA Clinical Sessions,* p. 309, New York, Appleton-Century-Crofts, 1968.

BOSANKO, L. A.: Immediate postoperative prosthesis, *Am. J. Nurs.* 71:280, February 1971.

BRADY, E.: Grief and amputation, *ANA Clinical Sessions,* p. 297, New York, Appleton-Century-Crofts, 1968.

BROWN, F.: Knowledge of body image and nursing care of the patient with limb amputation, *J. Psychiat. Nurs.* 2:397, 1964.

BROWN, W. A.: Postamputation phantom limb pain, *Dis. Nerv. Syst.* 29:301, May 1968.

BURGESS, E .M., et al.: *The Management of Lower Extremity Amputations,* Washington, D.C., Prosthetic and Sensory Aids Service, Department of Medicine and Surgery, Veterans Administration, August, 1969. (May be purchased from Superintendent of Documents, U.S. Government Printing Office, Washington, D.C. 20402.)

CAPP, A.: My well-balanced life on a wooden leg, *Life* 48(20):129-140, May 1960.

COMMITTEE ON PROSTHETIC-ORTHOTIC EDUCATION: *Amputees, Amputations and Artificial Limbs. An Annotated Bibliography,* Washington, D.C., National Research Council, 1969.

————: *Review of Visual Aids for Prosthetics and Orthotics,* Washington, D.C., National Research Council, 1969.

DIETZ, J. H., JR.: Rehabilitation of the cancer patient, *Med. Clin. N. Am.* 53:607, May 1969.

GERHARDT, J. J.: Immediate post-surgical prosthetics rehabilitation aspects, *Am. J. Phys. Med.* 49:3-105, February 1970.

GIERMAN, R. L.: Two medals for heroism, *Am. J. Nurs.* 72:1810, October 1972.

GORMAN, J. F., and ROSENBERG, J. C.: Dry ice refrigeration for above-knee amputations, *Am. J. Surg.* 113:241, February 1967.

HAMPTON, F.: A hemipelvectomy prosthesis, *Artific. Limbs* 8:3, Spring 1964.

HIGINBOTHAM, N. L.: Amputation: Crippling help, *J. Rehab.* 32:14, May-June 1966.

HODKINSON, M. A.: Some clinical problems of geriatric nursing, *Nurs. Clin. N. Am.* 3:675, December 1968.

*Hospital Resources for a Quality Amputation Program,* Report of Intersociety Commission for Heart Disease Resources, *Circulation* XLVI:A-293, July 1972.

HULL, P., and THOMAS, E.: Nursing regimen for the care of the amputee with contracture, *ANA Clinical Sessions,* p. 103, New York, Appleton-Century-Crofts, 1968.

JEGLIJEWSKI, J. M.: Target: Outside world, *Am. J. Nurs.* 73:1024, June 1973.

KAHN, K. H., et al.: A multiphasic study of lower extremity amputees, *JAMA* 199:537, February 1967.

KIRKPATRICK, S.: Battle casualty: Amputee, *Am. J. Nurs.* 68:998, May 1968.

LARSON, C., and GOULD, M.: *Calderwood's Orthopedic Nursing,* ed. 7, St. Louis, Mosby, 1970.

LEONARD, B. J.: Body image changes in chronic illness. *Nurs. Clin. N. Am.* 7:687, December 1972.

LOWMAN, E., and KLINGER, J.: *Aids to Independent Living: Self-Help for the Handicapped,* New York, McGraw-Hill, 1969.

MARTIN, N.: Rehabilitation of the upper extremity amputee, *Nurs. Outlook* 18:50, February 1970.

MAZET, R., and HENNESSY, C. P.: Knee disarticulation, *J. Bone Joint Surg.* 48A:126, January 1966.

MITAL, M., and PIERCE, D.: *Amputees and Their Prosthesis,* Boston, Little, Brown, 1971.

MOURAD, M., and CHIU, W.: Marital-sexual adjustment of amputees, *Med. Asp. Human Sexuality,* VIII:47, February 1974.

MURRAY, R.: Principles of nursing intervention for the adult patient with body image changes, *Nurs. Clin. N. Am.* 7:697, December 1972.

NADLER, S. H., and THELAN, J. T.: A technique of interscapulothoracic amputation, *Surg. Gynec. Abst.* 122:358, February 1966.

Overlapping roles of nurses and therapists, *Nurs. '72* 2:45, May 1972.

PLAISTED, L. M., et al.: The nurse on the amputee clinic team, *Nurs. Outlook* 16:34, October 1968.

RUSSEK, A.: Immediate postsurgical fitting of the lower extremity amputee, *Med. Clin. N. Am.* 53:665, May 1969.

RUSSEK, A. S., et al.: *Investigation of Immediate Fitting and Early Ambulation Following Amputation in the Lower Extremity,* Monograph No. XLI, New York, Institute of Rehabilitation Medicine, 1969.

SHEWCHUK, M., and YOUNG, L.: The amputee and immediate prosthesis, *Canad. Nurse* 65:47, May 1969.

SOKOLOW, J.: Management of the amputee in practice, *Med. Clin. N. Am.* 53:659, May 1969.

STERNBACH, R.: *Pain—A Psychophysiological Analysis,* p. 117, New York, Academic Press, 1968.

THOMAS, B.: Nursing care of patients with cancer of the bone, *Nurs. Clin. N. Am.* 2:459, September 1967.

WARREN, R.: Early rehabilitation of the elderly lower extremity amputee, *Surg. Clin. N. Am.* 48:807, August 1968.

WILEY, L.: Traumatic amputation, *Nurs. '72* 2:240, November 1972.

ZILM, G.: Hyperbaric oxygen units—high pressure nursing, *Canad. Nurse* 65:37, February 1969.

# UNIT FIVE

## Disorders of Cognitive, Sensory, or Psychomotor Function

# The Patient with Neurologic Disturbance: General Nursing Considerations

## CHAPTER 22

Nursing care for patients with nervous system disorders challenges the nurse's judgment and initiative to carry out the nursing process. Assessment of these patients involves identification of their specific problems and needs in order to develop and implement plans of care and to allow for goal-directed evaluation. These patients may display some impairment of intellectual and/or emotional function that may range from slight to an apparent psychotic episode. The patient with a neurologic lesion or injury can have altered states of consciousness and sensory and motor disturbances that require accurate appraisal to establish the nursing diagnosis.

An individual's nervous system is subject to a variety of insults that change his physical function and influence his concept of body image, and his abilities to walk, to talk, and, in general, to perform the activities of daily living. The nurse must be able to combine suitable knowledge, and interpersonal and technical skills in order to plan and implement individualized care and to follow through with evaluation based on the patient's responses to the formulated objectives. Nursing care for the patient with a neurologic disorder must be concerned with the patient's wholeness and his interaction with the environment. Only then can the patient and his family be helped to achieve the maximum level of wellness that is possible, or supported as they cope with the process of dying.

The material in this chapter is intended to serve as a guide for the nurse and as an introduction to the methods of assessment needed to plan and carry out the neurologic patient's care. More detail may be found by referring to the bibliography at the end of the chapter.

Nursing Assessment

Increased Intracranial Pressure

Diagnostic Evaluation

365

## NURSING ASSESSMENT

This phase may precede or be concurrent with other parts of the nursing process. Patient appraisal may be carried out in the home or the clinic or the patient may need to be evaluated after he is admitted to the hospital. The nurse's role is to assess the patient's levels of wellness and illness in order to identify problems which will allow her to make a nursing diagnosis and to develop the nursing care plan.

**History Taking.** History taking provides a means for obtaining the information needed to evaluate the patient. The following facts should be included in the pertinent neurologic data secured from the patient during the interview:

1. **Confirmation of his reliability as the informant. It may be necessary to establish whether he understands the questions. If the patient has possible brain pathology, several questions should be asked to evaluate his reliability. If he is unable to communicate effectively, or if he is extremely ill, another person, preferably a family member, should be asked to supply the information relevant to the patient's mental and physical health.**

2. **Comprehensive personal, medical, family, and social data which could supply factors needed for the nursing diagnosis. Certain cerebrovascular diseases are related to the patient's age and sex. The patient's occupation and place of residence may be of significance in infectious diseases of the nervous system and injuries to the vertebrae and peripheral nerves.**

3. **The patient's statement of why he is seeking help and elaboration of the details are essential data for the nurse to obtain. He may have trouble with his balance as can be seen with cerebellar and cranial nerve disturbances, or he may have difficulties with voluntary movement in his lower extremities as evidenced in both upper and lower motor neuron diseases. Planning nursing care must include establishing priorities based on patient needs. Coping mechanisms vary greatly and the neurologic patient, by the nature of his illness, faces a very stressful situation.**

Assessment of the patient involves appraisal of his intellectual and emotional status, as well as his physical condition. It is essential to evaluate such factors as the patient's orientation to his surroundings, his understanding of his illness and of what is happening to him in the treatment situation, his emotional response to the illness, and his ways of coping with the stress of the experience. The patient's ways of relating to others, such as close friends and family, and any recent changes in these relationships, as noted by the patient or by others, are significant.

**Physical Assessment.** The physical examination helps to validate the patient's history and includes observation, inspection, percussion, palpation, and auscultation. When assessing the patient to determine possible neurologic disorder, the nurse should observe and investigate for alterations in:

**Levels of Consciousness.** The following classification of *levels of consciousness* applies to altered consciousness from any cause, including increased intracranial pressure; cerebral vascular accident; edema; effect of a drug, such as alcohol; anesthesia; fever; and disorders of brain physiology that may be brought about by such deviations as hypoxia and hypoglycemia.

ALERT WAKEFULNESS. The patient responds immediately, fully, and appropriately to visual, auditory, and other stimulation.

SOMNOLENCE OR LETHARGY. This is a state of drowsiness in which responses to stimulation are delayed or incomplete and in which increased stimulation, usually by verbal or manipulative means, is necessary to get the patient to respond. He may be delirious and restless, or quiet, falling asleep again when left alone. Although he can answer questions, he may be confused.

STUPOR. The patient can be aroused only by vigorous and continuing stimulation, usually by manipulation or perhaps by strong auditory or visual stimuli. Such stimulation may arouse him enough to answer simple questions with one or two words, or his response may be only restless motor activity or purposeful behavior directed toward avoiding further stimulation.

SEMICOMA. The patient is unresponsive except to superficial, relatively mild painful stimuli to which he makes some purposeful motor-avoiding response. Spontaneous motion is uncommon, but the patient may groan or mutter.

COMA. The patient is unresponsive to all but very painful stimuli to which he may make fragmentary, delayed reflex withdrawal or, in deeper stages, may lose all responsiveness. There is no spontaneous movment and respirations may be irregular.

**Cranial Nerves.** (See Table 22-1.)

**Posture, Station, and Gait.** ROMBERG'S SIGN. The patient is unable to stand with heels and toes together and eyes closed. He may exhibit abnormal findings, such as swaying, or he may fall with eyes closed although there is no difficulty with his position when the eyes are open. (When the nurse is assessing the patient, it is important to prevent his falling, if this appears imminent. She should have assistance, and stand close to the patient ready to support him as necessary.)

**Table 22-1. Cranial Nerves: Major Functions and Examples of Pathology**

| NERVE | MAJOR FUNCTION(S) | SIGNS OF POSSIBLE NERVE DISTURBANCE |
|---|---|---|
| I. Olfactory | sense of smell | hypersmia—acute sense of smell<br>parasmia—abnormal sense of smell<br>anosmia—loss of sense of smell |
| II. Optic | vision | defects of visual acuity<br>defects in the visual fields<br>papilledema—choked disk |
| III. Oculomotor<br>IV. Trochlear<br>VI. Abducens | movement of eyes and eyelids<br>pupillary reactions | impaired pupillary reaction<br>nystagmus—involuntary movement of eyeballs<br>diplopia; ptosis—drooping eyelid and inability to elevate eyelid |
| V. Trigeminal | mastication<br>sensation for face, nose, and mouth | disturbances of facial sensation<br>inability to chew<br>facial pain syndromes (trigeminal neuralgia) |
| VII. Facial | facial expression | paralysis of muscles of facial expression<br>inability to blink or close eyelids |
| VIII. Acoustic | hearing and equilibrium | tinnitus—ringing in the ear<br>hearing deficit<br>vertigo—lightheadedness with disorientation in relation to space |
| IX. Glosso-pharyngeal | taste in the posterior third of tongue<br>swallowing<br>salivation | loss of taste in posterior third of tongue<br>loss of gag reflex<br>dysphagia—difficulty in swallowing |
| X. Vagus | laryngeal control<br>inhibit heart rate<br>stimulate peristalsis | dysphonia—impairment of voice<br>abnormal heart rate<br>abdominal distention |
| XI. Accessory | movements of head and shoulders | difficulty in rotating head and raising chin against resistance<br>atrophy of muscles |
| XII. Hypoglossal | movements of the tongue | when protruded, deviation to affected side<br>fasciculations (coarse involuntary movements) of tongue |

OBSERVATION OF WALKING. The patient should be observed for his type of gait, his ability to coordinate movements, and his ability to walk a straight line (tandem walking). Examples of abnormalities include circumduction, broad-based ataxia, scissoring, short shuffling steps, and footdrop.

**Motion and Strength of Extremities.** The patient should be asked to perform active movements against resistance. Strength can also be assessed by comparing both sides of the patient (e.g., bilateral handgrips). Special consideration should be directed to regions where the patient may complain of a weakness.

**Sensation (Pain and Temperature).** This testing requires the patient's cooperation and should be performed with his eyes closed. Temperature can be tested with a warm or cold object. Superficial pain can be elicited with a pin. The patient should be asked about any unusual sensations, such as numbness, tingling, or "pins and needles."

## INCREASED INTRACRANIAL PRESSURE

The brain is enclosed in a sealed bony vault, the skull (Fig. 22-1). Expansion intracranially can be caused by edema, hemorrhage, neoplasm, progressive obstruction of the cerebrospinal fluid pathways, and infections such as meningitis, encephalitis, or abscess. Even though the etiology may vary, permanent brain damage may result from increasing intracranial pressure (Fig. 22-2).

### Signs and Symptoms

The nurse should diligently assess the patient for headache with or without vomiting, vital signs, which include level of consciousness, pulse, respirations, pupillary response, and motion and strength of extremities, and unusual bodily movements which could be indicative of a seizure.

The comparison of signs and symptoms of increased intracranial pressure with those of shock are summarized in Table 22-2.

### Nursing Intervention

Nursing intervention for the patient with increased intracranial pressure will vary, depending on the cause. There must be ongoing evaluation to estimate the patient's current state, because any deterioration or improvement will require a revised plan of care. The following nursing actions provide the means for assessment.

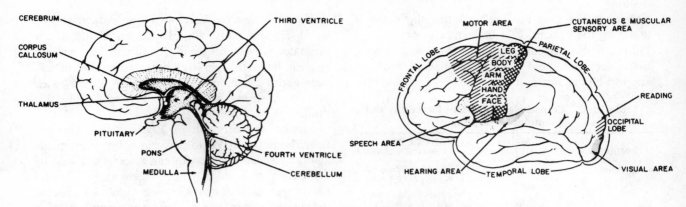

**Figure 22-1.** (*Left*) A diagram of the major structures of the brain. (*Right*) Diagrammatic representation of approximate areas of the brain that control various functions.

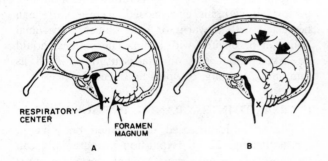

**Figure 22-2.** (A) The normal brain. (B) Herniation of the lower portion of the brain stem (medulla) through the foramen magnum, caused by increased intracranial pressure. Note the position of the respiratory center.

**Check Vital Signs Every 30 Minutes.** As with all disease conditions, the vital signs tell a story to the observer. A rapid increase in the pulse rate usually occurs initially. The rate may vary as much as 10 to 20 beats from the original reading; then, there is usually a drop. If the pulse becomes slower than 60 beats per minute and bounding, the physician should be notified immediately. Accompanying this change in pulse rate is an increase in the pulse pressure, and respirations may be variable. As the pressure on the cerebrum increases, there is usually an associated hypoxia. To compensate for this, the heart again beats faster. Tachycardia is one of the

**Table 22-2. Comparison of Signs and Symptoms of Increased Intracranial Pressure with Those of Shock**

| INCREASED INTRACRANIAL PRESSURE | SHOCK |
| --- | --- |
| 1. The pulse rate is increased initially; later, it is slow and bounding, 40–60 beats per minute. If hypoxia develops, the pulse becomes rapid again. | 1. The pulse rate is rapid, weak and thready, 100–160 beats per minute. |
| 2. Widening pulse pressure, i.e., the difference between the systolic and the diastolic blood pressure becomes greater than normal—example, 180/90. | 2. Both the systolic and the diastolic blood pressures drop. |
| 3. The respirations are irregular. | 3. The respirations are rapid and shallow; they may be as high as 40–50 per minute. |
| 4. The skin is dry and warm. The color may be pink or red. | 4. The skin is cold, clammy and moist; there is pallor due to peripheral vasoconstriction. |
| 5. The pupils may be unequal or unreactive. | 5. There is no pupillary change. |
| 6. There are decreasing levels of consciousness, progressing to coma. | 6. The patient usually is stuporous. |
| 7. There is increasing loss of motor power, such as hemiparesis. | 7. Loss of motor power is present only as it is related to low blood pressure. |

first homeostatic mechanisms to go into action when there is an oxygen lack for any reason.

As the sensorium becomes more depressed, respirations become more stertorous and wet due to the fluid collecting in the lungs and the lack of tone in the organs of respiration.

The widening pulse pressure is a compensatory mechanism. A gap of more than 30 points indicates increasing intracranial pressure if the original pressure was within normal limits.

**Check the Levels of Consciousness and Pupillary Reaction.** The brain stem has a great deal to do with the maintenance of the conscious state. Any direct trauma or associated pressure on the brain stem will cause a change in the level of consciousness. If a person is hit on the back of the head, he is likely to lose consciousness much more quickly than if he is hit on the forehead; however, if there is edema, hemorrhage, or increased production of cerebrospinal fluid, the brain substance itself will press down on the pons and cause progressive stupor.

If the temporal lobe is displaced medially by a mass, it may press on the third cranial (oculomotor) nerve, with the result that the muscles of the eye become paralyzed, and the corresponding pupil dilates and no longer reacts to a beam of light, such as that from a flashlight. Damage to the nuclei in the brain stem may result in constricted pupils, which also are unreactive.

**Check for Paralysis.** Loss of motor function is another valuable yardstick in ascertaining the amount of increased intracranial pressure. On admission of the patient, it should be determined whether or not he can move all four extremities. If the patient is asked to move his arm or hand, the nurse can determine not only the amount, kind, and type of motion, but also whether the patient understands and responds to requests. If he is semicomatose, he will respond only to a pinch or other painful stimuli. If he is able to move initially and later begins to lose this ability, the physician should be called immediately. Tests for motor function should be made as frequently as the vital signs are checked; if they are ordered every 15 minutes, the motor function should be checked every 15 minutes. During the time that the patient does not move himself, the nurse should position him in good body alignment, turn him from side to side to help to prevent pneumonia and decubitus ulcers, and start passive exercises to help to prevent contractures.

**Give Nothing by Mouth.** The previous three nursing actions have been concerned with the recognition of increased intracranial pressure. This action is directed toward its prevention. If the patient is given food or fluid by mouth, he runs the risk of vomiting. Vomiting, sneezing, coughing, and hiccoughing cause an increase in pressure. This must be guarded against, since any sudden increase in the pressure may precipitate herniation of the cerebellar tonsils through the foramen magnum, with medullary compression. The vital cardiopulmonary center is contained in the medulla. Pressure on this center will cause irregular respirations, or apnea. An unconscious patient is never given fluids by mouth, because he may aspirate them.

Although intake is prohibited by mouth, fluids are given intravenously. If the patient has been perspiring profusely, vomiting, or bleeding, additional fluid will be given. When there is marked increase in intracranial pressure, the fluid intake may be restricted. Overhydration or an infusion run too rapidly can increase intracranial pressure. The fluid should be administered at approximately 40 drops per minute.

**Elevate the Head of the Bed 30 Degrees, and Maintain the Patient's Head to the Side.** Patients with cerebral lesions are usually positioned with the head of the bed elevated to promote the return of venous drainage of blood and cerebrospinal fluid. Patients with basal skull fractures may be kept flat. In no instance should the patient's head be allowed to rest below the level of the rest of his body. Just as important is the maintenance of a patent airway.

Turning the patient on his side does not automatically result in a patent airway. He also may need suctioning. The principles of positioning of the patient with any cerebral lesion are (1) maintaining a patent airway, (2) avoiding increasing cerebral pressure by promoting, or at least not inhibiting, venous return from the brain, (3) preventing pressure sores, and (4) preventing deformities.

If positioning and suctioning do not result in an airway clear of secretions, a tracheostomy may be performed. Respiratory obstruction causes retention of carbon dioxide, which causes cerebral vasodilation and consequent swelling and congestion of the brain.

Oxygen is used frequently to combat the hypoxia associated with increased intracranial pressure. If oxygen is ordered by catheter, the patient's mouth and nose should be cleaned out frequently with a mild antiseptic solution and lubricated with some type of water-soluble lubricant, since oxygen has a dehydrating effect on the mucous membrane. The catheter should be removed and cleaned at least every four hours. The comatose patient who cannot swallow has increased oral and nasal secretions. In addition, he may have bleeding from the naso-pharynx, causing a clogging of the catheter with dried blood.

An emergency oxygen mask, nasal oxygen equipment, a suction machine, and an emergency tracheostomy tray should always be kept at the bedside for any patient who has an acute cerebral lesion of any type.

Concentrated, prompt, accurate action by the nurse is imperative. Any alteration in the patient's condition must be acted upon immediately.

## DIAGNOSTIC EVALUATION

Laboratory and radiologic studies provide useful data for the nursing diagnosis of the patient with a neurologic disorder. The subsequent nursing care plan and its implementation must be viable, and the laboratory and radiologic studies are essential to reassessment and replanning. The nurse must be able to explain the studies to the patient in order to answer his inquiries, and be sensitive to his expressions of fear and concern. Because patients frequently require a number of studies, priorities must be established to diminish threats to safety, fear of the unknown, and the amount of energy the patient must expend to cope with each given situation.

### Lumbar Puncture

Cerebrospinal fluid surrounds the brain and the spinal cord. By acting as a cushion it protects them and helps to maintain a relatively constant intracranial pressure.

Lumbar puncture is performed to obtain specimens of cerebrospinal fluids for examination, to inject medication (e.g., in spinal anesthesia), to measure the pressure of the cerebrospinal fluid, to withdraw the fluid for the relief of pressure, and to inject dye or air before taking roentgenograms of the brain and the spinal canal.

Normally, cerebrospinal fluid is crystal clear and colorless. It contains small amounts of protein, sugar, and, occasionally, a few lymphocytes. The normal pressure is 80 to 200 mm. of water; compressing the jugular veins increases the pressure of cerebrospinal fluid, if the circulation of the fluid is unobstructed (Queckenstedt's sign).

Changes in cerebrospinal fluid occur in many neurologic disorders. For example, meningitis (inflammation of the membranes that surround the brain and the spinal cord) causes a marked increase in the number of leukocytes in the cerebrospinal fluid, making it appear cloudy or even purulent. Often in a cerebral hemorrhage blood will be present in the spinal fluid, causing it to contain many red blood cells and to appear reddish. When a spinal cord tumor completely obstructs the flow of the fluid, no rise in pressure will occur during the Queckenstedt test. A partially obstructing tumor causes an unsatisfactory rise or fall. Fluid pressure is increased when intracranial pressure is increased, whether the cause be an abscess, a blood clot, a tumor, or any lesion that takes up space.

Bacteriologic tests on specimens of spinal fluid may reveal the presence of pathogenic organisms, such as the tubercle bacillus. Serologic tests for syphilis may be performed on spinal fluid.

Glucose will be decreased in bacterial meningitis. Protein usually is elevated when there is a spinal cord tumor or a brain abscess. Special analysis of the cerebrospinal fluid proteins (electrophoresis, immunophoresis) are frequently helpful in multiple sclerosis and other diseases.

A lumbar puncture is performed by inserting a hollow needle into the subarachnoid space of the spinal canal below the level of the spinal cord. (The cord extends to the region of the first and the second lumbar vertebrae; the needle usually is inserted between the third and the fourth lumbar vertebrae.)

The following points are important for the nurse to remember when she assists with a lumbar puncture:

- **Find out where the test is to be carried out and what position the patient is to assume. The test may be performed at the bedside or in the treatment room. Usually, the patient lies on his side, with his knees drawn up to his chest and his head drawn down to his knees. The arching of the back separates the vertebrae, so that the needle may be inserted more easily. Sometimes the test is performed with the patient sitting up on the treatment table.**

- **Help the patient understand the reasons for the test and why a written consent is needed. Emphasize the importance of lying still during the test. (Movement while the needle is in place may cause injury.) Some-**

times patients experience a shooting pain in one leg. Explain to the patient that he may experience some pain during the procedure, and that the pain does not indicate nerve damage. Knowing this possibility will help him to avoid sudden movement.

- Prepare the necessary equipment. An atmosphere of haste and confusion can be very upsetting to the patient.
- Help the patient to assume and to maintain the desired position, reassure him, and observe his reactions during the test.
- Help the patient to minimize headache. Headache occurs sometimes after lumbar puncture. Its exact cause is unknown, but it is thought to be associated with the loss of the cerebrospinal fluid. Patients may be asked to stay flat in bed for several hours after the test, because this position may minimize the likelihood of headache. The degree of ease and quickness with which the test is done, and the kind of preparation that the patient has had undoubtedly influence his emotional reaction to the experience, and that in turn may affect his symptoms afterward.

## Myelography

A lumbar puncture is performed in myelography, and a radiopaque substance is injected through the spinal needle into the spinal canal. X-ray films then are taken to demonstrate abnormalities of the spinal canal, such as tumors or a ruptured intervertebral disk. When the roentgenograms have been taken, the dye is removed via the spinal needle to prevent irritation of the meninges by the dye. Movement of the spinal needle is necessary in order to remove the dye. This movement sometimes causes pain, due to the contact of the needle with the nerve roots. If the patient is told before this test that some pain commonly is felt, and that it does not indicate any untoward response, it will be easier for him to tolerate the discomfort. Afterward he should rest flat in bed for a few hours. He should be watched for signs of meningeal irritation (stiffness of the neck and pain when an attempt is made to bend the head forward).

The term *diskography* refers to the injection of a radiopaque substance into an intervertebral disk, followed by taking x-ray films that reveal abnormalities of the disk. Diskography is used particularly in the diagnosis of ruptured intervertebral disk.

## Pneumoencephalography

A pneumoencephalogram is performed to visualize lesions of the brain by the use of roentgenograms. In this diagnostic test a lumbar puncture is performed with the patient sitting upright, cerebrospinal fluid is withdrawn, and filtered air is injected into the subarachnoid space through the spinal needle. The air rises in the spinal canal and fills the ventricles of the brain so that their size, shape, and position can be seen; then x-ray films are taken. If there is a brain lesion nearby that occupies space, such as a tumor, the contour of a ventricle may be distorted. Since the brain is held within the inflexible skull, abnormalities that take up space cannot cause herniation outward (except into the upper cervical spine via the foramen magnum) but can cause distortion of the surrounding tissue inside the cranial vault.

The preparation of the patient for pneumoencephalography is similar to that of a preoperative patient. The patient must give written permission for this diagnostic study. A sedative usually is ordered the night before, and often it is repeated the morning of the test.

Other aspects of preoperative care that are applicable to patients being prepared for pneumoencephalography include:

- Attention to personal cleanliness
- Removal of hairpins and dentures
- Noting and recording vital signs on the patient's chart
- Omission of food and fluids for six hours before the test

Patients usually experience a severe headache after pneumoencephalography. Some also have nausea, vomiting, and fever, and they may have shock, convulsions, respiratory distress, or symptoms of increased intracranial pressure. The patient may hear a splashing noise when he turns his head. This reaction is due to the presence of air in the ventricles. The symptoms gradually subside over a period of about two days, as the air is absorbed gradually, and cerebrospinal fluid is produced to replace that which was removed during the test.

After a pneumoencephalogram has been taken, the patient is placed flat in bed, at complete rest. The movement of his head tends to increase the severity of the symptoms. An ice cap to the head, codeine, and aspirin may be ordered. The patient should be fed, bathed, and given assistance when he turns. Fluids are encouraged to increase production of cerebrospinal fluid. Level of consciousness, state of pupils, pulse, respiration, and blood pressure are observed and recorded frequently, on the basis of the physician's order. Usually, these observations are taken every 15 minutes or every half-hour at first. On the second or the third day after the test, the patient is assisted to get up. He should sit up first and then slowly assume a standing position. If he experiences headache, he may be placed on bed rest for another day.

## Ventriculography

The procedure for ventriculography is similar to that for pneumoencephalography, except that the air is injected into the ventricles of the brain through burr holes made in the skull. Ventriculography is used when pneumoencephalography is not possible. For example, obstruction of the spinal canal may make it necessary to secure a ventriculogram rather than a pneumoencephalogram. Since the air injected during a lumbar puncture could not rise to the ventricles if the spinal canal were blocked, the air is injected into the ventricles. Ventricular puncture is the procedure preferred by many neurosurgeons when increased intracranial pressure is known or suspected, because lumbar puncture may permit shifts of brain tissue downward through the foramen magnum from loss of fluid below.

Hair that covers the area where the burr holes are to be made must be shaved before the ventriculography is performed. Other preparation is similar to that for pneumoencephalography. Ventriculography is performed in the operating room under local or general anesthesia.

The care of the patient after ventriculography is similar to that of a patient after pneumoencephalography. However, the former patient is less likely to suffer headache, because during ventriculography there is less chance the air will enter the subarachnoid space. Sterile ventricular needles should be kept at the patient's bedside. If there is a sudden increase in pressure after the ventricular puncture, the patient may require an immediate tap.

## Cerebral Angiography

In cerebral angiography, a radiopaque substance is injected into the cerebral circulation for x-ray studies of the extracranial and intracranial circulation. This test can reveal abnormalities of the blood-vessel walls, such as aneurysms or displacement of blood vessels by a tumor. The injection can be made into the carotid artery to outline the anterior, middle, and posterior cerebral arteries and returning nervous circulation; and the vertebral artery to outline the vertebral-basilar system. A brachial artery injection may also be performed for the purpose of visualizing cerebral circulation.

After angiography, ice is usually applied to the sites of the injections to lessen edema and to help prevent oozing of blood. To lessen edema around the sites of carotid injections, which may cause pressure on the trachea and so cause respiratory difficulty, an ice collar is applied to the neck.

Although most patients experience few complications after having an angiogram, there may be serious aftereffects, including fibrillation, hemiparesis, aphasia, and respiratory distress due to edema or a hematoma near the trachea. Patients should be watched for signs of muscle weakness on the side of the body opposite the injection; these would appear if trauma to the brain had occurred during the test. Any weakness of the extremities or of facial muscles should be recorded and reported. Blood pressure, pulse, and respirations should be taken frequently. After brachial or femoral artery angiography, peripheral pulses should be checked. If the pulse is not palpable in the extremity on which the test was performed, the physician should be notified. Because of the possibility of respiratory difficulty, a tracheostomy set should be kept handy. The patient may have difficulty in swallowing. Ice chips may be offered first, and then sips of water until the patient can be graduated to his usual diet.

## Electroencephalography

The electroencephalogram is a record of the electrical impulses generated by the brain. Electrodes are placed on the patient's scalp, and the graph is recorded by a machine called an *electroencephalograph*. Usually, the patient is taken to a separate room, where a technician carries out the test. The procedure is not painful, and it does not cause aftereffects. The patient is instructed to sit comfortably in a chair, or to lie on a bed or a stretcher, and to relax while the machine makes the recording. The test is run for varying lengths of time (one-half to two hours). It is important to explain the test to the patient before it is begun, so that he will not fear that the wires and the machine will give him a shock. The patient follows his usual activities after the test. No special care or observation is necessary.

## Echoencephalography

By using ultrasonic apparatus it is possible to record the echoes of sound waves from intracranial structures; these echoes are transmitted into the brain from the scalp surface. Shifts of brain tissue caused by space-occupying lesions may be seen on the graph. The test is not painful, and there are no aftereffects.

## Brain Scanning

Because certain brain lesions have a tendency to accumulate radioactive substances more readily than healthy tissue, a radioisotope may be given intravenously. A scanner is passed over the head in search for isotopic concentrations.

*Isotope cisternography* is a modification of brain scanning involving injection of the isotope into the subarachnoid space by either lumbar or cisternal puncture. Serial brain scans are taken over a period of 48 hours to observe the circulation of cerebrospinal fluid around the cerebral hemispheres. This provides information in questions of obstruction to flow or inadequate absorption, as in hydrocephalus.

## REFERENCES AND BIBLIOGRAPHY

CARINI, ESTA, and OWENS, GUY: *Neurological and Neurosurgical Nursing,* ed. 6, St. Louis, Mosby, 1974.

CHUSID, JOSEPH: *Correlative Neuroanatomy and Functional Neurology,* ed. 14, Los Altos, Calif., Lange Medical Pub., 1970.

FOWLES, WILLIAM, and HUNN, VIRGINIA: *Clinical Assessment for the Nurse Practitioner,* St. Louis, Mosby, 1973.

GARDNER, M.: Responsiveness as a measure of consciousness, *Am. J. Nurs.* 68:5:1034-1038, May 1968.

JUDGE, RICHARD, and ZUIDEMA, GEORGE (eds.): *Physical Diagnosis: A Physiologic Approach to the Clinical Examination,* ed. 2, Boston, Little, Brown, 1968.

KING, IMOGENE (ed.): Symposium on neurologic and neurosurgical nursing, *Nurs. Clin. N. Am.* 4:2:199-300, June 1969.

KINTZEL, KAY (ed.): "Nursing Intervention for the Patient with Central Nervous System Dysfunction," in *Advanced Concepts in Clinical Nursing,* Philadelphia, Lippincott, 1971, Chapter 16.

KORTE, MARY: Intensive care of the neurologic patient, meeting the challenge, *Nurs. Clin. N. Am.* 7:2:335-348, June 1972.

LITTLE, DOLORES, and CARNEVALI, DORIS: *Nursing Care Planning,* Philadelphia, Lippincott, 1969.

MERRITT, H. HOUSTON: *A Textbook of Neurology,* ed. 5, Philadelphia, Lea and Febiger, 1973.

NOBACK, CHARLES, and DEMAREST, ROBERT: *The Nervous System: Introduction and Review,* New York, McGraw-Hill, A Blakiston Pub., 1972.

Patient assessment: Taking a patient's history (Programmed Instruction), *Am. J. Nurs.* 74:2:293-324, February 1974.

TATE, GAYLE: Assessment and direction of nursing care for patients with acute central nervous system insult, *Nurs. Clin. N. Am.* 6:1:165-171, March 1971.

WEBB, KENNETH: Early assessment of orthopedic injuries, *Am. J. Nurs.* 74:6:1048-1052, June 1974.

YURA, HELEN, and WALSH, MARY: *The Nursing Process,* ed. 2, New York, Appleton-Century-Crofts, Educational Division, Meredith Corp., 1973.

# Patients with Common Neurologic Disorders

## CHAPTER 23

## NURSING MANAGEMENT OF THE PATIENT WITH SELECTED PATHOLOGY OF THE BRAIN

### The Patient Undergoing Cranial Surgery

When the patient enters the hospital for possible brain surgery, both he and his family may be extremely apprehensive, and both require skilled professional nursing care. The nurse must demonstrate both patience and a deliberate and unhurried pace to insure this comprehensive care. When the patient is admitted, the nurse assesses his physical and mental status and notes his symptomatic complaints. She records his blood pressure, temperature, pulse rate, respirations, and pupil reaction to use when· monitoring changes in the patient during the postoperative period.

After the initial assessment, and with knowledge of the physician's plan of care, the nurse plans to meet the patient's needs. She regularly makes neurologic nursing assessments, and notes and reports changes in the patient's condition to avert complications which may slow recovery or even cause death.

If immediate surgery is not necessary, the patient is given a complete physical and neurologic examination. Treatments and procedures are carefully explained to him in terms that he can understand in order to alleviate his fear about the probable diagnosis and the anticipated surgery.

Because brain surgery is so threatening to the patient and his family, every effort is made to inspire confidence in the surgeon, members of the nursing staff, and the hospital. It is especially important to explore with the patient his understanding of and his feelings about the

Cranial Surgery

Brain Tumor

Trigeminal Neuralgia

Myasthenia Gravis

Multiple Sclerosis

Parkinson's Disease

Epilepsy

374

surgery, thus supporting him in his preoperative experience. As before any other major surgery, the patient is encouraged to have his spiritual advisor visit.

Morphine (and other narcotic analgesics) generally are not given to the patient with any type of brain lesion. A mild analgesic may be given for the relief of headache or headache may be eased by such nursing measures as changing the patient's position or applying a cold compress. Measures which relieve the patient's discomfort should be noted carefully and recorded.

### Preoperative Care

Preoperatively, the patient's hair is shaved. Sometimes the shaving is done after he has gone to the operating room and is anesthetized. If it is done on the unit, the patient should be given privacy. The hair should be saved because the patient may wish to have it made into a wig that he can use while his hair grows back. The nurse should explain to the patient why shaving is necessary, that his hair will grow back, and that in the meantime a wig or turban can be worn.

The patient's bowel habits should be observed and measures instituted to prevent constipation. An enema may not be ordered because of the danger of increasing intracranial pressure. If an enema is necessary, the patient is instructed not to strain, and the nurse should stay near him while he is expelling it.

Most brain operations take between two and four hours—a long and anxious time for the family. The nurse should provide them with a place to sit, show them where they may get a cup of coffee, and see that they are informed of the patient's condition as soon as there is news.

### Surgery

Cranial surgery is performed to remove pathology, such as brain abscess, a hematoma, a cerebral aneurysm, or a brain tumor (Fig. 23-1). An opening is made in the skull in order to perform surgery on the brain and cranial nerves. The bone may be removed (craniectomy) or a bone flap may be turned back (craniotomy).

**Craniectomy.** The size of the craniectomy varies depending on the pathology. It may be only a small burr hole or trephine which is used to evacuate a hematoma or biopsy a lesion. A larger opening is used to attempt complete removal of a tumor and

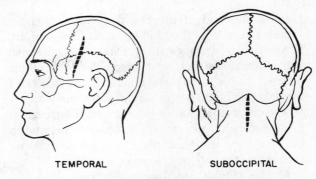

**Figure 23-1.** Common cranial incisions.

for removal of pathology in the posterior fossa (brain stem and cerebellum and fourth ventricle). A craniectomy may also be used to remove a large hematoma or tumor located in the cerebrum.

**Craniotomy.** In a craniotomy a series of burr holes is made in the skull. The skull between the holes is then cut with a flexible wire saw, or gigli. The bone remains attached to the muscle and is turned back. After surgery is completed, the bone flap is sutured back in place. This procedure is used for surgery on the cerebrum.

**Ventricular Drainage.** Ventricular drainage may be used preoperatively and postoperatively to reduce increased intracranial pressure. Ventricular fluid is withdrawn automatically by means of special equipment that maintains intracranial pressure at a desired level. After a burr hole is made, a catheter is inserted into the lateral ventricle, and a connecting tubing with a drainage bottle is attached to the catheter. The head of the bed is elevated, and the tubing is attached to it at a predetermined level.

### Postoperative Care

The postoperative bed is made with a turning sheet to facilitate moving the patient. Based on her knowledge of the patient's pathology, the nurse should be aware of possible complications, and have the equipment on hand to meet emergencies. Thus, the room should be equipped with a mouth gag, side rails on the bed, a ventricular puncture tray, an airway, a tracheostomy tray, a tray with emergency drugs (including stimulants and depressants), syringes and needles, and suction apparatus.

Immediately after the patient returns from the operating room, he is placed on his side to allow for adequate ventilation. If the bone has not been replaced in supratentorial surgery (surgery on the cerebrum), the patient is kept off the operative site.

Usually the head of the bed is elevated to assist venous return from the head and to aid respirations. If ventricular drainage is in place, the physician will establish the height at which the head of the patient's bed is to be maintained. The placement of the drainage bottle is also carefully determined.

The observations of the patient's neurologic status made before surgery are continued routinely when the vital signs are checked. These assessments are essential to the patient's recovery.

**Fluids.** Fluids are usually restricted after surgery; thus it is necessary to monitor carefully the patient's oral and intravenous intake. After supratentorial surgery, the patient generally tolerates fluids quite well. If vomiting occurs fluids are withheld because the associated straining may increase intracranial pressure. Intravenous fluids are given at this time. Hypertonic glucose is given slowly to nourish the patient and to reduce postoperative cerebral edema. Before the patient who has had surgery on the posterior fossa is given fluids by mouth, the presence of the gag and swallowing reflex should be determined. Because of edema or trauma, the function of the glossopharyngeal and vagus nerves are disturbed, resulting in loss of gag reflex and marked difficulty in swallowing. Diet is slowly progressed for all patients.

**Urinary Output.** Urinary output is carefully monitored. An indwelling catheter may be in place in the immediate postoperative period so that the patient's urinary output can be accurately monitored. After the catheter is removed, the patient's pattern of voiding should be observed. Incontinence or urinary retention may be a problem after brain surgery.

**Drainage.** The dressing is checked frequently for drainage. If drainage appears on the dressing, the nurse should outline it and report the amount and color. A yellow stain may be cerebrospinal fluid. Areas of drainage should be covered with a sterile barrier. If a drain is in place, the amount and color of drainage should be noted frequently. The patient may wear a cervical collar if a posterior fossa craniectomy is performed. Care should be taken to prevent the restless or disoriented patient from disarranging the dressing, putting his fingers underneath, or even removing it.

Frequently after the dressing is removed the scalp is covered with crusts. The application of yellow petroleum jelly will soften these crusts. Most female patients are very self-conscious about their shaved heads and must be reassured frequently.

Perhaps such a patient's family could be asked to bring a pretty turban to the hospital for her use. If the bone has been removed leaving a defect in the skull, the patient is informed about this and taught how to protect the area.

For the first 48 hours the patient's activity should be closely supervised. He should be assisted to change his position frequently, without jostling or jarring his head. By the third day he will become progressively more independent and more interested in his environment. Normal activities should be established as soon as possible. The patient may be allowed out of bed the day after surgery. To reduce the possibility of untoward reactions, the nurse should gradually elevate the head of the bed and allow the patient to dangle his legs over the edge of the bed under supervision. If no adverse reaction occurs, he should be allowed out of bed. The time out of bed should be gradually increased until the patient begins to walk. By the end of two weeks, if all has gone well, the patient is usually ready for discharge from the hospital.

**The Family.** Family members must be prepared to see the patient postoperatively. They should know that he will return from the operating room with a helmetlike headdressing, and that edema may distort his features. If he is unconscious or has any noticeable limitations, such as aphasia, they should be told of this. If a supratentorial incision is made, family members should be warned that when they see him on the day following surgery he may be unable to open one or both eyes, may have generalized facial edema, and may have discoloration of the skin about the eyes. Periocular edema is caused by postoperative cerebral edema, and usually improves in three or four days. It is important to allow time for family members to ask questions and to express feelings.

**Complications.** The nurse must be aware of postoperative complications that may occur so that she may intelligently observe the patient and plan appropriate nursing actions. *Shock* may result from an excessive loss of blood during or following surgery. Close observation of the patient should be made with careful assessment of the vital signs at frequent intervals.

Intracranial hemorrhage, cerebral edema, or meningitis may cause *increased intracranial pressure.* The patient should be closely observed with careful checking of vital signs. Elevation of the head should be maintained. Fluids should be limited and intake measured. Straining when vomiting or when at stool should be minimized. Dehydration is the conservative treatment. If other measures are not effective, further surgery is indicated.

An *elevation in temperature* may be caused by a disturbance in the heat regulating center in the hypothalamus, local or general infection, marked dehydration, or thrombophlebitis. Rectal temperature should be frequently taken. The cause must be found and treated symptomatically. Contamination at surgery or wound infection may cause *meningitis*. The signs and symptoms of meningitis are: headache, fever, increased sensitivity to light (photophobia), delirium, nuchal rigidity, soreness of skin and muscles, focal or generalized convulsions, and increased cells in the spinal fluid. Strict aseptic technique should be maintained when doing dressings or lumbar puncture. Early symptoms should be recognized and reported.

*Respiratory collapse* may be due to compression of the respiratory center after surgery in the posterior fossa. Early signs of respiratory embarrassment are manifested by changes in the rate and depth of respirations. *Respiratory infections* may be caused by the aspiration of mucus, food or vomitus, shallow breathing, or prolonged lying on the back. This complication can be prevented. The nurse should maintain a clear airway for the patient, assist him to cough and deep breathe frequently, and change his position at regular intervals.

The extent of *focal neurologic deficits* will depend upon the location and extent of the surgery and pathologic condition being treated. Accurate assessments of the patient's neurologic status are frequently performed; appropriate nursing measures are planned and executed.

Postoperative needs vary. The nurse must understand what neurologic deficit may occur when certain areas of the brain are affected. Her aim is to prevent disabling complications and maintain functioning of uninvolved parts. The patient is assisted to return to his highest level of function. His family is supported, assisted to understand the implications of surgery, and given the opportunity to be involved in all aspects of the patient's care.

## The Patient with a Brain Tumor

The patient with a brain tumor may be admitted to the hospital with only slight symptoms, or he may be acutely ill. The symptoms may have slowly progressed over several months, or they may have developed suddenly without warning. The diagnosis of brain tumor is frightening for both the patient and those close to him, and fears of death or the unknown, and the loss of ability to control his own body and mind are paramount. Brain tumors can occur at any age. However, they occur most frequently in early adulthood or in middle life when the individual is most active and productive.

Intracranial tumors arise from the cells of structures found within the cranial cavity. They can arise from the meninges, the blood vessels, the nerve cells, or glia. Metastatic tumors and those originating from the skull are also encountered. Brain tumors may be either benign or malignant, but because of their relationship to vital structures, tumors classified as benign may have malignant effects.

*Gliomas* arising from the glia, the supporting structure of the brain, account for 50 per cent of all primary intracranial tumors. These tumors are locally invasive and may metastasize within the central nervous system by seeding. *Meningiomas* are benign tumors accounting for 5 per cent of primary intracranial tumors. They are attached to the dura which covers the brain, compressing underlying structures without invading them. *Metastatic* tumors account for 10 to 20 per cent of all intracranial tumors. The commonest tumor to metastasize to the brain is carcinoma of the lung, followed by carcinoma of the breast, the gastrointestinal tract, and the urinary tract.

### Signs and Symptoms

The clinical manifestations of intracranial tumors are due to the local destructive effects of the tumor, and increasing intracranial pressure. Convulsions may be the first symptom. The focal symptoms vary depending upon the area of brain tissue compressed or destroyed. Tumors of the frontal lobe can cause changes of mood, personality, and behavior. The patient may be euphoric, irresponsible, and his behavior may be contrary to social norms. Tumors extending to the motor region will cause motor changes on the opposite side of the body.

Tumors of the parietal lobe can cause numbness or weakness of the opposite side of the body. The patient may drop things or fail to recognize by touch, a common object, such as a key or coin. Damage to the speech areas in the cerebral hemispheres can cause difficulty in the patient's ability to communicate.

Temporal lobe tumors can produce episodes in which the patient smells or tastes something that is not present. Tumors along the visual pathways in the temporal and occipital lobes can cause a visual disturbance in which the patient sees only half a visual field. The condition is known as hemianopsia.

Tumors of the cerebellum can cause disturbances of equilibrium and gait. Gait is slow, broad-based, and staggering, and the patient may fall to one side.

Pituitary tumors also produce visual problems, in some instances blindness, because they exert pressure on the optic chiasm. A chromophobe, the most common type adenoma of the pituitary, can cause hypopituitarism, manifested by amenorrhea in women, impotence in men, and hypothyroidism and hypoadrenalism in both sexes. Less common is the eosinophilic adenoma, which may secrete growth hormone and cause acromegaly in adults. The basophilic adenoma, the most rare type, involves an overgrowth of pituitary cells producing ACTH and results in Cushing's disease.

When the intracranial pressure is such that the brain stem is forced through the foramen magnum, the patient is in grave danger, since the vital structures are compressed, stretched, and become ischemic. Respirations become deeper, labored, and noisy, and then slow and periodic. Unless the condition is relieved, the patient dies of respiratory failure. With increasing intracranial pressure, the pulse slows (bradycardia) and the blood pressure elevates (Cushing's reflex or sign). This combination usually has a grave prognosis. Hyperthermia may occur as the temperature-regulating center in the brain is affected. Coma progressively deepens.

Treatment

Some brain tumors are easily removed without damage to nearby brain tissue; others can be excised only with the result of residual permanent brain damage; and some cannot be reached at all without fatal results. If healthy brain tissue has to be removed, some of the patient's postoperative symptoms will be determined by the location and function of the damaged tissue. Brain tissue does not regenerate. When an inoperable tumor obstructs the flow of cerebrospinal fluid, a shunting procedure may be performed to relieve the increased pressure.

Radiotherapy is effective in treating some types of brain tumors, particularly gliomas and metastatic tumors, and it is common for treatment to include both surgery and radiotherapy. Chemotherapy of malignant gliomas is still in the experimental stage. Corticosteroids are administered to alleviate symptoms due to increased intracranial pressure, and for a period of time their use may cause complete remission of focal symptoms.

The earlier the tumor is recognized and surgery performed, the better are the chances for recovery. The patient's prognosis depends on the type of tumor and its location. For example, benign meningiomas, pituitary tumors, and eighth-cranial nerve tumors, as well as some cerebellar tumors, can be cured. But the average time of survival with a glioblastoma, the most common tumor, is about one year.

Nursing Care

The nursing care of the patient with a brain tumor is determined by the patient's symptoms, his emotional response to the hospitalization and diagnosis, his socioeconomic situation, and the reaction of his family and friends. He may be alert with a slight neurologic deficit, such as diplopia (double vision), or he may be unaware of time and place with hemiplegia. The role of the nurse is to support him through the multiple diagnostic procedures and recommended treatment, maintain function, prevent complications, and return the patient to the highest functional level of which he is capable.

When the patient is admitted to the hospital with a diagnosis of brain tumor, the nurse makes a neurologic nursing assessment, which is used to initiate the nursing care plan, and later to determine if there are any changes in the patient's neurologic status. If not medically contraindicated, and if he can tolerate it the patient should be encouraged to be out of bed. If bed rest is to be maintained, the head of the bed should be kept elevated to help relieve cerebral edema. The patient's position should be changed frequently and active and passive exercises of his extremities should be performed regularly. While the patient is undergoing the necessary diagnostic procedures, the nurse should continue making frequent neurologic nursing assessments. The patient and his family should be given frequent explanations of the diagnostic procedures.

The patient's medical therapy is an important consideration in planning nursing care. Surgery may be indicated, in which case the nurse should perform the necessary pre- and postoperative care. Radiotherapy may be the treatment of choice. If so the patient should be told that he will lose his hair, and the nurse should observe any untoward reaction to the therapy. If the patient loses his appetite, small frequent meals should be offered. The nurse should administer corticosteroids as ordered and note any side effects of the medication.

Nursing care is influenced by the patient's residual neurologic deficits. Rehabilitation should be started as soon as the patient's physical condition stabilizes. Occupational and diversional therapy should coincide with each patient's needs and abilities, and the nurse should collaborate with the rehabilitation team in assessing the patient's responses. Some patients will require more guidance and retraining than others. The patient and his family will need help in adjusting to any residual disabilities, and the family should be encouraged to participate in the patient's care. The patient should be allowed to be as independent as possible within his limitations, and his capabilities should be emphasized. The patient with an inoperable tumor and a poor prognosis should also be encouraged to be independent, not only for his own morale and self esteem, but also to assist his family to cope with his care. Plans for discharge should be started early, with all members of the health care team involved in the patient's care, the patient, and his family participating in the planning. When possible the patient is discharged home with his family, or other significant persons. In some instances long-term care in an institutional setting is required. The nurse's role does not end with the patient's discharge from the hospital. She can assist with plans for the patient's care in a long-term facility, or work with the patient and his family in his home to promote maximum rehabilitation.

## The Patient with a Head Injury

Injuries to the head occur frequently in both civilian and military life. Automobile and motorcycle accidents are the most common cause of head injuries in civilian life.

Head injuries are classified according to the amount of damage to the skull. In a closed head injury there is no brain injury or only a linear fracture of the skull. When the skull fracture is depressed, fragments of fractured bone are depressed inward to compress or injure the underlying brain tissue. In this instance the bone is elevated to relieve the pressure on brain tissue. In a compound fracture of the skull there is a direct communication between the lacerated scalp and cerebral tissue through the fractured bone. In this instance the wound is cleaned and fractured bone removed. The prognosis for life and recovery of function depends upon the severity of damage to the underlying brain tissue. The injury to the brain may be directly beneath the site of the blow or it may be directly opposite.

The amount of damage to brain tissue is related to the force of the blow to the head. A severe blow can cause contusions, lacerations, and edema. Concussion results from violent jarring of the head and is associated with a period of loss of consciousness.

### Symptoms

Altered level of consciousness is the most common symptom of head injury. Coma may be prolonged, lasting for days or weeks. Duration of coma depends upon the site and severity of the injury. On recovery of consciousness the presence of headache, dizziness, vertigo, and other focal neurologic signs depends upon the severity and site of damage to brain tissue. There may be loss of memory for events immediately preceding the injury and amnesia for events occurring immediately after recovery of consciousness. When there is extensive damage to brain tissue there may be signs of permanent brain damage such as seizures, impaired intellect, speech difficulties, paralysis, impaired gait, and continuing alteration in level of consciousness.

### Complications of Head Injury

**Epidural (Extradural) Hematoma.** A rare complication of head injury, an epidural hematoma is usually caused by arterial bleeding which occurs very rapidly and separates the dura from the skull. Usually the hematoma is quite large. Characteristically, the patient will have a momentary lapse of consciousness, after which he may appear perfectly alert and clear. Within an hour or so he may relapse to coma with the development of hemiplegia. This is a true surgical emergency. Epidural hemorrhage may be treated by trephining the skull (perforating the skull with an instrument called a trephine), removing the clot, and ligating the bleeding artery. Extradural hemorrhage is the most fatal complication of head injury. The mortality rate is nearly 100 per cent in untreated cases and over 50 per cent in treated cases. The high mortality rate is related to the severity of associated brain damage.

**Subdural Hematoma.** This condition is a result of venous bleeding in the space below the dura.

The blood which collects in the subdural space is organized and encapsulated by the dura. The cerebral cortex is compressed by the clot. The symptoms of an acute subdural hematoma usually develop within the first few days after the injury. In some cases, symptoms may not develop for as long as two months after the injury. There is usually a change in level of consciousness accompanied by hemiplegia. The treatment of subdural hematoma is removal of the clot through a trephine opening or craniotomy.

### Nursing Care

When a patient with a possible head injury is seen in the emergency room, the nurse should ascertain how, when, and where the blow to the head was sustained; whether there was loss of consciousness and if so its nature; the position and movement of the patient after the injury; whether there was vomiting; and, any pupillary changes. All patients who have received trauma to the head should be watched for the development of signs of increased intracranial pressure. A patient with a minor injury and perhaps no loss of consciousness may be treated in the emergency room, and then he may return home. Before he leaves her care, the nurse should make sure he knows that he should return to the hospital if he develops any symptoms of increased intracranial pressure, such as becoming sleepy at an odd time, dizziness, vomiting, increasing pain, or double vision. The instructions should be given to the patient without frightening him. When it is possible, the patient should leave the hospital with a friend or a relative who is also alerted to the symptoms that require medical attention.

**Observation.** The patient who is admitted to the hospital with a diagnosis of head injury is observed frequently by the nurse for changes in the status of his nervous system. If he must be disturbed frequently for assessment of his level of consciousness, he should be aroused gently and slowly. The blood pressure cuff should remain in place on the patient's arm, so that he is not disturbed by having it replaced every 15 to 30 minutes. Because the nurse has the most contact with the patient, she is in an excellent position to determine changes in the functioning of his nervous system. Is he harder to arouse at 4:00 A.M. than he was at 3:30 A.M.? Is there a slight facial weakness starting on either side? Does the pulse seem to be more bounding?

The recognition of small changes may bring the physician to the bedside before serious brain damage has occurred.

Because the patient is unconscious in both sleep and coma, the only way to differentiate between the two is to rouse him periodically. Awakening the well-oriented but tired patient every half-hour to differentiate sleep from coma may make him angry, but an explanation of the importance of how this seemingly cruel practice protects him may help him to accept it. Determination of level of consciousness is the most significant indication of the status of the nervous system. Changes should be reported immediately.

**Vital Signs.** Frequent check of vital signs is essential in caring for the head-injured patient. Bradycardia, an increasing blood pressure, and restlessness may be signs of deterioration of the nervous system. The patient's eyes should be checked for pupil size and reaction to light and for eye movements. Convulsions or any involuntary movement of the body should be carefully noted. Strength and movement of the extremities are also evaluated.

**Adequate Ventilation.** Establishment of a clear airway with an adequate supply of oxygen is of prime importance in the emergency treatment of a patient with a head injury. For this reason, proper positioning, insertion of an oropharyngeal airway, aspiration of secretions by oropharyngeal suctioning, and removal of dentures are performed. Nursing measures are directed toward maintaining adequate ventilation, which may require the use of mechanical support.

**Fluid Balance.** Fluids are given intravenously during the acute phase of the patient's illness, but are usually restricted to decrease or control cerebral edema. An osmotic diuretic, such as mannitol (Manicol), and corticosteroids may be given intravenously to control cerebral edema. Head trauma can cause a variety of fluid balance problems, depending upon the area of the brain involved. For this reason the patient's intravenous and oral fluid intake and urinary output must be accurately monitored.

**Restraints.** The patient with a head injury may be restless. Restraints are used only if required for the patient's safety because they may make a restless patient more irritable. Narcotics are contraindicated because their actions may mask the signs of increased intracranial pressure.

**Leakage of Cerebrospinal Fluid.** After a head injury cerebrospinal fluid may leak from the ears (otorrhea) or nose (rhinorrhea). When cerebrospinal fluid otorrhea occurs there is danger of infection. Antibiotics may be given.

To determine if the fluid that is leaking is cerebrospinal fluid, the nurse should check for the presence of sugar. She should caution the patient not to blow his nose, and she should not suction him through the nose. She should not obstruct the leakage of fluid from either nose or ears, but instead should note the amount and characteristics of the drainage frequently.

Nursing intervention will depend upon the severity of the injury and the extent of the neurologic deficit. After a complete nursing assessment, appropriate nursing actions will be planned and executed. The patient may exhibit a reduced level of consciousness, hemiplegia, and aphasia. Nursing measures will be utilized to maintain the integrity of the skin and to prevent joint deformities. In addition, to meet the patient's need for communication, his family will require reassurance and explanation of procedures and equipment during this stressful experience.

## THE NURSING MANAGEMENT OF THE PATIENT WITH A CRANIAL NERVE DISORDER

### Trigeminal Neuralgia (Tic Douloureux)

The fifth (trigeminal) cranial nerve has three major branches: mandibular, maxillary, and ophthalmic (Fig. 23-2). It is a major sensory and motor nerve, important to mastication, facial movement, and sensation. For reasons not fully understood, it occasionally becomes exquisitely painful, particularly in people over 50 years of age.

### Symptoms

The pain comes in paroxysms, each lasting about 2 to 15 seconds, which are so painful that patients have been driven to suicide. During a spasm the face may twitch, tears come to the eyes, and the hand rises to the face, without touching it. The patient has learned that a certain facial expression helps to shorten the bout, and he maintains the grimace as long as the pain lasts. After the paroxysm he is left with a dull afterglow, a tongue that feels furry, and the fear of the next attack.

Certain trigger spots cause an attack when they receive the slightest stimulus: the vibration of music,

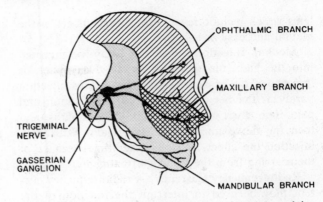

**Figure 23-2.** Diagram of the areas innervated by the three branches of the trigeminal nerve. These are the areas that become painful in trigeminal neuralgia.

a passing breeze, or a change of temperature. Patients are understandably reluctant to wash that side of the face, and men remain unshaven. The forehead over the eyebrow is a common trigger spot when the ophthalmic branch of the nerve is affected. If the trigger zone is in the angle of the mouth, the patient gulps a mouthful of food, has a paroxysm, and pauses while he gathers courage for the next swallow.

### Treatment

**Drug Therapy.** The pains are frequently so severe that they are not relieved by analgesic drugs. Diphenylhydantoin (Dilantin) injected intravenously will stop an acute attack, and the daily administration of the drug orally will prevent recurrence of the pain in many patients. However, the dose required, 0.4 to 0.7 Gm. daily, cannot be tolerated by most patients.

Recently another drug, carbamazephine (Tegretal), has been found to be more effective than diphenylhydantoin in the treatment of the pain of trigeminal neuralgia. This drug produces a complete remission of symptoms in many patients. The average dose is 400 to 800 mg. daily given with meals. During the initial phase of therapy, the patient may experience dizziness, drowsiness, unsteadiness on feet, nausea, and vomiting. Carbamazephine has been shown to cause severe bone marrow damage. Aplastic anemia, agranulocytosis, thrombocytopenia, and leukopenia have occurred. Complete blood and platelet counts are done prior to the start of therapy and at frequent intervals thereafter. The patient should be informed of the early signs and symptoms of potential hematologic problems which include fever, sore throat, ulcers in the mouth, and easy bruising.

**Alcohol Injections.** Alcohol may be injected into the gasserion ganglion in the dura mater or into one of the branches of the nerve. This injection paralyzes the nerve, causing loss of sensation and pain. The effect wears off in about six months, and then the nerve may be injected again. With each injection the effect lasts a shorter time because of the scarring from the previous treatments.

**Radiofrequency Current.** A radiofrequency current may be used to interrupt the function of the appropriate branch of the trigeminal nerve, with loss of sensation and pain. The use of this method of treatment is relatively new. It is hoped that it will produce a permanent relief of the patient's symptoms.

**Surgery.** At one time surgery was the treatment of choice. Partial section of the root of the ganglion was the standard operation. The effect is the same as that produced by injecting alcohol into the ganglion, but it is permanent. This method of treatment requires an extensive neurosurgical procedure. With the development of new drugs and techniques, this operation is rarely performed.

Nursing Care

The patient who enters the hospital for treatment of trigeminal neuralgia is severely distressed by the symptoms of the disease. On admission the nurse should note the characteristics of the attack-precipitating factors, frequency, duration, description of the pain, and the area involved.

Since temperature extremes stimulate the trigger zone, food and fluids should be tepid. The patient should be given food that is easy to swallow; perhaps he can take only semiliquids. The patient is in danger of becoming dehydrated and malnourished. After he eats, he may not be able to rinse his mouth. He may be able to use an applicator, but the nurse should not attempt to give him mouth care if this will stimulate pain.

The patient should talk as little as possible, since facial movement can start the pain. The nurse should avoid causing a breeze near his face, and ventilate the room in such a way that no draft will hit him. She should put a sign on his bed saying that it is not to be jarred, and avoid touching his face in any way. Hair brushing on that side may have to wait until after treatment. The patient may be exhausted from fighting the pain and need as-

sistance with bathing, dressing, and other personal hygiene.

After treatment, the patient will experience numbness in the affected area, and will require assistance to adjust to this altered sensation. If the ophthalmic branch is destroyed, the patient should be taught to care for and protect his eye by irrigating it three times a day and whenever he comes inside from out-of-doors. He must also inspect his eye daily. Redness may be the first sign of irritation that can result in a corneal ulcer and blindness. The patient should shield the eye whenever he goes out, or whenever he is in danger of catching a foreign particle in it, such as during house cleaning.

After he eats, the patient should check the inside of the mouth for particles of food that may remain and set up a site of infection. He should be instructed to rinse his mouth and brush his teeth after eating, and to make regular visits to the dentist, because he will not feel the warning pain of a dental cavity.

## THE NURSING MANAGEMENT OF THE PATIENT WITH A NEUROMUSCULAR DISORDER

### Myasthenia Gravis

Myasthenia gravis is a comparatively common disease characterized by pronounced muscular weakness, particularly after exercise of the affected muscles. Although it may occur at any age, it appears most frequently during young adulthood and middle life. The increase in incidence in recent years is probably due to better diagnosis of the disease.

The cause of myasthenia gravis is unknown, but it is believed to be related to a defect in the production or release of enough acetylcholine to allow proper conduction of nerve impulses to the muscles. The symptoms may be due to a disturbance of acetylcholine metabolism.

The onset of the disease is usually insidious. After any activity of the affected muscles, the patient quickly experiences loss of power in those muscles; after he rests, he is again able to resume the activity for a short period. For instance, if the arms are affected, the patient may start to feed himself, but soon experience such weakness of his arms that he must stop to rest. The disease often affects muscles of the face and the eyes, and those muscles that are involved in chewing, coughing, swallowing, and speaking. The face gradually develops a sleepy, expressionless appearance due to drooping of the eyelids and weakness of the facial muscles. The patient may find it very difficult to chew and swallow. When the muscles of respiration are involved, the patient experiences dyspnea. Inability to cough up respiratory secretions can lead to respiratory complications, such as pneumonia.

Some patients live for years with myasthenia gravis, whereas in others the disease is rapidly fatal. In the past, the prognosis was poor for patients with involvement of the respiratory muscles, but with the introduction of respiratory care units, the prognosis for these patients has improved. The severity of the disease fluctuates considerably. Exacerbations are associated often with emotional upsets and respiratory infections.

## Treatment

There is no cure for myasthenia gravis, but neostigmine (Prostigmin), a short-acting anticholinesterase drug, gives symptomatic relief (Fig. 23-3). The usual dose is 15 to 30 mg., three to four times daily. The first dose is usually given in the morning before arising. The relief from muscular weakness is so dramatic and so typical of the disease that the response to neostigmine is used as one diagnostic test for myasthenia gravis. The dosage is determined for each individual patient, so that he receives the amount that most effectively relieves his symptoms. Side effects of neostigmine include visceral disturbances, such as salivation, abdominal discomfort, cramps, and diarrhea. Tincture of belladonna may be administered to relieve the discomfort of the side effects.

Pyridostigmine (Mestinon), similar in action to neostigmine, is usually given in doses of 60 mg., orally. Some patients have better results and fewer side effects from pyridostigmine. Ambenonium chloride (Mytelase) is also given for relief of myasthenia gravis. The usual dose is 10 mg. orally.

An acute exacerbation of the disease accompanied by paralysis of respiratory muscles is considered a "myasthenic crisis." The patient usually requires a tracheostomy with mechanical control of respirations. Drug therapy is reinstituted as the patient is weaned from the respirator.

The relationship of the thymus to myasthenia gravis is not yet clear. Thymectomy has produced beneficial results in selected patients.

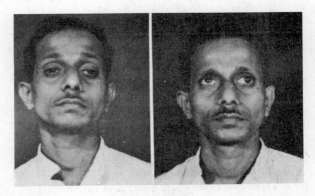

**Figure 23-3.** The facies of myasthenia gravis. (*Left*) Before Prostigmin. (*Right*) After Prostigmin. (Vakil, R. J., and Golwalla, A.: *Clinical Diagnosis,* Bombay, Asia Publishing House)

The use of corticotropins and immunosuppressive drugs in the treatment of myasthenia gravis is now being investigated. The use of cortisone has resulted in the remission of symptoms. Transient severe weakness may occur during the course of treatment. While the patient is undergoing steroid therapy he is placed in special respiratory units. Because corticotropins are not always effective, the use of immunosuppressives is now being studied.

## Nursing Care

If the patient's symptoms are mild, nursing care will involve helping him to plan his activities to avoid excessive fatigue. Concentrating on the most important activities and providing frequent rest periods are important in conserving his strength. Drugs must be administered on time. The nurse should note carefully the effect of the medication and observe for toxic effects. The patient should be taught how to avoid factors which could lead to respiratory infection. Since involvement of the muscles of respiration may occur, the patient's family must know how to perform pulmonary resuscitation.

When the disease is severe the patient is unable to do anything for himself. He will need to be fed, bathed, and turned. If he is unable to swallow, tube feedings may be necessary. The patient will require skilled nursing management to provide adequate ventilation. Respiratory function may need to be maintained by a mechanical ventilator. The patient may be placed in a special nursing unit.

It is helpful for the nurse to know of the Myasthenia Gravis Foundation which is a resourse for patients and families. The foundation has three goals: education, aid for and treatment of people with the disease, and research to find more effective methods of treatment.

## THE NURSING MANAGEMENT OF THE PATIENT WITH A CHRONIC NEUROLOGIC DISORDER

### Multiple Sclerosis

Multiple sclerosis is a chronic, progressive, disabling disease of the nervous system characterized by a variety of neurologic signs and symptoms.

### Cause and Pathology

The cause of the disease is unknown, but some theories implicate allergic reactions, viral infections, and chemical, metabolic, and enzymatic disturbances.

The symptoms of multiple sclerosis are due to a breakdown in the myelin sheath which surrounds the axons of the nerve fibers that comprise the white matter of the central nervous system. The myelin acts as an insulative covering and speeds transmission of nerve impulses. Multiple sclerosis is a demyelinating disease: there is patchy degeneration of the myelin sheaths in various areas throughout the nervous system and subsequent degeneration of the axons themselves. As a result, motor and sensory impulses are no longer transmitted and there is permanent dysfunction of the nervous system. Since the disease affects different areas of the nervous system, the symptoms may be quite varied and seemingly unrelated (e.g., blindness and paralysis may occur). Symptoms often subside during early phases of the illness, and the patient may appear perfectly healthy for several months or even years. But with each reappearance, the symptoms tend to be more severe and to last longer. These periods of remission and exacerbation form a characteristic pattern.

### Incidence

Multiple sclerosis is a disease of young adulthood and early middle life. The highest incidence occurs in persons between the ages of 20 and 40. Men and women are affected about equally. The disease is more common in cold, damp, and temperate zones than it is in warm, dry climates.

### Diagnosis

No single diagnostic test is specific for multiple sclerosis. For example, spinal fluid studies will show an increase in gamma globulin levels in most patients with the disease. Diagnosis is based upon the varied signs and symptoms of the disease, laboratory data, and the existence of remissions and exacerbations. Other possible diagnoses must be excluded; diagnosis of multiple sclerosis is one of exclusion.

### Clinical Manifestations

Characteristically, the signs and symptoms of the disease are multiple and vary greatly from patient to patient. Usually, symptoms appear gradually. There may be a slight weakness of an extremity or blurring or loss of vision, which is transitory. Often these seemingly minor symptoms are dismissed as a result of fatigue or strain. Later, when the physician questions the patient he may recall these episodes. Just as the symptoms themselves vary among patients, so do their intensity and duration. Some patients begin having severe, long-lasting symptoms early in the course of the disease, while others may experience only occasional and mild symptoms for several years after the onset of the illness.

Clinical manifestations depend upon the areas of the nervous system involved. Following are some of the common symptoms:

- Blurred vision
- Diplopia
- Nystagmus (involuntary movement of the eyeball)
- Weakness of extremities (paraplegia or quadriplegia [paresis])
- Intention tremor (the hand trembles when the patient uses it)
- Urinary disturbances (incontinence, frequency or urgency)
- Ataxia (motor incoordination)
- Slurred, hesitant speech
- Paresthesia (spontaneous feelings of numbness and tingling in extremities, face, or trunk)
- Mental disturbances (euphoria or depression)

### Prognosis

The prognosis for multiple sclerosis is decidedly variable.

Although many patients experience gradual worsening of their symptoms, this is not invariably the case. Some patients have the disease in mild form, and do not experience increasing severity of the symptoms, and some people who have had the disease for 15 years are able to continue their usual activities. Living for 20 years after diagnosis has been established is not unusual. Of course, these patients are subject to the same kinds of accidents and illnesses as are other people.

## Treatment and Nursing Care

There is no cure for multiple sclerosis, nor is there any single treatment that reliably relieves symptoms. Research is being carried out in many parts of the country to try to determine the cause and to develop specific therapy for multiple sclerosis. Organizations like the National Multiple Sclerosis Society are active in programs of education and research. Steroid therapy has recently been recognized as an effective treatment for some patients; however, its ultimate value still remains to be evaluated.

Treatment is symptomatic based upon the individual needs of the patient and his family. The goal of treatment is to assist the patient to maintain a normal life style and occupation, and the best possible general health. Prevention of complications is essential. The patient is instructed to avoid factors which may precipitate an exacerbation. Thus he is encouraged to avoid fatigue and to eat a nourishing well-balanced diet. He is taught how to avoid infections. As far as possible, he is cautioned to stay away from situations that may be emotionally upsetting. Physical, educational, occupational, and recreational therapy may be indicated as the disease progresses.

A major aspect of nursing care involves helping the patient to cope with the realization that he has a long-term illness, and to support him as he experiences the exacerbations and remissions so characteristic of the illness.

The patient is helped to maintain normal activity as long as he can. There is no reason why he cannot work, provided the job is within his physical capabilities. If his condition declines, he may be helped to find part-time work that is less taxing. Throughout his illness, emphasis should be placed on developing hobbies that the patient can enjoy if he is no longer able to work. One woman became an avid bird watcher. When she was no longer able to be outdoors, a feeder was placed near her bedroom window, so that she could still enjoy the bright liveliness of the birds.

The patient is assisted to remain at home with his family whenever possible (Fig. 23-4). A home care program should be developed. The visiting nurse should assess the program and revise the nursing care plan accordingly. Physical therapy and speech therapy can be provided in the home if necessary.

The National Multiple Sclerosis Society is a voluntary, nonprofit organization which helps support centers for the evaluation and treatment of patients with multiple sclerosis. In addition it works cooperatively in nationwide research programs directed toward finding the cause of multiple sclerosis. Counseling, recreational programs, and special equipment are also provided. The program also includes public education and the raising of funds to carry on its many activities.

## Emotional Responses

Mood swings (emotional lability) are common among patients with multiple sclerosis. The patient may feel on top of the world one minute, and shortly later declare that life is not worth living. Two possible explanations have been given for this state. The patient may experience fluctuations of mood because of damage done to his nervous system or because of his deep anxiety about his illness and prognosis. Both may contribute to alternating euphoria and depression.

Sometimes multiple sclerosis patients suddenly burst into tears for no apparent reason. Often they themselves do not know why they are crying. When this kind of episode occurs, it is best not to make a fuss over it, but to accept it as a manifestation of the illness. For instance, the nurse can encourage family members not to respond to a sudden flood of tears with "Oh my, what's the trouble? Why are you so upset?" Instead, calmly give the patient some tissues, and when his tears are over, go on with whatever activity or conversation was interrupted. Of course, this approach is not appropriate if the crying is a reflection of sadness or frustration rather than a symptom of neurologic disturbance. If the patient is upset, like everyone else he needs a chance to cry and then a chance to talk with someone about his trouble.

## Complications

Some patients show symptoms of impaired intellectual functioning late in the course of the illness. For instance, loss of memory, difficulty in concentrating, and impaired judgment may occur. As the disease progresses, the patient is subject to many complications. With the knowledge that paralysis and incontinence often occur, it is not difficult to

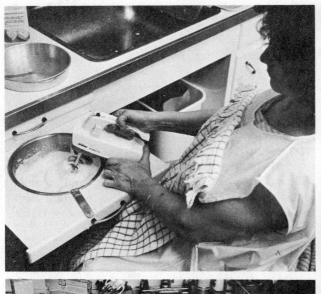
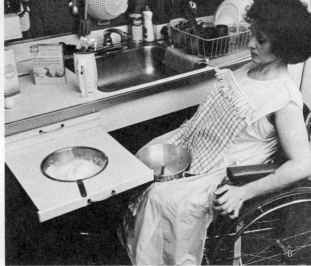
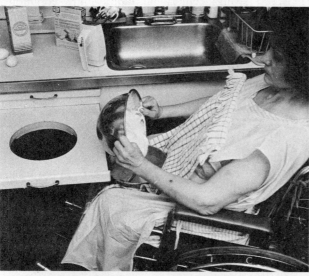
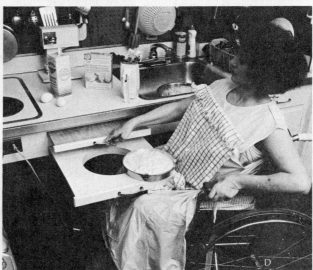
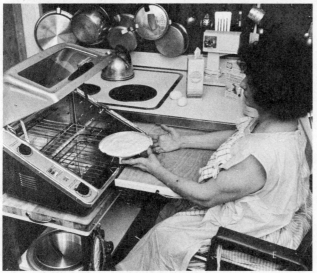

**Figure 23-4.** Kitchen equipment that has been planned to meet the needs of a homemaker who is severely disabled by multiple sclerosis. (A) Pullout board with hole for bowl lowers working height for heavy work such as beating, and the portable hand-beater can be rested on its surface for additional help. (B) and (C) Cake pan is stabilized in lap so that batter can be transferred using gravity as an assist. (D) and (E) Transferring the load gradually from lap to low pullout board, then to upper pullout board, eases lifting to height necessary for pushing pan into portable oven. (New York University Medical Center, Institute of Rehabilitation Medicine)

foresee the complications to which the patient is especially vulnerable:

**Genitourinary.** Either incontinence or retention of urine may be a problem. The perineal area and bed should be kept dry and clean. The patient should void at regular intervals. He should assume a normal position when voiding, and the nurse should apply slight pressure with the hand over the suprapubic area.

**Skin.** Incontinence and immobility, along with general body wasting (cachexia) make the patient an easy prey to decubitus ulcers. The diet should be high in protein with adequate fluid intake. Frequent change of position and massage over bony prominences helps to keep the skin in good condition. Devices such as an alternating pressure mattress, or sheepskin are used to prevent the development of decubitus ulcers.

**Respiratory.** Because the patient with multiple sclerosis is very susceptible to infection due to his limited activity, shallow breathing, and general debility it is not unusual for pneumonia to be the immediate cause of death. People with respiratory infections should be kept away from the patient. He should be encouraged to breathe deeply and to cough up mucus, and he should be helped to change his position frequently.

**Deformities.** These often occur because of weakness and paralysis. The nurse should put joints through full range of motion daily, paying careful attention to position and body alignment.

## Parkinson's Disease (Paralysis Agitans, Shaking Palsy)

Parkinson's disease is a slowly progressive disease of the central nervous system. It is primarily a disease of late adult life characterized by rigidity, akinesia (slowness of movement), and tremors. It is estimated that approximately 1.5 million people in the United States have Parkinson's disease, and every year one person in 1,000 over the age of 50 is newly affected. The disease affects both sexes.

### Cause and Pathology

Patients with Parkinson's disease have been divided into three groups: postencephalitic parkinsonism, symptomatic parkinsonism, and idiopathic parkinsonism, or paralysis agitans. Patients with postencephalitic parkinsonism developed the symptoms several years after having had encephalitis of the von Economo type. Symptomatic parkinsonism may follow injury to the nervous system by trauma, carbon monoxide intoxication, manganese and other metallic poisonings, intoxication with tranquilizing drugs. Frequently symptoms occur in elderly patients who have cerebral arteriosclerosis. In idiopathic parkinsonism symptoms appear in middle life without any obvious cause. In Parkinson's disease there is widespread, diffuse, degeneration of the basal ganglia and cerebral cortex.

The cause of the disease is unknown, but it is believed that the symptoms are due to a disturbance in the regulation of the nerve impulses sent to the nuclei of the basal ganglia from the substantia nigra. Research has demonstrated that the transmission of nerve impulses is mediated by dopamine. Studies have shown a decreased amount of the dopamine content of these structures, particularly in the substantia nigra in patients with Parkinson's disease.

### Symptoms

The symptoms of Parkinson's disease progress slowly. There may be a lapse of years between the time of the patient's first observation that something is wrong and the time of diagnosis. The symptoms may start on only one side of the body, and later may become bilateral. Within several years the patient may develop all the symptoms characteristic of the disease.

**Akinesia.** The first symptom to appear is usually akinesia, a generalized slowness of movement. The patient will have difficulty initiating voluntary movement, and the time required by him to perform activities of daily living will increase. He will have difficulty performing more than one action at a time.

**Rigidity.** Rigidity will be the next symptom to occur. Rigidity is limited to the muscles of the extremities in the early stages of the disease. The patient's posture and gait will be affected (Fig. 23-5). He will stand with his head flexed, shoulders stooped, and spine arched forward. The gait will be slow and shuffling without associated swinging of the arms. The patient will have difficulty starting to walk, but once started there will be a rapid increase in pace. He will break into a run with short steps and have difficulty stopping. Writing will be affected. It will appear tremulous and the letters will become progressively smaller. There will be loss of associated movements. For example, the patient will not cross his legs when seated. The facial expression will become fixed. The patient will blink infrequently, and will fail to twist a corner of his mouth into a quick smile or to show any of the thousands of expressions with which human beings communicate with each other. Speech will become impaired, with the voice becoming monotonous, and eventually unintelligible. Rigidity of trunk muscles will make it impossible for the patient to turn in bed or to arise from a sitting position. Due to the akinesia and rigidity swallowing will be affected. The time required to eat will increase. Normal involuntary swallowing will decrease causing drooling of saliva.

**Tremor.** Tremor will appear next. The rhythmic alternating tremor is rather coarse. It occurs in resting muscle, decreasing during activity and disappearing in sleep, except in the late stages of the disease. It may start in the fingers, spread to arms and then to the rest of the body, and become so

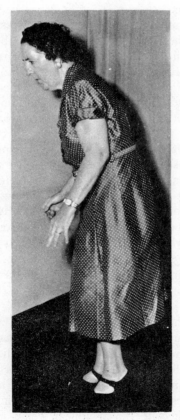

**Figure 23-5.** Typical posture of a person who has Parkinson's disease. Note the tense stance, the small step and the forward bend of the patient's body. (Dr. Lewis J. Doshay, New York, N.Y.)

severe that every movement is tremulous. It is a relatively slow tremor, with two to five shakes a second. Characteristically, the thumb beats against the fingers in a pill-rolling movement.

Intellectual faculties are usually not impaired. There may be mood disturbances, but these may be associated with any chronic disease. The loss of facial expression places the patient at a social disadvantage; he cannot respond appropriately because his face remains masklike.

Anxiety can produce an exacerbation of symptoms.

### Prognosis

Parkinson's disease progresses slowly. A patient may have the disease 20 years or more. Because of their disability, these patients are susceptible to respiratory disease, which may prove fatal.

### Treatment and Nursing Care

**Drug Therapy.** Drug therapy is aimed at the control of the symptoms. Until recently drug therapy was mainly the belladonna alkaloids or synthetic compounds with belladonnalike effects including trihexyphenidyl (Artane), benztropine mesylate (Cogentin), ethopropazine (Parsidol), and others. These drugs quiet the tremor and relax the rigid muscles. Toxic reactions to be aware of are excessive excitement, restlessness, and glaucoma. The nurse should observe for changes in pulse rate and blood pressure, for dizziness and mental confusion. Dryness of the mouth and blurred vision may occur. Atropine dries the skin, impairs bladder function, and may cause heat collapse by preventing perspiration.

Antihistamines decrease rigidity, with a resultant improvement in spontaneous movement, gait, and speech. They do not affect the tremors. Diphenhydramine (Benadryl), and phenindamine (Thephorin) may be given. The maximum effect is expected in about ten days. The nurse should watch for dryness of the mouth, gastrointestinal disturbances, drowsiness, and dizziness.

LEVODOPA. At the present time the preferred treatment is with levodopa (Larodopa, Dopar, L-dopa). Levodopa, a precursor of the neurohormone dopamine, is converted to dopamine in the basal ganglia. It helps correct the dopamine deficiency in the brain of patients with Parkinson's disease. Levodopa helps relieve symptoms of parkinsonism, particularly rigidity and akinesia, and controls tremor and postural difficulties. The drug is administered orally, and the dosage must be individually determined. It is given three to six times daily with meals or some food. Side effects include anorexia, nausea, vomiting, postural hypotension, and involuntary movements of the choreiform or dystonic type. The nurse caring for the patient undergoing levodopa therapy must guide and support him, supervise his activities, monitor his vital signs, and observe him for side effects of the drug.

The patient admitted to the hospital for treatment with levodopa has probably been suffering from the disabling effects of Parkinson's disease for many years. He probably will be frightened by the new surroundings but hopeful that this new treatment will relieve some of the symptoms of the disease. He will need help to adjust to his surroundings. Orientation to the hospital routine and explanation of procedures are essential. He has a great need to be accepted. The mannerisms and tone of voice of the nurse influence the patient's feelings about himself.

Because levodopa is administered with meals and the patient may have difficulty eating, it is important to notice what the patient eats. The patient requires time to eat slowly. The nurse should be aware that pyridoxine HCL (vitamin $B_6$) reverses the antiparkinsonian effects of levodopa.

The nurse should carefully observe and record the patient's daily progress, and assess his ability to perform daily activities. Any side effects of the drug should be reported. Since fluctuating blood pressure is a frequent reaction to levodopa, blood pressure should be checked frequently. The patient and his family should be instructed in the use of the medication.

**Surgical Therapy.** Surgical therapy attempts to destroy a small area of brain tissue in the thalamus or basal ganglia; when successful this gives the patient relief of symptoms of tremor and rigidity. This type of surgery is called stereotactic because the surgeon is guided to the desired location in the brain by elaborate mechanical devices. The patient is awake during the procedure. The surgical lesion may be made mechanically with a wire loop, by electrocoagulation, radiofrequency current, or freezing. At present, freezing the tissue with a liquid nitrogen probe is the surgical method of choice.

Thus far, surgery has been most successful in the younger patient with symptoms on only one side of the body. A decrease in tremor is the desired result. Some patients also have some lessening of rigidity. Because of the risk of hemorrhage and other complications, the older patient with bilateral symptoms is operated on more rarely.

POSTOPERATIVE CARE. The postoperative nursing management of this patient is the same as for any patient who has had brain surgery. The extent of the transient neurologic impairment which may occur will influence the patient's nursing care. Some patients may suffer hemiplegia, visual field impairment, and aphasia. The patient also may have weakness, decreased mentation, and headache for a day or two after surgery, during the time in which the brain is edematous. The nurse should make frequent neurologic nursing assessments. The patient's temperature should be taken frequently, as the temperature control center in the brain may be affected temporarily. If surgery is successful in controlling the patient's tremor and rigidity, he will need help to practice walking and swinging his arms, feeding and dressing himself.

**Rehabilitation.** Although it cannot halt progression of the disease, rehabilitation principles and techniques can result in the patient's maintaining greater ability for self-care than would otherwise be possible. Here, as always, early and consistent treatment is most beneficial. Gait training and transfer activities are included in a rehabilitation program. Unfortunately many patients in this country, because of distance, expense, or lack of facility, still do not obtain the therapy that could help them.

If there are no rehabilitation facilities, the nurse can teach the patient exercises such as the following for the specialized purpose indicated:

- **Speech. Practice using the lips with such twisters as "Massachusetts electricity" and "Methodist Episcopal." If a recording machine is available, reading into it may help the patient to identify the speech errors that he is making.**

- **Fingers. Type, play the piano, press the fingers backward against a door, squeeze a rubber ball. While the patient is watching television, have him button and unbutton a shirt. If buttoning is really impossible, put zippers in wherever it is possible. Have the patient massage cold cream every night into the muscles of his face and his neck.**

- **Goose stepping. The patient should keep the knee straight and let the heel be the first part of the foot to touch the ground. Patients should be encouraged** to keep lifting their toes instead of scraping along. Lacking a normal swing to the arms while he is walking makes the patient look odd and may make him feel odd. If he clasps his hands behind his back while he is walking, his appearance will be more normal.

- **Knee suspension.** While the patient is watching television, have him support the feet but not the knees. Gravity will pull the knee into a straight position and help to lengthen the hamstrings at the back of the knee joint.
- **Balance.** Teach the patient to walk with his feet wide apart. A broad base is steadier than a narrow one. Concentrate on swinging the arms. Taking walks is good exercise for the patient with Parkinson's disease. Put blocks of wood on the floor, and have the patient practice stepping over them. If his legs become "frozen" when he is walking forward, have him take a step backward. Patients may find it easier to walk in individually molded space shoes.
- **Turning.** Teach the patient not to try to cross his legs when he is turning. Rather he should turn in a series of small steps. Try it yourself first.
- **Chairs.** Rigid chairs are easier to get out of than soft ones. Have the patient move to the edge of the seat, press his feet tightly against the floor, and get up all at once, with as much speed as possible. If the legs are "frozen" while sitting, have the patient cross and uncross them two or three times before attempting to stand. Instruct him to sit on the left side of a bus, because it is higher on that side when the driver pulls over to the curb.
- **Blinking.** Teach the patient to blink consciously to protect his cornea and to prevent him from appearing to stare. Watching a tennis match or ping pong game is good exercise for the eye and the neck muscles.

**The Long-Term View.** The patient should be helped by his family, friends or the nurses only when he really cannot perform a motion by himself. It is important that stress and anxiety and fatigue, all of which make the symptoms worse, be kept to a minimum, and in achieving this aim the family can help. The nurse should discuss with the patient's family his needs for serenity and peace of mind. The nurse who recognizes the patient's needs —for encouragement, to be wanted, to be useful, to speak slowly without impatience on the part of the listener; and the family's needs—for encouragement, for expression of worry and perhaps of anger—helps both patient and family to make the necessary emotional adjustments to a lifelong disability. Light massage, frequent exercise of the various muscle groups and carefully supervised medical treatment help to keep a patient self-sufficient.

Parkinson's disease is discouraging for patient, family and nurse. It is a long-term affliction without remission in its symptomatology. The drooling disgusts the patient, the blank face and the slowed movements make social interchange difficult, and the rigidity is fearful and frustrating. There are large areas in which treatment facilities are scarce or nonexistent.

Yet—and the nurse can point out some of these things to a discouraged patient—present-day drug therapy does control many of the symptoms in many of the patients, and research on new drugs is going on all the time. Who knows what improvements tomorrow will bring in chemotherapy or surgery? In due time research workers may find drugs that will work even better than those available now.

Two foundations have been established to aid parkinsonian patients. The Parkinson's Disease Foundation at 125 East 50th Street, New York City 10022, is devoted primarily to research into the cause, the prevention and the cure of the disease. The National Parkinson Foundation at 135 East 44th Street, New York City 10017, is concerned with basic research and a broad program of service to patients.

## THE NURSING MANAGEMENT OF THE PATIENT WITH A CONVULSIVE DISORDER

### Epilepsy

Epilepsy was described by Hippocrates as long ago as 400 B.C., but because of superstitions and attitudes about the disorder, modern study and treatment were delayed until about a century ago. Until recently epileptics were considered to be possessed by good or evil spirits, and fear of the disorder, rather than study of it, was the rule.

However, superstitions about epilepsy still prevail, and evidence abounds that even today it is held in special awe and dread. It is viewed quite differently from diabetes or heart disease. Although most people recognize that those with diabetes must receive treatment to be able to maintain usual activities, this disease is usually accepted for what it is, a long-term disorder for which most patients can compensate effectively by following their treatment. Epileptics, too, have a long-term disability, one that can be controlled in most instances by careful treatment. Nevertheless, epilepsy is still mentioned sometimes in hushed whispers, as if it were a disgrace instead of a disorder that affects some otherwise healthy, capable people.

Attitudes toward epilepsy are reflected by the reaction of many employers when they discover that a worker has epilepsy. One man was employed for two years by a large company. During that time he was never late or absent, and he received several citations for excellent performance of his work. One day he had a seizure; the following day he was dismissed.

### Definition

Epilepsy means a tendency to have recurrent seizures. A common lay term for seizures is "fit." The seizures are not always accompanied by convulsive movements, but they do involve a temporary interruption of consciousness.

### Cause

About four-fifths of all cases of epilepsy are termed idiopathic (of unknown causes). The remaining cases are called symptomatic epilepsy (the seizures are symptoms of some lesion in the brain). For example, injuries or tumor of the brain may cause symptomatic epilepsy.

The pathophysiology of the idiopathic type is unknown. The role of heredity has been widely studied, and is still disputed. It has been shown

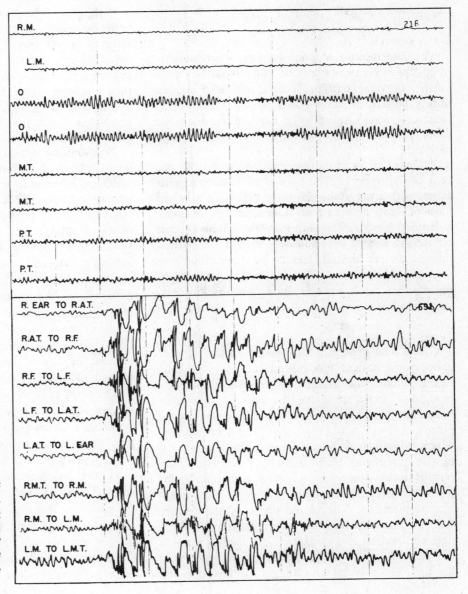

**Figure 23-6.** Contrast of a normal electroencephalogram with that of an epileptic patient during a grand mal seizure. Note the sharp, spiky waves recorded during the seizure. (Dr. Julius Korein, New York, N.Y.)

that epileptics frequently have abnormal electroencephalograms. Figure 23-6 contrasts a normal electroencephalogram with that of an epileptic. Note that the normal tracing has a regular, smooth pattern, where that of the epileptic looks jagged and irregular, with many abnormal discharges.

### Incidence

Over one million people in the United States have epilepsy. Usually, the seizures of idiopathic epilepsy appear during childhood and youth. When epilepsy appears late in life, it is often symptomatic of some trauma or disease of the brain. For example, arteriosclerosis may cause a lesion in the brain, which in turn causes seizures.

### Description

The interruption of consciousness characteristic of epilepsy may or may not be accompanied by convulsive movements. The seizure reflects a sudden unruly pattern of brain waves which is manifested in several ways. An epileptic may always have the same type of seizure; or he may experience a variety of types.

An aura or warning is experienced by 50 per cent of the patients. The aura is an ill-defined sensation which may take the form of seeing a bright flash of light, hearing a strange sound, or smelling a distinctive odor. The aura may occur long enough before the loss of consciousness to give the patient time to protect himself. He can lie down, thus preventing a fall, or he can get away quickly from objects that can harm him during unconsciousness, such as a hot stove.

### Types

**Grand Mal (The Big Sickness).** In this type of epilepsy the patient suddenly utters a cry and falls to the ground, unconscious. At first his whole body is rigid in tonic spasm of the muscles. Laryngospasm and spasm of the chest muscles cause a temporary obstruction of breathing. The patient's color, which initially may be pale due to the constriction of the superficial blood vessels, becomes bluish-purple during the moments when breathing is interrupted. Breathing resumes with deep, often irregular respirations. The clonic phase of the seizure follows. Jerky movements resulting from the alternate contraction and relaxation of muscles pervade the patient's entire body. Frothy saliva appears on his lips. He may bite his tongue. If he does, the frothy saliva will appear to be pinkish. The patient may be incontinent of urine during the seizure.

The patient may be aware that he has had an attack. He may have a headache and be exhausted afterward, and frequently he sleeps for several hours. After a severe seizure the patient may experience a period of mental confusion.

**Status Epilepticus.** Status epilepticus occurs when epileptic seizures follow one another so closely that the patient does not regain consciousness. If the repeated seizures are not stopped by treatment, the patient will die from brain damage. Fortunately, because of improved therapy, status epilepticus is much less common now than formerly.

**Petit Mal (The Little Sickness).** This type of epileptic seizure is characterized by brief interruptions of consciousness, sometimes accompanied by twitching of the head, the eyes, or the hands. The patient may pause suddenly in his conversation and then continue where he left off. He does not fall. Sometimes the seizures are so brief that they go unnoticed. Petit mal seizures are more common among children than among adults.

**Psychomotor Attacks.** Psychomotor attacks have been defined as "circumscribed and transient disturbances of mental or emotional functions." These attacks include a wide variety of clinical phenomena: automatic, purposeless movements that may seem voluntary, like hands fumbling at opening shirt buttons, licking, smacking, chewing, or swallowing movements around the mouth; perceptual distortions like hallucinations or illusions; emotional experiences like sudden intense fear or elation; memory distortions like feeling of familiarity of a place or event never actually before experienced (déjà vu). Some patients have only psychomotor attacks; in others these attacks occur sometimes instead of grand mal seizures.

The term *epileptic equivalent* is used to refer to seizure manifestations usually not looked upon as seizures, such as paroxysmal recurrent abdominal pain or vomiting, pallor and sweating, and palpitations, among others.

During psychomotor attacks the patient may show stereotyped behavior that is inappropriate for the situation. Attempts to make him stop what he is doing are unsuccessful, because he is not aware of his actions; nor will he remember them afterward.

Few patients who have psychomotor attacks become aggressive. The diagnosis of psychomotor attacks of epilepsy is of great legal as well as medical importance.

**Jacksonian Seizure.** Jacksonian seizures are usually a manifestation of symptomatic epilepsy. The seizure may originate in a lesion in the brain, such as a scar or a tumor. Convulsive movements usually start in one part, and may spread to involve the entire side of the body to which the part belongs. For instance, the seizure may start in the left hand and spread to the entire left side of the body. The brain lesion is on the side of the brain opposite to the side of the body having the convulsion.

## Diagnosis

Epilepsy may be the easiest or the most difficult disorder to diagnose, depending on the symptoms. Recurring grand mal seizures present a very typical picture. Irregular tracings on the electroencephalogram confirm the diagnosis. The history of the onset of the patient's illness, his family history, and a careful neurologic examination help the physician to differentiate between idiopathic epilepsy and symptomatic epilepsy.

The occurrence of a single convulsion is never conclusive evidence that a person has epilepsy. Convulsions may be caused by a variety of disorders, such as severe infections with high fever. It is especially important that a patient not be carelessly labeled epileptic, because he then, even without having epilepsy, may become subject to an array of restrictive laws and prejudices. For example, a truck driver suddenly had an attack of amnesia. Although it was thought at first that the symptom might represent psychomotor epilepsy, it was discovered that he had a perforated eardrum and a severe infection of his ear that in turn was causing increased intracranial pressure. Treatment with antibiotics relieved the symptoms. If a hasty diagnosis of epilepsy had been made, the man would have been deprived of his driver's license and thereby of his means of livelihood.

## Treatment and Nursing Care

There is no known cure for idiopathic epilepsy, but the underlying cause of symptomatic epilepsy is treatable. Thus if a brain lesion is causing the attacks, it is surgically removed. Drug therapy can often reduce the number and severity of the attacks, and in some patients it can actually prevent the occurrence of attacks.

Counseling is an integral part of therapy. It helps the patient and his family understand the nature of the disorder. It aids them in planning for as normal a life as possible. The need to utilize their resources is emphasized. The patient is encouraged to remain active by participating in social activities and moderate exercise.

## Drug Therapy

**Anticonvulsants.** Anticonvulsants make the patient less susceptible to seizures. Just how the drugs work is not fully understood, but it is known that they increase the resistance of the patient to seizures.

*Phenobarbital* is effective as an anticonvulsant in the treatment of grand mal seizures but it has the disadvantage of causing drowsiness when it is given in large enough doses to control seizures. The average daily dose is 0.1 to 0.3 Gm. *Mephobarbital* (Mebaral), similar to phenobarbital, is given in doses of 0.3 to 0.6 Gm.

*Diphenylhydantoin* (Dilantin), an effective anticonvulsant in treatment of grand mal seizures, does not have the hypnotic action of phenobarbital. Although the dose needed to control seizures varies widely, many adults are given 0.1 Gm., three times daily. If their attacks are not controlled, the physician may increase the dose to a total of 0.4 to 0.6 Gm. daily. The toxic effects of this drug include unsteady gait, nausea and vomiting, skin rash, and hypertrophy of the gums. Weight loss, fatigue, hyperchromic anemia, and adenopathy occur occasionally. This drug is usually given orally, but preparations for parenteral use also are available.

*Trimethadione* (Tridione) is used in control of petit mal seizures. Tridione is a dangerous drug, and for this reason is rarely given. It can cause severe aplastic anemia, and most physicians recommend frequent examinations of the blood while the patient is taking the medication.

*Ethosuximide* (Zarontin) is the drug of choice in petit mal and is safer than trimethadione. Starting dosages in children may begin at 0.25 Gm. once daily. Gastric distress from the drug may be avoided by giving it with meals.

*Mephenytoin* (Mesantoin) is similar in action to diphenylhydantoin. It is used primarily for the control of grand mal and psychomotor seizures. The dose is similar to that of diphenylhydantoin, 0.1 Gm. three or four times a day. The toxic effects include drowsiness, fatigue, skin rash, and, occasionally, aplastic anemia.

*Primidone* (Mysoline) is an anticonvulsant used in the treatment of grand mal and psychomotor epilepsy. The usual adult daily dose is 0.75 to 1.5 Gm. The toxic effects include nausea and vomiting, dizziness, somnolence, headache, and minor psychic disturbances.

**Diazepam.** Diazepam (Valium), usually used as a tranquilizer, has been found to be very effective when given intravenously in the control of status epilepticus. The dose is individualized on the basis of patient's age and general condition. The physician may request pulse and blood pressure be monitored closely during administration. The drug is generally less effective when given orally in long-term therapy, but may be used in combination with other drugs.

Patients need instructions concerning these drugs. They must understand that the drug is not a cure, but that it controls symptoms when it is taken regularly. When some patients have been symptom-free for a time, they decide to discontinue the medication, or they grow careless about taking it regularly. Most of these patients require medication for years. Since most of the anticonvulsants can cause severe toxic symptoms, patients should remain under close supervision while they are taking them.

**Relapse.** Patients who have had successful control of their seizures by drugs sometimes experience a sudden reappearance of seizures. The four most frequent causes of such recurrences are:

- Irregularity in taking prescribed medication
- Use of alcohol
- Increase in age and body weight (particularly of children), which requires adjustment in drug dosage
- Severe emotional strain
- Febrile illnesses

Patients with epilepsy are advised to abstain from all alcoholic beverages. Some patients, unable to follow this suggestion, are advised to use alcohol as sparingly as possible. As far as possible, the patient should be helped to lessen sources of emotional strain. In light of society's attitudes toward the illness, this poses a difficult problem.

### Care of a Patient During a Seizure

Witnessing a seizure, especially for the first time, can be an upsetting experience, whether one is a nurse or a layman. Knowing what to do and what to observe will enable those with the patient to protect him from injury and to contribute information about the seizure that may be very important in helping the physician to make a diagnosis. The same points that the nurse herself learns can serve as a guide for teaching the patient's family, friends or business associates. No one can predict just when or where a seizure will occur. Regardless of where it occurs, or who observes and assists the patient, the same principles are applicable. Learning what to do and, equally important, what not to do, before the situation arises will help to prevent injury to the patient and panic among the observers.

The first and perhaps the most important rule is: *stay with the patient.* There are several reasons for staying with the patient:

- **Most convulsions last only several minutes. (What seems like an hour to a terrified onlooker is usually about three minutes by the clock.)**
- **If you leave the patient to seek help, the attack often is over before you return. The patient may have injured himself, because no one was there to protect him.**
- **Unless you stay with the patient, you will be unable to observe and to report the necessary information concerning the seizure.**

Place a padded tongue depressor between the patient's back teeth to prevent him from biting his tongue. Insert the depressor quickly, before the patient's teeth become tightly clenched. Do not try to force the teeth apart to insert the tongue blade, because you might loosen or even break his teeth. If the seizure is already in progress when you arrive, it may be impossible to insert the mouth gag safely. Never place your fingers in the patient's mouth. (You probably will be bitten.) If a padded tongue depressor is not available, substitute something like a clean folded handkerchief. Fold it several times, so that it will form a thick, soft cushion. Avoid using hard or sharp objects that might cause further injury. For instance, a table knife would not make a good mouth gag, but a folded table napkin would. If you know that a hospitalized patient is likely to have a convulsion, keep a padded tongue depressor at his bedside.

Of course, the safest environment for the patient who is having a convulsion is his own bed, particularly if it is equipped with padded side rails to prevent him from falling. Usually, the convulsion starts so abruptly that if the patient is up and about, there is not time to help him into bed. Have him lie down —on the floor, if necessary—to prevent him from falling. Place a pillow or any soft object, such as a folded coat, under his head, and turn him on his side to allow saliva to run out of his mouth rather than to be aspirated. If he has fallen already when you arrive, do not try to move him until the convulsion is over, unless he has fallen on or near something dangerous, such as a hot stove or a radiator.

Do not try to restrain the patient's movements. It is impossible to stop the convulsion in this way, and both you and the patient are likely to be injured, if you try to hold him down.

Loosen any tight clothing, especially if it is around the patient's neck (ties, scarves, collars).

Protect the patient from being a spectacle. His problem is great enough without the added embarrassment of recovering to find himself surrounded by gaping spectators. Often one person can concentrate on observing and protecting the patient, while another screens the patient or—if screening is not possible—discourages onlookers.

Observe, report and record the following information:

- **Where the convulsion started (In Jacksonian seizure the part of the body first affected often gives the physician a clue about the location of the lesion.)**
- **The parts of the body involved (It may be just one extremity, one side of the body or the entire body.)**
- **Position and movements of the eyes**
- **The patient's level of consciousness during the seizure**
- **Skin color, diaphoresis**
- **Respiration (character and rate)**
- **The type of muscle response (clonic, tonic)**
- **How long the seizure lasted (Time the length of the seizure with a watch; most people greatly overestimate the duration of a seizure.)**
- **Any injury that occurred during the seizure, such as a bitten tongue**
- **The symptoms of the patient after the attack (e.g., somnolence, headache, orientation to surroundings)**

## Social, Emotional, and Economic Implications of Epilepsy

Many epileptics suffer more acutely from the stigma attached to epilepsy than from the symptoms themselves. Every life situation is tinged with the dread of an attack and the fear of what others will think. The family of the patient often is ashamed that a close relative has epilepsy. Family members often feel that the disorder of a relative is a reflection on them, and they make every effort to conceal it. The epileptic child may be denied admission to public school; or, if he is admitted, he may find that he is the object of curiosity, pity, or distrust.

Later the questions of marriage and child bearing may arise. The individual may be helped in making these decisions by personal counseling based on consideration of his particular condition.

Finding and keeping a job present tremendous problems for the person with epilepsy. Many people have the impression that epileptics are necessarily of subnormal intelligence. Although some persons with epilepsy experience alteration in their mental functioning, many of them are nevertheless coping satisfactorily with work, and with home and community responsibilities. The proportion of epileptics who have severe impairment of intellectual functioning, due to brain damage, and who are therefore unable to function adequately in work and other community situations is very small. Some people with epilepsy have unusual intellectual gifts, but all too often they lack the opportunity for advanced education and work commensurate with their talents.

Other misconceptions are that epileptics are unreliable, frequently absent, and a hazard to themselves and others. People with epilepsy are individuals; any sweeping statement concerning their abilities is bound to be untrue. To claim that epilepsy never poses an employment problem is just as fallacious as to declare that it always interferes with work. Epilepsy should not cause absenteeism or impair the quality of work, if the seizures are well controlled by medication. Persons with epilepsy who have frequent, severe seizures can be employed only in controlled situations, such as those afforded by sheltered workshops. It has been estimated that this group comprises only 15 per cent of persons with epilepsy.

Emotional strain often is a factor in precipitating seizures. Satisfying home and family life and suitable work are just as important to persons with epilepsy as to anyone else.

Drug therapy is but one part of the treatment. Helping the patient to live with the disability, particularly in light of the attitude of society, is a difficult but important part of therapy.

The following points about rehabilitation should be kept in mind:

- **The patient must recognize the importance of taking his medication and visiting his physician regularly. The control of the seizures is the foundation on which the rehabilitation program is built. The sudden withdrawal of medication can cause a seizure.**

- **People who associate closely with the patient in his everyday activities must understand the condition of the patient and know what to do if an attack occurs. They need help in overcoming their own fears and misconceptions about epilepsy.**

- **The condition and the capabilities of each patient must be evaluated individually, so that educational and vocational plans can offer him opportunities to contribute to society without jeopardizing his own safety or that of others.**

- **Some types of activity are unsuitable for any person who is subject to seizures. Society has a right and an obligation to protect its members; it cannot permit an epileptic to pursue activities that could become dangerous if they were interrupted by his loss of consciousness (for instance, piloting a plane). Such sensible restrictions do not constitute discrimination.**

Public attitudes have forced the epileptic to conceal his disability. Concealment has resulted in lack of help for many who could benefit from it. How can the epileptic receive help if he is afraid to admit that he needs help? A big job still has to be done in educating people about epilepsy. Nurses are in a strategic position to make a valuable contribution to this need.

Increasing public awareness of the needs of people with epilepsy had led to the development of organizations which are concerned with their problems, and which are involved in changing the attitudes of the public toward people with epilepsy and improving the life style of epileptics. There are four national organizations: American Epilepsy Foundation, National Epilepsy League, The Epilepsy Foundation of America, and the United Epilepsy Association. Free literature about epilepsy may be obtained from any of these associations.

## REFERENCES AND BIBLIOGRAPHY

BELAND, IRENE: *Clinical Nursing: Pathophysiological and Psychosocial Approaches,* ed. 2, New York, Macmillan, 1970.

CARINI, ESTA, and OWENS, GUY: *Neurological and Neurosurgical Nursing,* ed. 6, St. Louis, Mosby, 1974.

CAROZZA, VIRGINIA: Understanding the patient with epilepsy, *Nurs. Clin. N. Am.* 5:1:13-22; March 1970.

DILLON, ANN M.: Nursing care of the patient with multiple sclerosis, *Nurs. Clin. N. Am.* 8:4:653-664, December 1973.

ELLIOTT, FRANK: *Clinical Neurology,* ed. 2, Philadelphia, Saunders, 1971.

GARDNER, M.: Responsiveness as a measure of consciousness, *Am. J. Nurs.* 68:5:1034-1038, May 1968.

GLASS, JEAN S.: Nursing care of the neurosurgical patient: Head injuries, *J. Neurosurg. Nurs.* 5:2:49-55, December 1973.

JOHNSON, MARION R.: Emergency management of head and spinal injuries, *Nurs. Clin. N. Am.* 8:3:389-400, September 1973.

KINNEY, A., and BLOUNT, M.: Systems approach to myasthenia gravis, *Nurs. Clin. N. Am.* 6:3:435-454, September 1971.

KINTZEL, KAY (ed.): *Advanced Concepts of Clinical Nursing,* Philadelphia, Lippincott, 1971.

KORTE, MARY L.: Intensive care of the neurologic patient—meeting the challenge, *Nurs. Clin. N. Am.* 7:2:335-348, June 1972.

MCKENZIE, SHIRLEY: Stereotaxic radiofrequency coagulation: A treatment for trigeminal neuralgia, *J. Neurosurg. Nurs.* 4:1:49-60, July 1972.

MERRITT, HOUSTON, H.: *A Textbook of Neurology,* ed. 5, Philadelphia, Lea and Febiger, 1973.

METHENY, NORMA, and SNIVELY, W. D.: *Nurses' Handbook of Fluid Balance,* ed. 2, Philadelphia, Lippincott, 1974.

NOBACK, CHARLES, and DEMAREST, ROBERT: *The Nervous System: Introduction and Review,* New York, McGraw-Hill, A Blakiston Pub., 1972.

PARSONS, L. CLAIRE: Respiratory changes in head injury, *Am. J. Nurs.* 71:11:2187-2191, November 1971.

PERRINE, GEORGE: Needs met and unmet, *Am. J. Nurs.* 71:11:2128-2133, November 1971.

TATE, GAYLE: Assessment and direction of nursing care for patients with acute central nervous system insult, *Nurs. Clin. N. Am.* 6:1:165-171, March 1971.

# The Patient with
# Spinal Cord Impairment

## CHAPTER 24

Care of patients with spinal cord impairment presents a considerable challenge to the nurse. Injuries and diseases of the spinal cord often lead to paralysis, and to a multiplicity of problems in rehabilitation. Patients with spinal cord impairment have benefited particularly in recent years from advances in rehabilitation programs, and from nursing and medical care during the acute phase of illness which enables them to survive and which minimizes the incidence of such disabling complications as decubitus ulcers, pneumonia, and unresolved grief. Interdisciplinary collaboration is essential in the care of these patients, who require the services of various specialized therapists. Attitudes of the patient's professional and personal associates are also crucial in providing encouragement and support as the patient seeks to re-establish a satisfying life.

## THE SPINAL CORD

The spinal cord is continuous with the medulla oblongata and extends from the foramen magnum to the second lumbar vertebra. The spinal cord serves as the center for reflex action and provides pathways for afferent (sensory) impulses as they pass from peripheral nerves to the brain and for efferent (motor) impulses as they pass from the central nervous system toward the effector organ. It is composed of white matter (outer portion) and gray matter (inner portion). The white matter consists of myelinated fibers which link different segments of the cord and which link the cord to the brain. The anterior portion of the gray matter contains

397

the cell bodies from which efferent (motor) fibers of spinal nerves arise for voluntary and reflex activity of muscles. The sensory roots which consist of the afferent fibers that convey input from the sensory receptors in the body via the spinal nerves to the spinal cord are located in the posterior aspect of the gray matter. Thirty-one pairs of spinal nerves arise from the spinal cord.

## Symptoms

Clinical manifestations of spinal cord and spinal nerve disorders depend upon the level of the involvement of the cord and the rapidity with which the symptoms develop. Symptoms are due to either compression of nerve roots at the level of the lesion or interference with the transmission of nerve impulses within the cord.

Compression of nerve roots will cause pain and paresthesia followed by sensory loss, weakness, and wasting of muscles in the distribution of the affected roots. Specific symptoms depend upon the level of the lesion. For example, involvement of the upper cervical segments will produce phrenic nerve involvement with dyspnea on exertion, overactivity of accessory respiratory muscles, and difficulty coughing and sneezing. The early signs of spinal cord compression are spastic weakness and impairment of cutaneous and proprioceptive sensation below the level of the lesion and impairment of bladder control and, at times, of the rectum.

The nursing management of the patient with spinal cord dysfunction depends upon the location and extent of the patient's symptoms. After a careful nursing assessment and with knowledge of the patient's diagnosis and the physician's plan of care, the nurse determines the appropriate nursing actions.

## NURSING INTERVENTION FOR THE PATIENT WITH SPINAL SURGERY

Surgery on the spinal cord is performed when the lesion which is causing compression of the spinal cord (e.g., a herniated intervertebral disk, a tumor, a clot, and fractured bone fragments) can be removed without permanent damage to adjacent structures. In a laminectomy, the posterior arch of the involved vertebrae is removed to expose the spinal cord and allow further surgery. Sometimes a piece of bone is taken from another area, such as the iliac crest, and grafted onto the vertebrae. This is a spinal fusion. The fusion stabil-

izes the spine weakened by degenerative joint changes, such as osteoarthritis, and further weakened by the laminectomy. Fusion results in a firm union. When a portion of the lumbar spine is fused, the patient usually becomes unaware of stiffness after a short time because motion increases in the joints above the fusion. There is usually more limitation of motion when the fusion is in the cervical area. In the cervical area an anterior approach is used to remove damaged disks. The cervical vertebrae are exposed anteriorly, the disk and any bone spurs are removed, and the vertebrae are fused to prevent slipping.

## Preoperative Care

When the patient has spinal cord impairment from whatever cause, the nurse should assess motor and sensory function. She should also determine and record what activity and which position increase pain, and any gain or loss in motion and sensation since her last observation. Bladder and bowel function should be carefully observed and appropriate nursing actions initiated. Measures should be taken to prevent constipation.

The patient should be instructed in and encouraged to practice such exercises as deep breathing and coughing and "log rolling" (turning in bed) before surgery so that he has an experienced pattern to follow afterwards.

Immediately before surgery the patient's legs may be wrapped with elastic bandages to increase the circulating blood volume by decreasing the size of the vascular bed in the legs. This measure helps to prevent a drop in blood pressure. The surgery is performed with the patient in the prone position.

## Postoperative Care

**Laminectomy.** After a laminectomy the patient should deep breathe and cough at frequent intervals. Nursing assessment should be continued. A change in motor function or altered sensation may be the first indication of compression of the cord due to edema or hemorrhage at the operative site. The dressing should be inspected for leakage of spinal fluid as well as for hemorrhage.

Incisional pain usually can be relieved by narcotics. When there has been irritation of the nerve by pressure exerted by the herniated disk or by surgery, the pain may last for some time postoperatively. Heat and massage may be beneficial.

One of the most important principles of care after a lumbar laminectomy is to have the patient rest his back as much as possible. Twisting, turning, and jerking the back are not conducive to healing. Immediately after surgery the patient is kept flat on his back for four to six hours. He then can be turned "log fashion."

Before he is turned, the patient's bed should be flattened, and he should make himself stiff as a log, with his arms at his side. Then the nurse rolls him over all at once, without bending his spine. A turning sheet is helpful, especially early in the postoperative period. Usually patients feel safer when they are allowed to participate in the turning process. At first a patient may be limited to listening to the nurse explain just how the turning will be carried out, to be as comfortable and safe as possible. Later, he will be able to turn himself. It is essential to avoid any abruptness in the turnings, either in manner or the movement of the patient. Most patients greatly fear that they will be moved in such a way that the results of the operation will be compromised, or that they will suffer much pain. Therefore, the nurse should proceed slowly, with the patient's full knowledge, and his participation insofar as possible, in order to lessen anxiety. The nurse should support the patient's position in good alignment with pillows. The patient should be allowed a small pillow under his head.

The patient should not lift his hips to get on a bedpan, because this motion will bend his spine. Rather, he should roll onto the bedpan, and his back should be supported with pillows while he is on it. The nurse should anticipate what the patient will need, and put it close enough to him so that he can reach it without stretching.

When the patient gets up, there will be less strain on his back if he walks in shoes rather than in slippers. The patient's family should be asked to bring shoes, so that they will be available the first time he is to get up. Bedroom slippers are not advisable because they do not provide adequate support; and, by fitting loosely, they predispose to falls.

Of course, women should not wear high-heeled shoes. Only a shoe with a moderate heel that gives good support to the foot is desirable.

A brace or corset occasionally is prescribed and should be applied while the patient is still lying in bed. He should wear a thin cotton shirt under the brace, no part of which should contact the skin, and there should be no wrinkles to leave marks in the skin. If a shirt is not worn under the brace, there should be smooth padding where the brace touches the skin.

To help the patient into a brace, the nurse should have him lie on his side. She should center the stays on his back, and have him roll onto the garment. While he is still lying down, after the support has been snugly fastened in place, the nurse should assist him across the bed, so that when he sits up, his feet will be over the edge. She should help him to sit up, without straining or twisting his back. In such a support, the patient will have to keep his back straight. Also, the nurse should encourage the patient to maintain good posture with his muscles. The stronger the back muscles become, the more support they can give to the operative site, and the less the patient will need the external support of the brace.

Exercises in some form will be prescribed. Because swimming is effective in strengthening muscles and is enjoyable to many people, it may be recommended by the physician.

After a lumbar laminectomy patients are more comfortable and better supported when they sit in a straight chair rather than an easy chair.

The nurse should teach the patient not to bend over from the waist; instead, he should lower the body by bending the knees while keeping the spine straight.

**Spinal Fusion.** A patient who has had a spinal fusion is usually kept on postoperative bed rest longer than the patient who has had a simple laminectomy, and care must be taken so that he does not twist his back while the bones unite. The principles of care are the same as for the patient who has had a laminectomy. A patient who has had a spinal fusion may have two wounds: the wound in the spinal column and the wound in the donor site.

**Surgery of the Cervical Spine.** A patient with surgery of the cervical spine may wear a cervical collar to prevent neck movement. The patient may be turned from side to side with the aid of a turning sheet. A small pillow should be placed under his neck to keep his spine straight when he is positioned on his side. The neurologic nursing assessment should include evaluation of the patient's respiratory function.

**Surgery of the Thoracic Spine.** When surgery has been performed on the thoracic spine, a figure-of-8 dressing may be applied postoperatively. Because the dressing may constrict the axillary vessels, the radial pulse should be checked at frequent intervals. The patient is instructed not to stretch his arms until healing is well advanced.

### Resumption of Activities

When spinal fusion has been performed, the resumption of activities is gradual for six months to a year, after which the patient usually can resume full activity. After a laminectomy without spinal fusion, the patient is gradually allowed to do light work, but usually he should do no lifting for a year, and he may never be able to lift heavy objects. The light objects he does lift should be held close to his body to avoid back strain.

The restriction may be difficult for the patient. A farmer cannot pitch hay, a mother cannot lift her baby from his crib, and a clerk cannot carry a heavy stack of papers to the file. When caring for a convalescent patient, the nurse should review his daily activities with him, and help him to think through the ways of avoiding lifting for the period designated by his physician. Intelligent planning can help him to avoid a "just this once" exertion that may be damaging. If the patient's position requires heavy lifting, perhaps a different job can be found for him. The industrial nurse will be interested in this patient and will coordinate his care and return to work with the employer. Similar restrictions often are placed on patients with herniated disks who are treated medically.

### NURSING INTERVENTION FOR A PATIENT WITH A SPINAL CORD TUMOR

Spinal cord tumors may be primary arising from the substance of the cord itself, its roots, meningeal covering, vascular supply, and vertebral column, or, more commonly, they may be metastatic. The clinical manifestations of spinal cord tumors are produced by irritation and compression of nerve roots, obstruction of the cord's vascular supply, and compression and displacement of the cord. The symptoms become progressively worse as the lesion grows. Pain, spasm, motor and sensory changes, and urinary incontinence appear as the compression builds up. Patients with spinal cord tumors are treated surgically and with radiotherapy. They may also benefit from a rehabilitation program Nursing care is symptomatic directed toward the patient's physical and psychological needs. The

nurse institutes measures to prevent complications, such as pressure sores, contractures, and respiratory difficulties.

### NURSING INTERVENTION FOR THE PATIENT WITH BACK PAIN

Back pain is a condition which affects a large number of people in the United States. It probably is one of the major causes of absenteeism from work. Back pain can be caused by a variety of conditions, such as acute lumbosacral strain, unstable lumbosacral mechanism, osteoarthritis of lumbar segments, herniated intervertebral disk, and emotional conflict and tension.

### Herniated Intervertebral Disk

Disks of cartilage act as cushions between the vertebrae. Their spongy center (nucleus pulposus) is encased in a fibrous coat (annulus fibrosus). When stress, age, or disease weakens an area in the coat or in a ligament attachment to the vertebrae, and as the nucleus pulposus becomes thickened and hardened, the disk herniates causing pressure on the nerve roots. Disk protrusion occurs most frequently in the fourth to sixth decade of life and is found more commonly in men. The most common cause is trauma. The patient strains with the back in an odd position or lifts with the back flexed. The most common site of protrusion is at the level of the fifth lumbar to the first sacral vertebrae and the fourth to the fifth lumbar vertebrae. Pain along the distribution of the sciatic nerve is a common symptom. The patient complains of pain in the lower back radiating down the posterior surface of one or both legs. Paresthesia in a foot or leg may be present. Anything, such as straining, coughing, lifting a heavy object, that causes increased pressure within the spinal cord intensifies the pain. Pain is more severe when the nerves are stretched, such as when the patient, while lying flat on his back, tries to lift his leg without bending his knee. Pain is also worse when sitting or bending than when standing. The symptoms tend to be recurrent rather than steady, at least in the beginning of the disease. Ruptured disk may also occur in the cervical area.

### Treatment and Nursing Care

The patient with a herniated intervertebral disk is often treated first with conservative measures. For perhaps several weeks he is put to bed on a firm mattress, supported by a bed board. Pain is relieved by drugs, heat, massage, and rest. Since part of the pain is due to muscle spasm, heat to the back and muscle relaxants are often prescribed.

Traction by Buck's extension or a pelvic girdle for a lumbar herniated disk may be used to decrease muscle spasm. Traction also increases the distance between adjacent vertebrae. It may be continuous or intermittent, with 5 to 30 pounds of weight. The traction keeps the patient in bed in good alignment, and some patients find that it relieves their pain. Treatment with traction can be continued at home.

The following factors are important aspects of nursing care: relief of pain; relief of boredom; intervention (for personal hygiene, comfort) in bed rest and traction; maintenance of mobility in unaffected limbs. The patient is cautioned to avoid sudden movements that strain or twist his spine. Instruction in proper body mechanics is essential. The patient is taught the correct methods of bending and lifting. He may need to wear a lumbosacral corset. If conservative therapy fails to relieve symptoms of a ruptured intervertebral disk, surgery is considered.

## NURSING INTERVENTION FOR THE PATIENT WITH A SPINAL CORD INJURY

Much of the interest and knowledge concerning the treatment and rehabilitation of patients with spinal cord impairment has developed as a result of injuries to servicemen during World War II. Although many soldiers during World War I also suffered from spinal cord injuries, most of them died of pneumonia, shock, or urinary-tract infections shortly after the injury. Since then, the discovery of antibiotics and the improved treatment of shock have made it possible for these patients to survive the initial treatment and therefore to become candidates for rehabilitation. The civilian population has also benefited from the knowledge gained in the treatment of injured veterans. The patient with a spinal cord injury will require the skills of many members of the health care team to return him to his highest functional level.

### Etiology and Clinical Manifestations

The spinal cord and nerve roots may be injured by stab wounds, gun shots, shrapnel and other penetrating missiles, and by fracture and fracture dislocation of the vertebrae and their processes. Vertebral injuries result from excessive flexion or extension of the spine in falls, and in diving and automobile accidents.

Spinal cord trauma which is not direct may cause a concussion of the cord. This is usually a temporary and reversible disorder. There may be compression, contusion, or laceration of the substance of the cord causing irreversible damage. Hemorrhage into the cord (hematomyelia) and compression of its vascular supply may occur. The usual sites of injury to the cord are at the level of the fifth to sixth cervical vertebrae and the eleventh to twelfth thoracic vertebrae.

The manifestations of injury to the spinal cord are related to the level and extent of the injury. Paraplegia is paralysis of both lower extremities, and quadriplegia is paralysis of all four extremities.

### Course and Prognosis

The mortality rate for persons with spinal cord injuries is 80 per cent in military life and is lower in civilian life. The immediate prognosis for life is poor when the injury is in the upper cervical area because of the development of respiratory problems. Injuries below the fifth cervical vertebra initially have a better prognosis, but death may follow after a period of weeks or months as a result of severe infection arising from decubitus ulcers, urinary infection, or septicemia.

Except in cases of complete transection of the cord some degree of improvement in the patient's neurologic status can be expected. Incomplete transection of the cord results in a variable amount of motor and sensory loss below the level of the injury. Bladder and rectal paralysis may also be present.

In complete transection of the cord the motor and sensory loss is permanent below the level of injury. Immediately following the injury, a period of spinal shock develops during which there is absence of reflex activity and atonic paralysis of the bladder and rectum. There is also loss of vasomotor control causing orthostatic hypotension, paroxysmal hypertension on filling of the bladder or rectum, and disturbance of sweating and heat regulation. The patient is usually depressed and withdrawn. The length of this period is variable. Recovery from spinal shock is retarded by the presence of decubitus ulcers and urinary infection and by grief and depression. With recovery there is return of deep reflexes and improvement of bladder and rectal function. Bladder and bowel training may be possible at this time.

Prognosis depends upon many factors: the level of the cord injury, the occurrence of complications, the patient's motivation and perseverence, and the quality of care he receives. Many paraplegics are able to go home, to care for themselves, and in some instances to resume work.

### Early Treatment and Nursing Care

**First Aid.** Suppose that someone has been hurt in an automobile accident, and an injury to the spine is suspected. The patient should be placed without flexing his back or neck, onto a firm, flat surface, such as a door that has been removed from its hinges. He should not be moved until help is available, and a firm, flat support on which he can be carried has been obtained. Bystanders should never be permitted to pick up a patient hastily, thus flexing his spine, and to toss him into the back seat of an automobile. Such careless moving may damage the cord further. Proper first aid may mean the difference between the patient's being able to walk and having to spend the rest of his life in a wheelchair. Treatment for shock or hemorrhage may also be required as first-aid measures.

**Physical and X-ray Examinations.** After the patient has been admitted to the hospital, the physician will determine the extent of the injury by physical and x-ray examinations. If the vertebrae are so injured that they are compressing the cord, measures are taken to relieve the pressure of the fractured vertebrae on the cord. Traction may be applied to the head by a cervical halter or by skeletal head traction. For the care of the patient in traction, see Chapter 19 on care of patients with fractures. Laminectomy may be necessary to relieve the pressure of the vertebrae on the cord.

Nursing management is directed toward identifying the patient's specific needs, recognizing and preventing complications, assisting the patient to adjust to his disabilities, and preparing him for the active rehabilitation program which will follow. The patient and his family should be included in all aspects of care. The use of special equipment and devices should be explained. The patient will gradually assume responsibility for his own care.

**Assessment.** The patient's neurologic status is carefully assessed. Does he have sensation in the affected parts? Can he feel that water during his bath is warm or cold? Can he feel the pressure of the nurse's hand? Can he move the part? During spinal shock, the paralysis is flaccid (limp) and after resolution of spinal shock it becomes spastic. Observation of respiratory function is essential.

**Positioning.** During the period immediately after spinal cord injury the patient is seriously ill and requires a great deal of care and observation. When nerve impulses to the skin are interrupted, the skin's normal response to injury is diminished. The paralyzed patient cannot engage in the almost constant movement that is normal, even during sleep, and that protects the skin from pressure sores. Decubitus ulcers form easily in these patients, become infected easily, and heal very slowly. Unless his position is changed frequently by the nurse, decubitus ulcers will result. Eventually, the patient is taught to inspect his own skin. The Stryker or the Foster frame and the CircOlectric bed make it easier to turn helpless patients. The patient is positioned in proper body alignment with care taken to distribute his weight to avoid pressure on devitalized areas. Special equipment, such as an alternating pressure mattress or a sheepskin, is utilized. The skin should be kept dry and clean.

**Joint Mobility.** Deformities readily develop unless special precautions are taken. Footdrop is a frequent complication because of paralysis of the lower extremities. A footboard must be used from the very beginning of the patient's illness to prevent footdrop. Passive exercises to maintain range of motion, prevent contractures, improve circulation, and prevent atrophy of muscles are performed at regular intervals.

**Respiratory Function.** Because the patient is unable to move about, his breathing is shallow, and he fails to cough up respiratory secretions. Therefore, he is predisposed to the development of respiratory complications, such as pneumonia. Changing position frequently and encouraging the patient to breathe deeply and to cough up respiratory secretions are important in preventing respiratory complications. Chest physiotherapy is performed, and the nurse works closely with the respiratory therapist to maintain adequate respiratory function. The patient may require mechanical means to maintain adequate ventilation.

**Pain.** Many patients have pain in the affected area, even though sensation in the usual sense has been lost. The pain is associated with scar formation or irritation around a nerve root. In most patients the pain decreases gradually with recovery from the initial injury. Morphine sulfate for the relief of pain is contraindicated.

**Spasm.** Severe reflex spasms that the patient cannot control are frequent. The muscle movement is spasm and not the return of voluntary function. Physical activity helps to decrease spasm. Passive exercises and changes of position, when they are used regularly, also reduce spasms. The reason for these spasms should be explained to the patient and family.

**Elimination.** Cord compression can interfere with the patient's control over the bladder and the bowel. There may be incontinence or retention of feces, and fecal impactions are frequent. At first there usually is retention of urine; later the patient voids involuntarily. Even when the patient is incontinent, there is often some retention of urine. After a certain volume is reached in the bladder, the sphincter opens, but because the muscle tone of the bladder wall is poor, only a small amount of urine is voided. This condition is known as *overflow incontinence*. The bladder remains partially full, even though the patient has urinated. Stasis of urine in the atonic bladder is dangerous, because it invites infection, which travels up the urinary tract into the kidney pelvis. A retention catheter is used in the bladder. Enemas may be given daily or every other day to evacuate the bowel and to lessen the problems of fecal impaction or incontinence.

**Fluids and Food.** The fluid intake and the nutrition of the patient must be maintained. High-fluid intake helps to lessen the possibility of urinary-tract infections and calculi. High-protein foods are important in controlling decubitus ulcers, because they help to keep the tissues healthy, and they increase the ability of the tissues to heal. It is recommended that the patient have 200 Gm. of protein daily. When the patient is too sick to take a normal diet, parenteral administration of fluids and nutrients may be necessary.

## Psychological Impact

As the patient begins to recover from the overwhelming physical injury, he gradually becomes aware of what has happened to him. He finds that he is unable to move part of his body. Because he can no longer feel these parts, he must look to see if they are still there. Psychological trauma is intense. The body image must be changed. Now, instead of viewing himself as a whole, healthy person, the patient must recognize that part of his body is permanently useless. At first, most patients react with depression and withdrawal. They lie and stare into space, and they show no interest in people and events around them. During this period it is better to emphasize quiet presence, empathy, and attention to physical needs, than it is to adopt a cheer-him-up campaign. It will take time for the patient to recover from the psychological as well as the physical hurt of so devastating an experience.

**Dependence.** The patient recognizes his complete dependence on others, and he is fearful because he can no longer help himself. He wants someone near him day and night. Particularly, if he is a quadriplegic, his helplessness is extreme. He must be bathed, toileted and dressed—just like an infant. His mind is active, though, even if his body is not.

The patient and his family are anxious concerning prognosis. "Will he ever walk again?" is a question that looms large, and it must be dealt with realistically. If the degree of injury has been so great that there is little hope for any return to function, the patient should be helped to understand this prognosis early in the course of the illness. It is not a kindness to encourage false hopes that later will be dashed, and that meanwhile will keep the patient from accepting the need for rehabilitation. The major return of function can be expected to occur during the first year or year and a half after the injury.

It is impossible for an able-bodied person to fully understand what it means to have a severe and permanent disability like paraplegia; the simplest task becomes an insurmountable problem. Tying one's shoelaces or going to the bathroom may be almost impossible; if these acts are accomplished, they require the greatest effort and planning. The nurse cannot make this adjustment for the patient; he must do it himself.

The nurse may be able to help the patient by being a good listener. When he is ready to talk about how angry or discouraged he is, he does not need advice or cheering up. He needs someone who can help to lift the burden by accepting how he feels. A patient who tells a nurse that he wishes only for death may not tell her that again if her response is, "Oh, you have lots to live for. You can read, and you have two lovely children." The patient will still feel as hopeless as he did; he just will not discuss that subject with that nurse again.

The nurse who can reply, "You feel pretty discouraged," or "You don't see much purpose in life now," by implication is telling the patient that she understands how deeply he is discouraged, and that there is nothing wrong about feeling as he does. If she accepts his feelings, the patient may be able to express himself further, and afterward he may be able to give the nurse some clue as to how she can help him. He may mention tentatively and cautiously that he loves gardening, or that feeding himself is more important to him than walking. At this point the nurse can help him to develop a window-box garden, or redouble efforts to help him to feed himself.

Neither activity completes his care, but every small step forward is a point of encouragement. With understanding, the patient may be able to slowly restore his damaged psyche, so that he can be better able to rehabilitate his body.

**Incontinence.** Incontinence poses a tremendous problem. Very early in life human beings are taught to maintain high standards of personal cleanliness. Much is made of the shamefulness of not controlling excretory function. Frequently, threats and punishment are used to make the little child conform to these standards. During this process definite and strong feelings about proper excretory habits are acquired. An adult who becomes unable to control these functions often feels shamed and disgraced—even though intellectually he understands the reason for the lack of control. Incontinence poses a social problem, too. Patients are very sensitive to the reaction of others. Many paraplegics are constantly fearful that an embarrassing accident will occur while they are with others, or that other people will detect odors from catheters and urinals. Hence, the rehabilitation, when possible, of the bowels and the bladder is highly important, not only for physical reasons, such as preventing decubitus ulcers, but also for its effect on morale: it helps the patient to overcome the threat of embarrassment, and so it helps him to feel more like his adult, independent self.

**Disturbances in Sexual and Reproductive Functions.** Many men paraplegics are impotent, and these patients suffer a severe blow to their manhood. They may feel that they are being regarded with scorn and derision. Some women patients are able to have children. Questions about sexual functioning must be answered individually, since the degree of normal function will be determined by the particular nature and the extent of the illness. Both the patient and the wife or the husband should have an opportunity to discuss this subject.

**Social Implications.** In addition to disturbances of the sexual and the reproductive function, opportunities for meeting people usually are curtailed and opportunities for marriage decreased. The patient does not conform to the ideals of masculine or feminine attractiveness made fashionable by society. For instance, women must wear braces, use crutches and wear low-heeled oxfords to walk. A tall, well-built man who develops paraplegia no longer appears tall when sitting in a wheelchair.

The paraplegic is subject to a great deal of frustration. He cannot move about freely, and in many situations he must rely on others to help him. A quadriplegic may be unable to light his own cigarette, but he may have an even greater desire to smoke than he did before his injury, when his attention was absorbed by many activities.

Because of his disability the patient is less able than most other people to get away from situations that are irritating or frightening or to "work off steam" by physical activity. With his mobility decreased and his frustration increased, it is not surprising that the quadriplegic often flies into a rage over apparent trifles. Sometimes the frustration of not getting someone to light his cigarette is just too much after all the other discouraging situations.

The following is a brief summary of the findings of a nurse's study of the subjective experience of paraplegic patients.*

1. The dependency of the paraplegic patient is frequently the "object" that elicits pity in the nonhandicapped for the handicapped person. When perceived in another person, pity validates the handicapped person's sense of nonworth or uselessness.

2. The paraplegic is acutely aware of interpersonal relationships in his environment. Consequently, he and those who care for him require opportunities for help in becoming more skillful in these relationships.

3. The paraplegic suddenly finds himself in an entirely new relationship to the world with no immediate probability of reversing the situation beyond a fixed point. It is therefore necessary to help him to resolve the grief process. This need may not be recognized by other significant persons in his life. In fact, they

* Materials are used with permission of Sister M. Stella Haan, R.N., O.S.B., who at the time of her study was a graduate student at Rutgers, The State University of New Jersey. Title of study: "An Exploratory Study of the Subjective Experience, in Hospitals, of the Paraplegic Patient," unpublished, June, 1970.

may need to experience grief and mourning themselves, in dealing with the change in the paraplegic. Professional people can help both the patient and his close associates to deal with grief.

4. The paraplegic experiences his changed body image as overwhelming in terms of the effect this has upon his perception of himself and his relationship to others. Unless he is provided an opportunity to observe, describe, and explore his current experiences, he may fall victim to drugs or alcohol (or to other self-defeating responses) in an effort to obliterate the psychological pain.

5. The paraplegic is faced with the need for personal strengths that he now may be able to uncover or develop, perhaps for the first time in his life. The process of developing latent strengths requires effort. He will need to become convinced that this process of growth ultimately is worth the effort. The other significant persons in his life have a responsibility to reinforce positively the value of this effort.

6. Paraplegics, along with their families, need to be included in the evaluation of and the treatment-planning sessions for their particular rehabilitation program. Including the patient in interdiscipline planning sessions helps him to understand that his welfare is of concern to those caring for him.

## Rehabilitation

The aim of rehabilitation is to help paraplegics and quadriplegics to use their remaining capacities to the fullest and to avoid complications resulting from the disability. For example, decubitus ulcers seriously interfere with the program of rehabilitation. The patient who develops a large ulcer on the sacrum must return to bed and lie on his abdomen to relieve pressure on the part. Deformities such as footdrop interfere with the efforts of the patient to walk with braces and crutches. The patient who is withdrawn and depressed is unable to profit from the rehabilitation program, however elaborate the facilities. The patient who develops bladder infection must interrupt his program of

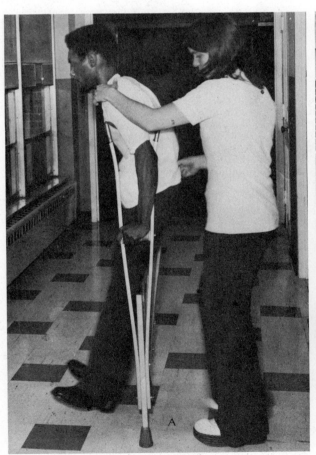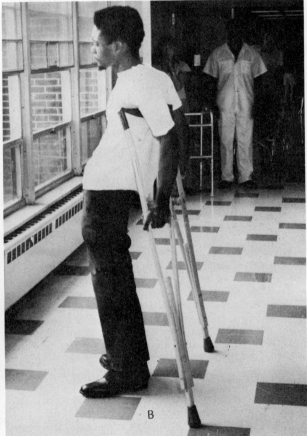

**Figure 24-1.** (A) Work phase of swing through gait. (B) Recovery phase of swing through gait. Crutches in reverse stance. (The Kessler Institute for Rehabilitation)

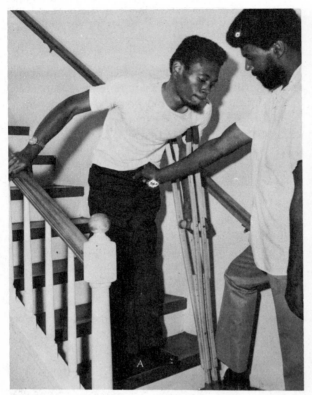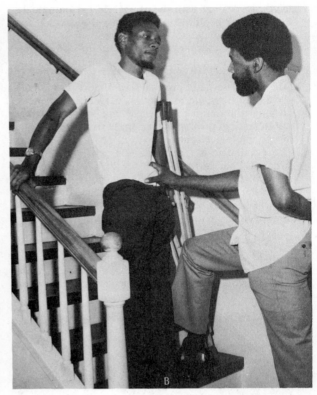

**Figure 24-2.** (A) Paraplegic patient initially descending stairs using handrail and crutches. The therapist provides physical and emotional support. (B) Recovery phase of patient descending stairs. (The Kessler Institute for Rehabilitation)

activities and receive intensive treatment to bring the infection under control.

The nurse plays an important part in the patient's rehabilitation by helping him to avoid complications, so that he can profit from the rehabilitation program. For example, she can help by:

- **Giving good skin care; being alert for beginning signs of pressure sores; placing a foam-rubber cushion in his wheelchair to help to relieve pressure.**
- **Teaching the patient about skin care, change of position, massage, and the importance of inspecting paralyzed areas daily. Because the patient cannot feel the discomfort caused by a beginning decubitus ulcer, he must be especially observant. Patients should use a mirror to inspect parts that they cannot see.**
- **Maintaining good body alignment; putting joints through a full range of motion: flexion, extension, abduction, adduction, internal rotation, external rotation, pronation, supination.**
- **Encouraging high-fluid intake; using careful aseptic technique when irrigating catheters.**
- **Showing sensitivity to the emotional needs of the patient; encouraging but not forcing him toward self-**care; allowing him to express his feelings concerning the disability.

**Mobility.** Paraplegics can learn to put on their own braces and to move from the bed to the wheelchair. Because of the tremendous effort required to walk (the patient must raise the entire weight of his body, plus the weight of the braces, with his arms), most paraplegics use the wheelchair most of the time and walk only short distances. However, it is important for the patient to assume upright posture at intervals during the day, whether or not he is able to walk. Quadriplegics who cannot stand or walk may be placed in an upright position with the aid of a tilt table or by using a CircOlectric bed. This position helps the patient to breathe more deeply, relieves pressure on the sacral region, relieves spasms, and helps to prevent urinary calculi and osteoporosis. The patient often feels dizzy and faint the first few times that he assumes an upright position. He must be watched carefully and protected, so that he does not fall. The pooling of blood in the abdominal area is a factor in causing postural hypotension. The application of an abdominal binder and elastic stockings to the legs before the patient gets up helps to prevent dizziness and faintness. When a tilt table is used, patients are strapped to it, and it is tilted gradually until the patient is standing erect.

Parallel bars help to support the patient whose upper extremities are unaffected. Therefore, he can support his own weight by grasping the bars. With the help of parallel bars, paraplegic patients can learn to balance themselves and to practice skills that later will be useful in crutch walking (see Chap. 19).

**Self-Care.** Paraplegic patients can learn to care for their own needs independently. Quadriplegics may attain varying degrees of self-care according to the function left in their upper extremities, but they require considerable assistance from others.

A quadriplegic must be bathed by the nurse, but he can shave himself with the aid of an electric razor that fits over his hand if he has enough function remaining in his arms to move the razor to his face, even though he cannot grasp it with his fingers.

**Bladder and Bowel Rehabilitation.** The rehabilitation of the bowels and the bladder is of crucial importance in helping the patient to move toward independence. Many patients can achieve self-controlled emptying of the bowels and the bladder, provided that they and those who care for them exert the persistent effort required to achieve this goal. Control of the bowels usually is easier to

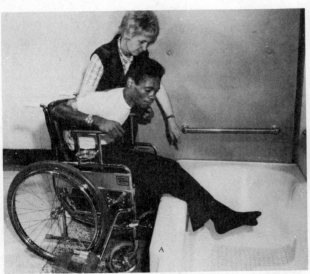
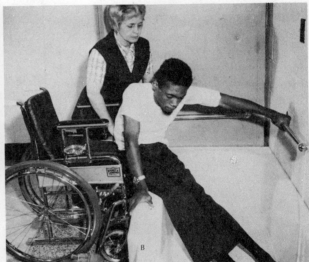
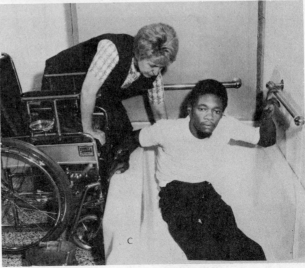

**Figure 24-3.** (A) Paraplegic patient transferring from wheelchair into tub; feet in tub, pedals swing away. (B) Patient moves forward to edge of tub, hand over grab bar. Feet and legs are headed forward in tub. (C) Patient lowers himself to bottom of tub using grab bar and side of tub for support. Procedure is reversed for getting out of tub. (The Kessler Institute for Rehabilitation)

achieve than control of the bladder. The following steps are useful in helping patients to achieve self-controlled emptying of the bowel:

- Encourage the patient to drink plenty of liquid and to eat foods that produce bulk, such as fresh fruits and vegetables. Teach him not to eat foods that normally cause him to have loose stools.
- Help the patient to plan to go to the toilet at a certain time each day. Select a time that will fit later into his own schedule for self-care.
- Allow the patient privacy and sufficient time to have a bowel movement.
- As soon as he is able, encourage the patient to go to the bathroom rather than to use the bedpan. The physical activity involved in getting out of bed often helps the patient to move his bowels. Using the bathroom has psychological value, too, with its indication of self-help rather than helplessness.

**Enemas and suppositories may be needed at first. For example, the patient may be given a small enema each day at the same time. He later may find that inserting a suppository just before the time for defecation will result in a normal bowel movement. Later his bowel function may become regulated so well that he has normal bowel movements without the aid of enemas or suppositories.**

Figures 24-1 to 24-6 show how two young men are coping with the experience of paralysis of the lower parts of their bodies. One patient is shown during his treatment at a rehabilitation institute; the other at home. Skilled assistance and concerned interest of others, plus the courage and perseverance conveyed by these two young people, are essential in rehabilitation.

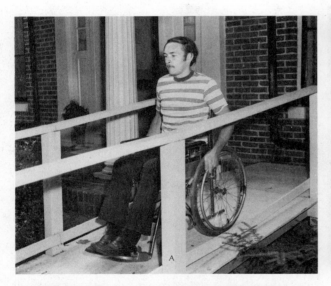

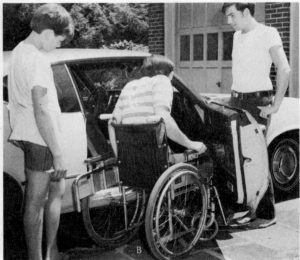

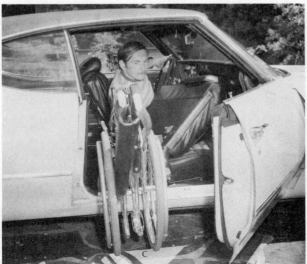

**Figure 24-4.** (A) The ramp enables this young man, paralyzed from the lower thoracic region, to enter and leave the house, and thus to engage in activities, such as attending college, which would not be possible otherwise. Note handrails which he uses to propel himself up and down the ramp. (B) With his brothers watching, he gets into his car unassisted. The car has been manually equipped for operation. (C) Once inside, he pulls his wheelchair in and places it behind the front seat.

The control of the bladder is more difficult to establish, but many patients can achieve it. (See Chapter 48 on the urologic patient.)

**Nursing Guidelines.** Helping paraplegic and quadriplegic patients to resume living that is as normal as is possible presents a tremendous challenge and equally great rewards. It is not an easy kind of nursing. The following are some suggestions that may help the nurse to avoid some common pitfalls when caring for the patient:

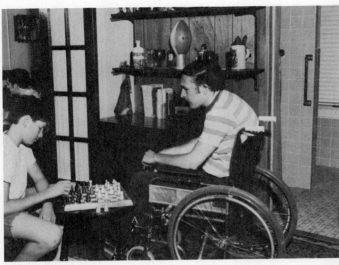

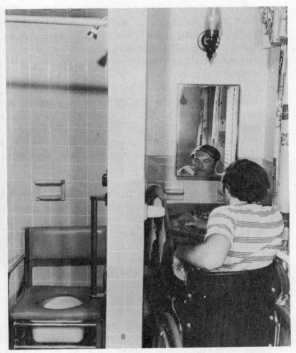

**Figure 24-5.** (A) The young man's room with adjacent bathroom is located next to the family living room. Note connecting doors which may be closed to provide privacy when needed. (B) In the bathroom, the sink is raised so the wheelchair fits under it. Cabinet and handrails are conveniently placed. The shower stall has no lip or "curb" so the bath-commode chair rolls right into it. The floor slants to a drain in back, keeping the floor dry even while the shower is being used.

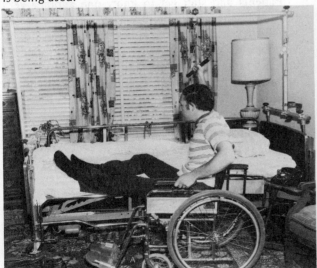

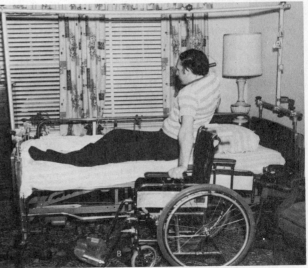

**Figure 24-6.** (A) When getting into bed, the young man first draws his wheelchair close to the bed and places his legs and feet on the bed. Note the trapeze. The casters on the bed are locked, and the brake on the wheelchair is set to keep it motionless. (B) Next, the young man raises his body onto the bed, pushing on the arm of the wheelchair with one hand and pulling on the trapeze with the other.

- Let him do as much as he can for himself. Arrange the environment so that self-care is encouraged (feeding devices, keeping belongings handy, and so on). It will take him longer to do it himself, so try to arrange the schedule to allow him extra time for such activities as feeding himself.
- Avoid pushing the patient. Great sensitivity is required to know when he is ready to attempt something new. Activities of daily living (ADL), such as feeding, bathing, and dressing, may seem elementary to a nonhandicapped person. Do not be surprised and try not to show disappointment on days when he seems to regress.
- Encourage the patient to be up and about, to get dressed, to go to the dining room, the bathroom, the recreation rooms. Try to help him to achieve as nearly normal living as is possible. Remember that these activities are very fatiguing, especially at first, when the patient is not used to them, and plan for rest periods as well as activity.
- Rigid insistence on self-help can waste time and energy. If, for example, it would take a quadriplegic an hour to mark his menu himself, but only five minutes to do it with help, it may be wise to help him with it, so that he can use the time and energy for eating.
- Partial self-care may not be as dramatic, but it is just as important a goal as the more complete rehabilitation of a less disabled person. Think what a difference it makes to the patient and his family if he can feed himself or pick up a telephone to call for help. Learning these skills may mean the difference between having to have a family member stay with him constantly and being able to be left alone. Whether the patient must remain in a hospital the rest of his life or can be cared for at home may hinge on his ability to perform simple tasks like feeding himself. Every step toward independence, however small it seems, is a giant step for the patient.
- Emphasis on activity and on being with others often makes patients long for a few moments to themselves. Do not insist that the patient be busy and with other people every minute. Everyone needs a balance of solitude and companionship.

## The Environment

**The Hospital.** The environment of the patient is important. Whether he is at home or in the hospital, his recovery is slow, and he is less free to move from one place to another. Some paraplegics are hospitalized four or five years. The significance of the ward environment is much greater for these patients than for those who return home after a few days.

Because physically disabled patients need special facilities, they often are grouped together in hospitals. Paraplegics, quadriplegics, and amputees may share a ward. Each patient compares his disability with that of others. "I can use my arms; that

poor fellow can't." "Losing a leg isn't very much. He'll be able to walk again." Envy of the amputee is common among paraplegics. Besides being able to walk with an artificial leg, the amputee usually does not suffer the problems of impotence and of the loss of control of the bowels and the bladder.

Relationships among these patients affect rehabilitation. Attitudes are contagious, and the role of the nurse involves working not only with individuals, but also with groups of patients. The depression or sarcasm of one patient may upset the whole ward. The cheerful good humor of one patient may help his buddies to laugh. Being around 20 to 30 severely disabled people can be like sitting on a powder keg: one spark, and the emotionally charged atmosphere can explode. Each individual is facing severe emotional strain. Patients find various ways of expressing their feelings about the disability. Joking is one; sarcasm is another. Often people say things in jest that they are unable to express in any other way. The patient may joke about his own awkwardness or helplessness or that of his companions. He may also vent some of his feelings on the staff in this way. It is not unusual for patients to resent the amount of help that they must seek; along with each request for help goes the possibility of refusal. "Wait a minute" and "I'm too busy now" are familiar remarks by members of a staff who face the huge task of caring for many helpless or partially helpless people.

Patients and staff get to know one another very well over the many months, and even years, in which they are together. This can be a rewarding, valuable experience—really knowing the patient and his family and home situation and having the opportunity to work with him and to see his progress over a long period of time.

However, there are pitfalls in caring for long-term disabled patients. Identifying some of them may help the nurse to avoid them.

- Do not play favorites. These patients are very sensitive to any show of favoritism, and they are quick to resent it. Treat all alike in the sense that they have equal call on your knowledge and skill. Treat each differently in the sense that each patient has his own unique needs.
- Remember that you are the patient's nurse, not a family member or a pal. (The relationship of nurse and patient may become confused when the nurse has cared for the patient over a long period of time.) If you concentrate on your own role as a professional nurse, this part of the patient's care will be well car-

ried out. The emphasis should be on helping the patient.

- Note how the patients get along with one another. Place them near those whose company they seem to enjoy.
- Avoid regimentation. For some the hospital is now the only home that they have. Avoid the use of uniform expressions that detract from the patient's sense of being an individual. Always refer to the patient by name, and never as "the quad in room 4."

**The Home.** In one way the home environment is less restricted than that of the hospital; in other ways it may be more so. At home the patient can have visitors at any hour, and he can arrange his own schedule for sleeping and waking, and so on. On the other hand, if his home does not have facilities that help him to get about, he may spend all his time in one room. One man found that he had to stay in one room all day while his wife was working, because the doorways were too narrow to permit his wheelchair to pass through. No one ever came to see him, and he found life in the hospital freer and pleasanter. "There were people to talk to, and I could get around in my chair," he said. Neighbors and friends sometimes avoid the disabled. They may be curious and stare because the person looks different, or they may try to do everything for him, assuming that if he is in a wheelchair, he must be completely helpless.

Yet home is the usual environment—and usually the best one—provided that the patient has a home and a family who want him. Going home is a major step in rehabilitation. It presents the challenge of helping the disabled patient to adjust to his home and his community. What may be some of the problems that the patient faces?

- How will his family feel about him?
- Will he be a burden to them?
- Will his friends forget him?
- Will he be able to manage without physicians and nurses around?
- What if he is alone in the house and something happens—like a fire? In the hospital there was always someone to help.

The patient and his family will need help in planning for his homecoming. The home situation will need to be evaluated; often a community health nurse or a social worker makes this evaluation. She notes the physical environment—the stairs, the bathroom, and so on—as well as the attitude of the family toward the return of the patient. Recommendations can be made concerning changes that

may be necessary before the patient goes home. The person who evaluates the home can talk over plans with the family and help them to find answers to some of their questions. The wife or the husband of the patient can go to the hospital, observe and help with the care of the patient, watch his activities in physical and occupational therapy, and confer with physicians, nurses, and therapists. It is one thing for the wife to be told that her husband can get in and out of his wheelchair; it is quite another thing to see him perform this seemingly impossible feat.

The wife will need to plan for the care of her husband and to be with him. One of the greatest challenges will involve continuing her own interests, not being made a prisoner by the dependence of the other person.

After the patient returns home, continued medical and nursing care and supervision will be needed. The community health nurse may continue the teaching begun in the hospital, showing the family how to adapt care to the home situation, as well as carrying out treatments, such as injections or dressings. In some communities physical therapists are available who come to the patient's home and continue the program started in the hospital.

It is important to continue planning for vocational rehabilitation after the patient gets home. All too often the plans begun in the hospital lapse, because no one in the community assumes the responsibility for continued planning. The patient may need training in addition to that received in the hospital, and he may need assistance in finding suitable employment.

What are the patient's chances for vocational rehabilitation? Are most occupations closed to these patients? What proportion of patients actually obtain work? A survey of 318 paraplegic and quadriplegic members of the Paralyzed Veterans of America revealed that 84.3 per cent were studying, working or seeking work; 47.8 per cent reported steady employment. Among the many different occupations reported were those of physician, postmaster, teacher, accountant, typist, editor, clinical psychologist, bookkeeper, and insurance agent (Frost).

The greater the intelligence, the education, the industry and the motivation of the patient, the greater is the likelihood that he will succeed with a program of vocational rehabilitation. Intelligence and education are especially important in the reha-

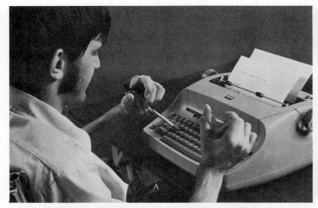

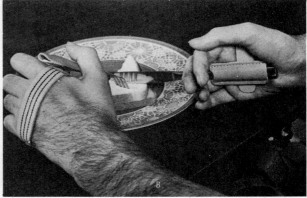

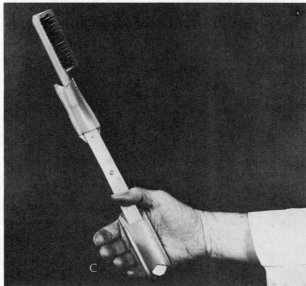

**Figure 24-7.** Devices for quadriplegics. (A) When partial grasp is present, Universal built-up handles provide functional use of the hand while performing various ADL (activities of daily living). (B) A Universal, C-clip, swivel ADL cuff on the right hand holds a regular knife in position for cutting and offers good stability. The Universal Vertical Holder, inserted into a universal ADL cuff is used on left hand to assist cutting. These devices are a substitute for grasp only and are indicated when forearm rotation is present. Equipment may be reversed for those desiring to cut with the left hand while eating with the right. (C) The Universal Extension Handle extends reach and accommodates various standard utensils. It is shown here with comb/brush for combing hair. It can be inserted into an ADL cuff when grasp is weak or absent.

bilitation of the physically disabled, because work requiring much physical stamina is closed to them. It is important to take the interests and the abilities of the patient into account. A patient who disliked school, and who has seldom read anything weightier than comic books, is not likely to show enthusiasm for going to college after he has become a paraplegic.

Continued interest, the services of professional persons and the full use of appropriate mechanical devices help paraplegic patients to live full lives and to become more independent (Fig. 24-7).

## REFERENCES AND BIBLIOGRAPHY

BELAND, IRENE: *Clinical Nursing: Pathophysiological and Psychosocial Approaches,* ed. 2, New York, Macmillan, 1970.

CARINI, ESTA, and OWENS, GUY: *Neurological and Neurosurgical Nursing,* ed. 6, St. Louis, Mosby, 1974.

CHALK, BARBARA A.: Anterior approach to cervical fractures, dislocations and herniated nucleus pulposus, *J. Neurosurg. Nurs.* 5:2:56-62, December 1973.

ELLIOTT, FRANK: *Clinical Neurology,* ed. 2, Philadelphia, Saunders, 1971.

FROST, R.: Success or Failure in the Economic Rehabilitation. Paraplegics and Quadriplegics, New York, Paralyzed Veterans of America, (n.d.).

HENDERSON, GLORIA M.: Teaching—learning for rehabilitation of the spinal cord—disabled individual, *Nurs. Clin. N. Am.* 6:4:655-668, December 1971.

JOHNSON, MARION R.: Emergency management of head and spinal injuries, *Nurs. Clin. N. Am.* 8:3:389-400, September 1973.

KINTZEL, KAY (ed.): *Advanced Concepts of Clinical Nursing,* Philadelphia, Lippincott, 1971.

Korte, Mary L.: Intensive care of the neurologic patient—meeting the challenge, *Nurs. Clin. N. Am.* 7:2:335-348, June 1972.

Merritt, Houston H.: *A Textbook of Neurology,* ed. 5, Philadelphia, Lea and Febiger, 1973.

Metheny, Norma, and Snively, W. D.: *Nurses' Handbook of Fluid Balance,* ed. 2, Philadelphia, Lippincott, 1974.

Noback, Charles, and Demarest, Robert: *The Nervous System: Introduction and Review,* New York, McGraw-Hill, A Blakiston Pub., 1972.

Ransohoff, J., and Sadik, Rasul A.: Spinal cord injury: Current status and some recent advances, *J. Neurosurg. Nurs.* 4:1:49-60, July 1972.

Trigiano, L. L.: Independence is possible in quadriplegia, *Am. J. Nurs.* 70:12:2610-2613, December 1970.

Tudor, Lea L.: Bladder and bowel retaining, *Am. J. Nurs.* 70:11:2390-2391, November 1970.

# The Patient with Cerebrovascular Disease

**25**

Cerebrovascular disease is a major health problem and includes disorders of any of the vessels which furnish blood to the brain. An abundant blood supply is required to provide adequate oxygen and nutrition to the brain cells and to remove wastes from them. Whenever cerebral circulation is adversely affected, structure and function may be altered. The brain tissue can become infarcted when blood supply is markedly decreased or cut off; hemorrhage may result from the rupture of a blood vessel in the cranial cavity. Motor, sensory, and higher mental functions may be affected by the disease process resulting in physical and mental disabilities.

As a health professional the nurse must prepare herself with the knowledge and skills needed to help prevent, detect, treat, and rehabilitate people with cerebrovascular disease. Whatever the environment in which the nurse practices, she must be mindful of the high incidence of morbidity and mortality caused by this major health problem.

## CEREBRAL CIRCULATION

Briefly stated the brain receives its blood supply from the internal carotid and the vertebral arteries which enter the cranium through the base of the skull. Each internal carotid artery divides at the optic chiasm into an anterior and middle cerebral artery. The two anterior cerebral arteries are connected by the anterior communicating artery. The two vertebral arteries unite to form the basilar artery which bifurcates at the level of the midbrain to form two posterior cerebral arteries.

Cerebral Circulation

The Patient with an Intracranial Aneurysm

The Patient with a Cerebral Vascular Accident

Nursing Intervention

Special Problems of Patients with Cerebrovascular Disease

**414**

Each of these is joined to the corresponding middle cerebral artery by the posterior communicating artery. The two systems are thus connected at the base of the brain, and the arrangement is called the circle of Willis. The circle acts as a safety mechanism with the intercommunication decreasing the chances of impairment in the circulation of blood to the brain, provided there is no disease or occlusion. Extensive branching and anastomoses allow an abundant blood supply to all parts of the brain. After repeated branchings, the arteries form capillaries. Veins arise from the capillaries and drain into the superficial venous plexuses and the dural sinuses, ultimately draining into the internal jugular veins at the base of the skull by which the blood returns to the heart. To satisfy its oxygen requirements, the brain requires, and normally receives, a greater volume of blood flow than any other tissue. Any interference quickly leads to a loss of function specific to the area of involvement.

## THE PATIENT WITH AN INTRACRANIAL ANEURYSM

The nurse must be aware that a person may develop an intracranial aneurysm at any age. This weakness in the wall of a blood vessel may be caused by a congenital malformation or can be the result of disease such as arteriosclerosis or septic emboli. Aneurysms usually develop slowly, and signs and symptoms result from either compression of cranial nerves or brain tissue, and from hemorrhage. Pressure by an intact cerebral aneurysm may cause the patient to manifest focal neurologic changes in the normal functions of cranial nerves, and sometimes he may complain of headache or have seizures. Frequently patients are asymptomatic until the aneurysm leaks or ruptures. The patient may complain of head pain which usually becomes more generalized as the meninges become irritated and edematous. Neurologic assessment should include close observation of the patient for changes in level of consciousness, signs of increased intracranial pressure, and generalized convulsions.

Bleeding from a ruptured aneurysm is an ever-present danger. If the patient survives one episode of leakage, he may have others. He should be kept flat in bed and engage in little or no activity. The nurse must anticipate his needs, provide a restful environment, and administer analgesics for headache and restlessness as often as indicated.

### Treatment

Treatment for intracranial aneurysm may include a lumbar puncture. Findings include bloody fluid and increased pressure of the cerebrospinal fluid. Cerebral angiography usually is performed, and it can indicate the presence and location of the aneurysm. Depending on the patient's condition, cerebral angiographic studies are done immediately or after a few days.

**Surgery.** As the danger of further hemorrhage from the weakened aneurysmal sac is great, particularly in the first weeks after the initial hemorrhage, surgical repair is often necessary. The operation is not without hazard, because manipulation of the small cerebral vessels may result in increased vasospasm or thrombosis and cerebral infarction. Usually the risks of surgery are less than the danger of recurrent hemorrhage. If surgery is decided on, it may not be performed for several days or perhaps two weeks after the bleeding episode, the surgeon waiting until the intracranial vascular situation is somewhat stable. Preoperatively, the patient may be given a hyperosmolar solution, which is dehydrating and thus shrinks the brain and facilitates the surgical exposure of the aneurysm. During surgery, measures such as hypothermia to reduce cerebral oxygen needs and cerebral blood flow may be used. The surgical procedure may consist of evacuating a sac that already has thrombosed, clipping the neck of the aneurysm, trapping the aneurysm between two clips, or putting a plastic coat around the vessel so that the wall cannot balloon out at a weak point. An attempt may be made to induce thrombosis in the aneurysm. Some surgeons prefer to ligate the common or internal carotid in the neck.

If the patient is treated conservatively, rest is imperative. As the rupture heals the patient will be allowed to slowly resume activities of daily living. Nursing intervention with passive exercises can gradually give way to the patient performing self-directed activities. The patient should become more alert and have decreasing complaints of headache. He and his family frequently need constant reassurance, support, and guidance with discharge planning that may necessitate restructuring of former work and leisure living patterns.

When surgery is indicated, the patient, if able, and the family must be assessed to insure their comprehension of the situation and awareness of what will occur. Ongoing individualized neurologic assessment of the patient by the nurse will continue during the postoperative phase, relevant to the type of surgery the patient has. Changes in level of consciousness, impending increased intracranial pressure, and differences in motor and sensory functions are priorities the nurse must assess and with which she must intervene during the immediate postoperative phase. As the patient recovers he and his family must be reassured and helped to deal with the adjustments needed for the patient to return to the community capable of functioning at his highest capacity.

## THE PATIENT WITH A CEREBRAL VASCULAR ACCIDENT

A cerebral vascular accident is usually the end result of long-standing cerebrovascular disease which is the most common neurologic disorder found in adults.

The pathophysiologic basis for cerebrovascular disease involves the lessened ability of the arteries to carry blood to the brain cells. The cerebral nerve cells are extremely sensitive to lack of oxygen, which is carried to them by the blood. Complete ischemia leads in a few minutes to the destruction of those cells that have been deprived of the oxygen. These changes are irreversible; those cerebral nerve cells that have been destroyed do not regenerate.

**Atherosclerosis and Arteriosclerosis.** The pathologic processes which impair the ability of the blood vessels to nourish the brain are primarily atherosclerosis and arteriosclerosis. In *atherosclerosis* fatty plaques (*atheromas*) are gradually deposited in the intima of the artery, causing its lumen to become narrowed and in some instances occluded. This process roughens the normally smooth lining of the artery, making it more prone to the development of clots that adhere to the atherosclerotic plaques. Such clots may form gradually and increase in size until they occlude a vessel (cerebral thrombosis), or they may travel in the bloodstream and become lodged in a narrowed portion of the blood vessel, cutting off the flow of blood (cerebral embolism) (Fig. 25-1).

In *arteriosclerosis* there is loss of elasticity of the artery and thickening of the intima of the artery. The combined effects of arteriosclerosis and atherosclerosis lead to a reduction of the artery's ability to transport blood. When the blood supply is completely cut off to an area of the brain, the normal tissues are destroyed and replaced by scar tissue. This region of the brain is referred to as an *area of infarction*. The episode itself in which an area of the brain undergoes infarction is called a *cerebral vascular accident*. Such an episode usually occurs suddenly, with the prompt development of symptoms of brain damage. The lay term for the condition is *stroke*.

**Association with Hypertension.** Cerebral arterial disease is often, but not necessarily, associated with hypertension. Although the drop in blood pressure may be to levels found in normotensive

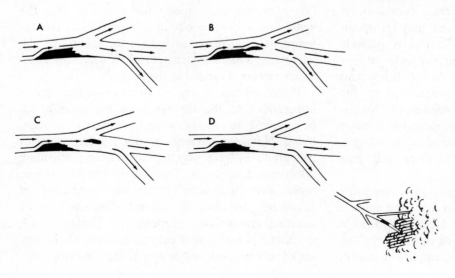

**Figure 25-1.** (A) A thrombus forms in a vessel. (B) The force of the flowing blood over the clot helps to break off a piece from it. (C) The embolus is loose in the bloodstream and can travel to any tissue fed by connecting blood vessels. (D) The embolus is pushed into a small terminal vessel, completely occluding it and causing anoxia of the tissue served by the occluded vessel.

persons, it constitutes a significant fall in persons with hypertension.

**Cerebral Hemorrhage.** When this hemorrhage occurs, there is interference with the supply of blood to an area of the brain, together with pressure on the brain substance from the pool of blood that has collected. Both factors damage the brain cells. Cerebral hemorrhage is more likely to be associated with effort and activity than is cerebral thrombosis. Arteries affected by arteriosclerosis and atherosclerosis are more vulnerable to rupture than normal arteries. A sudden rise in blood pressure, particularly in a patient who already suffers from hypertension, may lead to rupture of a cerebral blood vessel. Such a rise in blood pressure may occur in response to unusual physical exertion or emotional strain. However, in many instances no such precipitating incident can be identified; the hemorrhage occurs when the patient apparently is undergoing no unusual change in his activities and no unusual stress. Rupture of cerebral aneurysms is another significant cause of brain hemorrhage.

**Cerebral Thrombosis and Cerebral Embolism.** Cerebral thrombosis and cerebral embolism are more common causes of cerebral vascular accident than hemorrhage. Cerebral thrombosis is particularly likely to have its onset after unusual fatigue, or during sleep, when the patient's blood pressure is lowered. Cerebral emboli are sometimes a complication of cardiac arrhythmia, or of rheumatic endocarditis, conditions in which clots frequently form in the heart. They can enter the general circulation and become lodged in a cerebral artery, occluding it. These patients tend to suffer cerebral vascular accidents relatively early in life, for example, in their 30's or 40's.

*Transient symptoms* of cerebral ischemia may occur in patients who have cerebrovascular disease. Such episodes are often the first warning that the cerebral circulation is impaired, and they warrant prompt medical attention in the hope of preventing or postponing widespread brain damage. Although these patients may never experience a major cerebral vascular accident, they may, as the years go by, gradually exhibit considerable decrement of cerebral function. Symptoms of transient ischemia may include temporary weakness or paralysis of an arm, brief loss of consciousness, temporary loss or impairment of vision or speech. Unless the significance of such symptoms is recog-

nized, the fact that they may subside completely can lead the patient and his family to believe that no medical investigation is necessary.

**Extracerebral Blood Vessels.** The blood vessels responsible for impaired cerebral blood flow are not limited to those within the brain. For example, the importance of pathologic changes in the carotid arteries as a causative factor in cerebrovascular disease is being recognized increasingly. Arteriography has been a major factor in furthering the physician's knowledge of the location of occlusion of vessels; by making it possible in many instances to identify the location of the occlusion, the way has been opened for the development of surgical techniques to relieve these obstructions.

## The Onset of Cerebral Vascular Accident

The onset of a cerebral vascular accident is sudden. Whatever the patient's activity, he may fall into a shocklike state. Coma as a symptom of cerebrovascular disease is especially common after hemorrhage. It comes on suddenly, and it may be deep or light.

Immediately after a severe cerebral hemorrhage the patient is unconscious, his face often is brick red, and his breathing is stertorous and difficult. On the paralyzed side his cheek blows out with each respiration. His pulse usually is slow but full and bounding. Initially, blood pressure is likely to be elevated. The patient may proceed into deeper and deeper coma until he dies. He may remain comatose for days or even weeks, and then he may recover. However, the longer the coma is, the poorer the prognosis becomes. Pneumonia is the most common cause of death during prolonged coma.

When the accident is due to cerebral embolism, there are neurologic symptoms, usually without loss of consciousness, although the state of consciousness may be altered.

Sometimes cerebral vascular accidents occur without warning. In other instances the patient suffers from such symptoms as dizzy spells, headache, unusual fatigue, or disturbances of speech or vision. Usually, the significance of such premonitory symptoms is recognized only retrospectively, when the physician questions the patient or his family about his health just before the cerebral vascular accident.

If the patient survives a major cerebral vascular accident, his symptoms will depend on the extent and the severity, as well as the location, of the resulting brain damage. Some areas of his brain may have suffered from hypoxia and then recover as the supply of oxygen and other essential elements carried by the blood improves; other areas have died from anoxia. During the early stage it is not possible to tell whether the symptoms will be permanent or temporary. Improvement in neurologic symptoms can occur for at least six months after the accident—a point of encouragement for the patient, and a reason for the nurse's doing everything possible to prevent deformities and to help the patient to maintain and to improve his contact with other persons and his orientation to his surroundings.

## Special Problems of the Patient with a Cerebral Vascular Accident

**Hemiplegia.** The most common neurologic sequela of a cerebral vascular accident is hemiplegia. A hemorrhage or clot in the right side of the brain causes the patient to have a left hemiplegia, because there is a crossover of nerves in the pyramidal tract as they lead from the brain down the spinal cord.

The speech center is probably located in the left side of the brain. It is not uncommon for the hemorrhage or clot responsible for the patient's hemiplegia to cause aphasia by cutting off the blood supply to the patient's cerebral speech center.

**Hemianopsia.** This term refers to a condition in which the patient can see only half of his normal visual field. He cannot see, with either eye, what is going on to the right or to the left of him as he looks straight ahead. This is due to damage to the visual area of the cerebral cortex or its connections to the brain stem (optic radiations). This symptom is distressing and puzzling to the patient; and the reason for it should be explained to him. This symptom like other symptoms resulting from cerebral vascular accident may subside completely, or partially, or not at all.

**Aphasia.** The loss of the usual ability to use or to understand spoken and written language is called *aphasia*. Aphasia may exist without intellectual impairment.

Until aphasia is seen, it is a very difficult syndrome to believe. A patient with aphasia may know what a pencil is, if he is shown one. If it is handed to him, he will write with it; but he cannot think of the word "pencil." He may say, "Rag—sweater —miniature—wife." He may be able to conceive the symbol, but he cannot express the word "pencil." This type of aphasia is *expressive aphasia*.

SOME TYPES OF APHASIA
Receptive
  Auditory aphasia (symptom: difficulty in understanding the spoken word)
  Alexia (symptom: difficulty in reading aloud)

Expressive
  Motor (symptom: difficulty in speaking)
  Agraphia (symptom: difficulty in writing)

Any type of vascular disorder or tumor can cause aphasia if it involves the speech center in the brain. The patient may, to his horror, find that he has lost not only his speech, but, if he also has an auditory aphasia, that the words people speak to him are as garbled as an unfamiliar foreign language. He frequently does not realize that what he is saying is not what he thinks he says. He then is mystified, and sometimes becomes angry, at the seemingly strange behavior of others, who say, "What?" when he believes that he has asked a perfectly logical and intelligible question.

In the beginning the patient may perseverate (repeat) a great deal. Often the first speech to return is automatic (counting, the alphabet, responding "Fine" to "How are you?"). A native language that has not been spoken for years may be used by a patient who is powerless to speak or to understand English. Or a few words of special significance to the patient may be retained. Very common is the frustrating experience of having the correct word "on the tip of the tongue" and still stubbornly elusive. A patient may wish to ask for a drink of water and say, "My feet are cold . . . No, that's not right . . . I feel snow." (Pause) "I mean basket . . . No . . ."

**Psychological Impact.** The patient may manifest signs of depression, behavior such as crying for no apparent reason, and he may be anxious or confused. Distortion of body image due to motor and sensory disturbances is frequently of great concern to the patient, and close observation of his behavior will provide the data to establish the nursing diagnosis and needed intervention.

## Diagnostic Studies

In an attempt to identify the cause of the cerebral vascular accident, a lumbar puncture may be performed. A stroke caused by hemorrhage will show blood in the cerebrospinal fluid, whereas a stroke from a thrombosis will not.

Cerebral angiography may be done. An electroencephalogram and a radioactive brain scan may be indicated.

## NURSING INTERVENTION

Individualized assessment of the patient will provide the framework for intervention during the acute phase and throughout the long-term rehabilitation period. Initially the patient may be nonresponsive and in need of care that is applicable for anyone unconscious. Some physicians elect to have patients with a cerebral vascular accident receive adrenocorticosteroids, vasodilators, or anticoagulants, and the nurse must be alert for the patient's responses to these medications. Dehydrating agents may be indicated and occasionally a lumbar puncture is performed to remove cerebrospinal fluid to decrease increased intracranial pressure.

Sometimes the patient may have a surgical procedure to remove an intracerebral blood clot or an atheroma from the carotid or vertebral artery. However, the frequently grave condition of the patient may prevent intervention of such a traumatic nature.

The patient is usually placed on the critical list, and the family can visit at periods other than scheduled visiting hours. Family members make the decision on how long to stay in light of the patient's condition and their own reactions to the experience. Some wish to be present as much as possible. One consideration is that, if the patient's condition changes markedly, or if he dies, they will be with him at the critical time. Some family members do not undertake a prolonged vigil at the bedside, perhaps because of responsibilities for children or their need to get away from the stressful environment to regain their composure. The nurse should provide the reassurance that they will be notified if there is a change in the patient's condition. In every situation she should be perceptive of the family's reaction to the experience.

As the patient recovers from coma, the head of the bed may be elevated further. Although the patient may be allowed on his back, his affected arm still should be supported on a pillow. A roll of gauze or a rubber ball placed in his hand may help to prevent the clawlike contracture deformity that so frequently follows a cerebral vascular accident (Fig. 25-2). If the patient has any movement at all in his hand, he should be encouraged to squeeze the ball periodically for exercise. As the patient sits up more, special attention should be paid to the skin of the buttocks, in an attempt to prevent skin breakdown. Change of position and frequent massage continue to be necessary. The patient's feet should press against a footboard. The nurse should be alert for footdrop and outward rotation. A light splint may be used on an extremity if contractures seem to be forming.

### Recovery Phase

With continued improvement the patient may be able to eat and drink, although some of what he takes will run out of the paralyzed side of his mouth. He may not be able to swallow well (dysphagia). His embarrassment, when he feels that he is drooling like a baby, can be minimized by turning him on his unaffected side during meals and putting only small amounts of food in the side of his mouth that has the best control. This method

**Table 25-1. Guidelines for Feeding a Patient with Dysphagia**

| SUGGESTIONS CONCERNING FOODS |
| --- |
| Milk and milk products stimulate thick saliva that is difficult to swallow. Milk and milk products should be avoided. |
| Foods with some texture stimulate swallowing. Use toast instead of plain bread; boiled or baked potato instead of mashed potato. |
| Avoid difficult to swallow foods, such as plums, prunes, hamburger patties; consistency of the food depends on tolerance of the patient. |

| SUGGESTIONS FOR FEEDING THE PATIENT |
| --- |
| Help the patient sit upright for feeding, and one-half hour before and after feeding. |
| If the patient is hemiplegic, place food in the unaffected side of the mouth. |
| Instruct the patient to move the food around with his tongue. |
| In the initial stages, small amounts of food should be fed to the patient, with a gradual increase as the patient's ability to swallow increases. |
| Have the patient feel his laryngeal area during the act of swallowing. This demonstrates that he can swallow; often the patient is afraid that he cannot swallow. |
| Keep the environment quiet while the patient is eating. |
| Give liquids through a straw if the patient can suck. |
| Keep a daily chart of the amount and consistency of liquids and solid food that the patient takes. |

Prepared by John E. Buckley, M.A., CCC, Sp-A, Director of Speech and Audiology, Overlook Hospital, Summit, N.J. and Clinical Instructor, College of Medicine, State University of New York, Downstate Medical Center and Connie L. Addicks, M.A., CCC, Senior Speech Pathologist, Overlook Hospital, Summit, N.J.

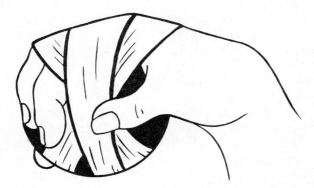

**Figure 25-2.** A ball placed in the spastic hand may help to prevent contractures and keep the hand more in a position of function. It may be necessary to bandage the ball lightly in place. If this is done, inspect the hand frequently to make sure that the fingers have not curled up between the gauze and the ball, causing the gauze to cut into the skin or to impede the circulation.

of feeding will also help to minimize the possibility of aspirating the food. Additional measures for helping the patient to swallow, and to eat, are included in Table 25-1.

As the patient recovers from a cerebral vascular accident, he should be taught not to strain while moving his bowels, as this may result in embolism or hemorrhage. A laxative or enema may be the treatment of choice to help him defecate. As the patient recovers he becomes aware of new limitations, and the discovery is frightening. Perhaps one reason that most people fear paralysis is that they have no assurance their needs will be met.

Diligent assessment can help to anticipate the patient's needs and indicate specific nursing intervention. Comfort measures will be greatly appreciated by the patient. If his mouth is dry, and he is allowed extra fluids, he may be given a glass of juice or a high protein drink. If he has diarrhea he will be fatigued and freshening the bed and providing quiet will help him to rest. If he vomits, his mouth will have a sour taste, and mouth care should be given without his asking for it. If his appetite is jaded, he should be given frequent snacks, attractively presented.

**Exercise and Ambulation.** Patients are usually encouraged to be as active as possible as soon as

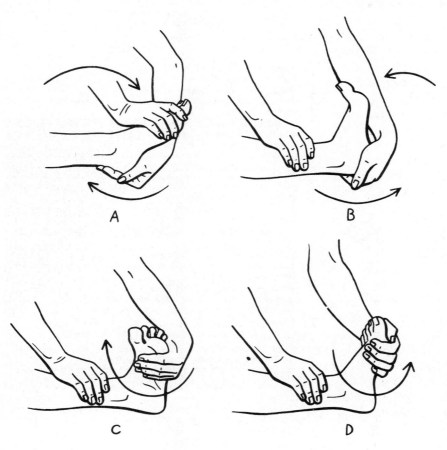

**Figure 25-3.** Range-of-motion exercises for the affected foot in hemiplegia. The motions should be conducted slowly and smoothly, with a momentary pause when spasticity causes resistance. As soon as the patient has movement, these exercises should be done actively rather than passively. In the beginning of the regaining of function, the patient may start the exercises, and the nurse completes the movements. As the patient gains strength, he should do them himself entirely.

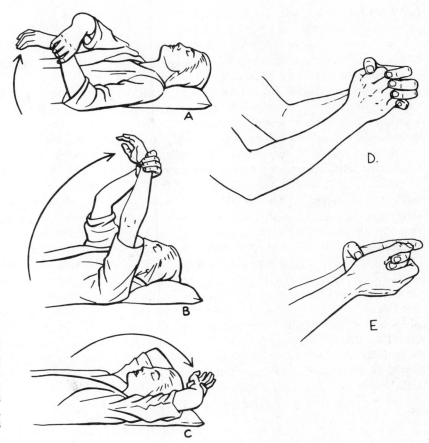

**Figure 25-4.** Exercises of the affected hand and the affected arm that the hemiplegic patient should learn to do himself. (A), (B) and (C): The affected arm is grasped at the wrist by the unaffected hand and is raised over the head. (D) and (E): The unaffected hand is slipped into the spastic hand, and slowly in turn each finger is extended.

possible. Consultation with the physical therapist should be effected. Written directions of the specific exercises will furnish data for intervention over the 24-hour period.

The patient should be taught to massage and to stretch the fingers of his affected hand with his unaffected hand several times daily, and should work toward passively exercising his affected arm with his good arm, thus exercising both arms at once. As soon as there is the slightest evidence of movement of either the affected arm or the affected leg, the nurse should rejoice with the patient, and capitalize on it. This change may be the beginning of the return of function. But because the patient is still weak, she should be careful that he does not become tired. Early use of exercise not only serves to prevent contractures and wasting of unused muscles, but also implies to the patient that he is not going to be a hopeless cripple (Figs. 25-3 to 25-5).

Helping the patient to walk requires application of safety and security measures. The patient who

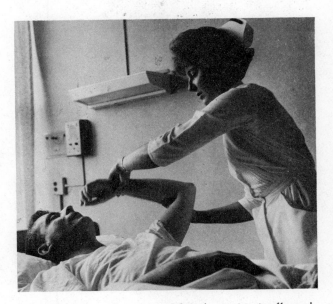

**Figure 25-5.** The nurse places the patient's affected arm through a full range of motion.

has lived for a while with his hemiplegia has found ways of moving that are effective for him, but the newly paralyzed patient does not know what he can do and what he cannot.

The patient should be allowed to sit at the edge of his bed for a minute, to become accustomed to the upright position. If dizziness is prolonged, he should be helped to lie down again, and the physician should be consulted. The nurse should tell the patient just what the sequence of movement will be, so that both she and the patient will be moving in the same direction. If the patient is not faint or dizzy, the nurse should put his robe on while he is sitting up. She should put the sleeve on his affected arm first (it would be much more difficult for him to maneuver his affected arm into the second sleeve). Later, in the same manner, the patient learns to get dressed (Fig. 25-6). The nurse should stand at the patient's unaffected side and support him from that side. It might seem logical to help him from his affected side, but this arrangement is not as effective. The nurse should support the side that helps the patient to steady himself. While she holds him firmly, she lets the patient step onto the footstool and then to the floor with his unaffected foot. The one or two steps to a chair are probably enough

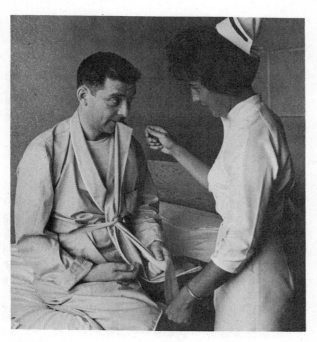

**Figure 25-6.** The nurse is teaching this hemiplegic patient to tie the belt of his robe.

for the first day. When helping the patient to go back to bed, the nurse should tell him to step up on the footstool with his unaffected foot. The other is still too weak to lift his entire body. Many hospitals have beds that are adjustable in height. If this type of bed is being used, it should be placed in the lowest position, and the patient helped to place both feet on the floor. This type of bed makes the use of a footstool unnecessary; the procedure is easier and safer for the patient.

Slowly, the patient may graduate to parallel bars, a walker, a crutch and a cane, and then to no aid. The goal of each day's activity should be one that is attainable, even if it is only one more step. Walking is a primitive activity, something that the patient doubtless has taken for granted for years. To lose it is disheartening. Every small success in regaining mobility is a point of great encouragement for the future; every failure may be a sign that the future is hopeless.

If the patient's arm on the affected side is completely paralyzed, a sling is recommended to keep the arm from dangling while the patient is out of bed. If a sling is used, the patient should be taught to remove his arm from it at intervals and to provide passive range-of-motion exercises for the paralyzed arm with his unaffected arm. It is usually recommended that the arm be left out of the sling if there is any function in the arm, no matter how feeble. Perhaps it will move in response to a need as the patient walks. It may start to open a door or to touch a chair as he passes. The patient should be encouraged to try to move. Any hint of movement should be persistently nurtured.

If the patient has lost sensation on the affected side, he will need to learn to protect himself from injury. A cut may bleed unnoticed. Heat in any form can lead to a painless, deep burn.

**Emotional Impact.** The emotional shock of losing the functions of an arm, a leg, or speech is severe. Intractable depressions are not uncommon, and often these patients become convinced that their productive life is over. Suddenly, they have lost the most fundamental abilities, abilities that were learned in childhood and have not been thought of consciously in years: how to write, to read, to walk; to tell a penny from a quarter; to know the difference between and the significance of a red and a green traffic light; to ask someone, "Which way is Main Street?" and to understand the answer. The disabilities of the patient may embarrass his family and him so much that contact with the outside world is dropped. This social isolation is unnecessary, but it happens over and over again. Social activities should be selected on the basis of what the patient enjoys, and what is within his capacity. A common mistake involves imposing on the older person the activities that others enjoy without finding out what the patient would like to do. Some patients are delighted with a chance to go to the movies; others find such a trip exhausting and would much prefer to join others in watching television at home.

It is no wonder that a constantly unhappy patient may make the members of an entire family feel guilty, helpless, and depressed. Attempts to rehabilitate many of these patients have been feeble, incomplete or nonexistent, and their residual ability has not been utilized.

## Rehabilitation

An early start at rehabilitation is one of the best ways to prevent depression. The patient should never be given the impression that there is no use in training his muscles up to their full capacity. It is also important for the patient to eventually take a realistic account of what he can and cannot do, so that he can plan his life; however, no one knows at the beginning how much function can be recaptured. Some patients recover completely. Every step forward is nurtured, encouraged, and enlarged. After about six to eight months, the patient's limitations, if any, will be more clear.

**Family.** Family attitudes are of the utmost importance. If family members become upset in the patient's presence, his newly labile emotions (based on the recent brain damage) will make him easily subject to depression. Then it will be more difficult to help him to recover from his depression and to work toward further function. A stable emotional environment is essential for the patient who is recovering from a cerebral vascular accident. His bouts of sudden, uncontrolled weeping should not be infectious to those around him.

The family should be encouraged and supported to help the patient with his retraining program. The emotional dependence of the patient on his family can be extremely taxing. If the family is large, and family members live near each other and typically come to one another's aid in crises, the patient's care can be shared in terms of both its emotional impact and its daily time-consuming activities, such as helping the aphasic patient read aloud. But in many instances such family assistance is not available, especially for elderly patients.

All patients should be assessed for their need of supplementary arrangements, such as the services of a visiting homemaker or a church worker. The nurse should seek the services of the social worker when possible. In some instances a severely disabled older person is sent home, to be cared for without guidance or assistance by an elderly wife or husband who has neither the physical stamina nor the knowledge required for so large a task. A common problem is finding someone to stay with the patient for a few hours while the spouse leaves to do errands. Such problems can be dealt with if the professional staff takes an active and responsible part in helping with arrangements for long-term care. If no assistance is given, one relative may become so overburdened that he reacts with anger to the patient, or becomes ill himself.

## Long-Term Treatment

It is necessary for most patients to make some changes in the pattern of their daily lives. Fatigue and the development of other illnesses must be avoided whenever possible, because they can lead to lowering of blood pressure and further brain damage from inadequate blood flow to the brain.

Patients with hypertension are sometimes given drugs to help lower their blood pressure. Such drugs are avoided when an infarction occurs, and are used cautiously at other times because of the possibility that a marked fall in blood pressure may precipitate cerebral infarction or increase the area of infarction. If the patient is overweight, he is advised to reduce. If he smokes, he is advised to stop, or if this is impossible, to decrease his smoking. Sometimes drugs which depress blood cholesterol levels are ordered in the hope of preventing additional atheromas. The long-range effect of such drugs in combating atherosclerosis has not been fully evaluated. Moderate exercise that does not lead to fatigue is recommended. Excessive use of alcohol is contraindicated.

For some patients only a part-time job is advisable, due either to problems of general fatigue or to residual disability. Others continue to work full-time, but curtail social and family activities to gain necessary additional rest.

Some patients find it impossible to accept necessary limitations. Older persons with cerebrovascular disease frequently have lost some of the adaptability that would make it possible to follow suggestions for changes in their way of living. They may reject a treatment regimen simply because it is not acceptable to them, although they recognize it may be ideal for most patients. Unfortunately, the patient's inability to follow a regimen is occasionally viewed as sheer stubbornness rather than as the result of years of gradually developing a way of life that he cannot suddenly relinquish, or possibly, of problems in adaptability due to brain damage. Most patients manage best when they have opportunity to consider the suggestions made to them without feeling undue pressure from others to change themselves or their way of living. Patients who have habitually overeaten, for example, ordinarily do not suddenly eat sparingly. The patient who has made work the center of his existence, and the means of helping to fill needs not met in other areas of his life, will not be likely to agree to give up his work until his condition forces him to do so.

The patient may decide that he would rather live in his accustomed way, however unwise it may seem in relation to his health, in order to fulfill other needs which for him may take precedence—such as the need to be self-supporting. In such instances he must be helped to carry out those aspects of treatment which he can accept.

Just as in retraining for arm movement and walking, speech rehabilitation is most effective when it is begun early. Ideally, the patient's speech problem is evaluated carefully and promptly by a speech therapist, and a program is developed in which the nurse can collaborate with the speech therapist.

Assessment should include the type of aphasia from which the patient suffers, whether the patient's intellectual functioning has been affected, and to what extent. The following suggestions may be helpful in obtaining a data base.

**To decide what speech areas need attention, the nurse should answer these questions about her patient:**
- **Does he have control over his breathing, his lips, and his tongue movements? If not, perhaps the place to start retraining is the control of these essentials.**
- **Can the patient blow out a match?**
- **Can he blow through a straw or into a balloon or a whistle?**
- **Can he stick out his tongue?**
- **Can he call a comb by its name when he sees it? Can he write the word? Copy it?**

**The nurse should help him with exercises to aid speech and swallowing. (See Table 25-2.)**

**Table 25-2. Guidelines for Exercises which Help the Patient to Speak and to Swallow**

| LIPS |
|---|
| Pucker lips and then smile widely |
| Whistle |
| Give a Bronx cheer, using only the lips |
| Round the lips in a pronounced "O" as if holding a straw between the lips |
| Suck on a straw; curl tongue around the straw and suck a small amount of water |
| Open mouth widely, and relax the lips |

| TONGUE |
|---|
| Lick the lips in a circular fashion, first clockwise; then counterclockwise |
| Protrude the tongue, from midline into the right interior cheek, and then into the left cheek. Move the tongue in circular fashion, using teeth as a guide. (If patient is hemiplegic, he should first push the tongue against the cheek on the unaffected side, and then to the affected side) |
| Touch each tooth with the tongue, slowly |
| Raise tongue to roof of mouth and click tongue |
| Protrude tongue from mouth and move laterally; protrude tongue and move it up toward forehead and down toward chin |

| BITING AND CHEWING |
|---|
| Open and close mouth slowly at first and then with increased speed |
| Bite down on tongue blade and hold it between teeth while nurse pulls gently on it. (If patient is hemiplegic, bite from unaffected side only) |
| Chew gum (closely supervised; gum can be swallowed) |
| Chew gum drops and move them into different positions in the mouth |
| Chew saltines and move tongue around to clean out the food |

Prepared by John E. Buckley, M.A., CCC, Sp-A, Director of Speech and Audiology, Overlook Hospital, Summit, N.J. and Clinical Instructor, College of Medicine, State University of New York, Downtown Medical Center and Connie L. Addicks, M.A., CCC, Senior Speech Pathologist, Overlook Hospital, Summit, N.J.

Intervention must be planned to make allowances for the patient's confusion, short attention span, and ability to be easily distracted. He usually is angry with his own incapacity, and he often is self-centered in his efforts to redirect his life. He may resent having words supplied to him, when he knows perfectly well what he means, and when someone understands what he means to say, he is grateful.

The following are ways that the nurse can help the patient with aphasia:

- **Because the patient has problems of association (between word and subject, between word and concept), talk to him and expect response from him (e.g., "Do you want a blanket, Mr. Jones? Here is a blanket. You say: Blanket."). Continuously strengthen asso-**

ciations. Do not tire him, but do not work in silence, guessing at what he wants and accepting only non-verbal communications, such as hand signals.

- Even if you are hurried, it is important to seem calm and unhurried to the patient. He is frightened by his loss of speech, and feels inadequate in not being able to talk as he could a few days ago, and any impatience or haste on your part will inhibit him even further. Wait quietly and pleasantly while he struggles with a word. Praise him if he succeeds, but do not show impatience if he does not.

- Never be tempted to treat him like a child, even though the tasks he must relearn are those that children learn.

- Capitalize on what speech he has. If he can say his dog's name, but not his own, build sentences that he can copy, using the dog's name, and ask him questions that he can answer with the dog's name. Point out his successes to him.

- Do not shout. He's not deaf.

- Set attainable goals. One sound may be worked on for weeks before it is mastered.

- Involve the family as much as possible in the early stages of rehabilitation. Show them how to help with retraining.

- Minimize distraction while helping the patient with his speech. Since he has difficulty concentrating due to his illness, working with him in an area where others are talking loudly, or where a radio is playing, adds unnecessarily to his difficulty and quickly leads to fatigue and frustration.

- Use any obtainable equipment that seems to be helpful. A large artist's pad and crayons may be easier for him in the beginning than a small pad of paper and a pencil. Later a recording machine may help him to recognize his errors in speech. Pictures with names printed beneath (cut out of magazines), a television set, a record player, a hand mirror, an illustrated book of the land or the state of his childhood may be helpful. Use pictures of objects that he commonly needs: a glass, a fork, a comb, a bar of soap. Emphasize what he needs to say, such as "I want water," rather than meaningless sentences, such as "The fox jumped over the fence."

- Be aware of your own reactions to the speech difficulty. Work with these patients can be taxing and frustrating for the nurse. If you work with the patient to a degree that exceeds your ability to tolerate the effort and stress, you will show impatience and frustration, which in turn can lead the patient to become discouraged or resentful. In general, both patient and nurse function best when speech practice periods are brief and interspersed with other activities.

- Because social isolation is such a common response to this disability, help both the patient and his family to feel that, his physical condition permitting, there is no reason for him to live without friends, parties, and outings. Group speech therapy often is the first contact that a patient has with others, but it should not be the only contact.

## SPECIAL PROBLEMS OF PATIENTS WITH CEREBROVASCULAR DISEASE

Cerebrovascular disease is typically a condition of later life; consequently, its incidence is rising sharply because of the increased number of older persons in the population. Many advances have been made in the care and the treatment of these patients. The importance given to rehabilitation after cerebral vascular accidents and the possibility of surgical treatment have made it possible for some of these patients to live fuller lives now than in previous years. A tendency exists, however, to ignore the needs of patients who, because of the extent of their disease or the unavailability of effective treatment, continue to have marked impairment of physical and mental functioning.

The number of such patients is growing rapidly. Many of them are in nursing homes; many continue to live in their own homes. Regardless of where they live, the problems involved in their care are difficult, and an increasing share of nurses' time is spent in caring for them. This is especially true of nurses employed in nursing homes and community health agencies. Efforts to care for these patients are often hampered because of the general apathy of many groups, both lay and professional, an apathy which may stem from feelings of hopelessness.

The first requisite in providing such assistance is a willingness to consider the problem realistically. It is not unusual for discussion to be held in professional meetings concerning the opportunities for employment of the handicapped. But many patients with cerebrovascular disease, especially those in their 80's and 90's, cannot qualify for gainful employment. Much discussion is held concerning advances in surgical treatment, but at this time many patients with cerebrovascular disease are not candidates for such surgery. While discussion of employment possibilities and of surgical treatment is essential and valuable, it is also necessary to consider the vast numbers of patients who in our economy are not employable, those whose disease cannot, with present available therapy, be markedly relieved. Failing to view this problem realistically constitutes a way of avoiding it rather than dealing with it.

This is understandable. People tend to avoid situations that provoke anxiety. It is common for individuals to fear the loss of self-control, dignity, or independence. Working with adults who have undergone brain damage may mean taking care of a man in his 60's who may suddenly burst into tears for no apparent reason or taking care of a 90-year-old woman who soils her bed and no longer recognizes her family. Such experiences can be distressing because they may trigger an individual's own fears concerning old age, or revive painful memories of the illness and the disability of older members of his family. In an institutional setting in which many such patients are gathered, the nurse sometimes feels overpowered by the helplessness of many of her patients, as well as by the fact that most of them suffer a progression of the illness.

Nurses who work successfully with these patients are able and willing to appraise the patient's condition for what it is. If it is unlikely that 98-year-old Ms. Winters will be gainfully employed, or that she ever will be able to care for herself again, what *is* possible? Instead of a bed bath, would it be possible to lift her into the tub? A tub bath would afford her the opportunity for stimulation of circulation, which might minimize the likelihood of decubitus ulcers, as well as provide her with relaxation and a feeling of personal freshness. Instead of dozing all day in her chair and spending restless nights, could she, by having someone to talk with and an interesting view to watch, be helped to remain awake part of the day and to sleep better at night? Is there a half-forgotten skill, such as knitting, which she could use if she were provided with the materials and simple directions?

Patients who have cerebrovascular disease are usually very much aware of the changes occurring in their abilities, unless their disease has progressed to the point that this awareness has been lost or blunted. For example, the patient's family may be talking and laughing together about an incident that occurred yesterday. The patient is painfully aware that he should know what the joke is about, but he doesn't. Observing that he is not laughing, his wife may say reproachfully, "Why, that happened only yesterday, Arthur. Don't you remember?" Nurses, too, can point up to the patient his lack of memory or his confusion by comments like "But it was only this morning that I asked you not to drink anything until the test was over. Now the test is ruined." Such small humiliations are common in the lives of those with cerebrovascular disease. In a sense they are being scolded for being ill. (Yet few people scold a person for having a fever.) The patient's symptoms by their very nature are

likely to be irritating to others. The impatience shown by others can increase the patient's feeling of being unwanted and a burden.

In caring for such a patient the nurse should make every effort not to demand of him abilities that he lacks. As she works with family members, she can help them to do likewise. For example, the patient's wife may tactfully mention to her husband, as the group begins to laugh and she detects a puzzled look on his face, the event that is the cause of the laughter. Such measures help the patient to feel more at ease in his relationships with others.

It is important to remember, however, that motivation for behavior is complex, and that it grows not only from conscious thought processes, but also from unconscious ones. If the patient's wife has been angry with her husband for many years, she may find ways to humiliate him, even though she is consciously aware of the kind or thoughtful thing to say in a given situation.

Nurses may also respond to patients in ways that are not wholly congruent with an intellectual grasp of their patients' needs. Recognition of the complexity of these factors does not lessen the need for their thoughtful consideration, but it does imply that one should not expect all problems to be solved by an intellectual approach.

The realization of these patients that they suffer some confusion and memory loss tends to intensify their feelings of insecurity and fearfulness. Since changes in environment or being alone in the dark may accentuate their fears and increase their confusion, it is important to keep their environment as unchanged as possible. For example, transfer from one room to another or contact with an entirely strange staff should be avoided when possible. Keeping a light on in the patient's room at night helps him to avoid the increased confusion that can result if he is left in a darkened room. Careful and, if necessary, repeated orientation to the location of the bathroom or his own room may help a patient who has been newly admitted to a nursing home.

Because of their infirmities, elderly persons with cerebrovascular disease tend to be emotionally and physically dependent on those who care for them. This tendency must be recognized and dealt with; otherwise, it engenders situations in which the patient clamors for more of the nurse's attention. For example, when a patient is newly admitted to a nursing home, it is important to recognize that his efforts to gain the nurse's attention are necessary to him to help him feel more secure and to assure him that those responsible for him care about him. By accepting and dealing with the patient's efforts to gain her attention, the nurse can help him gradually to feel safer. She can then slowly help him to increase his independence. For instance, she may help him to bathe and dress, if he states that he is unable to do this unaided. As she helps him, she can evaluate what aspects of self-care he seems capable of performing. As he begins to feel more at home in his new surroundings, she may encourage him to undertake aspects of care of which he seems capable, while stressing that she is available to help him if he requires her help. In the same way the nurse can help the patient to undertake recreational activities.

## Families

The families of patients with cerebrovascular disease are in particular need of the nurse's help. To a greater extent than many other disabilities, brain damage severely taxes interpersonal relationships. Sometimes these difficulties are avoided rather than faced. Many families fail to visit a member with cerebrovascular disease if he is in a nursing home; or if he lives at home, they find ways to exclude him from most of their activities. Too frequently, such reactions by the family are censured; instead, the family needs help in dealing with the problem.

The wife who has depended on her husband to make decisions and to provide financial and emotional support may find it overwhelming to cope with a husband who is confused and dependent on her. To the grown children of a parent afflicted with cerebrovascular disease, the illness can signify loss of the help and the support of a parent on whom they have relied. Adults who typically control their anger and their sexuality may, as a result of brain damage, behave in ways that are shocking to their families and friends. One elderly man with cerebrovascular disease who became disoriented at night talked of sexual matters in a manner far different from his usual restrained manner.

The family is usually doing the best that it can in the situation. Allowing family members opportunities to discuss, if they wish, some of the problems they are experiencing and showing them ways that can help to provide more satisfactory care for the patient often enable the family to be more understanding and to accept the illness better. The family should be helped to acquire information that is valuable in making decisions concerning long-term care. However, such decisions (e.g., whether to care for the patient at home or in a nursing home) should follow an appraisal by the family members of their own resources and the needs of the patient.

A difficult problem for families is the fluctuation in the patient's mental status. Some patients with cerebrovascular disease are well oriented at some periods and grossly confused at others. Those who care for the patient must become accustomed to evaluating his state of orientation and adapting their approach accordingly. If the patient typically is well oriented in the morning, the nurse should select the morning hours to talk over plans with him or to provide instruction or encouragement with a hobby. In evaluating the patient's orientation, it is important to distinguish between the ability to make stereotyped responses like "Hello, how are you?" and the ability to think abstractly. Many patients with brain damage are able to continue to respond in stereotyped phrases, but have impaired ability to think through current problems. Because a patient can smile brightly and say, "Good morning," it sometimes is assumed that he is more capable intellectually than he is. In such instances the patient may be expected to do things that actually are beyond his ability.

Another problem involves the patient's ability to perceive emotionally the significance of events. He may, for example, say without emotion, "My son was killed last week." Those who do not understand that he is ill may reproach him for being heartless, whereas actually the disease process has blunted his perception of the significance of events.

Care of the patient with cerebrovascular disease requires systematic use of the nursing process to provide patients with the means to attain their maximum level of wellness. The nurse must prepare herself to competently care for patients with this major health problem.

## REFERENCES AND BIBLIOGRAPHY

AMACHER, NANCY: Touch is a way of caring, *Am. J. Nurs.* 73:5:852-854, May 1973.

BEESON, PAUL, and McDERMOTT, WALSH (eds.): *Cecil-Loeb Textbook of Medicine,* ed. 13, Philadelphia, Saunders, 1971.

BELAND, IRENE: *Clinical Nursing, Pathophysiological and Psychosocial Approaches,* ed. 2, New York, Macmillan, 1970.

BURT, MARGARET: Perceptual deficits in hemiplegia, *Am. J. Nurs.* 70:5:1026-1029, May, 1970.

CARINI, ESTA, and OWENS, GUY: *Neurological and Neurosurgical Nursing,* ed. 6, St. Louis, Mosby, 1974.

CUICA, RUDY, et al.: Range of motion exercises, active and passive: a handbook, *Nurs. '73* 3:12:25-37, December 1973.

DREW, NANCY: How to cope with speech defects in stroke patients, *Nurs. '74* 4:2:20-21, February 1974.

ELLWOOD, EVELYN: Nursing the patient with a cerebrovascular accident, *Nurs. Clin. N. Am.* 5:1:47-53, March 1970.

FALKNOR, HELEN, and HARRIS, BEVERLY: Resocializing—through a club, *Nurs. Outlook* 21:12:778-780, December 1973.

FOX, MADELINE: Talking with patients who can't answer, *Am. J. Nurs.* 71:6:1146-1149, June 1971.

GAFFNEY, T. W., and CAMPBELL, R. P.: Feeding techniques for dysphagic patients, *Am. J. Nurs.* 74:2194, December 1974.

HACKLER, EMILY, and HOWELL, ANN: Resocializing the stroke patient—trained volunteers, *Nurs. Outlook* 21:12:776-778, December 1973.

JACOBANSKY, ANN: Stroke, *Am. J. Nurs.* 72:7:1260-1263, July 1972.

KELLER, MARGARET, and TRUSCOTT, LIONEL: Transient ischemic attacks, *Am. J. Nurs.* 73:8:1330-1331, August 1973.

KERN, FLORENCE, and POOLE, LAURA: Transfer techniques, *Nurs. '72* 2:7:25-28, July 1972.

KINTZEL, KAY (ed.): *Advanced Concepts in Clinical Nursing,* Philadelphia, Lippincott, 1971.

KORTE, MARY: Intensive care of the neurologic patient, *Nurs. Clin. N. Am.* 7:2:335-348, June 1972.

LARSEN, GEORGE: After stroke: Optokinetic nystagmus, *Am. J. Nurs.* 73:11:1897-1899, November 1973.

LEONARD, BEVERLY: Body image changes in chronic illness, *Nurs. Clin. N. Am.* 7:4:687-695, December 1972.

MACAWLEY, CECILIA, and ANDERSON, ALBERT: The nurse as a primary therapist in the management of the patient with stroke, *Cardio-Vascular Nursing* 10:2:7-10, March-April 1974.

MERRITT, H. HOUSTON: *A Textbook of Neurology,* ed. 5, Philadelphia, Lea and Febiger, 1973.

PFAUDLER, MARJORIE: After stroke: Motor skill rehabilitation of hemiplegic patients, *Am. J. Nurs.* 73:11:1892-1896, November 1973.

SCHULTZ, LUCIE: Nursing care of the stroke patient, *Nurs. Clin. N. Am.* 8:4:633-642, December 1973.

Symposium on neurologic and neurosurgical nursing, *Nurs. Clin. N. Am.* 4:2:199-300, June 1969.

# The Patient with a Visual Problem

Although modern methods of early detection and treatment of visual problems are preserving the sight of many people, thousands of others become blind or visually handicapped. Some of these disabilities could be prevented or minimized if patients were referred promptly for therapy.

Many of the serious diseases leading to blindness occur in middle life and old age. After age 40, an increasing number of people in the United States suffer from retinal disorders, cataracts, glaucoma, and other major causes of blindness. As the average age of the population increases, the incidence of these diseases also increases. The issue is not solely one of physical disability; visual handicaps take a psychological and economic toll which must be borne by individuals, their close associates, and society as a whole.

Working with the visually handicapped in clinics and hospitals which specialize in care of such patients is only one part of the nurse's role. In fact, in these settings it may be too late to institute primary prevention. Much of the health care effort goes into secondary prevention (dealing with the situation once disease has developed) due to limitations of knowledge, the chronicity of some conditions and their slow, insidious onset, and problems with the health care delivery system.

As citizens and health care professionals deal more effectively with these issues, the concept of health care broadens. For example, teaching about the importance of an adequate diet may include discussion of the relationship between adequate nutrition and healthy eyes. The breakdown of visual structures, such as the cornea,

429

due to A-avitaminosis is prevented by an adequate intake of vitamin A.

Teaching and early case finding and referral to the ophthalmologist can occur in varied settings: in industry, among the elderly residents of the community, many of whom live alone and have inadequate health care, and among persons who are institutionalized in such long-term care facilities as nursing homes and mental hospitals. Periodic screening tests of vision and eye examinations to determine possible pathology are essential, particularly among those over 40. Changing life styles have also affected the risk of eye disease. Some young parents who prefer home births are not aware of measures which are required to prevent gonorrheal infection of the eyes of the newborn. Careful instruction and use of prophylaxis are essential in order to lessen the risk of developing this condition.

When disease has already developed, it is important to minimize its possible effects upon vision. For example, diabetics commonly suffer from eye diseases, such as retinal hemorrhages. The nurse who cares for such a patient, whether in the hospital or community, should be aware of and alert for possible symptoms of visual disorder, refer the patient promptly, and plan with him whenever possible, care which limits the likelihood of complications which can impair vision. In addition, nursing measures among the very ill and elderly can prevent infection of and injury to the eyes. Scrupulous hand washing before carrying out any procedure involving the eyes, and protecting the eyes of unconscious patients who are unable to close them are examples.

## ANATOMY OF THE EYE

The eyeball is a spherical organ situated in a bony cavity called the orbit (Fig. 26-1). It is rotated in all directions by six muscles attached to its outer surface.

The eyeball may be divided into three coats. The dense white fibrous outer coat, or *sclera*, becomes continuous anteriorly with the *cornea*, the translucent structure that bulges forward slightly from the general contour of the eye. The cornea is innervated by sensory nerve fibers derived from the ophthalmic division of the trigeminal nerve. Posteriorly, the sclera has an opening through which the optic nerve passes into the eyeball. This nerve spreads out over the posterior two-thirds of the inner surface of the globe in a thin layer, or *retina*, which is composed of a pigmented outer layer and an inner sensory layer. The two layers are held very closely together; however, there is a potential space between them. The sensory layer receives visual stimuli that are then transmitted to the brain by the optic nerve. These impulses are interpreted as sight. The pigmented layer is in close contact with the choroid through which both layers of the retina receive their blood supply.

Between the sclera and the retina is the pigmented middle coat, or *uveal tract*, which is composed of three parts. The posterior part, the *choroid*, contains most of the blood vessels that nourish the eye. The anterior pigmented muscular part, the *iris*, gives the characteristic color to the eye. The circular opening at its center is the *pupil* which contracts or enlarges according to the intensity of the light. The muscular body located between the iris and the choroid is the *ciliary body* which is composed of radial processes arising from a triangle-shaped muscle. Between these processes and attached to them are delicate ligaments that pass centrally and become inserted into the capsule of the lens. The iris and the ciliary body play a role in the mechanism of accommodation and in bringing about changes in pupillary size.

The *lens* is a semisolid body enclosed in a transparent elastic capsule. The lens is capable of being modified to varying degrees of convexity by the contraction and relaxation of the *ciliary muscle*, thus changing the focus of the eye as it looks from one object to another.

The cavity within the eye is divided by the lens into two parts. The posterior part contains a jelly-like, translucent substance, the *vitreous humor*, which is the chief factor in maintaining the form of the eyeball. The anterior part contains the *aqueous humor* which is secreted by the ciliary processes. It bathes the anterior surface, or *anterior chamber*, of the iris and the cornea. Finally it is drained from the eye through lymph channels (the *canal of Schlemm*) located at the junction of the iris and the sclera. Normally a balance is achieved between the amount of aqueous humor formed by the ciliary body and the amount drained out of the eye. This balance helps to maintain normal intraocular pressure. Increased intraocular pressure may be a symptom of glaucoma (see below).

The *eyelids* are the protective covering of the eye. Lining the lid and entirely covering the

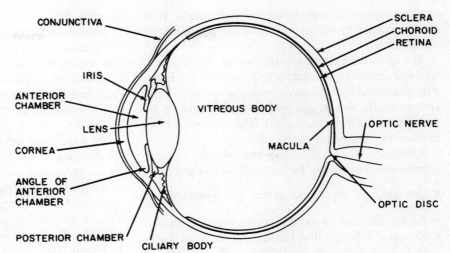

**Figure 26-1.** Diagram showing the location of some of the important structures of the eye. The cornea, aqueous humor, lens, and vitreous are the refractive media.

anterior portion of the eye is a transparent mucous membrane, the *palpebral conjunctiva*, which is reflected on to the sclera and up to the cornea as the *bulbar conjunctiva*. The reflections make cul-de-sacs known as the *lower and upper fornices*. The surface of the conjunctiva is kept moist by a constant flow of lacrimal fluid (tears). This fluid is excreted from the *lacrimal gland* and flows downward and inward across the eye and drains into tiny channels, or *lacrimal puncta*, whence it is conducted to the *lacrimal sac and duct* which pass downward and outward and open into the nasal cavity.

## ASSESSMENT

### History Taking

When taking the health history, it is important for the nurse to obtain information about the patient's background, including his present symptoms, if any, previous or current diseases, and treatment received. Family history is also important, especially in relation to such conditions as glaucoma, cataract, and diabetes. In addition, it is important to know something of the patient's concerns and his life style, for like all other symptoms, symptoms of eye disorders can be triggered by emotional stress. To obtain additional data, the nurse should ask the patient whether he has experienced any visual disturbance, such as discomfort from bright lights (photophobia), double vision, blurring or reduction of vision, and whether such reduction has been gradual or sudden, unilateral or bilateral.

The patient should be encouraged to describe the nature of his visual defect as he sees it.

If the patient complains of pain, the nurse should ask him about its location, character, when it is most severe, what symptoms, such as nausea and vomiting accompany it, and so on.

### Physical Assessment

External Inspection of the Eye

Before inspecting the eye, the nurse should wash her hands thoroughly. Dawson and others have implicated ophthalmic examining rooms as sources of nosocomial transmission of adenovirus type 8, resulting in a severe eye disease, epidemic keratoconjunctivitis. As the nurse assumes more responsibilities for inspecting eyes, she must use care that neither her hands nor her instruments become vehicles for transmission of pathogens. The main objective in inspection is to note deviation from normal; therefore knowledge of ocular anatomy is essential. The nurse should examine many normal eyes, with supervision, to become acquainted with normal characteristics, and also with variations within the normal. For example, yellowish spots (sebaceous glands in the lacrimal caruncle) located in the nasal corner of the conjunctiva become more prominent with age. However, when in doubt whether a finding is normal or not, it is important to consult an expert.

A useful system for the examiner to follow when inspecting the eye is to start from the outer parts and proceed inward. The physical appearance of the various ocular structures should be observed and their function assessed whenever feasible. When dealing with structures which are not visible, such as extraocular muscles, only their function can be observed.

The inspection begins with the lid, conjunctiva, lacrimal apparatus, cornea, sclera, anterior chamber, iris, pupil, and extraocular muscles of each eye. Differences in size, shape, position, and signs of inflammation or any anomalous findings which may indicate pathology are observed.

**Eyelids.** When inspecting the eyelids, the examiner should observe for the following signs:

- **Drooping of the upper eyelid (blepharoptosis or ptosis).**
- **Inadequate closure of the eyeslit (lagophthalmos).**
- **Excessive blinking (blepharospasm). Blepharospasm may be a symptom of fatigue, conjunctivitis, or anxiety.**
- **Edema. If bilateral, edema of the eyelids may cause temporary blindness, since the patient may not be able to open his severely swollen eyes. Edema may be associated with allergy or other systemic conditions involving the kidneys, heart, or thyroid gland, or with inflammatory conditions of the eyelids.**

    **The examiner should go no further in inspecting the eye than the edematous area, if following trauma, fracture of the bony orbit or perforation of the globe has not been ruled out. Immediate referral is also indicated if swollen eyelids are due to allergy or part of a larger picture including anasarca or congestive heart failure.**
- **Localized infection. Using a penlight, the examiner inspects for any evidence of localized infection, such as a sty, or crusting about the lashes.**
- **Cysts, tumors, and ulcerated areas. By palpating the lids and orbital margins, the presence of tumors which are not large enough to cause deformities can be elicited.**
- **Itching, rash, vesicles, cracks, or excoriations. These symptoms could be due to contact dermatitis from medications, cosmetics, or other substances.**

**Conjunctiva.** The lower fornix is examined by pulling down the lower lid and directing the patient to look up, down, and to each side. To examine the upper palpebral conjunctiva, the upper lid must be everted.

While examining the palpebral conjunctiva, the examiner looks for classic signs of inflammation or unusual appearance. Since there can be various manifestations of disease involving the conjunctiva, the examiner contributes to the diagnosis by describing accurately what she observes.

The bulbar conjunctiva should be inspected for subconjunctival pathology, such as edema which may result from trauma, allergy, trichinosis, and some types of conjunctivitis. In severe edema, ballooning folds of edematous conjunctiva may overlap the cornea. Other abnormal conditions to look for include air or blood which may collect between the bulbar conjunctiva and the sclera.

**Lacrimal Apparatus.** Malfunctioning of the lacrimal apparatus may be due to obstruction of the flow of fluid. A dry eye, resulting from tear deficiency may be presented by patients who suffer from such conditions as chemical burns, trachoma, or diseases which have caused conjunctival cicatrization (scarring).

**Cornea.** The cornea is inspected with a penlight and lateral moving illumination. A healthy cornea should be clear, bright, and glossy, and should reflect light without distortion from all parts of its anterior surface.

The examiner should inspect the profile of the cornea by viewing the cornea from above or by looking down from behind over the brow. A conical-shaped cornea points outward and results in diminished visual acuity and marked astigmatism, which prevents light focus at any point.

Corneal sensitivity can be tested by approaching the eye laterally, touching the cornea with a wisp of cotton, and observing for involuntary blinking. Sensitivity is reduced in some viral diseases affecting the corneal branches of the trigeminal nerve, such as herpes simplex keratitis. Vitamin C intake in the diet should be stressed for those suffering from corneal pathology and also to prevent its occurrence.

**Sclera.** When assessing the condition of the sclera, the examiner should observe for changes in color, keeping in mind that there are physiologic variants from the normal white (e.g., brownish sclera in the dark complexioned).

The examiner should observe for areas of thinning and bulging (staphylomas) which develop in the sclera because of increased intraocular pressure. She should also observe for dermoid cysts and for signs of inflammation.

**Anterior Chamber.** Under normal circumstances the anterior chamber should appear black (optically empty). The examiner observes for abnormal constituents of the fluid, such as blood in the anterior chamber (hyphema) or pus (hypopyon), which sink into the lowest part.

**Iris.** The examiner should observe the color of both irides. Differences in color (heterochromia) may indicate injury or disease.

The examiner should also look for irregularities in the shape of each iris. A notching of the iris (coloboma), usually present in the inferior portion, indicates that a part of this structure is missing, either because of surgery or congenital defect. Congestion and infiltration of the iris may cause it to adhere posteriorly to the capsule of the lens (posterior synechiae) giving an irregular shape to the pupillary edge of the iris. A tremulous iris (iridodenesis) indicates either displacement or absence of the lens (aphakia). (The lens is removed in treatment of cataract. See below.)

Because the uveal tract is pigmented and vascular, it is said to react more vigorously to the inflammatory response and immunologic process. It is also a major site for metastatic tumors and infections.

**Pupil.** The pupil normally has a round shape and a regular outline. Both pupils are equal in size (isocoric). There is, however, a normal variation among the general population which accounts for a 5 per cent incidence of unequal pupils (anisocoria) not associated with disease. In the other 95 per cent, anisocoria is an abnormal finding which may indicate disturbances in the innervation of the eye or intraocular disorders. The examiner should observe that the inequality is not due to synechiae in which case there would be an irregular shaped pupil as well. All patients with unequal pupils should be referred to the physician.

Dilated pupils (mydriasis) result from ocular injury, glaucoma, sympathomimetic drugs, and emotions, such as anxiety. Constricted pupils (miosis) are seen with inflamed irides, and in patients receiving morphine, pilocarpine, and parasympathomimetic drugs. Fixed, dilated pupils are seen with circulatory arrest and severe central nervous system damage. Before the pupils are examined, the nurse should inquire if the patient is receiving eye medications, since some medications affect the size of the pupil.

Examination for reaction to light is best performed in a darkened room, using oblique illumination. With increased illumination, the pupil should constrict (direct reaction to light). Constriction of the opposite pupil, even without increased illumination, is called consensual pupil reaction. When testing for accommodation, the pupil should dilate for far vision and constrict for near vision. The examiner may ask the patient to look at his finger placed about five inches from his eye and alternately to look at an object on the wall directly behind the finger. When the pupil reacts to accommodation but not to light, the finding is called the Argyll-Robert-son pupil and is associated with tertiary syphilis affecting the central nervous system.

**Extraocular Muscles.** The extraocular muscles are examined for possible deviations of conjugate gaze. Ocular movements may be tested by having the patient turn his eyes in the six cardinal directions of gaze and by having his eyes converge on a near point. The examiner may observe that in some patients the visual axes are no longer parallel in all directions of gaze and a strabismus, a squint, or crossed eyes are produced. These may be caused by weakness, paralysis, or some other anomaly of extraocular muscles.

The examiner also observes for the appearance of a rapid jerking motion of the eyes (nystagmus). This may be idiopathic, associated with disease of the nervous system, or due to long-standing poor vision, or anxiety. The nurse may carry out other aspects of eye inspection, such as testing intraocular pressure by use of the tonometer. (See pp. 435 to 436.)

Use of the Ophthalmoscope

Examining the fundus of the eye with the ophthalmoscope is done by nurses who develop this skill after considerable practice and with expert supervision. For nurses who are responsible for physical assessment, such extensive practice and supervision are essential. Here we shall present only introductory material which can assist the beginner.

It is essential to carry out the examination in a darkened room, and for the initial experience, to select patients with normal, healthy eyes. The examination is performed with the patient either seated or lying down. He is instructed to look at a distant object. This, and the darkness of the room, facilitate the examination by causing dilation of the pupil. To examine the patient's right eye, the examiner holds the ophthalmoscope in her right hand, in front of her right eye. She follows the same procedure using her left hand when examining the patient's left eye.

The examiner's head must come very close to the patient, with their foreheads almost, or actually, touching. The beam of light is directed into the pupil, at which time a red glow will be seen. Continuing to look through the scope, and approaching the patient more closely, the examiner will detect retinal blood vessels, the optic disk, which is round and pink, and the macula lutea, an avascular area near the disk, which is the point of greatest visual acuity. The condition of retinal blood vessels is significant, not only in relation to the eye, but also because it reflects the condition of vessels elsewhere in the body, and is therefore useful in noting such conditions as arteriosclerosis.

### The Color Sense

Because most human beings are capable of distinguishing colors, it is difficult to imagine that there are some people who lack the color sense. About 8 per cent of the men and 0.4 per cent of the women in the United States have some degree of color perception deficiency. Most deficiencies are inherited, and in the majority of cases the condition is transmitted as a sex-linked genetic defect. Occasionally color defectiveness may be a manifestation of acquired retinal or optic nerve disease, or the result of injury.

**Color Vision.** Color vision, like central vision, depends on an intact macula lutea. In this portion of the retina there is a central shallow pit, the fovea centralis, containing cones which hold photopigments capable of becoming stimulated by wavelengths of light. White light is made of all spectral colors, and each color corresponds to a given frequency.

Color vision and color blindness are explained by the Young-Helmholtz theory which postulates that there are three color-sensitive sets of retinal fibers or cones which respond selectively to red, green, and blue or violet, and that all complementary colors result from mixtures of signals from the three systems.

Individuals with abnormal color vision fall into several categories. Monochromats are totally color blind. They see the whole spectrum in shades of gray. Dichromats perceive only two primary colors. Anomalous trichromates constitute the less seriously affected among the color blind; they perceive the three primary colors, but there is a reduction in the sensitivity of one or more color systems in their fovea.

When testing for the color sense in the elderly, the examiner must remember that opacities in the ocular media (cornea, lens, vitreous humor) depress vision, including color vision. She should find out if the patient is taking any medications which may affect vision (e.g., chloroquine which may cause iridescent vision).

Because good illumination is essential, daylight is preferred for testing. Both eyes must be tested separately since color blindness could be unilateral.

There are various standard tests available for detection of color deficiency. One, the Holmgren test, involves the matching of yarns. The patient is given a set of yarns which includes the three primary colors with their many derivatives, and asked to match similar yarns according to color.

### Testing of Visual Function

**Visual Acuity.** In testing for visual acuity, the examiner aims to determine if the eye has the ability to perceive the shape or form of objects. When an object enters a person's field of vision and he focuses his gaze upon it, central or direct vision is taking place. This occurs when the visual image is received on the macula lutea. Thus testing for visual acuity is an assessment of central vision, or macular function, while looking at an object nearby or at a distance.

Measurement of visual acuity constitutes a relatively accurate clinical test of function and, when normal, indicates the following: (1) that myopia is not present or if present is of minor degree; (2) that any hyperopia present has been compensated by accommodation; (3) that the ocular media are relatively clear to permit an image to be formed in the retina; (4) that the fovea centralis is relatively intact, as are its nervous connections to the brain; (5) that perception by the higher visual centers is intact.

DISTANCE VISION (at 20 feet). Distance vision is tested with the Snellen chart. This visual screening device consists of a series of letters (or other symbols) of different sizes that have been standardized to indicate what people with normal vision can see at certain distances from the chart. For example, the largest letters can be read at a distance of 200 feet by those with unimpaired vision, and progressively smaller letters can be seen at 100 feet, 50 feet, and 20 feet. The patient is seated 20 feet from the chart. One eye is tested at a time, and the other eye is covered by a card. The acuteness of vision is determined by the smallest row the patient can read or identify.

The result of the test is expressed as a "fraction," the numerator being the distance of the patient from the chart, and the denominator the distance at which the letter can be seen by a person with normal sight. For example, if the patient can read at a distance of 20 feet letters no smaller than those that a person with normal vision can see at 40 feet, his visual acuity is described as 20/40. If the patient can read at 20 feet the letters that people with normal vision can read at 20 feet, his vision is described as 20/20. One way of recalling the significance of these figures is to remember that the larger the denominator of the fraction, the worse the patient's vision. Usually, vision that is reduced to 20/200 is considered legal blindness.

NEAR VISUAL ACUITY. Near visual acuity may be evaluated with the aid of a reading card using Jaeger test type. The test consists of different sizes of ordinary printer's types; the finest print is numbered 1, successive higher numbers indicating larger type. The patient should sit with his back to the light, so that the card is well illuminated. The standard distance recommended is 14 inches. Acuity of near vision is recorded $J^1$, $J^2$, the number corresponding to the finest print that can be read. Each eye should be tested separately.

**The Field of Vision.** The field of vision (the conformation of the area that the patient can see without turning his head or moving his eyes) is tested by the use of the tangent screen and the perimeter. One eye is tested at a time. The tangent screen, on which there are various markings indicating degrees, is used in testing the central visual field. The perimeter, an arc-shaped instrument, is used to measure the peripheral field of vision. Small test objects are moved from the side to outline the patient's field of vision. Reduction in the field of vision may indicate serious disorders, such as glaucoma and retinal detachment. Certain brain disease, such as tumor or stroke, may also cause visual field defects. Reduction in the field of vision below a certain limit constitutes legal blindness.

Examination of the field of vision can be carried out by the nurse by means of *confrontation testing*. This test is gross and is significant only when abnormal, but it is reliable as a screening device.

The patient is seated about three feet from the nurse, and instructed to cover his left eye and to look at the nurse's left eye. The nurse raises her hands from a position where she can barely see them in the two lower quadrants, and the patient indicates when he sees the moving hands rising in the lower quadrants. The upper quadrants are tested in the same manner with the nurse's hands moving downward. To test the left eye, the procedure is repeated, with the patient covering his right eye.

Normally, a patient should see about 60 degrees upward, 90 degrees temporally, and 70 degrees downward as measured from the anterioposterior axis of the eye (Havener, 1971).

Using the Tonometer

Routine tonometry should be done on patients over 35 years of age. The technique for tonometry, which can be carried out by the nurse as well as by the physician, should be learned under the supervision of an ophthalmologist. It consists of resting the tonometer, an instrument that measures the pressure within the eyeball, vertically upon an anesthetized cornea and observing the readings on the scale. As noted previously increased intraocular pressure is a sign of glaucoma.

Two types of tonometers are commonly used: the Schiotz and the Goldmann (Fig. 26-2).

**The Schiotz Tonometer.** First, the procedure and its purpose are explained to the patient, and he is instructed to look at a fixed spot on the ceiling and to avoid moving his eyes or eyelids while the

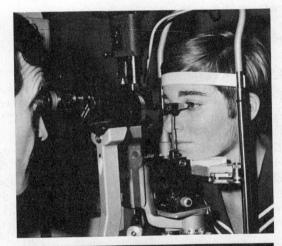
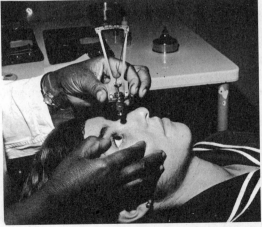

**Figure 26-2.** (*Top*) Tonometry using Goldman applanation tonometer. (*Bottom*) Tonometry using Schiotz tonometer.

readings are being taken. The patient is usually seated in a treatment chair which is then tilted to a reclining position, so that the patient is lying on his back facing straight upward. Each eye is anesthetized with a drop of 0.5 per cent proparacaine hydrochloride (Ophthaine) or some other suitable topical ophthalmic anesthetic. (The nurse will secure standing orders for each screening program she carries out.) One minute after instilling the anesthetic, the eyelids are separated gently and held open against the bony orbit. The footplate of the tonometer is immediately placed upon the cornea and held in a vertical position for a second or two while the scale is read. The procedure is repeated for the other eye. Because the footplate of the tonometer touches the eye, it must be sterilized with alcohol before use with each patient. The readings are recorded and checked against a table which transposes the readings from units to millimeters of mercury.

**The Goldmann Tonometer.** Applanation tonometry is another method which is increasingly being used by ophthalmologists because of its greater accuracy. This method uses the Goldmann tonometer which attaches to a slit-lamp microscope. A drop of anesthetic solution is instilled, followed by the application of fluorescein on the eye. The patient sits forward at the slit-lamp, where the instrument is placed on the cornea by the examiner who reads the pressure. Sterilization of the instrument is carried out with an antibacterial solution.

**Tonometer Weights.** It is important for the nurse to know that the tonometer may be used with three different weights (5.5, 7.5, and 10 Gm.). The tonometer plunger assembly alone weighs 5.5 Gm. Additional weights are added if more accuracy is desired when dealing with harder eyes. For screening purposes a 5.5 Gm. weight load is considered adequate.

Normal pressures are usually below 20 mm. Hg. An increase in intraocular pressure is not reported as glaucoma since the diagnosis of this condition involves at least two other diagnostic criteria.

**Tonography.** Tonography is a method of recording intraocular pressure over a period of four minutes during which time a specially sensitive Schiotz type tonometer is allowed to rest on the eyeball. The tonometer is attached to an electric recording device. This test is of value for diagnosing early glaucoma and for confirming that known glaucoma is being satisfactorily controlled by the prescribed method of treatment.

## EYEDROPS

Eyedrops are used for various purposes: for anesthesia, for dilating the pupil (mydriasis) to facilitate fundus examination, and for paralyzing the muscle of accommodation (cycloplegia) prior to examination for refractive errors, particularly in children and young adults. Cycloplegia, when induced by such medication, temporarily prevents activity of the ciliary muscle which alters the shape of the lens, thus interfering with focusing the eye on near objects, and causing the patient to experience a temporary loss of near vision. In middle and later life, considerable loss of power of accommodation makes the use of cycloplegics usually unnecessary.

Cycloplegics also dilate the pupil. All drugs that dilate the pupil are potentially dangerous in certain persons who are susceptible to angle-closure glaucoma. Drugs commonly used prior to refraction are cyclopentolate (Cyclogyl) 0.5 to 2.0 per cent solution, and tropicamide (Mydriacyl). These drugs produce cycloplegia in about one-half hour, and the effect usually wears off in six hours. In the past atropine and homatropine were widely used for this purpose, but they have the disadvantage of slower onset of action and prolonged effect, thus subjecting the patient to the inconvenience of loss of near vision for a day or longer. All of these drugs are ordered by the ophthalmologist specifically in each individual instance of their use.

In addition to medically prescribed eyedrops, many preparations are available in drug stores without prescription. Patients can be advised that such preparations are usually harmless in themselves, but that they may be harmful when used as a substitute for medical attention when the eyes are persistently irritated or uncomfortable. Those who experience itching, burning, tearing, or other discomfort of the eyes should consult an ophthalmologist.

INSTRUCTIONS TO PATIENT FOR PLACING DROPS IN THE EYE* (Fig. 26-3)

Wash hands thoroughly.
1. Sit down away from active people. This avoids the possibility of the hand being bumped.
2. With both eyes open, tilt the head back and look upward.
3. With the index finger of the free hand, pull the lower lid down gently to form a slight sac just below the eyeball.

---

*Adapted from "How to Place Medication in Your Eyes," Softcon Products Division, Warner-Lambert Company, Morris Plains, N. J.

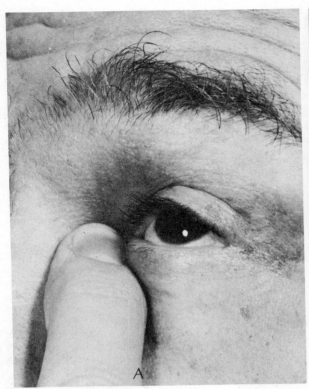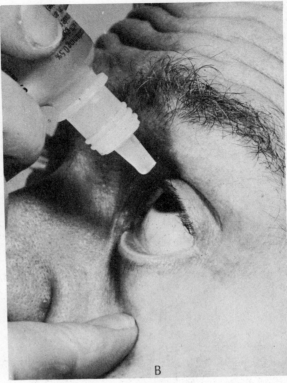

**Figure 26-3.** (*A*) When instilling eyedrops, the patient should press his forefinger against the corner of his eye to prevent medication from entering tear sac. (*B*) When inserting eyedrops, the patient should look up, evert the lower lid, and place the drop into the sac made by the everted lower lid. (Manhattan Eye, Ear, and Throat Hospital, New York, N.Y.)

4. Hold the bottle or dropper vertically over the eye, and squeeze gently until the correct number of drops fall into the small sac. Do not touch the eye with the bottle or dropper tip.
5. Release the lower lid so that the sac closes. Close the eye gently; do not squeeze it closed.
6. Replace the cap or dropper immediately so that neither contacts other surfaces.
7. Immediately press the forefinger against the corner of the eye to prevent medication from entering the tear sac. Hold the finger in place for two to three minutes.
8. Replace the bottle in refrigerator if required.

INSTRUCTIONS TO PATIENT FOR PLACING OINTMENT IN THE EYE (Fig. 26-4)
Wash hands thoroughly.

1. Sit down away from active people.
2. Lay the cap on a clean surface, and hold the container in the hand intended for use.
3. Look forward into a mirror. With the index finger of the free hand, pull the lower lid down gently so that it forms a slight sac just below the eyeball.

4. Place the correct amount of ointment in the small sac. Do not touch the eye with the tip of the container.
5. Release the lower lid so that the sac closes, and close the eye gently.
6. Replace the cap immediately so that neither cap nor container contacts other surfaces.

## PATIENT EDUCATION

Many people are confused by the terms *optician, optometrist, ophthalmologist,* and *oculist.* An *optician,* like a pharmacist, fills prescriptions given by the physician, such as those for glasses. In this case, the optician has the prescribed lenses made and sees that the glasses are properly fitted. An *optometrist* is trained to test vision for refractive errors and to prescribe and fit glasses to correct such errors. Because he is not an M.D., he is not permitted to prescribe medications for the eye or to diagnose or to treat eye diseases. The terms *ophthalmologist* and *oculist* are synonymous and

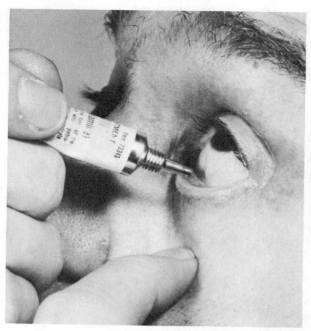

**Figure 26-4.** When applying ointment, the patient should look up, evert the lower lid, and place a "ribbon" of ointment inside the everted lower lid. (Manhattan Eye, Ear, and Throat Hospital, New York, N.Y.)

refer to a physician who has had special training in the diagnosis and the treatment of eye diseases, including refraction and the prescription of glasses. He also performs surgery.

**Glasses.** Nurses frequently are asked about the use of sunglasses. Glasses that are ground carefully and cause no distortion of vision are considered safe. People who need corrective lenses at all times should have dark glasses made to their prescription, or wear dark lenses that clip over their regular glasses.

Plastic lenses, which are lighter in weight and unbreakable, are often used instead of glass. However, they scratch more easily, and, when not in use, they should always be carried in a case, rather than being left unprotected in a purse or a pocket.

All glasses should be kept clean. Smudges and specks of dirt cut down vision, just as a dirty windshield does, and they also are unattractive. Glasses should be washed with warm water and soap and dried with a soft cloth at least once daily. Many people, particularly the elderly, sometimes borrow each other's glasses. This practice should be discouraged. People with visual difficulties should be advised to visit an oculist and, if glasses are needed,

to have them individually prescribed. People who need corrective lenses continuously should keep an extra pair in reserve in case of loss or breakage.

U.S. government regulations require glass lenses to be specially hardened to prevent breakage—an important safety factor.

Particularly in recent years, relatively low cost establishments for making glasses have become common in some areas of the country. The nurse can help her clients by advising them to check carefully the qualifications of those who make corrective lenses. Referral to a well-qualified optician is important.

### Daily Care of the Eyes

The following are simple rules for the daily care of the eyes:

- **Have a good light when reading, writing, or doing other close work. Place the light so that a shadow is not cast by the hands. The light source should be shielded to prevent direct glare on the eyes.**
- **Rest the eyes periodically when prolonged fine work is being done. Looking out of a window at intervals rests the eyes by allowing them to focus on distant objects (relaxation of accommodation).**
- **General health is important in maintaining the health of the eyes. For example, a form of night blindness is related to a deficiency of vitamin A. (The adjustment of the eye to see in the dark, called dark adaptation, involves a complicated photochemical process in the retina.) Epithelial tissues of the eye also are affected by vitamin A deficiency, and, if the deficiency is severe, the cornea may be so damaged that blindness results. Another example is diabetes mellitus, which predisposes to cataract formation and to pathologic changes in the retina.**
- **Get plenty of sleep. Lack of sleep is a common cause of irritation and discomfort of the eyes, as well as visual difficulties.**
- **Keep hands away from eyes. Rubbing the eyelids causes irritation and may introduce infection, leading to blepharitis and conjunctivitis.**
- **Do not use eyecups (fortunately now less popular). They can spread infection or cause injury.**
- **Avoid direct exposure of the eyes to sun lamps. They can burn the lids and the cornea, as can excessive exposure to sunlight at the beach or on snow-covered ground. Ultraviolet rays can cause painful burns that are not apparent for several hours after overexposure.**

### FIRST AID

**Removing a Foreign Body from the Eye.** Almost everyone has suffered the exquisite discomfort of a foreign body in the eye. A cinder barely large enough to be seen feels like a boulder. A foreign body may be removed by the nurse if:

- It is not on the cornea.
- It has not penetrated the eyeball (e.g., a sharp splinter of metal or wood that has pierced the eyeball).
- It is displaced readily by a sterile applicator.

The first requisite is a good light. The patient should be reminded not to rub the eye. This is an urge that is hard to resist when a foreign body is present, but it may lead to further injury and irritation or to imbedding the particle. The nurse's hands should be washed thoroughly. With the patient seated, the eye should be examined, including the inside of the upper and lower lids. To evert the upper lid, the nurse lays a toothpick swab just back from the edge of the upper lid, grasps the lashes gently but firmly with her other hand, pulls the upper lid slightly outward from the eye, and turns it upward to expose the underside of the lid.

When she locates the tiny particle, she touches it gently with a sterile swab moistened in clear water or sterile saline. (The latter is preferable, if it is available.) If the particle is not readily removed in this manner, further attempts to remove it should be avoided. Picking at it with the swab can push it into the tissues and may injure the eye. The nurse should explain to the patient that the services of an ophthalmologist are needed, and help the patient to make arrangements for further care, either in the physician's office or at an eye clinic. She should assure the patient that this referral does not necessarily mean that there is anything seriously wrong, but only that the physician's skill is needed to remove the particle safely. A similar explanation can be made if the foreign body is on the cornea. Attempts to remove it could lead to scarring of the cornea and to diminished vision. The physician uses the slit-lamp microscope and other delicate instruments to remove the particle with the least possible injury to the cornea.

Irrigating the eye with sterile saline is also effective in removing a foreign body. An irrigating tip attached to a flask of sterile saline may be used for this purpose, in a manner similar to that used when acids or other irritants are splashed unexpectedly into the eye.

After the particle has been removed, the patient usually continues to feel some irritation. An oval eye pad applied over the closed lids with Scotch tape affords relief. The patient should be instructed not to rub his eye, and, if it is not completely comfortable within a short time, he should be instructed to visit an ophthalmologist.

**Irrigation.** Splashing an irritating chemical, such as bleach, into the eye is another common emergency. The eye should be flushed copiously with water to remove the chemical as promptly as possible. If sterile saline is available, it should be used, but the irrigation should not be delayed to obtain it. Plain tap water should be used instead. If the accident occurs in the home or at work, the patient should be taken to the nearest sink or water fountain, where he should hold his eyelids open while the water cleanses the eye. The importance of speed cannot be overemphasized, because the longer the chemical is in contact with the eye, the more damage it does. The same procedure is followed if an eyedrop is instilled into the wrong eye, or if the wrong kind of medication is used. After irrigation, the patient is instructed to close his eye, and an eye pad is applied over the lid and held in place with Scotch tape. The patient is taken immediately to an ophthalmologist or to a hospital emergency room for further treatment.

Usually, further irrigation with sterile saline is carried out at the physician's office or the clinic. A flask of sterile saline is hung on an infusion pole about six inches above the eye, and, by means of rubber tubing and an irrigating tip, copious amounts of the solution are used to flush away the harmful chemical. The patient may be draped with a plastic apron like those used in beauty parlors to prevent wetting his clothing. The return flow is caught in a large emesis basin. The patient lies on a cot or is seated in a chair that can be placed quickly in a reclining position. The flow of solution is directed from the inner canthus to the outer canthus, so that it does not flow into the opposite eye. If both eyes must be irrigated, it is preferable to have two nurses, or a nurse and an assistant, work simultaneously. If this is not possible, the person performing the irrigation switches the flow from one eye to the other frequently, so that both eyes are irrigated as quickly and thoroughly as possible. The upper lid is everted and any solid particles, such as lime, are carefully washed out.

## SOME EYE DISORDERS

### Refractive Errors

The cornea, the aqueous humor, the lens, and the vitreous humor constitute the *refractive media* of the eye. Ocular refraction is the process by which rays of light are "bent" so that they will focus on

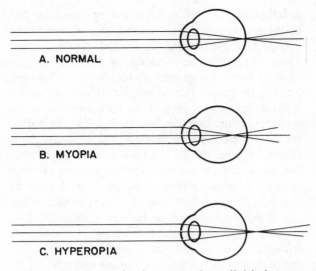

**Figure 26-5.** Ocular focusing of parallel light rays.

the retina. Normally, all the refractive media are transparent.

Refractive errors are the most common type of eye disorder, resulting when the refractive media do not converge light rays to a focus on the retina (Fig. 26-5). Many refractive errors have a tendency to be inherited.

**Myopia (Nearsightedness).** Myopia usually results from elongation of the eyeball. Because of the excessive length of the eyeball, light rays focus at a point in the vitreous humor before reaching the retina.

**Hyperopia (Farsightedness).** Hyperopia results when the eyeball is shorter than normal, causing the light rays to focus at a theoretic point behind the retina.

**Astigmatism.** Astigmatism results from unequal curvatures in the shape of the cornea or, sometimes, of the lens. Vision is distorted. For example, a straight object may appear to be slanted to the patient. Often a patient has both astigmatism and myopia or hyperopia. Astigmatism is corrected by cylindrical lenses.

Myopia, hyperopia, and astigmatism can cause diminished and blurred vision. The individual with myopia must bring things close to his eyes to see them, whereas in hyperopia objects are seen better at a distance. These conditions are corrected by lenses that bend light rays in a way that compensates for the patient's refractive error.

The shape of the lens is changed by the action of the ciliary muscle, thus providing the eye with a focusing mechanism. This process is known as *accommodation.* The lens is elastic and pliable in youth and early adult life.

**Presbyopia.** Presbyopia is caused by the gradual loss, during middle life and old age, of the elasticity of the lens which leads to a decreased ability to accommodate for near vision. As a result, small objects and print must be held farther and farther away to be seen clearly.

This loss begins in youth and progresses gradually. By the time the person is in his 40's the loss is sufficiently marked to interfere with reading and other close work. These presbyopic symptoms are noticed earlier by hyperopes and later by myopes. The latter may read comfortably without glasses even during old age.

CORRECTIVE GLASSES. To alleviate this condition bifocals are often prescribed. They are really two

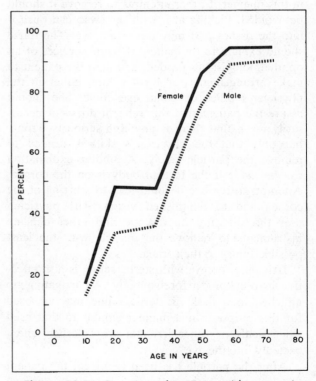

**Figure 26-6.** Per cent of persons with corrective lenses, by sex and age. Note the marked increase with advancing age. (U.S. Department of Health, Education, and Welfare: *Characteristics of Persons with Corrective Lenses,* Washington, D.C., U.S. Government Printing Office)

pairs of glasses in one: the lower part is for near vision; the upper part, for distance vision. The glasses permit the patient to see both near and distant objects clearly. A further refinement is the use of trifocals (three strengths of lens in one glass), which some patients find even more effective for viewing objects at various distances. Bifocals with a plain upper portion are used sometimes for those who need no distance correction, so that glasses do not have to be removed and replaced constantly. Halfmoon or "half-eye" lenses serve the same purpose.

Unlike other refractive errors, presbyopia is a normal condition that occurs in all people who live long enough to develop it. Like graying hair, presbyopia is an obvious indication of aging. The need for glasses may be ignored or denied, sometimes to the inconvenience or even the hazard of the individual and others. Nurses in industry should encourage older workers to compensate for their loss in accommodation by obtaining corrective glasses and by wearing them whenever they are needed. This makes the disorder less conspicuous, and permits the worker to maintain his efficiency with added safety.

In all types of refractive error, the nurse has an obligation to encourage the patient to wear his glasses as directed. Leaving them off lessens his efficiency as well as his comfort (headache and a feeling of strain are common), and may lead to accidents. The nurse can also be alert for signs that may indicate a need for glasses (squinting, wrinkling the forehead, holding objects too close or too far away), and she can advise the individual to consult an ophthalmologist.

CONTACT LENSES. Contact lenses are tiny, almost completely invisible plastic lenses that fit directly over the cornea, separated from it only by the tear film. They are worn by people who object to the appearance of conventional glasses, or by those with special needs that can be met more adequately by contact lenses. Often patients who have had cataracts removed see very well with contact lenses, and the new soft lens is useful in the treatment of corneal disease and in cases of intolerance to hard conventional lenses.

Contact lenses are expensive, and require patience and effort to wear successfully. Because not all people who desire contact lenses can or should wear them, patients who are interested in them should be referred to the ophthalmologist. If it is decided that the patient is a suitable candidate, he is carefully fitted with lenses and instructed in their use. Since they are foreign bodies, and at first may cause discomfort, the patient wears them for only a short period at first and gradually for longer intervals. Eventually most patients can wear them all day without discomfort.

The most common dangers involved in the use of contact lenses are injury and infection of the cornea.

A special type of contact lens, the scleral lens, fits the entire front of the eyeball. Scleral lenses are sometimes prescribed for treatment of certain diseases of the cornea or conjunctiva, and are occasionally worn by athletes.

## Cataract

Many people think of a cataract as a "growth over the eye," perhaps because of the strange whitish appearance of the pupil, which is sometimes seen in this condition. Actually, a cataract is a condition in which the lens of the eye becomes opaque (no longer transparent). Normally, the lens is not visible; only the pupil is seen. When the patient's lens becomes opaque, it may become visible as a white or a gray spot behind the pupil.

Vision diminishes as the lens becomes opalescent. The process usually advances slowly, eventually leading to loss of sight. When both eyes are severely affected, the patient becomes blind. Cataracts are the most common cause of legal blindness.

Cataracts may be congenital, caused by injury to the lens, or secondary to other diseases of the eye. When they occur in response to injury, they usually develop quickly. Most cataracts, however, are caused by degenerative changes associated with the aging process, and they tend to develop slowly. Although some people develop cataracts in earlier life, the incidence of the condition rises steadily with advancing years. Cataracts are especially common among persons in the seventh, eighth and ninth decades of life. A high incidence of cataracts occurs among patients with certain diseases, such as diabetes. A family history of cataracts is often pronounced.

**Treatment.** The treatment of cataracts involves removing the lens when vision is sufficiently impaired; changing eyeglasses does not cause improvement. No way has yet been found to restore the lens to its normal transparency. Removal of the lens is necessary, because its opacity prevents light rays from reaching the retina. The lens may be removed by the intracapsular method (removal of the lens within its capsule) or by the extracapsular method (removal of the lens, leaving the posterior portion of its capsule in position). The choice of method is made by the surgeon after considering the patient's age and the degree of opacity (often called "ripeness") of the cataract. The intracapsular extraction is the most common method. The operation is often done under local anesthesia, but general anesthesia is sometimes used and has certain advantages especially in the case of a very apprehensive patient. An enzyme, alpha-chymotrypsin, is often used to dissolve the lens ligaments, thus facilitating removal of the cataract. A recent development has been the use of a probe cooled to very low temperatures. The cataract is partially frozen and extracted in contact with the cold probe. This technique is known as cryosurgery. Implantation of intraocular lenses (i.e., substituting a plastic lens for the lens that has been removed) is being done in certain centers.

Modern techniques of cataract surgery result in success in over 95 per cent of cases. Most surgeons are using the operating microscope to attain excellent results.

After his lens has been removed, the patient must wear a strong lens (eyeglass) to take its place. The correcting lens causes the patient to see objects about one third larger than a normal eye sees them. If both eyes have had the lens removed, the patient can continue to use both eyes simultaneously. However, if only one eye has had the lens removed, the patient must use only one eye at a time. Contact lenses usually solve this problem. Some patients can be fitted with a contact lens for the aphakic eye (the eye from which the lens has been removed). The use of the contact lens lessens the difference in the size of the image perceived by each eye and makes binocular vision possible.

Two major complications of cataract extraction are loss of vitreous humor and hemorrhage. Loss of vitreous humor can occur during or after surgery; it is serious, because vitreous does not regenerate, and its loss may cause serious damage to the eye. Hemorrhage can injure the delicate structures of the eye. Special care is taken during the postoperative period to prevent straining, such as straining at stool, and sudden movement or jarring of the head, which might lead to hemorrhage or opening of the incision. The details of nursing care are discussed later in this chapter.

Nurses can encourage elderly people with cataracts to seek treatment. Often elderly patients and their families have the belief that "nothing can be done because of age." Loss of vision is thus added to other restrictions imposed by advanced age. Cataract extraction usually can be performed safely on even the very old. The operation restores useful vision to many older persons, enabling them to maintain their interests, independence, and contact with others. The elderly are especially vulnerable to the isolation and the dependence that can result from loss of vision. Being able to see may mean the difference between the patient's continued ability to live in his own home or having to live in an institution or with relatives.

The hospital stay after cataract extraction has been reduced to a few days. However, after the patient returns home he requires assistance for a time with such tasks as shopping and cleaning. It is important to plan with the patient for this period of convalescence.

## Glaucoma

Glaucoma is the term for a group of conditions that result in increased intraocular pressure due to a disturbance of the normal balance between the production and the drainage of the aqueous humor that fills the anterior chamber of the eye. Sometimes, this disturbance is caused by a narrowing of the angle leading to the drainage channels around the anterior chamber (closed-angle glaucoma). In other instances the angle appears to be open, but the drainage channels are obstructed (open-angle or chronic simple glaucoma). This latter form is more common. Glaucoma may also arise as a complication of other eye disease such as injury, inflammation, tumor, or detached retina. This form is termed secondary glaucoma.

If the increased intraocular pressure is not relieved, the eye will be damaged. The optic nerve is especially vulnerable to injury from increased pressure, and if it is damaged, it does not regenerate. Partial or total blindness can result from an acute attack of closed-angle type glaucoma. Visual impairment due to an injury of the optic nerve is permanent, even though pressure in the eyeball later may be relieved by treatment. Open-angle glaucoma is more insidious, because it progresses slowly and often painlessly.

Although glaucoma can occur at any age, it is most common in people over 40. Anatomic abnormalities and degenerative changes play a part in causing glaucoma, and commonly there is a family history of glaucoma.

Prompt diagnosis and treatment are essential in preventing loss of vision. Everyone should be examined regularly for early indications of glaucoma. Anyone who experiences symptoms that might indicate glaucoma should promptly consult an ophthalmologist.

### Acute Glaucoma

**Symptoms.** Symptoms include severe pain in and around the eyes, blurred vision, and the appearance of halos (colored circles), around lights. The attack also may be accompanied by nausea and vomiting, and a steamy appearance of the cornea. Acute attacks can occur suddenly, with little or no warning. Emotional stress sometimes triggers an attack.

**Drug Therapy.** Miotics (drugs that constrict the pupil) are given at once to pull the iris away from the drainage channels, so that drainage of aqueous humor can resume, thus reducing the intraocular pressure and relieving the symptoms. Acetazolamide (Diamox) or other carbonic anhydrase inhibitors are given to slow the production of aqueous humor, thus helping to decrease the intraocular pressure. Urea and mannitol are given intravenously for the same purpose. Glycerol, given by mouth with orange or lime juice, is also effective. Such agents are likely to be used just before surgery, in order to lower intraocular pressure, thus rendering the operation safer. Analgesics are given to relieve pain.

**Surgery.** Early surgical intervention is usually indicated to relieve acute glaucoma and to prevent further attacks. *Iridectomy* is performed to relieve the symptoms of acute closed-angle glaucoma: a section of iris is removed, thus preventing it from bulging forward, crowding the chamber angle, and obstructing the drainage of aqueous humor. Thus, a permanent entrance to the drainage canal is achieved. Two types of iridectomy are the *peripheral,* in which a small section of iris is removed at the periphery, and sector or *keyhole iridectomy,* in which a larger segment of iris is removed (Fig. 26-7). Local anesthesia is usually sufficient for both types of iridectomy. The operated eye is covered with a patch postoperatively.

Continued medical supervision is essential after the patient has had surgery. Nurses can help to prevent visual loss by emphasizing the need for con-

tinued medical care, and by participating in planned health supervision.

### Chronic Glaucoma

**Symptoms.** Chronic glaucoma occurs more frequently than acute glaucoma. Often, symptoms are absent, or they are not as dramatic and therefore are more readily disregarded. The patient may have occasional periods when he sees halos around lights, has blurred vision, and experiences some discomfort or aching of the eyes. These mild symptoms are sometimes precipitated by prolonged watching of TV or moving pictures, or by emotional upsets. These subacute attacks are transient, but are warnings of angle-closure.

Sometimes, a reduction in the field of vision is the first indication of chronic glaucoma. The patient may fail to see things on either side and appear to be awkward or clumsy by bumping into doors or furniture. The impairment of peripheral vision is a hazard if the person drives a car, because he is unable to see pedestrians or vehicles that are off to the side. Sometimes the patient's family is the first to notice this visual defect, perhaps after a near miss on the highway.

**Drug Therapy.** Patients who exhibit such symptoms should seek medical attention promptly. Miotics, such as eserine, pilocarpine, or carbamylcholine chloride (Carbachol) are used. Newer long-acting miotics include echothiopate iodide (phospholine iodide) which requires instillation only once or twice in 24 hours. Epinephrine is also used as eyedrops in open-angle glaucoma.

Carbonic anhydrase inhibitors, such as acetazolamide (Diamox), are often prescribed. When medical treatment is no longer effective, surgery is considered. Some of these patients require iridectomy if chronic angle-closure is present.

**Surgery.** Surgery for glaucoma is usually carried out under local anesthesia. Drainage operations frequently performed for chronic glaucoma include

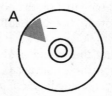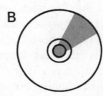

**Figure 26-7.** (*A*) Appearance of the eye after peripheral iridectomy. (*B*) After keyhole (sector) iridectomy.

sclerectomy, trephination, iridencleisis, and thermal sclerostomy. In trephining, a button of cornea and sclera is removed to allow aqueous humor to seep under the conjunctiva. In iridencleisis the iris is cut and inverted to form a wick that provides a filtering tract under the conjunctiva. Scleral lip and limbal lip cautery are procedures that also involve establishment of a permanent filtering tract between the anterior chamber and the subconjunctiva.

Only the operated eye is covered with a patch after surgery. A new microsurgical procedure known as trabeculectomy is now also being performed. These operations are not always successful. A common complication is the development of cataracts.

### General Measures

All patients with glaucoma (even those who have had surgery) require continued care and examinations as recommended by the ophthalmologist. Certain general measures also can help to control the condition. The patient should be instructed to:

- Avoid wearing a too tight collar.
- Avoid drinking too much fluid at one time.
- Avoid emotional upsets.
- Avoid heavy lifting. (This, too, can raise intraocular pressure.)
- Limit activities that make the eyes feel strained or fatigued (e.g., prolonged reading).
- Keep an extra supply of prescribed drugs on hand for vacations, over holidays, or in case of loss.
- Carry a card stating that he has glaucoma, so that necessary therapy can be continued even if he is sick or hurt.

Extreme care must be taken in administering eyedrops to any patient and especially to patients with glaucoma. If through error a mydriatic, such as atropine, is given, the resulting dilation of the pupil can further obstruct drainage of aqueous humor, precipitating an acute attack that could result in permanent blindness. *No amount of caution is too great to prevent such a tragedy*. Notice carefully which eye is to receive the medication, read the physician's order and the label on the bottle carefully, and identify the patient before instilling the drop in his eye.

There is less danger of using the wrong medication at home than in the hospital, because the patient usually possesses only the medication prescribed for him. Hospitalized patients should keep their own eyedrops at the bedside to avoid the possibility of receiving the wrong medication, and to reduce the possibility of transmitting infection.

### Detached Retina

In detached retina the sensory layer becomes separated from the pigmented layer of the retina. The separation of the two layers of the retina deprives the sensory layer of its full blood supply. Vision is lost in the affected area, because the sensory layer is no longer able to receive visual stimuli. Fluid from the vitreous flows between the separated layers of the retina, holding them apart and causing further separation.

Retinal separation is usually associated with a hole or a tear in the retina, which results from stretching or from degenerative changes in the retina. Sometimes, retinal detachment follows a sudden blow, a penetrating injury, or surgery on the eye (especially cataract removal). Loss of vitreous is particularly liable to lead to retinal detachment. It may be a complication of other disorders, such as myopia or advanced diabetic changes in the retina. Retinal separation occurs more commonly among those over 40.

**Symptoms.** Symptoms may occur gradually or very suddenly. The severity of the symptoms and the speed of their onset depend on the size of the area affected, as well as its location. The destruction of vision at the macula causes far greater visual loss than damage to an area of comparable size on the periphery of the retina. The patient often notices definite "gaps" in his vision or areas in which he cannot see. Sometimes, he has the feeling that a curtain is being drawn over his field of vision, and he commonly sees flashes of light. The sensation of spots or moving particles before the eyes is common. Complete loss of vision may occur in the affected eye. The patient has no pain, but he is usually extremely apprehensive.

Although the prognosis is guarded, it is now more favorable because of advances in surgical treatment. This is especially true when the patient comes for treatment immediately after the occurrence of detachment.

**Diagnosis and Treatment.** Prompt diagnosis and treatment are essential. After examining the patient's retina with the ophthalmoscope and establishing the diagnosis, prompt admission to the hospital is usually recommended. The physician's orders on admission usually include bed rest and the use of mydriatics to dilate the pupil, thus facilitating further examination.

The aim of surgery is to reattach the retina to the choroid by removing the subretinal fluid and sealing retinal holes. This is done under general anesthesia.

SURGERY. An operation often used is *scleral buckling.* This operation is performed on the section of the sclera that overlies the retinal detachment. A section of sclera (about two thirds of its depth) is removed surgically. Diathermy is applied to this raw area of sclera. The fluid separating the layers of retina is drained off. A piece of polyethylene tubing is placed over the raw surface of the sclera, and the two edges of the incision are drawn together (over the tubing) by sutures. The portion of sclera that has been thinned buckles (bends) inward as the sutures are drawn together. The diathermy applied to the denuded sclera causes inflammation of the deeper tissues, which helps to seal the holes in the retina by causing the formation of adhesions. The surgery accomplishes two objectives: draining the fluid that lies between the layers of the retina, and inducing inflammation of the choroid that overlies the hole(s) in the retina.

Another type of operation, is called *retinopexy,* in which diathermy is applied to the sclera, without thinning the sclera and making it buckle inward. The subretinal fluid also is drained off, and the hole is sealed by diathermy. Cryosurgery is replacing diathermy since it is less damaging to the sclera.

When retinal holes have been detected, but the retina has not yet been detached, the holes may be sealed with a process like "spot welding." This may be achieved by diathermy, cryosurgery, or using an intense light beam shone into the eye through the pupil (light coagulation).

**Postoperative Care.** After scleral buckling the patient returns from the operating room with both eyes covered. Although physicians' specific instructions vary, many patients who have scleral buckling are permitted out of bed the next day. Frequently, the patient may go home approximately one week after surgery. He is instructed to avoid jarring or bumping his head, and not to do any heavy lifting. He is advised to wear dark glasses for several weeks, thereby preventing the discomfort from bright light that occurs after treatment with mydriatics.

### Injuries and Diseases of the Cornea

Scarring and opacity of the cornea can convert it from a window that admits light to a barrier that excludes it. Any disorder of the cornea is potentially serious, and may lead to severe visual impairment or even blindness. Scars and opacification of the cornea can result from injury, such as might be caused by a foreign body or infection, or from inflammation of the eyeball, or diseases of the cornea.

Corneal lesions may be outlined by the instillation of fluorescein, a green dye. The use of this drug is potentially dangerous, because the solution readily becomes contaminated and can transmit infection from one patient to another. Extreme care must be taken (by hand washing and the use of a sterile dropper) to prevent contamination. Many hospitals now use small, single-dose sterile containers of fluorescein. The container is opened for each individual patient, and any unused drug is discarded. A fluorescein-impregnated sterile filter paper also is available and is considered safer than liquid fluorescein for staining the cornea. The filter paper is touched to the inner surface of the lower lid after the paper has been moistened with a drop of sterile saline. The technique is used in applanation tonometry.

Ulcers may form on the cornea in response to various types of physical or chemical injury, as well as local infections and systemic disorders such as dysentery. They are treated by resting the eye. Cycloplegic drops are usually used to dilate the pupil and rest the ciliary muscle. Antibiotic or sulfonamide eyedrops or ointments are employed to combat bacterial infection. Idoxuridine is used for herpes simplex ulceration. The eye is usually covered with an eye pad. Analgesics are often required since corneal ulcers are painful. The patient is cautioned not to rub or touch the eye, thus preventing further irritation. Ulcers leave scars. A tiny ulcer in the periphery does not affect vision significantly, but central ulcers or multiple ulcers can lead to scars that seriously impair vision. The soft contact lens is now used as a "bandage" to the cornea in treating certain types of chronic ulcerations.

*Keratitis,* an inflammation of the cornea, may result from local infection or from involvement by systemic disease (such as tuberculosis or congenital syphilis). Herpes simplex is a common virus disease that causes keratitis. Fungus infections of the cornea are also seen. The symptoms of keratitis include redness, tearing, photophobia, and pain. Treatment includes antibiotics, chemotherapeutic agents, and cycloplegics. Although steroids and chemotherapeutic agents may not cure the condition, they are sometimes useful in reducing the inflammatory reaction of the tissues, thus helping to prevent scarring while the patient's own resistance and other treatment bring the condition under control. Steroids used alone can be dangerous, because they relieve the symptoms but do not cure the disease. Topical steroids are very dangerous if herpes keratitis is present.

**Preventive Measures.** Prompt treatment of injuries or infections of the cornea is essential to prevent serious scarring. Some preventive measures include:

- Using protective goggles in hazardous occupations. For example, with metal workers, pieces of steel often become embedded in the cornea. Industrial nurses can help to educate workers to the need for compliance with rules for wearing the goggles. All persons who have lost an eye or have useful vision in only one eye, should wear protective goggles when exposed to possible injuries, or at all times if they have a refractive error requiring eyeglasses. The lenses may be specially toughened glass or plastic.
- Keeping the hands away from the eyes. If the eye must be touched, the hands should be washed first. (This rule has special relevance for nurses, who must often handle infectious material, such as soiled dressings.)
- Avoiding attempts to remove a foreign body on the cornea—one's own or another person's. Seek the services of an ophthalmologist.
- Seeking treatment promptly for any symptoms of injury or infection of the eye, such as foreign body sensations, scratchiness, or tearing.
- Not touching the eye with the nozzle of an eyedrop bottle when instilling drops.

**Emergencies.** The extent and nature of the injury caused by a chemical on the eye depend upon the duration of contact and the penetrability into the tissues as well as the chemical reaction with the tissues. The first essential in treatment is to remove the noxious agent as completely and rapidly as possible. In practice this is best achieved with the nearest water available. As an emergency measure thorough lavage is more effective than using a specific neutralizing agent if this involves loss of time, as is usually the case. For a complete list of groups of noxious chemicals and specific neutralizing agents, a textbook of ophthalmology should be studied. It should be emphasized that first-aid treatment must be immediate to be valuable.

**Corneal Transplantation (Keratoplasty).** When scarring of the cornea results in serious impairment of vision, sight can often be restored by transplanting a portion of a normal cornea to the eye of the patient whose cornea has become scarred. The possibility of using an artificial plastic cornea as replacement for the patient's cornea is being studied.

In this procedure, the opaque portion of the patient's cornea is removed, and a piece of the donor's cornea is sutured into its place carefully to ensure perfect fit. Some tissues of the graft are retained; others eventually are replaced by comparable tissues formed by the patient's own cornea. A proportion of corneal grafts become opaque. Often this happens because of an immunologic process called rejection.

The patient must stay flat and keep his head in one position for approximately one week after the operation. Any sudden movement, or the strain of coughing, vomiting, or sneezing might cause displacement of the graft before healing has had an opportunity to take place. The importance of helping the patient to remain quiet and to follow the physician's orders cannot be overestimated. The supply of donor eyes is very limited; this restricts the opportunities that the patient has for the restoration of his sight. When the period of strict bed rest is over, the patient must continue to be cautious and only gradually resume his activities.

Anyone may provide that, at death, his eyes be donated to restore sight to a blind person. Information can be obtained from each state's agency for the blind. Within a few hours after the donor's death, his eyes are removed and are promptly used to provide a corneal graft. Since fresh donor cornea often must be used promptly, special arrangements are necessary to see that the cornea from the donated eye is delivered quickly and in good condition to the patient who needs it. More recently, processes have been developed to preserve and store corneas for longer periods of time. Eye banks are located in various parts of the country. The supply of donor eyes is very limited. This restricts the opportunities that the patient has for restoration of his sight.

## Uveitis

*Uveitis* means inflammation of the uveal tract (iris, ciliary body, choroid). Any or all of these structures may be involved in the inflammatory process. Uveitis may be caused by injury or by local or systemic disease, but usually its cause remains undetermined. Symptoms include redness of the eye, photophobia, tearing, pain, and blurred vision. The pupil tends to be constricted.

Mydriatics, such as atropine, are used to dilate the pupil, thus helping to prevent the formation of adhesions between the iris and the anterior lens capsule. Analgesics are given to lessen pain. Steroids often are used to relieve the inflammation. Antibiotics may be given to control infection, and hot compresses are sometimes ordered to help to relieve pain.

Often uveitis is difficult to cure, and recurrences are common. It is a serious condition that can lead to cataract, glaucoma, or even destruction of the eye.

### Hordeolum

The term *hordeolum* means sty, an infection at the edge of the eyelid, which originates in a lash follicle. The sty starts as a red, painful swelling, which increases, and usually ruptures, releasing pus. After the pus has drained out, the pain diminishes, and the lesion heals spontaneously. Styes are treated by hot wet compresses that help to localize the infection. Often the causative organism is the staphylococcus. A single sty usually requires no treatment other than hot compresses. Occasionally, incision and drainage, the use of antibiotics, and immunization by vaccines are necessary. Often, people who have repeated styes have poor general health and lowered resistance to infection. Careful hand washing is important after any contact with exudate from the lesion. The patient should be cautioned not to handle the lid and not to pick or squeeze the sty, because this can result in the spread of the infection.

### Chalazion

Small, modified sebaceous glands called meibomian glands, are located within both eyelids, in the tarsal plates.

These glands secrete an oily substance that prevents the tear film on the eyeball from evaporating. A chalazion is an infection of a meibomian gland. It forms a firm swelling, which remains in the lid until it is excised. Sometimes a chalazion causes irritation of the cornea by constantly rubbing over it. It is usually removed surgically by the ophthalmologist. This procedure usually is performed in the physician's office or the clinic. Occasionally it is done in the operating room, especially for multiple chalazia.

### Conjunctivitis

Conjunctivitis is inflammation of the palpebral conjunctiva. The conjunctiva becomes red and irritated, and often forms an excessive secretion of mucus, which may become purulent.

*Pink-eye* is a term used to describe some forms of conjunctivitis. It may be due to a wide variety of causes, such as infection with the Koch-Weeks bacillus (which may be epidemic), or to the pneumococcus. Prevention involves hand washing before touching the eyes. Treatment depends on the cause (e.g., the type of antibiotic ordered is determined by the organism that causes the condition). Accurate diagnosis by the ophthalmologist is essential. Delay in seeking medical care and the use of self-medication should be strongly discouraged. Meticulous hand washing and the use of separate towels and bedding are essential in preventing the spread of infection.

Conjunctivitis can also be caused by allergy. Like other allergic reactions, it is treated by avoidance of the allergen, by antihistamines and occasionally by desensitization. Among the many other causes of conjunctivitis are viruses, chemical irritants, smoke, and dust. There is usually some degree of conjunctivitis in the presence of a corneal ulcer or keratitis.

### Ectropion, Entropion, Ptosis

These conditions usually are treated surgically. They are defined as follows:

*Ectropion* is a turning out of the eyelid. It is often seen in the elderly. Tearing often occurs, because the tears are not carried off in the normal manner, due to the abnormal position of the lid.

*Entropion* is a turning in of the eyelid, due to spasm. The lashes may rub against the cornea and irritate it. This occurs commonly among the elderly.

*Ptosis* is a drooping of the upper eyelid, due to congenital deformity, injury or neurologic disorder.

### Sympathetic Ophthalmia

Perforative injury of one eye sometimes results in the development of severe inflammation of the fellow eye. This rare condition is called *sympathetic ophthalmia*. Typically several weeks after serious injury to one eye, involving the ciliary body, the other eye develops severe uveitis that eventually may lead to loss of sight.

The cause of sympathetic ophthalmia is unknown. It is most likely to occur after penetrating injuries of the eyeball. Therefore, it is sometimes necessary to remove a severely injured eye (enucleation) without delay, to avoid risk to the unaffected eye and the possible loss of sight in both eyes. Recently, however, corticosteroids have proved to be so effective that enucleation is often avoided.

Frequently, enucleation is resisted by the patient and his family because they feel that while the patient still has the eye, there is hope that it will heal. In addition to the psychological trauma accompanying the loss of use of the eye, there is the loss of a part of oneself. Because the mechanism of sympathetic ophthalmia is mysterious, it is difficult for a patient to believe that such a thing could happen to the unaffected eye.

The nurse can help the patient and his family by letting them express their fears and disbeliefs and ask questions. It is essential that the nurse know just what the physician has told the patient and his family. She may discover that further discussion between patient and physician is needed to clarify information and to allay fears and doubts. The nurse develops her plan for teaching and emotional support in light of her assessment of the patient's requirements, and in collaboration with the physician.

### Enucleation

Removal of the eye may also be necessary when the eye has been destroyed by injury or disease. Such blind eyes sometimes develop malignant tumors. Fortunately these are not common. However, removal of the eye is necessary when a tumor is discovered, to prevent the spread of malignant cells to other parts of the body. Sometimes, the eye is removed to relieve pain, when it has been severely damaged by injury or disease, and is blind. It is a usual practice for a second ophthalmologist to examine the patient in consultation before enucleation is carried out.

The terms *enucleation* and *evisceration* have different meanings. *Evisceration* means that the contents of the eyeball have been removed, leaving the sclera in place. *Enucleation* means removal of the entire eyeball.

When enucleation is performed, a ball made of metal or plastic usually is buried in the capsule of connective tissue from which the eyeball has been removed. The eye muscles attach to this capsule and give movement to the ball that it now contains. After the tissues have healed, a glass or plastic prosthesis, shaped like a shell, is placed over the buried ball. The shell is painted to match the patient's remaining eye, and it is the part that sometimes is referred to as a "glass eye." The artificial eye thus consists of two parts:

1. A buried ball (called an *implant*) that moves and is invisible.
2. A visible shell-shaped portion that closely resembles the patient's other eye and moves when the buried ball is moved by the eye muscles.

Every patient whose eye must be removed needs help in understanding the necessity for the operation, as well as explanation concerning the use of a prosthesis. Artificial eyes now are made so skillfully that others are often unaware without close scrutiny, that the patient has lost an eye.

Depression is common after the operation. No amount of explanation or reassurance erases the fact that the patient has lost his eye, and that the loss is irretrievable. Most patients gradually are able to accept the result of enucleation, and become eager to acquire and learn to use the prosthesis.

After enucleation, a pressure dressing is applied for five days. The patient is observed carefully for any symptoms of bleeding or infection. The dressing is changed by the surgeon. Usually, the patient is allowed out of bed the day after the operation.

Although a temporary shell may be fitted much sooner, when healing is complete (approximately two to four weeks), the patient is fitted with the prosthesis. He learns to insert and to remove the prosthesis himself. He removes it before going to bed at night, and inserts it the next morning. When the patient is learning to insert and to remove the prosthesis, he should hold his head over a soft surface, such as a bed or a well-padded table, so that the shell will not be broken if it is dropped. The shell is cleansed gently after removal, and it is kept in a safe place where it will not be scratched or broken.

The patient removes the shell by placing one hand under his artificial eye, pulling the lower lid down, and slipping the lower edge of the prosthesis out, so that it is in front of the lower lid. He then places his finger on the upper eyelid and pushes down gently. This pushes the prosthesis down out of the socket and into his cupped hand. The shell is inserted by raising the upper lid, drawing it slightly outward, and sliding the prosthesis under the upper lid. One finger holds the shell in this position, while the lower lid is pulled down, and the lower edge of the prosthesis is slipped behind the lower lid. One side of the artificial eye is more pointed than the other. The more pointed side of the artificial eye is placed nearest the nose; the less pointed side is on the outside. The procedure is done quickly, and it is painless. A properly fitted prosthesis does not cause discomfort. Careful personal hygiene is important to maintain a clean socket. Thorough washing of hands is essential before inserting and removing the prosthesis.

The sudden loss of a nondiseased eye necessitates adjustment to the use of just one eye. At first the patient is very much aware of his "blind side." He can no longer see objects on that side without a conscious effort to turn his head. The field of vision is restricted, but the patient learns to compensate for this loss and soon can carry out his daily activities very well. Special care must be taken to prevent damage to the remaining eye. The patient needs help in achieving a balance between measures to prevent injury and the resumption of normal living. He should not deliberately take chances; on the other hand, he should not be afraid to go out of the house lest a cinder blow in his eye. The wearing of unbreakable glasses is recommended to protect the remaining eye.

## THE PATIENT WHO HAS HAD EYE SURGERY

Any eye disease, injury, or operation can be upsetting and even frightening because of its possible effect on vision. The patient can be helped by careful explanation of his condition and his treatment by both the physician and the nurse.

Some patients experience photophobia. Turning the bed so that it does not face the window and adjusting the blinds to keep out direct sunlight are important comfort measures. Often, the patient is instructed to wear dark glasses to protect his eyes from excessive light and glare.

### Preoperative Care

Many patients with eye disorders come to the hospital for surgery. At the time of admission the patient may have diminished or absent vision; sometimes, as in corneal transplantation, he enters the hospital in the hope that his vision will be improved by an operation. In other instances the patient has useful vision on admission, but, because of the kind of operation to be performed, both eyes may be covered during the immediate postoperative period. Since both eyes move together, it is often necessary to cover both eyes to provide rest for the eye that has had surgery (e.g., after detached retina surgery).

**Admission Procedure.** The admission procedure should be modified to help both types of patient. If the patient cannot see, a special effort should be made to help him become oriented to his surroundings. He should be introduced to the other patients in the room. If he is able, he should be allowed to walk about his room with assistance, noting the location of the furniture, the bathroom, and particularly the call bell, so that he knows how to call for help when he needs it. A walk about the ward, with the nurse showing him the location of other rooms, nurses' station, and lounge, also helps him to form a mental picture of his new surroundings.

If, on the other hand, the patient can see and later will have both eyes covered, he should be helped to use his sight to the greatest advantage in orienting himself to his room, his neighbors, and the ward as a whole. The next day, when his eyes are covered, he will be able to recall the layout of his new surroundings, and he will feel less lost and confused. If both eyes are to be covered, even though only one actually will have surgery, it is important that this be explained to the patient, so that later he does not fear that some injury or complication has befallen his unaffected eye.

**Sedation.** Usually, the preoperative preparation includes sedation to ensure rest the night before surgery, and relaxation before the patient goes to the operating room. Elderly patients should be observed carefully after sedatives have been administered. Sometimes, the patient becomes disoriented and restless after the administration of sedatives, particularly barbiturates.

**Eyedrop Technique.** Often, eyedrops, such as antibiotics or mydriatics, are ordered at specified intervals. When the nurse instills an eyedrop, the patient should be lying down or seated, with his head tilted backward. The hand in which she holds the dropper should rest against the patient's forehead. (The little finger and the side of the hand rest against the patient's forehead, while the thumb and forefinger grasp the dropper or the plastic squeeze bottle containing the medication.) This position helps to steady the hand and provides control of the dropper. The dropper should never be poked toward the patient's eye without resting the hand on the patient's forehead; if the patient moves suddenly, the dropper could be thrust into his eye. The patient is asked to look up, the lower lid is gently everted, and the drop is placed just inside the lower lid. The patient is asked to close his eye gently, allowing the medication to bathe his eye. The drop should not be allowed to fall on the cornea, which is very sensitive. Plastic squeeze bottles are often used in place of droppers. The medication is instilled into the eye directly from the bottle. The procedure for holding the bottle and inserting the drop is the same as that described for the dropper.

**Lash Clipping.** Sometimes, the nurse is asked to clip the patient's lashes before surgery. In other situations the physician does this. If the nurse is asked to clip the patient's lashes, she uses a small pair of sterile scissors with dull curved points. The patient should be seated and the light adjusted so that the nurse can see well. With a sterile cotton ball she applies a small amount of sterile petrolatum to the scissors. The lashes then will stick to the scissors instead of falling into the patient's eye. She supports her hand on the patient's face, making sure that the scissors are held pointed away from the patient's eye. She asks the patient to look down, and then she raises his upper lid and trims the lashes. Then she asks the patient to look up, draws the lower lid down, and clips the lower lashes. Lashes that stick to the scissors should be wiped off frequently, and fresh petrolatum should be applied to the scissors. The nurse should work slowly and steadily, cutting a few lashes at a time.

The lids and the skin surrounding the eye are washed carefully with soap and water or with a bacteriocidal preparation. In some hospitals the eye is covered by a sterile eye pad after the skin has been cleansed. In other hospitals the eye is left uncovered.

**Other Considerations.** Sometimes, an enema is ordered the evening before surgery, particularly if it is desirable for the patient to avoid the exertion of moving his bowels for the first day or two after surgery has been performed.

If the patient's head must be kept very still postoperatively, it is important to plan ahead, so that as much care as possible can be given before surgery, and preparations can be made that will permit the patient to lie quietly with the least possible discomfort. For example, the male patient should shave before his operation. The woman patient should have her hair carefully combed and held back from her face. Braiding the hair helps to keep long hair neat. A contour sheet fits better than an ordinary sheet, and stays smooth longer without frequent need for pulling and tightening it.

Any respiratory condition, such as allergy or infection, that might cause sneezing or coughing is treated before the patient has surgery to minimize the possibility of sneezing and coughing after surgery. Sneezing or coughing can cause hemorrhage postoperatively.

Eye surgery on adults is often performed under local anesthesia. Preoperative sedation helps to lessen the patient's apprehension during the procedure. However, he is able to respond and to cooperate with the surgeon. For example, he can follow directions, such as "Look up." The use of local anesthesia formerly had the advantage of lessening the likelihood of postoperative nausea and vomiting. Vomiting produces strain and may cause hemorrhage or separation of the incision. With modern anesthetic techniques and the use of new drugs however, there should be no nausea or vomiting after general anesthesia. This is especially advantageous in cataract surgery.

### Postoperative Care

Postoperative care is directed toward the prevention of hemorrhage or the disruption of the surgical wound. Pressure or trauma to the eye or the head, such as that resulting from jarring or suddenly turning the head, is avoided. The patient is encouraged to move his arms and his legs, but he is discouraged from raising his head or turning it suddenly.

**In Bed.** After surgery the patient is moved carefully and gently from the operating table to his bed. Placing him directly in his own bed means that he is moved only once, and that he does not have to be moved to a stretcher and then to his bed. The moving of the patient is supervised by the surgeon. Usually, he holds the patient's head steady. Other members of the staff, working in unison, gently lift the patient into bed. Usually, the head is kept flat. However, many surgeons permit the patient to have one pillow in the immediate post-operative period. Sometimes, a small pillow is placed on either side of the head to support it and to serve as a reminder to the patient not to turn his head. This position sometimes is referred to as "fixed head position." Sandbags no longer are used for this purpose, because they are hard, and the patient can easily knock his head on them and injure himself.

The patient is wheeled back to his room. If both eyes are covered, it is important that the nurse show him the location of his call bell and assure him that he is back in his own room. Whether or not both eyes are covered, side rails should be kept in place. Older people, especially, are likely to become confused and to attempt to get out of bed.

Keeping both eyes covered provides rest for the operated eye. Some older people, however, become restless and disoriented when they are unable to see. It is very important that the nurse stay with the patient as much as possible. A few words spoken frequently and the touch of her hand help the patient to realize that he is not alone, and they help to keep him in contact with his environment. Many patients need frequent gentle reminders not to touch the dressing or to lift the head. Often the assurance of someone's presence can help the patient to relax enough to fall asleep. Sometimes, a family member can help by sitting quietly at the patient's bedside and assuring him that someone is there.

When a patient with both eyes covered becomes extremely excited and disoriented, attempting to climb out of bed over the side rails, the unoperated eye is uncovered as an emergency measure. Usually, the ability to see helps the patient quickly to become oriented, and calms him enough to be able to co-operate again. Restraining the patient or giving him additional sedation often makes him more disoriented in such circumstances. It is important that the nurse check with the surgeon beforehand concerning the measures to be taken if the patient becomes disoriented.

If the patient vomits, his head should be turned gently to the side to prevent aspiration of vomitus, but the head should not be raised. Measures that help the patient to avoid vomiting, sneezing, or coughing should be used. For example, he should not be given anything by mouth if he feels nauseated, since this may lead to vomiting. Sometimes, taking a deep breath or sucking on an ice chip or a

piece of hard candy helps the patient to avoid coughing. If he experiences nausea, this symptom should be reported promptly to the surgeon. He may prescribe the injection of a drug, such as chlorpromazine, to relieve the nausea and to lessen the possibility of vomiting. Usually a p.r.n. order for an antiemetic drug is given.

The patient who must maintain a fixed head position has to be fed. Often the diet is restricted to fluids on the day of surgery to avoid nausea, vomiting and the facial movements required by chewing. Usually, a soft diet is permitted on the day after surgery. The patient is fed until the surgeon indicates that the fixed head position is no longer necessary, and until the unaffected eye is uncovered.

Specific postoperative orders differ widely, depending on the type of operation and the preferences of the surgeon. Before the nurse works with any patient who has had eye surgery, she should be able to answer each of the following questions. Most of the information can be obtained directly from the physician's order sheet and from conferences with the physician.

- May the patient have a pillow?
- May the head of the patient's bed be elevated? If so, how much?
- May the patient turn? If so, to which side may he turn?
- May he brush his teeth, or should mouth care be limited to rinsing his mouth with mouthwash?
- How soon may he be shaved?

Everything must be done for the patient in a slow, gentle way. Explanation is important, particularly if both the patient's eyes are covered. Saying her name helps the patient to learn who the nurse is by the sound of her voice. Jarring the bed should be avoided because sudden movements can startle the patient and may even injure his eye.

Diversion helps the long hours to pass more quickly. It also helps to keep the patient in contact with his environment. A radio becomes a real companion to a patient who cannot see. A volunteer or a member of the family can help by reading to the patient or chatting with him.

If the patient is unable to turn for several days, certain adaptations in his care will be necessary. The sheets are kept as clean and smooth as possible without changing them. If necessary, a small disposable pad may be placed under the patient's buttocks and changed as it is necessary merely by sliding it in and out when the patient raises his hips. Assistance with the use of the bedpan and the urinal is important, so that the patient does not raise his head. Cleaning after toileting is done by nursing personnel, because the patient is not permitted to move about. The sacrum may be massaged gently by slipping the hand under the patient's back when he raises his hips slightly off the mattress. Sometimes a small, flat piece of foam rubber helps to relieve pressure on the sacrum.

**Out of Bed.** The length of time that the patient must remain in bed varies. Often he is allowed out of bed a day or two after surgery, and the unoperated eye is uncovered. Sometimes, he must remain quietly in bed for as long as a week or even longer. Usually, his appetite returns to normal when he is allowed up and can feed himself. He also finds it easier to move his bowels when he can assume a more normal position on a commode chair or a toilet. Sometimes, the physician orders an enema or gentle laxative to help to re-establish regular elimination. Straining at stool must be avoided, because it may lead to hemorrhage or strain the wound in the operated eye. Stool softeners are often used.

The patient still needs considerable nursing assistance and supervision, even when he is permitted out of bed. He is cautioned not to stoop, to lift anything heavy, or to become excited and to laugh heartily or to cough. His movements must be slow and deliberate. Good posture helps to relieve muscle strain, and it makes the patient more comfortable. Special care is necessary to prevent falls in the aged. A fractured hip should never be a complication of an eye operation. Beds that can be adjusted to high or low position are ideal, since they eliminate the hazards of getting out of a high bed. A footstool is helpful. Very elderly people often require nursing assistance each time that they get into or out of bed, because they are too feeble to manage alone.

**Home Care.** Before the patient leaves the hospital, he is taught how to care for himself at home. Specific instructions, such as those concerning the use of glasses and the amount of activity that the patient may have, are given by the doctor. Repeated explanations by the nurse sometimes are needed; often, older people tend to forget details. Learning about the patient's home situation is important, to determine whether his living arrangements will permit him to carry out the physician's recommenda-tions. This point is of special significance, because many older people live in furnished rooms, without cooking facilities. Arrangements for care in a convalescent home or for community services, such as the visiting nurse service and groups that take a hot meal daily to the patient, may be necessary. Arrangements are made for the patient to return to the physician's office or clinic for continued care.

## THE VISUALLY HANDICAPPED

Visual disorders are extremely common. So many people wear corrective glasses that the need for them usually is not considered a disability. However, some individuals cannot have their vision improved by glasses or any other type of treatment. Their defective vision may have been caused by birth defects, injury or by a disease, such as glaucoma. Regardless of its cause, poor vision affects the individual's emotional, social, and vocational life. The incidence of visual handicaps rises markedly with increasing age.

The term *blindness* is used for many legal purposes when central visual acuity is 20/200 or less in the better eye, even when corrective glasses are worn. Those with severe restrictions in the field of vision also are referred to as "blind." For instance, the patient may be able to see only an area the size of a book page at a distance of 20 feet.

## THE PARTIALLY SIGHTED

The special needs of the partially sighted often are overlooked. These people do not fit into the category of either the blind or the normally sighted population. Although they are handicapped, they often are less likely to receive help through governmental and private agencies. When help is given, it may be the same kind of assistance offered the blind. But the partially sighted person requires a different type of assistance; placing him in a training program for the blind can cause him to become discouraged or even to panic. He may be led to believe that others consider him to be blind, or that they believe he soon will become blind.

Contrary to common beliefs, the use of the eyes by the partially sighted does not necessarily harm or strain them. Some refuse to read with a special magnifying glass for fear of further reducing their vision. The patient should be guided by his ophthalmologist's advice concerning how much to use his eyes. Practice in using a low vision aid, either as a hand lens or magnifying system fitted into eyeglass frames, can help the patient to make the most effective use of his remaining vision. The chief objectives in the rehabilitation of partially sighted individuals include:

- Preservation of the remaining sight by treatment, if possible, of the underlying disorder.
- Making the fullest possible use of the remaining vision by special lenses, large type, or holding the object closer to the eyes.
- Vocational training.

The patient's visual ability and the type of aids that might help him are evaluated carefully. Vocational preparation is undertaken in the light of the degree of visual disability. For example, a severe visual handicap would make driving a hazard for everyone concerned, whereas certain types of factory work could be performed efficiently and safely. The partially sighted individual should be assisted and encouraged to work at a suitable occupation and to help to take care of his home and his family. Ingenuity and willingness to try new ways of doing things can help the individual to maintain his independence. A diabetic patient with failing vision should not place himself in a position of dependence on a family member; instead, he can use a magnifying glass to help him to see the markings on his insulin syringe.

Emphasis on self-care and independence must be tempered with judgment and concern for the patient's welfare and that of others. For example, at what point should the patient be prohibited from driving his car? (In most states laws requiring tests of vision and setting minimum standards determine whether a patient may drive, but retesting, once an individual has a license, is often not required for renewal of the license.) These decisions are often difficult since the ability to drive may be crucial in the maintenance of independence, particularly when the patient has other disabilities, such as advanced age or neuromuscular disease. One patient with multiple sclerosis persisted in driving his car despite double vision. The nurse discovered that he lived alone, had no cooking facilities, and because of weakness in his legs was unable to walk to the nearest restaurant. The nurse contacted a community organization that brought one hot meal a day to the patient's home. He was able to manage the other two meals himself through the use of a hot plate.

## THE BLIND

### Misconceptions

For centuries blindness has been shrouded in mystery. Many myths have developed, such as that blind people develop extraordinary powers of hearing and touch to compensate for the loss of vision. Tests of these senses among blind and sighted people have not shown the blind to have unusual perception in the other senses. It is now believed that the sightless learn to make more effective use of other senses in their effort to interpret their environment. For example, the blind person learns to be especially aware of tones of voice, to recognize changes in other people's moods, although he cannot see facial expressions. Most people could learn to make greater use of auditory and tactile stimuli, but their ability to see makes this effort seem to be less necessary.

"Living in darkness" is another common misconception. Many blind people can perceive light shadows of some large objects. Some blind people describe blindness as being surrounded by fog, or by grayness, which is neither light nor dark.

### Living and Working in the Community

Pity is very much in evidence in attitudes toward the blind in contrast to the impatience and ridicule so often expressed toward the deaf. Blind persons often have been segregated in separate institutions, in the belief that they are unable to maintain themselves in the sighted community. Such institutions often provide opportunities for recreation and useful work, but contacts are limited almost exclusively to other blind people. Increasing emphasis now is being placed on helping blind people to live and to work in the community, although they may begin work in a sheltered workshop to gain confidence and skill.

An important early step toward the employment of blind persons among sighted people was the Randolph-Sheppard Act, which in 1936 provided government support for the operation of vending stands by the blind. Many such stands are now operated by sightless people throughout the country. Blind students are seen more and more frequently on college campuses, and blind people in increasing numbers are entering such occupations as teaching, farming and typing.

Numerous organizations exist to help the blind. The Federal Government offers such benefits as literature for the blind, which is made available through the Library of Congress, and a special income tax exemption. Each state has an agency to aid the blind. The name and the address can be obtained through the state's welfare department, or through the American Foundation for the Blind, Inc., 15 West 16th Street, New York City, 10011, a private agency that helps blind persons throughout the country by such services as research, counseling and the publishing of materials of interest to the blind and those who help them. For example, the Foundation publishes a directory of agencies serving the blind in the United States and Canada.

How can nurses help newly blind persons take their places in the community? Like others who have lost a part of themselves, these patients usually show sadness and depression, a natural reaction to loss. At this time they need support and encouragement—someone to listen when they feel like expressing their feelings, someone to guide their faltering steps, so that their clumsiness will be less embarrassing and less dangerous.

### Orientation and Aids to Self-Care

Gradually, the blind patient is helped to orient himself to his room in the hospital or at home. He is helped to form a mental image of his surroundings and gradually to move about his room without assistance.

At mealtime he is told where the food is on his plate. Likening the location of the food to the hands of a clock is helpful. In figure 26-8 the meat is at 9 o'clock, the potato at 3 o'clock and the

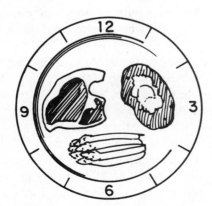

**Figure 26-8.** Telling the patient that his meat is at 9 o'clock, potato at 3 o'clock, and vegetable at 6 o'clock helps him to locate them on his plate.

vegetable at 6 o'clock. Placing the patient's food on his plate in the same position day after day will help him to become adept at finding it. Other articles should be kept in the same position at each meal (e.g., the napkin always on the left, near the fork, and the milk always on the right, near the knife). The patient is given as much help as is necessary to avoid repeated spilling and discouragement. At first he will need help in buttering bread, cutting meat, and pouring beverages. Gradually, he masters these tasks. Many blind people can eat with little or no assistance, once they have been oriented to the location of the food and the tableware.

It is important to tell the patient when something has been moved or is different from usual (e.g., that the easy chair has been placed on the other side of the room, or that he is having spaghetti instead of meat, potato, and vegetable). Doors should be opened wide or completely closed. The patient is likely to bump into a partly opened door.

The patient should be allowed to gradually assume responsibility for his own grooming. Bathing, combing hair, shaving, and brushing the teeth are all activities that he can learn to do himself. His toilet articles should be kept in the same place, and never moved without telling him. The patient at first will require tactful assistance. If he has missed part of his whiskers, he should be told so gently and helped to learn to feel his skin to make sure that his shave is complete.

The newly blind person needs contact with other persons who can help him become aware of, and correct, mannerisms which may interfere with his relationships with others. The blind person, particularly if he lacks such help from other people, may develop peculiarities of facial expression, gait, and posture of which he is unaware, but which make him appear awkward.

The community health nurse can help the patient and his family by familiarizing them with rehabilitation programs in their community. In New York City, for example, arrangements can be made for a specialist in rehabilitation of the blind to visit the patient's home and help him and his family develop a program of orientation to his home environment, and later, to the larger community.

Often, particularly when the services of a specialist are not available, the community health nurse can guide the family in this type of care. Frequently, the patient is cared for at home, and it is often his family who guides and assists him in his first efforts toward self-care. One patient's wife devised a system of arranging her husband's clothing so that he could differentiate colors. The suit closet had sections for each color, divided by large plastic garment bags. Similar arrangements were made for shirts and ties. Her husband could dress independently and with the confidence that he would not appear at the office wearing a green tie with a blue shirt.

Cooking utensils can be located by the blind housewife, if they are kept always in the same place. Canned goods can be labeled in Braille.

The patient's family and friends are encouraged to speak normally to him (remember, the patient is blind, not deaf). Awkward efforts to avoid the use of the terms "look" and "see" embarrass the patient and call attention to his disability because such expressions are a natural part of the language.

Other everyday activities with which the patient can be helped at home include seating himself in a chair and guiding him when he ventures out. The easiest and the least awkward way to offer a blind person a chair is to place his hand on the back of it. He then can seat himself. When guiding a blind person, let him take your arm. Walk slightly in front of him, so that the movement of your body when you stop or step up or down will give him advance warning of what to expect. Seizing the blind person's arm and pulling him along is a common mistake. It destroys his dignity and is likely to throw him off balance. Encourage the blind person to walk erect and to turn his head toward the person speaking to him.

Reading is an invaluable pastime for persons with all sorts of disabilities. Blind people can read, too, but by using Braille, a system of raised dots that the patient can feel with his fingertips (Fig. 26-9). The dots are arranged in different ways to signify letters of the alphabet and punctuation marks. The use of Braille requires learning and a great deal of patience. Information about securing Braille books may be obtained from the Library of Congress, Washington, D.C. Agencies for the blind, such as the American Foundation for the Blind, and state agencies for the blind can provide information about teachers of Braille, many of whom go directly into the patient's home. Braille watches also are available. They have no crystal, and the blind person feels the hands and the raised characters on the face of the watch with his fingertips.

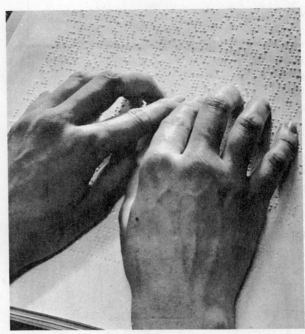

**Figure 26-9.** A page of Braille. Note the raised dots and the placement of the fingers on the page. Note also the special watch with dots in place of numerals. It has no crystal, and the user can tell the time by feeling the relationship of the hands and the dots. (American Foundation for the Blind, Inc., New York, N.Y.)

Talking books are long-playing records that allow the patient to listen to recordings of books and even some magazines. For instance, the *Review of the Week* section of the Sunday *New York Times* is recorded each week and mailed to blind subscribers. Talking books are available for purchase or loan. Information concerning talking books is available from the Library of Congress, Washington, D.C., and from state agencies for the blind.

Special Braille typewriters are available making it possible for blind people to write to one another. Blind people use a regular typewriter when they write to their sighted friends. They use the same touch system as sighted people. Also, handwriting is possible. Some blind people lay a ruler underneath the line of writing to keep it straight.

### Venturing into the Community

When the blind person has mastered techniques of self-care at home, he is ready to venture into the community. How can he get around safely? Modern city traffic poses a threat even to sighted persons! Small wonder, then, that the blind person usually is fearful of leaving his home. A guide is one answer to the problem. However, having someone to guide him makes the blind person depend on another and is a constant intrusion on his privacy. Also, it is very expensive, unless the guide is a family member who serves without pay. In that case the relative's freedom to lead his own life is severely curtailed.

Two methods, other than the human guide, are now widely used. One is the dog guide; the other is the cane. Both require training and practice.

### Measures to Assist in Locomotion

Training in use of a cane or guide dog is one aspect of a total program for assisting the blind person to get about independently. Other aspects include training in spatial orientation and in obstacle detection. For example, the blind person is taught how to use his sense of hearing to help him realize that he is approaching a wall, so that he can veer away from it.

Sometimes it is erroneously assumed that blind persons' abilities to compensate by their other senses, and their development of various skills in getting about spring miraculously into being due to the experience of blindness. Actually, as in so many aspects of living, success in learning to get about independently, despite loss of vision, requires many hours of instruction, often over a period of several months, and diligent practice on the part of the learner. Nurses can help blind and severely visually handicapped persons to realize that greater independence can be achieved with the help of competent teachers, a well planned training program, and the patient's own persistent effort.

Many factors affect rehabilitation. A slight degree of anxiety can be helpful in motivating the patient. However, severe anxiety interferes with learning and may actually immobilize the patient, making it impossible for him to use available resources. As in any type of learning, successful experiences are important in building the individual's skill and confidence. Many visually handicapped persons are in the older age groups; these older individuals are often further handicapped by hearing deficits and slow neuromuscular coordination, thus making it more difficult for them to compensate for their loss of vision.

The newly blind person typically reacts with depression to the loss of his vision. Gradually, with assistance and support, he may move through this grief reaction to the point where he is ready to learn to become as independent as possible. Some patients react initially with denial of their disability; these patients are especially disadvantaged, as they must first be helped to recognize the fact of their disability.

**The Dog Guide.** The Seeing Eye, Inc., Morristown, N.J., was the first center in the United States to train guide dogs for the blind. Now other centers also train guide dogs. Information about such centers can be obtained through state agencies for the blind. The dog is taught to recognize potential dangers, such as holes, obstacles in the path, and curbs (Fig. 26-10). Dog and person communicate through movements of the harness. The dog is permitted to go everywhere with the blind person—to work, in restaurants, and on public conveyances. When the dog is not actually leading the person, the dog lies quietly and unobtrusively (perhaps under a restaurant table or a chair in the theater) until he is needed. The blind individual is trained in the use and the care of his dog at the center that supplies the dog. However, other people need to learn how to behave with the dog. The following are some suggestions that the nurse can practice and teach.

- Do not coax or pat the dog while he is "on duty." He must give his undivided attention to leading the blind person.
- If you wish to pat or talk to the dog, ask first. If circumstances permit, the blind person will signal the dog that it is all right. This signal will enable you to show friendliness and interest, if you wish, without interrupting the dog's work.
- Show consideration for the individual and the dog in crowded places. Because he is close to the ground, the dog is easily stepped on in a crowd. Avoid jostling or pushing either the person or his dog.

Many who have adopted guide dogs find them not only invaluable guides but good company. Not every blind person wants or can use a dog; some do not like dogs, and others are unable to walk rapidly enough. This is especially true of elderly, feeble patients.

**The Cane.** The cane is a means of extending the patient's sense of touch into the environment. It becomes an extension of his arm, by means of which he learns to survey his surroundings so that he can walk safely. The cane, when painted white, further serves to identify the individual as visually handicapped.

The cane has other advantages:

- It is especially useful for elderly persons with a slow gait; in some instances such persons use an orthopedic

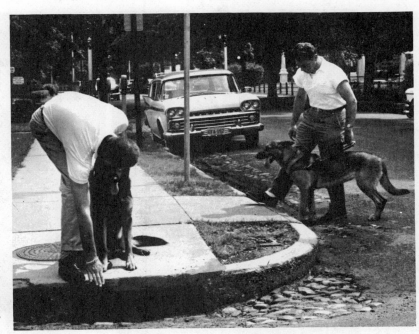

**Figure 26-10.** These Seeing Eye Dogs are being taught "curb stops" by instructors. Such training will enable the dogs to guide their blind masters safely. (The Seeing Eye, Inc., Morristown, N.J.)

cane which can provide physical support if they are feeble, as well as assistance in locomotion without vision, or with severely impaired vision.
- It is very inexpensive and requires virtually no up-keep or care.
- It is readily kept with its owner.

It is important for nurses to realize that individuals can become as independent by use of the cane as by use of a guide dog. The patient should be assisted to familiarize himself with the existence of both types of aids, so that, with the guidance of an expert teacher, he can evaluate which of these aids is best for him.

The cane is often referred to as a "prescription cane," since its measurements are prescribed for the individual patient, in relation to such factors as his height and the speed of his reflexes. The cane is usually long enough to extend from the floor to the base of the patient's sternum.

As part of his training program, the patient learns to use the cane to elicit information about his surroundings. He is taught to describe an arc in front of him, extending in width approximately three inches out from each shoulder. In this way he surveys the characteristics of the path he is about to travel, noting such obstacles as curbs, steps, and bumps in the pavement (Fig. 26-11).

**Aiding Blind Travelers.** Nurses can help and teach others to aid blind travelers by:

- Resisting the impulse to rush up and to try to help. If the blind person seems to be managing well, he will appreciate being allowed to continue to do so, rather than being whisked across the street, often opposite to where he wishes to go, by an impulsive "helper."
- Courteously asking the blind person how to help, if he seems lost or uncertain. If he requires directions, it should be remembered that he cannot see landmarks like "the big church on the corner." He can count the streets that he crosses and then turn left or right.
- Avoiding any fuss that would embarrass him and call attention to his disability. Unobtrusive, thoughtful help—offering him a seat in a crowded bus or preventing him from being pushed—is appreciated.

### Recreation and Skills

Like everyone else, blind persons enjoy and need recreation. The patient's former interests are the best guide to what he is likely to enjoy after blindness occurs. Someone who has always enjoyed reading will welcome talking books and Braille, whereas one who never cared for reading but was interested in sports may prefer listening to games broadcast on radio and TV. Those who love music will be able to continue to enjoy it. Blind people can continue to enjoy outdoor recreation, such as swimming and fishing. Although former interests serve as valuable guides, the patient can be encouraged to develop new interests, such as music, which do not depend on sight.

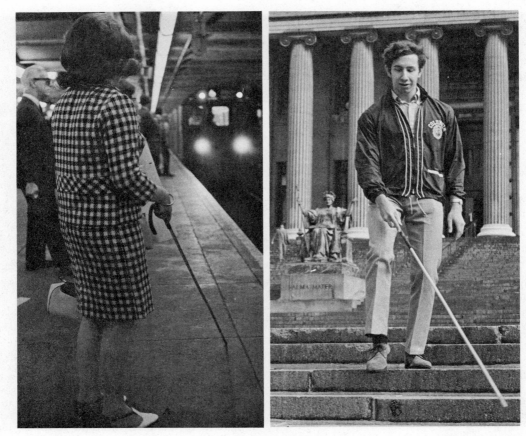

**Figure 26-11.** The long cane, especially prescribed to fit the individual's height and gait, has greatly increased freedom of mobility for blind persons. (The New York Association for the Blind)

Many skills that blind people have learned seem miraculous to the sighted observer. For instance, a blind man reaches into his pocket, takes out a dime, and makes a telephone call. How did he know it was a dime and not a penny? He felt the edge. Dimes have a serrated edge; pennies, a smooth one. Also, he can tell whether he is taking a one-dollar bill or a five-dollar bill out of his wallet by having someone fold them differently (e.g., the ones in half lengthwise, and the fives in half crosswise).

### Courtesies and Attitudes

Certain courtesies smooth the way for the blind person and his sighted companions. When addressing the blind person, especially when he is with a group, he should be called by name to save him the embarrassment of not knowing who is speaking to him. He cannot see that the speaker is looking in his direction. The nurse should speak to him before touching him, so that he will realize she is there, and what she is going to do. For example, the sighted hospitalized patient can observe the syringe in the nurse's hand, and he knows even before she tells him that he is about to receive an injection. The blind patient has no such way of preparing himself, and he is especially dependent on others for an explanation of what is about to happen, and what is expected of him. The nurse should tell the patient when she is entering or leaving the room, so that he is spared the uncomfortable realization that he has been talking to someone who has already left. She should teach the patient to turn on the light at a certain time each evening when he is alone. This will prevent others from the startling experience of unexpectedly finding him sitting in a dark room, when they were not aware that he was there.

Some people are afraid of the blind, and avoid contact with them. Perhaps they feel a certain eeriness in the lack of normal eye contact. Some blind people have learned that a handshake helps to overcome this when they meet people for the first time. Shake the blind person's hand when he extends it, but remember that he cannot see your hand if you initiate the handshake. In the latter instance, you will have to reach for his hand.

The only thing that blind people share in common is the inability to see. They differ from one another in other ways, just as sighted people do. The patient must be helped to maintain his individuality, and he must not, because of his handicap, be expected to conform to some nebulous personality considered appropriate for "the blind." Blind people rely on sighted people, not for pity, but for help in resuming independent lives despite the handicap. The one ingredient that often has been lacking, despite many charitable enterprises for the benefit of the blind, is true acceptance by the sighted community.

## REFERENCES AND BIBLIOGRAPHY

ALEXANDER, M. M., and BROWN, M. S.: Physical Examination: Examining the eye, *Nurs. '73* 3:41, December 1973.

ALLEN, J. H.: *May's Diseases of the Eye,* ed. 24, Baltimore, Williams and Wilkins, 1968.

AMMON, L. L.: Surviving enucleation, *Am. J. Nurs.* 72:1817, October 1972.

BAUMAN, M. K., and YODER, N.: *Adjustment to Blindness—Re-viewed,* Springfield, Ill., Thomas, 1966.

CHODIL, J., and WILLIAMS, B.: The concept of sensory deprivation, *Nurs. Clin. N. Am.* 5:453, September 1970.

CONDL, E. D.: Ophthalmic nursing: The gentle touch, *Nurs. Clin. N. Am.* 5:467, September 1970.

DUKE-ELDER, S.: *The Practice of Refraction,* ed. 8, St. Louis, Mosby, 1969.

ENSOR, G.: The sore eye 1, *Nurs. Times* 65:1479, November 1969.

————: The sore eye 2, *Nurs. Times* 65:1517, November 1969.

FOWKES, W. C., and HUNN, V.: *Clinical Assessment for the Nurse Practitioner,* St. Louis, Mosby, 1973.

GARRETT, J. (ed.): *Psychological Aspects of Physical Disability,* Washington, D.C., U.S. Government Printing Office, (n.d.).

GORDON, D. M.: Eye emergencies, *AORN* 11:78, January 1970.

GORLICK, H. S.: Glaucoma: The fight for sight, *RN* 31:44, February 1968.

GREISHEIMER, E. M., and WIEDEMAN, M. P.: *Physiology and Anatomy,* ed. 9, Philadelphia, Lippincott, 1970.

HADDAD, H.: Drugs for ophthalmologic use, *Am. J. Nurs.* 68:324, March 1968.

HAMILTON, M. J.: What the nurse should know about eye banks, *Nurs. Clin. N. Am.* 5:483, September 1970.

HAVENER, W. H.: *Synopsis of Ophthalmology,* ed. 3, St. Louis, Mosby, 1971.

HEVEY, L.: Vision and aging, *Nurs. Outlook* 12:61, June 1964.

HUGHES, W. F. (ed.): *The Year Book of Ophthalmology,* Chicago, Year Book Medical Publishers, 1973.

HUNT, L. B. (ed.): *Glaucoma: Epidemiology, Early Diagnosis and Some Aspects of Treatment,* Baltimore, Williams and Wilkins, 1965.

ISLER, C.: The world of transplants, work of the eye bank, *RN* 35:36, November 1972.

JACKSON, C. W., et al.: Sensory deprivation as a field of study, *Nurs. Res.* 20:46, January-February 1971.

JACKSON, G. D.: How blind are nurses to the needs of the visually handicapped, *Nurs. Outlook* 13:34, September 1965.

LERMAN, S.: *Basic Ophthalmology,* New York, McGraw-Hill, 1966.

McWILLIAM, R. J.: Infection of the eye, *Nurs. Times* 69:145, February 1973.

National Institute of Neurologic Disease: *Vision and Its Disorders,* Monograph No. 4, Washington, D.C., U.S. Department of Health, Education and Welfare, Public Health Service Publication No. 1688, 1967.

NEWELL, F. W.: *Ophthalmology,* St. Louis, Mosby, 1965.

OHNO, M. I.: The eye-patched patient, *Am. J. Nurs.* 71:271, February 1971.

RABB, M. F.: The present status of corneal transplantation, *Nurs. Clin. N. Am.* 5:477, September 1970.

RICHARDSON, F., et al.: Don't they know the blind are helpless?, *RN* 36:52, September 1973.

RUBEN, M.: Contact lenses, shells, and prosthetics, *Nurs. Times* 68:133, February 1972.

SAUNDERS, W., et al.: *Nursing Care in Eye, Nose and Throat Disorders,* ed. 2, St. Louis, Mosby, 1968.

SCHEIE, H. G., and ALBERT, D. M.: *Adler's Textbook of Ophthalmology,* ed. 8, Philadelphia, Saunders, 1969.

SEAMAN, F. W.: Nursing care of glaucoma patients, *Nurs. Clin. N. Am.* 5:489, September 1970.

SMITH, J. F., and NACHAZEL, D. P.: Retinal detachment, *Am. J. Nurs.* 73:1530, September 1973.

Symposium of the New Orleans Academy of Ophthalmology, *Industrial and Traumatic Opthalmology,* St. Louis, Mosby, 1964.

UFFENORDE, T. M.: Nurses view of eye surgery, *AORN* 16:45, December 1972.

WEINSTOCK, F. J.: Emergency treatment of eye injuries, *Am. J. Nurs.* 71:1928, October 1971.

————: Tonometry screening, *Am. J. Nurs.* 73:656, April 1973.

WHITEHEAD, K. P.: Chemical burns of the eye, *Nurs. Times* 67:759, June 1971.

# The Patient with
# Hearing Disturbance

CHAPTER 27

It has been estimated that 8.1 million adults in the United States have hearing impairments. Although hearing disability of various degrees of severity occurs at all ages, its incidence increases markedly after 50 years of age.

Not all people with hearing deficits are diagnosed and treated. The disadvantaged, especially the elderly poor, miss out on referral and corrective measures if nurses or the health care professionals providing for their primary care overlook hearing loss or dismiss the condition as part of the aging process. Notwithstanding that auditory perception diminishes with advancing age, ears with senescent changes are not immune to various otologic disorders.

All complaints of diminished hearing brought to the nurse's attention should be investigated by taking a careful history, examining the ears and the upper respiratory tract, and performing some hearing tests to determine hearing acuity. Patients showing deviations from normal should be referred to the otologist.

## ROLE OF THE NURSE IN PREVENTION
## OF HEARING LOSS

Severe hearing impairment may be associated with hereditary conditions such as agenesis of the inner ear, otosclerosis, and middle ear deformity.

Prevention of hereditary hearing disorders belongs in the realm of the genetic counselor. The nurse's preventive efforts will be implemented at the post-disease stage (see Chapter 7 for stages of disease). She will recognize anatomic deformities in the hearing apparatus and deficits or absence of the hearing function. Early detection and referral for diagnosis, treatment, and rehabilitation will prevent further social and educational deprivation of the individual. The nurse who cares for the newborn may detect such anomalies. On the other hand, some diseases such as otosclerosis may not become manifest until adolescence or the early twenties; there are no visible anomalies which the nurse can detect except the *Schwartz sign*, in which the drum membrane may show a reddish tinge during the active period of the disease.

Inability to hear in some individuals can be traced to developmental defects caused by maternal viral infections such as influenza, mumps, and rubella. Previously it was believed that the embryo was vulnerable to the rubella virus only during the first trimester, but it is now clear that the virus may persist and injure an embryo that is conceived weeks or even a few months after the infection, and injury to a fetus can occur at least as late as the seventh month of pregnancy (Davis and Silverman, 1970).

Other causes of deafness include birth injury, anoxia, prematurity, kernicterus, and the toxic effects of medications prenatally and postnatally from birth to senescence.

## Prevention

Prevention of developmental defects and peri-natal causes leading to deafness implies nursing efforts geared toward prevention of rubella and influenza epidemics, vaccination of children, and careful followup of expectant mothers at risk.

**Drug Therapy.** Control and prompt treatment of infectious diseases can prevent deafness caused by these infections. Upper respiratory infections that spread to the ear can affect an individual's hearing for the rest of his life. Fortunately, antibiotics are helping to control such infections. But, by the same token, there are several antibiotics and other drugs which cause serious ototoxic complications. Among these are included dihydrostreptomycin, gentamycin, kanamycin, neomycin, Coly-Mycin, and streptomycin. Other drugs having toxicologic action on the ear include phenylbutazone, quinine, and salicylates. Ethacrynic acid (Edecrin) has caused hearing loss within 20 minutes after administration and permanent deafness due to outer hair cell loss in the cochlea (Martin, 1971). The nurse must be knowledgeable about all the drugs she administers, particularly those which are known to have toxic effects. Observation for first signs of toxicity, as well as measures promoting good kidney function, are among the factors which may help mitigate toxicity.

Alertness, during work with parents and young children, can assist the nurse to note indications of child abuse. Loss or diminution of hearing can occur from a blow to the ear, and is a significant cause of hearing loss. Parents who exhibit such behavior require counseling to deal with their emotional problems.

Prolonged exposure to very loud noise causes hearing loss. Redesigning and soundproofing buildings, periodically testing workers who are in a noisy environment, encouraging the use of ear protection devices, such as individually fitted ear plugs, and rotating workers so that no one individual is exposed to loud noises for an extended period are important ways in which industry can help to prevent deafness. Industrial nurses can play a major role in such programs. Because exposure to loud noise as a cause of hearing loss is becoming more widely recognized, recent efforts to lessen noise and to protect individuals from existing noise have extended from industrial environments to home, school, and recreational settings. The aggregate of noise featured so prominently in modern life is now recognized not only as a nuisance, but also as a hazard. Nurses can play a part in alerting others to the hazard—for example, from a booming record player in a school lunch room.

**Community Agencies.** When dealing with patients whose hearing impairments have been diagnosed and who seek further assistance, the nurse may contribute to preventing social isolation and needless suffering by referring them and their families to appropriate national and community agencies. The American Hearing Society has branches in many cities. Local chapters of this society serve as information centers, employment bureaus, and clubs for social activities. Many chapters provide classes in speech reading and the use of hearing aids. Local chapters and the national society maintain lists of persons who are available to teach speech reading. The location of the nearest branch may be obtained by writing to the American Hearing Society, 919 18th St., N.W., Washington, D.C., 20036. The John Tracy Clinic, 806 West Adams Boulevard, Los Angeles, California, 90007, through correspondence offers services and in-

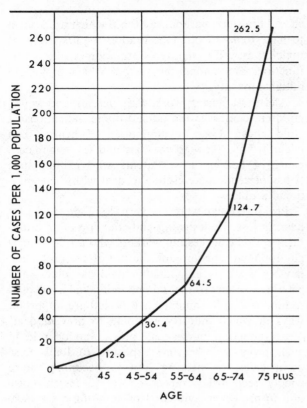

**Figure 27-1.** Hearing impairments in the United States. (U.S. Department of Health, Education and Welfare, Public Health Service: *Distribution and Use of Hearing Aids, Wheelchairs and Artificial Limbs,* Washington, D.C., U.S. Government Printing Office)

formation to people in all parts of the country. Hospital social workers and community organizations such as the United Fund headquarters often have helpful information concerning community facilities. State employment and rehabilitation services can help the deaf person find suitable work. The Veterans Administration operates audiology clinics for eligible veterans in many cities throughout the nation. To obtain information concerning the location of these clinics contact the nearest Veterans Administration Regional Office.

The National Association of the Deaf promotes the welfare of deaf persons in education, employment, and legislation and also assists individual deaf persons and local groups of deaf persons. Its official publication, *The Silent Worker*, is published monthly. For further information write to the Association, at 2495 Shattuck Avenue, Berkeley, California 94704.

The Alexander Graham Bell Association for the Deaf is another valuable resource. For information write to the Executive Secretary, Alexander Graham Bell Association for the Deaf, 1537 35th St., N.W., Washington, D.C. 20007. The Association's Volta Bureau has a large collection of books on deafness and is active in promoting the welfare of the deaf.

## HEARING IMPAIRMENT

Loss of hearing may be slight, moderate, or so severe that the sense of hearing is virtually nonfunctioning. Often, those with slight or moderate hearing impairment are said to be *hard-of-hearing*, whereas those with severe hearing loss are called *deaf*. Impaired hearing may be congenital (i.e., developing prenatally and being present at birth) or acquired (developing after birth). Hearing loss due to aging is called *presbycusis*. The incidence of hearing loss increases steadily with age and is a particular problem for those over 65 (Fig. 27-1).

Older people sometimes suffer from inability to understand what they hear. This type of disability may occur not only in association with hearing loss, but also in persons whose hearing is adequate. Failure or extreme slowness in understanding the words is due to changes in the brain, usually caused by arteriosclerosis. It is important to differentiate this type of disability from deafness. Persons suffering from difficulty in understanding words are not helped by hearing aids, but they can be helped by your speaking slowly, repeating what is said when it is not understood, and using short, uncomplicated sentences.

Hearing loss may be divided into two types: conductive and sensorineural. *Conductive hearing loss* is caused by any disease or injury that interferes with the conduction of sound waves to the inner ear. For example, an accumulation of cerumen in the auditory canal or the failure of the ossicles to vibrate may cause conductive hearing loss. *Sensorineural hearing loss* (formerly known as *perceptive* loss and sometimes called "nerve deafness") results from the malfunction of the inner ear, the auditory nerve, or the auditory center in the brain. The prognosis is better in conductive hearing loss because often its cause can be treated —for example, by removing excess cerumen from the auditory canal or by performing surgery to restore the ability of the ossicles to vibrate. Persons with conductive deafness benefit more from the use of hearing aids, since the organs that perceive sound, such as the auditory nerve and the brain, are able to function.

Sensorineural hearing loss of any degree is usually irreversible and thus far not amenable to surgical correction. Except when the loss is complete, the hearing may be improved to varying degrees with hearing-aid amplification. The hearing of those with a poor discrimination score (the measure of the ability to understand spoken words when amplified above the level of the individual's hearing) is difficult to improve with amplification.

Some patients have *mixed hearing loss*, a combination of conductive and sensorineural elements.

## ASSESSMENT

### Inspection

Inspection of the ear may begin with the auricle or pinna, the outermost portion of the auditory apparatus (Fig. 27-2). The reader is referred to anatomy texts, to become reacquainted, if necessary, with the names of the various eminences, depressions, and folds of the pinna, in order to facilitate naming the location of anomalies if any are found.

The nurse inspects the auricle for missing structures, malformations, accessory auricles, fistula, and occlusion of the external auditory canal. She observes the condition of the skin for evidence of infection, boils, ulcerated areas, and dermatitis.

Palpation of the auricle may reveal painful areas, nodules, or cysts. Forward displacement of the auricle because of edema over the mastoid process and marked tenderness over the same area strongly suggest mastoiditis (Foxen, 1968).

Examination of the external auditory canal is best carried out by means of an otoscope. When using this instrument the nurse must remember that:

- The otoscope and its batteries must be in good working order.
- The largest speculum which can be inserted without causing pain is selected for use.
- The speculum is inserted gently and not too far.
- The pinna is pulled upward and backward (in adults) to facilitate insertion of the speculum and visualization of the canal.
- The angle of visualization is changed by moving the speculum, allowing complete inspection of the tympanic membrane.
- The patient is asked to tilt the head to the opposite shoulder to facilitate inspection of the canal and tympanic membrane.
- Speculi are disinfected thoroughly between patients.

The external auditory canal is inspected for evidence of inflammation, edema, redness, discharge, foreign bodies, and tumors or any other lesions. The nurse must become familiar with normal ears in order to be able to recognize deviation. The external auditory meatus or canal is about one inch in length. It ends blindly at the tympanic membrane. The canal contains ceruminous glands and hairs in its cartilaginous portion, which ends about midway into the canal where the osseous part begins.

The tympanic membrane or eardrum has a dull bluish "pearly" gray and translucent appearance; when illuminated it may take on a pinkish or yellowish hue. The eardrum lies obliquely across the end of the canal cascading downward and medially. It is attached in its periphery to a bony ring, the annulus, which is continuous with the wall of the auditory canal. The tympanic membrane is

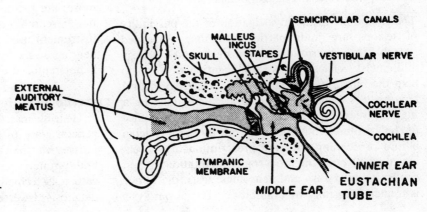

**Figure 27-2.** Diagram of a section through the ear.

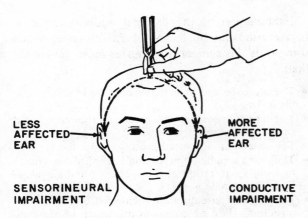

LESS AFFECTED EAR

MORE AFFECTED EAR

SENSORINEURAL IMPAIRMENT

CONDUCTIVE IMPAIRMENT

**Figure 27-3.** When a vibrating tuning fork is placed against the forehead, to the patient with conductive hearing loss the tone sounds louder in the more affected ear; whereas to the patient with sensorineural hearing loss, the tone sounds louder in the less affected ear.

also attached to the handle of the malleus, which draws the center of the drum inward. This area is called the umbo. From this point to the antero-inferior quadrant a cone of light is reflected forward and downward toward the annulus. These landmarks are important because they become distorted or disappear in otitis media and other conditions of the middle ear.

## Hearing Tests

Hearing tests are performed:

- To determine the ability to hear sounds by the use of the pure tone audiometer and recorded speech
- To test and compare the efficiency of the conductive apparatus by the use of the tuning fork and the audiometer
- To rule out retrocochlear lesions, especially an acoustic neuroma—a tumor arising from the acoustic nerve, located in the auditory canal

The tests done in the investigation of the possibility of lesions are audiometric pure tone, recorded speech for discrimination scores, and Bekesy audiometry. These tests are mentioned here to help the nurse realize that in cases of sensorineural hearing loss, especially unilateral, there must be a high degree of suspicion of tumor. The presence of such a tumor must be ruled out by the physician before proceeding with the prescription of a hearing aid and other methods of rehabilitation. When confirmed by x-rays and neurologic tests, the tumor is treated surgically by craniotomy. Facial paralysis

may be present before or may occur following the surgery.

Some types of hearing tests may be performed quickly, such as screening tests to determine whether impairment exists. For example, the nurse may have the patient turn his head, so that he cannot lipread, and repeat what she whispers. Tuning forks are also very useful. The nurse compares the patient's ability to hear the tone of the vibrating fork with her own ability, thereby ascertaining if there is hearing loss. Other tests with tuning forks help to distinguish between conductive and sensorineural loss. For example, a vibrating tuning fork may be placed against the patient's forehead; the patient is asked in which ear the sound is louder. The sound will be louder in the weaker ear if the hearing loss is conductive, and in the better ear if the loss is sensorineural. This is called the Weber or lateralization test (Fig. 27-3).

If hearing loss is suspected, the patient is referred to the otologist.

Audiometry is being used more and more frequently by schools and other institutions as a screening device to discover impaired hearing. The audiometer produces pure tones of controlled loudness (intensity, measured in decibels) and pitch (frequency of vibration of sound waves, measured in cycles per second). The results of the test are recorded on a graph called an *audiogram*. The audiometer is useful also in differentiating conductive and sensorineural hearing loss. Usually, audiometry is performed in a soundproof room, so that extraneous noise (such as the roar of traffic) will not affect the test results. The patient wears earphones and is instructed to signal when he hears the tone, and when he no longer hears it, by raising and lowering the index finger.

Automatic recording audiometers (Bekesy-Rudmose) are being used in hearing centers in diagnostic, research, and monitoring audiometry. The instrument uses the patient-control principle to test hearing at six frequencies in each ear. An operator is not required except to start the machine.

## Psychogenic Hearing Loss

Hearing loss can be psychogenic, due to a conversion state (a situation in which the patient expresses his anxiety through the inhibition of normal bodily functions, such as hearing or seeing). In this case it is termed *functional hearing loss*. Accurate diagnosis is essential, because the treatment involves psychotherapy rather than that of organic hearing disorders.

One test that differentiates functional from organic hearing loss is *psychogalvanometry*. This test is based on the fact that the reflex secretion of perspiration occurs when an electric shock is given to the hand. The shock (unpleasant, and yet not actually painful) is repeated until the patient consistently responds to it with perspiring hands. A tone then is sounded prior to the shock. This is repeated until the patient associates the tone and the shock, and responds to the tone in the same manner as to the shock. A person with functional hearing loss responds to the tone with perspiring hands, whereas one with organic hearing loss responds in this way only to the shock and not to the tone.

## The Patient with Hearing Loss

**Communication and Attitudes.** Hearing loss can seriously impair a person's ability to protect himself and to communicate with others; thus it can keep him out of touch with his environment. Perhaps most of us do not realize how often sounds warn us of danger. For example, the failure to hear the sounds of a fire or an approaching car could lead to serious injury. Listening to what others say is a vital element in all human relationships. Everyday life is accompanied by a background of sounds that we hear without being aware. The sound of others moving about the house or of traffic in the distance helps us to feel part of a dynamic world and to feel more alive ourselves. The loss of this aspect of hearing has a profound effect on the patient, who may describe having a feeling that "the world is dead." The loss of this auditory background is believed to contribute significantly to the depression that so commonly occurs after a patient loses his hearing. Besides serving to keep us in tune with the world, the auditory background noises serve as clues to changes that are occurring in the environment, thus helping us to become ready to meet and cope with these changes. Because he lacks these cues, the deaf person often feels vaguely insecure. While he is very keenly aware of his inability to hear conversation, he may be unaware of the reason for his feeling of insecurity. Explanation of this relationship can help the patient to cope with this reaction.

Whereas blindness usually is obvious to others, deafness usually is not. The person with impaired hearing looks very much like everyone else, and so his quizzical expression, his frequent requests to have statements repeated, and his inattention often are attributed to stubbornness, ill temper, or eccentricity. These attitudes frequently persist even after others become aware of the individual's disability. Such comments as "He can hear when he wants to" are common.

Such attitudes are unusual in relation to people who are blind or handicapped in other ways. Just why this difference exists is not clear. That hearing loss is not visible may be one factor. People may become irritated where one who seems to have no disability fails to join in a conversation or talks too loudly. (The inability to hear their own voices causes some deaf people to speak too loudly or in monotonous tones. This is a characteristic feature of sensorineural hearing loss.) Many people are offended when their voices do not command instant attention. Even our income tax reflects greater sympathy for blind persons, by offering them an extra exemption that is not offered to deaf persons nor to persons with other types of disability.

People with hearing impairment are very sensitive to these attitudes. Many flatly refuse to wear a hearing aid, because they feel it carries a stigma. On the other hand, glasses are well accepted by most people. Some persons with hearing loss refuse to admit that they have the disability and thereby they deprive themselves of the help that they require. For example, in addition to helping the patient hear, the hearing aid can serve useful purposes by calling attention to the disability, thus encouraging others to speak more slowly and more distinctly and indicating that problems in communication are due to hearing deficit rather than to intellectual impairment.

Hearing loss is a strain on both the patient and those around him. He must focus his attention to the utmost to catch as much as possible of what is said. Often the effort seems too great, and he simply ceases trying. Family and friends may find it tiring, and at times they may find it socially awkward, to raise their voices or to speak slowly and distinctly. Sometimes a mutual withdrawal occurs, when the patient and his associates cease exerting the necessary effort to communicate.

**Factors Influencing Rehabilitation.** The age at which hearing loss occurs, as well as the severity of the impairment, affects rehabilitation. If a person has been born deaf, his education and his opportunities for marriage, friendship, and career may be jeopardized unless he has had a great deal of help in learning to compensate for the handicap. Those who become deaf later in life have the advantage of having heard normally and of being able to become educated, start a home, and find a job before the onset of deafness. Older people may find it difficult to adjust to loss of hearing, especially if it occurs quite suddenly. Whereas the persons who develop hearing impairment early in life usually have become accustomed to the use of a hearing aid or have acquired skill in lipreading during childhood, the development of these capabilities entails considerable new learning and adaptation for older persons.

**How the Nurse Can Help.** The diagnosis of the cause and the extent of the hearing loss must precede any program of rehabilitation. Anyone with hearing difficulty should be urged to visit an otologist (a physician who specializes in diseases of the ear) or an otologic clinic. One old gentleman entered the ear clinic and said, "I can't hear, Doc. I'm getting deaf." After the physician had irrigated his ears and removed a large amount of impacted cerumen, the patient could hear well. A broad grin was on his face as he left the clinic—cured of his

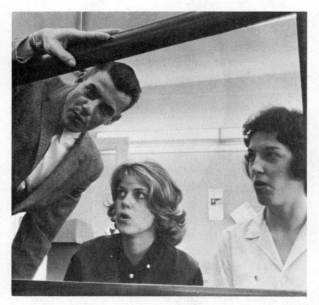

**Figure 27-4.** Using a large mirror, two students watch a lipreading instructor show them correct lip movements for words and sentences, at Gallaudet College, Washington, D.C. (a college for the deaf). (American Hearing Society, Washington, D.C.)

deafness in 20 minutes! Of course, many patients are not so fortunate. However, they may learn that surgery can restore their hearing—if not wholly, at least partially. Others, such as the large number of patients with presbycusis, learn that the hearing loss is permanent but that measures can be taken to increase their ability to hear and to understand despite the disability. There are many ways of helping people with hearing loss. Many patients are taught speech reading. They learn to watch facial movements so closely and skillfully that they can understand what is said. Often the patient does not catch every word; however, he understands enough to enable him to follow the conversation. The term *speech reading* is preferred by many to *lipreading*, because the skill actually encompasses not only reading lips but also noting facial expressions and gestures. The person who uses speech reading can be helped if others face him when they speak, so that he can see their lip movements and facial expressions. Adequate light is important. One patient appeared much deafer to the night nurse than to the day nurse, until the night nurse discovered that the patient used speech reading. Thereafter, she turned the light on before trying to talk with him.

Another way of helping people who use speech reading is to mention briefly and tactfully the topic of the conversation that he is following. For example, if a lively discussion about baseball is taking place among the patient's wardmates, turning to him and saying distinctly, "We are discussing baseball" will help him to follow the conversation. If the patient does not understand, the thought should be restated in different words. Some words are more difficult to "read" than others, and changing the wording often helps the speech reader to understand what is meant. The nurse should avoid dropping her voice at the end of a sentence. She should pronounce new or unfamiliar words with special care. People should try not to talk to the patient when they have something in their mouths, and avoid placing their hands over their mouths while they are speaking.

Shouting is seldom a help. Often it only confuses and embarrasses the patient. It is important to speak somewhat more loudly, but to emphasize slowness and distinctness of speech. Above all, the nurse should try not to show excitement or impatience when the patient fails to understand. She should treat the disability as she would any other—

accept it, and do everything that she can to help the patient to compensate for it. If he speaks too loudly, he should be told so tactfully, so that he can learn to modulate his voice.

If the patient is with others, and the nurse enters the room to speak with someone else, she should mention matter-of-factly that she has come in to speak with another patient. Sometimes the nature of the conversation can be stated briefly without violating the privacy of the other patient. For instance, she might say, "Hello, Mr. Brown. I stopped in to talk with Mr. Jones about his test tomorrow." Such a statement helps the patient with hearing loss not to feel ignored, and it indicates that the conversation does not concern him. Some people with impaired hearing become suspicious that others are talking about them. Many everyday matters can arouse their curiosity and suspicions because they can hear only part, or none, of what is said.

Whenever possible, the patient with hearing loss should be included in conversations and ward activities. He needs—and often he is denied—these opportunities for contact with others.

**Employment.** As is the case with any disabled person, finding suitable employment is a challenge. Prejudice against persons with hearing impairment prevents some of them from obtaining jobs that they are capable of performing. Vocational training and careful placement are essential. Both the requirements of the job and the deaf person's ability to perform it must be evaluated carefully. Contrary to popular belief, work in a very noisy environment is not always suitable for the deaf, because some deaf persons are very sensitive to noise, even though they lack sufficient hearing to follow conversation. However, some deaf persons can work in noisy situations more comfortably than persons with normal hearing. Switching off the hearing aid can protect them from the din and clatter that those with normal hearing find very distressing. Some deaf people also suffer from poor balance (because the vestibular portion of the inner ear, concerned with equilibrium, is affected). Persons who have problems with balance and equilibrium should not work in high or dark places. Community agencies, such as those discussed above, can help the deaf person to learn of opportunities for vocational training, counseling, and placement.

## Hearing Aids

In years past, some people with hearing impairment cupped a hand about the ear, or they held up to the ear a trumpetlike tube into which the other person spoke. Such crude devices helped to intensify

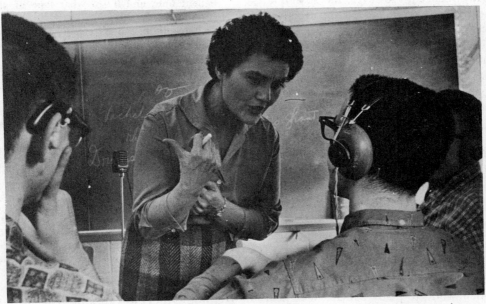

**Figure 27-5.** The lipreading instructor goes over a vocabulary list with several students. The microphone and the earphones help the students to hear maximum sound in accordance with their hearing capabilities, thus making lipreading and their own enunciation easier. (American Hearing Society, Washington, D.C.)

the sound reaching the patient's ear by channeling it directly into the ear.

Modern hearing aids are battery-operated sound amplifiers with a transistor circuit. Adjustable volume and tone controls are provided, so that the wearer can adapt the aid to changing conditions. For example, everyone wondered how one woman managed to display such patience with an employee who recited endless details of her minor illnesses and discomforts, until one day someone saw the woman flick off her hearing aid after listening to the employee's first few complaints. Some hearing aids have been designed as parts of glasses or hairbands. These inconspicuous aids appeal to people who ordinarily would shy away from a more conventional type.

Although hearing aids have helped many people, they do not restore normal hearing. In general, they do not provide as good a correction for the hearing loss as glasses provide for faulty vision. And unlike glasses, hearing aids require considerable time and effort to learn to use. The failure to understand these facts has led many persons to become discouraged and to abandon the use of the aid.

Because sound is considerably modified as it passes through the aid, it will approximate—but not duplicate—the sound that the patient remembers hearing before he became deaf. The range of tones is greatly reduced. However, the sounds are sufficiently similar to be interpreted correctly by most patients. The aid has the disadvantage of amplifying background noise as well as the sounds that the patient wants to hear. Amplified background noises are distracting, particularly to patients who have not become accustomed to the aid. For example, the roar of a passing truck when it is amplified by the aid can be very distressing. The inability to localize the source of the sound is another difficulty. When the individual is with a group, it may be hard for him to recognize which person is speaking to him. Wearing an aid in each ear may help to overcome this problem. Binaural (both ears) hearing aids are becoming more common, now that the aids are so small and so easily worn. Binaural aids sometimes are built into a pair of ordinary-looking glasses.

Despite these disadvantages, the modern hearing aid opens a new world to many patients with hearing loss. Constant improvements are being made in these instruments, making them not only less conspicuous but more efficient. Their very efficiency

poses a problem in adjustment. Patients sometimes find that the sudden increase in their ability to hear is quite startling. They must become accustomed to the sounds of everyday experiences all over again. (However, this is an adjustment that most people are delighted to make!)

The patient must learn to use his aid. He cannot slip it on and find that all his hearing problems are solved. Patience and careful attention to the instruction of the physician, nurse, and of the manufacturer of his instrument will help him to derive the maximum benefit. Wearing the instrument for short periods at first and gradually increasing the length of time that it is worn help the individual to become accustomed to it. However, persistence is important. Usually, the patient who tries the aid sporadically will have difficulty getting used to it. He should handle the instrument carefully, and avoid dropping it. The portion that fits into his ear should be cleaned daily with mild soap and water and dried thoroughly. A pipe cleaner is useful for cleansing the cannula. An extra cord and battery should be kept on hand for replacement purposes.

The following are some ways that nurses can help patients to obtain the best possible results from hearing aids:

- **Direct the patient to an otologist or an otologic clinic for help in determining whether an aid is likely to benefit him, and if so, what type of aid would be most useful for him.**
- **Avoid building up unrealistic hopes about the help that a hearing aid can give. Stress the need for patience and training in the use of the aid.**
- **Encourage the patient to follow the directions given him by his physician or by the manufacturer of his instrument.**
- **If a patient with hearing difficulty is admitted to the hospital, find out whether or not he uses an aid. If he does, ask his family to bring it to him. In the stress of illness the aid may be forgotten, and its absence can make the patient's adjustment to the hospital all the more difficult.**
- **Give the patient time to adjust his aid, if he needs to, before speaking with him.**
- **Remember that the aid is very valuable to the patient, besides being expensive. Protect it from loss or injury when the patient is unable to do so—for example, when his illness is severe, or when he is in the operating room.**

## Helping Others to Communicate with the Deaf Patient

Opportunities to talk over the particular problems that others have in dealing with the deaf person are important. They should be allowed to express some of their impatience and frustration to the nurse, who helps them to learn what they can do to make communication easier. The person with impaired hearing tends to be left out of more and more activities. He becomes more and more isolated. No one shares with him the latest news, jokes, or stories. Consequently he becomes less interesting to others—and he may be considered a bore.

What can be done to minimize the isolation of a person with hearing impairment and to help him to remain part of the family circle, or a part of the many other groups that are important in his life?

- **Help the person and those about him to recognize that he has a disability. For instance, an industrial nurse can help the individual with hearing loss and his coworkers to acknowledge that the problem exists.**
- **Urge diagnosis and treatment. For example, the industrial nurse can help to arrange for referral to determine the cause and the severity of hearing loss.**
- **Help the person with hearing loss to compensate for it by such measures as speech reading and the use of a hearing aid.**
- **Encourage both the person and others to "give a little"—to make adjustments that in the long run help everyone. Perhaps the family can encourage father to turn the television up for a few of his favorite programs, and to sit nearer the set, or obtain TV earphones. Family and friends can develop the habit of speaking slowly and distinctly to the person with a hearing loss. Why not save a front seat in the lecture hall for a student with impaired hearing, so that he can hear better or use speech reading? The willingness of others to help in these ways means as much as or even more than the assistance itself to the person with impaired hearing.**

## CONDITIONS OF THE MIDDLE EAR

The middle ear is a small, air-filled cavity in the temporal bone. Stretched across the middle ear cavity from the tympanic membrane to the oval window lies a chain of small bones called *ossicles*— the malleus, the incus, and the stapes—joined together by small ligaments and attached to the tympanic membrane by the handle of the malleus. The footplate of the stapes fits into the oval window, held in position by a ligament that allows free motion for the transmission of sound. The medial wall of the middle ear has two openings that communicate with the inner ear, the oval window (*fenestra ovalis*) and the round window (*fenestra*

*rotunda*). Sound waves pass into the external ear and its canal and strike the tympanic membrane, causing it to vibrate. The vibrations are transmitted by way of the mechanical linkage of malleus, incus, and stapes to the oval window. The motion of the footplate of the stapes in the oval window agitates the perilymph and the endolymph, thus stimulating the sensitive sound receptors of the organ of Corti, in the inner ear.

### Otosclerosis

Otosclerosis is a common cause of hearing impairment among adults. It is estimated that about 5,000,000 people suffer from otosclerosis in the United States today. It results from bony ankylosis of the stapes, which interferes with the vibration of the stapes and the transmission of sound to the inner ear. Fixation of the stapes occurs gradually over a period of many years. The hearing loss usually becomes apparent to the patient during the second and the third decades of life. Otosclerosis is more common among women. Heredity is an important causative factor; the majority of patients have a family history of the disease. The underlying cause of otosclerosis is unknown.

The progressive loss of hearing is the most characteristic symptom. The patient notices this symptom when it begins to interfere with his ability to follow conversation. The patient has particular difficulty in hearing others when they speak in soft, low tones, although he can hear adequately when the sound is loud enough. *Tinnitus* (a ringing or buzzing in the ears) may appear as the loss of hearing progresses. Tinnitus, which can occur in any type of hearing loss, is noticeable especially at night, when the surroundings are quiet, and it can be very distressing to the patient. Characteristically, the patient with otosclerosis speaks very softly, as the conductive loss allows him to hear his own voice more loudly. This phenomenon can be illustrated by plugging your ears with your fingers, thus creating a conductive hearing loss; now when you talk your voice will sound much louder to you, and you will tend to speak softly.

The diagnosis is made by an otologist after noting the family history, examining the ears, and testing the hearing. Although the hearing loss in otosclerosis is of the conductive type, often with progression of the disease, involvement of the cochlea supervenes and the hearing loss becomes a mixed type.

Although at present there is no cure for oto-sclerosis, the hearing loss can be corrected by surgery and the use of a hearing aid. The potential success of surgery, as well as the ability to wear an aid, depends greatly on the severity of the sensorineural involvement; the prognosis is best when the hearing loss is purely conductive. An otosclerotic patient has a choice between wearing an aid or undergoing surgery. With a hearing aid there is some electrical-mechanical quality to the amplified sound, whereas the hearing achieved by successful surgery is more physiologic. On the other hand, surgery is not always successful, and in fact may (though rarely) result in a deterioration of the hearing.

**Fenestration Operation.** *Fenestration* means making a window, in this case a new window through which vibrations can pass from the external auditory canal to the inner ear. Since the fixation of the stapes renders the patient's oval window useless, a new window about the size of the head of a pin is made. The sound waves strike directly against the new *fenestra*, causing vibrations in the perilymph of the inner ear. Because the structures are so tiny, the operation is done under special magnification.

The fenestration operation is seldom done today for reasons stated below. However, because the nurse works with patients who have already undergone fenestration, a description of the fenestrated ear cavity and its management are included. An entrance to the ear, about four times normal size, is created by excising skin and cartilage from the outer ear. This allows access to the lateral semi-circular canal where the new oval window (*fenestra novovalis*) is made. The bony wall which normally separates the ear canal from the mastoid is removed; the canal skin covering that wall is laid back into the mastoid cavity over the lateral semicircular canal and the new window. As a result, the ear canal and the mastoid bowl become one cavity. The eardrum is at the front of this cavity, and the semicircular canal with oval window covered by skin is in the back. From the nursing standpoint, it is important to know the following with respect to the fenestration cavity:

- Large amounts of wax and debris accumulate in the cavity.
- The material hardens and may produce dizziness by pressure on the oval window.
- The cavity requires cleaning by an otologist every six to twelve months for the patient's lifetime.
- Irrigation produces dizziness.

- If any medication or softening material is used in the ear it should be at room temperature to avoid dizziness.

The benefit of fenestration is limited by several factors:

- The incus is removed during the surgery to allow access to the horizontal canal and this interruption of the ossicular chain makes a later stapedectomy difficult.
- The operation leaves a modified radical mastoid cavity which must be cleaned by the otologist periodically. If this is not done, debris tends to accumulate in the cavity and may become infected.
- Since the ossicular chain is bypassed and since the sound vibrations are being delivered to a part of the inner ear other than the oval window, the maximum correction obtained is usually 15 to 20 db. less than that possible with stapedectomy.
- The *fenestra* shows a great tendency toward partial or complete closure; the patient's improved hearing is sometimes only temporary.

**Stapes Surgery.** During an exploratory operation on the middle ear of an otosclerotic patient, the stapes was manipulated to confirm its fixation, whereupon the patient proclaimed that he could suddenly hear. Because of the surgeon's keen awareness of what had actually happened (the stapes was freed and could vibrate) the "stapes mobilization" was born. Thousands of mobilizations have since been performed; but despite the superiority of the immediate results in hearing as compared with those of the fenestration operation, the duration of improvement was often disappointingly brief. However, recently a further advance has been made. Instead of merely breaking the fixed stapes free from the surrounding tissues, hoping that it would remain free to vibrate and not refix, surgeons remove the entire stapes, replacing it with a prosthetic device composed of such substances as fat or teflon. This procedure, known as *stapedectomy*, is generally accepted around the world as the procedure of choice in correcting conductive deafness due to otosclerosis (Fig. 27-6). This very delicate operation to remove one of the smallest bones in the human body is performed under the operating microscope. A small incision is made deep inside the external auditory canal behind the eardrum, and the drum is reflected to expose the middle ear. The surgery is carried out using very fine instruments designed specifically for minute tasks, and at its termination the patient is able to hear better. The hearing improvement is superior to that

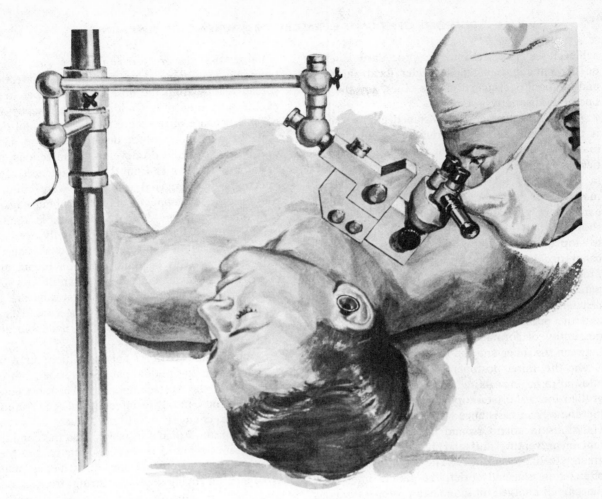

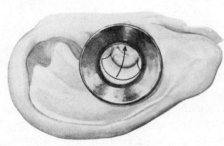

**Figure 27-6.** Operating microscope and line of meatal incision for Shea stapedectomy. In this operation the stapes is removed and a venous graft and plastic prosthesis are inserted to replace it. (*Top*) Microscope in place over patient (undraped to show detail). (*Bottom, left*) Incision (arrow indicates direction of reflection of meatal skin and eardrum over handle of malleus). (*Bottom, right*) Schema of completed operation. (Myers, D., Schlosser, W. D., and Winchester, R. A.; *Ciba Clinical Symposia* 14:2; medical illustrator Dr. Frank H. Netter.)

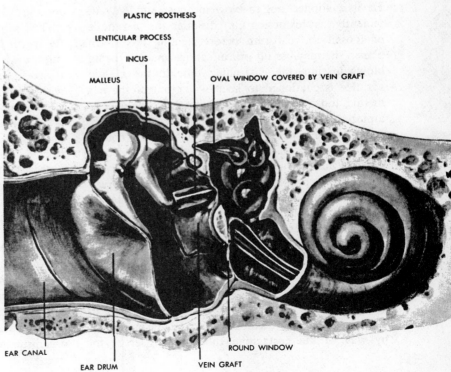

PLASTIC PROSTHESIS

LENTICULAR PROCESS

INCUS

MALLEUS

OVAL WINDOW COVERED BY VEIN GRAFT

EAR CANAL

EAR DRUM

VEIN GRAFT

ROUND WINDOW

achieved by fenestration, the procedure is easier on the patient (being done under local anesthesia and in about one-quarter of the time), and the post-operative disability is far less.

At the conclusion of the stapedectomy the ear is packed and allowed to remain so for approximately seven days. It is then unpacked and the patient is instructed to wear a piece of cotton loosely in the meatus to prevent dust and other foreign matter from getting into the canal. Occasionally the ear may ooze immediately after surgery. The nurse should notify the physician but should not attempt to stop the bleeding by additional pressure on the canal packing as this pressure may dislocate the prosthesis. For the first 48 hours after surgery, the patient is usually instructed to remain on strict bed rest with the head of the bed elevated 30 degrees and the operated ear up. This is to minimize the possibility of formation of a perilymphatic fistula between the inner and the middle ear.

On the third postoperative day the patient is allowed to begin walking about. He may have some vertigo for a short time postoperatively and should therefore have assistance when he begins walking. Handrails in corridors and bathrooms are important in preventing falls and in giving the patient a greater feeling of security. The total period of hospitalization is usually brief; the patient may sometimes be discharged on the fourth postoperative day. He is cautioned not to blow his nose suddenly or violently, as this action may dislodge the prosthesis or loosen the eardrum before healing has taken place, or may result in infectious matter being blown up into the eustachian tube to the middle ear. He is cautioned to keep water out of the ear as this, too, may lead to infection. He should keep a piece of clean dry cotton in the external auditory canal to help keep the canal clean. The cotton should be inserted gently and never pushed deeply into the canal. It is changed usually once or twice daily for approximately ten days after surgery. After healing has occurred the patient may shower, swim, and engage in practically all activities. Many surgeons restrict their patients from deep-water diving and caution against flying with a head cold, because severe pressure changes may dislodge the prosthesis.

## Infections

The middle ear connects with the nasopharynx by way of the eustachian tube, which serves to equalize the air pressure on either side of the tympanic membrane. Upper respiratory infections spread readily from the nose and the throat to the ear through this tube. Children are especially vulnerable because of the more nearly horizontal position of the eustachian tube during childhood. However, adults can and do develop ear infections, and in addition they suffer from the consequences of ear infections that occurred when they were children. Before the development of antimicrobial agents, ear infections often caused considerable damage before the patient's own resistance finally overcame them. Death from ear infections now is unusual, although it used to be quite common before antibiotics became available. However, antibiotics have created another problem: microorganisms are becoming resistant to them, and we are faced again with some infections for which the available antibiotics are of little benefit.

**Serous Otitis Media.** This condition, in which fluid forms in the middle ear, can result from obstruction of the eustachian tube. The obstruction itself may be caused by infection, allergy, tumors, or sudden changes in altitude, such as sudden descents in an airplane, in which case the condition is sometimes referred to as aero-otitis media. Measures that help to prevent aero-otitis media include avoidance of flying while suffering from a head cold, chewing gum, yawning, or repeated swallowing during descent open the eustachian tubes.

The symptoms of serous otitis media include a feeling of fullness, diminished hearing, and hearing one's own voice echoing in the involved ear. If allowed to remain, the fluid thickens and scars form, with resulting permanent hearing loss.

The treatment includes aspiration of the fluid after puncturing the eardrum (*paracentesis*). The underlying cause of the condition also may be treated. For example, antibiotics may be required to treat an infection; to treat an allergy, desensitization and/or antihistamines may be necessary.

Tonsils and adenoids should be removed when they are an etiologic factor. When the fluid in the middle ear is thick, a plastic ventilating tube is placed in the eardrum incision and left in place for a variable period of time. It is extruded spontaneously or removed by the otologist.

**Acute Purulent Otitis Media.** This acute infection of the middle ear (sometimes abbreviated OMPA) usually results from the spread of microorganisms to the middle ear through the eustachian tube during upper respiratory infections. Pus collects in the middle ear, causing increased pressure which, in turn, causes bulging of the eardrum.

The symptoms include fever, malaise, severe earache, and diminished hearing. The physician notes that the eardrum is red and bulging. Sometimes, it has perforated, and pus is present in the auditory canal. Prompt treatment usually can avoid rupture of the eardrum. Rupture often causes a jagged tear that heals slowly, sometimes incompletely, and with considerable scarring. Such scarring can interfere with the vibration of the drum, causing diminished hearing.

To prevent spontaneous rupture, the physician may incise the drum (*myringotomy*), letting the pus escape. This eases the pressure and relieves the throbbing pain. The incision heals readily with very little scarring. At first the discharge from the ear is bloody, and then it is purulent. The physician may order eardrops to facilitate drainage. He may ask the nurse to wipe the external portions of the canal with a dry sterile applicator. Cotton plugs should not be stuffed into the ear, because it is important for the pus to drain. The external ear must be cleaned frequently. Applying petrolatum to the skin helps to prevent excoriation. A small piece of cotton may be placed loosely at the meatus to help to absorb the drainage. It should be changed frequently. The drainage may continue for several days.

Culture and sensitivity tests are performed on specimens of the purulent materials to determine which antibiotics will be effective against the organisms. Antibiotics are given to control the infection. Fluids are encouraged. Rest and the avoidance of chilling are important until all symptoms of the infection have subsided.

The complications of acute purulent otitis media include mastoiditis (the middle ear connects with the mastoid process by complex passages through which infection can travel), scarring, and/or permanent perforation of the eardrum and hearing loss. The infection also may spread to the meninges, causing meningitis, or it may become chronic (chronic otitis media). Other complications include labyrinthitis, indicated by nystagmus, vertigo, nausea, and vomiting; and lateral sinus thrombosis (spread of the infection to the large veins at the base of the brain), causing clot formation and septicemia. Infection may injure the facial nerve and cause facial paralysis. Brain abscess may result from the extension of the infection to the brain.

Cholesteatoma can result from chronic perforation of the eardrum. The skin normally lining the external ear enters the middle ear, due to the perforation. Desquamation (shedding) of the skin occurs in this tiny space. The dead skin becomes trapped, collects, and becomes mixed with mucus. The collection gradually enlarges, grows into a ball, and becomes a medium for bacterial growth. Since it cannot escape, it causes damage by pressure on nearby structures. The cholesteatoma must be removed surgically.

Fortunately, these complications are less common than formerly, because of the prompt control of the infection with antibiotics. However, patients with perforated eardrums are prone to repeated infections throughout life. Often a chronic infection develops that is difficult to cure, and that spreads throughout the ear and the mastoid process. Patients who have perforated eardrums should avoid getting water in the ear, since this readily causes infection. Special precautions must be taken when they are bathing or swimming. Custom-molded ear plugs plus a bathing cap are sometimes recommended to keep water out of the ears. Some physicians advise their patients who have perforated eardrums not to swim at all, because of the risk of severe infection if water should enter the middle ear.

Plastic surgery (myringoplasty—see below) usually is successful in repairing the perforated drum. In one technique the edges of the perforation are cauterized, and a patch of bloodsoaked Gelfoam is used as a scaffolding over which new tissues grow until they have completely filled in the defect.

Subsequent repeated and chronic infections, with all their risk of spreading to the brain and the loss of hearing, may be avoided if the drum can be repaired.

**Chronic Otitis Media.** This preventable condition usually results from neglect or incomplete treatment of acute otitis media. The patient usually has a chronic discharge from the ear, a reduction of hearing, and sometimes a slight fever. Treatment with antibiotics may be effective in controlling the infection. However, when it has persisted for a long time, destruction occurs in the middle ear and the mastoid process. Such patients have marked loss of hearing, and often they are in danger of spread of the infection to the brain. Surgery usually is recommended to eradicate the disease and to prevent further complications. Often, a radical mastoid-ectomy is necessary to remove the diseased tissue.

**Mastoiditis.** The spread of the infection to the mastoid process can occur in either acute or chronic otitis media. The symptoms of *acute mastoiditis* include pain and tenderness over the mastoid process, chills, fever, malaise, and headache. The treatment includes prompt administration of anti-biotics and sometimes, if there is not a favorable response to medical treatment, simple mastoidec-tomy. Through a postaural (behind the ear) incision, the surgeon removes the infected mastoid cells. Hearing impairment usually does not occur.

*Chronic mastoiditis* carries a less favorable prog-nosis. Chronic infection in the mastoid process leads to destruction of the tissue, causing hearing loss. The infection usually involves the middle ear also, since chronic otitis media frequently causes chronic mastoiditis. Often, radical mastoidectomy (see below) is necessary to remove the diseased tissue. Usually, the hearing is reduced markedly be-cause of the necessity for removing important struc-tures. The diseased mastoid cells are removed, as well as the incus, the malleus, and the eardrum. The middle ear and the mastoid become one cavity. The stapes is left in position to protect the entrance to the inner ear. Just how radical the operation must be depends on the extent of the infection. The more extensive the surgery, the greater the hearing loss. Surgical procedures have been developed re-cently that preserve important structures. These delicate operations are performed under magnifica-tion, and they require a great deal of time, patience, and surgical skill. *Tympanoplasty* is the term used to describe the plastic reconstruction of the middle ear. Tympanoplasty may be performed with or after mastoidectomy in an attempt to rebuild the middle ear structures. Results of these efforts at restoration of middle ear function have been dis-appointing in the more severe cases. The patient may have to undergo several operations to achieve a minimal functional result.

The importance of prompt and adequate treat-ment of any ear infection cannot be overempha-sized. The prevention of chronic otitis media and mastoiditis is far easier and less disabling than the treatment of these infections.

## Examples of Middle Ear and Mastoid Surgery

The extent and variety of middle ear and mastoid surgery depends on the extent of the chronic dis-ease. All diseased tissue must be completely re-moved. The cavity may be closed or left open. The operations performed are as follows:

- Myringoplasty—repair of the eardrum perforation with a graft such as fascia or vein.
- Tympanoplasty—reconstruction of the ossicular chain.
- Modified radical mastoidectomy—removal of mas-toid cells, leaving the middle ear, eardrum, and ossicles intact.
- Radical mastoidectomy—surgical merging of the malleus, incus, drum, and posterior canal into one large cavity.
- Mastoid obliteration—filling of the mastoid cavity with muscle.
- Intact canal wall operation—the canal wall is not removed; it is drilled thin and left in place, and the surgery is performed by a combined anterior and posterior approach.

## Principles in the Care of Any Patient After Ear Surgery

Regardless of the specific nature of the operation, certain principles are applicable to the care of any patient after aural surgery. These may be summar-ized as follows:

- **Make sure that the external ear and the surrounding skin are meticulously clean. Excess cerumen will be removed from the canal by the physician.**
- **Injury to the facial nerve may occur during ear sur-gery. Note whether the patient can wrinkle his fore-head, close his eyes, pucker his lips, and bare his teeth. Report any inability to perform these move-ments. If these signs appear immediately after sur-gery, there probably has been damage to the facial nerve. If the paralysis appears after 12 to 24 hours postoperatively, it is probably due to edema; the physician may recommend loosening the ear dress-ing and administering anti-inflammatory drugs. Oc-casionally, the nerve is damaged permanently as a result of the surgery.**
- **Strict adherence to aseptic technique is essential. Because the ear is so close to the brain, any infection may endanger the patient's life. Antibiotics may be ordered to help to prevent infection. Instruct the pa-tient to keep his hands away from the dressing, which is changed only by the surgeon. Observe the dressing for drainage.**
- **Vertigo is common, due to the temporary effects on the body-balancing function of the semicircular canals. Special measures should be employed to pro-tect the patient from falling. Side rails and handrails should be used, and the patient should be helped out of bed. Vertigo is very distressing. Explain that this symptom is not unusual after ear surgery, and that it will subside gradually.**

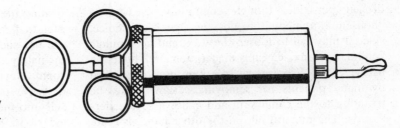

**Figure 27-7.** Pomeroy syringe, usually used in removing cerumen by irrigation.

• Instruct the patient not to blow his nose. During the postoperative period, nasal secretions should be wiped off the end of the nose without blowing it. Blowing the nose can permit infectious material to enter the operative area through the eustachian tube or may dislodge prostheses or grafts in the ear.

• Help the patient to realize what to expect as a result of surgery. If he seems not to understand, clarify with him and assist him to recall and to comprehend what the surgeon has explained. Additional explanation by the physician may relieve a great deal of worry and uncertainty. For instance, a patient who has had a fenestration operation may believe the surgery was unsuccessful if he does not hear better immediately.

• Protect the patient's hair from soiling. Braid it, or hold it away from the ear with a strip of bandage fastened by collodion.

## DISORDERS OF THE EXTERNAL AUDITORY CANAL

### Treatment of Disorders

The external auditory canal is subject to a variety of annoying disorders. Usually, these are discomforts rather than threats to life or hearing. However, if they are not carefully and adequately treated, these disorders may involve the middle ear and become serious problems. For instance, unskilled attempts at removing cerumen or foreign bodies may perforate the eardrum and push the material into the middle ear. Nurses often are asked to advise patients about apparently minor disorders of the external auditory canal. Therefore, it is very important to realize how patients may be advised about the care of their ears, so that disorders of the external ear can be prevented.

**Impacted Cerumen.** Sometimes, cerumen accumulates in the external auditory canal, causing a plug or obstruction. The chief symptoms are a feeling of stuffiness and discomfort in the ear, itching or irritation of the canal, and diminished hearing.

The ear is examined to determine the cause of the difficulty. If cerumen is blocking the canal, it is irrigated with warm water, using a Pomeroy syringe (Fig. 27-7). The patient, draped with a plastic apron, is given a large emesis basin to hold under his ear. Irrigation is continued until the canal is clear. The canal is dried thoroughly after the irrigation; leaving it wet predisposes to the development of infections. Sometimes, cerumen is removed with a curet or with suction.

Accumulations of cerumen do not necessarily reflect poor personal hygiene, since some people's ceruminous glands secrete an excessive amount, which accumulates inside the canal where the patient cannot remove it merely by washing his ears. Many patients are embarrassed by the condition, believing that others consider it an evidence of uncleanliness. The treatment of the condition must be handled gently. Care must be taken not to injure the ear when the cerumen is removed. The nurse also should avoid any remark that would reflect on the patient's habits of personal hygiene.

As indicated above, some nurses have preparation in examining the patient's ears and in the removal of cerumen from the canal. No irrigation should be undertaken before examining the tympanic membrane to make sure it is intact, and examining the canal, because:

• The cause of the discomfort may not be impacted cerumen. For example, a patient on a psychiatric ward may have pushed a dried pea into his ear; irrigation would make the pea swell and become more difficult to remove.

• The patient may have a perforated eardrum. This is a very common condition. Irrigation would be contraindicated, because the solution, as well as the cerumen, could enter the middle ear, causing infection.

The patient should be instructed not to pick his ear with his fingers or with applicators. He is unable to see how far he is inserting them. He may injure the canal, causing infection, or he may push the cerumen in farther. Patients who are troubled by accumulations of cerumen often are advised to instill a few drops of mineral oil at intervals. Hydrogen peroxide, though commonly used as a "household remedy," is not the agent of choice, since it may fail to loosen the wax, and accumulate behind the wax, causing maceration and infection in the canal. Proprietary solutions now purchased by many patients for removing cerumen may be irritating to the canal skin and cause a severe dermatitis. The mineral oil, on the other hand, is quite safe. It softens the hardened cerumen so that it more readily comes out of the meatus.

*Furuncles* (boils) are exquisitely painful when they occur in the auditory canal. Because the skin is tight and the lumen is narrow, the swelling caused by a furuncle causes pain out of all proportion to the size of the lesion. Most furuncles are caused by picking the ear in attempts to relieve itching or to remove wax. Bobby pins and matches sometimes are stuck into the canal, traumatizing it and leading to infection.

Antibiotics may be ordered to combat the infection. The local application of heat by a heating pad or a hot-water bottle is sometimes recommended. Salicylates and sometimes codeine may be necessary to lessen the pain. A wick soaked in aluminum acetate solution (Burow's solution) is sometimes inserted.

To prevent furuncles, it is important to keep the auditory canal dry and clean and avoid traumatizing it.

**External Otitis.** So-called fungus infections of the external auditory canal are common in warm, damp climates or when the canal is not carefully dried. Actually the organisms responsible are usually bacteria. Only a small percentage are due to fungi, but the term "fungus infection" persists. A preferable term for the condition is external otitis. Dead epithelium tends to collect in the canal, which has a brownish "moldy" appearance. Eardrops containing antibiotics, steroids, or copper sulfate, glycerin, and alcohol may be ordered. Infections sometimes are stubbornly persistent and require treatment for several weeks. The proper drying of the canal after swimming or bathing helps to prevent infections.

**Insects in the Auditory Canal.** Insects occasionally enter the canal. Although they usually fly out again, sometimes they remain inside. Their fluttering and buzzing are agonizing. Holding a flashlight to the ear often draws the insect out by attracting it to the light. A few drops of alcohol or mineral oil may be effective in killing the insect;

turning the head to the side may help the dead insect to float out of the meatus. If these measures are not successful, the patient should be taken immediately to an otologist or a hospital emergency room. Never try to remove the insect with forceps or tweezers. Sometimes the insect has fastened itself into the eardrum. Great care and skill are necessary to remove the insect without injuring the patient's ear.

## DISORDERS OF THE INNER EAR

The inner ear, or labyrinth, is a very complicated structure that lies deep in the temporal bone. It is surrounded, for protection, by the hardest bony substance in the body. The inner ear consists of a series of cavities and canals. The bony canals and spaces constitute the bony labyrinth. They are lined with periosteum and enclose the much smaller membranous labyrinth. The space between the two is filled with *perilymph*. The membranous labyrinth is filled with *endolymph*. The movement of this fluid stimulates the nerve endings of both branches (vestibular and cochlear) of the auditory nerve. There are two sections to the inner ear: an anterior portion, the cochlea; and a posterior portion, the semicircular canals.

The *cochlea* is formed like a snail shell. The end organ for hearing (the organ of Corti) is located within the cochlea. The three *semicircular canals* are placed in different planes: horizontal, vertical, and oblique. Each canal has at its end an enlarged portion, the *ampulla,* containing the nerve endings of the vestibular portion of the auditory nerve, which control the sense of balance. The movement of the head sets the endolymph in motion and stimulates these nerve endings. Each ampulla contains numerous hair cells that project into the endolymph. The motion of the fluid (started by moving the head) past these hair cells sets up stimuli that pass through the vestibular portion of the auditory nerve to the cerebellum, where the center of balance is located.

When the footplate of the stapes in the oval window moves, the perilymph and the endolymph become agitated and stimulate the sound receptors of the organ of Corti. The vibrations are converted to nerve impulses that pass over the cochlear nerve fibers to the auditory center of each of the cerebral hemispheres.

Disorders of the inner ear are difficult to treat. Inner-ear deafness is of the sensorineural type, which usually cannot be helped by surgery and only occasionally by hearing aids. As noted above, the auditory center in the brain, the inner ear, and the auditory nerve may be injured by drugs, tumors, systemic diseases, prolonged exposure to loud noise, and the aging process. The management involves the prevention of further injury, if this is possible, and training in speech reading.

**Meniere's Disease.** The cause of Meniere's disease is unknown, and the pathologic changes responsible for the symptoms are not entirely clear. Many theories have been stated. Among them are:

- Dilation of the endolymphatic spaces of the labyrinth
- Vasomotor changes resulting in spasm of the internal auditory artery

Also, it has been suggested that attacks of Meniere's disease may be related to an allergic response or to emotional or endocrine disturbances.

This condition is characterized by vertigo, tinnitus, and progressive hearing loss. It usually involves only one ear. An attack may last from a few minutes to weeks. The attacks occur with alarming suddenness. Often, the patient becomes afraid to leave his home lest he have an attack in public. Frequently, continued employment becomes impossible.

Symptomatic treatment includes the use of a low-sodium diet to lessen edema. Sedatives may help to relieve apprehension. Such drugs as dimenhydrinate (Dramamine) and eclizine (Bonine) may lessen the symptoms. Bed rest usually is necessary during an acute attack. Vasodilating agents, such as nicotinic acid, are prescribed sometimes. Some patients recover spontaneously from the disorder. On the other hand, it may be so incapacitating that the labyrinth is destroyed surgically to relieve the symptoms. Ultrasonic waves have been used to destroy the labyrinth. Recently, another type of operation has been developed that establishes permanent drainage of excessive endolymph from the inner ear into the subarachnoid space around the brain.

A third means of surgical treatment has been developed over the past few years. It is based on the fact that in an acute attack of Meniere's disease the increase in endolymphatic fluid pressure causes the saccule (one of the organs of balance) to balloon up. A small tack (1.3 to 1.9 mm. in length) is placed through the footplate of the stapes just over the saccule but not touching it. With any swelling of the saccule, it comes in contact with the tack and is punctured. This automatic, repetitive decompression relieves the excess endolymphatic pressure and aborts the attack.

It must be emphasized, however, that the surgical treatment of Meniere's disease is in its formative stages and results are not consistently good.

The nursing care of the patient with Meniere's disease is challenging. Every effort must be made not to aggravate the symptoms or to precipitate attacks by sudden movement. The patient should not turn over quickly or be jarred in his bed. All movements must be explained carefully beforehand and then carried out slowly. Protection from falls is essential when the vertigo is severe. It is important to use side rails when the patient is in bed and to give him assistance when he is out of bed. Foods and fluids are accepted better if they are offered frequently and in small amounts, and if the patient's preferences are considered.

## REVIEW OF SOME COMMON NURSING PROCEDURES

The following points will be useful in caring for patients with ear disorders:

**Straightening the Canal.** The canal should be straightened before any procedure such as instillation of drops or irrigation is attempted. This affords observation of the area and permits the medication or the solution to be directed into the canal. The nurse pulls the auricle upward, backward, and slightly outward to straighten the adult's auditory canal. She should never introduce anything into the canal farther than she can see after straightening it, because the eardrum may be damaged.

**Dry Wipe.** If the patient has a discharge from his ear, dry wipes are often used to keep the canal clean. The nurse should take a small, sterile, dry applicator, straighten the canal with one hand, and with the other insert and gently rotate the applicator to remove the drainage. A good light is essential, to enhance visualization of the canal and the position of the inserted applicator. Usually, several applicators are required, since the canal often must be wiped several times. The nurse should discard the soiled applicators immediately, and wash her hands thoroughly.

**Eardrops.** The patient should lie on his side with the affected ear uppermost. The nurse should straighten the canal, adjust the light, and look into the canal. If drainage is present, it should be removed with a dry wipe. The drops should be instilled as they were ordered. The hand should rest on the patient's head, to promote good control of the dropper if the patient should move suddenly. The amount and the strength of the solution to be used always are specified by the physician. Warming the medication to body temperature makes the procedure more comfortable for the patient. The patient should remain on his side for five to ten minutes, so that the drug will remain in the canal and produce maximum benefit. Cotton sometimes is inserted loosely into the orifice of the external canal to collect drainage.

**Irrigation.** When a nurse irrigates a patient's ear, she ordinarily uses a rubber bulb syringe, because it exerts only slight pressure. The solution should be warmed to body temperature. The patient should be draped with a plastic apron, and he should hold a large emesis basin under his ear. The irrigation usually is performed with the patient in a sitting position.

The nurse expels air from the syringe, and straightens the canal with one hand. With the other, she gently instills the solution, directing it either to the roof or floor of the canal, but not directly against the drum. She avoids obstructing the canal with the syringe; the solution should be allowed to flow back freely at all times. Failure to permit its return would cause too much pressure on the eardrum. The nurse notes the return flow. After the irrigation, the patient should lie on the affected side for a few minutes to allow all the solution to run out. The pillow should be protected with a piece of plastic and a towel, or with a disposable pad. The ear should be dried thoroughly.

## REFERENCES AND BIBLIOGRAPHY

BAILIE, R. W.: Deafness—a problem of communication, *Nurs. Times* 68:923, July 27, 1972.

BROWN, M. S., and ALEXANDER, M. M.: Physical examination: Hearing acuity, *Nurs. '74* 4:61, April 1974.

BURNSIDE, I. M.: Accoutrements of aging, *Nurs. Clin. N. Am.* 7:291, June 1972.

CARTY, R.: Patients who cannot hear, *Nurs. Forum* 11:290, 1972.

CHODIL, J., and WILLIAMS, B.: The concept of sensory deprivation, *Nurs. Clin. N. Am.* 5:453, September 1970.

CONOVER, M., and COBER, J.: Understanding and caring for the hearing impaired, *Nurs. Clin. N. Am.* 5:497, September 1970.

CORNFORTH, A. R., et al.: Deaf people in psychiatric hospitals, Part 1, *Nurs. Times* 68:101, January 27, 1972.

————: Disturbed and deaf, Part 2, *Nurs. Times* 68:139, February 3, 1972.

————: Subnormal and deaf, Part 3, *Nurs. Times* 68, February 10, 1972.

————: Progressive or sudden hearing loss, Part 4, *Nurs. Times* 68:205, February 17, 1972.

DAVIS, H., and SILVERMAN, S. R. (eds.): *Hearing and Deafness,* ed. 3, New York, Holt, 1970.

DeWEESE, D. D., and SAUNDERS, W.: *Textbook of Otolaryngology,* ed. 4, St. Louis, Mosby, 1973.

DUDLEY, J. P.: The cotton applicator: Friend or foe? *Community Med.* 37:187, April 1973.

FOXEN, E. H.: *Lecture Notes on Diseases of the Ear, Nose and Throat,* Oxford, Blackwell Scientific Publications, 1968.

HERTH, K.: Beyond the curtain of silence, *Am. J. Nurs.* 74:1060, June 1974.

JACKSON, C. W., et al.: Sensory deprivation as a field of study, *Nurs. Res.* 20:46, January-February 1971.

KUKK, A. C.: Traumatic deafness, *Nurs. Mirror* 134:36, January 28, 1972.

MARTIN, E. W.: *Hazards of Medication,* Philadelphia, Lippincott, 1971.

PAPARELLA, M. M., and SHUMRICK, D. A. (eds.): *Otolaryngology,* Vols. 1 and 2, Philadelphia, Saunders, 1973.

PERRON, D.: Deprived of sound, *Am. J. Nurs.* 74:1057, June 1974.

PRIOR, J. A., and SILBERSTEIN, J. S.: *Physical Diagnosis,* ed. 4, St. Louis, Mosby, 1973.

ROSEN, S., et al.: Presbycusis study of a relatively noise-free population in the Sudan, *Ann. Otol.* 71:727, 1962.

SATALOFF, J.: *Hearing Loss,* Philadelphia, Lippincott, 1966.

SAUNDERS, W., et al.: *Nursing Care in Eye, Ear, Nose and Throat Disorders,* ed. 2, St. Louis, Mosby, 1968.

ZATUCHNI, J.: *Notes on Physical Diagnosis,* Philadelphia, Davis, 1964.

# UNIT SIX

## Threats to Adequate Ventilation

# The Patient with Disease of the Nasopharynx or Larynx

## CHAPTER 28

Conditions of the nose, throat, and larynx vary from discomforting but benign chronic disorders such as sinusitis to life-threatening malignancies whose treatment sometimes involves radical facial disfigurement, change in normal airway, and loss of normal eating patterns and vocal communication.

Important aspects of the nurse's role are case finding and referral of patients for early treatment to help minimize losses, including loss of time from work, temporary or permanent interference with reception of stimuli of sound, sight, taste, or smell, or the social and aesthetic losses from radical facial disfigurement.

Nursing process for the clinical nurse specialist in an ambulatory care setting involves assessment of patient interview and laboratory data. She may become skilled at certain physical assessment techniques such as inspection of the nasal passages, mucous membranes, and sinuses, the oral cavity, soft palate and tonsils; palpation of cervical lymph nodes and salivary glands; examination of the neck for muscle symmetry and strength, blood vessel integrity, and abnormal masses; as well as indirect laryngeal examination. Detailed information on the physical aspects of assessment of patients with nose and throat disorders is found in nursing specialty literature on clinical diagnoses.

The nurse should also utilize opportunities for educating the public to seek prompt medical attention for a sore that does not heal, difficulty in swallowing, or persistent hoarseness. If detected early, oral or laryngeal cancer has one of the best prognoses of all sites of cancer.

Disorders of the
Sinuses and
the Nose

Laryngitis

Tonsillitis, Peritonsillar
Abscess,
Tonsillectomy

Cancer of the Larynx

The Patient with
Radical Surgery
of the Head
and Neck

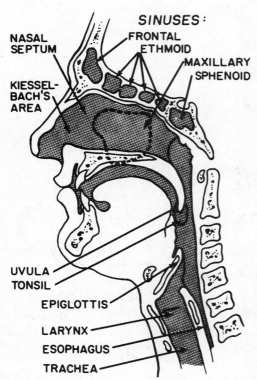

**SINUSES:**
NASAL SEPTUM
FRONTAL
ETHMOID
MAXILLARY
SPHENOID
KIESSEL-BACH'S AREA
UVULA
TONSIL
EPIGLOTTIS
LARYNX
ESOPHAGUS
TRACHEA

**Figure 28-1.** Some important structures of the nose and the throat.

## DISORDERS OF THE SINUSES AND THE NOSE

The lateral walls of the nasal cavity are formed by three bony protuberances on either side—the superior, the middle, and the inferior turbinate bones. Between the turbinates are grooves that contain the openings through which the sinuses drain. There are three pairs of openings (meatus)—superior, middle, and inferior—each beneath its respective turbinate. The entire nasal cavity is lined with a highly vascular mucous membrane, the surface of which is composed of ciliated columnar epithelial cells. Interspersed with the columnar cells are numerous goblet cells that secrete mucus which is carried back to the nasopharynx by the movement of the cilia.

The paranasal sinuses are extensions of the nasal cavity into the surrounding facial bones. The lining of these sinuses is continuous with the mucous membrane lining of the nasal cavity. These sinuses are located in the frontal, the ethmoid, the sphenoid, and the maxillary bones. Their functions are to lighten the weight of the skull, and to give resonance to the voice.

The two frontal sinuses lie within the frontal bone, extending above the orbital cavities. The ethmoid bone contains a honeycomb of small spaces known as the ethmoid sinuses, or cells, located between the eyes. The sphenoid sinuses lie behind the nasal cavity. The maxillary sinuses (antra of Highmore) are located on either side of the nose in the maxillary bones. They are the largest of the sinuses, and most accessible to treatment.

The olfactory area lies at the roof of the nose; directly above is the cribriform plate which forms a portion of the roof of the nose, and the floor of the anterior cranial fossa. Trauma or surgery in this area, therefore, carries risk of injury or infection to the brain.

### Sinusitis

Sinusitis is an inflammation of the sinuses. A maxillary sinus (antrum) most often is affected. Sinusitis is caused principally by the spread of an infection from the nasal passages to the sinuses and by the blockage of normal sinus drainage. Lessened resistance to infection is an important predisposing factor. Emotional strain, fatigue, and poor nutrition increase one's susceptibility to sinusitis. Sinusitis that accompanies or follows the common cold illustrates the role played by infection and obstruction. Because the mucous membrane lining of the nasal passages and the sinuses is continuous, infection spreads readily from the nose to the sinuses. Edema of the turbinates, which occurs in response to the infection, interferes with normal drainage of the sinuses by blocking their openings into the middle meatus, which lies under the middle turbinate (Fig. 28-3). Other common respiratory infections, such as influenza, often lead to sinusitis.

Anything that interferes with the drainage of the sinuses predisposes to sinusitis, because the trapped secretions readily become infected. Allergy frequently causes edema of the turbinates and therefore frequently leads to sinusitis. Nasal polyps and deviated septum are other common causes of faulty sinus drainage.

Sinusitis often is considered to be a minor affliction. However, although it usually does not cause death, it is a major cause of discomfort, particularly in northern temperate climates, where upper respiratory infections are common. Many people lose time from work, or they are less productive because

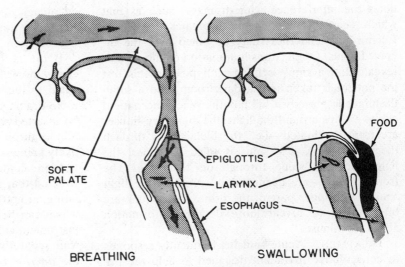

**Figure 28-2.** During swallowing, the soft palate is elevated to close off air from the nose. Breathing is interrupted momentarily. The larynx rises, and its opening is shut off by the epiglottis until the food has passed down into the esophagus.

of this condition. Sinusitis is very likely to recur in susceptible individuals—for example, among those who have frequent colds, allergy, or a deviated septum. Often the condition is neglected and becomes chronic. Chronic sinusitis leads to changes in the mucous membrane of the sinuses and makes the condition difficult to treat.

Sinusitis can lead to serious complications, such as spread of the infection by way of the eustachian tubes to the middle ear, through the thin bony walls of the maxillary and ethmoid sinuses to the eye, and retrograde through the venous channels to the brain. It can also lead to bronchiectasis and asthma. Nurses should encourage the prompt treatment of conditions that predispose to sinusitis, such as allergy and polyps, and should emphasize the importance of early medical attention when sinusitis occurs.

**Acute Sinusitis.** This condition frequently accompanies or follows upper respiratory infections.

It is characterized by pain and feelings of pressure over the involved sinuses—usually, the maxillary or the frontal sinuses. The pain from maxillary sinusitis typically occurs in the cheek. A characteristic sign of sinusitis is increased pain on bending down. Often, the upper teeth ache, due to the closeness of their nerve roots to the maxillary sinuses. The inflammation of the frontal sinuses is characterized by pain over the eyes, particularly shortly after arising in the morning. Swelling and redness also may occur over the involved sinuses. An appearance of puffiness and facial asymmetry is not uncommon. Low grade fever, malaise, fatigue, and lack of appetite are frequent. The nasal discharge usually is purulent. Postnasal discharge, often described by the patient as a drip or constant swallowing of mucus, may cause sore throat, cough, and pulmonary infections.

DIAGNOSIS. The diagnosis of sinusitis is made by history and physical examination. The physician

**Figure 28-3.** Edema can cause obstruction of sinus drainage. (A) Location of maxillary sinuses. (B) The maxillary sinuses normally drain through the openings that lie under the middle turbinates. Note that the opening for the drainage is nearest the upper portion of the sinus. (C) Edema, such as that which commonly accompanies upper respiratory infections, can obstruct the opening and prevent normal sinus drainage.

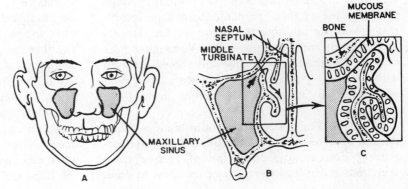

notes the interference with drainage, such as that which occurs from swollen turbinates or polyps. Edema and tenderness may be noted over the involved sinus. Often, transillumination of the sinuses reveals that a sinus is filled with pus. In this test the patient is taken into a dark room, and a small flashlight is placed in his mouth. When the patient closes his lips around the light, the maxillary sinuses are transilluminated—i.e., the light shines through them. However, if a sinus is filled with pus, the light does not shine through on that side. The frontal sinuses are examined by pressing the light against the upper part of the orbit. X-ray films are often taken to reveal more detailed information about the sinuses.

TREATMENT. Acute sinusitis frequently responds to conservative treatment designed to help the patient to overcome the infection. Bed rest, ample fluid intake, and salicylates for the relief of pain often are effective. Warm compresses sometimes soothe the discomfort. The use of vasoconstrictors is of great importance, in order to shrink the edematous turbinates, thus permitting drainage from the opening under the middle turbinate. Neo-Synephrine, 0.25 to 0.5 per cent, and Otrivin 0.1 per cent nose drops commonly are prescribed. The nose drops are used only during the phase when the discharge is thick, and the turbinates are swollen. When they are used at four-hour intervals over a period of several days, these drugs help to maintain drainage of the sinuses. Antibiotics usually are necessary to combat the infection.

The misuse of nose drops and other medicines can make the condition worse. When nose drops are applied too frequently or over too long a period, they provide shorter and shorter periods of relief, and are followed by "rebound" swelling of the turbinates, making the problem of obstruction worse. Many preparations may be purchased without prescription. The nurse who observes prolonged indiscriminate use of these preparations can perform a real service by advising the person of the dangers and referring him to a physician. Vasoconstrictors may be absorbed systemically and should be used with caution. Patients with hypertension should seek their physician's advice before using these preparations.

Many "cold tablets" contain antihistamines which thicken nasal secretions; while this action may temporarily decrease the discomfort of profuse nasal secretions it can lead to failure of the sinus to drain adequately, due to the thickened secretions. Secretions thus trapped readily form a focus for continuing infection.

If the lack of drainage has resulted in the accumulation of pus, the maxillary sinus often is irrigated to remove the purulent material and to promote drainage. Occasionally, a special catheter can be inserted through the normal opening under the middle turbinate. This particular procedure is relatively painless.

More commonly the normal opening is so obstructed that a catheter cannot be inserted, necessitating an antral puncture for irrigation of the sinus, which can be performed in the office or clinic. An instrument called a *trocar* is used to pierce the bony wall separating the nose and the antrum beneath the *inferior* turbinate where the bone is thin, and the irrigating fluid can be introduced into the base of the maxillary sinus where most of the purulent material has collected.

Pain, pressure and, sometimes, faintness accompany antrum puncture and irrigation. Local application of cocaine to the nasal mucosa is used before the procedure to lessen the discomfort. It is sometimes helpful for the nurse to support the patient's head with her hands during the brief interval when the physician is applying pressure with the trocar. The hands are placed at the back of the patient's head. Supporting the head makes the pressure less distressing to him. Support of his head as a means of lessening discomfort should be briefly explained to the patient so that he does not, in the apprehension of the moment, interpret it as restraint.

Warm normal saline usually is used for the antrum irrigation. The patient holds a basin under his nose, with his head tilted forward, and the irrigating fluid and pus drain into the basin. The nurse may assist the physician during the procedure in addition to supporting the patient by explaining the procedure to him. Sometimes the physician inserts the cannula and the nurse does the actual irrigation, while the physician is holding the cannula in place. The first few milliliters of irrigating solution should be injected slowly to assure that the cannula is actually in the sinus and not in the orbit. If it is in the latter, the periorbital tissues will swell immediately and the irrigation should be stopped.

Antrum irrigation is an uncomfortable and sometimes a frightening experience for the patient. The nurse can support him by such actions as placing her hand on his shoulder, handing him tissues as he needs them, quietly reminding him to breathe through his mouth, quickly supplying him with a clean drainage basin when it is needed, and helping him to a comfortable chair or cot where he may rest for a few moments when the procedure is over. The patient treated by antrum puncture and irrigation should be observed carefully for faintness and dizziness during and immediately after the procedure.

Trephine of the frontal sinus is used in treatment of refractory acute frontal sinusitis. This procedure, performed in the operating room, involves insertion of a tiny tube into a drill hole made into the frontal sinus. This allows drainage of secretions from the sinus, and a route through which medications can be instilled directly into the sinus. The tube remains in place until normal sinus drainage has been re-established.

**Chronic Sinusitis.** This condition responds more slowly to treatment. All of the measures previously described may be used. Particular emphasis is placed on increasing the patient's resistance by adequate rest, a nutritious diet, and the relief of worry. Underlying disorders, such as polyps and allergy, that predispose to recurrent attacks of sinusitis must be treated. Infected teeth are a frequent cause of chronic sinusitis. Typically these patients have a profuse nasal discharge with bad breath. Treatment of these patients is usually short-term and successful, and consists of eradication of the tooth infection —either through use of antibiotics or through tooth extraction.

Surgery may be indicated in treatment of chronic sinusitis. A new opening may be made in the inferior meatus to provide sinus drainage. This relatively simple operation is called an *antrotomy*, or antrum window operation. A more radical procedure occasionally is done through the mouth, above the upper teeth. This is called the Caldwell-Luc operation. The diseased mucous membrane lining of the sinus is removed, and a new opening is made into the inferior meatus of the nose, so that adequate drainage can occur. The nursing care after nasal surgery is discussed later in this chapter.

Nurses can avoid, and help others to avoid, the attitude that sinusitis is something to "put up with," and that nothing can be done about it. Modern treatment can prevent much needless misery, as well as help to avoid chronic sinusitis and serious complications such as bronchiectasis.

## Deviated Septum

The nasal cavity is divided into two passages by a septum consisting of bone and cartilage. Few people have an absolutely straight nasal septum, and some have a markedly crooked one. Sometimes the crookedness is congenital; often it is caused by trauma. When the septum is crooked, one nostril may be much larger than the other. Marked septal deviation can result in complete obstruction of one nostril and interference with sinus drainage. Surgical correction is necessary to restore normal breathing space and to permit adequate sinus drainage. Patients who have septal deviation due to injury should seek medical advice, so that the deformity can be corrected, and chronic sinusitis can be avoided.

The operation performed for deviated septum is called a *submucous resection,* usually simply abbreviated as "SMR." After a local anesthetic has been administered, the surgeon makes an incision through the mucous membrane and removes the portions of the septum that are causing obstruction. When the surgery is completed, both sides of the nasal cavity are packed with gauze, which usually is left in place for 24 to 48 hours. A mustache dressing (a folded piece of gauze applied under the nostrils and held in place with adhesive tape) is applied to absorb any bloody drainage.

## Polyps

Polyps are grapelike tumors that are believed to result from chronic irritation, such as that caused by infection or allergy. When polyps grow in the nose, they obstruct nasal breathing and sinus drainage. They are removed under local anesthesia. Unfortunately, polyps tend to recur, and the patient often must undergo surgery more than once for the same condition. The excised tissue is examined microscopically to determine whether it is benign or malignant.

## Nursing Assessment and Intervention in Nasal Surgery

Regardless of the particular operation performed on the nose, the principles of nursing care are similar.

● **Preoperatively the patient should be told what to expect postoperatively. Surgery on the nose, or on any part of the face, may arouse considerable anxiety over the possibility of a changed appearance. Any surgery done under local anesthesia may lead to fear** that pain will be experienced during surgery. Though nasal surgery is usually relatively painless, mentioning to the patient preoperatively that he can have pain medication if he needs it may help allay his fear of pain.

- An enema sometimes is ordered preoperatively to empty the lower bowel, so that swallowed blood will pass through the gastrointestinal tract more quickly after surgery. Cathartics may be ordered postoperatively for the same purpose.

- Postoperatively the patient is observed closely for the major complication of nasal surgery—hemorrhage. Vital signs are checked at regular intervals. (It is not unusual to saturate two or three mustache dressings after submucous resection—there is considerable bloody drainage after this type of surgery.)

The back of the throat should be observed with a flashlight to note whether blood is trickling down. The patient is instructed to spit out any drainage, so that its amount and character can be observed. (However, some swallowing of blood is usual after nasal surgery, and the patient may even pass a tarry stool postoperatively.)

- The patient is positioned on his side initially to facilitate the drainage of any blood or mucus from his mouth and nose. Later the head of the bed is elevated to a 45-degree angle to decrease edema and to promote more comfortable breathing.

- Nasal packing is uncomfortable and the patient may require a narcotic for relief of pain, apprehension, and restlessness during the early postoperative period. Occasionally, nasal packing slips back into the throat causing gagging and discomfort. The surgeon should be advised of the situation. In emergency treatment for packing that has slipped back into the throat and obstructs breathing, the patient is instructed to open his mouth, and the packing is grasped with forceps and pulled out through the open mouth.

- The environment should be kept neat—there is no need for a blood-stained gown, a soggy mustache dressing, or soiled tissues to be in view.

- Since the patient with nasal packing must breathe through his mouth such procedures as taking the temperature must be adapted accordingly.

- The patient must be protected from falling by the use of side rails until the effect of the sedatives has worn off and by having someone assist him the first few times that he gets out of bed.

- The patient is encouraged to help himself as soon as he is able—for example, by applying cold compresses to his nose.

- The importance of mouth care and oral fluids must be recognized. Old blood can give a foul odor and taste to the mouth, and dryness of the mouth is inevitable during mouth breathing.

- The patient is not forced to try more than liquids and soft foods until after the packing has been removed. This period lasts only a day or two, and afterward the patient quickly resumes a normal diet.

## Epistaxis (Nosebleed)

Most nosebleeds occur in Kiesselbach's area (see Fig. 28-1), a plexus of capillaries located on the anterior part of the nasal septum. Epistaxis may result from picking the nose or from local trauma, such as any kind of blow. Also it may result from diseases, such as rheumatic fever, hypertension, or blood dyscrasias. Epistaxis resulting from hypertension is likely to be especially severe and difficult to control.

Nosebleed is a common occurrence and is usually not very serious, but it is often a very frightening one for both the person experiencing it and those who witness it. Every nurse should be familiar with simple first aid for epistaxis. Merely applying pressure by holding the soft parts of the nose firmly between thumb and forefinger for several minutes often is effective in controlling bleeding. The patient should sit with his head tilted slightly forward to prevent the blood from running down his throat. He is instructed to breathe through his mouth, and then firm pressure is applied. The sitting position usually is preferable, because it lessens the possibility of fainting, as well as the fatigue and the discomfort caused by standing. Also, the flow of blood to the head is lessened by keeping the head elevated while the patient is sitting. The patient can be shown how to apply pressure, and often he can control the bleeding himself if it occurs while he is alone. If the bleeding is severe, a basin must be provided to catch the blood. The patient should be instructed not to swallow blood that may run into his mouth and throat, but to spit it out. If the bleeding is slight, tissues or a handkerchief may be sufficient to prevent soiling the clothing. Applying cold compresses to the bridge of the nose sometimes is helpful.

If the bleeding is profuse, or if it does not stop within a few minutes, the physician should be called. He may place cotton pledgets saturated with epinephrine 1:1,000 inside the nostril, as well as apply pressure. If the bleeding cannot be controlled, the nasal cavity may have to be packed with gauze to apply continuous pressure for approximately 24 hours. Sometimes, the bleeding area is cauterized. Calmness on the part of the nurse and others who are with the patient is essential. Patients with epistaxis often look very bloody; occasionally blood will be seen at the corners of the eyes, having gone up the lacrimal ducts, or in the auditory canal, having gone up the eustachian tube and perforated the drum. Despite the patient's alarming (and alarmed) appearance, the nurse must move deliberately and speak calmly as she positions him, applies pressure to his nose, and cleans away the old blood. Particularly if the bleeding is refractory, sedation is often ordered, because restlessness and apprehension increase the bleeding.

## Common Nasal Treatments

**Nose Drops.** The drops must go up the nose rather than down the patient's throat. Therefore the patient is positioned in a way which helps the drops to flow to the location where they are most needed. For example, if the drops are to go toward the maxillary sinus, the patient hangs his head slightly over the edge of the bed, and turns slightly so that the drops flow toward the affected side. If the drops are to flow to the opening of the eustachian tube, the drops are inserted with the patient lying flat on his back. The patient is instructed to maintain the position for several minutes after the drops have been instilled. The nurse checks the label for the proper concentration of the medication ordered. For instance, Neo-Synephrine commonly is ordered in strengths of 0.25 to 0.5 per cent. When the physician wishes medication "aimed" at a certain place, he usually prescribes drops. When the medication is to be diffused over the entire area, a nasal spray is usually ordered.

**Nasal Irrigation.** Nasal irrigation is ordered sometimes to remove crusts of mucus from the nose. These crusts can interfere with sinus drainage, and they are especially likely to form when the patient has a purulent discharge from his sinuses. Before the irrigation is begun, the patient is instructed to breathe through his mouth during the procedure, and to avoid talking or swallowing while the irrigating solution is flowing. These measures are necessary to exclude fluid from the eustachian tubes, which might carry infectious material into the middle ear. Normal saline (105 degrees to 110 degrees F) is the solution ordinarily used.

The treatment is carried out with the patient in a sitting position. The patient holds a basin in his lap, and bends slightly forward, so that the return flow will run into the basin. The solution passes to the nasopharynx and flows out the opposite nostril. Often the patient feels more at ease if he can control the flow of the solution himself by pinching off the tubing that leads from the irrigating can to the irrigating tip inserted into the nostril. The patient is instructed not to blow his nose for half an hour after the irrigation, to avoid forcing any irrigating solution into the eustachian tubes. Nasal irrigation is less frequently used nowadays, because it can spread infection from one sinus to another.

**Nasal Spray Nebulization.** Usually, the patient is taught to use the nebulizer himself. Sitting in an upright position, with his head tilted slightly backward, he inserts the nebulizer into one nostril and closes the opposite nostril by applying pressure with his finger. This prevents the entrance of air and allows the medication to flow up into the nasal cavity. The procedure is repeated for the other nostril.

## LARYNGITIS

The larynx often is called the *voice box*. A valvular mechanism leading into the trachea, it is made of a more or less rigid framework of cartilages held together by ligaments. The interior of this boxlike structure is lined by ciliated mucous membrane that is continuous with the mucous membrane of the pharynx and the trachea. The cartilaginous framework of the larynx consists of the *thyroid,* the *arytenoid,* and the *cricoid* cartilages.

On each lateral wall of the laryngeal cavity are two horizontally placed folds of mucous membrane —the ventricular folds or "false cords" and the vocal folds or true vocal cords. The latter are the lower of the two. The larynx and the air passages of which it forms a part constitute an air column that produces sounds of varying pitch. However, the larynx cannot produce words. The sounds made by the vibrating vocal cords are molded into speech by the pharynx, the palate, the tongue, the teeth, and the lips.

Laryngitis is an inflammation and swelling of the mucous membrane lining of the larynx. Laryngitis often accompanies upper respiratory infections, and it is due to the spread of the infection to the larynx. Laryngitis also can be caused by excessive or improper use of the voice or by smoking. The symptoms include hoarseness or, sometimes, the inability to speak above a whisper. A cough and a feeling of throat irritation commonly accompany laryngitis.

The diagnosis sometimes is made by the patient on the basis of the symptoms alone. If the condition persists, the individual should seek the advice of a physician. Most physicians believe that hoarseness which persists more than two weeks warrants a laryngoscopic examination, whereby the larynx can be examined visually. Indirect laryngoscopy is the visualization of the larynx by means of a laryngeal mirror held in the pharynx while a light is directed onto the mirror. In direct laryngoscopy, a laryngoscope (a hollow instrument with a light at its distal end) is passed to the larynx after the patient's throat has been topically anesthetized with 0.5 per cent tetracaine (Pontocaine) or 2 per cent lidocaine (Xylocaine). Nursing care before and after direct laryngoscopy is similar to that of a patient having bronchoscopy. The prompt investigation of the cause of persistent hoarseness is essential, because this symptom may be due to cancer of the larynx.

The treatment of laryngitis involves voice rest and the treatment or the removal of the cause. The meaning of the term "voice rest" should be explained to the patient. It means writing what he wishes to communicate rather than speaking. It must be emphasized that whispering is as bad as talking. Voice rest facilitates the healing of the inflamed mucous membranes, and, when the condition is due to an upper respiratory infection or to brief overuse of the voice, it is usually the only specific treatment required.

## TONSILLITIS, PERITONSILLAR ABSCESS, TONSILLECTOMY

These conditions are encountered more commonly among children than among adults and therefore are not included in this text. The student is referred to a textbook on the nursing of children. Care of patients with tracheostomy will be included in the section which follows, on care of the patient with laryngectomy.

## CANCER OF THE LARYNX

Cancer of the larynx is most common among people over 45. Men are affected much more frequently than women. Although the cause is unknown, it is believed that chronic laryngitis (caused by excessive smoking, drinking of alcohol, or habitual overuse of the voice) and heredity may predispose to the condition.

**Symptoms.** Persistent hoarsness usually is the earliest symptom. Often this is slight at first and is readily ignored. Also, the patient may have a sensation of a swelling or a lump in his throat, followed by dysphagia and pain when he is talking. If the malignant tissue is not removed promptly, the patient develops symptoms of advancing carcinoma, such as weakness, weight loss, and anemia. The importance of consulting a physician for any persistent hoarseness or difficulty in swallowing cannot be overemphasized. Patients who seek treatment early have a good chance of cure, because cancer of the larynx usually does not metastasize as early as cancer in some other parts of the body.

**Diagnosis.** The diagnosis is established by laryngoscopy, biopsy, and x-ray films.

**Treatment.** The surgical removal of the tumor, and often of the entire larynx, is necessary. Radiotherapy also may be employed. If the tumor is discovered promptly, the surgeon sometimes can remove it without removing the entire larynx; this less radical procedure is called *laryngofissure*. Because laryngofissure does not involve a removal of the total larynx, but only a portion of it, the patient does not lose his voice. However, his voice is husky. Laryngofissure is now less commonly performed. Patients who would formerly have been treated by laryngofissure now tend to be treated by radiotherapy. In more advanced cases total laryngectomy is necessary. If the disease has spread to the cervical lymph nodes, radical neck dissection (removal of the lymph nodes and the adjacent tissues) also is performed. Patients who have total laryngectomy have a permanent tracheostomy, because after surgery the trachea does not connect with the nasopharynx. The patient no longer can speak normally. The larynx is severed from the trachea and removed completely. The only respiratory organs in use thereafter are the trachea, the bronchi, and the lungs. Air enters and leaves through the tracheostomy; the patient will no longer feel air entering his nose. The anterior wall of the esophagus connects with the posterior wall of the larynx, and consequently it must be reconstructed. Tube feeding facilitates healing by avoiding muscular activity and irritation of the esophagus.

### Nursing Care of a Laryngectomy Patient

**Preoperative Preparation.** The surgeon explains the need and the expected extent of the surgery to the patient preoperatively. If total laryngectomy is necessary, the patient often is shocked and dismayed at the prospect of losing his voice. (Even the temporary loss of the ability to communicate verbally with others causes a great deal of anxiety.)

A detailed explanation of the measures that will be used to help the patient to communicate with others is important before surgery is performed. For example, patients who know how to read and write can write messages immediately after surgery using a Magic Slate. For those who can't read or write a Flash Card system, functional and environmental pictures, or a flip chart of commonly used questions and responses or gestures may be designed. All patients should be assured that their call light will be answered promptly. The patient can be visited by the speech pathologist preoperatively for an evaluation of his usual speaking pattern and an explanation of the alternative methods he can learn after recovery from the surgical procedure, such as *esophageal speech,* a method of speaking by regurgitating swallowed air, or the use of an electronic larynx. A visit from someone who has undergone laryngectomy and has mastered esophageal speech frequently arranged prior to the surgery often does more to convince the patient that such speech is possible than all the explanations of his surgeon and his nurses.

Some patients may be ready to absorb considerable information concerning speech rehabilitation preoperatively. However, many are too apprehensive and therefore are unable to absorb a great deal of detail. It is important to convey to every patient before the operation that the surgery will not mean that he is cut off from communication with others—either in the immediate postoperative period or later.

The patient should understand that he will be fed through a nasogastric tube or other type of feeding tube postoperatively. It will remain in place until sufficient healing has occurred. The patient can look forward to eating normally after the tube has been removed.

The patient is told that he will have a permanent tracheostomy, and that he will be taught how to care for this opening, as well as how to camouflage it with scarves, collars, and the like.

Instruction and emotional support help the patient to mobilize his defenses and to begin to learn how to cope with the effects of the operation. Many cities have branches of the IAL (International Association of Laryngectomees), a group of people who have had laryngectomy and who help one another to cope with the disability. Many of the members visit others who are hospitalized for laryngectomy, and they distribute literature that offers practical help and encouragement to others with the condition. Patients can find out about the club nearest them by contacting the American Cancer Society, 219 East 42nd Street, New York City, 10017, or by contacting their local chapter of the Society.

### Care of a Patient with a Tracheostomy

The patient requires almost continuous nursing care immediately after surgery. Not only is he unable to speak, but he must breathe through a new opening in his trachea. A tube made of sterling silver or plastic material is placed in the tracheal opening. The tube used after laryngectomy is shorter than that inserted after tracheostomy for other causes. Often, it is called a *laryngectomy* tube, to distinguish it from the longer tracheostomy tubes (Fig. 28-4). The principles of care are similar to those of any patient who has a tracheostomy for any reason. (Note that some surgeons do not have their patients wear a tube in the stoma after laryngectomy, in the belief that not using a tube at all produces less irritation and a better stoma. However, the use of a laryngectomy tube postoperatively is more usual than the practice of not using one.) When a tube is employed, there is now a tendency for its use to be discontinued more promptly than was formerly the case. For example, many patients now have their tubes removed after only two days.

Tracheostomy without laryngectomy may be necessitated by any condition, such as allergy or infection, that causes edema and results in obstruction of the patient's airway. In such situations the tracheostomy is performed as an emergency measure to create a new opening through which the patient can breathe. The operation may be performed at the bedside, or even outside the hospital,

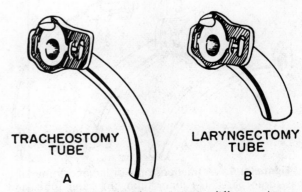

**Figure 28-4.** Both tubes come in different sizes.

when the patient's condition suddenly requires it. However, in most instances it is possible and preferable to prepare carefully for this operation and to perform it in a methodical way before the patient's respiratory distress is so acute that his life is in jeopardy. Nurses can help by promptly reporting respiratory difficulty to the physician, so that the needed care can be given immediately. Patients who have had tracheostomy without laryngectomy can speak by taking a breath, briefly covering the tube with a finger, uttering a word or two, and then removing the finger to resume breathing. A device called a Trach-Talk enables some tracheostomy patients to speak. A one-way valve diverts exhaled air through the larynx (Tyler, 1973).

After laryngectomy the trachea is sutured to the skin line; this procedure is not the case when a temporary tracheostomy is performed. Therefore, the removal of the entire tube usually is not followed by the prompt closure of the opening in laryngectomized patients, as it is in patients who have a temporary tracheostomy performed to relieve respiratory obstruction.

**The Tube.** The tube (cannula) has three parts —an outer tube, an inner tube, and an obturator (Fig. 28-5). Before the outer tube is inserted into the tracheal opening, the obturator is placed in the tube. The lower end of the obturator protrudes from the end of the tube to be inserted. The protruding end of the obturator is smooth, facilitating insertion. Since the obturator obstructs the lumen of the tube, it is removed immediately, once the tube is in place. The parts of the tubes are not interchangeable; they fit only one particular tube. If one part is lost, the entire set is useless. Therefore, each

part, including the obturator, is carefully accounted for, and accidental loss is avoided carefully. The obturator usually is taped to the patient's wrist when he returns from the operating room, so that it is returned to the unit with the patient.

Today many tracheostomy tubes or laryngectomy tubes are "cuffed," that is, an encircling balloon is attached or incorporated and when inflated provides a seal between the tube and the tracheal wall. This seal provides a closed system when the patient requires continuous positive pressure ventilation or IPPB treatments. The seal also prevents secretions from trickling down the trachea and can be used for hemostasis if bleeding occurs postoperatively. To prevent erosion of the tracheal mucosa and other complications the cuff should not be overinflated. The maximum pressure is most easily recognized when the patient is receiving IPPB, by listening closely and allowing a slight leak around the cuff. It must also be deflated at regular intervals ordered by the physician. Double-cuffed tubes are also available which provide alternate inflation sites. A small pilot balloon distal to the encircling balloon indicates whether the encircling balloon is inflated. (For pictorial technique of cuff inflation see Tyler, 1973, p. 29.)

**Care of the Tube.** The inner tube slides inside the outer tube. It is removed by the nurse as often as necessary, cleaned, and replaced. The inner tube must be locked securely in position after reinserting it. Various methods are used for cleaning the inner tube. Because dried mucus sticks inside, merely rinsing the tube with water is not sufficient. The lumen must be wiped as well. Some nurses use a piece of bandage threaded through the tube to clean the inside; others prefer a small brush. Soap and cold water, plus friction applied with a bandage or a brush, remove all the secretions. The tube always should be held up and inspected to be sure that it is clean and dry before it is reinserted.

In the immediate postoperative period, the inner tube may have to be removed as often as every half hour. Before the inner tube is reinserted, the outer tube is thoroughly suctioned. The inner tube should be cleaned promptly and reinserted. Otherwise, the outer tube will collect secretions. The outer tube is left in position. The entire tube usually is changed by the surgeon daily or several times a week.

An extra set always is kept at the patient's bedside, since immediate change may be necessary if the patient's tube becomes blocked with mucus that

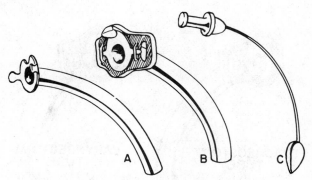

**Figure 28-5.** A tracheostomy or laryngectomy tube has three parts: (A) inner tube, (B) outer tube, and (C) obturator.

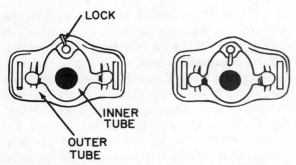

**Figure 28-6.** The inner tube fits snugly into the outer tube. Turning the lock up with the finger makes it possible to remove the inner tube for cleaning. Turning the lock down keeps the inner tube securely in place. The inner tube always is locked in place after it is reinserted.

cannot be removed by suction or removal of the inner cannula. Each time that the surgeon changes the patient's tube, the one that has been removed is scrubbed thoroughly with soap and water and sterilized by boiling. It is then ready for reuse. Often, the tube is placed in a jar and labeled with the patient's name. The tubes come in various sizes, and it is important that the patient always have the correct size at his bedside.

The outer tube is held snugly in place by tapes inserted in openings on either side of it and tied at the back of the patient's neck. These tapes always should be tied securely in a knot. A bow may be added if desired. If the knot is not tied securely, the patient can cough the tube out. This is a very serious occurrence if the edges of the trachea have not been sutured to the skin, as is the case in a temporary tracheostomy. If the outer tube accidentally comes out, the nurse immediately inserts a tracheal dilator to hold the edges of the opening apart until the surgeon arrives to insert another tube. The tracheal dilator is kept at the bedside at all times. If the tube should come out after tracheos-

tomy, it should never be forced back in. If force is used, the patient's trachea may be compressed (by pushing the tube alongside the trachea, thus compressing the trachea, rather than inserting the tube into the stoma). Such action could cause asphyxiation. It is essential for the nurse to try to remain calm if the patient's tube should come out, remembering to hold open the stoma with a tracheal dilator until the surgeon arrives, if the tube cannot be deftly and easily re-inserted by the nurse.

Many patients wear a "bib" of folded gauze or mesh over the tube as a camouflage. If the material is kept damp, it helps to humidify the inspired air. The bib never should be made of the kind of gauze that has a layer of cotton inside, since bits of cotton easily are sucked into the tube. It is important not to let any material hide the condition of the tube. Unless the nurse is alert to this possibility, a badly crusted tube much in need of being cleaned and changed may be overlooked. Commercially available devices which fit over the tracheostomy provide a continual flow of moistened air and supplemental oxygen if necessary.

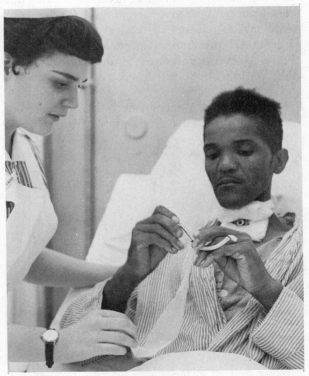

**Figure 28-8.** This patient is learning to clean the inner tube by threading a piece of bandage through it. Note the gauze dressings that fit snugly around the outer tube to absorb secretions.

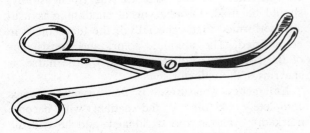

**Figure 28-7.** Tracheal dilator.

A gauze dressing is placed under the tube to absorb the secretions. Gauze squares usually are used for this purpose. A slit is cut halfway through the square, so that the gauze can fit around the tube. The cut edges can be bound with narrow-width smooth tape to prevent threads from frayed edges entering the wound or even the trachea. This piece of gauze should be changed as often as necessary (Fig. 28-9).

The patient's respiratory passages react to the creation of the new respiratory opening with irritation, excessive secretion of mucus, and formation of crusts of dried mucus. The inspired air passes directly into the trachea, the bronchi, and the lungs without becoming warmed and moistened by passing through the nose. The copious respiratory secretions that characteristically occur immediately after the new opening has been made are a threat to the patient's life. They may clog the only remaining breathing passage—the tracheostomy—and quickly cause death by asphyxia. The patient is usually very much aware of this possibility, and often he is terrified of being left alone even for a moment. Constant vigilance and care are necessary during the immediate postoperative period to keep the tube patent and to reassure the patient. He is taught to care for the tube himself as soon as possible; the ability to care for himself is the patient's most effective defense against the fear of a blocked airway.

**Suctioning.** A suction machine is placed in readiness before the patient returns from surgery,

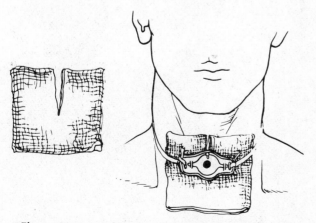

**Figure 28-9.** Gauze squares, slit halfway down, are placed around the tube to catch secretions. These dressings are changed by the nurse as often as necessary. Note the tapes that hold the outer tube in place. The tapes are tied in a knot at the back of the patient's neck.

and it is kept at his bedside at all times. After the nurse explains what she is about to do, mucus is gently suctioned from the tube by a No. 14 or No. 16 (F.) sterile catheter with a Y-valve attachment, inserted gently into the lumen of the tube. Suction is not applied while the catheter is on the way down the trachea, because this causes unnecessary irritation of the lining of the trachea. Instead, the suction is commenced once the catheter has been passed, and suctioning is continued while the catheter is withdrawn slowly. Newer disposable catheters have bypass ports that are kept uncovered as the suction catheter is passed so that no suction is applied. To apply suction the bypass port or open end of a Y-connector is covered by the thumb. As the catheter is withdrawn it is rotated, so that the openings in the catheter can remove mucus more effectively. This procedure may be necessary as often as every five or ten minutes in the immediate postoperative period. Routinely three to five ml. of sterile saline is introduced into the tube before suctioning to loosen mucous crusts and plugs and help maintain moisture deeper in the airway. The actual suctioning should not take longer than five to ten seconds. The catheter can be passed again if necessary after the patient has had a chance to breathe room air or oxygen or is assisted with deep breaths administered by a second person from a self-inflating bag. Cleanliness of all equipment used in caring for the tracheostomy is essential. The hands should be washed before suctioning the patient. An ample supply of disposable sterile gloves and suction catheters, sterile normal saline, and disposable cups for the catheter rinsing solution should be available at the bedside during the period of wound healing. Failure to observe these precautions results in the introduction of large numbers of harmful microorganisms. Poor technique may lead to postoperative pneumonia by spread of infection to the lungs. If it is necessary to suction through the nose or the mouth, another catheter (not the one used for the tracheostomy) should be used. Oropharyngeal suctioning is usually performed first, especially if the tube cuff is to be deflated. The amount, color, and consistency of the secretions should be noted by the nurse as she rinses the catheter.

**Emergency Measures.** If the airway becomes completely obstructed, the patient will become markedly cyanotic and frightened, and he will die within a few moments if the obstruction is not relieved. Therefore, first aid is of the greatest urgency, and, if the nurse is the one who happens to be with the patient, she promptly does everything in her power to remove the mucus, and simultaneously she has someone else call the physician. The removal of the tracheostomy tube followed by suctioning may be lifesaving. This first-aid measure usually may be undertaken safely after laryngectomy when healing has sealed the tracheal opening to the surrounding skin. Consultation with the physician ahead of time concerning the first-aid measures acceptable for the nurse to perform for each individual patient is essential. The nurse then will know which patients may have their tubes removed as an emergency measure.

### Immediate Postlaryngectomy Period

The patient is positioned on his side until he reacts from anesthesia. When he has reacted, and his blood pressure is stable, the head of the bed is elevated to a 45-degree angle. This position decreases edema and makes breathing easier. At first the patient is very apprehensive and restless. However, the constant presence of the nurse usually helps him to feel more secure. Frequent suctioning and cleaning of the inner tube and providing a means of communication also are reassuring. In the immediate postoperative period, writing messages is the only means of communication left to most patients. A Magic Slate is useful for this purpose, because the words can be erased promptly by raising the plastic cover, and the tablet is ready for reuse. The patient should not be left unattended during this early postoperative period, because he is unable to care for his own tube, and he could quickly experience respiratory obstruction from

copious secretion of mucus. Leaving him alone may lead to panic, if not suffocation, and may frighten him so much that later rehabilitation will be difficult.

Opiates usually are ordered sparingly, because of their tendency to depress respiration. Fortunately, this type of surgery does not ordinarily cause a great deal of postoperative pain. When narcotics are given, the nurse should note carefully their effect on respiration and report any respiratory depression. The patient is observed for cyanosis and dyspnea, as well as for other postoperative complications, such as shock and hemorrhage. Often, the patient returns from surgery with a Hemovac apparatus for collection of drainage. The Hemovac device must be watched carefully and not allowed to become plugged.

Usually, the patient is allowed out of bed on the first postoperative day. By this time he can be taught to suction his own tube, aided by a mirror so that he can see what he is doing. The patient can safely be left unattended when he is able to use his call light and to suction his own tube. He is also taught how to remove and clean the inner cannula. The patient's call light always should be answered immediately. The realization that someone will come right away if he needs help is tremendously important in helping the patient to develop enough confidence to stay alone.

After laryngectomy the patient is fed through a tube, usually for about a week (Fig. 28-10). However, some surgeons now discontinue the tube feedings and begin oral feedings as early as the second postoperative day.

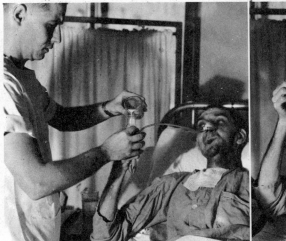
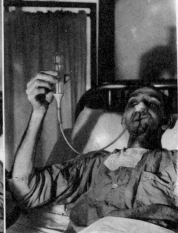

**Figure 28-10.** (*Left*) The nurse is shown pouring the tube into an Asepto syringe, which is being used as a funnel. The tube is kinked while the syringe is being filled. Note the damp mesh square that the patient is wearing over his tracheostomy tube. Facial deformity has resulted from the extensive surgery that was necessary to treat his condition. (*Right*) The feeding is permitted to flow through the tube by gravity. Before the syringe is empty, more of the feeding will be added. The patient is encouraged to help with the procedure.

When the patient can swallow, he is allowed sips of water. When he is able to swallow fluids without difficulty, the feeding tube is removed. The patient is permitted soft foods and fluids. Gradually, he is permitted to resume a normal diet.

Occasionally, an esophageal fistula forms, which delays the resumption of normal eating and prolongs hospitalization. Fistulas are especially likely to develop in patients who have had radiotherapy, since irradiated tissues do not heal readily. Infection of the operative area is not infrequent. Careful oral hygiene preoperatively and postoperatively, as well as the administration of antibiotics, helps to prevent infection.

### Care of the Patient with Levin (Nasogastric) Tube Feedings

Patients unable to swallow but able to digest foods placed in the stomach may be fed liquids through a Levin tube passed through the nose to the stomach. A patient fed this way can be kept alive for years, in good water and electrolyte regulation and well nourished. The amount and the type of tube feeding is ordered by the physician. The food passed through the tube is a liquid form of an adequate diet. The patient does not taste the mixture (fortunately, since such mixtures are usually unpalatable). Feedings may be ordered at one-, two-, or four-hour intervals.

Caution must be used to avoid aspiration, especially when tube feedings are given to a comatose patient, or one who is disoriented or restless. Before feeding, the tube is checked to make sure that the end is well situated in the stomach. Some tubes are marked with black lines. When the black line is at the nose, the end of the tube is in the stomach. Even if the tube has no such line, one can tell if it has pulled out by seeing whether or not the adhesive tape that holds it in place has been disturbed. The end of the tube can be placed in a glass of water. If bubbles appear as the patient exhales, do *not* feed. The end of the tube may be in the respiratory passage.

Tube feedings are warmed to body temperature and are allowed to flow in by gravity through an Asepto syringe, a funnel, or a 50 ml. syringe. After the feeding is finished, the tube is rinsed with a syringe full of clean water to prevent food particles from lodging in the tube and turning sour. Mouth care is given and the patient observed for irritation of the nostril through which the tube passes.

Oral medications may be crushed thoroughly, mixed with water, and administered through the nasogastric tube. Water is always rinsed through the tube after instilling the medication. Otherwise, the patient will not receive the entire dose, because part of the medicine will remain in the tube.

The patient is taught to administer his own tube feedings as soon as he is able. He is instructed never to let the funnel become empty during the feeding (since this would allow air to enter his stomach) and to clamp the tube carefully after administering the feeding. Many patients fold the tube over on itself, and secure it with an elastic band. A heavy metal clamp is not desirable, because its weight is uncomfortable and tends to pull the tube out. The feeding tube is kept anchored to the patient's face; some patients wear them fastened behind the ear. In any case, the tube should be well supported so that it does not dangle and annoy the patient. Intake is noted and charted.

### Later Postlaryngectomy Period

The patient is allowed up and about as much as he wishes after the fourth or fifth postoperative day. He bathes himself, administers his own feedings, and suctions and cleans his inner cannula using clean rather than sterile technique. From this point on, the nurse spends less time in direct physical care and more in teaching the patient to care for himself. Besides the techniques of suctioning and cleaning the inner tube, the patient must learn what foods he may eat when he returns home. (At first, soft foods and liquids are easier to swallow; gradually he resumes normal diet.) There is frequently a problem with constipation. Following the loss of his vocal cords, the patient is unable to build up as much intra-abdominal pressure (grunt) to assist his bowel movements. He also may learn acceptable ways of camouflaging his tube if he wishes. A scarf helps to keep dust and dirt out of the trachea, as well as to make the tracheostomy less obvious. A scarf made of smooth material, such as silk or rayon, may be worn loosely; fabrics that have fuzz must be avoided, since small fibers can be drawn into the tube.

Most patients no longer require suctioning when they return home; some do, and a suction machine must be provided. Many patients learn to change the entire tube each day at home. By the time that they are permitted to do this, the stoma is so well formed that there is no chance of its closing when the tube is removed. The patient purchases two tubes, since those he has used in the hospital are the property of that institution. Silver tubes cost over $25 apiece. Many patients eventually are able to go without any tube.

The patient with a permanent tracheostomy must prevent water from entering the tracheal opening, since it would flow down his trachea to his lungs. He never can go swimming, and he must be careful to prevent entrance of water into the tracheostomy during a bath. He may shower if he wears a special stoma shield and uses a shower hose attachment to direct the spray of water below his neck.

## Methods of Artificial Speech

Laryngectomy changes drastically a person's ability to speak, to cough, to eat, smell, bathe, lift, cry, and laugh, as well as his way of breathing. The patient becomes impatient and frustrated at his inability to communicate normally; the process of writing everything he has to say is tedious and time-consuming and it suffices only for a bare minimum of communication. Most patients are eager to have some alternate for normal voice.

**Esophageal Speech.** The speech pathologist may visit the hospitalized patient about one week post-operatively to demonstrate the three methods for achieving air intake for esophageal speech (injection, inhalation, and swallow methods). Actual speech therapy may begin about two to four weeks

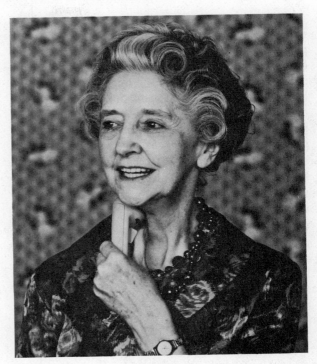

**Figure 28-12.** Telephone usage of the artificial larynx. (Courtesy, American Telephone & Telegraph Company)

postoperatively when healing and physical condition permit. Adequate esophageal speech levels are usually not acquired for seven to twelve months. Learning esophageal speech is not easy. The patient must practice between sessions with the speech pathologist and be willing to keep trying until he masters the technique. He needs the encouragement and support of family, physician, nurse, and other members of the health care team. The patient needs privacy for his practice sessions so that he does not feel embarrassed over an unusual maneuver such as swallowing and regurgitating air. Gradually, he is able to make himself understood in normal conversation.

**Artificial Larynx.** A small electronic device operated by batteries offers another means of speech to the patient. The artificial larynx is held in the hand with the vibrating surface placed against an optimum site on the neck, usually arrived at by trial and error. The surface of the instrument transmits vibrations to the pharynx and oral cavity where the articulators (tongue, lips, teeth) transform the vibrations into intelligible, amplified speech.

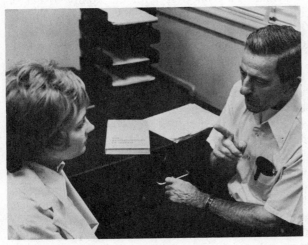

**Figure 28-11.** Speech therapist assisting patient who has undergone a laryngectomy. (Overlook Hospital, Summit, N.J.)

495

During the time the patient is learning esophageal speech, the artificial larynx may be used as a supplement. If a laryngectomee finds that his esophageal speech does not provide sufficient volume for speaking on the telephone, he may use the artificial larynx for telephone conversations or other supplementary purposes. It can also be used by those persons who, for various reasons, are unsuccessful in learning esophageal speech.

**VoiceBak Prosthesis.** In recent years, surgical techniques have been developed for restoration of voice after laryngectomy, though their use is not widespread (Asai, 1972; Taub, 1973). One technique involves a single-stage surgical procedure prior to the use of the LaBarge VoiceBak prosthesis. A surgical fistula is created from the side of the neck to the esophagus (cervical esophageal fistula). The VoiceBak is connected by the patient to the tracheostoma and is removed for sleeping (Fig. 28-13). This prosthesis permits normal breathing through an air bypass valve at the tracheostoma and also provides for the shunting of air from the lungs to the esophagus. The flow of air over the esophageal mucosa provides a sound source which is articulated by the mouth, lips, and tongue as speech.

Some advantages of the VoiceBak prosthesis are that it restores effortless speech immediately without any training with a quality equal to high quality esophageal speech and it can be concealed under a shirt and tie or dress. It is not used in patients who have had bilateral radical neck dissection because of inadequate protection of the carotid vessels nor in patients having other limiting conditions (Taub, 1973; LaBarge, 1973).

Despite advances in techniques of esophageal speech and the development of surgical procedures, supplementary devices, and prostheses, the patient who has had total laryngectomy inevitably has a change in the tone and the quality of his speech, and he faces the task of dealing with this change in himself and with the reactions of others to the change in his voice.

## THE PATIENT WITH RADICAL SURGERY OF THE HEAD AND NECK

Radical surgery of the head and neck may be performed in cancer arising in such structures as the lip, tongue, tonsil, nasopharynx, maxilla, mandible, thyroid gland, and larynx. Metastasis from primary tumors is to the cervical lymph nodes whose enlargement may interfere with the ability to eat or breathe. Erosion of major blood vessels by the tumor or metastasis to vital centers in the brain can also occur.

The primary tumor may be treated by irradiation followed by surgery or by surgery alone, depending upon the location and size of the tumor. Temporary or permanent tracheostomy may be necessary due to the threat of airway obstruction from the tumor or the surgery.

Surgical procedures involving the larynx and pharynx leave little external deformity but change or remove the ability to speak or swallow. Operations to excise malignant lesions in the nose, sinuses, mouth, mandible, ear, and skin of the facial area frequently result in cosmetic deformity. In any situation the need for professional counseling and advice is of utmost importance preoperatively.

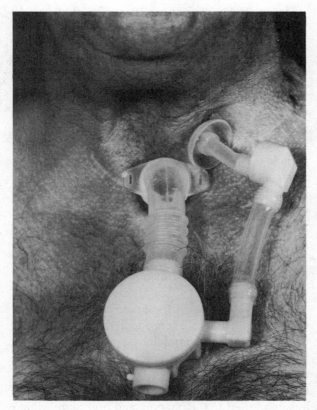

**Figure 28-13.** The LaBarge VoiceBak prosthesis for speech following laryngectomy. (LaBarge, Inc.)

Radical neck dissection is a part of head and neck cancer surgery if there are palpable lymph nodes in the cervical region, or without palpable nodes if the threat of metastasis is high. The second alternative varies with the type and size of the cancer. Without palpable cervical nodes or with slow-growing and early tumors, radical neck dissection may be avoided.

The surgery of neck dissection involves the removal of all cervical lymph nodes and channels. To accomplish this the internal jugular vein, fatty tissue, sternocleidomastoid muscle and other smaller muscles must be taken. It is often difficult for the surgeon to avoid the eleventh cranial nerve which travels through the sternocleidomastoid muscle. When this nerve is cut, weakness results in the trapezius muscle on that side, causing decreased shoulder elevation and sometimes pain in the shoulder region.

## Nursing Assessment and Intervention
### Preoperative Phase

Radical surgery for treatment of cancer of the head and neck is very emotionally stressful for the patient because it involves the threat or actuality of mutilating deformity of the face. It may also interfere with reception of stimuli of sound, sight, taste, and smell, and may change the normal airway and the normal patterns of mastication, swallowing, and speech. The patient must cope with these losses resulting from therapy at the same time that he must deal with the diagnosis of cancer and all that this portends for his future.

Because they are constantly exposed, the face and neck are in general assigned high social and esthetic value although the degree of emotional investment in these body parts will vary from individual to individual. Part of the role of the nurse who works with patients who require radical face and neck surgery is to be able to discuss the proposed changes with the patient preoperatively and to listen to the patient's expressions of his thoughts and feelings about his diagnosis and mutilation from radical therapy. She must be prepared to accept the patient with his changed body image and not be repelled by it since her positive attitude can assist the patient toward greater self-acceptance.

Many, though not all, patients with oropharyngeal cancer have used tobacco and alcohol to excess with consequent poor oral hygiene and un-

dernutrition. Nursing goals must be related to improving mouth care and nutrition to promote postoperative wound healing and prevention of infection. Assessment of the patient's smoking and alcohol intake habits is done on admission so that a plan can be devised to prevent delirium tremens in the postoperative period, and for continuing patient education.

The patient's and family's understanding of and response to the surgeon's explanation of the surgical procedure, and the anticipated cosmetic and functional defects and future plans for overcoming these should be a focus of communication. The patient's coping capacities need to be assessed. Denial, withdrawal, repression, or regression are not unusual responses to the threats produced by the diagnosis and prospective surgery. As support is provided the need for the patient to employ exaggerated defenses decreases. As this occurs, the patient can be expected to experience grief and go through a process of mourning the loss of his bodily integrity. The anger that accompanies grief may not be directed outward at the family or staff because of the patient's fear of abandonment. Unconsciously the patient may direct the anger against himself, with feelings of unworthiness, increased despondency, and self-debasement. Helping the patient work through the stages of grief toward acceptance of his condition is part of nursing intervention which continues into the postoperative phase. A primary nurse is most helpful for providing this continuity. A social worker can help with specific problems.

If the patient's normal speech pattern is to be disrupted temporarily or permanently postoperatively, an alternate method of communication must be devised. A Magic Slate or writing tablet may be satisfactory if the patient can read and write. An alternative is the use of Flash Cards or a flip chart with commonly used messages.

A feeding tube is usually necessary postoperatively, inserted either nasogastrically or via gastrostomy or cervical pharyngostomy.

Tracheostomy is usually performed if the patient has had previous surgery or radiation in the area or if intraoral resection is involved. The speech pathologist or International Association of Laryngectomees member can visit the patient for evaluative and social purposes. Since these procedures can usually be anticipated they are explained to the patient preoperatively. (See previous sections for principles of care of the patient with tracheostomy, laryngectomy, and tube feedings.)

Postoperative Phase

Nursing assessment, goals, and intervention are aimed at:

- **Maintenance of adequate airway.**
- **Maintenance of position, usually with head elevated 30 to 45 degrees to promote venous return, comfort, and ventilation. The patient may require assistance in lifting his head.**
- **Prevention of gastric dilatation and nausea and vomiting through gastric drainage (via feeding tube) until peristalsis returns.**
- **Provision for fluid and electrolyte balance.**
- **Relief of pain.**
- **Observation of drainage tubes under neck skin flaps to ascertain that they are functioning and the wound is free of blood, fluid, and air. Since a drainage system is used, bulky dressings are not necessary. However, drainage must be measured and inspected. It may be the nurse's responsibility to check that the skin flaps are down by palpating or rolling the flaps with a wide roll of gauze to help prevent drainage from accumulating. If this is not part of the nurse's role in a particular institution, she should call the surgeon if the skin flaps are up.**
- **Reduction of anxiety through attention to physiological needs such as suctioning.**
- **Acceptance of the patient with his functional and cosmetic defects.**
- **Maintenance of communication. Time and patience are required of the nurse when the patient must express his anger or fear through writing and other nonverbal methods. The patient must be assured of the privacy of his communication by destroying notes when their objective has been accomplished.**
- **Special mouth care, sometimes using a power spray after the immediate postoperative period.**
- **Physical therapy techniques to overcome functional loss from nerve and muscle interference, begun as soon as approved by the surgeon.**
- **Participation by the patient in all aspects of care such as tracheal suctioning or oral hygiene as soon as possible.**
- **Prevention and treatment of complications.**

*Hemorrhage* may occur in the immediate postoperative period due to inadequate hemostasis. Late hemorrhage (about eight to 20 days postoperative) due to wound breakdown, fistula, necrosis, or loss of the dermis graft is life-threatening. A small amount of bright red blood may be a warning signal of major vascular hemorrhage. This patient is considered seriously ill, and he is moved to a location where he can be constantly observed. Blood is drawn for typing and cross-matching.

*Carotid blowout* (carotid artery rupture) must be dealt with immediately by digital pressure with gauze pads or a bath towel, or application of a vascular clamp. These should be readily available at the bedside. A deflated tracheostomy cuff should be inflated and tracheal suctioning performed as necessary. The patient is moved as quickly as possible to the operating room for ligation of the carotid artery. This can result in neurologic deficit.

*Chyle leak* (lymphatic leak) is manifested by a large amount of clear opaque or milky drainage in the Hemovac, especially after the patient eats or when tube feedings are begun. A chyle leak usually arises from the thoracic duct in the left lateral neck, which may have to be ligated. The nurse should record the intake and output and the number of dressing changes. The surgeon may order that the lymph be returned via the nasogastric tube.

*Wound breakdown* or retarded healing can result in *salivary fistula formation*. The skin needs to be protected from maceration, and the patient provided with gauze pads for blotting. Fever, redness, and swelling of the neck are signs of the accumulation of secretions beneath the skin which can initiate a fistula. The patient should be observed for dehydration since a large amount of fluid can be lost.

**Preparation for Discharge.** Plans should include patient and family instruction in the care of wounds, tracheostomy, feeding tubes, and physical rehabilitation techniques. Necessary equipment must be in the home when the patient returns. Referrals are made for community nursing services, speech and swallowing therapy, prosthetists' services, specialized emotional support when indicated such as to a psychiatric nursing specialist, and to the state department of vocational rehabilitation or other agency for job placement if necessary. Patients with radical facial disfigurement or laryngectomy may have difficulty returning to their jobs, particularly if they involve sales or other types of prolonged public contact work. There is also a prejudice on the part of some employers to subject patients with a diagnosis of cancer to early retirement.

Most people have difficulty accepting the need for and adjusting to radical surgery. Many health professionals join together in a team effort to help the patient and family focus on what is left rather than on what is lost and to use appropriate community resources for optimal rehabilitation.

(For nursing care of the patient undergoing plastic or reconstructive surgery, see Chapter 57.)

## REFERENCES AND BIBLIOGRAPHY

ADLER, S.: Speech after laryngectomy, *Am. J. Nurs.* 69:2138, October 1969.

ASAI, R.: Laryngoplasty after total laryngectomy, *AMA Arch. Otolaryngol.* 95:114, 1972.

DeWEESE, D., and SAUNDERS, W.: *Textbook of Otolaryngology,* ed. 4, St. Louis, Mosby, 1973.

FENTON, M.: What to do about thirst, *Am. J. Nurs.* 69:1014, May 1969.

FOWKES, W. C., JR., and HUNN, V.: *Clinical Assessment for the Nurse Practitioner,* St. Louis, Mosby, 1973.

HAVENER, W., et al.: *Nursing Care in Eye, Ear, Nose, and Throat Disorders,* ed. 3, St. Louis, Mosby, 1974.

KEOUGH, G., and NIEBEL, H.: Oral cancer detection—a nursing responsibility, *Am. J. Nurs.* 73:684, April 1973.

KING, P., et al.: Rehabilitation and adaptation of laryngectomy patients, *Am. J. Phys. Med.* 47:192, August 1968.

KOMORN, R. M.: Laryngectomy and surgical vocal rehabilitation, *AORN* 17:73, June 1973.

LaBarge VoiceBak Prosthesis Product Literature Bulletin, St. Louis, LaBarge, Inc., September 1973.

Laryngectomy: paving the way to successful adjustment. *Nurs. '74* 74:60, June 1974.

MILLER, R.: Psychological problems of patients with head and neck cancer, in *Rehabilitation of the Cancer Patient,* Proceedings of the Annual Clinical Conferences on Cancer, sponsored by the University of Texas, M. D. Anderson Hospital and Tumor Institute at Houston, Chicago, Year Book Medical Publishers, Inc., 1972.

MYERS, E.: Rehabilitation after radical surgery of the tongue, *AORN* 11:55, February 1970.

Nursing management of patients with head and neck tumors, in BEHNKE, H., ed., *Guidelines for Comprehensive Nursing Care in Cancer,* New York, Springer, 1973.

O'DELL, A.: Objectives and standards in the care of the patient with a radical neck dissection, *Nurs. Clin. N. Am.* 8:159, March 1973.

———: The administration of airway humidification, *Nurs. '74* 74:66, April 1974.

PITORAK, E.: Laryngectomy, *Am. J. Nurs.* 68:780, April 1968.

Rehabilitation. Sound the way for laryngectomees, *Patient Care* 6:58, August 15, 1972.

TAUB, S.: Air bypass voice prosthesis for vocal rehabilitation of laryngectomees, *Am. J. Surg.* 125:748, June 1973.

TAUB, S., and SPIRO, R.: Vocal rehabilitation of laryngectomees, *Am. J. Surg.* 124:87, 1972.

TYLER, M.: Artificial airways, *Nurs. '73* 73:22, February 1973.

WELTY, M. J., et al.: The patient with maxillofacial cancer, *Nurs. Clin. N. Am.* 8:137, March 1973.

WHITE, H.: Tracheostomy care with a cuffed tube, *Am. J. Nurs.* 72:75, January 1972.

# The Patient with Acute Respiratory Disorder

Respiratory disorders are the most frequent type of acute illness. Who has not experienced the "common cold"? Much of the time in the basically healthy person, milder respiratory infections result in unpleasant symptoms and the inconvenience of loss of time from work, school, or social activities. However, a similar infection which develops as a complication of another disease, or in the elderly person, or in a person with chronic respiratory impairment may make the difference between life and death. If such a patient recovers, convalescence is prolonged and costly.

Acute respiratory disease is the most frequent cause of absence from work. Because of its physical, social, and economic effects on employers and employees, as well as its effect on the economy as a whole, the prevention as well as the prompt diagnosis and therapy of acute respiratory disorders is of paramount importance in the area of occupational health.

One of the most vital needs of man is a continuous supply of oxygen. Severe disease in the network of the respiratory passages can interfere with the oxygen supply. Because many respiratory conditions can be prevented to a certain extent, the nurse needs to know what causes them to develop, how they are spread, how their severity can be reduced, and how to care for the patient who becomes acutely ill.

## DIAGNOSTIC TESTS

**Physical Assessment.** Today knowledge and skill in basic techniques of physical assessment of the chest are a component of nursing care in many settings. For example, the nurse who cares for the patient in the respiratory intensive care unit develops the ability to judge the effects of various therapeutic modalities on the respiratory system, using physical assessment skills. Although the nurse is not responsible for the diagnosis of disease, the progress (or lack of progress) of all patients with respiratory disorders must be continuously assessed by the nurse specialist, and any changes discussed with the physician. While the respiratory rate is of unquestioned significance, the depth of breathing, character of chest cage movement, quality of breath sounds, and presence or absence of abnormal breath sounds are of much greater importance. The hospital nurse, with her close direct patient contact over an eight-hour period, can develop the ability to discern subtle changes in these parameters so that appropriate intervention can be planned and implemented at an early stage, preventing crises from occurring.

Although the bedside techniques required for assessment of lung function are simple, requiring only a stethoscope and a few moments' time, a certain amount of practice is necessary in order to develop skill and self-confidence. The neophyte nurse must first become proficient in assessing the normal person; then, through an association with a clinical preceptor, she can learn to recognize abnormalities. The skilled nurse can conduct her own assessment of pulmonary function at the time of admission and compare findings with the physician.

The four methods of the physical examination of the chest are: inspection, palpation, percussion, and auscultation. (See Chapter 2 for basic principles of these methods.)

INSPECTION. With the patient's chest completely exposed, the nurse should observe the expansion of the rib cage to determine the symmetry of respiration. Splinting of the chest occurs in response to pain as in pleurisy or trauma while lagging on inspiration may be due to regional alteration in air entry. Retraction of the intercostal spaces during inspiration is seen in pulmonary fibrosis and foreign body aspiration. Bulging of the interspaces follows pneumothorax. The use of the accessory muscles of respiration (neck muscles) may be seen during an acute asthmatic attack or in chronic obstructive pulmonary disease. Inspection may also reveal the "barrel chest" of chronic obstructive pulmonary disease, or a funnel chest.

The examiner does not assume that ventilation is taking place simply on the observation of chest cage movement. Patients with obstruction to air-flow within the tracheobronchial tree may make violent chest cage movements without ventilation. A similar phenomenon may be associated with the use of an intermittent positive pressure breathing apparatus during which the patient fights the machine while he continues to be dyspneic. Under these circumstances the measurement of airflow (as with a Wright Respirometer) or the auscultation of airflow with a stethoscope is mandatory.

PALPATION. Palpation can delineate areas of pain or masses of the thorax. This technique is also used to elicit vibratory sense or vocal fremitus over the lungs (Traver, 1973).

The position of the trachea should be felt. Normally it is midline; deviation to the right or left may signify the occurrence of a pneumothorax. The observation of subcutaneous swelling with a sensation of crepitation on palpation may indicate the presence of subcutaneous emphysema following tracheostomy or pulmonary surgery.

PERCUSSION. In standard percussion of the chest, a finger of one hand is struck by a finger of the other hand while the examiner is listening to the generated note. An alternate technique for the nurse clinician would be to strike the chest wall directly with the fingertips or tap the chest with the balls of the fingers. Although fine changes in percussion note cannot be detected by this method, much useful information may still be obtained. Hyperresonance is the excessive vibration of chest structures secondary to an excess amount of air within the lung or chest cavity. Examples of disease states resulting in a hollow percussion note are chronic obstructive pulmonary disease and pneumothorax. Decreased resonance occurs with consolidation of the lung in pneumonia. When pleural effusion is present the percussion note loses all resonance and can be described as flat. One can duplicate this sound by tapping with the balls of the fingers on the knee. Daily percussion can be a valuable guide to the resolution of a pneumonic infiltrate or pleural effusion.

AUSCULTATION. The most important auscultatory variable for the nurse clinician to identify is the change in intensity of breath sounds. Reduction or absence of breath sounds may signal the presence of marked airway obstruction due to a mucous plug or foreign body. As mentioned previously, the simplest way to assess air exchange is by listening to airflow within the lung. The visual observance of chest cage motion is of limited value and may lull the examiner into false security regarding a patient's ventilation. For example, the introduction of an endotracheal tube beyond the tracheal bifurcation into the right main stem bronchus may result in normal chest excursion but no ventilation of the left lung. Auscultation immediately identifies the problem. Other causes of diminished or absent breath sounds are hyperinflation of the lung from any cause, pneumothorax, and pleural effusion.

Adventitious sounds of many different types may be heard on auscultation. Examples of such sounds are the fine rales noted in congestive heart failure, the bubbly rales of acute pulmonary edema, and the friction rub of pleurisy and pneumonia. Careful auscultation should always be conducted if a patient is in the acute asthmatic state since disappearance of the wheeze may signify severe bronchospasm with very limited air entry and impending disaster.

While the above is an oversimplification of the thorough physical examination of the chest which is described in specialized textbooks, the nurse who masters the above techniques increases her ability in nursing assessment of the respiratory patient.

**Roentgenography.** The roentgenogram of the chest is secondary only to the physical examination in the diagnosis of acute respiratory disorders. Often, when the physical examination of the patient fails to reveal a respiratory disorder, small lesions may be noted on the chest x-ray film. A routine screening chest roentgenogram may reveal disease before the patient has symptoms. The chest roentgenogram is therefore a necessary adjunct to the physical examination in the assessment of respiratory disorders. The posteroanterior (PA) view with the patient's back facing the x-ray tube is the film usually ordered. A lateral view of the chest is often taken at the same time and various oblique views may also be ordered. A three-dimensional (stereoscopic) x-ray picture may help better to define spacially a suspicious shadow. A tomogram (body section roentgenogram) may be taken to delineate a lesion or thoracic shadow that ordinarily is hidden by overlying anatomic parts. In this technique, multiple films are taken at different planes of the chest until the area in question is in sharp focus. The tissues anterior and posterior to the desired area are blurred.

The x-ray examination under normal circumstances is performed in the radiology department. The patient may be transported to the radiology department either by wheelchair or stretcher depending on the severity of the disease. Before the x-ray examination, the patient should remove anything that will obstruct the view of his chest. For example, a religious medal should be removed from his neck and stored safely or taped to his wrist. A light blanket placed around the patient's

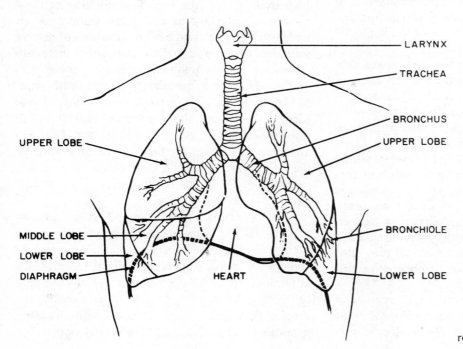

**Figure 29-1.** Diagram of the respiratory tract.

shoulders may be necessary to protect him from drafts in the elevator or the halls.

While it may not be necessary for the hospital chart to accompany the patient for routine studies, it is mandatory that the patient's records be available for more complex radiologic procedures. Most roentgenograms of the chest are taken with the patient in a standing, motionless position after a maximal inspiration. The deep breath fills the lungs with air, expands the chest, and separates pulmonary structures so that fine detail can be analyzed. Should the patient be unable to stand, films can be taken in the sitting position or if necessary while supine. When the patient is too ill to be transported to the radiology department, a chest film may be obtained at the bedside with the use of portable x-ray equipment. Modern portable x-ray equipment has reduced unnecessary patient radiation exposure to a minimum.

The nurse may help to position the patient according to the directions of the x-ray technician. The film holder (cassette) can be slipped into a pillow case to avoid having its cold surface touch the patient's skin. Ordinarily, the nurse leaves the area while the roentgenogram is being taken to protect herself from unnecessary exposure, unless her presence is required to help the patient to maintain the position in which the roentgenogram is to be taken. In this instance she should wear a lead-lined apron. If more than one patient requires help during x-ray exposure, or if one patient needing help has a series of portable x-ray pictures taken, other personnel should hold the patient.

In the acutely ill patient there is no need to shut off oxygen if fire safety standards are adequate.

**Fluoroscopy.** This examination enables the physician to view the thoracic cavity and all its contents in motion. Usually, the patient sits or stands in front of the machine, and he may need help in moving to the machine from the wheelchair. Currently, many hospitals are equipped with special image intensifiers on their x-ray equipment which are capable of displaying a continuous motion study of the chest on a television screen. Darkening of the room is usually not required and x-ray exposure has been reduced by this technique to an extremely low level. The most modern of the image intensifier units are also equipped with special motion picture cameras. With this equipment it is possible to record on film the entire fluoroscopic examination which can then be studied repeatedly

with no further exposure of the patient. Equipment using special television tape recorders is in the developmental stage and will provide instant playback when available. Although the exposure to x-rays is minimal, the physician performing the procedure and the nurse, if she is to observe the procedure, should be protected by light lead-lined aprons.

**Bronchoscopy.** The physician may elect to use a bronchoscope for direct visual examination of the trachea, the two major bronchi, and multiple smaller bronchi in both the diagnosis and therapy of acute respiratory disorders. The bronchoscope is a hollow instrument which can be passed readily into the trachea under local anesthesia. The newer fiber optic bronchoscope is a flexible instrument with a smaller diameter than the rigid metal bronchoscope. If necessary, it can be passed through the nose. Inspection of smaller bronchi is possible with the fiber optic bronchoscope. Tissue from lesions in the formerly inaccessible subdivisions of the bronchial tree can be obtained for study with tiny forceps at the tip of the bronchoscope. Through the lumen of the bronchoscope the physician may pass suction tubes in order to obtain secretions for culture and Papanicolaou cell studies. If required, special biopsy forceps can be introduced and specimens obtained for direct pathologic evaluation. In life-threatening circumstances such as when a foreign body has been aspirated or when a very sick patient with an obstructing mucous plug is too ill to be moved, bronchoscopy can be performed anywhere in the hospital. However, the location of choice is the operating room.

Before bronchoscopy the patient should have mouth care and any dentures removed. He is usually given nothing to eat or drink for eight to 12 hours before bronchoscopy to avoid the danger of vomiting and aspiration. Lights in the bronchoscopy room are dimmed, and a towel often is placed over the patient's eyes. If the procedure has been explained to him, he may be better able to help by keeping his neck muscles relaxed and breathing through his nose.

It is not unusual for the patient to fear this unpleasant procedure, and especially to feel as if he cannot breathe when the bronchoscope is in place. Prior practice of breathing through the nose with his mouth open may help him to relax during the time in which the bronchoscope is in place. An understanding of the diagnostic importance of the procedure may make it easier to bear. Some patients wish to hear more details about what to expect than do others, and the nurse uses the patient's reaction as a guide. Emphasis should be placed on what the patient is expected to do, and how he can help to make the procedure less uncomfortable. Sedation usually is ordered before the examination to help him to relax.

After the procedure the patient may have increased secretions due to irritation. Because the gag reflex has been temporarily abolished, he is given nothing by mouth for several hours. The return of the gag reflex may be tested by touching the posterior pharynx with a cotton swab. Supplied with a sputum cup and tissues, the patient should be encouraged to expectorate and to clear the secretions as often as necessary. Following bronchoscopy, his throat may feel irritated for several days and he is advised to smoke and talk as little as possible. Some bloody mucus usually is expectorated after the test.

COMPLICATIONS. These include laryngeal edema —which may be so severe that the patient requires a tracheostomy—and bleeding, if a biopsy has been taken. Red streaks of blood may be expected after biopsy, but frank bleeding requires the immediate attention of the physician.

**Bronchography.** After the pharynx and larynx have been anesthetized by spray, the physician introduces a catheter into the trachea by either the nasal or oral route and it is positioned above the bifurcation. A radio-opaque oil is then injected into the trachea via the tube and the patient is tilted in various positions so that the dye flows throughout the bronchial tree. X-ray films (bronchograms) are then taken that reveal the now radio-opaque outlines of the bronchi and bronchioles. The airways of both the right and the left lung can be studied at one session. However, the physician usually prefers to perform a complete evaluation in two sessions because, with different views of the chest, opacified airways may overlie each other and confuse the diagnosis. If tracheobronchial secretions are profuse, postural drainage may be necessary before the examination to clear mucus and to enable better visualization of smaller bronchi. The patient should be informed of the discomfort that he may experience during the procedure and should be advised not to cough during instillation of the contrast material since this may drive the dye into the alveoli.

Sedation may be ordered. Following bronchography, postural drainage may again be required to remove excess oil. The newer contrast media, however, are absorbed by the body and the lungs are usually clear within a 12- to 24-hour period. Frequently, bronchography follows bronchoscopy, and the care of the patient is similar.

**Pulmonary Function Tests.** These studies may be divided into two components. The first is the analysis of the physical phenomena involved with the movement of the air in and out of the chest. The second is a measure of the effectiveness of the mechanical processes. The first group includes the vital capacity, maximum breathing capacity, timed vital capacity, and the forced midexpiratory flow rate. These measurements are obtained during various respiratory maneuvers. The *vital capacity* is a measure of the amount of the air a patient can expire following a maximal inspiration. The normal range is 3,500 to over 5,000 ml., but is dependent significantly upon age and sex. The pattern of the vital capacity as recorded by the respirometer can then be related to time, permitting measurement of the *timed vital capacity* and the various flow rates. Edema, pain, fibrosis, and space-filling lesions, such as cancer, can lower vital capacity. The *maximum breathing capacity* (MBC) is the most air that a patient can voluntarily move in and out of the lungs within a period of one minute. This study is a measure of the airway resistance within the lungs and is reduced in patients with asthma and chronic obstructive pulmonary disease. The MBC, however, is a very strenuous test and many patients with acute respiratory disease perform poorly due to fatigue. Clinical nursing specialists in respiratory care may make some of these measurements or at least use the results in order to plan and evaluate nursing intervention such as training in deep breathing and coughing (Traver, 1974).

The primary tests for the assessment of the effectiveness of *ventilation* (the movement of air in and out of the lungs) are measures of the partial pressures of oxygen and carbon dioxide in the arterial blood. The analysis of arterial blood in the normal subject results in the following range of values: pH, 7.39 to 7.45; $P_{CO_2}$, 35 to 45 mm. Hg; $P_{O_2}$, 96 to 100 mm. Hg breathing room air; and arterial oxyhemoglobin saturation, 96 to 100 per cent. Nursing specialists in the care of patients critically ill from a wide variety of conditions commonly use the results of arterial blood gas analysis in planning patient care and in monitoring the results of therapy. (See Chapter 60 for care of the patient with deviations from these norms.)

**Sputum Examination.** Samples of bronchial secretions frequently are collected and sent to the laboratory. The microscopic examination of appropriately stained smears may reveal casts, cancer cells, or pathogenic organisms. If an attempt is to be made to grow the organisms in a culture, the collecting receptacle must be sterile, and both the nurse and the patient should be careful not to contaminate the inside. Because negative smears do not indicate necessarily the absence of disease, repeated examinations may be ordered on successive days. Sometimes 24-hour specimens are collected. Sputum specimens should be raised from deep in the bronchi, such as the sputum first expectorated in the morning. The patient's mouth should be cleaned first, so that no saliva or old food particles are expectorated into the collecting receptacle. Color, consistency, odor, and quantity of sputum should be noted and charted. The appearance of blood should be reported promptly. A waterproof, waxed sputum cup or a wide-mouthed bottle should be used. The patient is instructed to keep the outside of the container free of contamination by the secretions. The cup or bottle should be covered to keep airborne organisms and odor inside and to prevent the contents from being easily viewed. The specimen is refrigerated if there is a delay in sending it to the laboratory.

Patients who have difficulty raising sputum for specimens may be helped by inhalation of 10 per cent saline in distilled water from a heated nebulizer. Condensation of the vapor on the tracheobronchial mucosa stimulates the production of secretions which are then more readily mobilized. The patient needs to be taught the use of the heated aerosol apparatus as well as how to cough effectively so that an adequate specimen can be obtained (Ahlstrom, 1965).

**Analysis of Gastric Contents.** Because pathogenic organisms causing lung disease frequently are swallowed, the fasting contents of the stomach may be examined. This diagnostic procedure is used sometimes when tuberculosis is suspected in a debilitated or aged patient who is not expectorating sputum (see Chap. 40).

## PNEUMONIA

Pneumonia is the fifth leading cause of death in the United States, and from 9 to 10 per cent of some large community hospital annual admissions have been for the treatment of pneumonia (McHenry, 1974). Because organisms identified as causing pneumonia are different in the population whose infection is acquired in the community as compared with hospital-acquired infection (nosocomial infection), the diagnostic, therapeutic, and nursing care problems vary for these two groups (Mostow, 1974; McHenry, 1974). Typical bacterial pneumonia is an acute illness caused by inflammation or infection of the lungs, and is characterized by a productive cough, chest pain, and fever.

### Pathology

Coarse hairs at the entrance of the nose filter larger particles from the inspired air. The mucous membrane that lines the respiratory passages has an outer layer of ciliated epithelium, and its tiny, hairlike projections trap debris and microorganisms that enter with air. A sticky mucous secretion gathers these foreign bodies together. Then the motion of the cilia carries the foreign particles into the pharynx, where they either are swallowed or are eliminated through the nose or the mouth. Irritation of the respiratory passages due to noxious gases or large foreign particles stimulates additional secretions, sneezing, and coughing—all of which help to expel foreign particles and accumulated mucus. The defenses of the respiratory tract against infection are so efficient that not until the body is weakened, or the noxious stimuli are overwhelming, do the lungs become infected.

When bacteria enter the alveoli they act as irritants and cause the exudation of edema fluid filling the alveolar sacs. The fluid is an excellent culture medium and, as organisms grow in the fluid-filled alveolar sac, the body responds, as it does to all infections, by pouring more fluid into the area. The previously filled alveolus spills some fluid into the adjoining sac, and pneumonia spreads. The infected fluid moves into the bronchioles, and as the patient breathes and coughs, more alveoli become filled.

The final stage of the process, consolidation, is a filling of the alveoli with thick exudate, so that an exchange of gases is impossible in these areas of

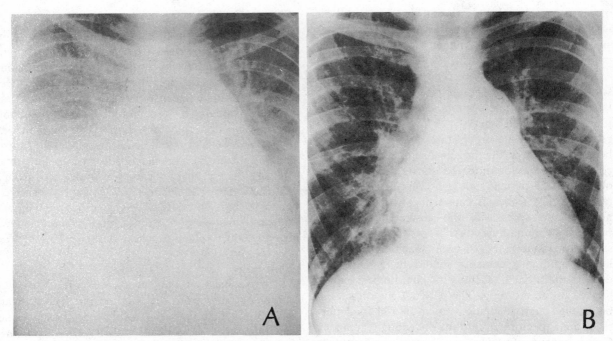

**Figure 29-2.** (A) Right lobar pneumonia. Note the consolidation of the right lower lobe. The left lung field is essentially normal. (B) Complete resolution of the pneumonia after two weeks of antibiotic therapy. (Department of Radiology, Methodist Hospital of Brooklyn)

the lung. When the pleura becomes infected, the patient has a severe, stabbing chest pain as the inflamed tissues rub over each other with each inspiration.

As the disease spreads, the mucous membranes of the nose, the pharynx, the trachea, and the bronchi become inflamed, as are the alveoli of the lungs. Secretions containing mucus, serum, fibrin, and cast-off cells exude from the membranes. As inflammation proceeds, blood oozes from the membrane and colors the sputum to the characteristic rusty color. Irritation of the mucous membrane with the collection of secretion causes coughing. At first, the cough may be dry and unproductive, but later the secretions are mucopurulent, and then they are rusty. Coughing and expectoration help to prevent clogging of the bronchi with mucous plugs.

When the inflammation is confined to one or more lobes of the lung, it is called *lobar pneumonia* (Fig. 29-2). Patchy and diffuse infection scattered throughout both lungs is called *bronchopneumonia*. Pneumonia caused by the pneumococci usually leads to lobar rather than bronchopneumonia.

## Etiology

Pneumonia can be caused by many different types of organisms, such as viruses, rickettsiae, streptococci, staphylococci, fungi and Friedländer's bacilli (Fig. 29-3). However, the most common causative organism is the pneumococcus (*Diplococcus pneumoniae*). This bacterium is common in the air. It often can be cultured from the throats of healthy persons. It causes illness when the resistance of the individual is lowered, or when the person is exposed to an extraordinarily large concentration of the organisms or to particularly virulent organisms. *Staphylococcus aureus* is responsible for 1 to 5 per cent of bacterial pneumonias (Fig. 29-4).

Pneumonia can be caused by a group of organisms called *Mycoplasma pneumoniae*. For many years bacteria could not be cultured from secretions of patients with this type of illness. The disease was then called primary atypical pneumonia or "virus" pneumonia. It is now known to be caused by the mycoplasma, one of the smallest organisms that can be grown in cell-free media. The disease is also known as Eaton's agent pneumonia.

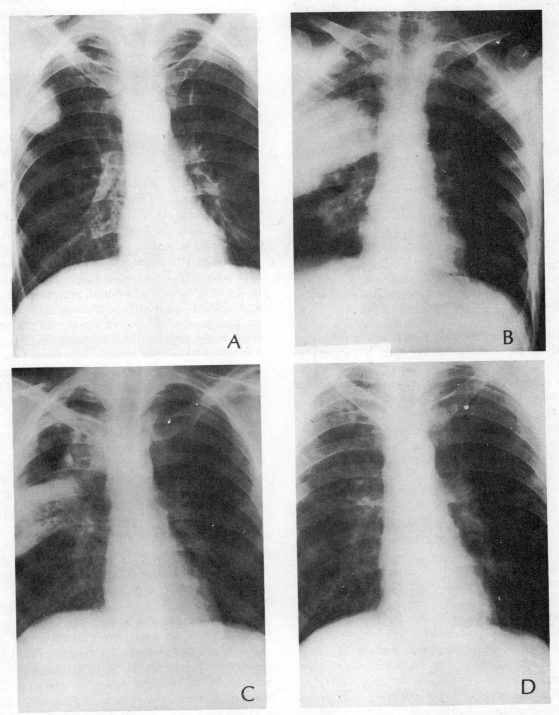

**Figure 29-3.** Friedländer's pneumonia. (A) Right upper lobe circumscribed infiltrate observed on admission to hospital of an alcohol addict. (B) One day later the pneumonia, lobar in type, has spread significantly. (C) Partial resolution after several weeks and (D) return to normal three months later. (Department of Radiology, Methodist Hospital of Brooklyn)

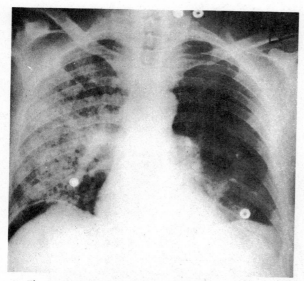

**Figure 29-4.** Staphylococcal pneumonia. The x-ray reveals a patchy pneumonic process involving the right lung. (Department of Radiology, Methodist Hospital of Brooklyn)

Hypoventilation of lung tissue over a prolonged period of time—as happens when a patient lies quietly in bed, breathing with only a part of his lungs over a prolonged period—can result in the accumulation of bronchial secretions and cause hypostatic pneumonia.

Pure oxygen, if inhaled for a period of several days, can result in atelectasis or collapse of the lung. The collapsed segment then becomes susceptible to bacterial invasion and can be the site of a pneumonic infiltrate.

Smoke particles and other air pollutants such as nitrogen dioxide can cause irritation of the linings of the air passages and create the setting for bacterial invasion.

If the epiglottis does not close completely on swallowing, and fluid or other food particles are aspirated into the bronchial tree, an acute chemical pneumonitis can result followed by bacterial infection and classical pneumonia.

People who are unconscious because of anesthesia, coma, sedation, or alcoholic intoxication are prone to pneumonia because the epiglottal reflex is slowed and because hypoventilation with retention of fluid occurs.

### Prevention

Nurses have a particular responsibility to prevent hypostatic pneumonia. Every patient on bed rest is a candidate for this disease, especially the heavily sedated, comatose, and elderly patients. All patients should move or be moved regularly, and they should take several deep breaths at least every hour during the day. The bed-rest patient must be taught to cough adequately. Since effective coughing requires a forward flexion motion it cannot be done while the patient is lying flat in bed (Lagerson, 1973).

Some patients may follow a regular preventive schedule after initial instruction; many will need frequent reminders and encouragement; others may need the direct presence and assistance of the nurse. The patient's needs should be written down on his nursing care plan so that all who care for him will follow the nursing orders to prevent complications of bed rest.

Nurses must ascertain that equipment used for respiratory therapy, tracheostomy care, and suctioning is cleansed according to recommended standards. Breaks in sterile suctioning technique can result in pneumonia as can trauma to the trachea and bronchi produced during suctioning.

When suctioning is indicated, it should be done promptly, before the mucus is aspirated. Levin tube feedings to a comatose patient are dangerous if the tip of the tube should slip up above the epiglottis, or if the patient regurgitates.

Oral fluids never should be poured into the mouth of an unconscious person.

The thin, slippery secretions of a head cold (unlike bacteria breathed in with dusty air) are less likely to be rejected from the body by the cilia, and, therefore, they may reach the alveoli, establishing an initial infection. Likewise, oily substances are not easily passed upward by ciliary action and may fill alveoli with fluid in which bacteria can grow. This is the reason that saline nose drops are preferable to those in an oil base.

### Incidence and Prognosis

From 1870 to 1910 the mortality rate from pneumonia climbed from 4.4 to 19.9 per 10,000 population (Lewis, 1910). In 1900, pneumonia and influenza were the first cause of death; in 1963 they ranked tenth. Pneumococcal pneumonia shows a 95 per cent recovery rate when it is treated (Beeson and McDermott, 1971). It may be rapidly lethal in untreated cases or when treatment has been started too late. Prognosis is grave also when there are other complicating factors—for example, aging or the presence of pulmonary or circulatory disease and alcoholism, which lower the general resistance.

The mortality rate of staphylococcal pneumonia prior to 1942 ranged from 50 to 95 per cent. With the discovery of specific antibiotics against the staphylococcus organism the mortality is now 15 to 20 per cent. Much higher mortality rates are seen in the elderly and when the organism is acquired in a hospital setting. Staphylococcal pneumonia frequently follows an influenzalike respiratory infection.

Pneumonia occurs most frequently during the change of seasons, fall and spring, and during the winter, when other respiratory diseases are at their peak. It is sporadic in nature, except for such rare epidemics as may occur after a widespread outbreak of influenza.

## Signs and Symptoms

The onset of bacterial pneumonia is sudden. Without warning symptoms, the patient is struck with severe, sharp pain in his chest, rapid prostration that sends him to bed, and often a shaking chill that gives way to a fever going as high as 106 degrees F. In untreated bacterial pneumonia in the days before antibiotic therapy, the temperature stayed high until sometime between the second and the ninth day, when it dropped as rapidly as it first rose. This period was called the "crisis," and it was anxiously awaited by all who attended the patient.

Irritation of the tissues of the respiratory tract produces a cough that is painful, since it causes movement of the chest wall and a consequent rubbing together of the two pleural layers. The sputum often is rusty in color. Breathing also causes pain, and the patient tries to breathe as shallowly as possible.

In bacterial pneumonia the alveoli become filled with exudate. Bronchitis, tracheitis, and spots of necrosis in the lung may follow. In pneumonia caused by mycoplasma there is thickening of the alveolar septa and partial filling of the alveoli with exudate. A hyaline membrane may line the alveoli. As the inflammatory process continues, there is more interference with the exchange of gases between the bloodstream and the lungs. With an increase in the carbon dioxide content of the blood, the respiratory center in the brain is stimulated, and breathing becomes more rapid and shallow.

The nostrils flare with each inspiration. Often there is dyspnea, and the patient is more comfortable and better able to breathe while he is sitting up. Although the cheeks are flushed, cyanosis may appear, especially around the mouth and in the nail beds. The normal arterial oxygen saturation is 96 per cent. If it falls to 85 per cent, the patient experiences symptoms due to hypoxia, such as confusion, dyspnea, cyanosis, and delirium (Morrow, et al., 1964). In an attempt to get blood to the lungs more quickly and in response to the fever, the heart rate increases.

If the disease process is not halted, the patient becomes sicker and perhaps delirious. If the circulatory system is unable to maintain the burden of decreased gaseous exchange, the patient may die from heart failure or asphyxia.

The fever of mycoplasmal and viral pneumonia does not resolve by crisis but by lysis; that is, it slowly returns to normal. Viral pneumonia also differs from bacterial pneumonia in that the blood cultures are sterile, the sputum may be more copious, the chills are less frequent, and the pulse and the respirations are characteristically slow.

The course of viral pneumonia usually is less severe than that of bacterial pneumonia, although the patient is far from comfortable. In viral pneumonia the mortality rate is low, but it rises when bacterial pneumonia occurs as a secondary infection. Often, the patient with viral pneumonia is weak and ill for a longer time than the patient with successfully treated bacterial pneumonia.

## Diagnostic Assessment

The diagnosis of pneumonia is made usually through the clinical signs and symptoms, including physical examination of the chest. Sputum and blood cultures are done immediately to identify the causative organism. Since the organism may not be present in early cultures, several cultures usually are ordered. Sputum for culture should be collected before antibiotics are given, since the choice of the antibiotic will depend on the positive identification of the organism. If antibiotic therapy is started before the specimen is taken, it may mask the organism. If a physician has ordered that an antibiotic be given after the collection of a sputum specimen, and difficulty is encountered in obtaining the specimen, the physician should be consulted concerning whether or not the antibiotic should be started.

Cultures of the sputum require at least 24 to 48 hours to grow.

A chest roentgenogram will be ordered. Knowledge of the pattern and extent of pulmonary infiltration is valuable in the diagnosis and treatment of the pneumonia. A consolidated lobe of the lung may be characteristic of a pneumococcal pneumonia while the presence of multiple pulmonary abscesses is the hallmark of staphylococcal pneumonia.

Gram stain of a sputum smear will separate gram-positive from gram-negative organisms and frequently the specific organism can be tentatively identified on the microscope slide pending culture. The white blood cell count is useful because it is most often normal or below normal in mycoplasmal infection while the elevation may be dramatic (30,000 per cu.mm.) in staphylococcal pneumonia. Viral and mycoplasmal pneumonias can occasionally be identified by the presence in blood of an elevated cold agglutinin titer. The cold agglutinin is an abnormal antibody that causes agglutination of red blood cells at temperatures below normal body temperature.

## Treatment
### Antibiotic Therapy

At present less than two days of treatment with antibiotics usually brings about a reduction of fever to normal and a marked improvement in the other symptoms.

The specific antibiotics chosen for treatment depend on the sensitivity of the causative organism to their action. Sometimes, tragically, an organism will be encountered that does not respond to any available antibiotics. If the infecting organism has not been identified, broad-spectrum antibiotics, i.e., antibiotics that are effective against a large number of organisms, may be ordered.

Antibiotic medication may be ordered by the intravenous route and added to the IV bottle, sparing the patient repeated injections. The intravenous flow must be at the rate ordered to maintain an adequate blood level of the antibiotic, and the patient must be observed carefully for side effects and toxic effects.

*Penicillin* often is used in pneumococcal and streptococcal pneumonia. Aqueous solutions of the potassium or the sodium salts of penicillin may be ordered in doses of 300,000 to 600,000 units given intramuscularly every three to six hours. This type of penicillin is absorbed into the blood in 15 to 30 minutes, and it is excreted in the urine in three to six hours. Procaine penicillin is absorbed and excreted more slowly. It is given intramuscularly in doses of 300,000 to 600,000 units once or twice a day. Penicillin may also be given intravenously if the rapid attainment of high blood levels is mandatory in the treatment of the extremely ill patient. The antibiotic is usually continued for approximately one week or until the patient is afebrile for from two to three days.

Penicillin is harmless for the majority of people. However, some persons, usually those who have had penicillin previously, develop an allergic reaction that manifests itself in a mild or severe urticaria, ulcerated mucous membranes, and fever. Some people die from anaphylactic shock caused by allergy to penicillin. Patients should be observed closely for signs of an allergic reaction, and these signs should be reported promptly to the physician.

Pneumonia due to *Staphylococcus aureus* may be treated with methicillin (Staphcillin), oxacillin (Prostaphlin), or cephalothin (Keflin). Oxacillin and cephalexin monohydrate (Keflex—a derivative of cephalothin) can be given orally with effectiveness. Methicillin is rapidly destroyed by acid solutions and by gastric secretions while cephalothin is poorly absorbed by the oral route. Toxic reactions are common, including thrombophlebitis at the site of the infusion, depression of renal function, fever, and rash.

*Ampicillin,* a synthetic penicillin, is active against most organisms that cause pneumonia. In addition to its penicillinlike activity, it is effective against gram-negative organisms such as *E. coli* and *H. influenzae.* The usual dose for adults is 250 mg. four times a day. The physician may increase the dose significantly (2 to 4 Gm. daily in divided doses) in the presence of severe infection. A contraindication to its use is a previous hypersensitivity reaction to any of the penicillins.

*Streptomycin* is an intramuscularly administered drug that is effective against both gram-positive and gram-negative organisms. It is particularly effective against the tubercle bacillus. Side effects, which include skin rash, fever, nausea and vomiting, loss of appetite, and pain at the site of injection, should be reported. Anaphylaxis can occur. A most dangerous toxic effect is eighth cranial nerve damage resulting in dizziness, ringing in the ears, loss of equilibrium, or hearing loss. The drug is stopped should these occur. The usual dose is 0.5 to 1 Gm. twice a day which is ordered reduced after one or two weeks.

*Tetracycline* is effective against mixed bacterial infections of the respiratory tract, penicillin-resistant and some staphylococcal infections, and *Mycoplasma pneumoniae*. Tetracycline is absorbed readily from the gastrointestinal tract and is excreted in feces and urine. It is usually given orally, although it may be given intramuscularly or intravenously. The dosage usually is 250 to 500 mg. four times a day. It is relatively nontoxic, although some patients experience nausea, vomiting, diarrhea, or pruritus of the anus or scrotum, and some may be allergic to the drug. It is not given to pregnant women in the third trimester when fetal tooth development is under way because it may cause discoloration of the teeth (yellow-grey-brownish).

*Chloramphenicol* (Chloromycetin) is a potent antibiotic that is effective against a wide variety of organisms. The response of patients with rickettsial infections is often dramatic. It is, however, a very toxic drug used only in serious infections for which less dangerous drugs are ineffective or contraindicated. The principal use for the drug is in the treatment of *Salmonella typhi* infection (typhoid fever). The adult dose is 50 mg. per Kg. per day in divided doses. The main toxic reaction is the development of bone marrow depression. Serious and fatal blood dyscrasias such as aplastic anemia are known to occur. It is desirable for patients to be hospitalized while on this medication in order to facilitate blood examination for signs of toxicity, although bone marrow depression may occur weeks or months after the drug treatment is completed.

*Erythromycin* is effective against most gram-positive organisms. It is absorbed readily from the gastrointestinal tract. The oral dose is 250 to 500 mg. every four to six hours. It has few toxic effects. This drug often is used when the patient is sensitive to penicillin.

*Cephalothin* (Keflin) closely resembles penicillin in its chemical structure and mechanism of action. It is useful against many gram-positive and gram-negative organisms. The value of this medication is in the treatment of infection when the organism is resistant to other agents. The drug must be given by intramuscular or intravenous route. The usual dose is 4 to 6 Gm. daily in divided doses but up to 12 Gm. daily may be ordered for severe infections. It is administered with great caution to penicillin-sensitive individuals because of partial cross-allergenicity. This drug causes a false-positive reaction for glucose in the urine with Benedict's solution or with Clinitest tablets, but not with urine sugar analysis paper (Tes-tape).

*Cephalexin monohydrate* (Keflex) is a semisynthetic cephalosporin antibiotic similar to Keflin but intended for oral use. Keflex is acid stable and may be given without regard to meals. Thus, Keflex is a logical follow-up to Keflin which can be given only intravenously or intramuscularly and presumably for serious illness. All the indications and contraindications of the cephalosporin family apply to Keflex. The dosage of Keflex is 1 to 4 Gm daily in divided six-hour doses depending on severity of infection.

*Gentamycin* (Garamycin) is effective against a variety of organisms many of which are resistant to other antibiotics. This drug is administered intramuscularly in a dose of 3 to 5 mg. per Kg. daily in divided doses (about 75 to 125 mg. three times a day). The patient requires close observation as it is potentially nephrotoxic and ototoxic. Urinary output is recorded. Dizziness, loss of equilibrium, ringing in the ears, or hearing loss which may indicate involvement of the vestibular or auditory branches of the eighth cranial nerve must be promptly reported and the drug withheld.

**Supportive Therapy.** Other treatment of the patient is primarily supportive, including bed rest to enable the body to use all its powers for fighting the disease. Fluids in large quantities are ordered to replace those lost through increased respiration and perspiration. If the patient cannot tolerate them by mouth, intravenous fluids are given.

For cough and chest pain, codeine, 30 mg. or 60 mg., may be ordered orally or subcutaneously every four to six hours. Codeine depresses respirations less than does morphine. Side effects include nausea, vomiting, constipation, and excitement.

### Nursing Assessment and Intervention

The patient admitted to the hospital with pneumonia usually is very sick and very uncomfortable. He is likely to be frightened. He not only has fallen ill suddenly, but also may be having great difficulty in breathing. Some severely ill patients are exhausted and have to struggle through pain for every breath.

**Environment.** In some hospitals patients with pneumonia (particularly staphylococcal pneumonia) are isolated during the acute phase.

Some physicians believe that the spread of pneumonia is prevented by this measure; other physicians believe that hand washing and ordinary cleanliness are sufficient to prevent the spread of infection. In either case, medical asepsis is enhanced if an isolation gown is worn over the uniform when giving direct care. The patient needs to be protected from secondary infection. The nurse should wash her hands before caring for him, as well as before leaving the unit. Visitors with head colds should be excluded from his room.

The room should be well ventilated so that the air is as fresh as possible. The nurse works with the Admitting Office so that the patient acutely ill with pneumonia is placed in a room as close to the nurses' station as possible. If isolation is not used, care should be taken that the patient's roommates are not in a high-risk group, such as the aged, postsurgical patients, or those with chronic obstructive pulmonary disease.

**Position.** The head of the bed should be elevated with the pillow placed lengthwise so that it supports the patient's entire back and helps to expand his chest. A pillow across the upper portion of the back will tend to bend him forward and lessen the expansion of his chest.

**Patient Monitoring.** The patient's color, facial expression, and body posture are noted on admission and frequently thereafter. Vital signs are taken on admission and every four hours, except during chills and sponges, when they are recorded more frequently. An increase of temperature to over 103 degrees or below 98.6 degrees should be reported to the physician immediately, since these signs are warnings of a drastic change in the patient's condition. Temperature is taken rectally, since coughing and oral breathing render oral readings grossly inaccurate. Alcohol sponges may be ordered for fever over 102 degrees or 103 degrees. During a sponge exposing the patient to a draft or chilling him must be avoided. A sharp increase or a sharp decrease in pulse rate as well as pulse irregularity warns of circulatory complications and also is reported. If the patient is on a cardiac monitor, the nurse observes for serious cardiac arrhythmias which could be manifestations of hypoxia. (See Chapter 61, The Patient with a Cardiac Arrythmia.)

The prepared nurse auscultates the lungs on admission and regularly to determine quality of breath sounds and presence or absence of abnormal breath sounds. Inspection, palpation, and percussion are indicated also.

The rate and character of respirations are observed closely. Increasingly labored respirations (dyspnea, orthopnea) indicate very rapid progress of the disease and are often a sign that more drastic treatment measures are required. It is characteristic for the patient to grunt with each expiration.

Arterial blood gases may be ordered. The nurse reviews the report immediately and consults with the physician since oxygen therapy is planned accordingly.

RESTLESSNESS. The patient is observed closely for restlessness and confusion which may indicate hypoxia. Clinical evaluation is necessary since restlessness can be due to other causes and appropriate intervention must be chosen. The patient should be asked about his perception of the reason for his restlessness. Depending on the cause, relief of pain, helping him to cough up a mucous plug, giving oxygen, changing his position, changing dampened bed linen, or listening to his thoughts and feelings about his situation may afford relief.

Restlessness may be a prelude to delirium. If it does not abate after nursing measures, the situation should be discussed with the physician. The restless patient needs to be protected by side rails and mild restraint if ordered.

REST. During the early phase of the disease, the patient is kept as quiet as possible.

Some patients feel that even when they are exhausted, they must do their part to establish a relationship with their nurses through talking. If the patient attempts to make small talk while he is acutely ill, he can be asked to conserve his strength. It is a challenge to show interest in the patient without stimulating him to excessive talk. When the acute phase is over the patient can be encouraged to express his thoughts and feelings about the illness, what led up to it, aspects of care, postdischarge plans, and whatever else he wishes to talk about.

**Medications and Treatment.** These are planned so that the patient is disturbed as little as possible. Antibiotics should be given on time to maintain consistent blood levels. Nursing care is planned, for example, so that medication, mouth care and fluids, position change, and physical assessment are done at one interval thus allowing for uninterrupted rest periods. During the acute phase, bathing should be planned to avoid tiring the patient. To avoid chilling, the gown and linen are changed every time that they become wet with perspiration.

**Fluid and Electrolyte Balance.** Oral fluids are generally ordered for the acutely ill patient as soon as they can be tolerated.

When it is fatiguing to drink fluids, they should be offered in small quantities at frequent intervals and in variation to promote appetite. Fruit juices, broths, consommé, milk, and eggnogs may be used. Since the ingestion of food may stimulate coughing, fluid should not be offered after a coughing spell. Ice chips may be used to moisten the mouth if fluids are not tolerated orally. Because the sputum is foul, mouth care is always given before offering the patient anything to eat or to drink.

Records of intake and output are kept. Any discrepancy should be called to the physician's attention. Since abdominal distention and paralytic ileus are complications of pneumonia, bowel movements should be observed and recorded, and the abdomen should be observed for distention, An enema or suppository may be ordered. A rectal tube aids in the expulsion of flatus. Distention pushes the diaphragm up, so that it presses on the base of the lungs at a time when they are especially in need of space for expansion.

**Expectoration.** When the patient is approached for medications or for treatment, he is encouraged to cough up mucus, using effective cough techniques (Lagerson, 1973). Whenever he coughs, whether voluntarily or by reflex, firm pressure with the hands can be used to splint the chest where it hurts. This will decrease the pain a little and help the patient to be more willing to cough. Some patients are shy about expectorating in the view of another person, but the infected sputum should not be swallowed. Tissues are provided and the patient in instructed to "cover his cough" and to dispose of the tissues in the paper bag provided. He is given a sputum cup with a cover if the sputum is to be saved for inspection or measurement. This equipment is kept within easy reach, so that the patient does not have to exert himself to reach it. The sputum cup or paper bag is changed at least twice a day; they are handled with great care and sealed so that the infection is not spread.

**Mouth Care.** Frequent mouth care is essential to prevent stomatitis. The lesions of herpes simplex often appear around the mouth and are a source of great discomfort for the patient. Camphor ice, cold cream, or tincture of benzoin may be applied.

**Oxygen and Humidification.** If the inflammatory process is far advanced, the patient may have considerable respiratory difficulty and may or may not be cyanotic. Oxygen should be prescribed as drugs are prescribed and may be given by a nasal catheter, cannula, or Ventimask. Oxygen therapy is monitored by arterial blood gas studies whenever possible.

The humidification of the inspired air is usually very helpful in liquefying secretions and is best administered by cool-mist vaporizer. In the presence of severe infection with thick, abundant secretions, the physician may perform endotracheal intubation or tracheostomy. These techniques make suctioning easier, and in addition, permit more effective ventilation by a positive pressure breathing apparatus. (See Chapter 60 for care of the patient with respiratory insufficiency or failure.)

**Shock.** If the combination of specific and supportive treatment, nursing care, and the patient's own body defenses are insufficient response to the infection, he can go into shock. Since shock must be treated early and rapidly if the patient is to survive, he must be closely monitored and signs or symptoms of shock reported promptly to the physician. (See Chapter 59 for care of the patient in shock.)

**Convalescence.** Generally with the administration of antibiotics, symptoms usually subside rapidly during the first 48 to 72 hours, and the patient feels much improved. However, he will be weak and tired. He is kept at rest for several days after his temperature has returned to normal. He then is helped gradually to resume self-care activities. The patient is encouraged to increase activity slowly, because the disease is exhausting, the antibiotics have disturbed the bacterial equilibrium of his body, and his resistance to secondary infection is low. A follow-up roentgenogram usually is ordered to make sure that the disease process is clearing. The importance of having this examination performed, and also of following instructions for postdischarge convalescence, are emphasized to the patient. A nourishing diet and gradually increasing levels of activity to optimal functioning are the usual recommendations.

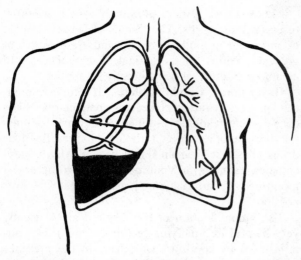

**Figure 29-5.** Fluid in the pleural space can compress the lung.

## Complications of Pneumonia

Complications of pneumonia are seen more rarely today than previously, since antibiotics usually reverse the disease process early. Congestive heart failure is a serious complication. On occasion a patient's temperature may fall within two days, but his pulse may remain fast. This is a pseudocrisis; even though the fever is gone, the lung pathology and the other symptoms remain. The patient is still acutely ill.

*Empyema,* the collection of pus in the pleural space, and *pleurisy* (see below) may occur. Both are becoming increasingly rare, as pneumonia is treated more effectively with antibiotics. Symptoms include continued fever and there are other signs of infection. The pain in the chest is usually at the site of infection. Empyema is treated with the antibiotics that are specific for the invading organism. This is determined through thoracentesis and bacteriologic examination of the fluid obtained.

The invasion of the bloodstream by organisms, which occurs during periods of *septicemia* while the patient is having a chill, makes all the body accessible to the organisms. Rarely, a secondary focus of infection may be established, resulting in endocarditis, meningitis, or purulent arthritis.

*Atelectasis,* or the collapse of a lung segment, is caused by the plugging of a bronchus with mucus. Encouraging the patient to cough and changing his position frequently will help to prevent this particular complication.

*Otitis media, bronchitis, or sinusitis* may complicate recovery, especially from atypical pneumonia, by the spread of the organisms to these organs.

## PLEURISY

### Pathology

Pleurisy is an inflammation of the *pleura,* the membrane that covers the lungs in two layers. Pleurisy occurs as a complication of pulmonary disease. Two forms are seen: acute fibrinous or dry pleurisy, in which only small amounts of exudate are formed during the inflammatory process; and *pleurisy with effusion,* in which large amounts of fluid are secreted and collect in the space between the pleural layers (Fig. 29-5). There may be so much fluid that the lung is collapsed partially on that side, and there is pressure on the heart and the other organs of the mediastinum. Dry pleurisy is seen most commonly in pneumonia, in which the inflammatory process spreads from the lung to the parietal pleura. Pleurisy with effusion may result from tuberculosis, carcinoma of the lungs, cardiac and renal disease, systemic infections, pneumonia, and pulmonary embolism. The pleura becomes thick, swollen, and rigid. The visceral pleura has no pain fibers, but the parietal pleura does. Very sharp pain occurs when the two surfaces of the pleura rub over each other during respiration. As fluid is formed, this pain gradually subsides; but the patient has a dry cough, fatigues easily, and may get out of breath.

A diagnostic thoracentesis may be done. On the specimen of fluid withdrawn, counts of erythrocytes and leukocytes are performed, as well as tests of specific gravity, glucose level, cytologic examination for malignant cells, and a bacteriologic examination. Occasionally, a pleural biopsy is taken with a needle designed for this purpose or by means of an open thoracotomy. After the latter the patient returns from the operating room with an intercostal catheter for temporary drainage.

### Treatment and Nursing Care of Pleurisy Patients

The care of the patient with pleurisy is similar to that of the patient with pneumonia. Bed rest is required. The room should be warm and well ventilated. The patient needs encouragement to cough. The nurse can help by firm pressure at the painful spot. Positioning the patient on the side of the effusion helps to splint the painful area and also encourages the expansion of the other side of the rib cage. A heating pad or hot-water bag to be applied to the painful area may be ordered for comfort.

If there is a great deal of fluid with respiratory embarrassment, the fluid may be removed by thoracentesis. The nurse observes the patient closely during thoracentesis for signs of weakness, excessive diaphoresis, increased respirations or dyspnea, pain, chill, nausea, coughing, or shock. Any such symptoms or signs are called to the attention of the physician, who then proceeds more slowly or discontinues the treatment. It may be necessary for the nurse to support the weakened patient in position. He should be comfortable so that he can remain immobile during the procedure. Leaning forward over a pillow-padded bed table is generally a helpful position.

If pleurisy is a complication of another disease, it usually heals spontaneously when the primary disease is treated successfully. Pleurisy due to metastasized cancer tends to recur. Repeated thoracentesis may be performed. Sometimes radioactive gold, mechlorethamine hydrochloride or nitrogen mustard is instilled into the pleural space.

## EMPYEMA

Empyema, pus in the pleural space, is a rare complication of pneumonia or chest trauma since the introduction of antibiotic therapy. Its presence is characterized by chest pain, fever, and evidence of a pleural effusion. The physician confirms the diagnosis by a diagnostic thoracentesis with culture of the withdrawn fluid. Usually he inserts a surgical drain in order to empty the empyema cavity. (If this cavity is not emptied, fibrosis of the pleural linings can occur which may require surgical removal at a later time.) The care of the patient is similar to the care of any patient with an infection and a draining, infected wound. He is observed for signs of pneumothorax. (See also Chapter 30 for further discussion of empyema.)

## INFLUENZA

### Pathology and Incidence

Influenza is an acute respiratory disease of short duration caused by one of several related and yet distinct viruses.

Influenza occurs chiefly in epidemics, although sporadic cases appear between epidemics. Some of the viruses that have been identified have been named with letters. Widespread epidemics caused by influenza A occur about every two to three years, whereas those caused by influenza B occur in a cycle of three to five years (Davenport, 1969). Influenza C rarely is seen. Another group designated type D refers to the para-influenza viruses. There are four major subtype A viruses. Pandemic or worldwide outbreaks of influenza have been recorded at intervals since 1743. The 1957 outbreak, which was first recognized in Asia and spread rapidly throughout the world, was studied widely. The illness has been labeled Asian influenza and the virus $A_2$. In the United States the mortality was highest among people over 65 years of age.

In January 1963, $A_2$ influenza started in the eastern section of the United States and spread throughout the country, sparing only the West Coast. It was a true epidemic: in 35 counties of Arkansas alone there were 45,000 patients.

Most patients recover. Fatalities usually are due to bacterial complications, especially among pregnant women, the aged or debilitated, and those with chronic pulmonary or cardiac disease. During an epidemic, the death rate from pneumonia and cardiovascular diseases rises.

### Signs and Symptoms

The incubation period is two to three days, and the onset is sudden, with considerable individual variation in symptoms. The patient looks acutely ill and complains of chilliness, severe headache, muscular aching, and fever. There may be anorexia, weakness, and apathy, as well as respiratory symptoms, sneezing, sore throat, dry cough, nasal discharge, and herpetic lesions of the lips and the mouth. Severe disease causes prostration and may lead to vasomotor collapse. Fever, 100 degrees to 103 degrees, persists about three days, but other symptoms usually continue for seven to ten days. Cough may persist longer.

Complications include tracheobronchitis, caused by damage to the ciliated epithelium of trachea and bronchi; bacterial pneumonia; and congestive heart failure. Staphylococcal pneumonia is the most serious complication, exhibiting a fulminant, often fatal course.

### Treatment and Nursing Care of Influenza Patients

Bed rest in a warm, well-ventilated room is recommended until the temperature is normal and for one or two days afterward. Temperature, pulse, and respirations are taken every four hours during the elevation. Copious amounts of fluid, given frequently, may include fruit juices, milk and egg drinks, and broths; a regular diet is given as soon as the patient's appetite returns. Sponges and back rubs promote the patient's general comfort and may help him to sleep. Acetylsalicylic acid (aspirin), 0.3 to 1.0 Gm., may be given every four to six hours for headache and muscular aching. Steam or cool vapor inhalation eases a dry cough. The physician may order codeine 30 to 60 mg. every six hours, as needed, to control the coughing.

The patient should be taught to use paper handkerchiefs once, to fold them carefully to avoid spreading infection, and to discard them in a paper bag. The viruses that cause influenza are transmitted through the respiratory tract. Hospitalization is not recommended in uncomplicated cases, because of the possibility of exposing the patient to a secondary bacterial infection.

The patient is observed carefully for signs of increasing fever, elevated pulse rate, chest pain, difficulty in breathing, change in the amount and the quality of the sputum—particularly, whether it is purulent or rusty—and for marked pain anywhere. A prompt report of any of these is made to the physician.

The return to normal activities should be gradual, because of the amount of prostration typical of influenza. Overexertion and chilling should be avoided. The patient should not return to work until all symptoms have subsided, including the cough.

### Prophylaxis Against Influenza

Epidemics can be predicted, and vaccines are available, but significant protection against influenza epidemics is not yet a reality. For example, although the vaccine against Asian influenza evokes an antibody response in 90 per cent of the people vaccinated, it is not highly effective in preventing the disease. Another problem is that there is not enough time between the identification of the virus of an epidemic and its spread to produce a sufficient amount of the vaccine and then give it to a sufficient number of people. Since immunity is of very short duration (about six months) and specific for only one type of virus, it is not possible to vaccinate far in advance. In 1962, 42 million doses of vaccine against $A_2$ influenza were given (Langmuir et al., 1964), but the 1963 epidemic was not prevented.

This problem has been approached by the production of polyvalent vaccine, which is capable of inducing simultaneous antibodies against several types of influenza. The antigenic composition of the vaccine for the 1964–1965 season included A, $A_1$, $A_2$, and B. The Surgeon General's Advisory Committee on Immunization Practices suggests that first attention be paid to giving the vaccine to high-risk groups: pregnant women, the elderly, and those with chronic illness. Vaccine also is given first to individuals vital to community welfare, such as health personnel, communication and utility workers, and military personnel. Hospitals usually admit only those patients who have the disease in very severe form and prohibit visitors during an epidemic. People are encouraged to remain at home at the first signs of disease and to avoid crowds as much as possible.

## COMMON COLD

The nurse should be familiar with the symptoms of this viral infection in order to protect her patients and herself. It is highly prevalent, with an average of three annual colds per person in urban communities in the temperate zone. The majority of colds occur during the cold weather and at the times of temperature change, i.e., the spring and the fall. Respiratory diseases, such as the common cold, which are insignificant medically, are important socially and economically because of the interruption they cause in daily living. It has been estimated that in the 12 months of the year 1958–1959, respiratory conditions caused almost half of the total of all days of restricted activity due to acute illness. The average was 4.1 days of restricted activity due to respiratory disease for every person in the country.

A large number of filterable viruses cause colds. Immunity is of very short duration, and incubation is short. Extraneous factors, such as fatigue, chilling, emotional upset, exposure to irritating gases or allergens—all of which affect the nasal mucosa—are believed to lower the natural resistance, facilitating invasion by the virus.

### Signs and Symptoms

Although there is considerable individual variation in the symptoms, they may include sneezing, chilliness, headache, watery eyes, and a dry scratchy throat, followed by copious nasal discharge, sore throat, hoarseness, and cough. There may be a slight fever. The cold lasts from four to 14 days, with symptoms gradually subsiding.

## Treatment

Bed rest, since it restricts contact with the public (and limits the spread of the cold), is particularly important for the individual who may be susceptible to complications—infants, aged and debilitated individuals, and those whose temperature is elevated. Ordinarily, the otherwise healthy adult does not remain confined to bed, although he should get extra rest and avoid contact with others. Fluids in large amounts are helpful. Petroleum jelly around the nose and the mouth will relieve chapping. Visitors should be restricted, and the patient should be instructed in the proper use of paper handkerchiefs and in hand washing.

Strict isolation precautions are out of the question with such a widespread infection. However, it is important that persons with colds avoid others, especially those likely to be susceptible.

Antibiotics are useless in the treatment of the common cold, because they are ineffective against the viruses, and the person is subject to the unfavorable side effects of the antibiotics without the likelihood of benefiting from them. Individuals who have a tendency to develop a secondary bacterial infection may benefit from prophylactic antibiotic therapy. In this group are patients with asthma, chronic obstructive pulmonary disease, and other chronic lung ailments. Aspirin, 0.3 to 0.6 Gm., may be given every four to six hours for the relief of general discomfort. Although nose drops or inhalers obtained commercially may help to relieve some of the nasal congestion, indiscriminate use of them is harmful. Many of them contain drugs that affect the body systemically, or they cause local irritation of the mucous membrane of the nose. Work is in progress to develop vaccines that would offer protection against at least some of the viruses that cause colds.

## INJURIES OF THE CHEST

**Fractured ribs** are a common form of injury to the chest. They may be caused by a hard fall or by a blow on the chest. Automobile accidents are a frequent cause. Although rib fractures are very painful, they usually are not serious unless injury to other structures results. For example, the sharp end of the broken bone may tear the lung or blood vessels. If the injury involves fractured ribs without other complications, the patient often is permitted to return home after treatment. The usual treatment includes supporting the chest with an Ace bandage or adhesive strapping to minimize the pain, and the administration of analgesics. Sometimes a regional nerve block is necessary to relieve the pain. If the patient is treated on an outpatient basis, it is important for him to understand that:

1. He should breathe as deeply as possible; his natural inclination will be to take very shallow breaths to minimize pain.
2. He should take the analgesic as ordered, in order to minimize the pain, to promote rest, and to permit more normal breathing.
3. He will probably breathe more comfortably in a sitting position than when he is lying flat.
4. If he experiences sudden, sharp chest pain or difficulty in breathing, he should call his physician at once.

**Blast injuries,** such as those which result from compression of the chest by an explosion, cause serious injury to the lungs by rupturing the alveoli. Death often results from hemorrhage and asphyxiation. The treatment includes the provision of complete rest and the administration of oxygen.

**Penetrating wounds** of the chest are also very serious. An open wound may permit air to enter the thoracic cavity, causing *pneumothorax*. If the wound is large, it may cause a sucking noise as air enters and leaves the chest cavity. Applying an airtight dressing is an important first-aid measure to prevent the entrance of more air into the chest cavity. Air also may enter the pleural space from an injury to the lung tissue. For example, the sharp end of a broken rib may tear the lung tissue, permitting air to enter the pleural space. Many chest injuries involve both pneumothorax and *hemothorax* (blood in the pleural space).

When medical aid has been obtained, the air and the blood are aspirated from the pleural space by thoracentesis. Sometimes a chest catheter is inserted and attached to closed drainage. Later it may be necessary to perform a thoracotomy to repair or to remove injured tissues. Foreign bodies that have entered the chest should be removed only by the physician. Their presence in the wound may prevent the entrance of air, and their removal without medical aid may cause pneumothorax.

## REFERENCES AND BIBLIOGRAPHY

AHLSTROM, P.: Raising sputum specimens, *Am. J. Nurs.* 65:109, March 1965.

AMBIAVAGAR, M., et al.: Intermittent positive pressure ventilation in the treatment of severe crushing injuries of the chest, *Thorax* 21:359, July 1966.

BEESON, P. B., and MCDERMOTT, W. (eds.): *Cecil-Loeb Textbook of Medicine,* ed. 13, Philadelphia, Saunders, 1971.

DAVENPORT, F. M.: Prospects for the control of influenza, *Am. J. Nurs.* 69:1908, September 1969.

GOODMAN, L. S., and GILMAN, A.: *The Pharmacological Basis of Therapeutics,* ed. 4, New York, Macmillan, 1970.

GRIFFIN, J. P., and CRAWFORD, Y. E.: *Mycoplasma pneumoniae* in primary atypical pneumonia, *JAMA* 193:95, 1965.

HARRISON, T. R., et al. (eds.): *Principles of Internal Medicine,* ed. 7, New York, McGraw-Hill, 1974.

HINSHAW, H. C.: *Diseases of the Chest,* ed. 3, Philadelphia, Saunders, 1969.

HUNTER, D.: *The Diseases of Occupations,* ed. 4, Boston, Little Brown, 1969.

HUSE, W.: The least you should know about chest injuries, *Consultant* 8:42, September 1968.

LAGERSON, J.: The cough—its effectiveness depends on you, *Resp. Care* 73:434, July–August 1973.

LANGMUIR, A. D., HENDERSON, D. A., and SERFLING, R. E.: The epidemiological basis for the control of influenza, *Am. J. Pub. Health* 54:563, 1964.

LEWIS, H. E.: *Pneumonia—A Symposium on the Occurrence, Etiology, Diagnosis, Prognosis and Treatment of Pneumonia,* New York, American Medical Publishing, 1910.

MARICI, F. N.: The flexible fiberoptic bronchoscope, *Am. J. Nurs.* 73:1776, October 1973.

MCHENRY, M., et al.: Hospital-acquired pneumonias, *Med. Clin. N. Am.* 58:565, May 1974.

MORROW, G. W., ANDERSON, H. A., and GERACI, J. E.: The diagnosis and management of acute infectious pneumonia, *Med. Clin. N. Am.* 48:829, 1964.

MOSTOW, S.: Pneumonias acquired outside the hospital, *Med. Clin. N. Am.* 58:555, May 1974.

SARTWELL, P. E.: *Maxcy-Rosenau Preventive Medicine and Public Health,* ed. 10, New York, Appleton-Century-Crofts, 1975.

SWEETWOOD, H.: Bedside assessment of respirations, *Nurs. '73* 73:50, September 1973.

TRAVER, G.: Assessment of the thorax and lungs, *Am. J. Nurs.* 73:466, March 1973.

———: The nurse's roles in clinical testing of lung function, *Nurs. Clin. N. Am.* 9:101, March 1974.

TURNER, H. C., JR.: The anatomy and physiology of normal respiration, *Nurs. Clin. N. Am.* 3:383, September 1968.

# The Patient with Chronic Respiratory Disease

CHAPTER **30**

Any change in the size, shape, or function of the body is apt to stir up anxiety. When the usual automatic function of breathing enters awareness and becomes a struggle, a vicious cycle often ensues. The dyspneic patient is anxious because he can't breathe normally, and the more anxious he becomes the more difficult it is for him to breathe. When the nurse skillfully facilitates the patient's breathing such as by providing oxygen therapy, teaching breathing exercises, supplying humidification, helping the patient to cough, giving drugs, explaining an intermittent positive pressure breathing (IPPB) treatment, or using therapeutic interpersonal skills in a counseling relationship, she reduces his anxiety and her own anxiety as well.

## EPIDEMIOLOGIC ASPECTS

The incidence of serious chronic respiratory disease is increasing. Between 1962 and 1966 the increase in death rate from respiratory diseases as a group was greater than that for any other cause of death. Although all factors leading to this increase are not understood, two important factors are cigarette smoking and air pollution.

The most current statistics from the U.S. Department of Health, Education and Welfare estimate that 10 million Americans are affected by emphysema, chronic bronchitis, and asthma. One half of the total 181,000 man-years lost due to lung disease is attributed to emphysema. The death rate between 1958 and 1967 has increased 80 per cent for chronic bronchitis and 172 per cent for emphysema. The mortality rate during the acute respiratory distress syndrome is approximately 40 per cent of 150,000 adult cases. A 6.3-billion-dollar-per-year cost factor is estimated for these diseases.

The nurse demonstrates her concern with the contributing factors to chronic respiratory disease by participating in screening and prevention programs and other educational efforts to eradicate or minimize personal air pollution (smoking) as well as environmental air pollution.

## ALLERGIC RHINITIS

**Definition.** Allergic rhinitis is a term used to describe the reaction of the nasal mucous membrane to various allergens commonly found in the environment. The allergic response is characterized by swelling of the nasal mucous membrane, sneezing, and increased nasal secretions. Other terms such as hay fever or rose fever have been used to describe the allergic response secondary to specific allergenic substances. Allergic rhinitis may occur seasonally and be specifically related to pollens or on a perennial (nonseasonal) basis where the reaction is due to other environmental antigens such as dust or feathers.

**Etiology and Pathology.** The condition is caused by allergy to a specific antigen (see Chapter 9 on allergy). When the symptoms are seasonal, allergic rhinitis usually is caused by pollens from weeds, trees, or grasses. In the United States three distinct allergic seasons can be described: in the early spring tree pollen is prevalent, the grasses pollinate in the early summer, and weed pollen, principally ragweed, in the early fall. Mold spores are another common cause of allergy and are most numerous in the summer. Perennial allergic rhinitis may be caused by dust, feathers, and animal danders. The allergen-antibody reaction occurring in the nose causes immediate release of histamine that affects the local tissues of the nose by causing edema, itching, and a watery discharge. The eyes and the pharynx also may be affected.

**Incidence.** Allergic rhinitis is common in persons who have an allergic background. Often there is a family history of allergy, although the specific allergen may vary among different members of the same family. Not uncommonly, persons with allergic rhinitis will exhibit other allergic symptoms such as eczema or asthma. It has been estimated that approximately 10 per cent of the population have a hereditary disposition to allergy. Allergic rhinitis can occur at any age. Although it tends to recur in the same individual for an indefinite period, its course over a lifetime is variable. One person may have the onset of symptoms at puberty; another may develop symptoms for the first time in middle life. It is possible for the symptoms to subside without apparent cause or to subside and be replaced by other allergic manifestations such as asthma.

**Symptoms.** The patient usually experiences itching of the nose, eyes, throat, and roof of the mouth. This is accompanied by sneezing, a profuse watery discharge, and tearing of the eyes. Marked swelling of the nasal mucosa may cause complete obstruction of the nasal airway, making breathing difficult. During a full-blown episode of allergic rhinitis a feeling of malaise accompanies the episode. Symptoms due to pollen are more severe on clear, windy days and during early morning and evening hours.

**Diagnosis.** Allergic rhinitis is diagnosed by securing a careful history concerning the events related to the attacks. Symptoms may appear only a few weeks at the same season each year, leading the physician to suspect pollen, or they may have their onset when a new pet or a new feather pillow is acquired. Skin testing is helpful in determining which substance is causing symptoms and, frequently, the patient may be allergic to several different substances. Physical examination and microscopic examination of nasal secretions are also helpful in diagnosis. The nasal mucous membrane usually appears edematous and pale. An abundance of eosinophils is found typically in nasal secretions.

**Treatment.** For the majority of patients, treatment centers around desensitization, antihistamines, and diminishing contact with the allergen.

Contact with pollen can be diminished by remaining indoors, away from open windows on windy days, and by using an air conditioner. Should the allergic rhinitis be of the perennial type and due to animal danders or feathers, the use of a foam rubber pillow and a new home for the pet may result in complete remission of symptoms. For those persons whose interest in the outdoors or love of a pet outweighs the desire for total relief, desensitization will often diminish the symptoms. Antihistamines frequently give temporary relief. ACTH and cortisone are not used except under life-threatening circumstances such as laryngeal edema. Symptoms are lessened by maintaining good general health.

**Course and Prognosis.** Allergic rhinitis is most severe when exposure to the allergen is at its height. Fatigue and emotional strain tend to aggravate the symptoms. Because the edema may block the drainage of the sinuses, sinusitis sometimes complicates allergic rhinitis. Obstruction of the eustachian tube results in middle ear infection, a common finding in allergic rhinitis. Should infection of the nasal mucosa intervene during an acute episode, nasal polyps may develop. These polyps further tend to obstruct the nasal air passages, resulting in difficult breathing. Some patients may go on to develop asthma as a consequence of their disease. Although allergic rhinitis is not a threat to life, it is a major cause of discomfort. Effective treatment, usually desensitization, cannot eradicate the condition, but can greatly add to the patient's comfort and decrease the likelihood of sequelae.

## BRONCHIAL ASTHMA

**Definition.** Asthma is derived from the Greek word for panting and is used clinically to mean shortness of breath. Many conditions which have as their main clinical feature shortness of breath have been referred to as asthma. Coal miners' asthma, cardiac asthma, and allergic asthma or bronchial asthma are but a few examples. Since "all that wheezes is not asthma," the diagnosis of asthma should be limited strictly to the allergic type. Other forms of shortness of breath would then be called congestive heart failure, not cardiac asthma, and anthracosilicosis, not coal miners' asthma. Bronchial asthma is typified by paroxysms of shortness of breath, wheezing, cough, and the production of thick tenacious sputum. The onset and the duration of the acute episode vary markedly between individuals. The duration may be brief, lasting less than one day, or extend into prolonged periods of several weeks.

**Symptoms and Pathophysiology.** The triad characteristic of the acute asthmatic state consists of spasm of the smooth muscle of the bronchi and larger bronchioles, swelling of the mucosal lining, and thick bronchiole secretions. The degree of airflow obstruction is directly related to the severity of the above mechanisms. In the presence of marked airway obstruction, the inspiratory effort to move air into the alveoli is great and may require the use of the accessory muscles of respiration. The increase in the negative intrapleural pressure re-

flects itself by marked retraction of the supraclavicular, suprasternal, and intercostal spaces. Once the air has entered the alveoli, air trapping takes place since the bronchioles and bronchi narrow during the expiratory effort. The attempt to move air across a narrowed orifice results, as in the playing of any reed instrument, in the production of musical tones. This is the classical wheezing that is heard on auscultation of the chest and which may be audible even without the stethoscope.

The patient is often aware of the wheezing and reports it as one of his symptoms. Every breath becomes an effort and during the acute episode the work of breathing is greatly increased. The patient may suffer from a sensation of suffocation. Frequently, a classical sitting position is assumed with the body leaning slightly forward and the arms at shoulder height. This position facilitates expansion of the chest as well as more effective excursions of the diaphragm. Because life depends on the power to breathe, fear accompanies the symptoms. Unfortunately, fear and anxiety tend to intensify the symptoms.

The effort to move trapped air within the alveoli is accompanied by a marked prolongation of the expiratory phase of respiration. Coughing commences with the onset of the attack, but is ineffective in the early stage and only as the attack begins to subside is the patient able to expectorate large quantities of thick, stringy mucus. Usually, the patient's skin is pale; however, if the attack is very severe, mild cyanosis of the lips and nailbeds may be noted. Perspiration is usually profuse during an acute attack. Following spontaneous or drug-induced remission of the episode, examination of the lungs commonly reveals normal findings; it is frequently impossible to diagnose bronchial asthma by physical signs without observation during the acute attack. Occasionally, however, the acute state can intensify and be resistant to all therapy, progressing into "status asthmaticus."

**Etiology.** Prominent among the causes of asthma are antigen-antibody reactions as seen in allergy, infection, and emotional stress. These factors vary in importance in different patients, but with careful observation all three components may be found active at the same time.

Bronchial asthma is classified according to etiology into three types. The first is extrinsic asthma, which occurs chiefly in response to allergens such as pollen, dust, spores, or animal danders.

Intrinsic asthma is the second type and has been associated with upper respiratory infection or emotional upsets. The third type is mixed (extrinsic and intrinsic).

**Incidence and Course.** Asthma may occur at any period in life. Approximately 50 per cent of all asthma occurs prior to the age of 10. A significant relationship between bronchiolitis in the first year of life and the development of bronchial asthma in early childhood has been noted. When the illness starts in early childhood, the symptoms tend to become less severe as the child grows older. Extrinsic asthma is the most common form noted in the childhood and young adult types. Intrinsic asthma due to recurrent infection frequently related to chronic sinusitis or chronic bronchitis is most frequently seen in patients beyond the age of 40. Asthma may be limited to occasional attacks and the patient is usually symptom free in the interim. Extensive long-term studies have been conducted that reveal normal pulmonary function studies during remission in asthma. For the average individual, other than the occasional acute episode, there is no progression of the disease, and pathologic examination of the lung during the asymptomatic state reveals normal structure. Occasionally, however, frequent and prolonged attacks, particularly those related to recurrent infection, tend to lead to chronic bronchitis and, if inadequately treated, may progress to emphysema.

### Treatment of Patients with Bronchial Asthma

Symptomatic treatment is given at the time of the attack and includes systemic hydration and humidification of inspired air, as well as bronchodilators and mild sedatives or tranquilizers. Oxygen therapy is prescribed on an individual basis and expectorants may be ordered in the convalescent stage.

If an acute attack is not treated promptly and aggressively, "status asthmaticus" can occur. "Status asthmaticus" is a medical emergency because it is potentially life-threatening. As many as 8,000 fatalities occur each year. Treatment includes intravenous fluids, aminophylline, oxygen therapy prescribed according to results of blood gas analysis, and corticosteroid therapy. Cardiac monitoring is done because blood gas and pH abnormalities can cause cardiac arrhythmias. Sympathomimetic drugs can cause arrhythmias also and are usually not given in status asthmaticus.

If hypoxemia cannot be controlled and/or if the $P_{CO_2}$ rises above 50 mm., ventilatory assistance is provided with an endotracheal tube (or rarely with a tracheostomy) and a volume-cycled respirator (Petty, 1971). (See Chapter 60 for care of the patient with respiratory insufficiency and failure.)

Long-term treatment for asthma is based on a patient education program so that the individual can recognize early symptoms and vary his therapeutic regime to bring an asthmatic attack under quick control. Hydration, drugs, and inhalation therapies form the major part of the long-term treatment plan. Treatment of allergy, infection, and emotional disorders may also be part of the therapy.

### Therapy, Nursing Assessment, and Nursing Intervention

**Acute Attack.** Observation is made of the patient's color, diaphoresis, cough, sputum, audible wheezing, rhonchi and rales on auscultation, rate and depth of respirations, use of accessory muscles, temperature, pulse and blood pressure, position assumed, degree of restlessness, anxiety level, and any subjective complaints. Included in the nursing history are specific questions regarding self-treatment of the current episode and usual long-term management.

It is wise not to ask the acutely distressed patient to answer any unnecessary questions, because respiratory difficulty is made worse by an attempt to talk. Only essential information is elicited. Answers might be provided by the person accompanying the patient and former charts can be requested.

The nurse must recognize that the patient's entire concern is with his breathing, and that nursing care must involve nothing that would increase the patient's difficulty in breathing. Measures should be taken to make the patient as comfortable as possible. Routine admission procedures may need to be modified temporarily. For instance, it would be most unwise to place an oral thermometer in the patient's mouth for an admission TPR, since the patient needs to breathe through his mouth. Recognizing that a sitting position makes breathing easier during an asthmatic attack, the nurse would not insist that the patient lie in bed, but she would assist the patient to assume the position that is most comfortable for him.

**Humidification** of the inspired air is extremely important in the therapy of the bronchospastic state. It has been shown that dehydration of the respiratory mucous membrane may by itself lead to attacks of bronchial asthma. The importance of adequate hydration of the mucous membrane can be demonstrated by the termination of an acute asthmatic attack by the simple infusion of a liter of 5 per cent dextrose and water over a two-hour period. During this time the patient is made comfortable in the emergency room and, other than mild sedation, no other therapy is given. Steam or cool vapor humidifiers have proved effective as therapeutic modalities. The value of the humidification becomes evident as the attack subsides and the patient brings up thick, stringy sputum. The liquefication of the secretions promotes more effective clearing of the airways and a rapid return to normal. Humidification is often inadequate in the hospital as well as in the home. The nurse can help by ordering a humidification device for the patient's hospital bedside or room at home, by teaching the family and patient the importance of humidification, and by finding out about commercially available humidifiers for the home, as well as possible sources of financial aid to obtain one of these for patients who find the cost prohibitive.

If plenty of fluids are provided within easy reach of the patient having an acute attack and the patient is encouraged and assisted as necessary to drink them, the increased fluid intake will help the secretions to become less tenacious and will help to replace fluids lost through perspiration. Tissues and a sputum cup should be provided, and the patient should be encouraged to expectorate the mucus.

The initiative for increasing fluid intake rests with the nurse. She must keep going to the patient and offering fluids. The exhausted dyspneic patient often cannot reach for and take them himself.

**Oxygen Therapy.** Oxygen is usually not necessary during an acute attack. This is because most patients with bronchial asthma are actively hyperventilating. The process of hyperventilation is necessary to compensate for the marked increase in airway resistance due to obstruction. Thus, the arterial oxyhemoglobin saturation is maintained at normal levels. Rarely, particularly after a long bout of asthma, some patients require oxygen which may be given by nasal catheter, mask, or intermittent positive pressure. Thus, the nurse does not automatically reach for oxygen for the patient in the acute asthmatic state unless cyanosis is present. Oxygen administration should be prescribed for each patient, as drugs are prescribed, and should

be monitored by arterial blood gas studies. The nurse can play a negative part in the patient's care if she does not insist on the physician prescribing what is to be done in the event of an acute attack and if oxygen is to be given, as well as ascertain what technique and liter flow are to be used, for example, $O_2$ per nasal cannula at 2 liters.

The nurse should explain to the patient the reason for the mask or the catheter. This explanation, as well as remaining with the patient initially until he gets adjusted to the oxygen and equipment, is necessary to allay the patient's anxiety and reduce the fear of suffocation.

**Bronchodilators.** The bronchodilator preparations are usually divided into two groups: the sympathomimetic drugs and the theophylline preparations. The sympathomimetic medications are those most commonly used in the treatment of acute bronchial asthma and include such drugs as epinephrine (Adrenalin), isoproterenol (Isuprel), and ephedrine. These agents tend to reduce bronchospasm by causing relaxation of the smooth muscle lining the bronchi and larger bronchioles.

*Epinephrine* is usually administered to the adult in a subcutaneous dose of 0.3 to 0.5 ml. of a 1:1,000 solution. The dose may be repeated at 30-minute intervals if required. The drug, however, is a potent stimulant and affects not only the smooth muscle of the tracheobronchial tree, but the entire body. The side effects of the drug are common and include tachycardia, palpitation, tremors, pallor, and anxiety. Frequently, a sedative medication such as phenobarbital may have to be administered concurrently in order to reduce the side effects. Since epinephrine is such a powerful and potentially dangerous drug, it is important for the nurse to recognize that it is given in very small, carefully measured doses. Preparations of epinephrine in oil providing prolonged action are also available. While the relief afforded the patient by epinephrine may be dramatic, repeated use of the drug may result in tachyphylaxis (rapid immunization to a toxic dose of a substance by previously injecting minute doses of the same substance) or epinephrine fastness during which time the drug is ineffective.

The nurse observes the patient for drug toxicity and side effects, and especially the anxiety and tachycardia and other cardiac arrhythmias possible with epinephrine. There is a need for sound nursing judgment when epinephrine is ordered on a p.r.n. basis. The physician should be consulted if the patient is becoming more anxious and tachycardic, or has chest pain, trembling, nervousness, insomnia, or other systemic effects of epinephrine. Patients vary greatly in their response to this drug and need close observation. When the nurse is in doubt about a further dose, the physician should be consulted.

*Epinephrine* and *isoproterenol* are extremely effective bronchodilators when given by nebulizer in solutions of 1:100 and 1:200. The advantage of delivering the bronchodilator by nebulizer directly into the lung is that the effect is maximal on the bronchial musculature and although side effects do occur, they are limited as compared with the subcutaneous injection. Since the effectiveness of the nebulized bronchodilator is dependent on the dose and proper delivery of the drug into the lung, specific instructions must be given to the patient. The usual dose is 0.5 ml., of the drug placed in the nebulizer reservoir. This should not be diluted by the addition of water or any other agent. It has been shown that the effectiveness of the nebulized bronchodilator is dependent solely on its concentration. Therefore, if the 0.5 ml. of drug is diluted with 2 ml. of saline, the overall effectiveness of the therapy will be one-fifth of that expected. It is important that the nurse understand the rationale of drug administration. Otherwise she may unwittingly reduce the effectiveness of a drug by carrying out an institutional routine (such as unwarranted dilution of a drug) without question. If the nurse receives an order to dilute the drug, she should discuss this with the physician.

When a hand-bulb nebulizer is used, it will take approximately 15 minutes to deliver the bronchodilator drug. In order to simplify delivery, many drug companies prepare the bronchodilator in pressurized aerosol form. The pressurized container is small and can be carried everywhere with the patient. The major advantage of the aerosol is the elimination of the fatigue factor that frequently occurs in the older patient attempting to use the hand-bulb nebulizer. The pressurized aerosol form also eliminates the microbiologic hazard associated with the use of a nebulizer. When inhalation therapy equipment is used, it is an urgent nursing concern that the patient have his own nebulization equipment, that it be cleaned thoroughly between use, disinfected daily, and sterilized between patients. Otherwise, bacterial contamination of the patient's lungs with resultant infection can occur.

Hospital policy and surveillance committees should reflect this concern.

The usual dose of the aerosol is one or two sprays delivered to the tracheobronchial tree every four hours. The tip of the nebulizer, whether hand-bulb or aerosol type, should be placed into the open mouth. The nurse instructs the patient not to close his lips around the nebulizer. Then, while breathing in, the patient should squeeze the bulb or press on the aerosol can. In this manner, the nebulized material will be carried with the airstream into the trachea, bronchi, and bronchioles. If not so instructed, many patients will close their mouth around the mouthpiece and while breathing through their nose, deliver the drug. This results in deposition of the bronchodilator in the oral cavity and absorption by the mucosa of the mouth. The principal effect will then be on the cardiovascular system with very little relief of respiratory symptoms. Because the pressurized aerosol form is so readily available, overmedication can become a problem. Obviously, these agents must be used with great caution in individuals who have cardiac disease.

The nurse explains to the patient and family the purpose of the drug, when and how it should be used, and why it should not be overused. They should be aware of the harmful, systemic side effects of the drugs and when to report these to the physician. The physician should also be informed when the usual dose of the aerosol seems to be ineffective. The community health nurse can give overall health supervision and specific instruction in the use of drugs at home to the patient. Especially when the patient is elderly or has other handicaps, the family needs both instruction and support to assist him.

*Ephedrine* acts similarly to epinephrine, but its effects are not as strong. Its principal usefulness is that it can be given orally in doses of 25 mg., repeated every four hours as needed. Sedatives may be required to counteract unpleasant side effects such as nervousness, trembling, and insomnia.

*Aminophylline* is the most effective of all the theophylline derivatives in reducing bronchospasm. It is most useful when administered intravenously in a dose of 0.25 to 0.5 Gm. The physician injects the drug slowly over a period of approximately 10 minutes in order to avoid a sudden drop in blood pressure, with dizziness, faintness, palpitation, and headache. If the drug is given rapidly, death may ensue. To avoid the risk of complications, aminophylline is often given as a small infusion consisting of 100 ml. of normal saline into which the dose of medication has been added. This may be given over a period of one-half hour. The risk of hypotension is minimized, but the patient should be carefully observed and his blood pressure checked frequently. For prolonged in-hospital use, the dose of aminophylline may be given over an eight-hour period in 500 ml. to 1,000 ml. of intravenous fluid. The use of aminophylline as a rectal suppository is valuable and effective. Most patients develop anorectal irritation, however, if the dose exceeds 0.5 Gm. every 12 hours. The nurse observes whether and to what extent symptoms are relieved and whether there is anorectal irritation. While the oral administration of theophylline and its derivatives would be the route of choice, to the present date, the oral preparations have not been effective.

**Expectorants.** These are not effective in the therapy of acute bronchial asthma. They may be used during the postacute stage to raise the thick respiratory secretions that are further obstructing respiration. Saturated solution of potassium iodide (SSKI), 10 drops, diluted in milk or water, frequently is given several times daily. Many patients, after several weeks of therapy, develop an allergic reaction to the iodine. The patient is observed for evidence of iodine reaction, which is frequently characterized by a skin rash, and this is reported to the physician. Gastric irritation and painful swelling of the parotid gland sometimes develop but are less likely to occur if the patient receives plenty of fluids.

Terpin hydrate, though not as effective as SSKI, may prove useful in some patients. Expectorants in general, however, are not used as a substitute for active inhalation forms of humidification. When ordered with other oral medications, expectorants should be given last instead of being followed by pills and the ingestion of water, so as not to shorten their desirable local effect on the pharyngeal mucosa.

**Sedatives and Tranquilizers.** These drugs are frequently used to control anxiety during the acute attack. However, care must be taken to avoid depression of respiration and the cough reflex. The anxiety that accompanies the acute attack is related to the patient's inability to breathe. To sedate the patient simply to relieve anxiety prior to relieving the respiratory distress may intensify the symptoms and, if the respiratory center is sufficiently depressed, death may occur. Narcotics, because of their respiratory depressant effects, are not used unless preparations have been made for mechanical support of respiration.

There is a great need for nursing judgment in the carrying out of p.r.n. orders for sedatives and tranquilizers for the dyspneic, asthmatic patient. The nurse should be aware that there can be a very human tendency to want to calm the patient down for one's own benefit and comfort, or out of kindness for the patient, and thus administer sedation unnecessarily. The nurse who works with dyspneic patients needs to develop an awareness of her own reactions to the patient's condition. If severe dyspnea makes her fearful, she can readily increase the patient's anxiety.

**Antibiotics.** If the acute asthmatic state is complicated by an infection, the physician orders antibiotics. Because most infections of this type are gram-positive, penicillin or one of the penicillin derivatives is the drug of choice. Many allergists believe that bronchial asthma is always complicated by infection and prescribe antibiotic therapy even in the absence of clinical signs and symptoms of infection.

**Steroids** are not generally used in the treatment of the patient with uncomplicated bronchial asthma. Medical opinion holds that bronchodilators, when used promptly, can be as effective as steroids but without the serious side effects. Should the disease progress, the physician may order steroids by the oral route. During status asthmaticus intravenous steroids in massive doses greater than 3 Gm. of hydrocortisone daily in divided doses have been effective and life-saving.

## Emotional Support

Seeing a patient in extreme respiratory distress may be a frightening experience for the nurse and it might be necessary for her to have help and support with her own responses if she is to be effective with dyspneic patients.

The patient is very anxious and looks to those who care for him for support and reassurance. Since it is the nurse who spends the greatest amount of time with the hospitalized patient, a large measure of this support and this reassurance become her responsibility.

Although the extreme dyspnea, the wheezing, and the struggle for breath make it appear that the patient will not survive, most patients who have acute asthmatic attacks do recover from them. Most attacks are temporary and short; thus the nurse on the basis of this understanding may help the patient to feel that his attack will subside. Through her understanding that the spasm of the patient's bronchi is causing marked interference with a vital function, the nurse will avoid giving glib and superficial reassurance. She will recognize that, although emotional factors may precipitate attacks in some patients, the patient who is having an attack is very ill, regardless of what may have caused the symptoms. Such attitudes as "It's all in his mind—he could snap out of it if he wanted to," betray a gross misunderstanding, and they seriously interfere with the nurse's ability to care for patients with asthma.

When asthmatic attacks are very prolonged or recur in rapid succession (status asthmaticus), the patient often fears that each breath will be his last. He may describe a feeling of suffocation or of drowning. Although most patients do not die during an asthmatic attack, nevertheless it is true that death sometimes occurs.

Because she recognizes the patient's anxiety during the attack, the nurse by her manner and her actions must convey to the patient that she is there to help him. There are many ways in which the nurse can demonstrate this:

- **Simply staying with the patient, if possible.**
- **Indicating by words and actions that his condition does not unduly alarm those caring for him.**
- **Being technically skilled so that her actions demonstrate self-confidence.**
- **Recognizing that improving the patient's breathing pattern can reduce his anxiety. Respiratory nursing clinical specialists may assist the patient to do breathing exercises during an attack. As the patient learns more control of his breathing, his sense of helplessness diminishes (Moody, 1974).**
- **Providing him with a way to signal for help when she cannot stay with him, answering calls promptly, and observing him when he does not call.**
- **Doing nothing to indicate within the patient's hearing that his attack is unusually severe or not responding to treatment.**
- **Checking with the physician if there is doubt regarding administration of sedatives for securing mental and physical rest so that anxiety resulting from the nurse's indecision is not transferred to the patient.**
- **Replacing the patient's moist nightgown and his bed linen with dry ones.**

- **Listening to the patient's concerns when he is able to express them and recognizing that all people have reasons to be angry and afraid. The skilled nurse leaves the door open for the expression of these emotions. She is a listener par excellence.**

It is not unusual for the hospitalized patient with asthma to signal the nurse repeatedly, often for apparently insignificant requests. Frequent use of the call bell is particularly likely at night or when the patient has had a recent attack and usually indicates that the patient is anxious and wants someone to stay with him. It is often true that the nurse has many patients to care for and cannot spend as much time with the patient as might be desirable. Regardless of how much time the nurse has, she can spend it more effectively by accurately assessing the situation and devoting her care to what the patient really seems to need. Spending 10 to 15 minutes with the patient, allowing him to express some of his fears and to ask questions concerning his condition may require no more time than answering the call light a dozen times to adjust the window, and it is often much more effective in helping the patient to rest. In his requests for attention the nurse can recognize the patient's anxiety about being alone. By understanding what the patient is really saying, the nurse can serve him better. These fine nuances of understanding make nursing an art.

The community health nurse can use these same principles to help the family be less frightened and more supportive of the patient at home.

**Environment.** The asthmatic patient's environment should be as free as possible of factors which contribute to respiratory infection. Nurses or visitors with upper respiratory infection should avoid contact with the patient in the home or hospital. When family or friends express a desire to send gifts to the patient, the nurse should tactfully suggest something other than flowers. The patient's living quarters should be damp-dusted daily and he should be protected from exposure to allergens that may have set off his attacks or that may continue to perpetuate them. Thorough cleanliness of all inhalation therapy equipment is urgent.

Since most patients with asthma already feel closed in, it is important to avoid intensifying this sensation by drawing curtains around the hospital bed or closing the doors and the windows in the patient's room.

In the hospital it would be wise to leave a dim light in the patient's room at night and to encourage him to signal the nurse whenever it is necessary.

**Chest Physical Therapy.** After the acute distress subsides, postural drainage along with vibration and percussion within the patient's tolerance may be given. After bronchodilator therapy, these maneuvers help the patient bring up the thick sputum which is then measured and observed for color and viscosity. Deep breathing and effective coughing maneuvers are also used on a regular schedule to clear the airways. The effectiveness of therapy is monitored by chest auscultation.

## Long-Term Care

As the patient's condition improves, the nurse may assist with and help the patient to understand various diagnostic procedures such as pulmonary function studies and skin testing. If it is the patient's first asthmatic attack, helping with his instruction concerning the attack itself, the treatment, and the preventive measures will be an important part of the nursing care. The role of infection, allergy, and the social and the emotional factors that may have played a part will be evaluated.

Long-term measures in the care of the patient with asthma are very important in preventing future attacks and lessening the likelihood of complications, such as chronic emphysema and cor pulmonale (pulmonary heart failure). Efforts to determine the cause of the attacks and to educate the patient to prevent recurrences are joint tasks of physicians and nurses.

If the patient's history and his diagnostic tests indicate that allergy is an important causative factor, treatment by the avoidance of the allergen, by desensitization, or by antihistamines may be used.

Common inhalants that may cause asthma are dust, feathers, pollens, and animal danders. It is important to keep the patient's environment as free as possible from substances to which he is allergic. Careful damp-dusting of his room daily helps to keep dust at a minimum. The use of draperies, rugs, and upholstered furniture is unwise, since they can be cleaned less readily. Careful attention should be given to the removal of dust from less obvious places, such as the mattress and the rungs of the bed and the chairs. Air conditioners are very helpful in eliminating pollen as well as in controlling temperature and humidity. Feathers and down frequently cause symptoms. Pillows made of synthetic fibers or foam rubber are preferable. Flowers also may aggravate the symptoms.

The control of infection plays a major role in the care of patients with asthma. Frequently, the patients are susceptible to respiratory infections, and these infections tend, as the patients say, "to go to the chest." Patients should avoid factors that predispose to respiratory infections, such as exposure, fatigue, personal air pollution (smoking), and contact with persons who have colds.

Respiratory infections, when they do occur, should be treated promptly. Antibiotics are often necessary. Sometimes patients who acquire repeated respiratory infections with serious consequences are given daily prophylactic doses of antibiotics, particularly during the winter.

Emotional stress is often a causative factor in asthmatic attacks. Adjustments in home or job situations may be helpful in relieving stress.

If the patient's attacks seem closely related to emotional factors, individual or group psychotherapy by a clinical nursing specialist or other therapist may help the patient to understand and to handle his emotional reactions in a more positive way.

The maintenance of good general health is important in reducing the frequency of attacks and in helping the patient to achieve the maximum benefit from his treatment. Rest, optimum diet, and a balance of work and recreation are important.

Specific components of the patient education program are incorporated into a teaching plan developed by the physician and nurse and based on an individual cognitive, affective, and psychomotor assessment, and may include:

- **Knowledge of the drugs prescribed including purpose, dosage, time of administration, and side effects.**
- **The correct usage and dose of the nebulizer or metered-dose device for bronchodilator inhalation.**
- **Precipitating factors and how to avoid them.**
- **Action to be taken when an episode begins.**
  **Selected patients may be taught to inject epinephrine subcutaneously at home if oral drugs, inhalation therapy, or rectal aminophylline do not successfully abort an attack. A usual dose is 0.3 ml. of 1:1,000 epinephrine, but patients may vary their regimen with appropriate instruction and ongoing medical supervision. Maximal dose and frequency of dose are taught as well as a plan for the next phase if treatment with epinephrine is unsuccessful.**
- **A plan for obtaining medical advice and further care when necessary. (See also Chapter 9 for nursing care of the patient with allergy and asthma.)**

## ACUTE BRONCHITIS

Acute bronchitis is a disease characterized by inflammation of the mucous membranes lining the major bronchi and their branches. Frequently, the inflammatory process also involves the trachea, and is then referred to as tracheobronchitis. The most common cause of acute bronchitis is viral infection. Frequently starting as an upper respiratory infection (URI), the inflammatory process extends into the tracheobronchial tree, with direct involvement of the mucous linings. This involvement takes the form of inflammatory change with the production of increased amounts of mucus by the secretory cells of the mucosa. Usually the disease is self-limiting, lasting approximately three to four days, with symptoms that initially include a dry, nonproductive cough that later becomes productive of a mucopurulent sputum, fever, and malaise. It is treated simply by bed rest, salicylates, and a light, nourishing diet with plenty of liquids. Humidifiers are used, because dry air aggravates the cough. Occasionally, secondary bacterial invasion takes place and the previously mild infection may then become a serious bacterial infection with the production of a thick purulent sputum and a cough that may persist for several weeks. While antibiotics are not generally ordered for the treatment of acute bronchitis of viral etiology, secondary invasion of the tracheobronchial tree is an indication for culturing the sputum and starting antibiotic therapy. A period of two to three days will be required prior to the sputum culture report. During this time period, a broad-spectrum antibiotic such as tetracycline may be ordered. The antibiotic medication may be changed later depending on the sputum culture report. Acute bronchitis may be complicated by laryngitis with hoarseness and occasionally loss of voice, and sinusitis. These secondary areas of infection will usually subside as the bronchitis subsides.

Although acute bronchitis is most often related to an infectious process, chemical irritation due to noxious fumes (sulfur dioxide, nitrogen dioxide, smoke, and other air pollutants) can also cause acute bronchitis. The disease may be further complicated by the development of bronchial asthma. Nursing care of the patient with acute bronchitis is similar to that in any acute respiratory infection with emphasis on rest and prevention of the secondary infection, as well as on preventing the spread of infection to others.

## CHRONIC OBSTRUCTIVE PULMONARY DISEASE (COPD) OR CHRONIC AIRWAY OBSTRUCTION

The term "pulmonary emphysema" has been used for many years to define the *clinical* triad characterized by marked shortness of breath with persistent breathlessness even at rest, a chronic cough productive of large quantities of mucoid sputum that may be purulent, and intermittent episodes of expiratory wheezing. This triad of symptoms is nonspecific and can be seen in patients suffering with bronchial asthma as well as chronic bronchitis.

Currently, any patient presenting the above symptoms is diagnosed as having chronic obstructive pulmonary disease (COPD). This title was selected in order to provide a more suitable term for the clinical labeling of this group of patients. Chronic obstructive pulmonary disease can be subdivided into two groups: (1) chronic bronchitis, and (2) generalized obstructive lung disease. The latter is further subdivided into reversible obstructive lung disease, such as asthma, and irreversible or persistent obstructive pulmonary disease of the type pathologically described as pulmonary emphysema. Since the symptoms in asthma, chronic bronchitis, and other obstructive disease may all be present concurrently, the term COPD can encompass the symptoms of all three disease states. Further subdivision is unnecessary for the treatment of the disease, and a definitive diagnosis must often await thorough morphologic examination.

### Chronic Bronchitis

Chronic bronchitis is the disease characterized by the hypersecretion of mucus by the bronchial glands as well as a chronic or a recurrent respiratory infection. It is a serious health problem with symptoms that develop gradually and go untreated for many years until the disease is well established. A chronic cough, often attributed to smoking, may persist and gradually grow worse. The cough is frequently disregarded and early treatment delayed.

An important nursing role, particularly for the community health nurse and occupational health nurse, is to act as a case finder and urge early treatment to prevent chronic bronchitis from advancing. The seemingly healthy patient who expends a large amount of energy every morning on a coughing spell and the mobilization of secretions is apt to forget about his condition once his morning routine is completed. It is this type of patient who can benefit from early nursing referral for treatment.

**Etiology and Incidence.** Multiple factors in the causation of chronic bronchitis have been recorded. The development of the disease may be insidious or may follow a long history of bronchial asthma or an acute respiratory infection, such as influenza or pneumonia. Air pollution is a major cause of chronic bronchitis, as evidenced by the extremely high incidence of disease in Great Britain.

The role of cigarette smoking cannot be overemphasized. In one study of 150 patients with chronic obstructive pulmonary disease, it was found that 143 were cigarette smokers (Mitchell et al., 1964). In fact, the advanced stages of chronic bronchitis are usually never seen except in smokers. Smoking characteristically causes hypertrophy of the mucous glands and hypersecretion. The mucosal surface of the tracheobronchial tree is lined by uncountable numbers of small hairs called cilia. These cilia play a significant role in clearing the air passages of the lung of mucus and secretions. Their function is specifically to propel excess secretions to the trachea, where a cough or other method of clearing the throat will rid the body of this material. Many air pollutants, such as sulfur dioxide and smoke, have been shown to significantly alter cilial activity with retention of secretions the end result. These secretions form plugs within the smaller bronchi and are excellent culture media. Infection readily ensues. A chronic infection of the ariway can then result in further increases in mucus secretion and ultimately areas of focal necrosis and fibrosis.

Those individuals who are exposed to large amounts of irritating dusts and chemicals are very likely to develop chronic respiratory diseases such as bronchitis. For instance, coal miners are especially prone to develop chronic bronchitis. Although the disease may occur at any age, chronic bronchitis is most frequently seen in middle age, and it is usually the result of many years of untreated, low-grade bronchitis.

**Ecologic Aspects.** The role of the nurse with regard to chronic respiratory disease does not end with her tour of duty. She is an important health resource as an individual, or as a member of organized nursing or community groups in efforts to decrease air pollution. The occupational health nurse needs to work closely with safety engineers in planning and implementing programs to employ safety devices such as protective masks in the prevention of chronic pulmonary disease in workers in high-risk industries. Early detection through regular physical examination and referral for job relocation if necessary are additional ways of providing nursing assistance.

**Symptoms.** A cough is usually the earliest symptom, and is accompanied by the expectoration of thick, white, stringy mucus that is usually attributed to cigarette smoking. The cough is ordinarily most marked on arising in the morning and just prior to going to bed. Acute respiratory infections are frequent during the winter months and all colds tend to "settle in the chest" and may persist for several weeks or more. As the disease progresses, the sputum may become purulent, copious, and occasionally streaked with blood after a severe paroxysm of coughing. Although the patient may have a sensation of heaviness in the chest, dyspnea is usually not a symptom of uncomplicated chronic bronchitis. In fact, pulmonary function tests are frequently normal. The general health is usually maintained and the physical examination may be remarkably normal.

**Diagnosis.** The patient's history is very important and the diagnosis usually can be made by evaluation of the duration of symptoms, circumstances under which they started, type of employment, previous respiratory diseases, and smoking history. Physical examination, x-ray films of the chest, fluoroscopy, and pulmonary function tests may all be normal. Examination of the sputum, particularly the volume expectorated per day, may be helpful in assessing the severity of the disease. Sputum culture may be of therapeutic interest. All the above studies must be obtained in order to exclude other diseases such as bronchogenic carcinoma, bronchiectasis, tuberculosis, and other diseases where cough is a predominant feature.

## Treatment

Management of patients with chronic bronchitis requires long-term planning and attention to detail. Patients may be disappointed to learn that there is no miracle drug that can wipe out chronic bronchitis. If chronic infection is present, all treatment is usually palliative in nature. However, careful treatment can do much to minimize symptoms and prevent complications.

In general, the essence of treatment is directed toward the prevention of recurrent irritation of the bronchial mucosa either by infection or chemical agents. The smoking of tobacco in any form should be immediately discontinued as it is virtually impossible to prevent exacerbation and progression of the disease during active smoking. The patient must be helped to realize that even one cigarette may cause marked irritation of the mucosa and can by itself lead to bronchospasm.

Since most patients who smoke become quite anxious at the prospects of discontinuing smoking, the physician may prescribe tranquilizers to reduce tension and the craving for tobacco during the withdrawal period. One study suggests that smoking behavior is conditioned directly by social and psychological factors, and that the psychological factors are importantly influenced by conditions in the family and other social groups during childhood and adolescence. Thus, efforts of education and persuasion to assist the patient to stop smoking must take into account the possible complexities of its roots (Srole, 1968). The American Heart Association, the American Cancer Society, and other groups sponsor programs and offer literature for the support and instruction of people in their efforts to become nonsmokers. (See Chapter 11 for further discussion of methods of helping patients to stop smoking.) With only slight readjustment in the diet, most individuals do not gain any additional weight following cessation of smoking, and the anxiety that accompanies the discontinuation of tobacco usually diminishes with substitution of other appropriate outlets for tension relief, such as knitting or hobbies which involve small but repetitive motor actions.

If the patient's work involves exposure to dust and chemical irritants, a change of occupation may be necessary. It is impossible to escape from the air pollution of our urban areas. However, in the patient's home air conditioning with filtration of incoming air often can result in marked reduction of sputum production and cough. The maintenance of optimal general health and the avoidance of other respiratory infections are very important in maintaining the patient's resistance. A diet that contains adequate protein, vitamins, and other nutrients is important as well as adequate rest and the avoidance of emotional strain. There is usually no need for any change of climate and, although some individuals may derive relief from living in a warm, dry climate, it is better that the patient live in an area where the relative humidity is maintained at a moderate level so as to assist in the liquefication of secretions and prevention of mucus plugs. In fact, the maintenance of a high relative humidity between 40 and 50 per cent in the home is considered a prerequisite for good treatment, especially in the winter months.

The specific therapy is directed toward the prevention of recurrent infection and the suppression of chronic infection. In the late stages of chronic bronchitis the infection is usually persistent and antibiotic therapy may become a lifelong therapeutic measure. It has been shown that it is impossible, once chronic infection has set in, ever to eradicate the bacteria from the lung. The suppression of infection is therefore of paramount importance and can be done by several techniques. The preferred method is to give antibiotics, usually tetracycline, on any two consecutive days of the week at a dose level of 250 mg. four times daily. Most men who are employed prefer to have their medication on Saturday and Sunday to avoid the embarrassment of carrying pills to work. This intermittent therapy has proved highly successful because effective suppression of the bacterial growth occurs on the two days of therapy, followed by a period of five days of slow bacterial growth, and then resuppression. In this manner the level of infection is always held at a low point and an acute exacerbation of the disease does not occur unless an overwhelming bacterial infection takes place. Should this occur, the antibiotic dosage may be increased to a daily program or a different antibiotic may be given as treatment for the acute infection. The occupational health nurse can exert her influence in the provision of relief breaks for such employees as assembly-line workers who must pause to take a scheduled medication.

Bronchospasm can be a feature of chronic bronchitis and, as in patients with bronchial asthma, drugs such as ephedrine, aminophylline, and epinephrine may be helpful in reducing the spasm. Expectorants such as potassium iodide are helpful in liquefying secretions and clearing the respiratory passages of mucus. Postural drainage, particularly in the morning, is usually very effective in clearing the respiratory tree of mucus (Fig. 30-1).

**Course and Prognosis.** With adequate control many patients can be maintained for the rest of their lives without further progression of the illness. The aim of the treatment is to arrest the disease and to prevent the further destruction of tissue.

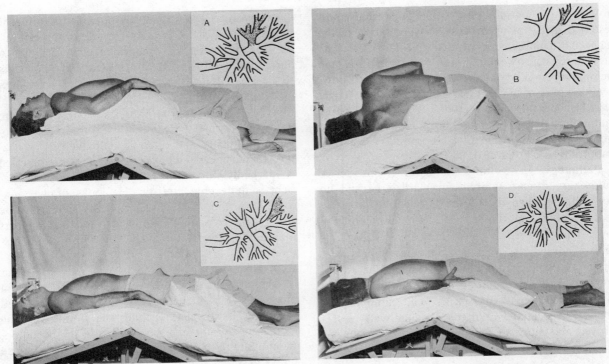

**Figure 30-1.** (A) Postural drainage of the right middle lobe of the lung. (B) Postural drainage of the lateral basal segment of the right lower lobe. The patient is placed on the unaffected side. (C) Postural drainage of the anterior basal segment of the right lung and the anterior and medial basal segments of the left lung. (D) Drainage of the posterior segments of the right or left lower lobe bronchi. (Ayers, S. M., and Giannelli, S.: *Care of the Critically Ill*, New York, Appleton-Century-Crofts)

Although the disease commences with the hypertrophy in the mucous glands in the bronchi, it frequently progresses to chronic inflammatory changes with fibrosis and structural damage. If adequate treatment is not requested or given, chronic bronchitis may progress into a more severe form of chronic obstructive pulmonary disease with progressive destruction of the alveolar linings of the lung and the capillary bed.

## Pulmonary Emphysema

The term "emphysema" refers to a specific irreversible morphologic change in the lung that is characterized by overdistention of the alveolar sacs, rupture of the alveolar walls, and the destruction of the alveolar capillary bed.

**Etiology.** The exact cause of irreversible chronic obstructive pulmonary disease (emphysema) is unknown. The frequent association of chronic bronchitis with the development of severe COPD suggests more than a casual relationship. Those factors previously listed in the section on chronic bronchitis are of obvious importance. These include smoking, respiratory infection, air pollution, and allergy. Although a direct relationship between cigarette smoking and chronic obstructive pulmonary disease has not been established, over 90 per cent of all individuals with this disease are heavy smokers. The constant irritation of the tracheobronchial tree and the suppression of normal cilial function in the respiratory airways predisposes the respiratory tract to chronic infection. The repeated pulmonary infection can result in alteration of lung structure and destruction of pulmonary tissue. Inner pollutants such as nitrogen dioxide and sulfur dioxide result in chronic irritation of the tracheobronchial linings and may cause permanent changes. Industrial exposure to coal dust, asbestos, cotton fibers, and molds and fungi has resulted in COPD. Hereditary factors have also been incriminated in the causation of COPD. The disease is more prevalent and of greater morbidity and mortality in men than in women. Aging may play a role. A normal manifestation of the aging process is overaeration of the lung and enlargement of the alveolar sacs. The destruction of alveolar walls and change in the pulmonary capillary bed has not been noted, however, as part of the aging process. The previously discussed nursing care regarding early detection of pulmonary disease and measures to help decrease smoking and environmental air pollution are very important in COPD also.

**Pathology.** The lungs in chronic obstructive pulmonary disease (emphysema) are large and do not collapse when the thorax is opened. Large air sacs or bullae may be seen over the surface of the lung. The cut surface of the lung reveals large air spaces everywhere, giving a moth-eaten appearance. On microscopic examination, the walls of the alveoli are broken down, resulting in one large sac rather than multiple small air spaces. The capillary bed previously located within the alveolar walls is destroyed and much of the tissue replaced by fibrous scarring as illustrated in Figure 30-2.

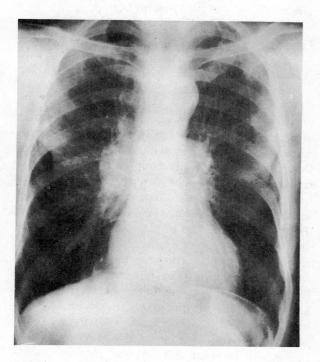

**Figure 30-2.** Typical chest x-ray of a patient with chronic obstructive pulmonary disease (COPD). Observe the widened interspaces, flattened diaphragms, and engorged pulmonary arteries (suggestive of cor pulmonale). (Department of Radiology, Methodist Hospital of Brooklyn)

**Symptoms.** Exertional dyspnea is usually the first symptom of COPD. As the disease progresses, the breathlessness may continue even at rest. A chronic cough is invariably present and is productive of mucopurulent sputum. Inspiration is difficult because of the rigid chest cage, and the patient must use the accessory muscles of respiration to maintain normal ventilation. Expiration is prolonged, difficult, and often accompanied by wheezing. In advanced emphysema, respiratory function is markedly impaired. The appearance of the patient is quite characteristic. He looks drawn, anxious, pale, and speaks in short, jerky sentences. He sits up, often leaning slightly forward, and appears markedly dyspneic. Often the veins in his neck distend during expiration.

In advanced COPD, the patient may have loss of memory, drowsiness, confusion, and loss of judgment. These changes are due to the marked reduction in oxygen reaching the brain, and the increased amount of carbon dioxide in the blood. If untreated, the level of carbon dioxide in the blood may reach toxic levels, resulting in lethargy, stupor, and finally coma. This is called carbon dioxide narcosis. (See Chapter 60 for care of the patient in ventilatory insufficiency and failure.)

Approximately 30 per cent of all patients suffering with chronic obstructive pulmonary disease will develop a peptic ulcer at some time during the course of the illness. When this occurs, the patient often complains of epigastric pain, abdominal soreness, and may have frank episodes of hematemesis. Because of the abdominal pain, the appetite may be significantly reduced and marked weight loss may ensue. The nurse who cares for patients with COPD should be alert to symptoms of peptic ulcer and report early symptoms so that treatment can be instituted before serious complications occur.

**Diagnosis.** A thorough history will usually reveal many of the symptoms of chronic obstructive pulmonary disease. The disease can be diagnosed on the basis of the history alone. Physical examination may reveal classical signs that can be confirmed on x-ray films and fluoroscopy. Tests of pulmonary function may indicate characteristic changes. The *maximum breathing capacity* (a measure of the greatest amount of air that the patient can move in and out of the lungs with maximal effort) is always reduced. This test reflects the degree of obstructive change that is present in the airways. While the *vital capacity* (the maximum amount of air that can be expelled following a maximal inspiration) may be normal, the *timed vital capacity* or the percentage of the vital capacity that the patient expels in the first, second, and third seconds will invariably be reduced. The normal values for the timed vital capacity are 83, 94, and 97 per cent in the first, second, and third seconds, respectively. Other measures, such as the *forced midexpiratory flow rate* and the *forced expiratory flow rate,* are extremely sensitive as screening tests and can be performed in the physician's office or in the clinic with very simple equipment. *Residual volume* (the volume of air remaining in the lungs at the end of maximal expiration) is always increased.

Blood gas studies, including the measurement of arterial pH, $Po_2$ (partial pressure of oxygen), $Pco_2$ (partial pressure of carbon dioxide), plasma bicarbonate concentration ($HCO_3^-$), and arterial oxyhemoglobin saturation, are useful in assessing the state of blood gas exchange across the lung. The more severe the chronic obstructive pulmonary disease, the higher will be the $Pco_2$ and the lower the $Po_2$ and arterial oxyhemoglobin saturation. Other tests such as the direct measurement of lung compliance (distensibility) and airway resistance are useful but require expensive equipment and highly trained personnel for their performance.

Prevention, Treatment, and Control

The prevention of COPD is directly related to the cessation of cigarette smoking as well as more effective public health measures against air pollution. Prompt and effective treatment of conditions that predispose to pulmonary obstructive disease is essential. The education of the public in the necessity for medical evaluation of minor respiratory symptoms, such as "morning cough" or "smoker's cough," is important in breaking the chain of events leading to emphysema.

Symptomatic treatment is similar to that in chronic bronchitis. Efforts to increase pulmonary ventilation by reducing bronchospasm include the use of such medications as epinephrine, ephedrine, and aminophylline. Unfortunately, as patients develop advanced states of the disease, the bronchospastic component may be negligible and not responsive to bronchodilator therapy. The use of expectorants, humidity control, and a program of bronchial hygiene including postural drainage is necessary in order to remove the excess respiratory secretions.

The control of infection is important. This may be achieved by measures to increase the individual's resistance, by the avoidance of contact with those suffering with respiratory infection, and by the use of antibiotics. The lung in COPD is chronically infected. Attempts to eradicate the infection by continuous long-term antibiotic therapy in single or multiple drug combinations are useless. As described in the section on chronic bronchitis, some physicians prefer to give antibiotics on only two consecutive days of the week for suppression of the infection. Because of its broad spectrum nature, tetracycline has been found to be extremely effective for chronic therapy at a dose level of 250 mg. four times daily. During acute exacerbations of the illness continuous therapy on a daily basis with tetracycline alone or additional drugs may be ordered.

Oxygen may be necessary in severe obstructive disease if the arterial oxyhemoglobin saturation is significantly reduced. However, the use of oxygen in high concentrations can be dangerous if the level of carbon dioxide in the patient's blood has increased. The respiratory center of the brain is usually sensitive to a level of carbon dioxide in the blood and if the level increases slightly, the respiratory rate and the depth increase so as to eliminate the carbon dioxide. If, however, the carbon dioxide level is chronically elevated, the respiratory center becomes insensitive to carbon dioxide changes. Under these circumstances the level of oxygen in the blood becomes a regulatory factor—the hypoxic drive to respiration. As long as the oxygen saturation of the blood is at a low level, the patient will tend to breathe effectively in order to maintain oxygenation. Should the patient suddenly be given 100 per cent or any other high concentration of oxygen by mask or other means, the hypoxic drive to respiration is lost and the respiratory rate will drop. This leads to the further retention of carbon dioxide, apnea, and death. Safe methods for the administration of oxygen for the patient with COPD include nasal catheter or cannula, with the oxygen flow rate set at no more than 2 or 3 liters per minute. The "Ventimask" (Venturi mask) is designed to deliver oxygen of predictable concentration. This is of great importance in the patient with chronic airway obstruction. It must be observed that the vent holes in the plastic face mask are not occluded in order to prevent accumulation of carbon dioxide and change in oxygen concentration.

There is danger in the routine administration of oxygen to patients whose medical history is unknown. If the patient's color improves but he becomes increasingly somnolent, he may be approaching respiratory arrest (see Chap. 60).

Intermittent positive pressure with compressed air or oxygen is frequently used to provide a more adequate aeration of the lungs. The many different types of equipment available are divided into two groups. *Pressure-cycled* equipment is regulated by a gauge on the face of the machine which registers the pressure developed by the onrushing air in the trachea and the major airways. When the inflow pressure equals the pressure set at the machine, the machine shuts off and expiration starts. The volume of air delivered to the patient is dependent on the generated pressure and may vary from minute to minute in a very sick patient. The *volume-cycled* respirators do not rely on pressure as a sensing device and are not pressure regulated. A decision is made regarding the volume of air to be delivered during each respiratory cycle. This technique insures the continued delivery of a known quantity of air under all circumstances. Volume-cycled equipment is expensive to purchase, requires skill in its maintenance, and is occasionally dangerous to the patient's health. It is, however, the most useful equipment for the effective in-hospital therapy of severe chronic obstructive pulmonary disease. While the pressure-cycled apparatus may be used with either mask or mouthpiece, volume-cycled equipment can be effectively applied only via a tracheostomy or an endotracheal tube. The nurse must know how the equipment functions before undertaking the care of the patient.

### Nursing Care of Patients with Chronic Pulmonary Insufficiency

The nursing care of patients with chronic pulmonary insufficiency requires a high level of clinical judgment and technical skill, patience, attention to detail, and the ability to maintain interest and hope when progress is slow.

An approach that emphasizes the day-to-day progress, however slight, often helps these patients to continue to follow their treatment. For example, noting that the patient walked to the bathroom this week, whereas last week he found it impossible to do so, can be a point of encouragement. Patients who are highly motivated are better able to profit from whatever treatment is available and, despite their severely damaged lungs, are able to make the best possible use of their remaining pulmonary function.

Because the illness is a discouraging one and one that is believed to be closely linked to smoking, it is essential for the nurse to guard particularly against:

- **Adopting an attitude that implies that the patient has, by his smoking, willfully brought the condition on himself.**
- **Becoming enveloped in the patient's discouragement and, therefore, becoming unable to help him.**

Many of these patients express sadness and bitterness at not having been able to stop smoking before illness became incapacitating. Helping such patients to believe that there is some use in trying to stop smoking now and that it is worthwhile to follow a rehabilitation program can, in some instances, result in greater symptomatic relief than was originally thought possible.

**Assessment.** The nursing history emphasizes the effect of the patient's symptoms on his life style and his use of coping mechanisms as well as other usual aspects of the nursing history. Inspection, palpation, auscultation, and percussion as well as participation in the evaluation of pulmonary function studies are valuable skills which require specialized preparation.

Observation of the patient's symptoms and signs is necessary. It is important to note the amount of coughing, the amount and the character of sputum, the degree of dyspnea and/or wheezing, as well as the patient's color, weight and appetite, and response to activity.

The nurse must carefully observe the patient for *complications and progression of his illness,* whatever the care setting. Increased dyspnea, cough, and sputum are important factors, as are chills and fever. Right heart failure (cor pulmonale) may occur because of the increased resistance in the pulmonary vascular bed, which in turn increases the work of the right ventricle. Symptoms of heart failure include edema and cyanosis, as well as dyspnea, orthopnea, and cough.

**Patient Education.** As in other long-term conditions, a patient education program based on the individual's cognitive, affective, and psychomotor capacities and needs is essential. A large part of nursing the patient with chronic pulmonary insufficiency requires expertise in the teaching and counseling roles. One major objective is to prevent crisis episodes requiring hospitalization.

GENERAL HEALTH. The patient's general health is important in his struggle with chronic respiratory illness. It is important to review with him and his family the principles of optimum nutrition and the maintenance of normal weight, and to help plan for rest, recreation, and satisfying work. Often patients feel there is little use in trying these measures, and an important aspect of nursing care involves communicating the belief that such considerations are worthwhile.

Helping the patient to establish a regular routine, whether he is cared for in the hospital or at home, is important in maintaining therapy over long periods. It is not unusual for these patients to follow treatment carefully for a few days or weeks and then gradually to abandon it when dramatic improvement does not ensue. Most of the gains will come about slowly.

SMOKING. The cessation of smoking is an absolute necessity. The patient needs to know why he should stop smoking as well as to be given support in how to stop (see Chap. 11).

HYDRATION. Adequate hydration helps to keep tracheobronchial secretions loose and easy to cough up. Adequate fluid intake (10 to 12 glasses daily) and room humidification, especially when central heating systems are operating, are important measures. The mouth breathing of the dyspneic patient causes air to bypass the nasopharynx which normally adds humidity to inspired air.

ACTIVITY. The patient should be as active as his cardiopulmonary status permits. Patients with advanced COPD have severe limitations on their physical activity. Even moving from bed to chair can cause extreme dyspnea.

Some of the limitation might be due to the high energy cost of an ineffective breathing pattern and to muscle deconditioning as a result of the mistaken notion that "taking it easy" somehow rests the lungs.

Newer techniques such as blood gas studies at rest and after exercise and other measurements of pulmonary function can be made so that an activity program, including conditioning exercises, can be prescribed on an individual basis. Before attempting to increase exercise tolerance the patient must learn energy conservation through techniques of muscular relaxation and breathing control. The patient who

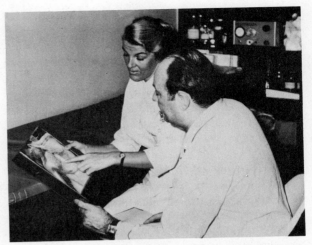

**Figure 30-3.** For the patient with COPD, education is an essential part of nursing care. Visual aids are most helpful.

is untrained in such techniques uses considerable energy in ineffective breathing which only increases dyspnea and fatigue.

Bed rest or physical inactivity leads to stasis of secretions, muscle deconditioning, diminished cough reflex, and hypoventilation, among other hazards. Thus, bed rest should be prescribed just as medication or oxygen is prescribed. Excessive napping during the day should be discouraged, particularly if the patient doesn't sleep well at night.

The patient with COPD who has bed rest prescribed must also have a program of preventive activities prescribed, such as frequent deep breathing, positioning, muscle conditioning activities (active or passive), effective coughing, and diversion.

Through the teaching of bronchial hygiene measures and reconditioning techniques, the nurse may help the patient to increase his activity tolerance though the pathology in his lungs is not reversed.

Adjustments in the patient's schedule can help him to continue some of his accustomed activities. For example, one man arranged to work from 10 A.M. to 6 P.M. rather than from 8 A.M. to 4 P.M., because the early morning hours were especially difficult for him. He almost invariably experienced prolonged, severe coughing and some dyspnea for an hour or two after arising. Starting work later gave him an opportunity to recover from these symptoms before going to work as well as to avoid rush-hour traffic. Had he not been able to adjust his hours of work, he could have gone to bed earlier, and arisen an hour or two earlier each morning, to allow time to get over the coughing. Although it is undesirable for the patient to undertake strenuous exertion, neither is it wise for him to abandon all his interests and his activities. The latter course rapidly leads to invalidism. Activities which offer diversion should be strongly encouraged as long as they are within the patient's tolerance.

MEDICATIONS. Patients with chronic airway obstruction may receive prescriptions from various classes of drugs such as bronchodilators, expectorants, steroids, tranquilizers. Coexisting heart disease may necessitate digitalis and diuretic preparations.

An essential part of the patient education program is learning the precise name and nature of all of his medications (which should be labeled by name) and their expected effects and side effects, and the timing and spacing of drug administration. If the patient cannot learn this, another responsible person must be instructed. It is easy for the patient receiving large numbers of oral drugs to make a self-medication error.

Precise instructions concerning aerosols for bronchodilator therapy as well as rectal aminophylline should also be given.

**Oxygen Therapy.** When necessary, oxygen is given as a supportive measure to correct tissue hypoxia caused by inadequate pulmonary gas exchange resulting in decreased oxygenation of arterial blood (hypoxemia). Simultaneously, physical measures are necessary to relieve the cause of the hypoxemia when this is possible (such as retained secretions).

Tissue hypoxia is often initially manifested by behavioral changes such as confusion and disorientation. Cardiac arrhythmias may also be manifestations of tissue hypoxia.

Oxygen should be ordered in a specific amount to treat a specific need. Analysis of arterial blood provides optimum monitoring.

Some patients, especially those who continue to be hypoxemic despite good respiratory care, are advised by their physicians to continue to use intermittent positive pressure inhalations with air or oxygen after discharge from the hospital. Although the initial cost of the equipment is high, its long-term use makes it a worthwhile investment. The apparatus is attractively packaged and usually comes in a suitcase fitted with a small air compressor for total portability. Nurses, physicians, or inhalation therapists can teach the patient and family the use of the equipment at home. The community nurse provides overall health supervision as well as advice in seeking financial assistance if this is necessary for the patient to purchase or rent equipment.

**Removal of Secretions from the Airways.** Mobilization of secretions from small airways to the main stem bronchi where they can be coughed out is necessary to prevent complications. Systemic as well as local airway hydration aids in this effort as do effective coughing and postural drainage.

Effective coughing emphasizes a forward flexion motion and slow expiratory flows. A teaching program is designed for the individual patient based on his disease state, age, and ability to generate an adequate expiration (Lagerson, 1974).

Postural drainage helps to remove secretions by gravity. The exact position of the patient during the treatment will depend on the location of the lesions to be drained. (See Fig. 30-1.) Usually recommended is 5 to 15 minutes three times a day in each prescribed position while inhaling slowly and blowing the breath out through the mouth.

For some patients postural drainage may require the headdown jackknife position, but a number of other positions in bed are designed to drain a specific bronchopulmonary segment. For example, the upper lobes are drained in the sitting position. Leaning 30 degrees forward drains the posterior upper lobe segments. A backward lean of 30 degrees drains the anterior segments. If the bed is gatched in the center or two pillows are placed under the patient's hips so that his head is about 30 to 45 degrees from the general body axis and he is positioned on his abdomen, the posterior lower lobe segments can be drained. Lying on the back in this position drains the anterior lower lobe segments, and lying on either side drains the lower lateral segments.

Before positioning, patients are encouraged to breathe deeply, or their ventilation can be assisted with a breathing bag such as the Ambu, or with an intermittent positive pressure ventilator. They are then assisted as necessary to assume each position and are encouraged to cough between positions. A sputum cup, tissues, and a call bell should be available. *Pulmonary physical therapy* measures by a nurse or therapist include gently shaking or vibrating during expiration the segment being drained and gentle but firm clapping or percussion with cupped hands on the chest wall over the segment. These measures help to loosen secretions which are then moved by gravity to the trachea where they can be coughed up or suctioned.

Patients vary in their tolerance for postural drainage. Aged and debilitated patients may need the procedure modified, so that the head is not placed too low, and the length of time that the position is maintained is shorter. Some may not be able to tolerate a lowered head position at all. Special care and frequent observation of elderly or weak patients are important during and after postural drainage. The patient is assisted to resume normal position when the treatment is over, and encouraged to rest afterward. Dizziness and falling are especially likely to occur if the patient gets up rapidly and if these precautions are not taken. Younger, more vigorous patients may be able to carry out the procedure with little or no assistance after they have done it a few times with the nurse's guidance.

Mouth care is important after the treatment, because sputum leaves an unpleasant taste and an odor in the mouth. The amount, color, and viscosity of sputum that the patient expectorates during and immediately after the treatment is observed and recorded.

Postural drainage should not be attempted after meals, because nausea and vomiting may result from the position and the coughing.

**Breathing Retraining.** Anxiety, apprehension, and muscular tension markedly increase oxygen consumption and carbon dioxide production. The struggling dyspneic patient uses almost every muscle in his body, wasting much energy. A more effective pattern of breathing emphasizes patient control, slow expiratory flow with lips slightly parted but not tightly pursed, and a slow respiratory rate. When the pattern is acquired the patient is encouraged to perform his activities in rhythm with his breathing (Lagerson, 1974). Muscle relaxation techniques are taught initially.

A therapeutic breathing pattern emphasizes the effective use of the diaphragm, thus relieving the compensatory burdens on the muscles of the upper thorax. The patient is taught to let his abdomen rise as he takes a deep breath and to contract the abdominal muscles as he exhales. He can feel whether he is doing the exercise correctly by placing one hand on his chest and the other on his abdomen. During abdominal breathing his chest

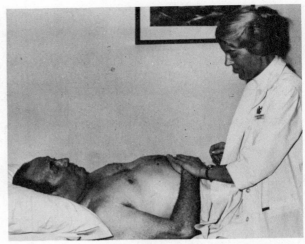

**Figure 30-4.** The nurse teaches methods of abdominal muscular relaxation and breathing control before attempting to help the patient increase his exercise tolerance.

should remain quiet, and his abdomen should rise and fall with each breath. Other maneuvers include practice in blowing out candles at various distances and blowing some small object, such as a pencil or a piece of chalk, along a table top. Patients are encouraged to exhale more completely by taking a deep breath and then letting the body move forward at the waist while they exhale as fully as possible.

## Psychosocial Aspects

Prolonged breathing difficulty often causes feelings of helplessness and despair. Patients who have formerly been active and self-sufficient often feel severely crippled by their inability to walk up a flight of stairs without gasping for breath. The fact that the disability is less immediately obvious than the amputation of a limb makes it no less distressing to the patient.

Many patients with COPD are elderly; they are simultaneously involved in the developmental changes, needs, and tasks of this age group.

Breathing difficulty can arouse anxiety in family members who can respond by withdrawing support from the patient when he needs it most. The patient can also withdraw from his usual cultural supports for fear of alienating key people in his life or from fear of becoming a burden on others.

Patients with COPD together with their families can benefit from group sessions led by a specially prepared nurse with the focus on the affective dimensions of the disease with the participation of other members of the respiratory care team as indicated.

Nett and Petty (1970) also note that therapy for the emphysema patient involves not only a physiologic orientation, but measures to support the associated psychological burden which accompanies the disease. The emphysema patient suffers from the labor of breathing and the forced relinquishing of his usual pleasurable and work activities. He faces a long-term, unrelenting disease while he is undergoing metabolic burdens such as altered blood gases which affect the functioning of his tired and frustrated mind. He may react with fear or excessive demands, turn his anger inward and experience depression, or direct his anger at others who often are trying to help him.

As the disease progresses, the patient is forced to curtail more activities and may have to retire early with less pay; often the male patient may have to relinquish his role as breadwinner to his wife. Impotence due to physical inability or loss of self-esteem or both occurs often in the male, and the female may lose interest in sex. Fear of death and fear of the unknown predominate. If the patient is not helped by competent medical and nursing care, there is progressive failure of sleep and appetite, loss of weight and physical strength, and lack of interest in activities. These symptoms of depression, a heightened degree of somatic complaints, and diffuse anxiety based upon fear of suffocation are the type of psychopathology manifested by the emphysema patient.

In contrast with asthmatic patients, whose attacks usually are interspersed with periods of relative well-being, patients with far-advanced pulmonary emphysema receive little respite from their respiratory distress. For many of these patients the severe curtailment of their daily activities and their enforced dependence on others are made more difficult by the realization that their condition is not likely to undergo marked improvement. Helping such patients to live with their disability without resorting to false promises such as, "You'll be fine in a month or two—spry as ever," demands sensitivity, tact, and knowledge. It is essential that the nurse understand what the physician has told the patient concerning his condition and prognosis, so that the patient is spared the added anxiety of receiving conflicting information.

## BRONCHIECTASIS

Bronchiectasis is a chronic infectious disease in which structural changes in the bronchial walls result in saccular dilations of the bronchi. Purulent material collects in these dilated areas. The expulsive power of the affected areas is diminished, and the purulent material tends to remain in the dilated bronchi.

**Etiology.** Infection is the principal cause. Bronchopneumonia and chronic sinusitis may be precursors of bronchiectasis. Congenital weakness of the bronchi may be a contributing factor. The disease often begins in early adulthood and frequently has a long slowly progressive course.

**Symptoms.** Patients with bronchiectasis cough and expectorate foul, greenish-yellow sputum. Coughing is most severe when the patient changes position, as on arising in the morning or lying down at night. The amount of sputum produced in one paroxysm varies with the stage of the disease. It may be 200 ml. or more. The expectoration of the foul sputum leaves an unpleasant odor in the mouth and on the breath, making frequent oral hygiene especially necessary. Fatigue, loss of weight, and anorexia are common. *Hemoptysis* may occur. Usually, the symptoms develop gradually.

**Diagnosis.** The diagnosis of bronchiectasis requires bronchography.

**Treatment.** The treatment of bronchiectasis includes drainage of the purulent material from the bronchi. Antibiotics are used to control infection. These may be administered parenterally, orally, or by aerosol. The maintenance of the general health by rest and nutrition and the avoidance of further infection are important. If bronchiectasis is confined to a relatively small portion of the lung, a cure may be achieved by surgical removal of the diseased portion. Medical treatment is palliative, since the damaged bronchi do not return to normal. For patients with extensive disease of both lungs, this is the only treatment possible.

## EMPYEMA

*Empyema* is a general term used to denote pus in a body cavity. However, it usually refers to pus within the thoracic cavity (thoracic empyema). Empyema results from infection, which causes the formation of pus. Infection may follow trauma or pre-existing diseases, such as pneumonia, tuberculosis, or lung abscess. Before the introduction of antibiotics, empyema was a frequent complication of pneumonia. Symptoms of empyema include fever, pain in the chest, dyspnea, and malaise. Diagnosis is made by roentgenogram and by aspiration of purulent fluid during thoracentesis.

Initial treatment often consists of antibiotics, given both parenterally and into the pleural space, and aspiration of pus by thoracentesis. Sometimes closed drainage of the empyema cavity is used. Open drainage may be used when pus is very thick, and when the walls of the empyema cavity are strong enough to keep the lung from collapsing during the time that the chest is opened. One or more soft rubber tubes may be placed in the opening to promote drainage. The wound then is covered by a large absorbent dressing that is changed as it is necessary. The drainage of the pus results in a fall in temperature and general symptomatic improvement. If empyema is inadequately treated, it may become chronic. A thick coating may form over the lung, preventing its expansion. Decortication (removal of the coating) allows the lung to reexpand.

## LUNG ABSCESS

An abscess, a localized area of suppuration, may occur in the lung as a result of the aspiration of a foreign body or of respiratory secretions after surgery. Lung abscesses also may follow pneumonia or a mechanical obstruction of the bronchi, such as that due to cancer. The prevention of lung abscess involves the avoidance of the aspiration of secretions by patients who are unconscious and the avoidance and the prompt treatment of obstructions and infections in the respiratory tract.

Symptoms of lung abscess include chills, fever, weight loss, and cough productive of purulent or bloody sputum. Clubbing of the fingers often occurs in chronic cases.

The treatment of lung abscess involves the drainage of the abscess, the control of infection, and measures to increase the body's resistance. Sometimes, postural drainage and the use of antibiotics prove sufficient; in other instances, surgical drainage of the abscess may be necessary. The portion of the lung containing the abscess may be removed surgically.

## PNEUMOCONIOSIS

Pneumoconiosis is an inclusive term used to describe any disease of the lung caused by the inhalation of dust. It usually refers to diseases caused by inhalation of silica (silicosis) or asbestos (asbestosis). Pneumoconiosis is common among persons who work in industries in which exposure to these substances is prolonged, such as mining, stonecutting, and manufacture of products using asbestos. The manifestations of the disease may not occur until 20 years after exposure.

Only the tiny particles of dust reach the lung; the larger ones are trapped in the respiratory passages. Therefore, the tiny particles are the most hazardous; they cause irritation and gradual fibrosis of the lung tissue. The lung tissue loses its elasticity; reduced vital capacity, with dyspnea and cough, results. Tuberculosis has a very high incidence among persons who have silicosis. The diagnosis of pneumoconiosis is based on the history of exposure (usually over a prolonged period), roentgenography, and pulmonary function studies.

The prevention of the condition is an important problem in industrial health. Removal of dust from the air, the wearing of protective masks, and careful examination of workers for early symptoms of pneumoconiosis and tuberculosis are important preventive measures. Workers who show beginning symptoms of pneumoconiosis should be helped to find another occupation.

## CANCER OF THE LUNG

**Incidence.** It is estimated that in 1974 approximately 60,000 men and 15,000 women will die of lung cancer. New cases for 1974 are estimated to be 83,000. Lung cancer is the leading cause of male cancer deaths with an increase of the disease in men continuing at an alarming rate—14 times greater than 40 years ago ('74 *Facts and Figures*, American Cancer Society).

More accurate diagnosis, increasing numbers of older persons in the population, the popularity of cigarette smoking, and increasing air pollution in industrial centers may be factors explaining increased incidence. Most patients are over 40 when the disease is discovered, and unfortunately lung cancer is difficult to diagnose in time for cure. The

American Cancer Society estimates that only about 9 per cent are being saved. It has been noted that the incidence of carcinoma of the lung is especially high among those who suffer from chronic bronchitis, and that many of these chronic bronchitis sufferers have been heavy smokers for many years. The question of the relationship of cigarette smoking to cancer of the lung is discussed more fully in Chapter 11.

**Pathology and Symptoms.** Bronchogenic carcinoma, a malignant tumor arising from the bronchial epithelium, is the most common type of lung cancer. The tumor usually produces no symptoms at first; however, as it enlarges, the patient may experience cough productive of mucopurulent or blood-streaked sputum. The cough may be slight at first and be disregarded or attributed to smoking. As the disease advances, the patient experiences fatigue, weight loss, and anorexia. Dyspnea and chest pain occur late in the disease. Hemoptysis is not uncommon.

**Diagnosis.** An early diagnosis of cancer of the lung is difficult, since symptoms often do not appear until the condition is well-established. Routine chest roentgenograms, particularly in persons over 40 and those who are heavy cigarette smokers, are recommended as part of the annual physical examination to detect carcinoma of the lung in the early, asymptomatic stage. Other diagnostic measures include bronchoscopy, biopsy, examination of sputum, and surgical exploration.

**Treatment.** Surgical removal of the malignant tissue offers the only type of cure and usually is successful only in the early stages of the disease. Depending on the size and the location of the tumor, lobectomy or pneumonectomy may be performed. (Chemotherapy or radiotherapy may be used to slow the course of the disease and to alleviate symptoms. See Chapters 17 and 18 for further discussion of the treatment of cancer by chemotherapy and radiotherapy.)

**Course and Prognosis.** The prognosis is poor unless the condition is treated early. Metastasis occurs to the mediastinal and cervical lymph nodes, the esophagus, and the opposite lung. The patient with advanced carcinoma of the lung with metastases is very ill. Marked wasting of tissues, pain, dyspnea, and cough are present. (See Chapter 12 for care of the dying patient.)

## REFERENCES AND BIBLIOGRAPHY

BARSTOW, R.: Coping with emphysema, *Nurs. Clin. N. Am.* 9:137, March 1974.

BASS, H., et al.: Exercise training: therapy for patients with chronic obstructive pulmonary disease, *Chest* 57:116, 1970.

BEAMONT, E.: Portable I.P.P.B. machines, *Nurs. '73* 3:26, January 1973.

BRANNEN, P.: Oxygen therapy and measures of bronchial hygiene, *Nurs. Clin. N. Am.* 9:111, March 1974.

Breathing reconditioning exercises for your COPD patient, *Patient Care* 8:140, February 15, 1974.

DIRSCHEL, K.: Respiration in emphysema patients, *Nurs. Clin. N. Am.* 8:617, December 1973.

DUDLEY, D. L., et al.: Psychosocial aspects of care in the chronic obstructive pulmonary disease patient, *Heart Lung* 2:389, May–June 1973.

EGAN, D.: *Fundamentals of Respiratory Therapy,* ed. 2, St. Louis, Mosby, 1973.

FAGERHAUGH, S.: Getting around with emphysema, *Am. J. Nurs.* 73:94, January 1973.

FOSS, G.: Postural drainage, *Am. J. Nurs.* 73:666, April 1973.

GIBBON, J. H., JR., et al.: *Surgery of the Chest,* ed. 2, Philadelphia, Saunders, 1969.

GLOOR, E. M.: Chronic obstructive pulmonary disease and the role of the public health nurse in instituting a programme of home care services, *Int. J. Nurs. Stud.* 10:111, May 1973.

HARGAVES, A.: Emotional problems of patients with respiratory disease, *Nurs. Clin. N. Am.* 3:479, September 1968.

KASS, I., et al.: Sex in chronic obstructive pulmonary disease, *Med. Asp. Human Sexuality* 6:32, February 1972.

KUDLA, M.: The care of the patient with respiratory insufficiency, *Nurs. Clin. N. Am.* 8:183, March 1973.

LAGERSON, J.: Better breathing for all! A nursing challenge, *ANA Clinical Sessions, 1972,* New York, Appleton-Century-Crofts, 1973:157.

————: Nursing care of patients with chronic pulmonary insufficiency, *Nurs. Clin. N. Am.* 9:165, March 1974.

————: The cough: its effectiveness depends on you, *Resp. Care* 18:434, July–August 1973.

LAGERSON, J., et al.: Chronic airway obstruction: essentials of care, *Hosp. Med.* 9:38, September 1973.

MASFERRER, R.: Role of patient instruction in improving IPPB treatments, *Inhal. Therapy* 14:17, 1969.

MITCHELL, R. S., et al.: Cigarette smoking, chronic bronchitis and emphysema, *JAMA* 188:12, April 1964.

MOODY, L.: Asthma—physiology and patient care, *Am. J. Nurs.* 73:1212, July 1973.

————: Nursing care of patients with asthma, *Nurs. Clin. N. Am.* 9:195, March 1974.

MUSHIN, W., et al.: *Automatic Ventilation of the Lungs,* ed. 2, Philadelphia, Davis, 1969.

National Tuberculosis and Respiratory Disease Association: *Chronic Obstructive Pulmonary Disease. A Manual for Physicians,* ed. 3, 1972.

NETT, L.: The use of mechanical ventilators, *Nurs. Clin. N. Am.* 9:123, March 1974.

NETT, L., and PETTY, T. L.: Why emphysema patients are the way they are, *Am. J. Nurs.* 70:1251, June 1970.

NIELD, M. A.: A nurse-directed chest clinic, *Nurs. Clin. N. Am.* 9:147, March 1974.

OAKES, A.: Understanding blood gases, *Nurs. '73* 3:14, September 1973.

PETTY, T. L.: *Intensive and Rehabilitative Respiratory Care,* Philadelphia, Lea & Febiger, 1971.

———: A new simple IPPB device for hospital and home use, *JAMA* 203:871, March 1968.

PETTY, T. L., et al.: A comprehensive care program for chronic airway obstruction, *Ann. Intern. Med.* 70:1109, June 1969.

Pointers on bronchial hygiene, *Patient Care* 8:106, February 15, 1974.

RICHARDS, W., et al.: Status asthmaticus, *Emerg. Med.* 6:294, February 1974.

RIE, M. W.: Physical therapy in the nursing care of respiratory disease patients, *Nurs. Clin. N. Am.* 3:463, September 1968.

SCHWAID, M.: The impact of emphysema, *Am. J. Nurs.* 70:1247, June 1970.

SROLE, L.: Social and psychological factors in smoking behavior: the Midtown Manhattan Study, *Bull. N. Y. Acad. Med.* 44:1502, December 1968.

TRAVER, G.: The nurse's role in clinical testing of lung function, *Nurs. Clin. N. Am.* 9:101, March 1974.

———: *Nursing the Patient with Respiratory Insufficiency,* The League Exchange Number 96, New York, National League for Nursing, 1972.

U.S. Department of Health, Education and Welfare, Public Health Service: *National Heart, Blood Vessel, Lung and Blood Program, Vol. I,* DHEW Publ. No. (NIH)73-515, National Heart and Lung Institute Summary, May 1, 1973.

———: *Smoking and Health,* Public Health Service Publ. No. 1103, Washington, D.C., U.S. Government Printing Office, 1964.

# The Patient with Pulmonary Tuberculosis

## CHAPTER 31

Nurses in almost every practice setting become involved in aspects of the prevention, treatment, or follow-up care of patients with tuberculosis. In schools, industries, mobile or stationary community health centers, hospital clinics, or medical offices, nurses participate in tuberculosis screening programs.

Nurses in community health practice support patients and their families or close associates in their homes through the lengthy treatment process which includes ascertaining that the treatment prescription is adhered to, monitoring for side effects of drugs, instructing individuals and groups, and seeing that public health standards for control of the disease are being met. Nurses in acute care hospitals, extended-care facilities, or specialized chest hospitals may give bedside care to acutely symptomatic patients and also prepare them for going home, including referral to appropriate community agencies.

In all settings and in all phases of care of patients with tuberculosis much emphasis is placed on the teaching and counseling roles of the nurse since successful control of tuberculosis depends on the willingness and ability of the patient and his close personal associates to complete long-term drug therapy.

## THE NATURE OF TUBERCULOSIS

Tuberculosis is often described as a "sociocultural disease with medical overtones." Though it is true that infection with the tubercle bacillus is necessary to the development of the disease, it is not a sufficient cause. Many people at some time become infected with the tubercle bacillus but only a small proportion ever become ill from tuberculosis. The incidence of tuberculosis is closely related to the consequences of social and economic deprivation—crowded and inadequate housing, poor nutrition, poor sanitation, poor education. Often tuberculosis victims have associated health problems such as alcoholism or drug addiction. Since these conditions are most commonly found in large urban areas in industrial societies, tuberculosis morbidity and mortality are higher among residents of such areas.

In few other diseases is the biopsychosocial concept of health and illness so clearly manifest. Clearly evident also is the bitter fact of all the injustices of our health and social systems, for despite the successes of modern chemotherapy, tuberculosis remains a very serious problem among the deprived urban poor. Nursing care and medical treatment, to be successful, must be predicated on an assessment of the many factors underlying the disease process, and must help the patient to cope with them.

While at one time treatment involved isolation in a sanitarium-type facility, recent advances in chemotherapy enable the patient to be treated in most cases within his home environment. The exceptions are those patients (mostly from inner-city ghetto areas) who are basically homeless, family-less and penniless, without education or job skills and with additional health problems. For these patients the provision of temporary shelter, food, clothing, health supervision, and teaching in an atmosphere of respect and concern is considered essential to secure compliance with drug therapy.

A team approach to care of the patient is most likely to be successful. Such a team might be comprised of nurses associated with clinics, schools, community health nursing associations, industries, or hospitals as well as physicians, specialists in TB contacts, social workers, alcoholism and drug addiction counselors, and home health aides. The last are carefully trained and supervised residents of the same area as the patient population, who usually share the same racial and cultural background. They are notably more often successful with the patients than other health team workers because of their first-hand knowledge and concern for the special needs of patients and their families, such as the urban black poor (Saltman, 1973), or the Spanish-speaking groups.

Since tuberculosis is a communicable disease and public health authorities are responsible for tuberculosis control, confirmed cases, and in some places suspected cases, must be reported by the physician. This report activates a health department epidemiological investigation to determine the source of the patient's infection and initiates the screening and surveillance of the patient's contacts.

## HISTORY

Tuberculosis has existed since ancient times; archeologic investigations have found skeletons that showed signs of tuberculous infection. In earlier times it was called "phthisis" and also "consumption" because of the bodily wasting associated with the disease. During the latter part of the 19th century, knowledge of the disease accelerated greatly; during the 20th century, major advances have been made in treatment and control of tuberculosis. Among the outstanding persons who have contributed to these advances during the latter part of the 19th century were:

- Robert Koch, who discovered the tubercle bacillus, and how to prepare tuberculin.
- Villemin, in France, who proved for the first time that tuberculosis can be transmitted.
- Forlanini, in Italy, who suggested the use of pneumothorax in therapy of tuberculosis.
- Brehmer, in Germany, who was the first to institute sanitarium care.
- Edward Livingston Trudeau, who established a well-known sanitarium at Saranac Lake, New York.

When, in 1895, Roentgen discovered the use of x-rays, an extremely valuable aid in the diagnosis of tuberculosis became available. In 1904, the National Association for the Study and Prevention of Tuberculosis was founded. Its name later became the National Tuberculosis and Respiratory Disease Association (NTRDA), which today has become the American Lung Association.

The year 1944 initiated the era of chemotherapy for tuberculosis which has almost totally replaced collapse therapy or excisional surgery. The discoveries of para-aminosalicylic acid (PAS) by Waksman of the United States were milestones in the treatment of the disease. Continued drug developments such as isoniazid (INH) (1951), ethambutol (EMB) (1967) and rifampin (RIF) (1971) further increase the potentiality for successful prevention of the spread of disease within the affected individual, as well as to other persons. Emphasis today is on early and sustained chemotherapy for the affected individual patient, and on INH chemoprophylaxis for infected close contacts.

## EPIDEMIOLOGY

### Mortality

Dramatic improvement in the mortality rate from tuberculosis has taken place within our own lifetimes. In 1902, tuberculosis was the leading cause of death in the United States; and in 1953 there were 19,707 deaths from tuberculosis, a death rate of 12.4 per 100,000 population; whereas in 1972, there were 4,550 deaths from tuberculosis, a death rate of 2.2 per 100,000 population (1972 Tuberculosis Statistics: States and Cities).

### Morbidity

The marked reduction in mortality has led some people to the false assumption that tuberculosis is no longer an important health problem. However, tuberculosis continues to be an important cause of sickness and disability, and a bitter personal problem when it strikes.

Case rates have declined much more slowly than death rates. In 1972, there were 32,882 new cases of active tuberculosis reported in the United States, a case rate of 15.8 per 100,000, a 7.6 per cent decline from a rate of 17.1 in 1971 (Fig. 31-1). Due to the increase of the U. S. population by almost one-third since 1953 when new case data were first reported, case *rates* have shown a more rapid decline than actual cases. Since the advent of chemoprophylaxis and chemotherapy, incidence of disease

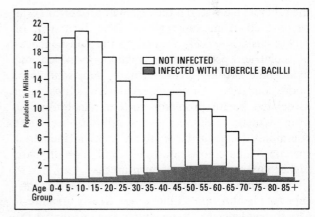

**Figure 31-2.** TB infection in the United States by age group. (Farer, L. S.: Preventive treatment of tuberculosis, *Basics of RD,* Vol. 2, No. 2, November 1973)

particularly among children 5 to 14 years old and young adolescents has been reduced steadily whereas case rates for persons 45 years and older have been dropping very slowly during the past 10 years.

Regardless of the continuing reduction of the incidence of tuberculosis, there are persistent characteristics: four out of five new cases in 1972 were reported from age groups 15 to 24 and above, and two out of three new cases were males. The case rate for other than the white races in all age groups was five times that for whites (Fig. 31-2). Tuberculosis has been reduced among all races but in the nonwhite population there continues to be a growing proportion of the total number of new cases amounting to 40.6 per cent in 1972 as compared with 26.2 per cent in 1953.

For many years pulmonary tuberculosis has accounted for about 90 per cent of all new cases of active tuberculosis. However, during the past five years while new cases of pulmonary tuberculosis have declined, the number of cases of extrapulmonary disease has remained almost constant. Thus the proportion of extrapulmonary cases has increased from 8 per cent in 1966 to 11.8 per cent in 1971.

Provision was made in 1970 to report separate counts of new active tuberculosis and reactivated cases. Although data on reactivations is not precise, a comparison of new and reactivated cases shows that persons with reactivated disease tend to be older, having a median age of 55 compared with 49 for new cases; 95 per cent of reactivated cases were pulmonary as compared with 88 per cent for new cases, and the advanced stage of the disease

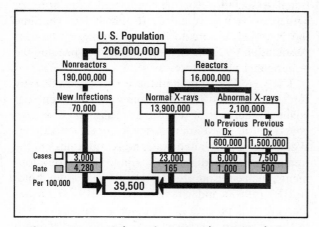

**Figure 31-1.** Tuberculosis in the United States, 1971 (schema). (Farer, L. S.: Preventive treatment of tuberculosis, *Basics of RD,* Vol. 2, No. 2, November 1973)

was slightly greater for reactivated cases—40 per cent compared with 36 per cent for new cases (Reported Tuberculosis Data 1972).

## Geographic Distribution

In 1972 the tuberculosis case rate for big cities in the United States, i.e., 59 cities with over one-quarter million population, was 28.3 per 100,000 as compared with 15.8 per 100,000 for the country as a whole. Case rates are highest in the Appalachian region and surrounding counties, in counties close to the Mexican border, and in a few isolated enclaves where there is a concentration of Indians. The highest state case rate was in Hawaii with 38.9 per 100,000; the lowest was in Iowa, 4.1 per 100,-000. In 1972 the highest new active case rate in cities of over 250,000 was in Newark, New Jersey (69.6 per 100,000) (Reported Tuberculosis Data, 1972).

## Socioeconomic Factors

Mobility of population in the United States has played a major role in the growing concentration of poor nonwhite families in big cities. Many leave rural areas for job opportunities in the big cities which do not materialize, while at the same time there has been an outward migration of whites, as well as a shift of jobs, to the suburbs. The central cities of metropolitan areas account for 29 per cent of all poor whites and 53 per cent of all poor blacks. Lack of access to primary health care, marginal income, high unemployment, larger average family size, a higher percentage of high school dropouts, substandard housing and sanitation, undernutrition, and crowded living conditions increase the risk of contracting an infectious disease such as tuberculosis and influence the difficulty of controlling it.

The incidence of tuberculosis is especially high among alcoholics because of health and social problems associated with alcoholism, for example, malnutrition. Diabetics have a higher incidence of tuberculosis than do nondiabetics, presumably due to their diminished resistance to this infection.

## ATTITUDES TOWARD TUBERCULOSIS

Fear and shame were common reactions to tuberculosis in the past, as were feelings of being "unclean," and of guilt over the possibility of spread of the disease to others. While such reactions still occur, they are not as widespread today. These changes in attitude stem from the vastly improved outlook for tuberculosis patients, and from changes in therapy. For instance, it is no longer necessary for most patients with tuberculosis to have extended care in a sanitarium, nor is it common nowadays for them to give up their usual jobs. Most patients can resume their accustomed activities and relationships promptly enough to avoid the major upheaval in personal and vocational life which used to be common among patients with tuberculosis, who were sometimes confined to a sanitarium for several years. Changes in protective techniques have had an effect, too, on attitudes toward this disease. No longer need patients be cared for by staff swathed in cap, mask, and gown, nor are the letters they have written and the books they have read required to be placed on a window ledge to air for several days, since the disease is not transmitted by bed linens, dishes, books, letters, or other fomites.

Nevertheless, the recollection of older forms of treatment and of a less hopeful outlook for recovery remains vivid among some older people, who in turn influence attitudes of younger people. It is not unusual, therefore, for the nurse to find that her patients' and their families' attitudes toward tuberculosis may be related more to past experiences (either their own, or those of others) than to current realities. An important task of the nurse involves listening to the views of patients and their families concerning tuberculosis, and helping them obtain up-to-date information about the disease and its treatment. A similar appraisal of her own attitudes is necessary for the nurse, too, so that she does not unwittingly convey to patients an attitude of unwarranted pessimism, and an overconcern with future restriction of life patterns and goals, which may not become necessary, and so that she does not burden herself with exaggerated fears of contracting the disease. The genuine fear of contracting the disease experienced by nursing and medical personnel and other contacts of patients can be alleviated by an effective tuberculosis surveillance program (Weg, 1972) and the knowledgeable application of techniques to reduce the concentration of airborne organisms, whether in the hospital, clinic, or home.

## ETIOLOGY

### Predisposing Factors

Active tuberculosis results when the body's resistance, influenced by many biopsychosocial factors, is insufficient to defend against the causative organism, *Mycobacterium tuberculosis* (the tubercle bacillus).

In relation to tuberculosis the word *infection* is used to indicate that the organisms have entered the body and the body has reacted to them. This may or may not lead to active disease. It is estimated that 25 million Americans would be tuberculin positive if tested, which would indicate that they had been exposed to the tubercle bacillus and acquired tuberculosis infection; but fortunately, most do not become ill from active tuberculosis. Ordinarily, tuberculosis is not contracted from brief exposure (as measles can be, for example). Particular danger exists in family groups in which one member has undiagnosed active tuberculosis and, also, in work settings where a coworker has active but undiscovered disease. The danger is intensified if ventilation and sanitation are poor and if crowding exists.

Many factors predispose to the development of tuberculosis. When the body's resistance is lowered, such as through inadequate rest and poor nutrition, or when the organisms are sufficiently virulent and numerous, the clinical disease may develop.

Other conditions which lower resistance to tubercle bacilli in an infected person include pregnancy and the stresses of the first few months after delivery; occasional virus infections such as influenza; gastrectomy, which contributes to undernutrition; and steroid therapy. Diabetics have about three times the incidence of active tuberculosis as do nondiabetics. Workers with diseases of the lungs such as silicosis and related diseases (from the inhalation of silica dust in mining operations) have an increased risk for active tuberculosis and may be treated prophylactically for one year with INH and remain under surveillance for the rest of their lives.

Emotional factors also may play an important part in lowering the body's resistance to disease. Anxiety, tension, and unhappiness may contribute to the development of tuberculosis by upsetting the body's metabolic and physiologic balance. It was formerly believed that a certain "personality type" was most likely to get the disease. More recent studies suggest that although no one specific personality type is linked to tuberculosis, psychological factors are related to the onset and the course of this illness as well as of many others. For some persons, for example, tuberculosis may satisfy an unconscious desire to be dependent and cared for, or it may represent an escape from an intolerable situation at home or work. Reactions to emotional stress may take the form of irregular eating, or loss of sleep, and they may prevent the individual from carrying out reasonable measures in personal hygiene.

Alcoholism as a response to the inability to cope with various stressors is the most common predisposing factor for tuberculosis in the United States today. In addition to the nutritional deficiencies and gastric and liver complications associated with alcoholism, alcohol has a paralyzing effect on the mucociliary system of the bronchi (as does tobacco), which limits the capacity of the lungs to trap and expel inhaled germs.

Though drug addiction may play a role similar to alcohol, to date it does not appear to involve as many patients as alcohol does.

## Population Testing

In areas of high incidence of tuberculosis it is essential to identify infection early in order to prevent disease. Certain age groups are selected for skin testing in order to provide an *index of tuberculosis* in a given population. National experience shows that tuberculin reactor rates in very young children are low, even in ghetto areas. Although the American Academy of Pediatrics' *Red Book* has recommended tuberculin testing of small children, this is not accepted by the Tuberculosis Division of the Center for Disease Control as desirable for entire population groups. The tuberculin test is done at the discretion of the individual pediatrician. If reactor rates in grade-school or high-school children are less than one per cent, retesting is not indicated. For example, in a school district where children in specific grades are tested and the reactor rate is less than one per cent, the State Department of Health might direct that the testing need not be repeated in those grades in future years. Of course, the presence of active tuberculosis in a school would be reason for testing additional grades, or an entire school population.

## The Tubercle Bacillus

Although predisposing factors in the physical and the emotional life of the individual are important, it is still true that infection with the tubercle bacillus is necessary to the development of the disease. Some understanding of this organism and of the ways of controlling its spread is essential to the nurse in protecting herself and others.

The tubercle bacillus is aerobic, varies in shape, virulence, and chemical characteristics, and has acid-fast staining characteristics, which allow microscopic demonstration of the organism on direct smear.

Bacilli are borne in tiny particles called "droplet nuclei." Inhalation of droplet nuclei is the way in which pulmonary tuberculosis is transmitted. A person with active tuberculosis who is not on chemotherapy expels large droplets of respiratory secretions which become airborne with the acts of coughing, sneezing or spitting, laughing or singing. These large droplets may evaporate to form droplet nuclei of one to ten microns in size. Droplet nuclei are not filtered out in the upper respiratory passages but can pass beyond the protective mucociliary barrier into the alveoli.

When inhaled by persons in close, continuous, and prolonged contact with the diseased individual, droplet nuclei may reach the alveoli where they settle out, survive, and multiply, and the *infection* is established. If resistance is poor, eventually the *disease* may start.

Contrary to previously held beliefs, tuberculosis is not hereditary and it is not spread by fomites such as bed linen, clothing, books, or eating utensils. Tubercle bacilli lodged on such fomites die quickly through the action of drying, heat, or sunlight. Airborne particles which arise from such fomites are too large to penetrate into the alveoli.

Because the discharges from body areas affected with nonpulmonary tuberculosis do not become airborne, the risk of infection from such sources as these is remote.

Although tuberculosis occurs in many species, including birds, cattle, and swine, the types of organisms that are important sources of human infection are the human, and to a lesser extent, the bovine. Infection with the bovine type was once quite common, but it is now relatively rare in many countries, including our own, due to the eradication of tuberculosis in cattle and to the pasteurization of milk and milk products.

The existence of a typical or opportunistic species of mycobacteria has been noted. Some of these species are pathogenic; others are not. Different mycobacteria are distinguished mainly by cytochemical tests.

The fact that there are different strains of *Mycobacterium tuberculosis* has relevance to drug therapy, since differences in the organisms lead to differences in their response to chemotherapeutic agents.

## CONTROL OF TRANSMISSION OF DROPLET NUCLEI

Control of the disease involves preventing the patient known to have active tuberculosis from excreting bacilli into the atmosphere. Transmission of droplet nuclei can be minimized by the following measures (National Tuberculosis and Respiratory Disease Association, "Infectiousness of Tuberculosis," 1967):

### Prevention of Contamination

**Chemotherapy.** Antituberculosis drugs reduce the number of bacilli in the sputum, the amount of sputum, and the amount of coughing within a matter of days. The excretion of tubercle bacilli is rapidly reduced and usually halted within a few weeks. At this point, the classification of the disease as "active" is not to be interpreted as meaning communicable.

**Covering of Nose and Mouth** by the patient when coughing or sneezing prevents atomized secretions from becoming airborne. Raised sputum should be expectorated into tissues, placed in special containers, and burned or flushed into the sewage system.

The use of a mask by the patient is only indicated when intimate face-to-face contact with staff members is necessary and the patient is unable to control or unwilling to cover his cough. A fresh well-fitting high-efficiency disposable mask is required. The conventional surgical mask is not effective in preventing the transmission of droplet nuclei. Gowns are unnecessary and ineffective. The use of a mask by the physician and nursing staff during bronchoscopy of a tuberculosis patient is important because the provoking of a cough reflex can expose team members to a large inoculum of infectious material.

### Decontamination

**Room Ventilation.** Adequate ventilation reduces the concentration of droplet nuclei in room air and thus the risk of inhaling them. The use of "one way" or nonrecirculating air conditioning is most effective; open windows are not as effective but are of some help.

**Ultraviolet Light.** Studies have shown that irradiation with ultraviolet light can rapidly make the air of the tuberculosis patient's room noninfectious. Installation should be close to the ceiling and in heating and air ducts if air is being recirculated. Ultraviolet lights should be placed in areas such as clinic waiting rooms, emergency or observation wards, offices where ill people with unsuspected or undiagnosed tuberculosis may congregate, and in the rooms of patients in the early phase of chemotherapy.

## PATHOLOGY

Tubercle bacilli are inhaled into the respiratory passages, or they may be ingested and travel by way of blood and lymph to the lungs. Transmission of the human-type tubercle bacillus is primarily through the respiratory passages; transmission of the bovine-type tubercle bacillus occurs mainly by ingestion of contaminated food, such as milk from infected cows. Tuberculosis most frequently affects the lungs, and sometimes the organisms may be carried by the circulatory system to other organs, such as bones, kidneys, or fallopian tubes. Tissue sensitivity or allergy, manifested by a positive tuberculin reaction, develops in two to ten weeks after the initial infection. Although the intensity of the allergic response is not a measure of immunity, these two factors are believed to be related closely.

When the tubercle bacilli enter the lung, and the person's resistance is not adequate, they start to multiply and create an area of pneumonitis called a *tubercle* or lesion. This small focus of infection is often referred to as a primary infection. Usually, healing occurs by fibrosis and calcification; subsequent roentgenograms may reveal such calcified nodules. With a primary infection, germs are carried by lymphatic channels to lymph nodes around the hilum of the lung which become enlarged. Hilar lymphadenopathy may last for several months after the primary infection has cleared, even though chemotherapy is given. The combination of the initial pulmonary infection and the hilar adenopathy is called a "primary complex" (or Ghon complex). The individual may experience no symptoms during this process, or he may experience briefly malaise, chills, and fever. The fact that primary infection has occurred may be discovered later by a routine tuberculin test or a roentgenogram.

A second way of evolvement of the tubercle is to persist as a *granuloma* which may result in endogenous reactivation at some future time.

If treatment is inadequate, if individual resistance is low, if the organisms are very virulent or numerous, or if contact is repeated and prolonged, the tubercle may enlarge and undergo caseation, a form of necrosis with a cheeselike appearance. This area of caseation may slough away, leaving a cavity in the lung. Caseous material carrying tubercle bacilli can be disseminated throughout the bronchial tree, especially under the influence of cough (bronchogenic spread).

The caseating process may occasionally involve a blood vessel. In this instance massive infection of the bloodstream (hematogenous spread) can result in the development of many small foci of infection throughout the lungs and other organs. This massive seeding is known as miliary tuberculosis. Erosion of the wall of a blood vessel may also cause blood to escape and become mixed with the sputum (hemoptysis). This is not necessarily a sign of more severe disease. In fact it may be beneficial if it results in early diagnosis of the disease.

Unlike many other infections, which result in prompt symptoms and subsequent elimination of the infection, infection with the tubercle bacillus may remain dormant for many years. Organisms may remain within the body and, for reasons not fully understood, later cause active disease. It is thought that activation of a dormant infection may be related to stress with its heightened secretion of adrenocortical hormones. A person with an inactive infection may develop active tuberculosis years later, perhaps in response to fatigue, malnutrition, or emotional strain.

Reinfection, or *secondary infection,* may occur from a new infection entering the body from outside (*exogenous*), or it may result from the reactivation of a previous infection within the body (*endogenous*). It is possible for live tubercle bacilli to continue to exist within an apparently healed lesion for long periods. A patient who has seemed to recover from the disease may have another outbreak if his resistance is decreased.

In countries where tuberculosis is widespread, opportunities for dissemination of infection abound and a large proportion of reinfection is believed to be exogenous. In countries where tuberculosis is less prevalent and opportunities for spread are fewer, the majority of reinfections are believed to be endogenous. In countries such as the United States, the greatest danger of developing active, clinical tuberculosis exists among the population previously infected by the tubercle bacillus, and it is believed that, even though a previous infection confers some increased resistance to subsequent exogenous infection, this advantage is more than offset by the increased risk of developing endogenous tuberculosis.

The disease affects the upper lobes of the lung more frequently than the lower, and the posterior lobes more than the anterior. This may be a result of gravitational stress in upright man. The growth of mycobacteria are favored in the upper posterior lungs because their alveoli are stretched to four to five times the lower lobe size with resultant poorer blood perfusion, reduced local immunity, and increased ventilation and oxygen tension.

The more the disease spreads, the more difficult and prolonged the treatment is, and the more uncertain the prognosis. Lesions of tuberculosis heal slowly. Pulmonary cavitation is one consideration in determining the communicability of tuberculosis.

## CLASSIFICATION OF TUBERCULOSIS

In 1974 new classifications of tuberculosis were developed by the American Thoracic Society, the medical arm of the American Lung Association. An explanation of the classifications published in *Diagnostic Standards and Classification of Tuberculosis and Other Mycobacterial Diseases,* New York, American Lung Association, 1974 is as follows:

**O.** No tuberculosis exposure, not infected. No history of exposure, negative tuberculin skin test.

**I.** Tuberculosis exposure, no evidence of infection. History of exposure, negative tuberculin test.

**II.** Tuberculosis infection, without disease. Positive tuberculin skin test, negative bacteriological studies (if done), no x-ray findings compatible with tuberculosis, no symptoms due to tuberculosis.

**III.** Tuberculosis: infected, with disease. The current status of the patient's tuberculosis is described by three characteristics: location of the disease (e.g. pulmonary, bone, genitourinary, etc.), bacteriological status, and chemotherapy status. For some patients additional characteristics—x-ray findings and tuberculin skin test reaction—would be included.

The term *tuberculosis suspect* may be used until diagnostic procedures are complete but not for more than three months.

## DIAGNOSTIC ASSESSMENT

### Signs and Symptoms

The onset of tuberculosis is insidious, and early symptoms vary somewhat from person to person. For a long time the patient may have no symptoms at all; indeed, he may feel well. The problem of early diagnosis is made more difficult by the widespread belief that people with tuberculosis always look sick—thin, pale, gaunt. Actually, these symptoms often do not appear until the disease is well advanced.

The early symptoms of tuberculosis are often vague, and they may be readily dismissed. Fatigue, anorexia, weight loss, and slight, nonproductive cough are all symptoms that can be attributed to overwork, excessive smoking, or poor eating habits; however, they are also early symptoms of tuberculosis. Elevation of temperature, particularly in the late afternoon and the evening, and night sweats are frequent as the disease progresses. The cough often becomes productive of mucopurulent and blood-streaked sputum. Hemoptysis, the coughing up of blood, may occur. Occasionally, it is the first symptom of the disease. Marked weakness and wasting are characteristic of later stages of the illness; dyspnea may be a late symptom. Chest pain may result from the spread of infection to the pleura, which reacts by producing large amounts of fluid.

### Diagnostic Tests

Diagnostic tests for tuberculosis consist chiefly of tuberculin tests, chest roentgenograms, and examinations of sputum and other body substances.

#### Tuberculin Tests

The use of tuberculin tests is based on the fact that, after the body has been invaded by tubercle bacilli, tissue sensitivity or allergy to the protein components of the bacilli develops gradually in about six to eight weeks. When a small amount of filtrate from dead tubercle bacilli is injected into the skin of a person infected by tuberculosis, some redness and induration will develop at the injection site. Depending on the size of the area of induration, this may be classed as a positive reaction and, if so, is evidence that a tuberculous infection has existed at some time somewhere in the body. Since most such infections with the tubercle bacillus do not result in disease, a positive test is not necessarily an indication of active clinical disease, either

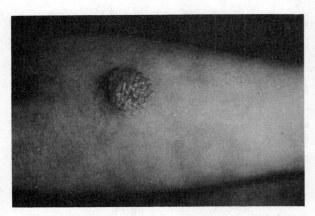

**Figure 31-3.** A positive reaction to tuberculin following a Mantoux test. (Medichrome—Clay-Adams, Inc., New York, N.Y.)

past or present. A common misconception concerning the significance of a positive tuberculin test is that the individual with a positive reaction to tuberculin has merely been in contact, at some time, with someone with active tuberculosis, rather than that the organisms have actually entered his body and caused infection. One reason for this misunderstanding may be a natural reluctance to admit the possibility of infection.

The chief value of tuberculin testing lies in case finding and control of tuberculosis. By means of tuberculin tests it is possible to discover which persons have been infected by the tubercle bacillus and to perform further tests to determine whether clinical disease is present. Tuberculin tests can also be of value in prevention, because those persons who have had recent conversion from a negative to a positive tuberculin reaction can be given a year of chemoprophylaxis to prevent the development of tuberculosis disease.

In the past, a positive tuberculin test was looked upon favorably since it indicated a certain state of immunity, and only nursing personnel with a positive tuberculin test were permitted to work with tuberculosis patients. Today the view is that positive reactors have a greater risk of developing the disease than nonreactors because the bacilli can remain dormant and cause active disease in the future. Therefore, today it is desirable and also possible (since many people do not come into contact with a tuberculosis patient) to be tuberculin negative.

False negative tuberculin tests are a possibility due to interference with the capacity to respond on an allergic basis to the test. *Anergy* or failure to react to tuberculin may be due to the aging process, intercurrent infections, measles during the first two or three weeks after onset of infection, hypothyroidism, late pregnancy or puerperium, viral infections, the administration of adrenocorticosteroids or immunosuppressive agents, sarcoidosis, and concurrent or recent immunization with live viral vaccines such as measles or influenza. Accordingly, the tuberculin test should be given and read before the administration of any live virus vaccine (Figs. 31-3 to 31-5).

**The Mantoux Test.** Tuberculin may be administered in several ways. The most accurate, since an accurately measured dose of PPD (purified protein derivative) can be given, is the Mantoux test. The intradermal injection is usually given into the flexor surface of the forearm about four inches below the bend of the elbow. The skin is first cleansed with alcohol or acetone and allowed to dry. The test material is usually administered with a 1 ml. syringe calibrated in tenths and fitted with a three-eighths or one-half inch 26- or 27-gauge needle. With the needle bevel up, the tip is inserted into the most superficial layers of the skin and 0.1 ml. is injected. A definite bleb about 10 mm. (⅜ inch) in diameter will rise at the needle point and disappear in minutes. A separate sterile needle and syringe must be used for each injection to prevent the possibility of the spread of homologous serum hepatitis or other infectious agents from one person to another.

The test is read 48 to 72 hours after the injection. The transverse diameter of the area of distinctly palpable induration (firmness) is measured and recorded in millimeters. Induration 10 mm. or more in diameter constitutes a positive reaction. Standard procedures for administering the test and interpreting the result are very important.

Stabilized tuberculin PPD for the Mantoux test first became available commercially in 1973. It contains a detergent, Tween, which prevents PPD adsorption loss on the glass or plastic of a vial or syringe and assures more accurate results (no false negatives due to decreased strength of PPD) than those of early test solutions such as the Old Tuberculin (OT), prepared by Robert Koch as a filtrate of dead tubercle bacilli, or the later purified protein derivative (PPD) prepared by Long and Siebert in the United States in 1931 and used until the Tween-stabilized product became available.

Stabilized PPD is available in three strengths—1 Tuberculin Unit, 5 TU, and 250 TU. The 5 TU (or intermediate strength PPD) is the standard TU referring to biologic activity rather than to micrograms of protein contained in the 0.1 ml. dose, which was the previous definition. The 1 TU strength is used for persons suspected of being highly sensitized, to minimize necrotic reactions, and the 250 TU is used only when the 5 TU test is negative. Tween-stabilized PPD comes in vials as a ready-to-use solution which is stable for one year under refrigeration. However, once withdrawn into a syringe the product should be used promptly to avoid the possibility of even a slight loss of potency.

The administration of the test should always be preceded by an explanation of its significance; in the period between the administration of the test and its reading, the patient often is separated from medical personnel. If during this period a positive reaction develops, and the patient believes that this is certain evidence of active clinical disease, he may become extremely and unnecessarily apprehensive.

**Other Tuberculin Tests.** Tuberculin tests using multiple-puncture technique have replaced the patch and the scratch tests. Various companies manufacture equipment for multiple-puncture tests. Those commonly used in this country include the tine, the Sterneedle (Heaf), and the Mono-Vacc tests, all based on the principle of multiple small prongs advocated by Heaf in England in 1956. The advantage of these tests for mass screening is that the equipment comes individually sterilized, packaged, and ready for use. No syringes or needles are necessary. The tuberculin is already incorporated in each individual packet. These tests are administered by pressing a small disk firmly against the palmar surface of the patient's forearm. Impregnated prongs or tines pierce the skin. The test causes scarcely any discomfort. Tine and Mono-Vacc tests use OT (Old Tuberculin). Sterneedle uses a special PPD solution (two-year stability) which must not be used for the Mantoux test.

A more costly test is the hypo spray jet which is able to inject either OT or PPD beneath the surface of the skin by high pressure. Several hundred tests per hour can be performed, but slight bleeding occurs in a significant percentage of cases.

Regardless of technique used, the test must be read from 48 to 72 hours with the exception of the Sterneedle (Heaf) test, which may be read in three to seven days. This is helpful in school and clinic

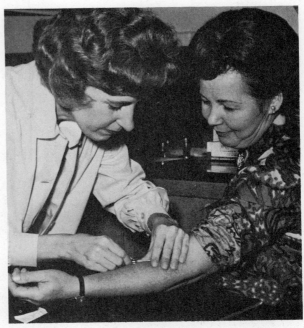

**Figure 31-4.** Nurse administering Mantoux test. (Photo courtesy American Lung Association, formerly National Tuberculosis and Respiratory Disease Association)

situations where individuals might not be able to be present for reading of their reactions within the usual 48- to 72-hour period.

Multiple puncture tests, although frequently used for mass screening, are less accurate than the Mantoux test. For this reason, the Mantoux test should be used to verify results of multiple puncture tests with one exception. Vesiculation (blistering) means that the individual is a tuberculin reactor and a Mantoux is not required.

## Roentgenography

Chest roentgenograms are used to determine whether the disease is present in persons who have a positive Mantoux test and to follow the course of the disease in those who do develop tuberculosis. Because of time limitations, routine chest x-ray of all newly admitted patients is used as a screening procedure rather than the Mantoux test in many general hospitals. In addition to changes in the lung, hilar lymphadenopathy is a characteristic of the "primary complex." Chest x-rays have been used in selected groups without prior tuberculin testing to discover new cases of tuberculosis; however, it is recommended that the intradermal Mantoux test

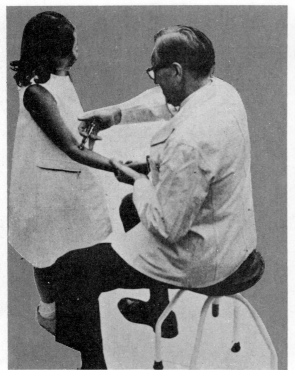
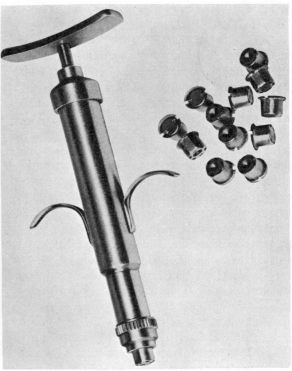

**Figure 31-5.** (*Left*) The doctor is administering a tuberculin test using the Sterneedle device, which is suitable for children and adults. (*Right*) On the Sterneedle a different attachment is used for each patient. (Panray Division, Ormont Drug and Chemical Co., Englewood, N.J.)

be used first, particularly in children and young adults, to avoid unnecessary exposure to radiation. A special group or industrial survey should be done only if there is a specific reason for it, i.e., a known case of newly diagnosed active tuberculosis. Even in this instance, chest x-rays should be reserved for those who are positive reactors to the Mantoux test.

A survey should not be undertaken with a commercial x-ray company without first checking with the state department of health or environmental protection to see that the equipment has been made as safe as possible.

Roentgenograms continue to be indispensable in the diagnosis of tuberculosis. Their judicious use by qualified medical personnel in the diagnosis of tuberculosis and other diseases should not cause alarm over excessive radiation.

### Sputum Examination

Microscopic examinations of sputum to detect acid-fast bacilli are often carried out when tuberculosis is suspected.

First a smear of treated sputum is studied by direct microscopy ("smear," "slide," or "spread" examination). Then specimens of sputum are placed on a suitable medium in test tubes for culture of the organism. This growth takes four to six weeks to complete.

Acid-fast bacilli seen on slide examination are not diagnostic for tuberculosis, even if the chest x-ray is highly indicative of tuberculosis. There is the possibility of other types of mycobacteria, which would be later identified growing on culture.

Absence of acid-fast bacilli on slide examination is not conclusive because the organisms present may not be numerous enough to be seen. After the patient has received chemotherapy, a few organisms may be seen by microscope when a smear is studied. However, the organisms may be too weak to grow on a culture medium. Therefore the patient may have a negative culture and a positive smear before both tests become negative as a result of chemotherapy. In such cases a nongrowing tubercle bacillus is considered for practical purposes a nonvirulent one.

A definite diagnosis of active tuberculosis can be made when a culture of sputum grows *Mycobacterium tuberculosis.*

Since it is possible that tubercle bacilli, although present, may not be recovered from a single specimen, serial tests of sputum are often ordered by the physician. A frequent order reads: "Sputum for acid-fast bacilli x 3." It is important to explain to the patient the necessity for repeated tests, so that he will not become irritated or apprehensive by the request for more than one test.

To obtain a suitable sputum specimen, the patient is instructed to cough deeply, so that the specimen will not consist merely of saliva. Most patients find that they are most likely to expectorate sputum when they first get up in the morning; therefore, this is the best time for them to obtain a specimen. A wide-mouthed specimen bottle is used for this purpose. It is important to see that the outside of the bottle is free from contamination and to avoid contamination of the specimen with other organisms.

Gastric lavage or gastric aspiration may be used to determine the presence of the organisms, particularly among patients such as young children who have difficulty raising a sputum specimen for examination. Tubercle bacilli reach the stomach from the lungs when sputum is raised and is not expectorated but swallowed. The specimen of stomach contents is obtained when the patient awakens in the morning, before he has taken food or liquid. Only a positive culture of tubercle bacilli from a gastric specimen is considered diagnostic.

Gastric aspiration is used less commonly than it was previously. Instead, many patients who have difficulty producing a sputum specimen are asked to inhale a heated vapor (aerosol) of saline or saline mixed with propylene glycol. After inhaling the vapor for 10 minutes, the patient is asked to cough. The vapor helps to loosen secretions, making it easier for the patient to produce sputum for the examination. This procedure is much less uncomfortable for the patient and less time-consuming for the staff. It is effective for many patients, thus decreasing the number who have gastric analysis performed in order to obtain a specimen for examination.

A variety of cytochemical tests are performed to identify the organisms and their characteristics (including atypical forms). Of particular importance in relation to therapy is the sensitivity of the organism to various chemotherapeutic agents.

To insure quality control the culture should be done by the laboratory of the state department of health (or a laboratory approved by the department), which performs sensitivity tests or antibiograms on a routine basis. Culture results and sensitivity test results are generally available within six weeks.

Increasing recognition is being given to the importance of atypical species of acid-fast bacilli. Often these atypical species are resistant to drug therapy. Infection caused by one of these species should not be reported as tuberculosis.

## NURSING ASSESSMENT

Before planning care for the tuberculosis patient, the nurse gathers data from appropriate sources regarding some or all of the following points, depending upon the care setting:

- **Age, sex, and developmental needs and tasks.**
- **Living conditions. What is "home" for this patient? A room in a boarding house? Who lives at "home" with the patient? If no one lives with him, is there a caring person who can act as a surrogate family member and help with the therapeutic plan? Are the present living facilities reasonably safe for the prevention of spread of infection? What are the family's or friends' feelings about the patient, the disease process, the therapeutic plan? What eating arrangements are available?**
- **Occupation and income. What are the employer's and coworkers' attitudes about the patient and the disease process? Does the occupation carry increased risk for tuberculosis?**
- **Race.**
- **Ethnic origins and ties.**
- **Religion.**
- **Historical factors such as family history of tuberculosis, geographic history including place of birth to present residence, and occupational history.**
- **Extent and clinical activity of the disease process.**
- **Bacteriologic results of sputum smear and culture.**
- **Length of illness.**
- **Symptoms.**
- **Prescribed treatment regime and possibility of drug contraindications.**
- **Additional health problems and how they are being treated, e.g., alcoholism, malnutrition, drug abuse.**
- **The patient's knowledge of the disease process and treatment plan.**
- **The patient's feelings about his diagnosis and treatment plan and his acceptance of these.**
- **Tuberculin skin test and chest x-ray results of family or other close personal contacts, their knowledge and acceptance of the proposed treatment plan for the patient and the preventive program for themselves.**

Weg (1971) notes that a stable living situation with interested and cooperative household members who can accept their own involvement in the therapeutic plan is one of the most important factors in maintaining the patient's commitment to complete his treatment. But many patients do not have the advantage of such ideal circumstances. The community health nurse as the patient's advocate can help by assisting the patient to identify and solicit the help of surrogate family members such as neighbors who care, by seeing that the patient knows what to expect from the therapeutic plan, by explaining his rights regarding health care and how to go about obtaining care, and by following through to see that the health care delivery system does not prevent the patient from getting what he needs and what is his right. Patient advocacy extends beyond medical treatment; it may, for example, include prevailing upon a welfare department to give a better food allowance to the patient, reporting housing and sanitation violations such as rats and vermin, or seeking better living quarters for the patient through appropriate channels.

## PATIENT'S RESPONSE TO DIAGNOSIS

As is true in any illness, the patient may at first deny that he has the condition. He may even refuse tests to confirm the diagnosis. Often it is the task of the community health nurse to support the patient during this period, and to help him recognize the need to seek tests and treatment. The problem is made more difficult when, as is so often the case, the patient's health practices have been poor and his business and family relationships have been unstable.

If the patient is not accustomed to accepting responsibility for his own health, it is difficult but extremely important to help him learn how to follow his treatment, and to assist him in adapting his mode of life as necessary in order to carry out his treatment. All the drug discoveries are of no use unless the patient can be helped to realize the necessity for taking prescribed medications over a long period.

Emotional reactions to the illness vary. A patient who is hard-driving and ambitious may resent having to take instruction from physicians and nurses. On the other hand, a passive person may be willing and in fact docile about following instructions, but may have difficulty accepting responsibility for carrying out his treatment. Experiencing any illness can be cause for anger, and more so in the minority group member already angry over his "second-class citizenship." Some are so emotionally drained from the wearying long-term struggle to meet the bare exigencies of daily life that they have little physical or emotional energy to deal with yet another crisis and may appear apathetic. Allowing the patient to talk about his feelings, especially with a trained health worker who shares the same sociocultural background, may help him to deal with them, and avoid letting them interfere with the treatment which is so essential to his welfare, and so important for the safety of those with whom he has contact.

Together with the nurse and other team members, the health aide can do or expedite for the patient what he is temporarily unable to accomplish for himself with regard to obtaining health care and the necessities of life such as food, shelter, clothing, money, instruction, and human concern.

## TREATMENT

### Chemotherapy for Active Tuberculosis

Chemotherapy is the most important aspect of treatment for tuberculosis. Data from worldwide studies under varied conditions document a success rate of over 95 per cent when chemotherapy is given the primary role in the treatment of tuberculosis (Weg, 1971). The usual plan is that the patient receives a minimum of two effective antituberculosis drugs for a period of two years. Successful treatment depends on completion of drug therapy.

All the drug discoveries are of no use unless the patient can be helped to realize the necessity for taking prescribed medications over a long period. Thus, an important role of the nurse who cares for tuberculosis patients in any setting is to offer sustained and individualized support to the patient and his family or friends which will promote a commitment to a full course of treatment and to be aware of factors in noncompliance with therapy and how to mediate them.

Characteristics of Antituberculosis Drugs

Drugs have made recovery more rapid, and they have provided a chance for the arrest of the disease for those with advanced lesions, but drugs do not provide a guaranteed cure. Their usefulness lies in their ability to decrease the growth and the multiplication of the tubercle bacillus (bacteriostatic), thus giving the patient's body a chance to overcome the disease. Two factors make drugs less than ideal: toxicity and the tendency of the tubercle bacillus to develop resistance to the drugs. Combined therapy with two or more drugs decreases the problem of drug resistance, because different drugs work in different ways on tubercle bacilli, thus decreasing the possibility of the growth of resistant organisms.

Positive response to chemotherapy is characterized by a decrease in cough and sputum, improvement in chest x-ray findings, and rapid conversion of sputum from positive for tubercle bacilli to negative, thus making the patient's disease noncontagious, a possibility in a matter of days after starting chemotherapy.

Antituberculosis drugs may be classified as *primary* or initial treatment drugs and *secondary* or retreatment drugs. The latter are used when resistance to primary drugs develops.

Drugs are prescribed by the physician on the basis of their initial and continuing sensitivity to the patient's organisms. When drug sensitivity tests indicate that an initial treatment drug is unsuitable for that patient, it is replaced by another. It is important that reliable laboratories for mycobacteriologic services be used to perform spreads, culture tests, and sensitivity tests on a routine basis. Generally such laboratories are operated by or approved by state departments of health and provide results within six weeks.

### Primary or Initial Treatment Drugs

In general, isoniazid (INH), streptomycin (SM), aminosalicylic acid, which is identical to para-aminosalicylic acid (PAS), ethambutol (EMB), and rifampin (RIF) are the most effective drugs. Some distinguish these as primary or initial treatment drugs and the remaining tuberculostatic drugs as secondary; others do not make such a distinction.

*Isoniazid (INH)* is considered the basic drug and is given in combination with one or two others depending on the clinical activity and extent of the disease, physician preference, and cost. INH and RIF are bacteriocidal; the remaining drugs are bacteriostatic. Isoniazid (INH) has the advantage of oral administration and relatively low toxicity.

Isoniazid may be given orally or parenterally when the oral route of administration is not possible. The usual adult dose is 300 mg. per day in one dose although a higher dosage sometimes is

used. In addition to hepatotoxicity, toxic symptoms and side effects include peripheral neuritis, muscular twitching, constipation, difficulty in voiding, fever, and rash. Since neurologic toxic symptoms may be related to pyridoxine deficiency, supplementary doses of pyridoxine (25 or more mg. daily) often are prescribed for aged, debilitated, or alcoholic patients. INH has been associated with hepatotoxicity and resultant death in rare instances. Liver damage with INH is believed to be a hypersensitivity reaction but the matter is still under study. Present national recommendations are that alcoholics who are only tuberculin reactors should not be given INH but should be kept under surveillance. On the other hand, alcoholic patients who require treatment for tuberculosis disease should be given INH, but their liver function should be monitored periodically including enzyme studies such as SGOT and LDH. Because all patients on INH, whether for treatment or prophylaxis, require close monitoring for side effects and toxicity, it is customary to issue INH on the basis of a one-month supply at a time. The patient is questioned regarding symptoms of liver damage such as anorexia, fatigue, or malaise. Dark urine, jaundice, or scleral icterus are signs of liver damage.

*Para-aminosalicylic acid (PAS)* is used in combination to increase primary drug effectiveness and to delay drug resistance. Para-aminosalicylic acid is not as effective a tuberculostatic agent as isoniazid, rifampin, ethambutol, and streptomycin. PAS is given as the sodium or other salt in doses of 12 to 15 Gm. daily (0.5 Gm. tablets), usually in three doses of 4 Gm. each. Toxicity includes diarrhea, nausea, and vomiting; some patients show hepatotoxicity or dermatitis. The drug is tolerated better when given after meals.

A highly purified form of aminosalicylic acid is available which requires a daily dose for an adult of 6 to 8 Gm. This has fewer side effects than any of the salts of the acid and is more expensive. It is useful for an individual whose organisms are sensitive to PAS because the patient is much more likely to maintain a regimen including 12 tablets of PAS than one involving 24 to 30 tablets daily.

*Ethambutol (EMB)* occasionally causes headache, dizziness, nausea, and reduction of visual acuity. The last must be guarded against by an initial ocular history and funduscopic examination and periodic monitoring of red-green color discrimination and visual acuity with a Snellen eye chart. If loss of visual acuity occurs, the drug is discontinued. The initial dosage of ethambutol may be 25 mg. per Kg. The recommended maintenance dose is 15 mg. per Kg. With the latter, ocular side effects are reportedly not a problem.

*Streptomycin (SM)* was the first antibiotic to be employed against tuberculosis. Initially, the physician may prescribe 1 Gm. of streptomycin intramuscularly daily. However, as soon as the most severe symptoms become controlled, the dose is usually reduced to 1 Gm. two or three times a week or the drug is discontinued in order to minimize its toxic effects. Toxic reactions may include vertigo, ataxia, deafness, nausea, vomiting, fever, and rash.

*Rifampin (RIF),* released in this country in 1971, is considered at least as effective as INH and is used for initial treatment or retreatment, usually in combination with INH. It has low toxicity, but can affect the liver, which limits its usefulness in alcoholic patients or others with liver disease. Rifampin's wholesale cost (1974) is about 65 cents per capsule and the usual adult dose is two capsules (600 mg.) daily, which means that the cost of treatment per patient over a two-year period for this one drug would be about $1,000. The retail cost would be very much greater. Cost is a factor limiting the availability of rifampin for treatment in state-supported clinics.

The effectiveness of rifampin is dependent upon the patient's taking the drug each day without interruption. If interruptions occur, the patient may show undesirable side effects and the organisms may develop resistance. Some physicians recommend that rifampin be used only during the period of initial hospitalization, and for retreatment of patients who have failed to respond adequately to other drug combinations. Studies are presently being monitored by the Tuberculosis Division of the Center for Disease Control to determine the effectiveness of rifampin if given in combination for a relatively brief period such as the period of acute hospitalization with subsequent use of other drugs.

## Secondary Drugs

Some other drugs are available when the patient has adverse reactions to the initial treatment drugs, and when the patient's mycobacteria become resistant to previously prescribed drugs. Use of secondary drugs is limited by their tendency to cause toxic symptoms. Bacterial resistance also occurs when secondary drugs are used. These "secondary drugs" include viomycin, pyrazinamide, cycloserine, kanamycin, ethionamide, and capreomycin. See Table 31-1 for dosage, side effects, and monitoring.

*Adrenocorticosteroids* (such as prednisone) can be prescribed for short periods (always in combination with antituberculosis drugs) to reduce complications and mortality in patients with tuberculous meningitis, tuberculous pleurisy, tuberculous pericarditis, tuberculous peritonitis, and far-advanced pulmonary tuberculosis. Because of the possibility of side effects of corticosteroids, such as diabetes, gastric ulcer, hypertension, fluid retention, and excessive potassium excretion, these drugs have to be used with special precautions under close medical supervision.

## Drug Administration

All of the tuberculostatic drugs should be given for long periods without interruption, since healing is slow and resistance to drugs may be increased by interrupted treatment. Lapses in the administration of these drugs can be serious, and the patient should understand the importance of taking his drugs regularly. If he refuses or is unable to take the prescribed medication, the nurse should consult with the patient to find out the reason. The problem can be an economic or psychosocial one rather than physical intolerance. For example, the ghetto dweller living a chaotic hand-to-mouth existence may relegate the daily taking of pills for an asymptomatic condition to a much lower priority than that desired by the health care team. Thus the patient advocate must find out what the basic problem is and must try to do something about it even though it may not be treatment-related, or the goals of treatment will not be met.

For example, a worker might be embarrassed to have to swallow a large number of pills at one time in front of his coworkers. In such a case the physician may allow him to take the entire daily amount of drugs at one time, before or after work.

Current medical opinion is that antituberculosis drugs should be administered once a day, rather than in divided doses three or four times a day. The rationale for this view is that the higher blood level which is achieved for a few hours after administration of the total daily dose (all at once) is more effective in arresting the proliferation of tubercle bacilli than is the use of divided doses. Use of the single daily dose makes it especially important to explain the purpose and value of this regimen to the patient, since it usually requires him to swallow a large number of pills at one time. The educationally deprived patient may not understand or appreciate this; he may require a much longer time period and a great deal of patience for minimal goals of patient education to be accomplished.

This patient may need someone to administer the drugs daily or to carefully monitor his self-medication routine. Since many patients also receive medicines other than tuberculostatic drugs, it is important to schedule administration of these drugs (such as vitamins) at some time other than the time when the patient must take his tuberculostatic drugs. This decreases somewhat the number of oral medications the patient must take at any one time.

### Table 31-1. Antituberculosis Drugs and Their Side Effects

| DRUG | DOSAGE (Adult-Daily) | SIDE EFFECTS (Usual) | MONITORING† | REMARKS |
|---|---|---|---|---|
| Isoniazid (INH) | 5-10 mg/kg 300-600 mg | Peripheral neuritis, hepatitis, hypersensitivity, convulsions | SGOT/SGPT (not as a routine) | For neuritis, pyridoxine 25-50 mg as prophylaxis; 50-100 mg as treatment |
| Ethambutol (EMB) | 25 mg/kg for 60 days, then 15 mg/kg§ | Optic neuritis (reversible with discontinuation of drug; very rare at 15 mg/kg); skin rash | Visual acuity, red-green color discrimination (Snellen Chart) | Ocular history and funduscopic exam before use; contraindicated with optic neuritis; use with caution if serious ocular problems |
| Streptomycin (SM) | 0.75 gram-1.0 gram (frequently given for initial 60 days with advanced disease) | Otic and vestibular toxicity, decreased hearing, vertigo, tinnitus (nephrotoxicity—rare) | Gross hearing (ticking of watch): if abnormal, audiograms; BUN and creatinine | More common in older patients (> 60); decrease dose or avoid drug if renal insufficiency |
| Para-aminosalicylic acid (aminosalicylic acid) | 12-15 grams | Gastrointestinal, hypersensitivity (rash), hepatotoxicity, sodium load | SGOT/SGPT | For GI irritation temporarily reduce dose or use Ca, K, ascorbic acid or resin combinations; avoid Na salt in elderly or patients with heart failure or renal disease |
| Rifampin | 600 mg once daily (children, 10-20 mg/kg to a maximum of 600) | Minimal; liver dysfunction rarely | SGOT/SGPT | Extremely effective |
| Ethionamide‡ | 750-1000 mg | Gastrointestinal, hepatotoxicity, hypersensitivity (rash) | SGOT/SGPT | Temporarily stop or reduce dose with GI irritation and hepatotoxictiy |
| Pyrazinamide‡ (PZA) | 20-35 mg/kg; not over 3 grams | Hyperuricemia, hepatotoxicity, arthralgia | Uric acid, SGOT/SGPT | Benemid or allopurinol to reduce serum uric acid |
| Cycloserine‡ | 750 mg | Psychosis, personality changes, convulsions, rash | Drug blood levels if poor renal function | Pyridoxine, 50-300 mg/day may help; mental problems more common with predisposition |
| Capreomycin‡ | 1 gram daily for 60-120 days, followed by 1 gram 2 to 3 times weekly | Nephrotoxicity, ototoxicity, hepatotoxicity, hypersensitivity | Same as streptomycin with SGOT/SGPT in addition | Effective, newly released drug; not for pediatric use |
| Viomycin‡ | 1 gram every 12 hours twice a week | Similar to streptomycin but nephrotoxicity more common | As for streptomycin, plus urinalysis | As for streptomycin |
| Kanamycin‡ | 0.5-1 gram | | | Rarely used |

† The most important monitoring device is an informed patient having ready access to medical care supplemented by a careful history and appropriate physical examination.

§ FDA recommends 15 mg/kg for entire treatment period except for re-treatment cases, when 25 mg/kg is recommended for the initial 60 days.

‡These are the so-called second-line drugs which have more frequent and more severe side effects; knowledge and experience in their use is a desirable prerequisite.

(Weg, J. G.: *Treatment and Control of Tuberculosis,* National Tuberculosis and Respiratory Disease Association, 1972)

## Additional Treatment Modalities

Rest and a nutritious diet are important also in the therapeutic regimen; however, because there is now more definitive treatment for the disease, the regimen of healthful living has now taken its place in a supportive role, leaving the primary focus on drug therapy. Special diets are used only for those patients with concomitant problems such as diabetes, malnutrition, or alcoholic liver damage. A well-balanced 2,500-calorie diet is usually prescribed with increases according to the caloric expenditure involved in work activities.

Many urban poor patients with tuberculosis are malnourished in a very basic sense. They may be admitted to the hospital for initial treatment because they need food as well as diagnostic tests and drugs. A meager welfare check, lack of mobility to do comparison shopping, lack of knowledge of what an adequate diet includes, and loneliness are factors which contribute to malnutrition.

While prolonged bed rest used to be typical, it is no longer considered necessary for most patients. Bed rest is usually prescribed only for seriously ill patients and for those who have had recent hemoptysis. Others are permitted to go to the bathroom, and to be out of bed for gradually increasing periods. Rest, in the sense of relief from worry and strain, continues to be important. If the patient is tense and anxious, and worried about his prognosis or his family, he will be unable to rest.

There is now also recognition that while special climates may offer enjoyable diversion and rest, relocation to such places is not necessary for effective treatment.

## Outpatient Care

Many factors determine the advisability of home or hospital care. The degree of the patient's illness, concomitant illnesses, his living situation, whether his sputum is positive, and his estimated capacity to carry out the full treatment program are important considerations. With the exception of those with multiple socioeconomic or psychological problems in addition to physical illness, today the greater period of drug therapy is carried out while the patient is at home. Patients receive their medical care at the physician's office, a hospital outpatient clinic, or a neighborhood health center. The visits of the community health nurse, or home health aide working under her direction, are important in assisting the patient to carry out his treatment and to adapt to his living situation as necessary.

It is an unfortunate fact that many patients who need continuous community health nursing support live in neighborhoods characterized by a high incidence of crime, which makes it dangerous for a lone nurse to make home visits. Strategies must be developed appropriate to the locale which minimize the risk of harm to the health worker and maximize the patient's chances for sustained support. Such an approach might consist of a team of health workers traveling to a neighborhood by car and visiting patients homes in pairs or larger groups.

Providing ongoing evaluation of the patient's adherence to the treatment regime as well as individual or group instruction regarding the disease and its treatment are other important roles of the community health nurse in the clinic. As in other situations, patient participation in education or counseling sessions with others with the same disease can be a source of great sustenance and continuing motivation to stick with the treatment program. Social work services, individual counseling, and vocational guidance services should also be made available to the patient with tuberculosis.

It is important to emphasize to the patient the necessity for returning regularly to the clinic or office for overall health supervision, sensitivity testing of his organisms for the drugs he is taking, and monitoring for drug effectiveness and toxicity. Patients who do not keep their appointments must be contacted by telephone, letter, or personal visit. The cooperation of hostile or rebellious patients can often be secured when they are approached with compassionate firmness by a health worker who shares the patient's racial and cultural background rather than someone from the traditional societal authority structure (Saltman, 1973).

Systems of outpatient care which minimize the traditional long waiting times in clinics are more likely to secure the patient's cooperation, especially when clinic hours can more realistically be related to a patient's working hours so that time is not lost from the job or so that a mother who must bring small children with her does not become frustrated and exhausted. Nurse-managed neighborhood satellite clinics where patients can be more personally monitored and obtain drugs quickly, yet can be referred to a central clinic when medical services are necessary, are one means to encourage compliance with the therapeutic program.

Tuberculosis (in any site) is a reportable disease. Individualizing approaches to patients makes it less necessary to resort to legal sanctions for the control of persons deemed a menace to the health of the public or their household contacts.

Occasionally, especially among the very downtrodden, it is necessary to evaluate a patient's reliability in taking his drugs, by using urine tests to monitor medication ingestion. If the patient is unreliable in daily medication taking, a health team member or personal acquaintance must assume this responsibility, or the patient may require inpatient treatment for his own well-being as well as that of others.

## Hospitalization

Admission to a general hospital is primarily to establish a diagnosis quickly and efficiently, to combat infectiousness, to initiate drug therapy and evaluate the patient's response, and to educate the patient and close contacts about the long-term management of the disease and secure their commitment to the program. When the acute phase of the illness has subsided and the disease is considered noncontagious in response to chemotherapy, there is no longer a need for hospitalization in an acute care facility. The necessary referrals to appropriate community resources for outpatient care should be initiated prior to discharge. When tuberculosis is but one problem among many with which a patient cannot cope without a great deal more assistance than can be provided him as an outpatient, arrangements are made for transfer to a specialized intermediate or extended-care facility.

**Sanitarium Care.** Chest hospital care today is largely limited to those patients whose overwhelming sociocultural problems, concomitant illnesses such as alcoholism, or predictable inability to adhere to a treatment program necessitate the provision of supervised shelter and long-term attention to counseling, educational, and health care needs. Many of these patients are homeless, elderly, poor, and debilitated. The length of stay depends on an assessment of the patient's capacity to live in the community and continue care responsibly on an outpatient basis. Sanitaria specifically for the treatment of tuberculosis are considered by many to be economically impractical today because of the reduction in incidence of tuberculosis and in the length of confinement necessary to treat the disease.

## Care in the General Hospital

*Guidelines for the General Hospital in the Admission and Care of Tuberculosis Patients,* based on sound scientific evidence, has been published by the National Tuberculosis and Respiratory Disease Association (1969). Acceptance of these guidelines has been slow, possibly because of unfamiliarity with the rationale of the modern management of tuberculosis and fear based on recollection of earlier experiences with the disease rather than current realities. Hospital, medical and nursing practice based more on ritual than rationale still subjects patients to the often dehumanizing experience of isolation when it is not necessary. Within a few days after the institution of a full program of chemotherapy, communicability is markedly reduced. The greatest tuberculosis hazard in hospitals is from unrecognized disease in patients admitted for other reasons. Patients with diagnosed or suspected tuberculosis are admitted to private rooms in a special area or to larger rooms restricted to tuberculosis patients on respiratory isolation precautions until such time as the disease is shown to be noncommunicable. Grouping of patients in this way also facilitates the educational process.

Guidelines for infection control committees in general hospitals admitting tuberculosis patients, concerned with patient care as well as employee protection, have been approved by the American Hospital Association and the American Lung Association (*Statement on Care of Patients with Pulmonary Tuberculosis in General Hospitals,* 1972).

Nurses have a key role in helping the tuberculosis patient in the general hospital to have a positive experience which enables him to learn more about his illness, to understand the ways he can participate in protecting others from infection, and to establish a treatment regimen which he can later carry out at home. Unfortunately, it is not unusual for a tuberculosis patient treated in the general hospital to feel rejected, and to receive the impression that his illness is a menace to staff and to other patients. While the protective techniques employed may be elaborate, they may also be quite ineffective in preventing spread of infection. For instance, staff may don cap, gown, and mask to enter the patient's room to hand him an oral medication, but little attention may be given to ventilation and to use of ultraviolet light in the patient's room. Use of the latter measures plus emphasis upon careful hand washing, safe disposal of sputum, and education of the patient are effective in preventing spread of tuberculosis, whereas the use of gowns and masks is ineffective and not called for. Masks are indicated to be worn by the patient only during instances of intimate face-to-face contact when in the contagious phase, and when the patient is unwilling or unable to cover his cough (*Infectiousness of Tuberculosis,* 1967).

With regard to respiratory isolation precautions, patients with active tuberculosis who may have positive sputum should be placed in rooms with individual air-conditioning units or with exhaust ventilation. These rooms must not be connected with the general air-conditioning or ventilation system serving other parts of the hospital because infectious droplet nuclei could then be transported to other rooms.

Too often the tuberculosis patient in the general hospital is given the impression that others will take all the precautions, and that his role is to acquiesce passively in whatever protective techniques are employed. Fostering the patient's participation, by instructing him in such measures as covering his cough and disposing of sputum, can help increase his feelings of self-esteem and responsibility toward himself and others.

### Protection of Personnel

Various techniques have been established for protecting hospital personnel from infection. It is important for the nurse to familiarize herself with the details practiced in each particular setting, since protective techniques are ineffective unless they are consistently practiced by all personnel. In medical as well as in surgical asepsis each practitioner, whether physician, nurse, orderly, or maid, depends on the others for meticulous attention to such matters as hand washing and handling of sputum cups. Knowing whether the patient's sputum or other excreta contain tubercle bacilli forms the rational basis for the use of precautions. No protective technique is required, other than the usual hygienic measures employed with any patient, when the patient's body is not discharging organisms. Therefore, patients with arrested disease may mingle freely with others both within the hospital and later when they resume living in the community.

Routine chest x-rays of all patients on admission to a clinic or inpatient facility and in employee tuberculosis surveillance programs (Weg, 1971) is a method of providing for personnel safety. The American Hospital Association recommends that tuberculin-negative hospital employees have repeat skin tests at least annually, and more often if respiratory exposure of infectious patients is intimate or prolonged. Tuberculin-positive employees should have annual chest x-rays and it is strongly recommended that recent converters be given one year of chemoprophylaxis (*Statement on Care of Patients with Pulmonary Tuberculosis in General Hospitals,* 1972).

### Surgical Treatment

Surgical treatment in the general hospital may be required for patients with advanced disease or for those who do not respond to medical treatment. Resistance of organisms to chemotherapeutic agents is an important factor in lack of response to medical treatment.

Radical surgery, such as pneumonectomy (removal of an entire lung), is done less frequently than formerly, and there is increasing use of operations that remove only a portion of the lung. When the disease is located primarily in one section of the lung, that portion may be removed by *segmental resection* (removal of a segment of a lobe) or by *wedge resection* (removal of a wedge of diseased tissue). If the diseased area is larger, *lobectomy* (removal of a lobe) may be done.

Various procedures used to be employed to collapse portions of the lung in order to facilitate healing. These measures have been largely supplanted by newer therapies in this country.

## Complications

Two complications of pulmonary tuberculosis are hemorrhage and spontaneous pneumothorax. Careful observation for the signs of complications, as well as skilled care if they should appear, are important responsibilities of the nurse.

### Hemorrhage

Hemorrhage may begin with streaking or staining of sputum, or it may occur without warning. Patients may be restless and anxious before hemorrhage from any part of the body; however, these changes may be so slight as to be noted only in retrospect. The amount of bleeding may vary from a few drops to several ounces. Copious bleeding is extremely frightening to the patient and to the family members if they are present.

The nurse can be of greatest help to the hemorrhaging patient by staying with him and signaling for someone else to call the physician. If the nurse is the only staff member on the ward, she should explain to the patient that she must leave to call the physician, but that she will return promptly. She can reassure her patient better if she herself realizes that hemorrhage is seldom fatal. Death, when it occurs, is due more often to asphyxia than to actual blood loss. However, hemoptysis may cause the spread of the disease, as well as anemia, if the blood loss is severe or frequent.

The nurse's first action when hemoptysis occurs usually is to provide a receptacle into which the patient may expectorate and to help him to assume a position that prevents aspiration of the blood. The nurse's presence is a potent factor in reassurance, since being left alone at this time increases the patient's fear. Although she may not feel calm, an assured and confident manner will help to lessen the patient's apprehension.

It is important to note the amount of bleeding, the patient's color, pulse, and blood pressure and to be ready to report these to the physician. Blood that is expectorated, as well as the receptacles used, should be handled with careful medical aseptic technique.

The physician often will order sedation sufficient only to decrease apprehension and excessive coughing but not sufficient to abolish cough completely, thus permitting the retention of blood in the respiratory passages. Frequently, complete bed rest and nothing by mouth are ordered immediately after the hemorrhage. If fluids are permitted, sips of cold beverages are refreshing. Lying on the unaffected side should be avoided (the physician will determine the site of the bleeding), since it may increase the likelihood of spreading the disease. Nursing care should encourage rest and avoid factors that might lead to renewed bleeding.

Assisting with personal hygiene should be carried out with discretion; morning care should not become an automatic routine. For example, even though it may be time for the bath, it may be better for this patient to be allowed to rest. A little later a partial bath may be given. It is advisable to be very gentle when giving back care; this precaution may help to prevent further bleeding. Careful mouth care is important to remove the disagreeable taste and the odor of old blood.

Sometimes transfusions and infusions are necessary if the bleeding has been severe. Care must be taken to administer intravenous fluids slowly, so that bleeding is not reactivated. Surgical excision may be life-saving in severe cases if a surgical team can be rapidly mobilized.

### Spontaneous Pneumothorax

Occasionally, during the disease process air escapes from the lung and enters the pleural space, causing the lung to collapse. The collapse of the lung interferes with respiration and may lead to empyema by allowing inhaled bacteria to reach the pleural space. Spontaneous pneumothorax may occur in a variety of pulmonary conditions, including emphysema. It occurs infrequently in association with tuberculosis.

The first symptoms of spontaneous pneumothorax are a sudden sharp pain in the chest, dyspnea, and severe apprehension. Other symptoms include faintness, profuse perspiration, fall in blood pressure, and weak, rapid pulse. The color usually is pale or slightly cyanotic. As in the nursing of a patient with hemorrhage, it is desirable, if possible, for one nurse to remain with the patient to help to lessen his apprehension, while another nurse notifies the physician and prepares equipment for use in treatment.

The patient should be placed in a sitting position, since this makes it easier for him to breathe. Oxygen may be ordered. A thoracentesis is performed in order to remove air from the pleural space and to permit the re-expansion of the lung. If air continues to enter the pleural space, a catheter may be inserted and closed drainage of the chest instituted. After spontaneous pneumothorax, the patient should be allowed to rest and instructed to avoid physical exertion. Lessening the patient's apprehension will help him to breathe quietly and to avoid gasping and coughing. Re-expansion of the lung is checked by roentgenography and fluoroscopy.

## PATIENT EDUCATION AND REHABILITATION

The two earliest measures in rehabilitation are helping the patient and his family to accept the reality of the diagnosis and teaching them about the disease and its treatment. Unless the patient can accept the fact that he has tuberculosis, he will be unable to perceive the need for instruction and treatment.

If the patient is not accustomed to accepting responsibility for his own health, it is difficult but extremely important to help him learn how to follow his treatment, and to assist him in adapting his mode of life as necessary in order to carry out his treatment.

In initiating a teaching program, it is important to avoid overwhelming the patient by detailed instruction before he has had an opportunity to take in what has happened to him. Severe anxiety interferes with learning; therefore, it is unwise to attempt a vigorous instructional program at the onset of the disease, when the patient may be very anxious and perhaps not yet able to accept the fact that he has tuberculosis.

Due to limited opportunities to utilize sources of formal education, the degree of total or partial illiteracy among TB patients from metropolitan ghetto areas is high. The approach to patient teaching, including word usage and the selection of audiovisual materials, must take into consideration the educational level of the individuals involved. Assessment of the cognitive and affective capacities and responses and the psychomotor skills involved in multiple pill taking, especially for the aged, is a necessary component of any education program.

The main points to teach the patient and his family include: the nature of the illness, its course and its treatment; the prevention of its spread; the need for medical followup throughout therapy; and the gradual resumption of social, vocational and recreational activities.

The nurse can find many ways of helping the patient to bridge the gap between dependence on care during illness and independent living. The gradual resumption of independence as the illness improves is important.

The period of disability from tuberculosis is considerably shorter now than was the case a few years ago. It is therefore especially important to help the patient and his family participate in the plan of treatment as soon as they are able. Although drug therapy must be continued for an extended period, most patients are able to resume their usual activities including the same type of work (except where there is certain respiratory hazard) within a relatively short period.

For the patient in the sanitarium, the opportunity to go to the dining room, rather than having a tray brought to the bedside, the wearing of street clothes rather than night clothes, and the opportunity to participate in group activities are all part of rehabilitation, and help to restore self-confidence. Job retraining or the development of skills for gainful employment are important aspects of rehabilitation for the patients who cannot resume their usual work or who had limited employable skills prior to illness.

Stereotypes of the "good patient" and the "cooperative patient" frequently held by medical personnel bear little relation to the patient's chances for recovery. The passive, obedient patient who is often characterized as "good" may have difficulty in resuming independence. Positive relationships between the patient and the staff are extremely important. The patient naturally will seek the approval of those whose care is so important to his recovery. It is essential that the staff, by their own attitudes and their relationships with the patient, encourage his independence, self-respect and self-reliance.

## TUBERCULOSIS CONTROL

The ultimate goal is the eradication of tuberculosis from the community. In addition to treatment and followup of those persons with active tuberculosis, control of the disease depends on case finding and preventive measures, including chemoprophylaxis of individuals at high risk in areas with a high incidence of disease.

### Case Finding

The most sensitive means of identifying the disease is the intradermal tuberculin test (Mantoux). Mass chest x-ray screening programs have been largely discontinued because of the low yield of active cases of TB. An exception is routine chest x-rays of patients admitted to general hospitals.

Selective screening for tuberculosis infection with the aid of the Mantoux test involves such groups as household and close contacts of a patient with newly diagnosed TB; transients or residents of places with known or suspected high incidence such as skid-row areas or prisons; those in certain industries such as asbestos manufacture or mining operations; hospital or other institutional staff such as physicians, nurses, aides, or attendants in close and prolonged contact with diagnosed or suspected tuberculosis patients; those likely to infect others such as teachers in contact with children; and those in special clinical situations such as long-term steroid therapy, with diabetes, or who have undergone gastrectomy. It is recommended that positive Mantoux reactors from these groups have a complete diagnostic workup, including a chest x-ray.

## Chemoprophylaxis

Chemoprophylaxis, such as with INH 300 mgm. daily for 12 months for the adult, is recommended for positive reactors in certain high priority groups:

1. All household contacts of new and reactivated cases whether tuberculin positive or negative (especially children).
2. Those of any age whose skin test converts from negative to positive within two years.
3. Those with known inactive tuberculosis not previously treated with drugs or treated inadequately.
4. Positive tuberculin reactors with abnormal findings in the chest x-ray.
5. Positive tuberculin reactors under the age of 20 years.
6. Positive reactors in special clinical situations, e.g., those with unstable diabetes mellitus, gastrectomy (who may be undernourished as a result of malabsorption), silicosis, leukemia, Hodgkin's disease, or on adrenal corticosteroid therapy (*Preventive Treatment of Tuberculosis*, 1971)

There is no evidence to support the continuation of preventive therapy with INH beyond one year, even in silicosis or other chronic diseases.

## BCG Prophylaxis

In other countries, for people who are exposed to the disease frequently or who may be particularly vulnerable to it, or in areas where tuberculosis is widespread, BCG (Bacillus Calmette-Guérin) vaccine is often used. This vaccine is made from living, attenuated tubercle bacilli and is given to those who react negatively to tuberculin. Although it offers some protection, BCG cannot be relied on for the complete prophylaxis of the disease.

Because those who receive BCG develop a positive tuberculin reaction, the use of the vaccine negates the usefulness of tuberculin testing, which is one reason why BCG is not widely used in the United States.

Those who receive BCG are given periodic x-ray examinations to detect possible development of tuberculosis. However, in areas where the incidence of tuberculosis is high and where a considerable segment of the population is tuberculin-positive, interference by BCG with the use of tuberculin testing often is viewed as less important than the conferring of some degree of protection.

## Further Prophylactic Measures

The education of the public and improved living and working conditions have helped to reduce the incidence of tuberculosis. People in this country are better clothed, fed, and housed than they were at the turn of the century, when tuberculosis was a leading killer. Hours of work are shorter, and, as more active cases are detected and treated, fewer sources of infection exist within the community.

The American Lung Association (formerly the National Tuberculosis and Respiratory Disease Association) has been a powerful force in the control of tuberculosis. Though it does not give direct patient services, ALA has been active in public education and in cooperating with official agencies in detection and control programs through the provision of support services such as literature distribution and publicity. Local chapters are an excellent community resource with which nurses may wish to become familiar. Films and charts provided by the Association are available for professional groups, such as nursing students. Many of the Association's pamphlets are excellent teaching aids for patients and their families.

In addition, the combined resources of the National League for Nursing and the American Lung Association (ALA Nursing Department at NLN) facilitate the development of effective nursing services for persons with pulmonary disease through educational and consultative services to individuals, health care institutions, and educational institutions.

## REFERENCES AND BIBLIOGRAPHY

American Hospital Association: *Statement on Care of Patients with Pulmonary Tuberculosis in General Hospitals,* Chicago, 1972.

American Lung Association: *Diagnostic Standards and Classification of Tuberculosis and Other Mycobacterial Diseases,* New York, 1974.

————: *The Tuberculin Skin Test,* supplement to *Diagnostic Standards and Classification of Tuberculosis and Other Mycobacterial Diseases,* New York, 1974.

BARHAM, V. Z.: How I wanted to be treated, *Nurs. Outlook* 19:48, January 1971.

————: Tuberculosis care—1971. Changing the attitudes of hospital nurses. *Nurs. Outlook* 19:588, August 1971.

BUCHARDT, E. M.: Nurse-directed clinics in rural Kentucky. Without them, patients can't get there, *NTRDA Bull.* 57:6, June 1961.

Conference on Immunization in Tuberculosis, Bethesda, Md., U. S. Natl. Institutes of Health, 1972 (Supt. of Docs., U. S. Govt. Printing Office).

FAGERHAUCH, S. Y.: Mental illness and the tuberculosis patient, *Nurs. Outlook*, 18:38, August 1970.

FISHER, L.: Rifampin—new and potent drug for TB treatment, *NTRDA Bull.* 57:11, September 1971.

FREEMAN, R. B.: Practice as protest, *Am. J. Nurs.* 71:918, May 1971.

FREEMAN, S. O.: Tuberculin testing and screening: A critical evaluation, *Hosp. Pract.* 7:63, May 1972.

GALLAGHER, M.: Communicate, or else (#45-1477), NLN Publ. Nurs. Advisory Serv., NLN-NTRDA: 69, 1973.

GARRETT, J. F. (ed.): *Psychological Aspects of Physical Disability*, U. S. Department of Health, Education and Welfare, Washington, D. C., U. S. Government Printing Office (n.d.).

GATLING, I. W.: Tuberculosis nursing: A challenge to the metropolitan nurse, New York, National League for nursing, NLN Publ. (#45-1378):32, 1969.

GRASSO, M.: *Pulmonary Tuberculosis* (A Teaching Program for Student Nurses), Englewood, N. J., Panray Div., Ormont Drug and Chemical Co., Inc., 1973.

JOHNSON, J. E., III (ed.): *Rational Therapy and Control of Tuberculosis,* Gainesville, Univ. of Florida Press, 1970.

KELLY, H. B.: Tuberculosis care 1971, patient population and treatment choices, *Nurs. Outlook* 19:541, August 1971.

KOSIK, S.: Patient advocacy or fighting the system, *Am. J. Nurs.* 72:694, April 1972.

MARVIN, B. A.: Denver's nurse-directed TB clinic, *NTRDA Bull.* 57:2, June 1971.

MCINNIS, J.: Do patients take antituberculosis drugs? *Am. J. Nurs.* 70:2152, October 1970.

MOODIE, A. S., et al.: Baltimore uses inner city aides in a tuberculosis control program, *Pub. Health Rep.* 85:955, November 1970.

MURPHY, P. R.: Tuberculosis control in San Francisco's Chinatown, *Am. J. Nurs.* 70:1044, May 1970.

———: Satellite clinics for tuberculosis care, *Nurs. Outlook* 20:186, March 1972.

MUSHLIN, I., et al.: Big city approach to tuberculosis control, *Am. J. Nurs.* 71:2342, December 1971.

National League for Nursing: *Patient Care in Tuberculosis,* Publ. No. 45-1414, New York, 1973.

National Tuberculosis and Respiratory Disease Association: *Guidelines for the General Hospital in the Admission and Care of Tuberculosis Patients,* New York, 1969.

———: *Infectiousness of Tuberculosis,* Report of the NTRDA Ad Hoc Committee on Treatment of TB Patients in General Hospitals, New York, 1967.

———: *Introduction to Respiratory Diseases,* ed. 4, New York, 1969.

———: *Preventive Treatment of Tuberculosis,* New York, 1971.

Ormont Drug and Chemical Co., Inc., Panray Div., Englewood, N. J.: Information supplied on tuberculin testing with Sterneedle multiple puncture test.

PALMER, H. D., M.D.: Personal communication.

SALTMAN, J.: Health aides make the difference in Baltimore's TB program, *Am. Lung Assoc. Bull.,* 59:205, July-August 1973.

THORP, D.: Click, click, and Harry has his TB drugs, *Am. Lung Assoc. Bull.* 59:2, June 1973.

TIZES, R.: Tuberculosis in suburbia—new indices for an old disease, *Am. J. Pub. Health* 62:1586, December 1972.

U.S. Department of Health, Education and Welfare: *1972 Tuberculosis Statistics: States and Cities,* DHEW Publ. No. (CDC) 74-8249, June 1973 issue.

———: *Reported Tuberculosis Data 1972,* Publ. No. (CDC) 74-8201, December 1973 issue.

WEG, J. C.: Tuberculosis and the generation gap. *Am. J. Nurs.* 71:495, March 1971.

———: *Treatment and Control of Tuberculosis* (pamphlet), New York, National Tuberculosis and Respiratory Disease Association, 1972.

WRIGHT, M. G., et al.: Tuberculosis in the 70's, *Canad. Nurse* 68:27, June 1972.

## Film

*The Modern Management of Tuberculosis.* American Lung Association. Loan prints available from Dow Pharmaceuticals, The Dow Chemical Company, Indianapolis, Indiana 46206.

# UNIT SEVEN

## Insults to Cardiovascular Integrity

# The Patient with a Blood or Lymph Disorder

Many people with blood dyscrasias or related disorders are chronically ill. The term "chronic illness" is often used in our society synonymously with a disease of old age. But more than 75 per cent of protracted illness occurs between the ages of 15 and 64 years (Parets, 1967). Chronic illness taxes the patient's resources to the utmost. While his body is in the throes of physical illness, he must modify his beliefs, goals, interests, social contacts, and his usual daily habit of living. The chronically ill have fears based on fact and reality. Among these are the fear of death, incapacitation, abandonment, economic bankruptcy, and the fear of spreading disease to others. Loss of self-esteem and changes in family and social relationships add to the deprivation experienced by the patient.

When the patient's disease carries a fatal prognosis, as in leukemia, the nurse can provide support in many ways. Physical care and various therapies such as the use of chemotherapeutic agents exert heavy demands on knowledge, skills, and time. However, the emotional drain on the nurse who supports the patient during the experience is taxing. She becomes vulnerable to feelings of helplessness, frustration, anger, and sadness. So that she can be an effective support for the patient and family as they attempt to cope with their problems, it would be wise for the nurse who works with patients who have blood dyscrasias to seek help with her own feelings. This can be done, for example, through discussions led by a nurse counselor for a group of nurses experiencing similar clinical situations, or interdisciplinary group meetings dealing with the needs of specific patients. (See Chapter 12 for care of the dying patient.)

567

## BLOOD DISORDERS

The term *blood dyscrasias* often is used to describe a large group of disorders affecting the blood. (*Dyscrasia* is derived from Greek words meaning *bad* and *mixture*.) Although all blood dyscrasias affect the blood in some way, the disorders themselves are manifestations of many different pathologic processes. For instance, leukemia is believed to be due to malignant changes; anemia may be due to a variety of causes, such as blood loss, inadequate formation of red blood cells, or increased destruction of red blood cells. However, regardless of the pathology, disorders of the blood lead to many similar symptoms and nursing problems, and they necessitate many similar kinds of diagnostic tests. For instance, many of these patients exhibit a bleeding tendency that may be due, for example, to reduction in the number of platelets (as occurs in leukemia) or a disturbance of the coagulation of blood (as in hemophilia). Whether bleeding is due to leukemia or hemophilia, nursing problems involving care and observation of the patient with a bleeding tendency are similar.

### Common Diagnostic Tests

The most common type of diagnostic test involves the collection of blood specimens and the comparison of the various elements in the patient's blood with those normally found. Blood samples are obtained by pricking the end of the finger or the ear-lobe, or by venipuncture.

Samples of the blood often are examined for the number of cells and the amount of hemoglobin. The number of white blood cells, platelets and red blood cells per cubic millimeter is compared with the normal values. Frequently, the relative number of the different types of white cells is of diagnostic importance, and a differential count of white blood cells is ordered. The size and the shape of the cells, as well as their number, may be significant. Red blood cells of normal size are called *normocytic,* abnormally small ones are called *microcytic,* and abnormally large ones are called *macrocytic.* The amount of hemoglobin contained in the erythrocytes may be contrasted with the normal, using the terms *hypochromic* (less hemoglobin than normal) and *hyperchromic* (more hemoglobin than normal). Samples of the blood are examined also for the clotting time.

Usually, patients with blood dyscrasias must have repeated blood specimens taken. Often they comment jokingly, "You know, if you keep on taking my blood, I won't have any left." For some patients this is merely a joke, but for others it reflects real apprehension, which is increased by a lack of understanding of the relationship between the amount of the blood drawn and the total amount in the body, as well as the body's constant formation of new blood cells. The sensitive nurse often can detect when such remarks really reflect apprehension and misunderstanding, and she can help the patient by explaining the need for repeated specimens and by clarifying the manner in which the body compensates for small losses of blood. It is possible, however, for a patient in a large hospital under the care of different specialists whose blood specimens are required by different laboratories to suffer needlessly from repeated venipunctures. The nurse in the managerial role should initiate some means of coordinating the diagnostic workup.

Because the nurse frequently is not actually present when a specimen of the blood is drawn, she must make a special effort to remember the patient's need for explanation and reassurance. If the patient is very apprehensive or confused, his nurse can be very helpful by giving a few words of encouragement or by assisting with the procedure. Since many patients with blood dyscrasias have a bleeding tendency, the site of the puncture should be inspected frequently to make sure that there is no oozing. The patient usually is instructed to apply firm pressure to the site for a few minutes after the blood has been withdrawn, preferably with a sterile dry gauze after alcohol sponge.

Sometimes, patients who must have blood taken repeatedly become increasingly apprehensive each time the technician arrives at the bedside. The frequency of the procedure has made the patient dread something that used to seem little more than an inconvenience. Flinching or jumping when the needle is inserted must be recognized for what it is—a sign that the patient's emotional reserves have been worn down by the repeated discomforts of tests and treatments. The nurse's special care, skill, and support are needed by these patients when blood is drawn.

Some patients become more upset when they watch the needle, others when they do not. In any case, the nurse should not deliberately shield the patient's eyes but, instead, should give the patient the opportunity to look at something else or squeeze her hand if he wishes to do so. The nurse also can employ conversational techniques to help divert the patient's mind from the procedure.

**Sternal Puncture.** Specimens of bone marrow are very useful in studying the formation of blood cells. Although these specimens can be obtained from the sternum or the iliac crest, sternal puncture is performed most frequently. The patient lies on his back, either in bed or on the treatment table. The skin over the sternum is cleansed and anesthetized with procaine. A needle is inserted into the marrow of the bone. A dry, sterile 5- to 10-ml. syringe is attached, and specimens are withdrawn. The patient may feel discomfort when the specimen is taken, as well as apprehension and a feeling of pressure when the needle is inserted. (A special needle is used that is short and strong; there is generally a guard on the needle that will prevent it from being inserted too far.)

The nurse assists the patient by making him as comfortable as possible and by clarifying the explanation of the procedure. She positions and drapes the patient, and assists the physician if necessary. As with any test or treatment that is uncomfortable or upsetting, a few words or a smile of encouragement help the patient.

**Capillary Fragility Test.** This test is done to determine how easily the capillaries rupture. In some blood dyscrasias, capillary fragility is increased, leading to tiny hemorrhagic spots (*petechiae*) under the skin. The physician wraps a blood-pressure cuff around the patient's arm, inflates it to a point between the patient's diastolic and systolic blood pressure, and leaves the cuff inflated for five minutes. After he removes the cuff, the physician examines the skin distal to the area where pressure was applied. Normally, only one or two petechiae per square inch are noted. If the patient's capillaries are abnormally fragile, many petechiae will be found. The physician explains the test to the patient; the nurse reinforces this and may assist with the test. Usually, the patient is not told how many petechiae normally appear, since this information might cause him additional worry. He can be told that the development of some tiny red spots on the skin is to be expected when the cuff is removed.

## Importance of Accurate Diagnosis

Laboratory findings are carefully studied and correlated with the patient's history, his symptoms, and his physical examination. An accurate diagnosis is especially important in the light of the popularity of drugs that can be bought without prescription to "build up the blood." Frequently, such preparations are expensive and contain a variety of ingredients such as iron, vitamins, and liver extract. If the patient really is anemic due to the deficient intake of iron, he will be helped just as effectively and much more economically by taking an iron preparation, such as ferrous sulfate. Symptoms that the patient attributes to his blood may be due to some other condition that goes undiagnosed and untreated while he is taking a "shotgun" remedy—so named because of the belief that one of the variety of ingredients may do the patient some good.

Changes in the blood often accompany other disorders. Anemia may be the first warning of cancer, or it may be the first clue to the discovery of a peptic ulcer that has been causing the persistent loss of small amounts of blood. Finding an abnormal blood count is only the beginning. In order to treat the patient effectively, the physician must first discover the cause of the condition.

The nurse can help by explaining the nature of and need for diagnostic tests and educating the public and the individual patient regarding the folly of succumbing to the lures of advertising and trying remedies that can waste money or provide false assurance while a serious disease continues to be undiscovered.

## Anemia

The term *anemia* means that the patient has a decrease in the number of red blood cells and a lower than normal hemoglobin level. The number of red blood cells normally present varies with age, sex, and altitude. Infants have more red blood cells per cubic millimeter than adults. Women have fewer erythrocytes per cubic millimeter than men; normally women average about 4,500,000 red blood cells per cubic millimeter of blood; men average 5,000,000 per cubic millimeter. The difference between men and women in the number of red blood cells is most noticeable during the reproductive years. People who live at very high altitudes have an increased number of red blood cells. It is believed that this helps the body to compensate for the decreased solubility of oxygen at the low atmospheric pressure of high altitudes.

Erythrocytes perform the important function of carrying oxygen from the lungs to the tissues, and carbon dioxide from the tissues to the lungs. The red color of the blood is caused by hemoglobin, which is contained in the erythrocytes. Hemoglobin combines with oxygen to form oxyhemoglobin. The average amount of hemoglobin is 14.5 to 15.0 Gm. per 100 ml. of blood. Men have slightly more hemoglobin than women. As the blood passes through the lungs, oxygen is taken up and carbon dioxide is released. Oxygenated blood is bright red and is carried by arteries and capillaries to all tissues of the body. After the oxygen has been released from the hemoglobin for use by the tissues, the hemoglobin is called "reduced hemoglobin." The blood at this time looks dark red and is returned by the veins to the heart and to the lungs, where the carbon dioxide is released and the blood reoxygenated.

Anemia can be caused by loss, destruction, or faulty production of red blood cells and hemoglobin. Blood loss can occur suddenly and copiously, as in severe hemorrhage from a severed artery, or it may result from slow but persistent bleeding from hemorrhoids or a peptic ulcer. Bleeding also results in the loss of iron from the body, since iron is contained in the hemoglobin. Normally, the body saves and reuses the iron for the production of new hemoglobin after the worn-out red blood cells have been broken down. Because, by increasing its production of erythrocytes, the body can compensate for some degree of loss or destruction of erythrocytes, anemia becomes manifest only when the body is unable to increase its production of erythrocytes sufficiently to compensate for these losses. Normally, production can be increased up to six times when the body supply of erythrocytes has been depleted, as may occur after hemorrhage.

*Hemolysis* (the destruction of red blood cells) leads to a reduction of their number. It is believed that, normally, each red blood cell survives for about four months. Old red blood cells are destroyed in the spleen, the bone marrow, and the liver. The body constantly is making new red blood cells and destroying old ones, so that the number is kept fairly uniform. In hemolytic conditions the red blood cells do not survive as long as they normally do. They may survive only two weeks. The increased destruction of red blood cells leads to anemia. Hemolysis may be caused by infection,

abnormal red blood cells, transfusion of incompatible blood, or exposure to harmful chemicals.

Inadequate production of red blood cells can be due to an injury to the bone marrow (for example, by toxic effects of drugs) or to the lack of necessary materials (such as iron, folic acid, vitamin $B_{12}$) for the formation of red blood cells and hemoglobin. Anemia also may be caused by other diseases, such as cancer and rheumatoid arthritis.

Symptoms of anemia are similar, regardless of the cause, and are due largely to the inability of the blood to transport sufficient oxygen to the tissues. Fatigue, anorexia, faintness, and pallor are typical. The patient may faint, particularly when he is standing for long periods. Pallor may be noted in the nail beds, sclera, conjunctiva, lips, buccal mucosa, tongue, palms, and soles, as well as in the skin. The appearance of the mucous membranes is especially helpful in indicating anemia, since the skin color varies so much in different people. Usually, the patient feels cold, even when others find the temperature quite comfortable. A rapid pulse occurs, because the heart beats faster in order to circulate the limited supply of red blood cells and hemoglobin to the tissues. Since fewer red blood cells are available to carry oxygen, the body sends them around more quickly to supply the requirements of the tissues. Sometimes, the patient is made aware of a rapid heart rate by experiencing palpitations. Exertional dyspnea occurs when anemia is severe, because the ability of the blood to carry oxygen to the tissues is markedly reduced.

### Iron-Deficiency Anemia

Iron is necessary for the production of hemoglobin. Iron-deficiency anemia is frequent among persons whose need for iron is increased. Less than 10 per cent of the iron obtained from food is absorbed. During periods of rapid growth, at the onset of the menses, and during pregnancy there is increased need for iron, which often results in anemia unless additional iron is obtained. It is sometimes difficult to provide for these increased needs with dietary measures alone, although correction of a faulty diet, if it exists, is an important aspect of treatment. Iron-deficiency anemia is characterized by red blood cells that are microcytic and hypochromic.

**Symptoms.** Symptoms are similar to those of anemia from any cause: fatigue, pallor, anorexia, and a feeling of faintness.

**Treatment.** Treatment involves the administration of extra iron, such as ferrous sulfate 0.3 Gm., three times daily. Ferrocholinate is a preparation that is said to produce fewer side effects than ferrous sulfate. The dose of ferrocholinate is 330 to 660 mg. three times daily. Ferric ammonium citrate is sometimes used, in doses of 500 mg. three times daily. Also commonly prescribed is ferrous gluconate. Iron is usually given after meals to lessen the likelihood of gastrointestinal irritation, the most common side effect of iron administration. Some physicians now recommend that iron be given before meals, in the belief that better absorption results. Iron causes the stools to appear black, and patients are always informed of this fact, so that they will not fear that the color indicates gastrointestinal bleeding. Iron is given occasionally in liquid form. It should be taken through a straw; otherwise it will stain the teeth. Iron is given occasionally by injection, particularly when the patient has some intestinal disturbance, such as colitis, that impairs the absorption of iron from the gastrointestinal tract. A preparation for intramuscular use is iron-dextran complex (Imferon). Dosage is adapted to the patient's requirements; initial dose is often 50 mg. Deep intramuscular injection using the Z-track technique is recommended.

Foods high in iron are important in the diet. The patient may have to force himself to eat at first, because the anemia causes anorexia. This is especially important when the body's need for iron is increased, as it is during puberty and pregnancy. Conditions that can lead to chronic blood loss, such as hemorrhoids or uterine tumors, should be treated promptly to avoid the development of anemia.

## Pernicious Anemia

An intrinsic factor normally present in the stomach secretions is necessary for the absorption of vitamin $B_{12}$ found in food. Vitamin $B_{12}$ is necessary for the normal maturation of red blood cells. Patients with pernicious anemia have a lack of the intrinsic factor, which normally is contained in the gastric juice.

Pernicious anemia is a nutritional anemia in the sense that the body is unable to absorb the needed vitamin $B_{12}$ from the food. However, this condition is not the result of a deficient intake; rather, it is the result of the patient's lack of the intrinsic factor.

The body requires such small amounts of vitamin $B_{12}$ that most people have an adequate supply in their food. Animal proteins, such as meat, milk, eggs, and cheese, contain vitamin $B_{12}$, and even a small daily intake of these foods ensures an adequate supply of the vitamin. This point is stressed, because some patients mistakenly believe that pernicious anemia can be cured by diet, and that medication will no longer be necessary. Patients with pernicious anemia do need an adequate diet to maintain general health, and instruction in what constitutes such a diet is indicated if the patient's nutrition is poor. Yet dietary treatment alone is not sufficient. Everyone must help the patient to understand this. Probably, the crux of the problem lies in helping the patient to understand that different types of anemia require different kinds of treatment. The patient with pernicious anemia may have a neighbor with iron-deficiency anemia, whose condition responded quickly to the administration of iron and an improved diet, and who therefore could stop taking the medication.

In contrast, patients with pernicious anemia must have regular injections of vitamin $B_{12}$ to control the disease, because their lack of the intrinsic factor in gastric secretions prevents the adequate absorption of vitamin $B_{12}$ from food. Liver extract used to be given intramuscularly to these patients. It is now recognized that it was actually the vitamin $B_{12}$ in the liver extract that helped the patient. Consequently, vitamin $B_{12}$ is the sole treatment of choice for patients with pernicious anemia.

**Diagnosis** of pernicious anemia is established by the patient's history and symptoms and by studies of his blood and bone marrow. Gastric analysis is often useful, because patients with pernicious anemia usually have achlorhydria, even after the injection of histamine. In the Schilling test, radioactive vitamin $B_{12}$ is administered orally following a parenteral injection of $B_{12}$, and the amount subsequently excreted in the urine is noted. In pernicious anemia, vitamin $B_{12}$ is very poorly absorbed when given orally, and very little of the radioactive drug is found in the urine. The patient's response to parenteral administration of vitamin $B_{12}$ is also of diagnostic significance. A trial dose of vitamin $B_{12}$ is injected, and the patient's hematologic response is noted. Patients with pernicious anemia show definite improvement in the blood picture, as well as symptomatic improvement.

**Treatment.** Vitamin $B_{12}$ (cyanocobalamin) is given intramuscularly in a dosage that is adequate to control the disease. Although the dosage may vary, 100 mcg. once a month is the amount most often ordered. No toxic effects have been noted from the use of vitamin $B_{12}$. Occasionally, oral treatment is given, in the form of capsules or tablets containing both vitamin $B_{12}$ and gastric mucosa (containing the intrinsic factor) obtained from animals. The parenteral administration of vitamin $B_{12}$ usually is considered preferable, because there is greater certainty that the vitamin is absorbed.

**Other Considerations.** Pernicious anemia differs in other important ways from iron-deficiency anemia. The red blood cells, although they are few in number, are macrocytic. They may be hyperchromic or *normochromic* (of normal color). In addition to the usual symptoms of anemia from any cause, patients with pernicious anemia occasionally develop a sore tongue and a sore mouth, digestive disturbances, and diarrhea. The anemia may be so severe that the patient experiences dyspnea on the slightest exertion. Jaundice often occurs. Personality changes are not unusual, especially when the disease is severe. Often the patient is irritable, confused, and depressed. Such changes are most likely to be noted by the patient's family, who often observe that "He just isn't himself lately." Fortunately, personality changes usually disappear promptly with treatment.

If the condition is not treated promptly, the patient develops degenerative changes in the nervous system, sometimes referred to as *combined system disease.* Numbness and tingling of the extremities and ataxia are common. Vibratory and position sense may be lost. Symptoms of neurologic damage may improve somewhat, but permanent damage sometimes occurs before treatment is begun. The earlier the diagnosis and the more prompt the treatment, the greater is the likelihood of escaping permanent neurologic damage. Physical therapy may be of benefit.

Pernicious anemia is most common in the north temperate zones of Europe and the United States. Usually, the patients are over 35 years old. It is sometimes stated that the disease is more likely to occur in blond, blue-eyed people whose hair turns gray prematurely. However, the disease has been noted in persons with widely varied physical characteristics. Both men and women are affected.

**Nursing Care.** During the severe phase of the illness, nursing care involves keeping the patient warm and at rest. Despite anorexia, the patient is encouraged to take easily digested, nutritious foods and fluids. Soft foods that are not highly seasoned are preferable, especially if the patient's mouth is sore. Eggnog, gelatin, and creamed chicken are examples. Appetite usually returns promptly after treatment is begun. Gentleness and patience are important, because the patient is often irritable and apprehensive.

Neurologic symptoms should be watched for and reported if they occur. The prevention of falls is particularly important if the patient is ataxic. The extent of permanent neurologic damage often cannot be assessed at the beginning of the treatment. The physician should answer questions concerning the possibility of recovery from neurologic symptoms. Some of these symptoms may subside or improve after treatment, but the patient may need help in accepting some permanent residual disability. Because the patient is ill and weak he does not have normal resistance to other illnesses and infections. He should be protected from contact with those who have any type of infection.

Some patients are more likely to take the injections with the frequency recommended by the physician if a member of the family is taught to administer the medication. If such instruction cannot be arranged, the patient must return to the office or clinic or have the injections given by a community health nurse. If the patient has been hospitalized, plans for continued treatment should be made before he leaves the hospital. Whether the patient or his family administers the medicine, or whether he returns to the clinic or office, it is of paramount importance that he and his family understand the necessity for continued therapy. If the medicine is skipped, the patient will at first feel no ill effects and may, unless instructed otherwise, believe that the injections are no longer necessary. Teaching the family is particularly important because one of the symptoms of this disease is mental confusion and apathy. The patient who neglects his therapy (visits to the physician or nurse specialist; following treatment at home) may begin to have mental changes that make it impossible for him to recognize the need for treatment.

## Anemia due to Blood Loss

Blood contains cells and liquid (plasma) in approximately equal volume. It has been estimated that the total blood volume is approximately one thirteenth of the body weight. An adult weighing 154 pounds has about six quarts of blood. Normally, the quantity of blood circulating in the body is kept relatively constant at all times.

Blood loss, either acute or chronic, causes anemia. Sudden severe bleeding leads to *hypovolemia* (diminished volume of circulating blood) and shock. The most effective treatment involves the replacement of lost blood by transfusions. If blood loss is chronic, as may be the case in uterine tumors or hemorrhoids, the main treatment is that of the underlying condition causing the bleeding. Depending on the amount of the blood lost, the treatment may include transfusions and/or administration of iron to help the body to compensate for the blood loss. Continued care and observation are necessary for any patient who has experienced blood loss. Sometimes, the patient does not understand the reason for continued care, and, once the emergency is over, he continues to experience fatigue and weakness due to anemia that might have been readily corrected had he realized the importance of returning to his physician's office or to the clinic.

## Anemia due to Destruction of Red Blood Cells

A reduction in red blood cells and hemoglobin may be caused by hemolysis. The life span of the red blood cells is shortened; the cells die more rapidly than they normally should.

*Acquired hemolytic anemia* (sometimes called autoimmune hemolytic disease) is due to the development within the patient's body of substances harmful to his erythrocytes. These patients are treated by corticosteroids. In some patients the steroid can be withdrawn after several weeks; in others, not for several months. Sometimes splenectomy is performed. Transfusions may be necessary.

One group of hereditary hemolytic anemias is referred to generally as *thalassemia.* Thalassemia major, or Cooley's anemia, has a high incidence in the Po valley (Italy) and on islands of the Mediterranean. Treatment of the various forms of thalassemia is symptomatic. Transfusions may be required frequently.

Hemolysis often accompanies severe infections, such as malaria and subacute bacterial endocarditis. Rapid hemolysis is accompanied by chills, fever, prostration, headache, and gastrointestinal disturbances. Jaundice follows, due to the rapid destruction of erythrocytes and the escape of hemoglobin into the plasma. Hemolysis can be caused also by transfusions of incompatible blood and by administration of certain drugs, such as quinine.

The treatment of hemolytic anemia is that of the underlying condition—for instance, stopping the transfusion or the drug and giving supportive treatment, such as oxygen, or treating whatever infection may be present. Transfusions may be necessary to replace red blood cells and hemoglobin.

## Sickle Cell Disease

*Sickle cell disease* is a hereditary blood disorder occurring mostly in blacks. It exists in two forms. Carriers of *sickle cell trait* are usually symptomless but can pass the disease on to future generations. About two million black Americans carry the sickle cell trait. In *sickle cell anemia,* which is present in about 56,000 black Americans, red blood cells carry an abnormal type of hemoglobin (Hb-S instead of normal hemoglobin-A) which does not readily dissolve in fluids when oxygen supply is deficient. The normally round and disk-shaped red blood cell becomes crescent-shaped, or curved like the blade of a sickle. Hemoglobin levels of 7 or 8 mg. per 100 ml. are not uncommon, but most patients make the adaptation necessary to handle the stresses of daily living and minor infections. However, the thicker, heavier, and stickier blood does not flow through the capillaries as easily as normal blood does. Thrombosis and sludging in the capillaries reduces the flow of oxygen to body organs and tissues resulting in the swelling and pain of *sickle cell crisis.*

**Nursing Assessment and Intervention.** *Sickle cell crisis* may be precipitated by many stressors including hypoxia, dehydration, emotional tension, or infection. Under conditions of extreme low oxygen tension, even a carrier may experience sickle cell thrombi. A crisis lasts from about four days to several weeks. Treatment of crisis includes restoration of fluid balance, administration of oxygen to correct hypoxia, transfusion of packed cells, and relief of pain. Careful patient assessment is carried out because the symptoms of crises can mimic other diseases such as appendicitis or rheumatic fever. In the postoperative patient sickle cell crisis can first manifest itself as delayed reaction from anesthesia, tachycardia, or shock. The nurse should administer oxygen, take the vital signs, and notify the physician immediately.

Some hospitals (especially those in urban areas where the prevalence of the disease is higher) routinely screen newly admitted black patients for sickle cell disease. If this is not the case, the primary nurse who does the nursing history can inquire if the patient has been previously screened, and if not, if he has experienced joint swelling, aching bones, or leg ulcers. The physical assessment should include observation for jaundice, pale mucous membranes (Roach, 1972), joint swelling, and skin ulcerations. A history of or suspicion of sickle cell disease should be reported promptly to the physician. A major nursing goal for the hospitalized patient with sickle cell disease is the prevention of hypoxia through such measures as avoidance of upper respiratory infection, performance of pulmonary physiotherapy techniques, careful observation of the patient receiving medications, such as barbiturates, which can depress respirations, and careful monitoring of oxygen therapy.

Teaching the patient with sickle cell anemia and his family about the disease and how to prevent crisis episodes are additional important nursing functions. There is no cure for sickle cell anemia, but chemotherapeutic substances are currently being investigated. The patient's condition must be monitored by laboratory studies on a regular basis. The nurse in the ambulatory care setting has the responsibility for continued teaching and patient and family counseling.

## Aplastic Anemia (Bone Marrow Failure; Aregenerative Anemia)

Erythrocytes, granular leukocytes (granulocytes) and platelets are formed in the bone marrow. *Aplastic anemia* is the term used to describe a condition in which the activity of the bone marrow is depressed, and red blood cells, white blood cells, and platelets are not adequately produced. The formation of one or all of the three elements may be impaired, with varying degrees of severity. Aplastic anemia is a serious toxic manifestation of certain drugs, such as streptomycin, chloramphenicol, (Chloromycetin) and nitrogen mustard. This condition also occurs without known cause. It is believed sometimes to have a hereditary basis.

Anemia, leukopenia (decreased leukocytes), and thrombocytopenia (decreased platelets) result in fatigue, weakness, exertional dyspnea, lowered resistance to infection, and a bleeding tendency. Patients with aplastic anemia are very ill, and the death rate is high.

In treating the condition, every effort must be made to prevent infection. The patient should be in a private room. Meticulous hand washing and a clean gown worn over the uniform while caring for the patient help to prevent the transmission of or-

ganisms to him via the hands or the clothing. The use of a face mask also is recommended occasionally.

The causative agent, if it is known, is removed; for instance, the administration of a toxic drug is discontinued. Repeated transfusions are given to supply erythrocytes and hemoglobin. Usually, antibiotics are given to help to prevent infection. The objectives of treatment are to supply the missing elements of the blood and to prevent or to treat the infection or the bleeding, in the hope that the patient will recover his ability to produce the blood cells. If the bone marrow has been so damaged that this recovery is impossible, death will result. Nursing assessment and intervention for patients with a bleeding tendency are discussed below.

## Leukemia

There are three types of leukocytes (white blood cells): *lymphocytes, monocytes,* and *granulocytes.* Normally, there are between 5,000 and 7,000 leukocytes per cubic millimeter of blood. Fighting infection is one important function of the leukocytes, and they increase in number during most infections. This increase is called *leukocytosis.*

Lymphocytes are produced in the lymphatic tissue; granulocytes are produced chiefly in the bone marrow. It is believed that the different types of leukocytes survive varying lengths of time. Much remains unknown concerning the life span of various kinds of leukocytes. At the end of their life span the leukocytes die and are replaced by the new white blood cells that are constantly being formed.

Blood platelets (*thrombocytes*) are concerned with the clotting of the blood. Normally, there are about 300,000 platelets per cubic millimeter of blood. It takes blood about five minutes to clot in a test tube. This laboratory test is often referred to as "coagulation time" or "clotting time."

Leukemia is a fatal disease characterized by a marked increase in the number of the leukocytes (Fig. 32-1). This rampant increase in the white blood cells is not useful to the body. The patient is less, rather than more, able to cope with infections; although he has more leukocytes, they are immature and therefore are not effective in fighting infections. The rapid proliferation of the leukocytes and of the tissues that produce them results in the diminution of the number of erythrocytes and platelets. The patient eventually suffers from severe anemia, and the reduction in platelets leads to bleeding.

The cause of leukemia remains unknown. Some researchers believe that, rather than being one disease with one cause, leukemia may be a group of diseases of varied etiology. There are two main theories regarding the etiology of leukemia. One is that the disease is caused by infection; the other is that it is essentially a malignant neoplasm causing the unruly proliferation of the white blood cells. The latter theory is now most widely accepted. Recent studies concerning the role of a virus in the etiology of cancer could prove eventually that both theories are correct. Heredity and excessive exposure to radiation are other factors that are believed to play a part in causing leukemia.

The incidence of leukemia is increasing. It is not clear whether this is due to the increased life span that allows more people to live long enough to develop the disease, to improved methods of diagnosis, or to greater exposure to radiation. People whose work entails considerable exposure to radiation have a greater than average risk of developing leukemia.

Leukemia can be acute or chronic. Acute leukemia is more common under age 40, whereas chronic leukemia is more common after age 40. However, either form can occur at any age. Untreated acute leukemia usually causes death within four months, although some patients survive several months, a year, or even longer. Recent evidence has shown significant prolongation of survival in adults with acute leukemia receiving intensive chemotherapy. Prolongation of life has been more apparent in children who have acute leukemia. Chronic leukemia may cause death within two or three years after its onset, but, with treatment, some patients live eight to ten years after developing the disease.

An encouraging aspect of these therapeutic advances is that some patients' lives may not only be prolonged but also are made more comfortable and happy by the temporary remission of symptoms. Although these gains may seem insignificant in view of the ultimately poor prognosis, they offer patients and their families a few more precious months or years together. To those confronted with the loss of a loved one, this reprieve is a priceless gift. It also offers the hope that the life of patients with leukemia can be further prolonged, and that these added years someday will enable some patients to benefit from a cure for the disease.

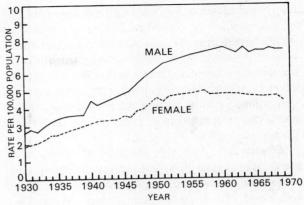

Source: Vital Statistics of the United States.

**Figure 32-1.** Leukemia death rates by sex in the United States, 1930-1969; standardized for age on the 1940 U.S. population. (American Cancer Society)

### Acute Leukemia

**Symptoms.** In acute leukemia, symptoms begin abruptly. The onset often coincides with an acute upper respiratory infection. Ordinarily, attention is directed at first to the symptoms of sore throat, fever, or rhinitis, whereas the seriousness of the underlying illness is unsuspected. Sometimes, the patient is admitted to the hospital for the treatment of the respiratory infection, and the discovery of an unusually large number of leukocytes in the routine admission blood count is the first clue to the existence of the disease. Sometimes unusual pallor, weakness, fatigue, or bleeding warn that the illness involves more than a cold or tonsillitis, and examination of specimens of blood and bone marrow confirms the diagnosis.

The patient's blood usually contains large numbers of leukocytes, with a predominance of immature white blood cells. At first the number of leukocytes may be normal or even below normal. However, as the disease progresses, their number usually increases, sometimes reaching over 100,000 cells per cubic millimeter. The type of leukemia is determined by the type of immature leukocyte that predominates—for example, lymphoblasts or myeloblasts.

Anemia is usually severe and causes pallor, weakness, and fatigue. The number of the platelets is reduced, causing a tendency to bleed. Bleeding may be from any part of the body; it may be internal or external. Common sites from which bleeding occurs include nose, mouth, gastrointestinal

575

tract, and vagina. The bleeding tendency also may be reflected by the persistent oozing of blood after such a minor injury as the administration of an injection. Usually, fever is present, particularly as the disease advances. Occasionally, the patient will develop a spontaneous temporary remission of symptoms, perhaps lasting several months. More often, the symptoms grow progressively and steadily worse.

**Treatment.** Although there is no cure, treatment gives respite from the symptoms. The patient is given repeated blood transfusions to increase his red blood cells and his hemoglobin. Antimetabolites, such as aminopterin, methotrexate (Amethopterin) and 6-Mercaptopurine, are given. Arabinosylcytosine and 6-Thioguanine is one of the most effective drug combinations in the treatment of the adult acute leukemia patient (Gee et al., 1969). These drugs interfere with the multiplication of cells, particularly of cells undergoing rapid proliferation, such as the leukocytes of patients with leukemia. Aminopterin and methotrexate belong to the group of folic acid antagonists, that is, they block (antagonize) folic acid that is needed for the multiplication of the cells. 6-Mercaptopurine and 6-Thioguanine act as antagonists to purines needed by cells that are rapidly growing and dividing. Arabinosylcytosine is a pyrimidine antagonist, blocking the synthesis of DNA which is necessary for proliferating cells. These drugs are highly toxic; they can impair the formation of all blood cells, including erythrocytes and platelets. Other toxic effects include anorexia, nausea, vomiting, and diarrhea. The patient's blood picture is watched very carefully while these drugs are being administered.

Vincristine sulfate is currently being used and is useful in acute lymphoblastic leukemia, but is more effective when used in combination with a corticosteroid like prednisone. Toxic effects include neurologic and neuromuscular disorders such as paralysis, confusion, and nervousness, as well as moderate to severe constipation. Patients should be cautioned to maintain normal bowel habits, with the aid of laxatives if necessary. If constipation occurs, the patient should be advised to let his physician know. Vincristine as well as other cytotoxic drugs may also cause severe partial or total alopecia (hair loss) because they affect the epithelial cells of the hair follicles. Some physicians attempt to reduce the effect of such drugs on the hair follicles of the scalp by tying a tourniquet around the patient's head when the agents are given intra-

venously. This side effect generally causes a psychological depression and patients should be reassured that if their hair does fall out, the hair will regrow after the drug is stopped. The regrowth will take three to four months. Selection of a wig may help the patient feel better during the regrowth period.

Vincristine is carefully administered intravenously generally once a week. If the drug is accidentally infiltrated subcutaneously, a painful inflammation and subsequent ulceration may appear at the injection site. Dosage is individualized; the smallest therapeutically effective amount is utilized. Peripheral neuropathy, adynamic ileus, and myopathy can occur.

Antibiotics are given to treat the secondary infections that so commonly are the complications of the illness. Corticosteroid preparations are used in the treatment of acute leukemia and often provide temporary relief of the symptoms.

The patient eventually becomes resistant to all forms of treatment, and he becomes severely ill with weakness, fever, bleeding and, often, secondary infections such as pneumonia. Often death occurs within a few weeks after the patient develops resistance to treatment.

### Chronic Leukemia

**Onset and Symptoms.** The two most common types of chronic leukemia are lymphocytic and granulocytic. Both conditions have an insidious onset. In chronic lymphocytic leukemia the total leukocyte count is increased, with the largest proportion of the increase in the lymphocytes. Often the disease commences with the painless enlargement of one or several lymph nodes in the neck, axilla, or groin. The patient develops anemia, characterized by fatigue, palpitation, pallor, and dyspnea. A decrease in platelets is reflected in a bleeding tendency. Often the spleen is enlarged (*splenomegaly*).

Marked splenomegaly is often the earliest symptom of chronic granulocytic leukemia. The patient may notice a swelling in his left upper quadrant and a sense of heaviness in his abdomen. The largest proportion of the increased leukocytes consists of granulocytes. The patient develops anemia and thrombocytopenia (symptoms arising from these conditions were discussed previously).

In both types of chronic leukemia the patient may, with treatment, live five years or longer. However, eventually he no longer responds to treatment, and he becomes very weak, has a tendency to bleed, and develops fever. Secondary infections such as influenza or pneumonia are common.

**Treatment.** The treatment of chronic leukemia includes radiotherapy, 6-Mercaptopurine, transfusions and antibiotics for the treatment of secondary infections, and corticosteroids, which provide some relief of symptoms. Chlorambucil (Leukeran) is used, particularly in chronic lymphocytic leukemia. It is a derivative of nitrogen mustard, a drug that is toxic to all tissues and especially so to rapidly growing cells. Severe depression of bone marrow may result from its use, causing aplastic anemia. Nausea and vomiting also may occur. Busulfan (Myleran), which resembles nitrogen mustard, is used, particularly in chronic granulocytic leukemia. Busulfan acts particularly on the cells of the bone marrow. It can cause severe depression of the bone marrow and the development of aplastic anemia. Chlorambucil and busulfan are administered orally. The usual dose of each drug is 2 to 6 mg. Radioactive phosphorus also is used in the treatment of chronic leukemia. The rapidly growing cells—those in the bone marrow particularly—take up the phosphorus. Its radioactivity helps to slow their unruly growth. Radioactive phosphorus is excreted in the urine; special precautions are necessary in the disposing of the urine. Cyclophosphamide (Cytoxan), another drug sometimes used in treatment, inhibits multiplication of cells. Toxic effects include depression of bone marrow, leading to aplastic anemia, nausea, vomiting, and diarrhea. The usual dose is 2 to 3 mg. per Kg. of body weight, daily, orally. The medication may be given intravenously, but generally the oral medication is more convenient and equally effective. (For further information on specific agents used in cancer chemotherapy see Table 17-3.)

### Nursing Assessment and Intervention for Patients with Leukemia

**Acute Phase.** Caring for patients with leukemia makes particular demands on the nurse's observational ability, insight, and adaptability. Newer drugs can cause dramatic changes in the course of the disease. A patient admitted to the hospital with acute leukemia may appear moribund—pale, weak, bleeding, and feverish. Weeks later, as a result of treatment, he may be up and about and ready to go home. But treatment with cytotoxic drugs can make the patient feel worse for a time due to the toxic side effects that sometimes result. And there comes the time when the patient reaches his terminal episode.

Because the hospitalized leukemia patient's condition is rapidly changeable, his nursing care plan is a dynamic one, requiring daily reassessment. Working from the initial data base, the primary nurse keeps the plan updated by anticipating complications, correlating nursing observations with laboratory results, and observing responses of patient and family to the course of illness.

DRUG THERAPY. Specific nursing responsibilities include:

- **Knowing the anticipated action, route of administration, and toxic effects of the various chemotherapeutic agents; when multiple drugs are ordered, the nurse should work with the pharmacist in devising a time and spacing schedule to avoid drug incompatibility.**
- **Administering antiemetics or tranquilizers as ordered.**
- **Observing for allergic reactions such as fever, chills, nausea, or liver and pancreatic dysfunction from toxicity.**
- **Observing for cushingoid features such as "moon" face in the patient on adrenocortical steroids; electrolyte disturbances can also result, such as fluid retention or hypokalemia.**
- **Monitoring blood uric acid lab results and the pH of voided urine. Hyperuricemia can occur from cytotoxic therapy; the nurse can assist the patient to increase his fluid intake.**

The patient may be sensitive about his appearance. Pallor, petechiae, and purpuric areas on the body as well as mouth and lip lesions and discoloration may be painful as well as disfiguring.

MOUTH CARE. Nursing responsibilities include:

- **Providing for frequent mouth rinses with a bland mouthwash such as saline or sodium bicarbonate is important. A mixture of hydrogen peroxide and water can help remove sloughing tissue and old blood.**

  **An effective irrigation device may be achieved by hanging a disposable irrigation container and tubing from an IV pole. The height is adjusted to permit the nurse or patient to direct a gentle stream of water into the mouth. The patient is instructed to keep the fingers out of the mouth.**
- **Vaseline or an emollient can be used to keep the lips from cracking. Orabase may be applied to ulcerated areas to relieve pain and afford protection.**
- **Mouth lesions can interfere with nutrition. The patient is helped to select bland but palatable foods and high-caloric liquids. The family can be encouraged to bring the patient his preferred foods if they are not rough or highly seasoned.**
- **Popsicles can be offered to maintain fluid intake and for cooling and soothing purposes when the patient has difficulty with swallowing or mastication.**

PREVENTION OF INFECTION. A major concern of patient and nurse is the prevention of infection. The myelosuppressant effects of drugs and leukocyte immaturity predispose leukemia patients to infection from organisms which are usually harmless or from opportunistic species. What would be a low-grade infection for the average person might be life-threatening for the patient with leukemia. Nursing intervention includes:

- **Providing for environmental infection controls. Personnel must wash their hands between patients. Visitors or staff members who have any kind of infection, such as colds or boils, should not enter the patient's room. The patient may require standard isolation precautions or be cared for in a life island setting.**
- **Inspecting the skin daily and reporting any unusual findings. The patient is taught to do this if able. Painful skin lesions can result from generalized infections such as Pseudomonas.**
- **Using bacteriocidal agent that may be ordered for bathing the patient.**
- **Knowing that frequent venipunctures and prolonged IV therapy necessitate special efforts to decrease microbial phlebitis (Schumann and Patterson, 1972).**
- **Taking the temperature, reporting any elevation, and assessing the possible causes. Because abscess formation in the anorectal area can easily result following thrombosis of small vessels, rectal temperatures, medications, and enemas are avoided to prevent trauma.**
- **Taking a culture of infected sites and sending this for sensitivity testing as well.**
- **Knowing that organisms from skin infection sites can enter the bloodstream. Gram-negative septicemia and shock are possible, with a fever of 104 to 105 degrees F. (40 to 40.5 degrees C.). Antibiotic therapy, adequate hydration, hypothermia measures, and an antipyretic drug such as Tylenol are ordered. Aspirin is contraindicated since it inhibits normal platelet aggregation and bleeding time is prolonged.**

BLEEDING. Bleeding is often a problem, particularly in subcutaneous and submucosal tissues such as in the mouth. The risk of hemorrhage increases as the platelet count falls to 30,000 per cubic mm. or less. Nursing management for patients with bleeding tendencies include:

- **Observing the skin for petechiae or purpura. Observing body discharges such as saliva, vomitus, urine, and feces for gross blood and testing for occult blood at times, as well as listening to the patient's complaint of painful joints.**
- **Reporting promptly to the physician any signs of bleeding.**
- **Observing the patient's color (Roach, 1972) as well as vital signs, especially increase in pulse rate and drop in blood pressure.**

- **Using or providing the patient with a soft-bristled toothbrush or dentifrice-impregnated tooth swabs to reduce the possibility of trauma.**
  Topical thrombin or Gelfoam is sometimes ordered for hemostasis.
- **Reducing the risk of epistaxis (nosebleed) by instructing the patient to avoid blowing the nose but in turn keeping his nostrils clean with moistened applicators in order to minimize the patient's need to manipulate them. If epistaxis occurs, the patient is placed in high Fowler's position. Hemostasis can be enhanced through the use of ice compresses, the application of a surgical glove filled with ice chips, or a nose clip for continuous gentle pressure if ordered; the physician may use Neo-Synephrine-saturated pledgets, or packing may be necessary.**
- **Assisting with the administration of packed red cells for anemia or a platelet transfusion (Becker, 1972). The labels must be checked carefully, to prevent the administration of incompatible blood. The patient is observed frequently during the transfusion. The blood runs at the rate recommended by the physician. If the patient shows any symptoms that might indicate an allergic reaction to the blood, or that possibly he is receiving the wrong blood, the flow of blood is stopped immediately and the physician notified. Chills, cyanosis, rise in temperature, dyspnea, orthopnea, pain in the lumbar region, restlessness, or urticaria are important signs of incompatibility or allergy.**
- **Keeping the patient at rest during bleeding episodes. Remaining with him is important in the management of the related anxiety.**
- **Observing and reporting complications at other sites. Splenic infarction is characterized by severe pain in the upper left quadrant. Cold applications, such as a large plastic bag filled with a layer of crushed ice, analgesics, and bed rest are ordered. Intracranial hemorrhage can be manifested by headache, irritability, confusion, disorientation. Supportive nursing measures are necessary to prevent further neurological damage. Falls are serious because they may precipitate further internal or external bleeding; side rails are necessary if the patient is confused.**
- **Avoiding the use of sharp instruments such as cuticle scissors or a blade razor by patients with acute leukemia. An electric razor is preferable and may be used with caution.**
- **Avoiding intramuscular injections, since the patient's skin will bruise easily. Medications are usually given orally or intravenously. If intramuscular injections are ordered, they should be kept to a minimum. And when compatible, drugs should be combined to avoid multiple punctures. However, large volumes should be avoided in intramuscular injections since they frequently cause sterile or pyogenic abscesses. Following an intramuscular or other injection, firm pressure should be applied over the site to control the bleeding after withdrawal of the needle. Needle punctures can cause oozing of blood and ecchymoses.**

578

HYGIENIC CARE of the patient is time-consuming and demanding. The patient needs to be kept clean and comfortable. Bathing and other physical ministrations must be accomplished with gentleness and care. Frequent turning and skin care are necessary to prevent pressure ulcers.

PATIENT EDUCATION is an ongoing process. Many patients can cope better if they know what the purposes of treatment are and how to participate in their care. The nurse and/or physician may include the following points in the teaching plan:

- **Inspection of the skin and hygienic care**
- **Taking and recording the temperature**
- **Recognizing signs and symptoms of infection and when to report these**
- **Oral hygiene**
- **Drug treatment and toxic effects**

PROVIDING EMOTIONAL SUPPORT for the patient and family is a major role of the nurse. Disfigurement, discomfort, pain, nausea, fear of hemorrhage, anorexia, weakness, behavior changes, fear of death, and hopelessness are just some of the problems which make care challenging for patient, nurse, and family.

Everything possible is done to help the seriously ill patient and his family. Does a member of the family want to stay all night? A lounge chair or cot with a pillow and a blanket can be provided. The quiet, reassuring presence of a loved one may mean more to the patient than anything else and should be permitted whenever it is possible.

The patient's clergyman often provides comfort and help, both for the patient and his family. By her courtesy and helpfulness the nurse can recognize his important contribution.

Patients often derive help from copatients with the same diagnosis. Though the relationship is supportive in many ways, the death of a friend/patient may cause the other to grieve and to become preoccupied with thoughts of his own demise. A supportive nurse can help by encouraging the patient to talk about his friend's death and listening to his expressions of thoughts and feelings about his own situation. (See also Chapter 12 for care of the dying patient.)

**Remission Phase.** The remission of symptoms in leukemia is often quite dramatic and poses somewhat different problems from those of the patient with cancer. For instance, a 20-year-old who feels well is usually active, busy, and very much involved in planning for his career and establishing his own home and family. If he has acute leukemia, such plans and activities will be short-lived. Most people who work with these patients believe that they should be helped and encouraged to live as full, normal lives as possible. Activity in itself is not harmful, and staying at rest will neither slow the course of the disease nor alter the eventual outcome. The patient should take every precaution to avoid infections, such as colds, and he should seek medical care promptly if he develops the symptoms of any illness. Sufficient rest and an adequate diet are important in preventing secondary infections. During remission meningeal involvement might be evidenced by nausea and vomiting, headache, papilledema, and cranial nerve dysfunction. These symptoms and signs warrant prompt medical attention.

Long-range planning is important. When the patient feels well, he is encouraged to continue his usual activities—at school, at work, or at home. The disease has been temporarily checked, but it has not been overcome. Often, the patient is aware of his diagnosis and prognosis; rarely, the family knows, but the patient does not. (The problems related to telling or not telling the patient he has a fatal disease are discussed in Chapter 12.)

To advise the patient to live as fully and as normally as possible gives no recognition of the agonizing decisions that face patients who know they have leukemia. If the patient is engaged, he may wonder whether going ahead with the marriage would be fair to his fiancée. One young man told his fiancée that he had leukemia. After they had discussed this problem together and had talked later with the physician, they decided that they would continue their plans for marriage, realizing that their period of happiness together might be brief. The patient and others intimately affected by his illness must make these decisions after learning as much as they can about the disease and its prognosis. For every patient, as long as he lives, there is the hope and the possibility that a cure will be found before death occurs.

Life expectancy is longer for patients with chronic leukemia. Because they tend to be older when the disease appears, concern is more likely to be with helping them to maintain their usual occupations and home life than with making decisions concerning career and marriage. Nevertheless, with both types of patients, there is the tremendously important need to help the patient to maintain his will to live and his determination to keep on trying despite an uncertain future.

The patient must understand the importance of returning regularly to the physician's office or clinic. Frequent examinations of the blood and sometimes of the bone marrow are essential, in the light of both his disease and the treatment that he is receiving. Emphasis should be placed on the importance of these examinations in helping him to stay well rather than on the possible complications from drug therapy.

Usually, the patient is admitted to the hospital several times over a period of a few years. Each time that he leaves, he is improved, although often he is not as strong as he was in the early phase of his disease. However, the time comes when his illness strikes for the last time—this time to win. Usually, the patient and his family are well aware when this time has come. Sometimes, the patient says something like this: "Well, it's caught up with me, I guess. I always hoped I'd be the one lucky one—but I suppose I really knew all along that it would be this way."

**During the Final Illness.** The nursing care during the patient's final illness is similar to that cited for the acute phase plus additional considerations for the dying patient (see Chap. 12). Sometimes the patient is cared for at home, so that he can remain with his family and in familiar surroundings. Community health nurses may help to provide care in the home.

Whether the patient is cared for at home or in the hospital, the nurse's role involves helping the family to endure the emotional and the physical strain of the patient's illness. Frequently, the family appreciates the opportunity to do things that help the patient or add to his comfort. Feeding him or bringing in a dish of his favorite food gives the family opportunities to express their love and their concern. The sensitive nurse can encourage such participation without giving the family any less support and help and without pushing them to become involved in the aspects of the care that are too upsetting or too emotionally taxing for them.

The death of a young person is usually harder to accept than that of an older person. Young people with acute leukemia are often surrounded by family members who are deeply grieved and shocked. The staff, too, feels the helplessness of watching a young person die. Usually, the physician and often the nurses have worked with the patient for several years and know him well. The care during the patient's last illness demands of them a high degree of compassion and an awareness and a control of their own feelings.

When death comes to an older person, solace is sometimes derived from the attitude "He led a full life." In the case of a young person, there is often the feeling, "But he was just starting his life." Frequently, family members recognize (even though they may never say it aloud) that the elderly person's life is drawing to a close, and they have time to acknowledge and, to some degree perhaps, accept this fact. But every expectation of the family and the friends of a young person is that he will have opportunity to live and to achieve and contribute according to his abilities and interests. Shock and disbelief are especially prominent when fatal illness strikes a young person.

Sometimes it is noted that family members, once they learn that death is inevitable, gradually withdraw their emotional involvement with the ill person, probably as a way of attempting to cope with a situation that makes overwhelming demands on them. It is especially important for physicians and nurses to recognize the burdens that families face in such situations. By helping the family to cope with the experience, physicians and nurses may make it more possible for the family to contribute to the patient's comfort during his last days, as well as to provide the family with support that can aid them, not only during the final days of illness, but afterward, as well, in dealing with their grief. Some ways in which such help can be given include:

- **Providing an atmosphere in which the family members can discuss, if they wish, some of their feeling and concern, and providing this opportunity not only in the patient's presence, but away from the bedside, as well.**
- **Making it possible for the family to participate in some aspects of the patient's care, but avoiding exposing them to situations (such as massive bleeding or care of incontinence) which can add greatly to their anguish.**
- **At all times demonstrating concern and compassion as well as skillful care of the patient.**

## Purpura

The term *purpura* refers to small hemorrhages in the skin, the mucous membranes, or the subcutaneous tissues. The hemorrhagic area may be tiny, as when petechiae occur, or it may be larger and result in ecchymoses of various sizes. Purpura results either from lack of platelets or from abnormality of the blood vessels. For example, certain diseases (e.g., leukemia) or the administration of x-ray therapy or certain drugs can depress the formation of platelets. Lack of ascorbic acid can damage the blood vessels, thus leading to bleeding. The treatment of all of these conditions involves discovering and treating the cause of the purpuric lesions. Often the purpuric spots are only one symptom of a bleeding tendency. The patient may suffer severe or even fatal hemorrhages in other parts of his body.

*Idiopathic thrombocytopenic purpura* is characterized by a reduction in platelets, the development of purpuric lesions (petechiae and ecchymoses), and bleeding from other parts of the body, such as the nose, the oral mucous membrane, and the gastrointestinal tract. It is believed that most cases are the result of an autoimmune disorder, in which the patient's body develops an antibody which harms and destroys the platelets.

Patients with idiopathic thrombocytopenic purpura often recover spontaneously. Corticosteroid preparations are often used to provide symptomatic relief until the patient recovers from the disease, and to induce an elevation in the platelet count. Subsequently, the corticosteroid preparation is very gradually tapered off. Often the platelet count will remain normal.

Transfusion of platelets as well as blood may be necessary to supply additional platelets in a hemorrhagic emergency, but generally are of limited usefulness. (Platelets cannot survive in stored blood.) If the patient does not recover spontaneously, splenectomy may be performed. This operation is useful because the spleen (for reasons not fully understood) may be destroying too many platelets. The removal of the spleen often results in a rise in the platelet count and relief of the symptoms. The patient is observed carefully postoperatively for any symptoms of hemorrhage.

**Nursing Care.** The nursing care of the patient with purpura is essentially the same as that for any patient with a bleeding tendency and has been discussed in relation to leukemia. It may be summarized:

- Watch for petechiae and ecchymoses. They are especially likely to occur following injury, however slight.
- Handle the patient gently. Help him to avoid falling or bumping himself. Keeping the bed crank turned

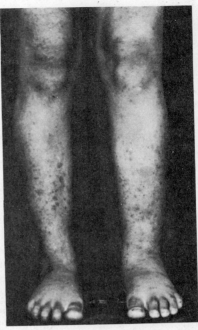

**Figure 32-2.** Petechiae in purpura. (Vakin, R. J., and Golwalla, A.: *Clinical Diagnosis,* Bombay, Asia Publishing House)

in, out of the way, is one way to prevent injury to ambulatory patients.
- Be alert for bleeding or symptoms of bleeding in other parts of the body. The patient may have epistaxis, a tarry stool, or a cerebrovascular accident due to hemorrhage into his brain. Blindness may result from retinal hemorrhage.
- Watch for unusual pallor, restlessness, fall in blood pressure, rapid pulse, and fainting. These symptoms may indicate internal bleeding.

### Hemophilia

Hemophilia is a hereditary disease characterized by prolonged coagulation time, which results in persistent and sometimes severe bleeding. It results from deficiency of the antihemophilic factor normally present in blood plasma. The disease is transmitted from mother to son as a recessive sex-linked characteristic. Although women do not develop the disease, they can inherit the trait, which, when it is passed on to a male infant, results in the development of the disease.

Hemophilia occurs with varying degrees of severity. Mild forms sometimes go unrecognized for years, until unusual bleeding is noted after an injury. Usually, however, bleeding is noted in infancy and childhood. There is persistent oozing of blood after slight injuries, such as a pinprick or a tiny cut. Often, bleeding occurs into joints, (hemarthroses) eventually damaging the joint and leading to deformity and limitation of motion. Relatively minor surgical procedures, such as tooth extraction, carry considerable risk and must be performed in a hospital setting.

Life expectancy and optimal functioning are reduced by the disease; many patients do not reach adulthood. On the other hand, those with mild hemophilia may lead full and productive lives despite the illness. Treatment includes avoidance of injury, the application of thrombin to a bleeding area, direct pressure over the site of the bleeding, and sometimes the use of cold compresses. Substances containing the missing AHF (antihemophilic factor) are used when bleeding does not respond to local treatment. These include fresh frozen plasma, cryoprecipitate obtained from slow thawing of fresh frozen plasma, and commercially prepared concentrates of normal human plasma. Selected patients and/or family members may be taught to transfuse the antihemophilic factor in the home with ongoing clinic and telephone supervision for overall management of the condition (Sergis and Helgartner, 1972).

## Polycythemia Vera
(Primary Polycythemia)

Polycythemia vera is a disease characterized by the excessive production of red blood cells and hemoglobin. The number of white blood cells also is increased. Its etiology is unknown. One theory is that it is a proliferative malignant disease of the blood-forming organs. The patient may have 10 million red blood cells per cubic millimeter rather than the normal 5 million. The increased number of cells in the blood makes it more viscous than normal and leads to increased blood volume and to a tendency to develop thrombi. When clots cut off the blood supply to the tissues, areas of infarction result. The thrombosis of cerebral vessels is common.

Polycythemia vera is more common in men than in women, and usually it occurs in middle or later life. Fortunately, it is quite uncommon.

The patient with polycythemia vera has an unusually florid complexion. Often the color of the face, and especially of the lips, is a reddish-purple. Fatigue, weakness, headache, and dizziness are common. The patient may bleed excessively after minor injuries, perhaps because of the engorgement of his capillaries and his veins. Splenomegaly commonly occurs. The condition usually has an insidious onset and a prolonged course.

The treatment involves measures to reduce the volume of the circulating blood, to lessen its viscosity, and to curb the excessive production of the red blood cells. Frequent medical examinations are important to determine the course of the disease and the patient's response to therapy.

Venesection (*phlebotomy*) may be performed at intervals. Usually 500 ml. of blood are removed from the vein at a time. This is one instance in which bleeding the patient still has a legitimate place in modern medical treatment.

Radioactive phosphorus is sometimes administered to decrease the production of the blood cells in the bone marrow. Antineoplastic drugs, such as nitrogen mustard and busulfan, may be administered to curb the excessive activity of the bone marrow.

The patient is encouraged to continue his usual activities as long as he is able. He is observed carefully for symptoms of thrombosis. The patient is advised to limit his dietary intake of iron, since this limitation may lessen to some degree the production of the red blood cells.

## Agranulocytosis

Agranulocytosis is a condition characterized by a decreased production of the white blood cells. Agranulocytosis may result from the toxic effects of drugs, such as sulfonamides, tranquilizers, aminopyrine, and barbiturates.

The symptoms of agranulocytosis include fatigue, fever, chills, headache, and the appearance of ulcers on the mucous membranes of the mouth, the throat, the nose, the rectum, or the vagina.

The prognosis is related to the cause of the condition. When the cause can be determined and promptly removed, and when the treatment can be commenced immediately, the patient usually recovers.

The treatment includes removing the causative factor—for example, stopping the drug that is producing the toxic effect. Infection usually occurs promptly and severely, and the patient, if he is untreated, is powerless to fight the pathogens. Antibiotics are given to control infection. Careful medical aseptic technique is important in preventing

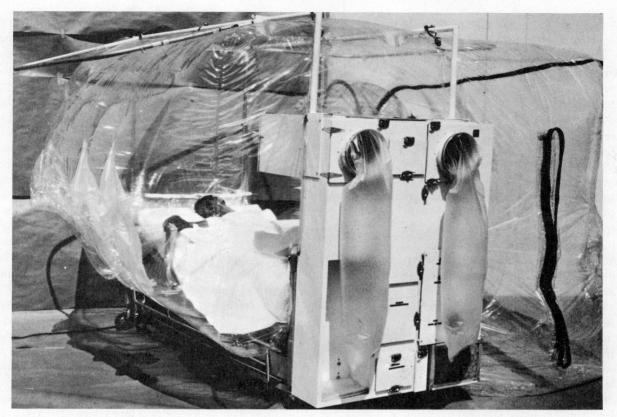

**Figure 32-3.** Inside the plastic isolator the patient is protected from contamination by organisms from the outside. Nursing care is accomplished through closed sleeves at the sides of the tent; the sleeves end in gloves. (Dr. Charles B. Beal, Stanford University School of Medicine, and *The Modern Hospital* 104:70)

the spread of pathogenic organisms to the patient. Meticulous hand washing and the wearing of clean gowns and masks while caring for the patient are necessary. The removal of the drug usually results in the resumption of the normal production of the white blood cells.

The prevention of agranulocytosis involves the careful medical supervision of the patients who are taking drugs that have been known to cause the condition.

**Self-medication.** A particular hazard is self-medication. It is not unusual to find a patient who has been taking tranquilizers for months without medical supervision. Often a person whose physician has prescribed the drug for him has with misplaced generosity kept a friend supplied with the medication. One man commented: "I didn't think it could do him any harm. After all, I take it, and it helps me to sleep, and so I thought it might help Joe, too."

When such sharing of prescriptions comes to the nurse's attention she should explain the necessity for professional supervision in the use of medications and the importance of accurate, individualized diagnosis. Since the people involved are trying to be helpful to one another, factual explanations are likely to be more effective in encouraging them to seek medical advice than scolding or blaming.

### RELATED DISORDERS

#### Lymphosarcoma

Lymphosarcoma is characterized by overgrowth of lymphocytes in lymph nodes, spleen, and lymphoid tissues in other parts of the body. As is true in other forms of neoplastic disease, the overgrowth of tissue (in this instance of lymphocytes) is unruly and, unless it can be completely eradicated, ultimately fatal. Lymphosarcoma is more common in later life than in the young.

**Symptoms** depend on the site of lymph-node involvement. Lymph-node enlargement typically occurs in cervical, axillary, and inguinal regions. For example, if cervical lymph nodes are enlarged, dyspnea and dysphagia can result from pressure on nearby structures. In the final stages of illness the patient develops fever, cachexia, bleeding, and vulnerability to infection.

**Treatment** includes primarily irradiation, corticosteroids, and chemotherapy with alkylating agents. Surgical removal of involved lymph nodes for histologic examination may be performed. The objectives of therapy are to control the growth and the spread of the disease and to provide symptomatic relief during the course of the illness, which may last from several months to several years. It is questionable whether patients are ever cured of this disease; it is considered likely that even patients who experience unusually long remissions will eventually succumb.

## Hodgkin's Disease

Hodgkin's disease is characterized by the painless enlargement of the lymph nodes. Usually, the cervical nodes are involved first; inguinal and axillary nodes usually are affected later.

The cause of Hodgkin's disease is unknown. There are two main theories concerning its etiology. One states that the disease is due to infection; the other states that it results from a malignant neoplasm of the lymphatic tissue. In light of the present views concerning the possibility that some malignant diseases are of viral origin, there is the possibility that both theories may eventually prove to be correct.

Hodgkin's disease is more common among men than women. It occurs most frequently during young adulthood. Like acute leukemia, Hodgkin's disease is a particularly tragic condition, because it so often claims the lives of young people. However, Hodgkin's disease is one of the few types of neoplastic disease which have a possibility of being curable upon early diagnosis. It is of utmost importance that this diagnosis be made early and treatment instituted upon establishment of the diagnosis.

The diagnosis of Hodgkin's disease is established by a biopsy of an affected lymph node. The pathologist notes the changes that are typical of Hodgkin's disease, including the presence of a particular type of abnormal cell called a *Reed-Sternberg cell.*

**Symptoms.** The early symptoms of Hodgkin's disease include the painless enlargement of one or several lymph nodes. As the nodes enlarge, they often press on adjacent structures. Enlarged retroperitoneal nodes can cause a sense of fullness in the stomach and epigastic pain. Marked weight loss, anorexia, fatigue, and weakness occur. Chills and fever are common. Sometimes the patient develops marked anemia and thrombocytopenia, which results in a bleeding tendency. The resistance to infection is poor, and staphylococcal infections of the skin and respiratory infections often complicate the illness. Pruritus is a common symptom. Patients who receive treatment usually have remissions that may last months or even years. However, symptoms recur, and eventually they cause death from respiratory obstruction, cachexia, or secondary infections.

**Treatment.** The treatment of Hodgkin's disease includes radiation therapy of the nodes, corticosteroids, and antineoplastic drugs, such as alkylating agents and vinca-alkaloids.

Alkylating agents are harmful to all living cells. The use of alkylating agents in Hodgkin's disease provides remission of the disease for varying lengths of time. The patient is also given several courses of treatment, and the drugs may be used in combination. However, some patients eventually fail to respond and the drugs are no longer effective in producing remission of the disease. Alkylating agents are highly toxic. Nausea and vomiting are associated with some of the drugs used. The marrow-depressing effect of the drugs used may result in severe anemia, leukopenia, and thrombocytopenia. If an intravenous form of an alkylating agent is given, the drug is introduced by the physician into the tubing of an infusion already running because this method helps to prevent the irritation of the vein as well as decrease the possibility of subcutaneous infiltration with the drug.

A frequently used alkylating agent is nitrogen mustard. Because nitrogen mustard is highly caustic upon contact with tissue, rubber gloves should be worn during preparation and administration. Sometimes, sodium phenobarbital and chlorpromazine are given with nitrogen mustard to lessen the nausea and the vomiting caused by the drug. Frequently, nitrogen mustard is given in the evening, and sedation is given to help the patient to sleep through the night. By morning the most severe gastrointestinal symptoms may have subsided. A meal tray should not be taken to the patient who is experiencing severe nausea after the administration of nitrogen mustard. Sometimes, in the busy routine of the ward, such a patient receives his usual tray. Usually, the sight and the smell of food precipitate severe nausea and vomiting. The patient should be permitted to rest quietly until the symptoms subside. Antiemetics may help. Because the drug is so toxic, it usually is prepared and administered by the patient's physician.

Antibiotics are given to fight secondary infections. Transfusions may be necessary to control anemia.

The nursing care of patients with Hodgkin's disease is similar to that of patients with leukemia.

## Infectious Mononucleosis

Infectious mononucleosis is a condition that affects lymphoid tissues primarily. Lymph-node enlargement is typical, accompanied by malaise, fever, sore throat, and headache. The cause of the disease is unknown, although viral etiology is suspected. Infectious mononucleosis seems not to be very contagious, since members of the same family and other close associates usually do not contract the disease, even when no special precautions are taken.

Infectious mononucleosis occurs most commonly among college students and students in medical and nursing schools. There has been a steady rise in the incidence of the disease since 1948 (Shapiro, 1969). The designation "kissing disease" is occasionally used as a synonym for infectious mononucleosis, due to the mode of transmission suggested by some investigators. Besides kissing, other forms of rapid indirect oral contact such as passing a soft drink or beer bottle from mouth to mouth are thought by some to spread the disease. The incubation period is about six weeks.

Diagnosis is based on the symptoms, the presence of lymphocytosis, and a positive heterophil agglutination test. The latter two diagnostic tests are performed on samples of the patient's blood.

There is no specific treatment for this disease which, fortunately, is usually self-limited. Rest, optimal diet, and prevention of secondary infection are important. Secondary infections, if they occur, may be treated with antibiotics. The average course of the disease is four weeks, after which most patients experience a period of weakness and fatigue of variable duration. Nursing care involves provision of rest and quiet recreation, measures to avoid secondary infection, and guidance in gradual resumption of activities after recovery. Young people who have missed schoolwork need help in planning their return to a full schedule gradually, instead of trying to resume school and make up what they have missed while still feeling below par.

## REFERENCES AND BIBLIOGRAPHY

AGLE, D., and MATTASON, A.: Psychiatric and social care of patients with hereditary hemorrhagic disease, in RATNOFF, O., et al.: *Treatment of Hemorrhagic Disorders,* New York, Harper and Row, 1968.

BALDY, C. M.: The lymphomas: Concepts and current therapies, *Nurs. Clin. N. Am.* 7:763, December 1972.

BECKER, G.: Platelet transfusion therapy, *Med. Clin. N. Am.* 56:81, January 1972.

DAMESHEK, W., and DUTCHER, R. (eds.): *Perspec. in Leukemia,* New York, Grune, 1968.

DOSWELL, W.: Sickle cell disease: how it influences preoperative and postoperative care, *Nurs. '74* 74: 18, June 1974.

DREIZEN, S.: Opportunistic gram-negative bacillary infections in leukemia: Oral manifestations during myelosuppression, *Postgrad. Med.* 55:133, April 1974.

EISENHAUER, L.: Drug-induced blood dyscrasias, *Nurs. Clin. N. Am.* 7:799, December 1972.

Fact and fancy about infectious mononucleosis, *Patient Care* 2:102, July 1968.

FOSTER, S.: Sickle cell disease: Pathophysiology and therapeutic approaches, *ANA Clinical Sessions 1972,* New York, Appleton-Century-Crofts, 1973: 163.

FRANCIS, G.: Cancer, the emotional component, *Am. J. Nurs.* 69:1677, August 1969.

GEE, T. S., et al.: Treatment of adult acute leukemia with arabinosylcytosine and thioguanine, *Cancer* 23:1019, May 1969.

JACKSON, D. E.: Sickle cell disease: Meeting a need, *Nurs. Clin. N. Am.* 7:727, December 1972.

Keeping up on infectious mononucleosis, *Nurs. Update* 4:11, February 1973.

KLAGSBRUN, S. C.: Cancer, emotions and nurses, *Am. J. Psychiat.* 126:1237, March 1970.

KORKOFF, I. H.: Cancer chemotherapeutic agents, *CA —A Cancer Journal for Physicians,* 23:208, 1973.

KUBLER-ROSS, E.: *On Death and Dying,* New York, Macmillan, 1970.

MANGAN, H.: Care, coordination and communication in the life island setting, *Nurs. Outlook* 17:40, January 1969.

NEBE, D. E., et al.: Lymography and patient's reactions, *Am. J. Nurs.* 73:1366, August 1973.

PARETS, A.: Emotional reactions to chronic physical illness, *Med. Clin. N. Am.* 51:1399, November 1967.

PATTERSON, P.: Hemophilia: The new look, *Nurs. Clin. N. Am.* 7:777, December 1972.

ROACH, L.: Assessment: Color changes in dark skins, *Nurs. '72* 72:19, November 1972.

RODMAN, M.: Drug therapy today. Drugs that affect blood coagulation, *RN* 32:59, June 1969.

SCHUMANN, D., and PATTERSON, P.: The adult with acute leukemia, *Nurs. Clin. N. Am.* 7:743, December 1972.

SERGIS, E., and HELGARTNER, M.: Hemophilia, *Am. J. Nurs.* 72:2011, November 1972.

SEWELL, R. L.: *Malignant Blood Diseases,* Baltimore, Williams & Wilkins, 1972.

SHAPIRO, S. L.: Some unsolved problems concerning infectious mononucleosis, *Eye Ear Nose Throat Mouth,* 48:594, October 1969.

Teaching transfusion for home care, *Am. J. Nurs.* 72:2079, November 1972.

VAZ, D. D. S.: The common anemias: Nursing approaches, *Nurs. Clin. N. Am.* 7:711, December 1972.

VOTAW, M., and BULL, F.: Drug therapy for neoplastic disease in adults, *Med. Clin. N. Am.* 53:1265, May 1969.

WARREN, B.: Maintaining the hemophiliac at home and school, *Nurs. '74* 4:75, January 1974.

WRICKWARE, D. S. (ed.): Sickle cell anemia: Improving the odds for your patient, *Patient Care* 6:104, February 15, 1972.

# The Patient with Heart Disease: Overview

## CHAPTER 33

## ATTITUDES

The diagnosis of heart disease causes fear and anxiety in most people. The heart has always been thought of as the central and most vital organ. This attitude is reflected in such expressions as "the heart of the matter." Somehow, to most people, it never sounds quite so grave to have gallbladder disease or a broken hip as it does to have heart disease. Nevertheless, an individual may live quite comfortably with heart disease for 20 years and then succumb to a seemingly less serious condition.

Everyone knows that the body has only one heart, whereas many other organs come in pairs. One lung or one kidney may be removed or badly damaged, and yet the individual survives because he still has another in reserve. The brain and liver are examples of other single vital organs.

People often have intense reactions to the diagnosis of heart disease. They may be frightened out of all proportion to the seriousness of the condition and become helpless invalids, when all that the physician has suggested is a slowing down of the hectic pace of their lives. Other people may verbally acknowledge the physician's recommendations and yet drive themselves all the harder, getting less sleep than ever and smoking twice as much. Such patients seem to be saying by their actions—and often they express the thought in words when they are given an opportunity—"What's the use? Nothing can be done for it anyway. When your heart goes, that's it, and I may as well get as much fun as I can out of life in the time that I have left."

It is true that tremendous advances have been made in the treatment of heart disease; particularly spectacular have been the advances in heart surgery. Not quite so dramatic, but just as important in helping cardiac patients to live more comfortably, are some of the new drugs. For instance, the newer diuretics are helping to relieve edema, thereby enabling many cardiacs to live longer and more comfortably. Despite these modern advances anxiety over heart disease persists, and it is not likely to be dispelled by such pat reassurances as "Oh, they can do wonderful things for heart disease nowadays."

All too often the patient is discouraged from talking about his condition—particularly his feelings concerning it. Nor are such discussions easy for those who minister to the patient. How to help the patient to understand his condition without frightening him and how to listen to him without catching some of his anxiety demand the utmost in skill, tact, and self-understanding. Such situations are difficult to handle. If a patient is told, "Now don't you worry about your heart! Just let us do the worrying," his anxiety will not be relieved and may even be intensified by the prevention of its expression. The patient should be encouraged to discuss his worries and to learn more about his condition and his treatment.

**Fear of Sudden Changes.** What are some of the things that patients and those who care for them fear most about heart disease? Sudden death or even a "sudden turn for the worse" is one. Such sudden changes are by no means limited to heart disease; nevertheless, almost everyone has heard and read about a person who was apparently in excellent health and then died suddenly of a "heart attack." (The term "heart attack" has no precise medical meaning, but it is often used to refer to myocardial infarction. However, it may be used to refer to any symptoms of heart disease and even to some that are unrelated to the heart.) The very unpredictability of some types of heart disease forms a basis for fear and uncertainty. Fear of sudden and dire symptoms may make the patient afraid to go on a trip or to continue with his job—even though the physician has assured him that his condition does not warrant curtailment of these or other activities.

**The Value of Accurate Knowledge and Reporting.** Those who care for the patient may wonder, "What if something happens? Will I know what to

do?" No one wants to feel that his inability to cope with an emergency can result in the death of a patient. The best insurance against this feeling—in any situation—is knowledge. Here are needed general knowledge about heart disease, its treatment and its complications, and specific knowledge about each particular patient's condition: what complications may occur, and, if so, what to do until the physician is available. This information is necessary for the family, too; it must be given to them in terms that they can understand, and it must be stated in a manner that does not cause undue alarm.

Thoughtful study can help the nurse to acquire general knowledge; conferences with the physician and nursing staff and thorough familiarity with the patient's chart can enhance understanding of each individual patient's condition. Any nurse who cares for the patient can initiate such conferences. They are worthy of the time spent, because they help the patient to receive better care.

When the physician anticipates certain types of complications, he often will leave specific written orders to guide the nurse until he arrives. For example, a patient who is likely to develop dyspnea and cyanosis may have an order on his chart for oxygen as necessary.

In reporting a sudden change in the patient's condition, the significant assessment data should be communicated clearly. "Mr. Brown suddenly has sharp pain in the left side of his chest. He is very pale and frightened. His blood pressure is 95/60, and his pulse is 100 and weak" is more helpful than "Come right away. Mr. Brown has gone bad." Clearly reporting concise, relevant data saves time, and often makes it possible for the physician to give directions for the patient's care until he arrives. Thus, in the example above, the physician might have responded to the report of severe chest pain by saying "Give him 15 mg. of morphine right away, and keep him quiet. I'll be right over." To give accurate information saves seconds that can be vital.

**Meeting Different Needs.** Despite the sudden onset of some types of heart disease, by far the largest proportion of patients find that their disease has become a lifetime companion. Many of these people continue to lead active, useful lives, though chronically ill, while others become incapacitated. The less dramatic needs of people are

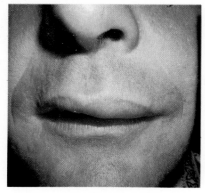

**Plate 1.** Giant swelling or angioedema of the upper lip during a systemic anaphylactic reaction. (David A. Mathison, M.D.)

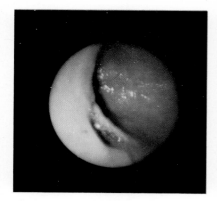

**Plate 2.** Peptic ulcer, viewed endoscopically. (Courtesy, Howard Shapiro, M.D.)

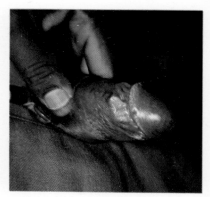

**Plate 3.** Chancre, the primary lesion of syphilis. (Courtesy, Dr. Neil C. Franzese, Cranford, N.J.)

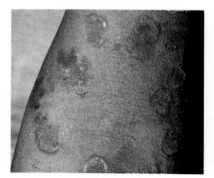

**Plate 4.** Skin eruption due to secondary syphilis. (Courtesy, Dr. Neil C. Franzese, Cranford, N.J.)

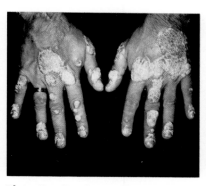

**Plate 5.** Psoriasis. (Courtesy, Dr. Neil C. Franzese, Cranford, N.J.)

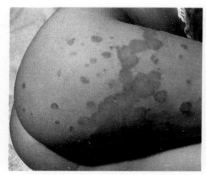

**Plate 6.** Impetigo. (Courtesy, Dr. Neil C. Franzese, Cranford, N.J.)

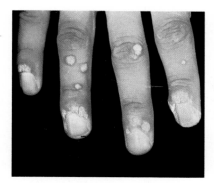

**Plate 7.** Warts. (Courtesy, Dr. Neil C. Franzese, Cranford, N.J.)

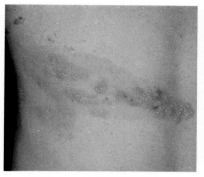

**Plate 8.** Herpes zoster. (Courtesy, Dr. Neil C. Franzese, Cranford, N.J.)

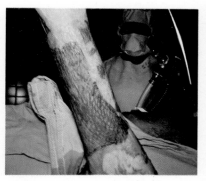

**Plate 9.** Mesh graft. In this procedure, the surgeon smooths a fragile strip of skin onto a sheet of plastic, tops it with another plastic sheet, and cranks the skin-and-plastic "sandwich" through a machine which spreads open the skin to a mesh, the "threads" of which are only 1/20 of an inch. (Courtesy, Dr. Robby Meijer, Livingston, N.J.)

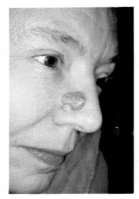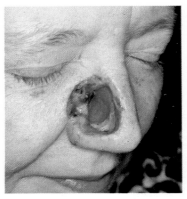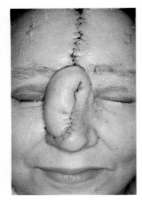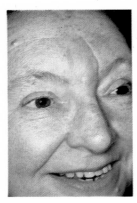

**Plate 10.** (A) Basal cell carcinoma. (B) "Through and through" excision. (C) Reconstruction with forehead. (D) End result after multiple stages. (Courtesy, Dr. Robby Meijer, Livingston, N.J.)

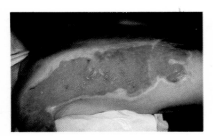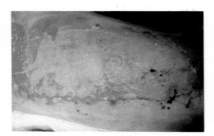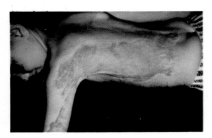

**Plate 11.** (A) Third degree burn of left chest, axilla, and arm. (B) Split thickness graft to chest. (C) Patient, three months, postoperative. (Courtesy, Dr. Robby Meijer, Livingston, N.J.)

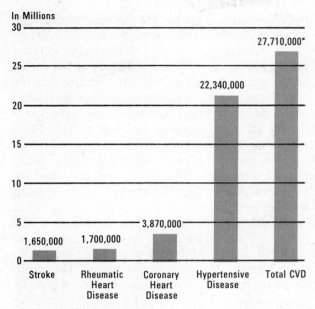

*The sum of the individual estimates exceeds 27,710,000 since many persons have more than one cardiovascular disorder.

**Figure 33-1.** Estimated prevalence of the major cardiovascular diseases in the United States, 1971. (Reprinted from "Heart Facts 1974" with permission of The American Heart Association)

often overlooked. Everyone is concerned about the businessman who has just suffered a myocardial infarction, but the older woman next door who forgets to take her digitalis and refuses to stay on a low sodium diet may be forgotten.

The care of chronically ill cardiac patients is difficult and, in a different way, demanding, too. Teaching the patient to care for himself and guiding him in planning his activities and following his treatment require patience and understanding. The nurse must be willing to work with a situation that may improve slowly and almost imperceptibly, or possibly not at all. Despite rapid progress in the treatment of heart disease, there are still some patients who cannot be helped by present medical knowledge. Some of them are older people whose failing hearts no longer respond to treatment. Others are young people whose hearts have been functioning under great handicap, such as the severe damage that results from rheumatic fever. These patients need our support and care as their independence and well-being gradually diminish. All too often the attitude of physicians and nurses

in working with patients who do not respond to treatment is pessimistic if not fatalistic. At such times our patients need us the most. Caring for the patient does not stop even when there seems little likelihood of cure.

## EPIDEMIOLOGY

In this country heart disease is the leading cause of death. The number of people succumbing to heart disease mounts steadily as age increases. So much emphasis has been placed on mortality from heart disease that its importance as a cause of disability is sometimes not fully understood. It has been estimated that there are in excess of 27,710,000 persons suffering from the major cardiovascular diseases—stroke, rheumatic heart disease, coronary heart disease, and hypertensive disease (The American Heart Association, *1974 Heart Facts*) (Figs. 33-1 and 33-2).

Although statistics point up the immense importance of heart disease among the adult population of our country, statistics are easily misinterpreted. Sometimes these alarming figures are viewed as evidence that "nothing can be done for it," and that people's hearts merely are growing weaker. Actually, these dire predictions are not true. Statistics can lead sometimes to unwarranted pessimism. Heart disease is an especially serious problem

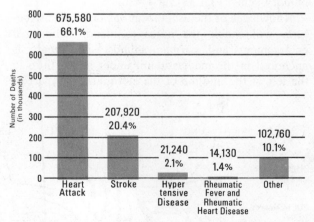

Source: National Center for Health Statistics, U.S. Public Health Service, DHEW and The American Heart Association.

**Figure 33-2.** Deaths due to cardiovascular diseases by major type of disorder in the United States, 1971 estimates. (Reprinted from "Heart Facts 1974" with permission of The American Heart Association)

among the aged, and because of the increased life span more and more people are living long enough to develop it. Improved diagnostic methods have indicated that deaths once attributed to "old age" now may be classified as deaths from heart disease. When old age has greatly weakened the body, and the time of death draws near, some one organ of the body must give way first, precipitating death. Often this organ is the heart. However, death at the age of 88, precipitated by a failing heart, does not mean the same thing in terms of life goals as sudden death from myocardial infarction at the age of 50 or disability from rheumatic heart disease during the entire span of an adult life.

All these are grouped together under the heading of "heart disease." Included in this category are not only a whole group of diseases, related in the sense that they all affect the heart, but also a variety of conditions that affect people's lives in quite different ways.

## STRUCTURE (ANATOMY) AND FUNCTION (PHYSIOLOGY) OF THE CARDIOPULMONARY SYSTEM

The heart is a four-chambered muscular pump about the size of a man's fist. It can be viewed as a master pump to which is attached a system of tubes for outflow and inflow, namely, the aorta and pulmonary arteries, and the venae cavae and pulmonary veins (Fig. 33-3).

Knowledge of the usual locations of cardiac structures will enable the nurse to identify abnormal enlargement and cardiac sounds. The heart is anchored in the mediastinum, under and a little to the left of the midline of the sternum. (The part of the heart directly under the sternum is the right ventricle; this is significant in the dynamics of external cardiac compression.) The heart's lower border lies on the diaphragm. The lower left corner of the heart, formed by the left ventricle and the ventricular septum, is known as the apex. In normal hearts this apex thrusts forward during systole, producing an impulse which can usually be felt by palpation. The point of maximum outward movement or maximal intensity (PMI) is usually in the fifth intercostal space, in the left midclavicular line. (The midclavicular line is a vertical line drawn halfway between the midsternal line and a vertical line dropped from the distal end of the clavicle.) The "base" of the heart refers to the region of the proximal aorta and pulmonary artery and is located beneath the upper sternal border. This seems an inappropriate use of the term, since the designated location is superior when the patient is in an upright position. Likewise, other topographic areas have been inappropriately identified to locate and identify heart sounds and murmurs (e.g., the mitral area, meaning the fifth intercostal space in the left midclavicular line). It is preferable to utilize a more exact description that is in relation to the sternum and the rib number, counting down from the suprasternal notch. The second intercostal space is at the level that the manubrium joins the body of the sternum. For example, "This sound is heard loudest at the second intercostal space, along the left sternal border" (Fig. 33-4).

Three distinct layers of tissue make up the heart wall. The bulk of the heart consists of specially constructed muscle tissue known as the *myocardium*. Covering the myocardium on the outside and adherent to it is the *pericardium*. Lining the interior

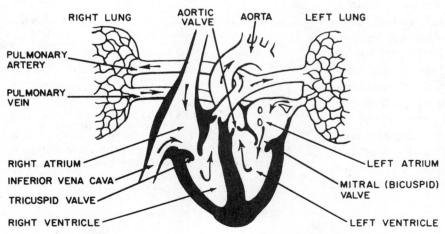

RIGHT LUNG
AORTIC VALVE
AORTA
LEFT LUNG
PULMONARY ARTERY
PULMONARY VEIN
RIGHT ATRIUM
INFERIOR VENA CAVA
TRICUSPID VALVE
RIGHT VENTRICLE
LEFT ATRIUM
MITRAL (BICUSPID) VALVE
LEFT VENTRICLE

**Figure 33-3.** Diagram illustrating the flow of the blood through the heart and the lungs. The path can be observed by starting at the vena cava and following the arrows through the right atrium, the right ventricle, the pulmonary artery, the lungs, the pulmonary vein, the left atrium, the left ventricle, and into the aorta.

wall of the heart is a delicate layer of endothelial tissue known as the *endocardium*. This is the layer that the blood directly contacts.

Of the four chambers, the ventricles are considerably larger than the atria, because they carry a heavier pumping burden. In addition, the wall of the left ventricle is about three times as thick as the right ventricle because of the amount of work that it does in pumping blood to the entire body. The right ventricle just has to pump the blood to the lungs. Notably, the systolic pressure in the left ventricle is approximately 125 mm. Hg whereas the systolic pressure in the right ventricle is only 25 mm. Hg.

To perform a basic examination of the heart or to understand the purpose and meaning of various diagnostic tests which are performed for cardiac patients, it is important to understand the sequence of events called the cardiac cycle (complete heartbeat). This cycle begins with the electrical stimulation of the atria, causing the atria to contract. This first phase, *atrial systole*, results in an increase in atrial pressure and increased blood flow from the atria to the ventricles. The increased volume causes the left ventricle to bulge forward, producing an outward motion which can usually be felt. As the electrical stimulation passes into and stimulates the ventricles, the ventricles contract, beginning the second phase of the cardiac cycle, *ventricular systole*. This rise in ventricular pressure closes the mitral and tricuspid valves, in that order. The composite sound produced by the closing of these valves is known as the *first heart sound*. When the pressure in the left ventricle exceeds the pressure in the aorta and the pressure in the right ventricle exceeds that of the pulmonary arteries, the aortic and pulmonic valves open and blood is thrust forward. Following the electrical discharge the ventricles must return to their resting state. As the ventricles relax and pressure falls within the aorta and pulmonary arteries, the aortic and pulmonic valves close, causing the *second heart sound*. When ventricular pressure is below atrial pressure the mitral and tricuspid valves reopen, initiating the third and final phase of the heart cycle, *ventricular diastole,* or the phase of ventricular filling.

While they work in unison, the left and right sides of the heart perform different functions. The left atrium receives newly oxygenated blood from the lungs via four pulmonary veins. This oxygenated blood flows during diastole into the left ventricle through the mitral valve, and during atrial systole

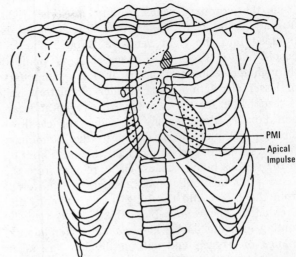

**Figure 33-4.** Surface projections of heart and blood vessels.

there is a squeezing down of additional blood into the ventricle before the valve closes.

Attached to the mitral valve are cordlike structures known as chordae tendinae, which in turn attach to two major muscular projections from the left ventricle known as papillary muscles. During contraction of the left ventricle these muscles also contract, thereby providing tension on the mitral valve and preventing prolapse or invagination of the mitral valve back into the left atrium. If this were to happen, as it sometimes does when the papillary muscles are involved in a myocardial infarction, then blood would flow not only forward into the aorta, but also backward into the left atrium through an incompetent mitral valve (mitral regurgitation).

The blood pumped through the aortic valve into the aorta flows under pressure into many smaller arteries, thence to arterioles. Arterioles branch into capillaries which permeate the tissues of each individual organ and are in intimate contact with the cells of those tissues. Oxygen and metabolic foods are delivered to the cells through this complex circulatory network. The thin walls of the capillaries, their tremendous surface area, and their tiny size, all allow for rapid exchange of gases and metabolic substances between the blood and cells. After this exchange takes place, deoxygenated venous blood is transported back to the heart under low pressure by the veins.

Veins from all organs of the body drain into the superior or inferior vena cava, and along with blood from the coronary veins, empty into the right atrium of the heart. Then this venous blood is pumped into the right ventricle through the tricuspid valve. From this chamber it is pumped through the pulmonary artery into the pulmonary or lesser circulation. This smaller circulatory unit is responsible for the exchange of oxygen and carbon dioxide. Blood leaving the right ventricle flows through the pulmonary artery to the pulmonary capillaries. Here, carbon dioxide, which has built up in the venous blood because of its release from the tissue as a metabolic end product, is transferred from the blood into the lung spaces (alveoli) and is exhaled. The venous blood takes on oxygen by coming in contact with inspired air. After this exchange of oxygen and carbon dioxide has taken place, the oxygenated blood is transported through four pulmonary veins to the left side of the heart.

Because the *arteries* are responsible for propelling blood forward under pressure through the cardiopulmonary system, they are called the "resistance vessels" of the circulatory system. The volume of blood in the arteries amounts to about 20 per cent of the total blood volume.

Because the *veins* are adapted to alter their capacity to store blood and redistribute the total volume according to body needs, they represent the major blood reservoir and are known as the "capacitance vessels." Approximately 75 per cent of the total blood volume is contained normally in the veins.

Because the *capillaries* allow for the rapid exchange of nutrients and metabolic end products, they are called the "exchange vessels." Approximately 5 per cent of total blood volume is found in the capillaries.

Though the structure of the pump itself and the complex lengthy system of arteries and veins are impressive, the entire cardiopulmonary system is designed to serve as a transport system to provide oxygen and other nutrients and to remove metabolic end products from the individual cells. The critical action occurs at the cellular level.

## ASSESSMENT OF THE PATIENT

When the nurse knows that the patient has heart disease, she assists in the diagnosis and treatment and evaluates the patient's condition by obtaining as much information as she can about him. To acquire this information she must develop the skills of observation, communication, and physical examination. The accumulation of knowledge about her patient begins as soon as she approaches him. She must observe him carefully for the following signs: his bodily position or posture, difficulty in breathing (Does this difficulty occur at rest, or when he is walking down the hall?), facial expression indicating pain, depression, or fear, and evidence of weight gain or edema.

### History and Symptoms

In heart disease the patient's history is very significant. Sometimes the diagnosis is dependent upon the history and subjective data (symptoms) which the patient describes. Sometimes there are few symptoms, and those which are present are difficult to elicit because of the patient's reticence to discuss them. For this reason, any information which the patient or his family offer must be carefully analyzed for recording and reporting. Certain symptoms should always be looked for: fatigue, dyspnea, pain, syncope, palpitation, and edema. Behavioral evidence of anxiety, fear, agitation, or indifference is also significant.

Physical activity and emotional turmoil further increase the work of the heart. If increased severity of symptoms is observed, this should be reported promptly and accurately. It is important to place the patient at rest, stay with him as much as possible, and provide reassurance and support. Insufficient blood supply to the heart is often indicated by pain in the chest, pallor, apprehension, and sweating. The location, intensity, and duration of the pain should be noted. The patient is placed at rest and the symptoms reported immediately.

Dyspnea is defined as an awareness of respiratory discomfort or breathlessness, and it may or may not be associated with signs of labored breathing. In the patient with heart disease it may be due to retention of sodium and water, inadequate venous drainage of the lungs, or fatigue of the respiratory muscles. Inefficient pulmonary circulation can lead to congestion of the lungs, causing dyspnea, cough, or audible, noisy breathing (rales). Inefficient oxygenation of the blood may be reflected in cyanosis, dyspnea, and orthopnea (difficulty in breathing in the supine position). If the patient shows respiratory distress, he should be placed at rest with his head elevated.

## Physical Assessment

The history which the patient and his family relate and the symptoms which he describes are revealing. In addition, the nurse can learn much about the patient through using the skills of physical assessment. These skills involve the use of the senses of touch, sight, hearing, and smell. Certain basic techniques can be easily learned and practiced. They can be used to form a baseline of information from which changes can be documented, they can increase the knowledge about the patient for the physician, and they can provide data to be used in determining the kind of nursing care which is needed.

Techniques of the physical examination which can be frequently used by the nurse who cares for the cardiac patient include inspection, palpation, and auscultation. The technique of percussion which is performed to estimate cardiac size and to examine the lungs, is used less often as a nursing tool. Examination of the heart is best done with the patient lying on his back, with the examiner at

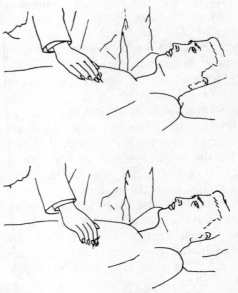

**Figure 33-6.** Palpation of the apex beat, supine position.

the patient's right side. Inspection and palpation are usually combined when examining the region overlying the heart and great vessels of the thorax. The thorax is inspected for bulging or deformities. Certain normal landmarks and functions can be identified. The normal apical beat (the forward thrust of the apex during systole) should be located. In the thin patient it can sometimes be seen as a faint impulse in the region of the left midclavicular line and the fifth intercostal space. The nurse should palpate for the cardiac apical impulse, using the tips of the index and third fingers, or the palmar surface of the fingers of the right hand. If the patient is a woman, the right hand is placed on the chest wall under the left breast. The location of the point of maximal impulse (PMI) is a measure of cardiac size, and should be recorded. It can be described as to the number of centimeters left of the midsternal line, or in relation to the midclavicular line. For example, "The apical impulse can be felt in the fifth interspace, 8 cm. left of the sternum." If the impulse cannot be felt, it can often be brought out by asking the patient to turn to the left lateral position, thus forcing the heart closer to the chest wall (Figs. 33-5, 33-6).

Auscultation involves listening with a stethoscope to the sounds within the body. The room should be as quiet as possible. The stethoscope should be

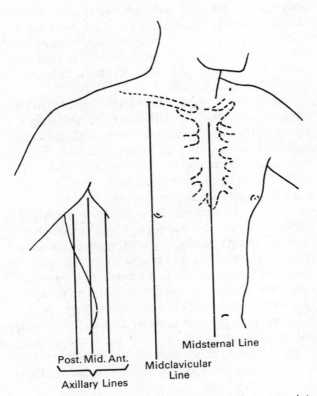

**Figure 33-5.** Thoracic lines of reference used in examination of the heart.

comfortable, with the earpieces fitting snugly, not too tight or too loose. Both a bell and diaphragm are needed. The bell, which accentuates the lower frequency sounds, is placed on the skin lightly. The diaphragm brings out the high frequencies, and is used for most of the cardiac examination. It is pressed firmly against the skin.

In listening to the heart, it is important to review and be thoroughly familiar with the events of the cardiac cycle previously described. It is good practice for the nurse to listen to her own heart in order to become familiar with the character of each sound and to learn the anatomical points at which these sounds are best heard. Before concentrating on the individual heart sounds, she should listen to the cardiac rhythm. Is it regular? Are there occasional beats that come early? Do some beats drop out? What is the rate? Sudden changes in rate are very significant, particularly if the patient is receiving a cardiac drug (e.g., digitalis).

When listening to the heart, four items are kept in mind: the first heart sound, the interval between the first and second heart sounds (systole), the second heart sound, and the interval between the second and first heart sounds (diastole). The first heart sound may be identified in any area by gently feeling the carotid pulse which occurs simultaneously with the first sound. The radial pulse may be used; however, there will be a slight delay after the first sound before the pulse is felt, due to the distance from the heart. The first heart sound is generally louder at the apex and the second sound is louder at the base. The systolic interval between the first and second heart sounds is shorter than the diastolic pause which follows the second sound. The actual cause of the first and second heart sounds is not clearly understood. They are generally associated with the closure of the atrioventricular and semilunar valves. However, they also appear to be related to acceleration and deceleration of blood flow, causing vibration of valvular and muscular structures.

After identifying the sounds, the nurse listens to their intensity. Age and physical build may alter the intensity of the sounds which are heard. They also vary with the position of the patient. Is there a splitting of the sounds? Are the intervals silent, or are there murmurs present? Heart sounds are particularly difficult to hear in the obese, thick-muscled individual, and are usually very clear in the thin-chested patient. Systolic murmurs occur during ejection of blood from the heart and are produced by the flow of blood across the pulmonic or aortic valve, or by regurgitation across the mitral and tricuspid valves. Blood flow across an interventricular septal defect will also cause a systolic murmur. Systolic murmurs are sometimes inconsequential. Diastolic murmurs, on the other hand, usually signify heart disease.

There are four classical areas for auscultation of the heart:

1. The second intercostal space just to the right of the sternum, where the second heart sound is usually the loudest
2. The second intercostal space to the left of the sternum
3. The fifth intercostal space, left midclavicular line, where the first heart sound is normally louder
4. The area to the left of the lower sternum

With experience in identifying the first and second heart sounds, the nurse caring for the acutely ill cardiac patient can learn to identify abnormal sounds, splitting of sounds, and arrythmias when they occur.

Observation of temperature, pulse, respiration, and blood pressure is also important. It is not necessary to have a specific order to make and record observations. Cardiac patients' symptoms often change suddenly. Significant signs, such as changes in heart rate and rhythm, may manifest themselves only at brief intervals. If the nurse who is with the patient fails to note and to report them, important information may be lost.

**Temperature.** Fever is characteristic in some types of heart disease, particularly in acute myocardial infarction, rheumatic fever, and bacterial endocarditis. Patients with these conditions should have their temperatures taken rectally, since this method provides the most accurate reading. Though a rectal temperature is more accurate, oral temperatures might be ordered in order to avoid vagal stimulation from the insertion of the rectal thermometer. Vagal stimulation can produce slowing of the heart (bradycardia) and other cardiac arrhythmias such as heart block, especially in the patient with acute myocardial infarction. If the more accurate rectal temperature is still desired, care should be taken that the thermometer is well lubricated and inserted gently. An eye on the electrocardiographic monitor or a finger on the patient's pulse will give evidence of excess vagal stimulation. This should be reported.

**Pulse.** When taking the pulse, the nurse notes not only its rate but also its rhythm and its quality. Is the rhythm regular? If not, does the irregularity have a pattern? (For example, she may note an unusually long interval after every fourth beat, or that weak and strong beats alternate.) Is the pulse strong, or does it seem weak and hard to detect? Can it be easily obliterated by the pressure of your fingers? Is the pulse bounding and jerky, so that it seems to be striking forcefully against the nurse's finger? All these observations are important, and they can help with diagnosis.

The pulse rate is not always the same as the heart rate. Some of the beats may be too feeble to produce a pulsation in the radial artery. Counting the radial pulse of such a patient is equivalent to counting only the strong beats. Listening to the heartbeat at the apex with the stethoscope may indicate that his heart rate is 90 per minute rather than the rate of 60 which was counted when the radial pulse was taken. The difference between heart rate and pulse rate is known as *pulse deficit*. It can be detected by taking an apical-radial pulse. One nurse counts the beats as she listens over the apex while another nurse counts the radial pulse. Both nurses count for at least a full minute; then they leave the patient's bedside and compare results. Both figures are charted (for example, $\dfrac{A90}{R60}$).

It should be remembered that if a pulse deficit exists, the number of beats at the radial artery is fewer than the number heard at the apex. If the results indicate that the radial rate is more rapid than the apical rate, a mistake has been made! The apical rate is most significant in a patient with pulse deficit. For example, when the nurse counts the pulse prior to administering digitalis, a pulse rate below 60 is not reported until the apical rate has been checked (Fig. 33-7).

The careful nurse, noting that the patient's radial pulse is very weak and irregular, counts the apical pulse. Instead of reporting, "His pulse is weak and irregular. I'm not really sure—I guess it's about 80," and then charting it as 80 on the graphic sheet, she reports: "The apical rate was 100, very irregular, and the radial pulse was 80." It is good practice to check the pulse bilaterally and to learn to palpate other peripheral pulses—the carotid, brachial, femoral, popliteal, dorsalis pedis, and posterior tibial—since they indicate patency of the arterial system. This is particularly important following a cardiac catheterization when an artery has been used.

Today many hospitalized cardiac patients receive continuous electrocardiographic monitoring. This

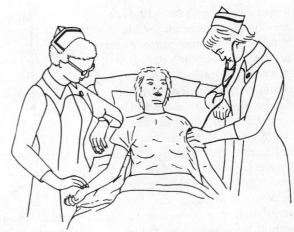

**Figure 33-7.** Taking the apical-radial pulse. One nurse listens to the heart with a stethoscope; the other feels the radial pulse. Both nurses count the beats simultaneously and compare their figures.

monitor will indicate the patient's heart rate and rhythm but not the quality of the beat. The quality of the beat can be ascertained by feeling the pulse. Correlating pulse quality with the cardiac monitor provides useful information. The cardiac rhythm on the monitor, for example, can look normal but the cardiac output, reflected in a weak, thready pulse, can be low. Also, the monitor pattern might be irregular but the pulse and other data show that the patient can maintain sufficient cardiac output. By correlating cardiac monitor data with the feel of the patient's pulse while the patient is on the monitor, the nurse is better able to detect arrhythmias by feeling the pulse when the patient is off the monitor.

**Blood Pressure Readings.** Blood pressure readings are important, because diseases of the heart often are closely associated with changes in blood pressure. For instance, a drop in blood pressure frequently follows acute myocardial infarction. The nurse should make certain that the patient is sitting or lying in a comfortable position, and she should note carefully and record the systolic and diastolic readings. The blood pressure is taken in both arms on admission and once a day, and any discrepancy should be reported.

**Respirations.** Careful observation of the rate and character of respiration is important. The average respiratory rate for the normal adult is from 16 to 20 per minute. However, the rate of respiration is not a valuable criterion for the adequacy of ventilation, since either fast or slow rates may be associated with other factors. Too often the nurse focuses only on rate, although other observations are equally significant. While counting the rate for a full minute, the nurse observes the quality of respiration. Is the patient's breathing easy or labored (dyspneic)? Are his respirations deep or shallow, wet or dry, wheezing or quiet? Does he use his neck muscles or abdominal muscles to help him breathe? Is the rate faster than normal (tachypnic)? Is he restless or confused? (This can indicate oxygen lack.) Does he have late signs of hypoxia, such as cyanosis or orthopnea? Does he have Cheyne-Stokes type breathing.

When examining the patient for adequacy of ventilation, the nurse can listen for normal breath sounds by auscultation. Either the diaphragm or the bell portion of the stethoscope may be used in listening to the lungs. If the patient is thin and the ribs prominent, she must be sure the entire surface of the diaphragm or the rim of the bell is in contact with the chest wall. Again, the nurse should practice listening to her own chest or those of her colleagues to learn to identify the different types of breath sounds: *vesicular* (soft, rustling), heard over the periphery and lower lung fields; *bronchial* (tubular, harsh, high-pitched), heard over the trachea; and *bronchovesicular* (a combination of the other two, resembling the vesicular inspiratory phase and the bronchial expiratory phase), heard over the lung near the major airways. With experience the nurse can learn to recognize abnormal breath sounds and adventitious sounds (sounds superimposed on the normal respiratory cycle). Rales, the name commonly given to these noisy extra sounds, generally refers to sounds which originate in the smaller bronchi or alveoli as air is forced through liquid, sputum, or other foreign material. Rales may be described in many ways: fine, coarse, moist, crackling, bubbling, and so on. Rales will sometimes disappear when the patient takes a deep breath or coughs. Rales are often present when the left side of the heart cannot pump blood out efficiently, causing fluid to accumulate in the lungs.

**Color.** Cyanosis is the blue coloration of the skin and mucous membranes due to an increased amount of reduced hemoglobin in the small blood vessels. It may be *central,* due to excessive loss of oxygen from the arterial blood, or *peripheral,* in which there is normal arterial saturation but regional slowing of the circulation. Cyanosis is best observed in the tongue. The earlobes, conjunctivae,

and nail beds are less reliable. It is difficult to detect in patients with anemia, because the amount of hemoglobin pigment is too low, and it may be falsely interpreted in patients whose hemoglobin is excessively high. Cyanosis may not be perceived with certainty until the arterial oxygen saturation is reduced to 75 to 85 per cent. Even then, this estimation is far from accurate. Blood gas analysis is the only reliable means of determining hypoxemia.

**Edema.** Edema should be noted, particularly in dependent parts of the body such as the feet and the ankles, and over the sacrum. Edema often accompanies congestive heart failure. The blood is not pumped efficiently, and venous blood that is being returned to the heart by the large veins cannot be received promptly and pumped by the right side of the heart. As a result the venous blood being returned to the heart dams up in the veins. The inefficient return of the blood to the heart causes congestion in the veins and the collection of extra fluid in the tissues.

Fluctuations in weight are important indications of edema. A gain in weight often means that edema is increasing, and not that the patient is growing "fatter," in the usual sense of the term. Loss in weight often reflects the desirable and needed loss of excess fluid that has collected in the tissues. If a daily weight measurement is ordered, the patient should be weighed at the same time each day and with the same amount of clothing. The recording of weight should be as accurate as possible. A pound more or less may indicate that edema is increasing or decreasing.

**Gastrointestinal Changes.** Occasionally the patient with heart disease may show signs and symptoms relating to the gastrointestinal system, due to decreased oxygenation of the abdominal viscera or distention of areas of vasculature (e.g., the portal system). When anorexia (loss of appetite), nausea, vomiting, bloating, or diarrhea occur, these should be reported. Some symptoms may indicate a toxicity to the level of medication being administered.

## DIAGNOSTIC TESTS

### Noninvasive Procedures

**Electrocardiogram (ECG).** Some laboratory tests administered to the patient with heart disease consist of external recordings of the events of the cardiac cycle. As the heart contracts it produces energy in the form of movement and sound which can be converted into graphic form (Fig. 33-8). The scalar electrocardiogram (ECG) is a graphic record of electric currents generated by the heart muscle. The record is made by a special instrument, called an electrocardiograph, which measures and records these currents. The 12-lead ECG is especially useful in determining the nature of myocardial damage and in interpreting arrhythmias. Connections are made between the machine and the patient by means of electrodes that are placed at various points on the patient's body. A special conducting jelly is rubbed on the points of contact. The leads placed on the extremities are strapped in place, and the chest lead is held in various positions on the chest by the technician, or by a suction cup. In the routine screening electrocardiogram, 12 leads are used.

No special preparation for the test is needed other than explaining it to the patient, but since the test does involve the heart the explanation should be individualized to prevent undue anxiety. The nurse should explain that the test is painless, and that it merely records the electrical currents of the heart. Otherwise, patients who are having it done for the first time may feel uneasy when they see wires being attached to them, and may wonder whether they are about to receive some kind of electric shock.

The nurse should make sure that the patient is comfortable and ready for the test. Even though a technician may do the test, the nurse may need to stay with the patient if he is very ill, anxious, or in pain. If there are any doubts about the electrical integrity of the machine, it should not be used. For example, a spark in the presence of oxygen quickly becomes a fire, and faulty wiring or improper grounding can lead to electrocution of the patient. The patient should be helped to understand that the ECG is often repeated in order to aid the physician in following the course of the patient's illness.

At the time of the test the patient is asked to remove clothing from the areas where the leads are to be placed, and to lie down and relax. In most hospitals the technician wheels the machine to the patient's bedside and performs the test there. In some intensive and coronary care units the nurse does the admission and daily ECG, or others as the patient's condition warrants. There are several advantages to this. The test can be planned to work in with the patient's rest or other activities and an additional person (technician) is eliminated from the many who normally confront the sick, hospitalized patient. To avoid electrical hazard to the patient his cardiac monitor must be disconnected when the 12-lead ECG is taken. If a nurse prepared in arrhythmia detection does the 12-lead ECG, she can continuously monitor the patient's rate and rhythm as the ECG is being taken. The patient may resume his usual activities immediately following the test. No special care or observation is necessary.

Nurses who work with cardiac patients often learn to interpret certain arrhythmias which are recorded by the ECG. After the complete tracing has been examined by a cardiologist it is returned to the patient's chart. In addition to the tracing there is usually a detailed explanation of the findings and a brief summary statement. All nurses should develop the habit of reading these summaries and interpreting them as they relate to the patient's

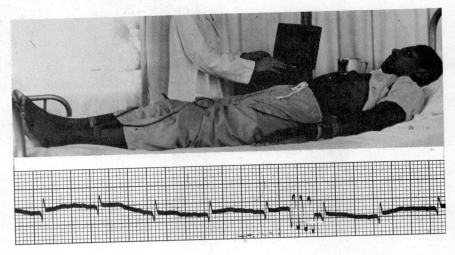

**Figure 33-8.** (*Top*) Technician taking an ECG. Leads have been placed on arms, legs, and chest. (*Bottom*) A sample of the graphic record obtained by electrocardiography.

care. For example, the statement may indicate recent damage to the myocardium as a result of coronary occlusion, or a disturbance in heart rhythm which should be carefully observed.

**Other Noninvasive Techniques.** These are used to record the events of the cardiac cycle. Most of these techniques are performed in the laboratory, since the equipment is more complex; a skilled technician is required, and sometimes a quiet environment is necessary. The preparation of the patient is the same as for the ECG. The nurse should be sure that he understands what will happen to him and accompany him if it seems indicated.

Heart sounds and murmurs are recorded on the *phonocardiogram.* Various locations over the chest are used, such as the area over the proximal aorta to best record the second heart sound. *Vectorcardiography* also records the electrical activity of the heart in reference to the body surface. It differs from the ECG only in the instrumentation used for recording and the format of the record (the heart's forces are represented by arrows and loops rather than waves and complexes). The changes in electrical potential are represented as vectors, that is, electrical forces with definite direction and magnitude. The vectorcardiograph displays the vectors of depolarization as they are referred to the body surface in all three dimensions: the frontal plane (left-to-right and head-to-toe), the sagittal plane (front-to-back and head-to-toe) and the horizontal plane (front-to-back and left-to-right) (Fig. 33-9).

Recently a new technique, *echocardiography,* has been developed for evaluating cardiac structure and function. Sound waves of very high frequency are transmitted into the chest of the patient. As these waves cross tissues or structures of differing acoustical density (e.g., the chest wall, valvular tissue), they are reflected back to a receiver which records these reflected waves, or "echoes." This procedure excels the x-ray because it reflects the motion of various tissues of the heart. The transmitter and receiver are contained within a small unit which the technician places on the patient's chest in order to direct the beam. There is no pain or damage to the tissues through which these sound waves pass. This procedure is helpful in measuring the size of various cardiac chambers, the thickness of cardiac walls, and the effectiveness of ventricular contraction. An expert technician is required, and a cardiologist experienced in echocardiography interprets the complex recordings.

*Fluoroscopy* is also used to observe the heart in action, and the *chest x-ray* provides a permanent record of heart size, evidence of early accumulation of fluid, and so on.

*Exercise testing* is used with cardiac patients to determine functional significance of anatomical lesions. One commonly used exercise test is the *Master Two-Step Test* in which the patient walks up and down two steps of specified height for a predetermined number of trips, varying with the age, weight, and sex of the patient. An electrocardiogram

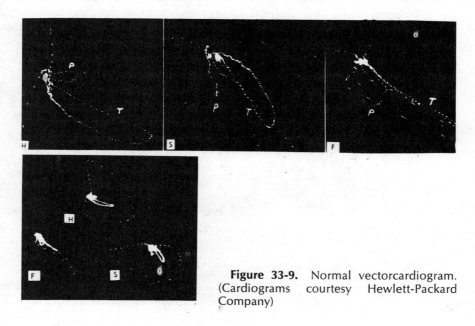

**Figure 33-9.** Normal vectorcardiogram. (Cardiograms courtesy Hewlett-Packard Company)

is recorded before and after one, three, seven, and ten minutes of rest and is examined for evidence of ischemic changes. The precise significance of this test is not known. Exercise testing has been modified in recent years to include increasing levels of exertion in order to quantitate exercise capability. During these more complex examinations of the patient during exercise the ECG may be recorded throughout the activity as well as afterward. Blood gases may also be examined concurrently. The nurse can help the patient understand the purpose of the test and the procedures which will be followed, and carefully observe him afterward for new or changed symptoms. Any change should be reported (see also Chap. 39).

## Invasive Procedures

Sometimes an examination of heart structure and function requires the invasion of the body with instruments, such as needles or catheters, and foreign materials, such as radiopaque dyes. An example of a common invasive technique is the drawing of arterial or venous blood for examination. If the samples are drawn for analysis of oxygen content, the procedure does not require that the patient omit breakfast before the blood is taken. The nurse must carefully check the diagnostic procedures planned for the patient each day and see that he is properly prepared, both physically and psychologically.

The more complex invasive techniques used in diagnosis of cardiac abnormalities usually take place in the x-ray department or the cardiac laboratory. Breakfast may be omitted, and sedative and antihistaminic drugs may be administered one-half to one hour before the patient is taken from his room. On certain occasions it is important that the patient is *not* sedated so that normal cardiac function can be observed. Therefore the preparation of the patient for the procedure, including answering any questions he might have, is very important. Some procedures are lengthy and sometimes uncomfortable. Every effort should be made to reduce the anxiety of the patient. This may require that the nurse accompany the patient and remain with him throughout the procedure. Severe anxiety can cause peripheral vasoconstriction and prevent a satisfactory examination.

The intravenous *angiogram* is a test in which a radiopaque dye is injected into a vein and its course from the right heart to the lungs and back to the left heart and out the aorta is recorded by a rapid series of x-ray pictures. This test is used in diagnosing certain congenital abnormalities of the heart and great vessels. In the *aortogram* dye is injected into the aorta and x-ray films are taken to outline the abdominal aorta and major arteries in the lower extremities. *Coronary angiography* provides radiographic visualization of the coronary arteries which have been injected with dye. In this procedure a catheter is introduced into a peripheral artery and advanced in a retrograde manner into the ascending aorta, the dye is injected into the coronary arteries, and serial films are taken. The physician looks for localized blockage of a coronary vessel which may be amenable to surgery. *Cineangiography* involves the recording of moving films after injection of a radiopaque dye. In this way the examiner can visualize valvular motion, shunts, and ventricular contractions. In *radiocardiography* a radioisotope is injected intravenously. The course and timing of the radioactive material through the heart is noted by the use of a Geiger-Müller counter and recorded on a graph.

When arteries are opened for diagnostic procedures there is a greater chance for bleeding than after a venipuncture. A pressure dressing is applied and patient activity is restricted for several hours. The nurse observes the patient for bleeding and loss of pulses. The pulse distal to the site of injection is checked in searching for a clot or spasm of the vessel. The absence of a pulse on that side requires immediate attention of the physician.

**Allergic Reactions.** During and after tests in which a dye is used, the nurse watches for allergic reactions to the dye, including urticaria, flushing of the skin, fall in blood pressure, nausea, vomiting, and less commonly, respiratory distress and anaphylactic shock. Before such tests a skin test may be performed to determine possible allergic reactions. Systemic allergic reactions are most likely to occur shortly after the dye is administered. However, when the patient returns to his room, the nurse should observe for any signs of delayed systemic reaction, and watch for adequate urinary output, as the dye may cause a temporary renal insufficiency.

The treatment of allergic reactions includes epinephrine, antihistamines, and oxygen for respiratory distress. Drugs needed to combat allergic reactions and equipment for giving oxygen should be available.

Other emergency resuscitation equipment such as a defibrillator, an "Ambu" or other breathing bag, and a tracheostomy set likewise is kept available for immediate use. The patients undergoing the tests are likely to have cardiac impairment. A continuous ECG is usually taken during the tests to monitor the patient's condition. Especially during an angiocardiogram a cardiologist may be present. The nurse keeps frequent check of the patient's pulse, remaining alert for any irregularity. Cardiac arrhythmia—ventricular fibrillation is the most common—and cardiac arrest may occur.

**Other Reactions.** Thrombosis and irritation of the vessel into which the dye was injected also may occur, and the dye may cause irritation if it leaks beneath the skin. The vessel used for the injection should be observed for pain and swelling. Tenderness over the vessel is usual and disappears in one or two days.

The tests are tiring. For example, an angiocardiogram may take two and a half hours. On returning from the x-ray department the patient should be given the opportunity to rest in a quiet atmosphere.

Operative permits are required for most of these procedures. After the tests patients usually are allowed to eat, to drink, and to ambulate as they desire. When anesthesia has been used, they may go to the recovery room before they return to their own beds.

### Cardiac Catheterization

*Cardiac catheterization* involves passing a long flexible catheter into the heart and the great vessels. As the catheter enters the various chambers, the pressures are measured, blood flow is calculated, and samples of the blood are obtained and analyzed for the content of oxygen and carbon dioxide. For example, the oxygen content of the blood in the right atrium is higher than normal when there is an atrial septal defect (a hole in the septum that separates the atria).

In right heart catheterization the catheter is introduced into a peripheral vein, such as the anticubital vein, and directed under fluorscopic control into the superior vena cava, the right atrium, across the tricuspid valve, into the right ventricle, across the pulmonary valve, and into the pulmonary artery. It is sometimes "wedged" into a distal arteriole, where much information about left heart function can be determined. Here the examiner can indirectly measure the pressure in the pulmonary capillaries, which is nearly the same as pulmonary venous pressure and left atrial pressure.

The left side of the heart is approached in several ways. Sometimes a needle is advanced through a catheter which has been introduced into the right side of the heart and then passed through the atrial septum into the left atrium, across the mitral valve, and into the left ventricle. At other times the catheter is passed in a retrograde fashion through a peripheral artery, the aorta, and into the left atrium.

Cardiac catheterization is a technique employed for the patient who is sufficiently disabled by heart disease to warrant consideration of corrective surgery. The clinical diagnosis can sometimes be confirmed and additional abnormalities can be identified. Ordinarily, the adult patient is not anesthetized (the walls of blood vessels have no fibers that transmit pain), but he may be given a sedative before the test. Breakfast is withheld on the morning of the test. The procedure is usually quite painless. The patient may have some slight discomfort at first from the cutdown and the insertion of the catheter. As the catheter enters the chambers of the heart, he may experience some irregularity of heart rhythm that resembles a feeling of fluttering or "butterflies in the chest." If this should occur, the patient is reassured that the sensation will pass, and that there is no cause for alarm. The patient may cough when the catheter is passed up the pulmonary artery. If so, he is told that the sensation will pass quickly. However, despite sedation the patient often is alert and apprehensive, and he is very much aware of the slightest sensation that is out of the ordinary.

When the procedure is over, the catheter is withdrawn gently, and the patient returns to the ward with a small sterile dressing over the site of the cutdown.

Cardiac catheterization is not without danger, although most patients experience no complications, except possibly transient arrhythmia during the actual procedure. The patient's pulse is checked frequently after the catheterization has been performed. The physician orders the frequency with which the pulse is to be taken (usually every 15 minutes for the first hour and less frequently for several hours thereafter). If the pulse is rapid or irregular, report this information to the physician. Occasionally, thrombophlebitis develops in the vein through which the catheter has been passed. The site of the cutdown should be observed afterward

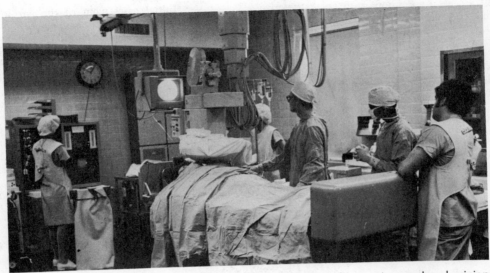

**Figure 33-10.** The cardiac catheterization team watches the monitor as the physician threads a catheter into the heart of a patient. (New Jersey Newsphotos)

for any tenderness or inflammation. Pulmonary edema and air embolism are rare complications. Sometimes the patient's temperature is elevated for a few hours after the test. Frequently, antibiotics are ordered before and after the test to prevent infection. Some physicians permit the patient to resume his usual activities after cardiac catheterization. Others advise that the patient should remain in bed, except for bathroom privileges, for the remainder of the day.

## THE INTER-SOCIETY COMMISSION FOR HEART DISEASE RESOURCES (ICHD)

Since 1968, representatives from 29 leading nursing, medical, and allied health organizations including the American Nurses' Association and the National League for Nursing have formed the Inter-Society Commision for Heart Disease Resources (ICHD) because of their mutual interest in the prevention of heart disease and in the quality of care being received by cardiovascular patients. Study groups have issued a series of reports on the major cardiovascular disorders emphasizing primary prevention, acute care, continuing care, long-term care, and rehabilitation. Attention has been given to the provision of resources (human and material) and guidelines for development of resources for optimal care (McIntyre and Betson, 1971). The reports have been published in *Circulation* and are available through the local chapters of the American Heart Association.

Nurses care for cardiovascular patients in all phases of illness and in many different settings. Patient care can be enhanced by knowledge and application of the recommendations found in ICHD reports pertinent to each nurse's area of practice.

## REFERENCES AND BIBLIOGRAPHY

AMERICAN HEART ASSOCIATION: *Examination of the Heart* (a series of four booklets). Part One: History taking, by Howard B. Sprague, M.D. Part Two: Inspection and palpation of venous and arterial pulses, by Noble O. Fowler, M.D. Part Three: Inspection and palpation of the anterior chest, by J. Willis Hurst, M.D. and Robert C. Schlant, M.D. Part Four: Auscultation, by James J. Leonard, M.D. and Frank W. Kroetz, M.D. New York, 1972. (Available from your local heart association.)

———: *1974 Heart Facts,* New York, 1973.

ARMINGTON, SISTER C., and CREIGHTON, H.: *Nursing of People wtih Cardiovascular Problems,* Boston, Little, Brown, 1971.

COGEN, R.: Cardiac catheterization: Preparing the adult, *Am. J. Nurs.* 73:77, January 1973.

FEIGENBAUM, H.: Clinical applications of echocardiography, *Prog. Cardiovasc. Dis.* 14:531, 1972.

GURNERT, C. F., et al.: Pulmonary artery catheterization (pictorial), *Am. J. Nurs.* 73:1182, July 1973.

KERNICKI, J., et al.: *Cardiovascular Nursing: Rationale for Therapy and Nursing Approach,* New York, Putnam's, 1970.

LAMBERTON, M. M.: Cardiac catheterization: Anticipatory nursing care, *Am. J. Nurs.* 71:1718, September 1971.

LAWSON, B.: Clinical assessment of cardiac patients in acute care facilities, *Nurs. Clin. N. Am.* 7:431, September 1972.

LEHMANN, SISTER J.: Auscultation of heart sounds, *Am. J. Nurs.* 72:1242, July 1972.

McINTYRE, H. M. (ed.): *Heart Disease: New Dimensions of Nursing Care,* New York, Trainex Press, 1974.

————: Initial assessment of the cardiovascular patient, *ANA Clinical Sessions 1972,* New York, Appleton-Century-Crofts, 1973:135.

————, and BETSON, C.: Unified approach to heart disease: Inter-Society Commission for Heart Disease Resources, *Am. J. Nurs.* 71:2369, December 1971.

MOORE, V.: In-bed weighing: Product survey, *Nurs. '72* 2:13, July 1972.

MORGAN, W. L., and ENGEL, G. L.: *The Clinical Approach to the Patient,* Philadelphia, Saunders, 1969.

RODBARD, S.: The clinical utility of the atrial pulses and sounds, *Heart Lung,* 1:776, November-December 1972.

SANDERSON, R.: *The Cardiac Patient: A Comprehensive Approach,* Philadelphia, Saunders, 1972.

# The Patient with
# Congestive Heart Failure

## CHAPTER 34

## CARDIAC PHYSIOLOGY

### Cardiac Output

The basic work of the heart is to pump blood. The left ventricle does the primary work of pumping, but the atria by their squeezing action contribute about 15 to 20 per cent of the total output of the pump.

Cardiac output is a term used to express the amount of blood the left ventricle pumps into the aorta each minute. The normal heart at rest, beating about 72 times a minute, ejects about 70 ml. of blood at each beat. The average cardiac output is then about 5,000 ml. or 5 liters a minute in a 150-pound man. The cardiac output varies widely; well-trained athletes can eject 30 liters per minute during exercise. Cardiac output is lower during sleep but increases during exercise, eating, or strong emotions such as fear in order to meet body tissue demands. How large the cardiac output is depends on how fast the heart beats, or the heart rate, and how much blood is ejected with each stroke of the heart, or the stroke volume. This can be expressed by an equation:

$$\text{Cardiac Output} = \text{Heart Rate} \times \text{Stroke Volume}$$
$$\text{CO} = \text{HR} \times \text{SV}$$

Since all the blood that fills the ventricle during diastole is not ejected during systole, the stroke volume represents the amount of blood in the left ventricle before ejection begins (the left ventricular end diastolic volume) minus the volume of blood remaining in the left ventricle at the end of systole (the left ventricular end systolic volume). The left ventricle normally holds about 130 ml. of blood. Since only 70 ml. are ejected

603

at rest, one way of increasing the cardiac output is to increase the volume of blood ejected with each stroke; another way is to increase the heart rate. The normal homeostatic mechanism which takes place in response to increased demands on the heart is to increase the heart rate. This mechanism can effect rapid changes in cardiac output particularly in untrained individuals under conditions of moderately increased demands. An increase in heart rate, by itself, may increase cardiac output threefold. There is, however, a point of no return. Since filling of the heart and myocardial perfusion occur during diastole, with very fast rates (like 170 in normal young individuals or 150 to 160 in those with myocardial disease) the diastolic filling period is very short. Therefore, cardiac filling is poor and cardiac output begins to actually fall off because of a decrease in stroke volume. At this point the heart rate must be slowed. Also, with increased heart rate, the oxygen demands of the myocardium are greater and the myocardium suffers from poor coronary perfusion at very fast rates.

In heart conditions characterized by very slow rates, cardiac output can fall unless there is a compensatory increase in the stroke volume. In acute myocardial infarction, for example, where there is actual damage to the pump (left ventricle), the stroke volume is lessened because the pump has lost some of its power. If a vagal response results in a slow heart rate, cardiac output will fall with resultant pain and arrhythmias due to poor perfusion of the myocardium. Cardiac output can be improved by increasing the rate to normal or through increasing the quality of the pump.

Cardiac output is distributed in the following manner:

4 per cent or 200 to 225 ml. goes to the coronary arteries
15 per cent goes to the brain
35 per cent goes to the liver, spleen, and other viscera
25 per cent goes to the kidneys

These are the critical body organs and when cardiac output is lowered these can be drastically affected by poor tissue perfusion.

## Heart Rate

Factors accelerating heart rate include rise in blood temperature, stimulation of skin heat receptors, and the emotions of anger, anxiety, and fear.

The hormones epinephrine and thyroxine also increase heart rate. Factors decreasing heart rate include a below normal body temperature, sleep, stimulation of skin, cold receptors, sudden intense pain, the emotion of grief, and overwhelming emotional shock. Pressoreflexes constitute the dominant heart rate control mechanism. These are located in the aortic arch, carotid sinus, and the proximal portion of the venae cavae. If blood pressure within the aorta or carotid sinus *increases* suddenly, it stimulates the pressoreceptors in these vessels. This leads to stimulation of the cardioinhibitory center in the medulla and reciprocal inhibition of the accelerator center, which in turn leads to more impulses per second over the vagus and fewer impulses per second over the cardioaccelerator nerves to the heart, causing reflex slowing of the heart. If pressure within the aorta or carotid sinus *drops* suddenly, pressoreceptors are stimulated less intensely. The cardioinhibitory center is therefore less stimulated and the accelerator center less depressed, and reflex acceleration of the heart occurs. Pressoreceptors in the venae cavae are stimulated by increased pressure. This leads to stimulation of the cardioaccelerator center with reciprocal depression of the inhibitory center. As a result more impulses travel to cord sympathetic centers and proceed via the cardioaccelerator nerves to the heart to bring about its reflex acceleration (Bainbridge reflex).

## Stroke Volume

Stroke volume depends primarily on systolic ejection and diastolic filling.

### Systolic Ejection

The volume of systolic ejection and the rate at which it is ejected are related to the strength of myocardial contraction and opposed by the outflow resistance to the ejection of blood from the left ventricle offered by aortic or arterial blood pressure. A change in the contractile characteristics of the heart mainly alters the fraction of the total blood in the left ventricle that is ejected per beat. The more vigorous the contraction, the more complete is the ventricular emptying per beat and the greater is any individual stroke volume.

The contractile force of the heart may be modified by the following:

**Sympathetic Nerve Discharge.** Some sympathetic nerve fibers terminate directly in the myocardial muscle fibers. When they are activated, they release small amounts of norepinephrine at their endings and increase the contractile force of the left ventricle. When sympathetic nerve fibers to the adrenal medulla are stimulated, epinephrine is released into the venous blood This neurohormone induces changes in the force of left ventricular contraction when it reaches the coronary circulation that are similar to those of norepinephrine. Epinephrine and norepinephrine are termed catecholamines.

**Drugs.** Norepinephrine (Levophed), epinephrine, isoproterenol (Isuprel), metaraminol (Aramine), and other sympathomimetic drugs increase the force of cardiac contractions. Calcium (chloride or gluconate) also causes similar effects.

**Coronary Blood Flow.** As the blood flow to myocardial tissue declines, for example, in coronary arterial narrowing or obstruction, the contractile properties of the heart and myocardial performance deteriorate.

Diastolic Filling

Some of the factors involved in diastolic filling are:

**Duration of Diastole.** As the diastolic filling period lengthens, the left ventricle fills with a greater volume of blood. Conversely, as the heart rate increases and the period of diastolic filling shortens, less blood fills the ventricles and the stroke volume decreases.

**Filling Pressure.** Blood flows from areas of higher pressure to areas of lower pressure. The greater the pressure head (atrial minus ventricular pressure) during diastole, the more rapid is ventricular filling.

**Distensibility of the Ventricle.** Increased diastolic distention contributes to stroke volume by increased diastolic filling and also by increased systolic ejection and more complete ventricular emptying (Frank-Starling relationship). Both these factors contribute to the decrease in stroke volume and cardiac output in patients who have impaired ventricular contractility due to heart disease when they develop a tachycardia.

## CONGESTIVE HEART FAILURE

The term "heart failure" usually implies to the layperson that the heart has stopped beating. ("She nearly had heart failure when she found out that her brakes wouldn't hold.") When the term is used medically, it has a quite different meaning. It describes the condition of a patient whose heart is unable to keep up with the job of pumping blood, and who therefore develops symptoms due to the derangement of the circulation. For example, the heart muscle may not be able to cope with the added burden placed on it by a damaged valve. The term *congestive* is often used in describing heart failure, because the inefficient circulation leads to the congestion of many organs with blood and tissue fluid.

Heart failure can occur with varying degrees of severity. When symptoms are slight, the patient may be able to be up and about without having any marked symptoms. In contrast, the patient in severe heart failure is critically ill. A patient can go through varying degrees of heart failure, and with treatment he often can recover from it. When the patient shows symptoms of heart failure, his condition is described as *decompensated*—that is, his heart is not able to compensate or to make up for the demands placed on it. When the treatment succeeds in enabling the heart to keep up with the circulatory load, the symptoms disappear, and the condition is described as *compensated*. Often, however, the abnormality of the heart that led to heart failure remains, and unless the patient has continued treatment, he may again develop the symptoms of congestive heart failure.

## Causes of Congestive Heart Failure

Congestive heart failure results from many different forms of heart disease. This condition usually develops gradually, as the result of strain placed on the heart by congenital defects, diseases of the heart and blood vessels, or other diseases that overburden the heart. For example:

- Rheumatic fever can damage the heart valves, and the strain of pumping a sufficient amount of blood through the damaged valves may cause heart failure.
- Cor pulmonale (or pulmonary heart disease) secondary to disorders of the lungs such as chronic obstructive pulmonary disease (COPD) causes excessive work for and consequent enlargement of the right ventricle which may reach a point of decompensation progressing to frank cardiac and pulmonary failure (see Chaps. 30 and 60).
- A branch of a coronary artery may become occluded and cut off the blood supply to a portion of the heart muscle, which then becomes necrotic (myocardial infarction). The efficiency of the heart may be impaired by this injury, and congestive heart failure may develop.

- The pericardium may become inflamed, and later scarred and constricted. Constriction can interfere with heart action by pressing on the heart and so lead to heart failure.
- Hyperthyroidism, if it exists for many years, can cause a normal heart to fail because of the excessive demands placed on the heart by the very rapid heart action that occurs in this condition.

The treatment of congestive heart failure involves locating the cause and, if possible, correcting it. Sometimes, cure of the underlying condition is impossible, and treatment consists entirely of measures designed to help the heart to continue to function as efficiently as possible despite the underlying disease. Thus, an abnormality of a valve damaged by rheumatic fever may be corrected surgically. If surgery is not possible, medical treatment designed to help the heart to function despite the valvular lesion would constitute the treatment. The treatment of hyperthyroidism can cure congestive heart failure due to the overactive thyroid. Combating hypoxia and maintaining adequate ventilation must accompany standard measures for cardiac improvement when a lung disorder is the underlying cause.

Particularly in older age groups congestive heart failure frequently is brought about by a combination of factors. The blood vessels may gradually lose their elasticity (a condition called *arteriosclerosis*), and the lumen of the arteries may slowly grow smaller due to the fatty deposits in the walls of the arteries (*atherosclerosis*). The elevation of the blood pressure is common among older persons. In time, these vascular changes can lead to congestive heart failure by interfering with the blood supply to the heart muscle and by causing the heart to pump blood through vessels that have become narrowed and inelastic. The heart itself is not exempt from the process of aging. Gradually, with advancing age, cardiac reserve is lessened, and the heart becomes less able to withstand the effects of injury or disease. Congestive heart failure, then, is not a separate disease; rather it is a pathologic state resulting from a variety of conditions that impair heart function. Although the immediate treatment of acute congestive heart failure is the same regardless of the cause, the treatment of the underlying condition can involve a variety of measures, both medical and surgical, designed to relieve or to cure the underlying disorder.

## The Process of Congestive Heart Failure

Disturbances of one part of the heart, if they are severe enough or last long enough, eventually affect the entire circulation. The following is one example of the process of congestive heart failure from mitral stenosis:

- The narrowing of the mitral valve impedes the flow of the blood from the left atrium to the left ventricle.
- The left atrium, because it cannot empty normally, becomes enlarged, and the pressure within it increases.
- This increased pressure, in turn, causes the lungs to become congested with fluid, because the distended left atrium cannot effectively receive the oxygenated blood coming to it from the lungs.
- This increased hydrostatic pressure and transudation of fluid into the pulmonary interstitial spaces causes a decrease in lung compliance and decreased diffusion of gases across the alveolar membrane. As a result, the patient develops dyspnea, cough, orthopnea, and sometimes hemoptysis. These are symptoms of left-sided failure.
- Because of the congestion in the lungs, it becomes harder for the right ventricle to pump blood to the lungs. The right ventricle must pump more forcefully to overcome the resistance of the lungs to the blood coming from this ventricle.
- The right ventricle eventually becomes unable to keep up with its work. It cannot pump the blood effectively, and the right side of the heart becomes congested with blood.
- Venous blood returning to the right side of the heart cannot be pumped to the lungs quickly and efficiently enough because of the failure of the right side of the heart. Congestion develops in the large veins leading to the heart and eventually in other organs and tissues of the body as the result of inefficient venous return.
- Dependent edema, such as that of the feet and the ankles on standing, appears. The abdomen may become distended with fluid (ascites). The liver, too, becomes edematous and enlarged. Presacral edema may be present in the patient on bed rest. The veins in the neck become distended. These are symptoms of right-sided heart failure.

This is only one example of the process of congestive heart failure. In each type of heart disease the process is somewhat different, depending on the location of the heart damage and its severity. Yet the process is similar in that, although one part of the heart and the circulation are primarily affected at first, the process, if it continues, eventually affects the entire circulation. The sequence in which symptoms appear reflects the sequence of physiologic disturbance. Symptoms of either right-sided or left-sided heart failure may appear first; eventually, symptoms of failure in both sides usually will be present.

Patients with congestive heart failure retain excessive amounts of sodium. This excess sodium contributes to the problem of edema by holding water in the tissues.

According to Guyton (1970), in cardiac failure there is an increase in aldosterone secretion by the adrenal cortices caused by the reduced cardiac output. Aldosterone increases the rate of reabsorption of sodium by the renal tubules.

## Assessment of the Patient

Signs and Symptoms of Congestive Heart Failure

Often the patient notices that he is unusually tired after work that previously had not caused fatigue. Some patients find that dyspnea on exertion is their first symptom. For instance, a patient who lives on the second floor may find that he becomes short of breath and has to rest on the landing before he attempts the second flight of steps. He may notice that he has difficulty breathing while he is lying flat, and he begins to use two or even three pillows. Cough, occasionally productive of blood-streaked sputum, may occur.

The patient may notice that his feet and his ankles are swollen, particularly at the end of the day, when he has been standing and walking. This swelling usually disappears during the night when his feet and his legs are elevated, but the fluid can shift to the lungs or sacral region.

Actually, the edema does not really disappear. It is just distributed differently due to the patient's posture and is therefore less noticeable. When he stands, his ankles gradually will swell again. By the time that the edema becomes noticeable, the patient

usually has retained 10 or more extra pounds of fluid in his tissues. These extra pounds, which actually are due to the retained fluid, show up on the scale when the patient is weighed. His apparent gain in weight is not in the usual sense of increased fat or muscle tissue. Although the patient's weight gradually increases, he usually is losing rather than gaining fat and muscle tissue. When this process has continued for a time, the patient often looks strangely out of proportion. The lower parts of his body (the ankles, the legs, and eventually the thighs and the abdomen) become swollen and heavy, whereas his face and the upper parts of his body look thin and wasted. When edema is relieved by treatment, his family and friends often are amazed at how thin and frail he looks.

Edema of the feet and the legs rarely causes pain, but it makes the patient's legs feel heavy, clumsy, and tired. It is described usually as "pitting edema," because when pressure is exerted, the part that has been pressed will become indented. The indentation gradually disappears after the pressure has been released (Fig. 34-1). Edema of other areas, though it is less visible, often causes symptoms of the dysfunction of the organs involved. For example, the distention of the liver and the other abdominal viscera may cause flatulence, anorexia, and nausea. The patient may have impaired renal function manifested by reduced urinary output. Impaired cerebral function may be manifested by memory loss, confusion, or difficulty in communication.

Some patients with congestive heart failure experience Cheyne-Stokes respirations. This symptom is believed to be due to poor circulation to the brain, causing the respiratory center in the brain to become less sensitive to the amount of carbon dioxide in the blood. According to Guyton (1970) there is a slow waxing and waning of respirations occurring repeatedly every 45 seconds to 3 minutes. When respiration is more rapid and deeper than usual the $P_{CO_2}$ (arterial blood carbon dioxide partial pressure or tension) decreases because more $CO_2$ is "blown off." When this pulmonary blood reaches the brain in a few seconds, the decreased $P_{CO_2}$ inhibits respiration and pulmonary blood $P_{CO_2}$ gradually increases. When blood with increased $CO_2$ arrives at the respiratory center in the brain, respiration is stimulated and the patient overbreathes again initiating a new cycle.

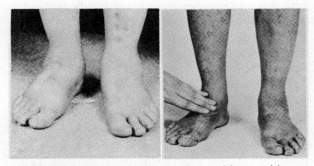

**Figure 34-1.** (*Left*) Pitting edema of feet and lower legs. (*Right*) The same patient after treatment relieved the edema. (CIBA Pharmaceutical Company)

Another type of periodic breathing is called Biot's breathing. This is characterized by several normal respirations followed by a period of complete cessation of respiration. A cycle can be as short as ten seconds or as long as a minute. It is thought that Biot's breathing results from abnormality of the rhythmical mechanism of the respiratory center. Irritability, restlessness, and decreased attention-span may occur when these conditions are very severe. These symptoms are due to impaired cerebral circulation, and they may progress to stupor and coma before death.

Physical Assessment

Through using some of the techniques of physical examination the nurse can detect signs of early or advanced heart failure. These physical signs are the result of cardiac dilatation or hypertrophy, pulmonary congestion, systemic venous hypertension, and fluid accumulation in the interstitial spaces of the pleural, pericardial, or peritoneal cavities.

In examining the heart, the nurse locates the ventricular impulse at the apex of the heart by palpation. (See Chapter 33 for the basic techniques of the cardiac examination.) This apical impulse, usually found in the fourth or fifth intercostal space at the midclavicular line, will be displaced to the left and downward if the left ventricle is enlarged. If the right ventricle is dilated, an impulse may be felt along the left parasternal area. When listening to the heart sounds with the stethoscope, the examiner can usually hear third or fourth heart sounds, or extra heart sounds.

Extra heart sounds are not usually heard in the normal adult, though they are sometimes present in children. The low-pitched, diastolic third and fourth heart sounds of ventricular failure assume a gallop or cadence rhythm when the heart rate is increased. This gallop rhythm can best be heard with the bell of the stethoscope placed at, or medial to, the cardiac apex, with the patient in the left lateral position.

The moist rales caused by pulmonary congestion are readily detectable by auscultation of the lungs. With the patient in a sitting position, the stethoscope is used to listen to the breath sounds at the posterior bases of the lungs. The rales, or adventitious sounds, may be moist, crackling sounds heard only at the peak of inspiration, or, if the failure is more severe, they may occupy more of the respiratory cycle. In severe failure they are heard throughout inspiration and expiration. When pulmonary edema occurs, the hoarse, gurgling rales are audible with the human ear when it is placed close to the patient.

Abnormal fluid within the lung spaces can also be detected by palpation and percussion. When the palms of the hands are placed on both sides of the posterior chest and the patient repeats "ninety-nine, ninety-nine" as the hands are moved slowly downward, the vibrations of the voice can be felt when the lungs are normally resonant. This is called *tactile fremitus*. These vibrations are decreased when fluid accumulates in the bases of the lungs.

The technique of percussion is performed in the following manner:

The plexor, or striking finger, is usually the third finger of the right hand. The nail of this finger must be kept short so that the end of the finger strikes briefly and sharply against the terminal phalanx of the pleximeter, or finger receiving the blow (usually the third finger of the left hand). The pleximeter finger is held firmly against the skin, with the other fingers of that hand held off the surface to avoid altering the percussion note. The plexor wrist should be held relaxed and free, striking lightly and briefly, somewhat like a piano hammer. This skill requires considerable practice. Through practicing percussion over the areas of the normal lung the nurse can learn to identify the resonant areas, which are increased over the anterior lung field. One can learn the position and function of the diaphragm by percussing progressively downward from the tips of the scapula until an area of dullness is reached, with the patient in deep inspiration and after expiration. With heart failure, if fluid accumulates in the pleural cavity, examination at the bases of the lungs will reveal a flat percussion note and decreased or absent breath sounds. Figure 34-2 shows the technique of percussion.

The increased pressure within the venous system, one of the early signs of right heart failure, can be identified by examining the jugular veins. The pulsations of the jugular veins may be seen in the normal individual at the base of the neck when that person is lying flat or with his head slightly elevated and turned slightly to one side (in a relaxed manner, not taut). External jugular distention is observed by raising the patient's head to a 45-degree angle. In the position the pulsations normally ascend only one to two cm. above the clavicle. Any distention of these veins indicates an abnormal elevation of central venous pressure. The pressure can be estimated by measuring the vertical distance in centimeters from the manubrium sterni, or suprasternal notch, to the upper level of the column of blood that is visible in the vein. This distance, plus normal central venous pressure (6 to 12 cm. of water), approximates the central venous pressure (Fig. 34-3).

## Tests for Circulatory Impairment

Because congestive heart failure is a disorder that can be produced by a variety of diseases of the heart, any test or combination of tests used for cardiac patients may be ordered in an effort to discover the underlying cause of congestive heart failure. For example, in addition to the history and the physical examination, the patient may have electrocardiograms, x-ray examination and fluoroscopy of his chest, or cardiac catheterization.

Two tests—measuring the venous pressure and the circulation time—are done especially to deter-

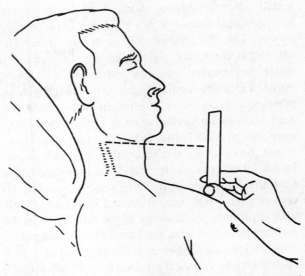

**Figure 34-3.** Central venous pressure is estimated by measuring the vertical distance in centimeters from the sternal angle to the upper level of distention of the right external jugular vein, with the patient's head and shoulders elevated at 45 degrees.

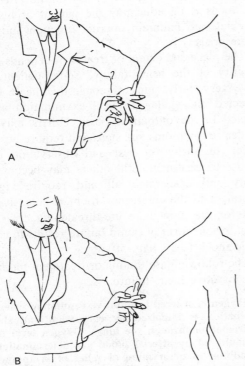

**Figure 34-2.** The technique of percussion. *A,* The third finger of the examiner's left hand is pressed firmly against the skin, while the other fingers are held off the surface. *B,* As the right hand swings freely at the wrist, the tip of the third finger strikes the underlying terminal phalanx sharply to produce a percussion note.

mine the congestion and the slowing of the circulation so typical of congestive heart failure.

**Measuring Venous Pressure.** The technique of indirectly measuring arterial pressure, which we usually refer to as "taking the blood pressure," is a familiar one. Measuring venous pressure is done less often, and it may be less familiar. The physician performs this test, and the nurse assists him and the patient when it is performed. First, the patient's arm is positioned at the same level as his heart by supporting the arm with a pillow or a rolled blanket. The physician performs a venipuncture, and to the needle and the syringe he attaches a water manometer that has had sterile normal saline placed in it. A three-way stopcock connects the syringe, the needle, and the manometer. When the manometer is in place, the stopcock is adjusted to allow the saline from the manometer to flow into the patient's vein. The pressure in the vein will permit only a certain amount of the saline to run in. When the saline stops entering the vein, the level of the saline left in the manometer is read. The normal venous pressure ranges from 60 to 120 mm. of water. It is increased in congestive heart failure.

**Measuring Central Venous Pressure.** A more accurate measurement of venous pressure is obtained when a catheter is inserted into a peripheral vein and threaded into the vena cava or right atrium. This is called central venous pressure. The catheter is connected via a three-way stopcock to a water manometer and an intravenous infusion bottle, and serial readings are taken. Central venous pressure is recorded as the height of the fluid column in the manometer when it is filled with fluid from the infusion bottle. When the venous pressure is not being read, the three-way stopcock is adjusted so that the intravenous fluid runs through to keep the catheter patent. Since venous pressure decreases slightly on inspiration and increases slightly with expiration, oscillations of the fluid level in the manometer occur with the patient's breathing (Fig. 34-4). Right atrial venous pressure is about 0 to 4 cm. of water. Vena cava pressure is about 4 to 10 cm. of water. Central venous pressure is increased in congestive heart failure. (See Chapter 59 for use of central venous pressure in shock.)

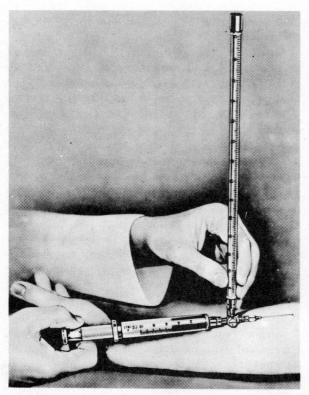

**Figure 34-4.** Equipment for the direct measurement of venous pressure. (Becton, Dickinson and Company, Rutherford, N.J.)

**Measuring Circulation Time.** The circulation time is determined by the intravenous injection of a substance that can be tasted by the patient when it reaches his tongue. Decholin, which causes a bitter taste, or sucrose, which causes a sweet taste, may be used. The substance is injected into a vein in the arm, and the time interval between the injection and the patient's tasting the substance is called the *arm-to-tongue time*. Normally, this is less than 15 seconds. The test is timed by a stopwatch, after careful instruction of the patient to signal as soon as he tastes the substance. In congestive heart failure the circulation time is prolonged.

## Treatment

The immediate treatment of congestive heart failure involves measures to help the heart function as effectively as possible in meeting the demands of the tissues of the body and to relieve the symptoms and signs produced by the inefficient circulation. When this is accomplished to the extent possible, the treatment focus is on the underlying disorder. If the congestive heart failure is chronic, the focus is on educating the patient or his close associates to maintain optimal function and avoid acute crisis.

The place and extent of treatment depends on the severity of the heart failure. Some patients may have very early signs of congestive heart failure detected on regular physical examination and be treated on an outpatient basis. Others may have moderate symptoms and signs and require hospitalization primarily for rest and observation of response to treatment. Still others may become suddenly and desperately ill and require vigorous treatment in the emergency room or intensive care unit for the immediate life-threatening crisis. The most serious form of pump failure results in cardiogenic shock (see Chap. 59).

The following are the major treatment modalities in congestive heart failure:

- **Oxygen is ordered to improve ventilation when oxygenation is impaired by congestion and sluggish circulation through the lungs. Oxygen level is best monitored by arterial blood gas determinations, in addition to observation of relief of symptoms and signs. An evaluation of the best oxygen delivery device is made for each individual patient so that the best tolerated method of administration is used.**

**Generally a nasal catheter or face mask is used. Oxygen is administered cautiously to patients with chronic obstructive pulmonary disease and to those**

who present themselves for treatment with no prior history. An increased oxygen content of the blood can remove the hypoxic stimulus which drives the respiratory center in some patients with COPD. This can result in decreased stimulation of the respiratory center and even respiratory arrest.

When oxygen is administered care must be taken to maintain the proper liter flow. Matches and electrical appliances are excluded from the environment to minimize the fire hazard.

- To reduce the oxygen need, the patient is helped to rest. His heart may be able to meet the demands of the body at rest, but be unable to cope with the demands placed on it by physical or emotional stress. Sedatives are sometimes necessary to help the patient to rest.

As a result of data gathered from clinical studies some physicians believe that chair rest, rather than bed rest, is more beneficial for the patient in congestive heart failure (Levine, 1966). The principle involved is that the heart works less in the sitting position than in the recumbent position. The patient in the chair does not engage in any more activity than he would if confined to bed. Only bradycardia or hypotension sufficient to interfere with cerebral circulation are contraindications to chair rest. The patient is assisted to sit in bed, then to touch the floor, and pivot into a chair. He is not lifted. He is returned to bed in the same manner. Because the legs are dependent, critics of chair-rest treatment state that increased incidence of thrombophlebitis is a sequela. However, proponents of chair rest deny this. The use of elastic stockings and foot and ankle exercises prevent stagnation of blood, whether the patient rests in bed or in a chair. A lounge-type chair in which the pelvis is lower than the patient's legs is not a recommended cardiac chair because blood can pool in pelvic veins.

- Diuretics are given to rid the body of the excess fluid and the sodium that have been stored in the tissues. Paracentesis sometimes is necessary to relieve ascites.

The predicted time of effect of the diuretic given the patient must be known. For example, with a diuretic such as ethacrynate sodium (Edecrin Sodium) given intravenously, diuresis can be observed in 15 minutes with the peak volume in 30 to 60 minutes. After a similar drug (ethacrynic acid, Edecrin) is given orally, the peak urinary volume occurs in about two hours. Patients, especially elderly ones, may be given sedation along with the diuretic on admission. Sudden diuresis can result in bed wetting or in acute urinary retention. The patient must be offered the bedpan or urinal, and his bladder must be checked for distention. Urinary frequency and urgency is very tiring especially on the first day of hospitalization. The female patient should be assisted on and off the bedpan and the male patient must have an empty urinal when he needs it.

Intake and output are carefully recorded. If the patient has an order to be weighed daily, preferably the same person should perform the procedure at the same time daily (before breakfast). Similar clothing or bed clothing should be incorporated each time the patient is weighed.

Careful observation of the patient for electrolyte imbalance should be made, especially when the patient is receiving a potassium-depleting diuretic. Weak pulses, faint heart sounds, hypotension, diminished tendon reflexes, and generalized weakness are signs of potassium deficiency (hypokalemia).

ECG signs of hypokalemia include S-T segment depression and a flattened or inverted T wave, as well as cardiac arrhythmias.

- The abnormal retention of sodium is also combated by limiting the patient's intake of sodium, whether in food or drugs. The term "low sodium" is preferable to "salt free" in describing the diet because salt is restricted rather than entirely absent, and in conveying the idea that all forms of sodium, rather than only salt, are limited, the patient is helped to recognize other sources of sodium, such as sodium bicarbonate.

The amount of sodium allowed varies from about 500 mg. to 3 Gm. daily.

- Digitalis is given to slow the heart rate and to strengthen its beat. These two actions help the weakened overburdened heart to pump blood more efficiently.

Digitalis enables the ventricles to empty themselves more completely after each systolic contraction (increased stroke volume). This reduces the diastolic size of the heart and the smaller, stronger heart pumps more efficiently than a large, flabby one.

There are many forms of digitalis. Table 34-1 indicates some of the more commonly used preparations.

Digitalis preparations vary in dosage from grams to milligrams. Digitalis is a very powerful drug, and in incorrect dosage it is a very dangerous one. The label must be read very carefully and the average dose of the particular preparation known before giving the drug.

Relatively large doses of these preparations are given at the beginning of therapy in order to accumulate therapeutic amounts of the drug in the body. This is called digitalization. A daily, smaller dose then is given that is sufficient to maintain therapeutic amounts of digitalis in the body. This is called the maintenance dose.

The apical pulse is checked before administering digitalis. Though signs of digitalis toxicity tend to appear gradually, severe potassium deficiency (hypokalemia) resulting, for example, from the use of potassium-depleting diuretics can provoke digitalis intoxication.

If signs of digitalis toxicity are present, such as bradycardia with an apical pulse below 60 per minute, increasing P-R interval, dropped beats, or premature ventricular contractions, the physician is notified before the drug is given.

## Table 34-1. Digitalis Preparations

| NAME | DOSE | ROUTE OF ADMINIS-TRATION | THERAPEUTIC ACTION AND USES | TOXIC OR SIDE EFFECTS |
|---|---|---|---|---|
| Digitalis | 0.1 Gm. | Oral | Digitalis preparations strengthen the heart's contractions and slow its rate, thus increasing cardiac output and leading to better circulation to all parts of the body. | Anorexia, nausea, vomiting, diarrhea, excessive slowing and irregular rhythm of pulse; headache, drowsiness, blurred vision. |
| Digitoxin | 0.1 –0.2 mg. | Oral Parenteral | | |
| Digoxin | 0.25–0.5 mg. | Oral Parenteral | | |
| Lanatoside A, B, C, mixed, Digilanid | 0.33–0.66 mg. | Oral Parenteral | | |
| Lanatoside C (Cedilanid) | 0.5 mg. | Oral | | |
| Deslanoside (Cedilanid-D) | 0.2 –0.6 mg. | Parenteral | | |
| Ouabain (G-Strophanthin) | 0.5 mg. | Parenteral | This drug works very quickly; it usually is given intravenously for rapid digitalization. It is not given if the patient has already been digitalized. | |

• **Though additional potassium is usually taken by liquid oral supplement, or by dietary means, in severe potassium deficiency with digitalis intoxication potassium may be given intravenously. The usual rate of administration is 40 mEq. every eight hours. The maximum rate is 40 mEq. every two hours. Cardiac arrest can occur with potassium excess.**

## SUMMARY OF NURSING ASSESSMENT FACTORS

Initial and continuing data specific to the patient with acute congestive heart failure are gathered by obtaining a nursing history from the patient if he is able, or from the person who accompanies him, by reviewing earlier records, by communicating with the physician and other team members, and by making careful note of the following aspects of the patient:

• **General appearance including color; facial expression; preferred position; restlessness, apprehension; location and degree of edema, such as ascites, presacral, or pedal; skin integrity; signs of dehydration in tissues; external jugular distention.**

• **Respiratory rate, depth, character, degree of effort, cough, secretions.**

• **Circulatory data obtained by systolic and diastolic blood pressure and discrepancies between arms; pulse quality, rate, rhythm, and apical-radial difference; temperature and color of extremities; intake and output, and specific gravity of urine; chest pain or discomfort.**

• **Special observations when indicated including auscultation, palpation, and percussion of heart and lungs; data from noninvasive techniques such as electrocardiographic monitor; data from invasive procedures such as central venous pressure or arterial blood pressure; laboratory data related to ventilatory and acid-base and electrolyte status including $PO_2$, $PCO_2$, pH, bicarbonate, BUN, Na, K, and Cl.**

• **Psychological data including anxiety level and responses such as denial, regression, depression.**
   **Sociocultural factors such as immediate religious needs, family and cultural supports, socioeconomic concerns, living accommodations.**

### Nursing Intervention

#### Acute Phase

When a patient is admitted to an emergency room or intensive care unit or to the general ward with acute congestive heart failure, nursing care involves participating as a team member in making a skillful rapid systematic nursing assessment, setting priorities, and quickly providing oxygen and medications, while supporting the patient and family through this very frightening experience. The need for reassurance is especially great. The nurse provides reassurance to the patient and family by her competent performance, her caring attitude, and her availability and response in meeting the patient's basic needs. The establishment of a sense of trust, which is vital to the future rehabilitation of the patient, is a major therapeutic goal. Patients experiencing acute congestive heart failure, especially repeated episodes, are often discouraged and even despondent. Forced into a position of helplessness and dependency and aware of the life-threatening nature of his cardiac illness, the patient needs from the nurse both physical and emotional comfort. The nurse also needs to have a sensitivity to the distress of waiting relatives or friends and their need to be informed of the progress of the patient. Assessment and decision must be made concerning the potential contribution of the visitors to the patient's care. In some situations a family member's presence during more than the usual visiting periods may be helpful, such as with a very elderly confused patient; in other situations the visitor may be too distressed to be able to be supportive to the patient.

Only essential components of the nursing history are dealt with during a crisis, for example, information concerning digitalis or diuretic intake. The remaining aspects of the history and detailed explanations are deferred until the patient improves. At first he is too sick to take in complicated explanations, and care must be given quickly. For example, instead of giving a detailed explanation of why oxygen is necessary, the nurse assures the patient that it will help his breathing, deftly applies it, and stays with the patient. A quiet, "All right, now just breathe in and out," until the patient becomes accustomed to the oxygen mask or other device, conserves the patient's energy and helps him to realize that it really does help him to breathe and will not smother him.

When there is acute crisis the nurse must move swiftly and expertly as she functions as a member of the emergency team. Providing for a position of comfort which takes respiratory demands into consideration, applying cardiac-monitoring electrodes, starting an intravenous line, obtaining an ECG, starting an intake and output record, providing for warmth and safety, and attending to spiritual as well as emotional needs are necessary aspects of care. Acting with awareness of the apprehension of the patient can help the nurse to focus on the distressed patient even while carrying out these numerous tasks.

Sometimes the failing heart will no longer respond to medical treatment, and the patient is in the terminal stage of life. Part of the nursing role is to offer support through her caring, listening presence and to foster the involvement of other psychological and sociocultural supports such as clergy, lawyer, friends, or family to help the patient to a peaceful dignified death.

### Recovery Phase

It is sometimes mistakenly thought that all the dramatic cardiac recoveries are reserved for surgical treatment. Actually, most patients with heart disease are treated medically, and many of them have spectacular relief of symptoms. However, after an acute crisis of chronic congestive heart failure, the patient does have some permanent impairment which requires adaptation for life to continue and for optimal cardiac function to be achieved. Listening to the patient as he attempts to cope with imposed limitations and life-style changes and helping him work through his feelings will assist him in the adaptations he must make to chronic illness.

## CHRONIC CONGESTIVE HEART FAILURE

As soon as the patient recovers from his most acute symptoms, plans are made to involve him and his family in a long-term program designed to promote optimum health by maximizing cardiac function. The same principles apply whether the patient is hospitalized during the recovery phase or whether he was able to avoid hospitalization for an acute crisis and is seen as an outpatient by a physician or a cardiac nurse specialist in a nurse-managed clinic.

One of the foremost roles of the nurse caring for a patient with chronic congestive heart failure is in the area of patient education therapy. This involves working collaboratively with the physician and patient in planning a regimen including the major areas of drugs, diet, and activity.

A comprehensive patient assessment is necessary in order to identify problem areas which impede the patient's progress in meeting his self-care needs or which maximize rather than minimize self-care deficits. Limitations in achieving optimal health are not necessarily due to the disease process alone, but also to cognitive, affective, or psychomotor factors. The nurse works with the patient, not for him, because solutions to problems must have personal significance to the patient if they are to be integrated into his daily living pattern.

### Patient Education

Many patients with congestive heart failure are in the geriatric age group and have coexisting medical defects as well. Problems related to cognitive, affective, and psychomotor domains of learning are intimately intertwined with the problems of aging and the developmental needs and tasks of the aged in our society.

### Cognitive Factors

**Assessment.** The patient's ability to understand and to carry out his responsibilities in the regimen of diet, drug, and activity regulation in the long-term management of CHF is influenced by such factors as basic intelligence, educational attainment level, memory loss or periods of confusion, failing vision or hearing, earlier exposure to a limited range of problem-solving behavior or failure to develop fully the ability to cope with problems, or a life style of dependency on another (such as a spouse) for providing health-care-related needs.

**Intervention.** After the problems or potential problems are diagnosed the nurse devises appropriate intervention strategies with the patient. For example, color-coding medications for the person who cannot see or read small type on labels, or designing a calendar with large date blocks to mark off when medication has been taken, can be helpful for the patient with memory loss. A poster with a sample of each pill or capsule taped on it with the name, purpose, dosage, and time to be taken is helpful for the person who has to take a number of drugs.

### Affective Factors

**Assessment.** Many aged patients with CHF live alone on subsistence income in substandard housing, including walk-up apartments. The effort expenditure involved in food shopping may overtax their reserves, particularly in inclement weather. Yet many would prefer to remain in familiar surroundings rather than go to a nursing home or custodial care environment. Older middle-aged patients may be forced into early retirement and change in living accommodations, such as moving from a house to an apartment; these individuals may have to adapt as well to the problems of role reversal when the primary breadwinner is the patient.

A seeming lack of motivation for assuming self-care responsibilities may result from lowered self-esteem. Periods of depression related to forced dependency and a feeling of hopelessness about the future can be anticipated in some patients whose chances for adaptation to chronic illness are not maximized by successful earlier life experiences or by the current support of family or friends. A most discouraging situation exists for the patient whose cardiac reserve continues to diminish and who becomes symptomatic despite his compliance with therapy.

**Intervention.** Nursing actions related to psychological or sociocultural problems in adaptation to congestive heart failure can include arranging for more frequent nursing supervision and involving family members, friends, or volunteers as surrogate "legs" so that the patient's business and personal affairs can be taken care of with minimal energy waste. Listening to the patient's expressions of feelings about his difficulties as he attempts to cope with changes in his life situation and giving positive direction when indicated, such as to other health and social or religious agencies in the community, are parts of the nursing role. Taking the position of the patient's advocate to obtain more welfare money for food, arranging for transportation for medical follow-up, or maintaining a "crisis" telephone service are ways nurses can respond. Following up when patients miss appointments demonstrates concern for the individual and is a key component in securing compliance with long-term therapy.

### Psychomotor Factors

**Assessment.** Other limiting conditions such as arthritis of the fingers or hand tremors must be considered since such factors make opening pill bottles difficult, especially with "childproof"-type containers. Ways in which energy may be wasted in the home should also be assessed.

**Intervention.** The nurse can make the pill-taking routine less complicated by suggesting alternative ways of safely packaging the drugs and storing them at home. Pouring doses of drugs for several days at a time and arranging these in a safe and easy retrieval system can help the patient with failing vision or physical handicap; suggesting ways of rearranging furniture, shelves, utensils, etc. can help the homemaker conserve energy.

### Activity and Rest

A prescription for rest and activity is an important part of the patient's regime. The nurse needs to have a broad perspective on the patient's daily needs and an ability to establish priorities of care. It is important to select aspects of care that help the patient to progress without undue strain. For the hospitalized patient, periods of rest should be provided for at intervals. For example, breakfast, bath, and bedmaking, along with nursing and medical rounds, x-rays, and ECG tests, are often scheduled to occur in one flurry of early morning activity, even though some aspects of hygiene could be delayed for the patient's benefit.

As new activities are added, the patient's response is closely monitored by counting the pulse rate and noting its rhythm and quality or by observing the cardiac monitor for rate and rhythm changes. The nurse can unobtrusively observe other parameters such as respiratory effort or degree of sweating, while she is engaged in other activities in the area; the patient's confidence increases and the nurse is nearby in case the patient becomes excessively fatigued and needs to rest.

The nurse has to be alert for possible complications and their prevention. Because she recognizes the danger of thrombophlebitis in patients who are confined to bed, she does not roll up the knee gatch to hold the patient up in bed and leave the gatch that way for days. This position places pressure behind the knees and discourages normal movement of the legs. A footboard is used so that by placing the feet against it the patient is kept from sliding down in bed. Use of a covered supply box is a simple method of extending a footboard to keep the short patient from sliding down in bed. The feet and legs must be maintained in good alignment.

Massage of pressure areas, clean dry clothing and bed linen, periodic change of position, and a sheepskin under the buttocks can be used to prevent decubitus ulcers. Because edematous tissues are not well nourished, special skin care is necessary to prevent breakdown.

Today there is a growing tendency to put activity prescription for the cardiac patient on a more scientific basis. Progression begins with basic self-care activities with gradual increments of other forms, especially walking. The basic considerations for activity prescription for the patient with compensated congestive heart failure are found in Chapter 39.

## Diet Therapy

**Dietary Potassium.** To guard against the development of hypokalemia, a complication of administration of potassium-depleting diuretics, patients on such drugs are instructed to increase their dietary intake of potassium. The patient needs to understand that the potassium ordered to be in-gested in foods is as important a prescription as a liquid potassium supplement. Foods high in potassium include many fruits such as bananas, apricots, oranges, grapefruit, prunes and their juices (canned or fresh), and fresh tomatoes. High-protein foods such as meat or fish, nuts, nonstarchy vegetables such as spinach, white and sweet potatoes, and whole-grain cereals are also high in potassium. Care must be taken not to add sodium when increasing potassium intake if the patient is on a sodium-restricted diet. The symptoms and signs of hypokalemia include weak pulses, faint heart sounds, hypotension, muscle flabbiness, diminished tendon reflexes, and generalized weakness.

The physician may prescribe an oral potassium supplement if dietary intake is insufficient. Since potassium solutions can cause gastric irritation, they should be diluted in water or fruit juice before being swallowed.

**Low-Sodium Diet.** Special diets are a necessary part of many therapies. It is often difficult for the patient to accept dietary restrictions, but it is nevertheless true that his future well-being partially depends on following the diet. The patient with edema, for example, cannot eat food with a high sodium content because sodium causes water retention. Many patients ask a question such as: "Why is it that I can't eat salt now? I always used to and it never bothered me." The nurse can answer, "Dr. Gray explained to you about how your body holds fluid, and that that was why you noticed swelling in your ankles. The sodium in salt helps to hold the fluid in your body. When you cut down on the salt, less fluid stays in your tissues."

An average diet contains about 4,000 to 6,000 mg. of sodium daily. One level teaspoon of table salt (NaCl) contains 2,300 mg. of sodium. Sodium is found naturally in nearly all foods, in cooking agents such as baking powder, in food additives such as monosodium glutamate, in drinking water, and in medications (such as sodium bicarbonate).

Successful diet therapy requires teamwork on the part of the physician, dietitian, nurse, patient, and family or associates involved in meal planning, shopping, and cooking.

The physician usually prescribes the diet in mg. of sodium according to what he thinks the patient's body can handle. For example, a standard diet without free salt would contain about 2,500 mg. sodium. A *mild* sodium-restricted diet simply reduces sodium intake to about half the usual amount by ruling out very salty foods such as potato chips, most cheeses, olives, and soy sauce as well as a few commercially prepared foods such as regular canned soups, stews, and casserole-type dishes which are particularly high in sodium, and by reducing table salt consumption by half.

A *moderate* sodium-restricted diet contains about 1,000 mg. of sodium. A *strict* diet contains only about 500 mg. of sodium, while a *rigid* diet contains less and requires even low-sodium milk. Commercial salt substitutes (which are high in potassium) require the physician's approval before use.

The following common foods are high in sodium and usually are excluded completely: salty or smoked meats, bacon, salted fish, salted nuts, potato chips, salted crackers, ketchup, mustard, peanut butter, frankfurters, luncheon meats, cheese (except washed cottage cheese), and foods prepared in brine such as pickles or sauerkraut.

The following foods also contain considerable sodium and may be excluded or restricted in amount: ordinary bread, butter, and milk (special preparations that limit sodium content of all these are available), cake and cookies, most shellfish, frozen peas, lima beans, and some frozen fish.

Dietetic foods prepared for sodium-restricted diets, such as ham or bacon, and low-sodium milk (Lonalac) are available in some supermarkets and specialty food stores. It would be helpful if such facilities in each community were listed and the list made readily available to cardiac patients to avoid the energy expenditure involved in looking around for such facilities.

For the hospitalized patient, written diets are helpful to take home, but it is almost useless to call the dietitian on the day of discharge and ask her to race right up "with a diet for Mr. Brownell," who has already packed his suitcase and is standing in the corridor with his wife. As soon as the nurse suspects that the patient will require sodium-restricted diet therapy, she confers with the physician about the prescription and then notifies the dietitian.

Although the dietitian usually carries out detailed instruction in low-sodium diets, the nurse may assist by contributing to the diet history, by reinforcing the instruction, and by evaluating the patient's cognitive and affective response to the instruction and his physiologic response to the diet, such as by daily weight measurement. In the home or hospital, the nurse can provide audiovisual educational materials and review these with the patient as one means of assessing the patient's comprehension. Eliciting his feelings about the diet may help him become more accepting of it and thus more open to further learning.

Will it be the patient who has the chief responsibility for food arrangements? In the hospital it may be the nurse who arranges for the spouse to visit when the dietitian makes her rounds, so that the person who does the cooking can have the opportunity to ask questions about the preparation of food. In the home the nurse might speak to several family members.

What cultural factors are involved? Often special diets are thought of as modifications of our own American diet. But, Spanish-speaking peoples, Egyptians, and Japanese go on special diets in their own countries. The special diet should be an adaptation of a normal diet for that patient. Unfortunately, attempting to change food patterns often seems like saying to the patient, "You must get over being Italian and be American."

Despite sodium restriction, the patient can still have many of his favorite dishes if he has a competent dietitian or nurse in the hospital or home figure the food values and show him how to plan menus, to use diet literature, and to make low-sodium foods palatable. The amount of sodium in snack foods must be considered as part of the patient's daily allotment. Foods that are virtually free of sodium such as fresh fruit are recommended snack foods.

The dietitian can talk with the patient or family member several times about the sodium content of various foods, the kind and the amount of food that he could have each day without exceeding the amount of sodium permitted, and the variety of other seasonings that can be used, such as a hint of onion on meat, a dash of lemon juice on fish, and pepper on an egg; she can also provide him with materials for ready reference. The patient and family can be shown various labels so that they can become accustomed to evaluating sodium content. Labels describing sodium may read salt, soda, sodium, or the symbol Na. A call-in service to a dietary counselor is a helpful measure in assisting the patient to assume the long-term responsibilities for his diet therapy.

The nurse who reviews the sodium-restricted diet with the patient and discusses what he is allowed to eat will be most constructive when her attitude is light in touch and sympathetic in nature, rather than punitive. Restriction of diet may be a true loss to a patient. Only anger and rebellion will be aroused in a patient if a nurse uses threats of readmission or demeaning comments in an attempt to secure his compliance with diet therapy.

The period when the patient is beginning to change food habits is the most difficult. This is the time he suffers most and needs the most support and encouragement. He especially needs to be encouraged by having his successes in managing his diet noted. He may be helped by direction to divisionary activities which offer new avenues for satisfaction, as well as by emphasis on the positive outcomes of the diet. When people following diets concentrate on the pleasure of looking better and feeling better, they may gain some satisfaction that helps to make up for not being able to eat such morsels as salted crackers, ketchup, potato chips, pretzels, or salty bacon.

Patients on very low sodium intake must be observed, especially in hot weather, for symptoms of sodium deficit. When the patient perspires a great deal, he may need more sodium than his diet provides and as a consequence develop weakness, apprehension, dizziness, headache, abdominal cramps, and diarrhea. Hypotension and a rapid thready pulse are signs of sodium deficit. If these symptoms or signs appear, the physician increases the allowance of sodium.

The nurse can help the family members to appreciate the difficulties the patient is experiencing with his diet and make suggestions for increasing their sensitivity, such as not buying potato chips or pretzels for family snack foods or at least not eating them in front of the patient.

The patient needs to know how and where to get help with his diet after he leaves the hospital and how to get his questions answered. The American Heart Association (44 East 23rd Street, New York City, 10010) and its local affiliates and the United States Public Health Service (write the Government Printing Office, Washington, D.C., 20025) have pamphlets available that describe the uses of sodium in the body, sample diets, and recipes in "Your 500 mg. Sodium Diet (Revised)," "Your 1,000 mg. Sodium Diet (Revised)," and "Your Mild Sodium Restricted Diet." Some states have regional diet counseling services, where patients and families can receive special help on an outpatient basis. Patients who require continued dietary supervision or help in other areas of congestive heart failure management should be referred to a community nursing agency for posthospital nursing care.

## Drug Therapy

Many cardiac patients take digitalis for years. It helps to control their disease and permits them to live comfortably. Patients especially need to know that they should not discontinue their digitalis when they feel well, or take more than the prescribed dose when they don't feel well.

Toxic effects can occur from digitalis. They tend to appear gradually. The patient is generally instructed to consult the physician if he experiences sudden loss of appetite for 24 hours, unexplained nausea or vomiting, unusual palpitation or change in pulse, or sudden disturbance in vision (LaDue and Burckhardt, 1967). If early symptoms are noted and reported to the physician or nurse, more serious toxic effects usually can be avoided.

The physician or nurse who sees the patient for long-term care questions the patient at each examination regarding what drugs he is taking. Drug interactions must be considered when an adverse reaction to drug therapy arises. Over-the-counter drugs as well as prescribed drugs can be involved. For example, calcium in a vitamin-mineral supplement can act synergistically with digitalis and cause more rapid toxicity (Lancour, 1973). A drug such as propranolol, taken for arrhythmia suppression, can aggravate existing heart failure. Careful questioning of the patient and a cardiovascular physical examination can point out early symptoms and signs.

Many patients on digitalis receive diuretics also. Observation of signs of hypokalemia and hyponatremia are part of the continuing patient assessment at follow-up visits.

## Patient Self-Monitoring

The patient who understands and accepts his condition can be instructed to monitor his response to therapy so that he can get medical help before a crisis occurs. If the patient is unable, a responsible person can be instructed. Points that may be discussed, depending on the individuals, include:

- Any recurrence of symptoms is to be reported to the physician or nurse promptly, for example, dyspnea on usual exertion, fluid retention manifested by swelling in legs or abdomen, paroxysmal nocturnal dyspnea, unusual fatigue or weakness.

- Patients on digitalis should report loss of appetite, nausea or vomiting, change in vision (especially yellow vision), change in usual heart rate (especially slowing, palpitations, or irregular heartbeat).
- Patients on diuretics are to take daily weight every morning before breakfast, always wearing similar clothing. Daily weight is to be recorded and shown to the physician or nurse each time a follow-up visit is made.
- Symptoms of electrolyte depletion are often vague, and a listing of all of them can unnecessarily alarm a patient. Generalized weakness, apprehension, and muscular or abdominal cramps should be reported. Since individuals are unique each can be encouraged to respect his own warning signals.
- Nonproductive cough, which may be due to pulmonary congestion, should be reported, as should upper abdominal discomfort, which may indicate liver congestion.
- Anxiety, confusion, or forgetfulness may indicate decreased cerebral circulation. These symptoms may also indicate that the patient's coping abilities are overtaxed, a condition which contributes to further cardiovascular stress. In either case, such symptoms or signs should be reported to the physician; the nurse plans with the patient for appropriate nursing strategies.

## ACUTE PULMONARY EDEMA

Pulmonary edema represents an acute emergency for the patient and often is associated with heart disease. The weakening of the left ventricle, which may be caused by such conditions as acute myocardial infarction, arteriosclerotic heart disease, or rapid cardiac arrhythmias, makes the left ventricle incapable of maintaining sufficient output of blood with each contraction. However, the right ventricle continues to pump blood toward the lungs. The pulmonary capillaries and the alveoli become engorged, because blood continues to flow to the lungs and is not adequately and promptly pumped into the systemic circulation by the left ventricle. Sometimes, the lungs become rapidly inundated with fluid. This inundation of the lungs can occur in patients who have congestive heart failure; it may be triggered by some unusual exertion or by slipping down in bed during sleep. (When the patient lies flat pulmonary congestion is increased by an increase in systemic venous return, an increase in capillary hydrostatic pressure in the lungs, and a decrease in vital capacity.) Acute respiratory distress develops. This condition is termed paroxysmal nocturnal dyspnea.

Acute pulmonary edema can result also from injury to the lung tissue, such as blast injuries causing many small hemorrhages within the lung, or by the inhalation of irritants, such as ammonia.

Patients with acute pulmonary edema experience prodromal anxiety, restlessness, sudden dyspnea, wheezing, orthopnea, cough (often productive of pinkish, frothy sputum), cyanosis, and severe apprehension. Respirations sound moist or "gurgling."

The relief of these symptoms is urgent. The patient literally can drown in his own secretions during an attack of acute pulmonary edema. Every effort is made to relieve the congestion in the lungs as quickly as possible.

The physician's orders may include measures to provide physical and emotional relaxation, to relieve hypoxia, to retard venous return to the heart, and to improve cardiovascular function.

- Provide physical and emotional relaxation.

Morphine or meperidine (Demerol) often is ordered intravenously to lessen apprehension. Morphine, particularly, seems to help to relieve the attack by depressing higher cerebral centers, thus relieving anxiety and slowing the respiratory rate. In addition, morphine promotes muscular relaxation to reduce the work of breathing. Very importantly, morphine dilates peripheral veins thus reducing venous return by a so-called internal or pharmacologic phlebotomy (Hultgren and Flamm, 1969). The patient should be permitted to stay in the position most comfortable for him, usually sitting up. Anything that would increase his feeling of breathlessness and choking should be avoided, such as pulling curtains around his bed or closing the window if the patient indicates he wants it open. If it is possible, have one nurse talk to the physician and family while another remains with the patient so that the patient is not left alone in his distress.

- Relieve hypoxia and improve ventilation.

To produce a pressure gradient sufficient to raise the rate of oxygen diffusion across the fluid barrier of edema in the alveoli, 100 per cent oxygen through a positive pressure, non-rebreathing type of mask may be ordered initially. This helps to prevent further engorgement of the lungs with fluid. Later, a nasal catheter or nasal cannula may be substituted. The mask must be applied quickly, but not without a brief word of explanation and reassurance to the patient, who is already afraid of suffocation, and who may be made more so by the sudden application of the mask. There should be a firm seal between the mask and the patient's face, but not so tight as to cause pressure damage to the patient's skin. Frequent drying of the skin will minimize this risk.

Oxygen must always be humidified to prevent the drying of secretions and further impairment to ventilation. In acute pulmonary edema the problem of humidification is somewhat different. The thin, watery fluid which accumulates in the alveoli and bronchioles often contains some blood. There is sufficient protein in this edema fluid to produce froth as air passes through it, and this froth severely obstructs the small airways and alveoli. Sometimes the physician will order ethyl alcohol as an aerosol. The alcohol mixes with the edema fluid and lowers its surface tension, causing the bubbles to lose their stability, rupture, and return to the liquid state. The liquid can then be more easily removed by the cough mechanism or through the circulation.

Aminophylline may be administered intravenously to dilate the bronchi and to make breathing easier, and to lessen pulmonary-capillary transudate. An intravenous drip of the drug in solution not to exceed a rate of 20 mg. per minute may be ordered.

- Retard venous return to the heart.

Measures may be taken to decrease the volume of circulating blood, thus helping to relieve the congestion of blood and fluid in the lungs. These measures consist of wet or dry phlebotomy, the use of an intermittent positive pressure ventilator, and the use of morphine. Wet phlebotomy of approximately 500 ml. of blood may be performed, or rotating tourniquets may be used to trap blood in the extremities, so that it is not returned to the already overburdened and congested heart and lungs, a so-called "dry" phlebotomy.

When rotating tourniquets are used, they may be applied clockwise or counterclockwise, provided that the tourniquets are always rotated in the same direction throughout the treatment. The tourniquet is applied tightly enough to interfere with venous return and not tightly enough to cut off arterial circulation. If a rubber tourniquet is used, the pulse in the extremity is taken after applying the tourniquet. If the pulse has been obliterated, the tourniquet has been applied too tightly, and it should be loosened. If blood-pressure cuffs are used, each cuff is inflated to a point between the patient's systolic and diastolic blood pressure.

The exact procedure to be used varies, and it will be specified by the physician. Tourniquets may be rotated every 15 minutes, although in some instances the physician may order more frequent rotation. If 15-minute intervals are used, each extremity will have had the tourniquet on it for 45 minutes and will have been free of the tourniquet 15 minutes (see Table 34-2 and Fig. 34-5).

### Table 34-2. Plan for Rotating Tourniquets

| TIME A.M. | RIGHT LEG | LEFT LEG | LEFT ARM | RIGHT ARM |
|---|---|---|---|---|
| 9:00 | off | on | on | on |
| 9:15 | on | off | on | on |
| 9:30 | on | on | off | on |
| 9:45 | on | on | on | off |
| 10:00 | off | on | on | on |

The patient's extremities will become swollen, mottled, and uncomfortable due to engorgement with venous blood, and the patient should be told that the

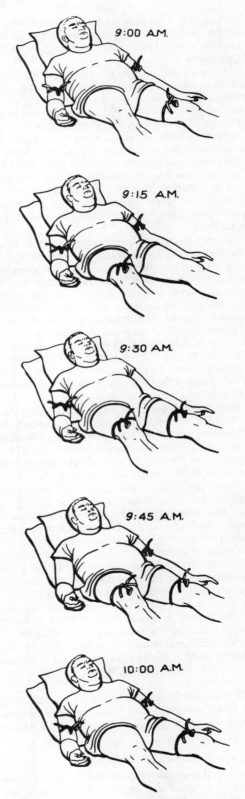

**Figure 34-5.** Rotation of tourniquets at 15-minute intervals. (See Table 35-2)

swelling will disappear when the tourniquets are removed. The pulse in the extremity must be palpated frequently, to be sure that the circulation to the part is adequate.

When the tourniquets are to be removed, the same rotation already established is followed and one tourniquet is removed every 15 minutes, so that by the end of 45 minutes all tourniquets will have been removed. Tourniquets are never removed all at once. To remove them all at the same time would cause a sudden increase in the amount of circulating blood, with a return of more blood to the heart and the lungs than they can handle, causing another attack of pulmonary edema. If the extremities do not return promptly to their normal appearance when the tourniquets have been removed, the physician must be notified.

Several models of electrically operated automatic rotating tourniquet machines are currently available (Fig. 34-6). The use of these machines saves nursing time since there is no need to change the velcro-fastened blood pressure cuff-type tourniquets once they are applied. Inflation and deflation time is automatically cycled. The machine is more efficient since it eliminates the variability in technique and skin pressure which results when more than one person manually applies rubber tourniquets. Human failure resulting from "forgetting" to rotate the tourniquets or not being able to get back to the patient on time is eliminated.

Blood pressure can be taken easily using the pressure gauge on some machines or, on others, by disconnecting an arm cuff from the machine and attaching a sphygmomanometer to it. The same observations relative to arterial circulation and discontinuance of therapy are necessary.

Some physicians advocate mechanical positive pressure breathing during inspiration (IPPB) to reduce venous return to the heart in the treatment of acute pulmonary edema. Normally, the intrathoracic pressure of spontaneous respiration is negative. When this negative pressure is replaced by positive pressure, venous return to the heart is reduced. The physician determines flow-rate, pressure, and inspiratory/expiratory ratio in order to arrive at an intrathoracic net positive pressure which will impede venous flow. (If the patient is hypotensive, further reduction of venous return to the heart is contraindicated.) IPPB has the additional benefit of assisting ventilation in all lung segments and is an effective means of administering oxygen. (See Chapter 60 for care of the patient on a respirator.)

Morphine sulfate, because of its property of pooling blood in peripheral vascular beds, is used to retard venous return as well as to decrease anxiety and relieve dyspnea.

- Improve cardiovascular function.

When the attack of pulmonary edema is due to congestive heart failure, other measures for the treatment of this condition may be begun promptly,

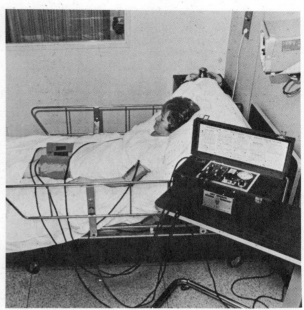

**Figure 34-6.** Patient receiving treatment with automatic rotating tourniquets. (Jobst Institute, Inc., Toledo, Ohio)

if the patient has not already been receiving them, for example, the injection of a rapid-acting, potent diuretic such as ethacrynate sodium (Edecrin Sodium) and digitalization with a rapidly acting preparation, like ouabain.

## REFERENCES AND BIBLIOGRAPHY

ABELMANN, W. H.: The cardiomyopathies, *Hosp. Pract.* 6:101, March 1971.

BETSON, C.: The nurse's role in blood gas monitoring, *Cardiovasc. Nurs.* 7:83, November-December 1971.

———, and UDE, L.: Central venous pressure, *Am. J. Nurs.* 69:1466, July 1969.

BROWSE, N.: *The Physiology and Pathology of Bed Rest,* Springfield, Ill., Thomas, 1965.

CHURCH, C. F., and CHURCH, H. N.: *Bowes and Church's Food Values of Portions Commonly Used,* ed. 11, Philadelphia, Lippincott, 1970.

CLARK, N. F.: Pump failure, *Nurs. Clin. N. Am.* 7:529, September 1972.

CREWS, J.: Nurse-managed cardiac clinics, *Cardiovasc. Nurs.* 8:15, July-August 1972.

EGAN, D.: Management of acute pulmonary edema, *Hosp. Med.* 2:20, February 1966.

———: *Fundamentals of Inhalation Therapy,* St. Louis, Mosby, 1969.

FISHMAN, A. P.: Chronic cor pulmonale, *Hosp. Pract.* 6:101, May 1971.

GANS, J.: Digitalis glycosides, *Nurs. '73* 3:59, June 1973.

GUYTON, A.: *Textbook of Medical Physiology*, ed. 4, Philadelphia, Saunders, 1970.

HANCHETT, E., and JOHNSON, R.: Early signs of congestive heart failure, *Am. J. Nurs.* 68:1456, July 1968.

HULTGREN, H., and FLAMM, M.: Pulmonary edema, *Mod. Conc. Cardiovasc. Dis.* 38:1, January 1969.

HURST, J., and LOGUE, R.: *The Heart*, New York, McGraw-Hill, 1966.

LaDUE, J., and BURCKHARDT, D.: Digitalis intoxication, *Hosp. Med.* 3:23, February 1967.

LANCOUR, J.: The nurse and cardiovascular drug therapy, *Cardiovasc. Nurs.* 9:19, July-August 1973.

LARSON, E.: The patient with acute pulmonary edema, *Am. J. Nurs.* 68:1019, May 1968.

LEVINE, S.: Chair rest versus bed rest, *Hosp. Med.* 2:2, January 1966.

MALANG, J.: The difference it makes, *Am. J. Nurs.* 72:276, February 1972.

McINTYRE, H.: Clinical nursing and the congestive heart failure patient, *Cardiovasc. Nurs.* 3:19, September-October 1967.

MORGAN, W. L., and ENGEL, G. L.: *The Clinical Approach to the Patient*, Philadelphia, Saunders, 1969.

OLSEN, E., et al.: The hazards of immobility, *Am. J. Nurs.* 67:779, April 1967.

Potassium imbalance: Programmed instruction, *Am. J. Nurs.* 67:343, February 1967.

RAMSEY, M. A.: The failing heart, *Nurs. '72* 2:18, October 1972.

REDMAN, B.: Client education therapy in treatment and prevention of cardiovascular disease, *Cardiovasc. Nurs.* 10:1, January-February 1974.

SCHWARTZ, D., et al.: *The Elderly Ambulatory Patient*, New York, Macmillan, 1969.

SPENCER, R.: Problems of drug therapy in congestive heart failure, *RN* 35:46, August 1972.

# The Patient with Rheumatic Fever; Rheumatic Heart (Valvular) Disease; Bacterial Endocarditis; Pericarditis

## CHAPTER 35

Patients with inflammatory cardiac diseases such as rheumatic fever or rheumatic valvular disease, bacterial endocarditis, or pericarditis share certain common features besides the often overwhelming awareness that they have been struck down by dreaded heart disease. These disorders often follow infection elsewhere in the body, mainly in the throat and the mouth, which has left the patient in a weakened condition to cope with additional physical and psychosocial threats. The treatment process is not dramatic but rather slow and tedious. The diseases are frequent among young adults who must forego their usual job, civic, and family and social responsibilities for a long period, sometimes with loss of income. Those who are economically at the poverty level are most often affected and despite some public programs (Medicaid, for example) frequently lack the quality of health care needed.

The chronicity of a condition such as rheumatic heart disease, or its prophylaxis, involves regular medication and frequent physical assessment, ECG's, and x-rays. The estimated costs of visits to physicians for rheumatic fever and rheumatic heart disease in fiscal 1969 was about 28 million dollars (Inter-Society Commission for Heart Disease Resources, 1970).

All of the diseases carry an uncertainty about the future. How much permanent heart damage, if any, has occurred is difficult to predict. Nevertheless, the question is there, though unanswerable, and the course of the patient's future life plans may be profoundly affected by heart damage. The extent of the damage often is not fully manifest during youth, but may lead to symptoms later in life when the individual experiences

Rheumatic Fever

Active Rheumatic Fever

Chronic Rheumatic Heart Disease

Rheumatic Heart (Valvular) Disease

Bacterial Endocarditis

Pericarditis

additional stressors, such as another illness, child bearing, or the aging process.

## RHEUMATIC FEVER

Today, a major cause of cardiovascular disease which is preventable is rheumatic fever. However the availability of effective preventive agents does not guarantee effective prevention. It is an unfortunate reflection on the delivery of health care in the United States today that rheumatic fever is predominantly a disease of the poor who live in slum areas and are least likely to seek or obtain health care (Markowitz, 1970).

Rheumatic fever often leads to permanent damage to the heart and valves with subsequent chronic valvular heart disease. *Rheumatic heart disease* refers to the cardiac manifestations of rheumatic fever, in either the acute phase or the later stage of chronic damage. This is the major reason that the condition is important among adults. In caring for adults, health care professionals are concerned primarily with rheumatic heart disease, but it is important to understand something about its original cause, rheumatic fever.

### Incidence

At one time rheumatic heart disease was the most common form of organic heart disease in persons under 50 in the United States. Between 1944 and 1965, however, the death rate from acute rheumatic fever in the United States showed a decline of 90 per cent, primarily due to vigorous treatment with penicillin (National Health Education Committee, 1966).

Approximately 100,000 new cases (first attacks) of rheumatic fever and rheumatic heart disease still occur each year. Since the 1930's new cases of rheumatic fever have been reduced only about 30 per cent, with the reduction occurring in middle- and upper-class populations (Inter-Society Commission for Heart Disease Resources, 1970).

Rheumatic fever is found most among those who are between the ages of 5 and 15. It sometimes occurs in late adolescence and young adulthood, particularly in persons with a history of the disease in childhood; it is rare after the age of 25. Under conditions favoring epidemic streptococcal infection, however, such as among new recruits in military installations during World War II, there was a high incidence of rheumatic fever. Penicillin prophylaxis

among such populations has resulted in a marked and sustained reduction (Stamler, 1967).

### Etiology

Rheumatic fever does not occur without a preceding streptococcal infection, but the manner in which these two events are connected remains unknown. Some physicians believe that rheumatic fever occurs in persons who have a hypersensitivity to the streptococcus or its products, and that rheumatic fever is essentially an allergic reaction to streptococcal infection.

Rheumatic fever is a systemic response found in 3 per cent of persons infected with group A hemolytic streptococci (Erb and Wilson, 1968). Why 3 people are affected and 97 escape is an unsolved mystery. A previous attack increases the risk of recurrent attack following streptococcal infection from 30/1,000 (3 per cent) to 500/1,000 (50 per cent) or higher (Stamler, 1967). It often follows such conditions as pharyngitis, tonsillitis, and scarlet fever. Some investigators have noted a strong familial tendency, but this is sometimes attributed to the spread of streptococcal infection within a family.

Environment plays a part, too. Rheumatic fever is most prevalent during cool, damp weather, and its incidence is greater in the northern sections of the United States than in the southern regions. These variations may be related to the higher incidence of streptococcal infections during cold, damp weather.

Substandard living conditions with inadequate heating and sanitation, overcrowding, and undernutrition seem to increase the incidence of rheumatic fever by lessening individual resistance to infection and increasing the likelihood of the spread of the streptococcal infection from one person to another.

Markowitz (1970) notes that two-thirds of the patients who develop rheumatic fever do so following asymptomatic or mild streptococcal throat infections. People in the lower socioeconomic group are the least likely to seek treatment for an overt upper respiratory infection.

## ACTIVE RHEUMATIC FEVER

### Symptoms

Rheumatic fever affects the connective tissue in many different areas of the body. Therefore, symptoms often are widely distributed, involving, for example, joints, heart, and nervous system. The manifestations of the disease vary greatly. In one patient most of the symptoms may be related to the nervous system, whereas in another patient the inflammation of the joints may be severe. Sometimes, the disease is so mild that it escapes detection, or it is so atypical in its symptoms that many and repeated tests, plus very careful observation of the patient, are necessary to confirm the diagnosis.

The disease may appear one to four weeks after a streptococcal infection. It may be gradual in onset, with slowly increasing fatigue, anorexia, weight loss, lassitude, and slight fever, or it may begin suddenly with acute swelling and inflammation of one or many joints, moderate fever, and malaise and pallor. Joint symptoms often are described as *migratory polyarthritis,* meaning that the condition moves from one joint to another, eventually involving many joints in the body. The joints later heal completely; even those which were very swollen and painful have no permanent deformity. A rash called *erythema marginatum,* characterized by wavy lines and circles or portions of circles which appear and disappear rapidly on the trunk and abdomen and do not itch, and firm, nontender *subcutaneous nodules* may be part of the patient's symptomatology.

Cerebral lesions can be associated with neurologic symptoms such as chorea. Chorea occurs in childhood, especially in girls, and it is characterized by uncontrollable, uncoordinated, purposeless movements. These symptoms usually disappear entirely after a period of rest and supportive care. Most children who have chorea develop other evidences of rheumatic infection. They should be observed carefully for such symptoms—especially those related to cardiac function.

Pulmonary and pleural lesions can also occur.

The amount of the cardiac involvement is of great concern in rheumatic fever, because the heart can develop permanent deformity as a result of the disease. The involvement of the heart varies from patient to patient. Typically, patients with rheumatic fever have tachycardia out of proportion to the degree of the fever. Some experience palpitation associated with rapid heart action. Pain over the heart sometimes occurs. Myocarditis (inflammation of the heart muscle) and pericarditis (inflammation of the sac enclosing the heart) account for most of the cardiac symptoms that occur during the acute phase of the disease. If the involvement of the heart

is severe enough, the function of the heart will be impaired, and the patient with active rheumatic fever may show symptoms of congestive heart failure or cardiac arrhythmias.

The endocardial involvement consists of inflammation of the endocardium and valve leaflets. Characteristic vegetations (verrucae) appear in the valves. There is edema and inflammation of the valve ring which heals with scar formation. This can seriously deform the delicate valve structures and result later in chronic valvular disease manifested by cardiac enlargement, congestive heart failure, and rhythm disturbances.

As a result of clots or a piece of valve breaking off and entering the general circulation, cerebral emboli or peripheral arterial occlusions can develop. (Valvular heart disease due to rheumatic fever is discussed below.)

**Diagnostic Assessment**

The diagnosis of rheumatic fever is primarily based on clinical judgment since there is no specific laboratory test to prove that a person has the disease. Nurses participate collaboratively with physicians in the diagnostic assessment. A nurse in a hospital or neighborhood "storefront" clinic, a mobile health unit, or a school nurse may be alerted to the possibility of rheumatic fever by a client's history of sore throat, fever, and joint pains; she can initiate or pursue referral for further workup. Diagnostic data is gathered from the following sources:

- History—the client is questioned about symptoms of streptococcal pharyngitis in the recent past, such as sudden onset of sore throat, fever, chilliness, enlarged and tender lymph nodes; and about contact with a person with streptococcal infection.
- Socioeconomic factors—the client is questioned about pertinent data such as housing, heat, food intake, number of occupants in household and their states of health.

Physical Assessment

- Examination of the heart—rheumatic carditis is a part of rheumatic fever, not a complication. The endocardium, myocardium, and pericardium can be involved. Auscultation can reveal cardiac valve involvement causing murmurs; myocardial inflammation, indicated by weakening of heart sounds, tachycardia, and cardiac dilatation may also be found. Pericarditis may cause accumulation of fluid in the pericardial sac simulating heart enlargement. The latter can occur due to stretching of weakened heart muscle or may represent the hypertrophy of heart damage from earlier attacks of carditis. Early signs of congestive heart failure should be given close attention. A fast sleeping pulse may be indicative of carditis. Prolongation of the P-R interval of the ECG is a diagnostic clue.

- Examination of the joints for arthritis.
- Examination of the skin for subcutaneous nodules and erythema marginatum.
- Examination of the nervous system for chorea.
- Chest x-rays for assessment of cardiac enlargement or pulmonary complications.

## Laboratory Tests

- Throat culture—a throat culture positive for group A streptococci is supportive of a diagnosis of acute rheumatic fever. However, a positive throat culture can also indicate a long-standing carrier state, while a negative culture does not rule out rheumatic fever since the streptococci may have disappeared from the throat or be difficult to detect by the time rheumatic fever appears.*

- Streptococcal antibody determinations—epidemiologic studies show the association of group A hemolytic streptococci with pharyngitis preceding rheumatic fever by one to three weeks. An immunologic response is seen in the antigen-antibody reaction to streptococcal infection. One measure of the antibody response in the patient's blood is the antistreptolysin-O titer (ASO titer). The level of the antibody response, or a rising antibody titer, gives an indication of the preceding streptococcal infection. With the measurement of other streptococcal antibodies (antihyaluronidase, antistreptokinase, for instance), it is now possible to demonstrate preceding streptococcal infection in 95 per cent of patients with acute rheumatic fever if they are studied within two months of onset (Stollerman, et al., 1956).

- CBC (complete blood count)—leukocytosis and anemia are characteristic during an acute rheumatic infection.

- C-reactive protein—this protein substance, which is not present normally in the blood, appears in the blood in a variety of inflammatory states, including rheumatic fever.

- Increased sedimentation rate—the rate at which the red blood cells settle to the bottom of a tube is increased in rheumatic fever, as it is in many other conditions characterized by infection or inflammation. The particular usefulness of this test in rheumatic fever lies in the tendency of the increased sedimentation rate to persist even after other evidences of active disease have subsided. The sedimentation rate is more useful in determining whether the patient's disease is still active than it is in indicating whether the disease is rheumatic fever.

- Aschoff bodies—this specific type of inflammatory lesion in the myocardium is considered definitely to be an indication of rheumatic fever. These microscopic bodies are noted on postmortem examination. The Aschoff body is a collection of polymorphonuclear cells and lymphocytes surrounding multinucleated giant cells found especially in the left atrial appendage in rheumatic myocarditis (Erb and Wilson, 1968).

The nurse can help the patient and his family during the diagnostic tests by explaining the reasons they were ordered and by encouraging the continuation of the tests recommended by the physician. Often it is hard for the patient to understand that there is no single definite test for rheumatic fever, and that varied and repeated tests are necessary to establish the diagnosis.

## Treatment

The aims of management of the acute attack are early detection of carditis and congestive heart failure and their symptomatic relief with anti-inflammatory and cardiotonic drugs, reduction of cardiac workload until the inflammatory process has subsided, and relief of other symptoms.

During the acute stage the patient must be under daily supervision of a member of the health care team in a hospital, day-care center, or in the home if the environment meets adequate health standards and a responsible adult is available to care for the patient. Unfortunately the severity of valvular deformities resulting from the acute attack bears little or no relation to treatment. Only avoidance of first attacks through effective prophylaxis can prevent valvular deformity, and only prevention of recurrent attacks can prevent the worsening of valvular deformities.

**Medication.** The first principle in the treatment of active rheumatic fever is said to be the eradication of the group A beta hemolytic streptococcus. Penicillin is the drug of choice. Erythromycin may be used if the patient is sensitive to penicillin. Throat cultures may be ordered at various times after the onset of treatment to confirm eradication of the organism. Various forms and dosage levels of penicillin may be ordered in the acute stage, and monthly intramuscular benzathine penicillin G may be administered indefinitely to keep low but effective levels in the blood of susceptible patients.

---

*To take a throat culture, the swab should be brought down across the tonsil on one side, the tip should touch the posterior pharyngeal wall as it crosses the throat to the other side, and then the swab should touch the other tonsil as it comes up. This is the "down-across-up" maneuver (Watson, 1966).

Salicylates are very effective and have been used for many years for the symptomatic relief of rheumatic fever. Usually, fairly large doses are necessary to control the symptoms. Some adults receive as much as 10 Gm. of acetylsalicylic acid a day, in divided doses. Often therapy is started with 0.6 Gm. (gr. 10) every four hours, and gradually it is increased and then maintained at a level that controls the symptoms without causing toxic effects, such as nausea, vomiting, and ringing in the ears (tinnitus).

ACTH and cortisone promptly and effectively relieve the symptoms of rheumatic fever; like salicylates, they do not cure the disease. Their effectiveness in decreasing the damage to the heart is being studied. It has been suggested that the prompt administration of these steroids, by decreasing the inflammation, may lessen the damage to the heart. The dosage of steroids in the treatment of rheumatic fever varies. Some investigators stress the importance of the prompt administration of steroids in a high dosage as a possible way of preventing heart damage. A daily total of 60 mg. of prednisone (Meticorten) has been recommended, given in divided doses. Toxic effects of steroids include edema, moon face, hirsutism, glycosuria, and sometimes mental disturbances. These symptoms usually disappear when the medication is discontinued.

**Rest** is very important during the active stage of rheumatic fever. The patient is kept in bed. Some physicians allow bathroom privileges if the disease seems mild. In recent years some physicians are allowing more flexibility than others in the strictness of bed rest after the second week of the onset of the disease, provided that there has been no evidence of carditis. If cardiac involvement occurs, it does so within the first two weeks of the illness in 80 per cent of the patients who develop this complication. However, the effects of activity beyond strict bed rest during acute rheumatic fever have not yet been well studied, and most physicians prefer that bed rest be maintained until all signs and all symptoms of active disease have subsided. The patient's emotional reaction is considered, too. If he becomes extremely restless and discontented after many weeks of strict bed rest, the physician may permit him to be taken to the bathroom once daily in a wheelchair. The activity of getting out of bed, carried out in such a way that it entails as little exertion as possible, may boost the patient's morale and may also help him to comply with the order for extended rest.

Rest is both facilitated and made more difficult by other aspects of treatment. Salicylates and/or steroids promptly and effectively relieve the symptoms, but they do not cure the underlying disease. The patient feels better, and although the lessening of the joint pain and the fever helps him to rest more comfortably, it also makes him wonder why he needs to rest at all. It is hard for him to understand that feeling well is not necessarily indicative of being well.

**Diet** is important in helping the patient to overcome the disease. Because patients with rheumatic fever tend to have poor appetites, frequent small meals may be tolerated better than three large ones. A liberal fluid intake is important. Sodium may be restricted to prevent edema due to steroids, or if the patient develops congestive heart failure.

### Nursing Assessment

When developing a nursing care plan for the patient with acute rheumatic fever, effective nurse-physician collaboration should yield data pertinent to the following points to be assessed:

- **The extent of carditis and congestive heart failure and cardiac manifestations such as tachycardia or edema.**
- **The degree and location of joint pain.**
- **Other symptomatic manifestations such as fever, chilliness.**
- **The medical prescription for rest and activity.**
- **The location of the therapeutic environment (hospital day-care center, or home) and the facilities and supportive persons available.**
- **The patient's (and family's or associates') understanding of and acceptance of the disease and restriction of activity.**
- **The diversional preferences of the patient permitted within the limits of the activity prescription.**

### Nursing Intervention

Skillful nursing care can make the difference between a fretful, restless patient who tosses and turns, one who seems to delight in finding new ways to defy the physician's recommendation of rest, and a patient who is able to tolerate the restricted activity. Ways in which the nurse can help follow:

- **Smooth, sure, unhurried movement by the nurse prevents any additional pain in the patient's swollen, painful joints. Reduction of the possibility of sudden jerky motions may be accomplished through the use** of temporary supporting splints or pillow support of the extremities, especially when the patient is turned.

- The nurse should not insist on unnecessary restrictions, or carry out in a punitive manner those which are necessary. Most patients with rheumatic fever are young people. They are accustomed to activity, and they need gradually increasing independence.
- She should find out from the physician the rest and activity prescription and what kind of diversion the patient is interested in within these limits. Reading and television help to while away the hours, as do hobbies, such as painting or handwork.
- The nurse adds her efforts to those of the physician in helping the patient and his associates understand the reason for the restriction of activity.
- She should not underestimate the importance of pleasant, cheerful surroundings. If the patient is in the hospital, he should be placed near others who are congenial.
- She should provide for all the devices for keeping bed patients comfortable: an extra long back rub; placing the patient's feet in the basin when they are bathed; a bottom sheet tucked in so that it stays smooth all day; attention to details of personal grooming.
- If the patient is allowed out of bed for a short time each day, the nurse should make these precious moments count by giving him a change of scene, perhaps wheeling him to a window or a porch.
- Housekeeping chores such as stripping and airing the bed should be done in the patient's absence, so that everything is fresh and clean when he returns to bed.
- Although young people are not as susceptible to pressure sores as older people, they can get them. The patient's gown and bedding should be dry. If he perspires freely, several changes a day may be needed. Careful massage over bony prominences should be given, and a frequent change of position should be encouraged.
- The nurse should be prepared for the patient's ups and downs. Any young person who has to curtail so many pleasures and so many of the normal experiences of growing up is bound to become discouraged and angry at times. It is important for the patient to keep in touch with his friends, even if it gives him a twinge of envy that he cannot see an exciting football game. He should be encouraged to keep up with his studies, if the physician permits. Instead of worrying about how far behind he is in his schoolwork, he may, with the guidance of teachers and friends, use his endless leisure for study and compensate somewhat for the loss of time from school.
- The nurse should help the young person to mature by expecting and assisting him to assume some responsibility for his care and to develop concern for others. A prolonged illness can interfere with the development of these abilities and attitudes, and as a consequence the patient's relationships with others may suffer.

## Prognosis and Rehabilitation

Many people recover from attacks of rheumatic fever with little or no permanent heart damage. However, the prognosis grows less favorable with each repeated attack. Some patients die during an acute attack; others may survive the acute attack but succumb shortly afterward. When death occurs, it is due usually to severe cardiac damage resulting in congestive heart failure. The later in life the first attack occurs, the better is the prognosis, since the likelihood of repeated attacks diminishes with age, and recurrence after the age of 25 is very unlikely. It has been estimated that approximately 25 to 50 per cent of the patients who have had rheumatic fever develop some degree of permanent heart damage (Beeson and McDermott, 1966).

The greater awareness of the problem of rheumatic fever, of the need for early diagnosis and treatment, and of the importance of prophylaxis has led to a more hopeful outlook for many persons with this disease. Although the lack of medical care and unawareness of the symptoms of rheumatic fever still exist, particularly among the underprivileged, greater recognition of the problem has led to earlier diagnosis and more thorough treatment for many children whose illness might once have been dismissed as "growing pains." Because of improved diagnosis and treatment, the outlook for people with rheumatic fever is more favorable than it was a generation or two ago. Recurrences of rheumatic fever have decreased markedly due to the prophylactic use of antibiotics among those who have had an attack.

Continuing nursing care for the patient involves:

- Education of the patient concerning his abilities and his limitations, in the light of the degree of heart damage, and helping the patient to learn to live within his limitations.
- Teaching the patient what symptoms to watch for and to report (for example, fever, sore throat, ankle edema, fatigue).
- Specific directions for obtaining and maintaining antirheumatic prophylaxis, as well as protection against bacterial endocarditis.

The plan of rehabilitation depends on the degree of heart damage and the patient's reaction to his experience with the illness. Those patients who do not develop heart disease after rheumatic fever are encouraged to live active lives. Their only reminder of the disease is the need for preventing further attacks. Because rheumatic fever so frequently results in heart disease, it is hard for some of these patients to believe that their hearts can tolerate normal activity. Very important is faith in the physician who has assured them that they may be more active, along with a willingness to cross the chasm caused by their own fear and to venture some new activity. Invalidism can become a way of life, especially in an illness like rheumatic fever and rheumatic heart disease that imposes prolonged restrictions on the patient's living. Some patients through fear are unable to break away from this pattern even when their physical condition no longer makes it necessary.

### Prevention of Rheumatic Fever

The programs for the prevention of rheumatic fever are based on its close relationship to streptococcal infections. The community health nurse as well as nurses employed in educational institutions, the military services, or industry have a major role to play in the prevention of rheumatic fever. Mass throat culture programs and appropriate antibiotic therapy result in a decreased incidence of acute rheumatic fever. The nurse acts as a case finder and also gives leadership to community efforts to prevent the spread of streptococcal infections.

The Inter-Society Commission for Heart Disease Resources recommends that each community decide which agency is to have primary responsibility for a prevention program. The local health department, Heart Association, medical society, or children's bureau are possibilities. The components of such a program should include:

- A streptococcal diagnostic service including low- or no-cost throat cultures.
- Maintenance of a rheumatic fever registry.
- Implementation of the necessary follow-up services to make the registry effective (such as drug dispensing and monitoring).

The nurse should find out what resources are available within her home or her work community.

Every possible measure is taken to prevent further streptococcal infections in patients who have had rheumatic fever, because every such infection carries with it the high possibility of the recurrence of rheumatic fever. Each new attack of rheumatic fever carries the threat of heart damage. Some physicians recommend that the siblings of patients with rheumatic fever also have prophylactic treatment. The prevention of this disease is extremely important, because there is at present no cure. It causes serious heart disease among many young people, often interfering with their plans for a career, marriage, and family life; and sometimes it results in severe illness and death during what should be their most productive years.

Work on a streptococcal vaccine to eliminate streptococcal respiratory infection and rheumatic fever as well as prevent glomerulonephritis is in progress (Fox, et al., 1966).

The following measures have been recommended for the prevention of rheumatic fever:

- Prophylactic medication. Oral penicillin (200,000 to 400,000 U.) or sulfadiazine (1.0 Gm.) is given daily to protect the patient from streptococcal infection. As noted above, an injection of repository benzathine penicillin G (one that is slowly liberated from the tissues after the injection) may be given once a month, particularly if the patient is not reliable in carrying out his daily oral treatment. This can be assessed by pill count or much more reliably by urine examination. Most physicians agree that prophylactic medication should be taken for at least five years following the most recent attack of rheumatic fever. Some believe that prophylactic medication should be continued indefinitely or be reinstituted prophylactically if the patient has to undergo dental surgery or other kinds of stressful experiences where the risk of streptococcal infection is increased. Toxic symptoms may follow the use of either drug; however, serious reactions are relatively infrequent, and the advantages of preventing streptococcal infections far outweigh the risks from drug toxicity. Toxic effects of penicillin may include urticaria and angioneurotic edema; sulfadiazine occasionally causes nausea, vomiting, fever, skin rash, and leukopenia.
- Avoidance of contact with persons who have upper respiratory infections. Although this cannot always be accomplished, the person who has had rheumatic fever should take reasonable precautions. For example, he may not know at first that a coworker has a severe sore throat; but once he does know it, he is not the member of the office force who should visit his sick colleague at home. It would be much safer for him to send a card or letter and to leave the visiting to those less vulnerable to illness.
- Reporting to the physician or nurse any symptoms, such as sore throat and fever, that might indicate a streptococcal infection.
- Following the physician's and nurse's recommendations concerning regular visits to the office or clinic for careful cardiac follow-up after the attack is over. The regimen for rheumatic fever prophylaxis has been outlined succinctly in the Report of the Inter-Society Commission for Heart Disease Resources, Prevention of rheumatic fever and rheumatic heart disease, *Circulation* 43 ,May 1970.

## CHRONIC RHEUMATIC HEART DISEASE

The nurse is often the initial member of the health care team to suspect rheumatic heart disease in a client through a nursing history and such symptoms as tachycardia, fatigability, or edema. Patients with chronic RHD may come to the attention of the health care team during a bout of acute rheumatic fever, or due to an attack of congestive heart failure as a complication of previously undiagnosed RHD; or they may be totally asymptomatic. The latter group are those recognized by cardiac changes found during routine physicals, mass screening, or school, army, or insurance examinations. It is recommended that all patients with confirmed chronic RHD be given antirheumatic prophylaxis as well as protection from attacks of bacterial endocarditis.

### Nursing Assessment

Nursing assessment and planning for the patient with rheumatic heart disease include:

- **Performing those elements of a standard cardiovascular examination which the nurse is prepared to do, in collaboration with the physician and depending on the practice setting. For example, the rural community health nurse may be proficient at cardiac auscultation, whereas the nurse in the obstetric clinic may refer the patient to the physician for this examination after observing signs such as dyspnea, tachycardia, and distended neck veins.**
- **Observing signs of recurrence of rheumatic infection or any streptococcal infection (fever, malaise, sore throat, joint swelling, and pain).**
- **Observing symptoms of congestive heart failure (dyspnea, cough, orthopnea, edema, fatigue, change in heart sounds).**
- **Seeking the patient's and family's understanding of the disease and the ways in which it affects their lives.**
- **Investigating those factors which interfere with compliance with recommendations for RF prophylaxis or treatment of heart failure, such as difficulty in reaching clinics or in attending during working hours, long waiting periods, the costs of care, lack of continuity of physician management, and lack of comprehensive health care.**
- **Clarifying to the patient the restrictions imposed by the disease and how activities such as work capability, leisure time preferences, sex, marriage, and child bearing are involved and can be managed.**
- **Assessing learning and counseling needs and facilitating direction of the patient to appropriate resources.**

Nurses can assist in securing compliance to an RF prophylaxis program when they recognize and act on the fact that patients with RHD, especially those from poor socioeconomic circumstances, face a great many daily stressors which tax their coping reserves. They are not liable to assign the same priorities with regard to preventive measures as is someone whose major concerns do not need to be with the exigencies of daily life. Noncompliance can also be based on hopelessness, when physical illness is but one recurring theme in a vicious cycle of poverty and disability for which the patient can envision no way out. Nursing intervention, then, may take the form of planning strategies with the patient so that he can cope more effectively with his social, economic, occupational, or housing problems if these are of first priority to him. With such support, and the availability of stable helpful resources, either dropping out or noncompliant staying in can be reduced. Patients who do drop out may best be approached by a trained health worker from the patient's own cultural milieu who can understand the patient's problems and relate to him more effectively.

## RHEUMATIC HEART (VALVULAR) DISEASE

A series of thin but strong valves ensures that the blood in passing through the heart does not seep back and reverse its direction of flow. A valve separates the atrium from the ventricle on each side of the heart, preventing blood from passing back into the atrium each time the ventricle contracts. Valves also prevent blood that is pumped into the aorta and the pulmonary artery from flowing back toward the heart. The name of the artery is used to describe its valve; these valves are the *pulmonary* valve and the *aortic* valve.

### Endocarditis

Endocarditis (inflammation of the lining of the heart, including the lining of the heart valves) is the type of the rheumatic involvement of the heart that leads to permanent scarring and deformity. As an end result of endocarditis, heart valves, particularly the mitral and the aortic valves, become scarred, and they function inefficiently. Damage to the valves can be found even after attacks of such mildness that the patient does not recall having had the disease. Often such lesions are detected many years later during a routine physical examination. While listening to the patient's heart with a stethoscope, the physician or nurse may discover the abnormal heart sounds that are associated with the deformities of the valves.

These patients may have been completely free of symptoms and leading active lives. If the deformities of the valves are slight, these patients may continue to be asymptomatic, requiring no treatment and no limitation of their physical activity. If the deformity of the valves is considerable, the patient's heart function may in time become sufficiently impaired that the heart can no longer keep up with the circulatory load, and the patient will develop symptoms of congestive heart failure. These symptoms may appear first when the patient encounters some unusual strain, such as a pregnancy, an infection, or an unusual physical exertion.

Patients whose hearts have been damaged by rheumatic fever are susceptible to subacute bacterial endocarditis, an infection of the lining to which deformed heart valves are particularly prone, which will be discussed later in this chapter. Atrial fibrillation is another disorder that may occur in patients with rheumatic heart disease.

### Mitral Stenosis

The mitral valve lies between the left atrium and the left ventricle (see Fig. 33-3). It has two leaflets. In the healthy heart these open with each pulsation of the atrium to allow the blood to flow from the left atrium into the left ventricle, and then they close as the ventricle fills.

The most common cause of stenosis (narrowing) of the valve is the inflammation and the scarring of the leaflets as a result of rheumatic fever. The leaflets stick together and are prevented from opening all the way, as a valve should. They tend to become progressively thicker. The opening narrows, so that the blood in the atrium does not have time to flow into the ventricle. The atrium cannot then empty to receive a new full load of blood from the pulmonary artery and veins. To compensate, the atrium contracts harder. It enlarges. Pressure is exerted backward through the blood vessels of the lungs. Pressure builds up in the pulmonary artery (pulmonary hypertension), which carries blood from the right ventricle to the lungs. Eventually, pressure also increases in the right ventricle. Because it usually takes less force to pump blood through the lungs than through the rest of the body, the walls of the right ventricle are thinner than the walls of the left ventricle. In long-standing mitral stenosis the walls of the right ventricle get thicker. When hypertrophy of the muscular walls no longer meets the demands of the increased work caused by the narrowed

mitral valve, pressure is passed to the right atrium, and to the entire venous system of the body. The liver and the lungs become congested; edema of the legs appears. Because the ventricles are not receiving a normal amount of blood to pump through the body, the organs are not getting sufficient nourishment. The patient tires easily and becomes dyspneic. He suffers the progressive disability of cardiac failure.

Another symptom of this condition is lowered systolic blood pressure. When the blood pressure of a patient with mitral stenosis is taken, it is possible to get a reading of 80/60! By checking the patient's chart to see what previous readings have been, it may be evident that this is the usual blood pressure for this patient. The patient often appears emaciated. Although he may gain weight due to edema, he has poor appetite, and is chronically tired and listless.

Mitral stenosis is the most common vascular aftermath of rheumatic fever. Two-thirds of all patients with mitral stenosis are females.

**Treatment.** Treatment of mitral stenosis used to be limited to the relief of congestive heart failure with such drugs as digitalis and diuretics. The symptomatic relief of congestive heart failure still forms a very important part of the treatment of some patients with mitral stenosis. In many instances surgical treatment is possible. However, not all patients with mitral stenosis are suitable candidates for surgery. Usually excluded are those whose condition is so slight that it does not cause symptoms, or so severe or of such long duration that profound changes in the heart and the lungs have occurred. The earlier the operation, the greater is the likelihood of cessation of symptoms. Patients who have had one episode of cerebral or peripheral embolization from a piece of clot or valve but are in good condition nonetheless are candidates for surgical correction.

The usual operative treatment of mitral stenosis is commissurotomy, valvuloplasty, or valve replacement. (See Chapter 63 for care of the cardiac surgical patient.)

### Mitral Regurgitation

Regurgitation of a valve means that it does not close completely, consequently allowing blood to return through it. An opening remains when the valve is supposed to be completely closed. Any heart valve may develop regurgitation.

Regurgitation of the mitral valve is caused most commonly by rheumatic fever. The left ventricle becomes overfilled with blood, because each contraction of the ventricle fails to empty the chamber through the aorta. Instead, some blood is pushed back through the mitral valve into the left atrium and then leaks back into the ventricle. The walls of the ventricle become distended, and the patient may suffer from left ventricular failure (Fig. 35-1).

The surgery for mitral regurgitation has a higher mortality rate and a poorer prognosis than the surgery for mitral stenosis. Frequently, patients with mitral regurgitation are disabled to a greater degree before the operation. Among the operations performed to correct mitral regurgitation are the suturing of loose valves and the implanting of a prosthetic valve to restore unidirectional blood flow (see Chap. 63).

### Aortic Stenosis

The three-leaf aortic valve is between the aorta and the left ventricle. The cusps may be thickened, stiffened, and eventually calcified after rheumatic fever, although the aortic valve is affected less commonly than the mitral valve. In older patients aortic stenosis may be caused by arteriosclerosis (Fig. 35-2).

When there is stenosis of the aortic valve, the work of the left ventricle is increased. More force is needed to push blood through the narrowed

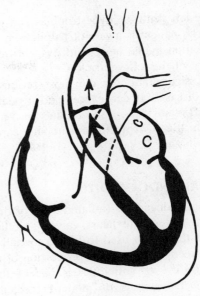

**Figure 35-2.** Aortic stenosis.

opening. A sufficient supply of blood may not be passing through the narrowed valve to nourish adequately the brain and the muscles of the heart. In this instance the patient will present symptoms of dizziness, fainting, and anginal pain from insufficient blood in the coronary arteries. Instead of being full, the radial pulse is weak. It seems to crawl against the finger rather than to hit it. Characteristically, angina and syncope occur before heart failure. Surgery should be considered before the patient reaches the late stages of the disease and suffers dyspnea, a congested liver, and dependent edema, as the left ventricle enlarges, and heart failure occurs. Mitral stenosis and aortic regurgitation may be associated with aortic stenosis.

### Aortic Regurgitation

Aortic regurgitation can be caused by rheumatic heart disease, by subacute bacterial endocarditis (especially when it is superimposed on a valve already damaged by rheumatic fever), and by syphilis. When the aortic valve is incompetent and does not close tightly, blood flows through it during systole, dropping back into the ventricle instead of moving forward through the aorta. This backflow results in a decrease in the amount of circulating blood and an increase in the amount of blood in the ventricle. The patient may have a "pistol-shot" pulse, which consists of a pronounced pulsation and then an extraordinarily long interval before the next sharp

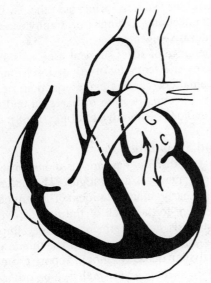

**Figure 35-1.** Mitral regurgitation. The inadequate valve allows blood to return to the left atrium.

beat. The left ventricle hypertrophies and goes into failure. The patient is aware of palpitation, a throbbing sensation in the head, and dyspnea related to the failure of the left ventricle.

Aortic regurgitation is the most serious of the valvular diseases. It can cause sudden death, even before left ventricular failure, due to ventricular fibrillation. (See Chapter 63 for nursing care of patients having aortic valve surgery.)

## BACTERIAL ENDOCARDITIS

Bacterial endocarditis (inflammation of the membrane that covers the heart valves and lines the cavities of the heart) used to kill almost all its victims. The recovery of a large proportion of patients through the use of antibiotics is one of the most dramatic achievements of modern medicine. Although the prognosis has improved markedly, bacterial endocarditis continues to be a serious and a relatively common health problem among adults.

Bacterial endocarditis may be acute or subacute. The acute condition has a more abrupt onset and a more rapid course, whereas the subacute form has a gradual onset, and the duration of the illness is usually longer. In subacute bacterial endocarditis the infecting organisms are usually less virulent, whereas the organisms causing acute bacterial endocarditis are usually more virulent. When the infecting organisms are sensitive to antibiotics, the prognosis of the patient usually is good. With other organisms the mortality rate is approximately 50 per cent (Mandel, 1970), and the disease often is crippling for those who survive. Modern therapy, with emphasis on prompt diagnosis and the control of the infection, has so altered the course of the disease that the terms "acute" and "subacute" are now less frequently used to describe it.

### Incidence

People whose heart valves have been damaged are most vulnerable to bacterial endocarditis. The majority of patients who develop it have had rheumatic fever. The relationship between rheumatic heart disease and bacterial endocarditis is so marked that bacterial endocarditis often is considered a complication of rheumatic heart disease. The condition also occurs in those who have congenital defects of the heart. Although it may occur at any age, bacterial endocarditis is most common during young adulthood and early middle life.

### Etiology and Pathology

*Transient bacteremia* occurs fairly commonly in the lives of most people—for example, after tooth extraction. In most instances the organisms are quickly overcome by the body's own defenses. However, patients with damaged heart valves are especially prone to develop bacterial endocarditis after such relatively safe experiences as the pulling of a tooth, cystoscopy, childbirth, or an upper respiratory infection. Organisms that invade the bloodstream after such occurrences tend to settle on damaged heart valves, where they multiply and produce vegetations (verrucae)—clumps of material composed of bacteria, necrotic tissue, and fibrin, which accumulate on the affected heart valves. These vegetations are *friable* (easily broken). Pieces of the vegetation tend to break off and travel in the bloodstream. They are then called *emboli,* and they may damage other organs by occluding blood vessels, thus interfering with the organ's blood supply.

A variety of bacteria can cause bacterial endocarditis. *Streptococcus viridans* is one of the organisms most frequently responsible (50 per cent of cases). *Staphylococcus aureus* is the culprit in 10 to 20 per cent of bacteremic cases. Fungi or rickettsiae can also be at fault.

Today the pattern of bacterial endocarditis is changing somewhat. An increased incidence is evident in such populations as those undergoing heart surgery with cardiopulmonary bypass and heroin and morphine addicts who use the intravenous route of injection. A fungus or staphylococcus can be the causative agent.

Maintenance of strict surgical asepsis is an essential task of the team involved in insertion of cardiac pacemakers, cardiac catheterization, or cardiac surgery if the complication of bacterial endocarditis is to be avoided (Rabinovich, et al., 1968).

### Signs and Symptoms

Often the disease has an insidious onset, with slight fever, malaise, and fatigue. The patient may ignore the early manifestations of the illness, attributing them to "a touch of the flu" or overwork. Early diagnosis and treatment are very important. Patients—particularly those with rheumatic or congenital valvular defects—should report promptly to their physician any fever, malaise, or other symptoms of infection, because they may have bacterial endocarditis or a recurrence of rheumatic fever.

As the condition advances, the patient often develops a muddy, sallow complexion, sometimes described as the color of *café au lait*. His fever becomes more marked and more frequent, and often it is accompanied by chills and sweats. Pronounced weakness, anorexia, and weight loss are common. Petechiae, tiny reddish-purple hemorrhagic spots on the skin and mucous membranes, are characteristic. Anemia and slight leukocytosis are common. Heart murmur is present in the vast majority of patients.

Embolism, resulting in the occlusion of a blood vessel by a clump of vegetation that has broken away from the heart valve, may cause sudden disturbances in many organs of the body. One patient with bacterial endocarditis suddenly developed excruciating pain, pallor, and coldness of one leg below the knee. An embolus had cut off circulation to his lower leg. Had it not been for the speed and the teamwork of the physician, the nurse, and the surgeon who was immediately called, the patient would have developed gangrene and therefore would have lost his leg by a necessary amputation. The prompt reporting of the condition and the surgical removal of the embolus saved the patient's leg. Another patient suddenly became dyspneic; she coughed and expectorated bloody sputum. She had suffered pulmonary embolism.

An embolus to the spleen may cause sudden pain in the left flank, whereas an embolus to a kidney may result in hematuria and flank pain. Emboli may affect the brain, causing neurologic symptoms, such as paralysis and aphasia.

Clubbing of the fingers and the toes may appear later in the course of the illness. The symptoms of congestive heart failure may appear, either during the active infection or afterward as a result of the damage to the valves during the illness. Often this development is best described as further damage to the heart valves, because many of the patients already have some valvular damage.

## Diagnosis

There is no single laboratory test for bacterial endocarditis. The patient's history is carefully evaluated, particularly in relation to rheumatic heart disease or congenital defects and in relation to any recent operation, injury, or illness, however minor, that may have resulted in bacteremia. When the history and the symptoms lead to the suspicion of bacterial endocarditis, blood cultures are ordered in an attempt to discover the organism circulating in the blood. Often several blood cultures are required before the organism is found. Occasionally, no bacteria are found despite repeated blood cultures, although the patient has a history and symptoms that are typical of the disease. In these instances the diagnosis is made as carefully as possible on the basis of other evidence, but the treatment with antibiotics cannot be as precisely planned when the sensitivity of the organism to various drugs is not known. Persistent negative blood cultures are found in 15 to 20 per cent of autopsy-proved cases of bacterial endocarditis (Rabinovich, et al., 1968).

## Treatment and Nursing Care

When the causative organism has been identified, the physician prescribes the appropriate type and dose of antibiotic. Every effort is made to eradicate the infection promptly and completely before serious complications occur. Large doses of the antibiotic to which the organism is sensitive are given. For example, a patient may receive 4 to 20 million units of penicillin daily in divided doses intramuscularly or via a continuous intravenous infusion. Treatment is continued for three to four weeks.

It is important to give the drugs on time, exactly as ordered, so that a sufficient amount of the drug will be maintained continuously in the patient's blood. The patient is observed carefully for any toxic reactions to the drugs, which are reported if they occur. Good technical skill in giving injections helps to minimize the patient's feeling of being a "dart board." Rotating the site is essential when so many injections are given, so that one area does not become traumatized from repeated injections. The nurse's attitude can convey to the patient that drug therapy is very important, and it will be carried out in a way that causes the least discomfort possible. One nurse said, "Oh, Mr. Jones is so good; he never complains about the injections." One day Mr. Jones disappeared from the hospital. He had gone home because he was "tired of being a pincushion." Even the most stoical patients grow weary of repeated injections. Skill, patience, and encouragement can help them to continue with the treatment that is lifesaving.

If the patient is receiving his antibiotics intravenously, he will have an intravenous line inserted for the duration of treatment to avoid frequent venipunctures. The antibiotic may be given either in divided doses with a "keep-open" infusion running between doses, or the drug may be given by continuous drip. The venipuncture site is observed for signs of infiltration or inflammation. The level of fluid in the bottle is checked to see that it is sufficient to keep the fluid from running out and that the flow rate is that ordered for achievement of drug blood level. Often patients fear that air will enter their veins if the fluid is all absorbed. They also dread the necessity of needless needle reinsertion. Since the patient may become ambulatory after seven to ten days of therapy, his IV pole should have casters incorporated.

In some institutions with progressive nursing care services the patient may be discharged after seven to ten days and the community health nurse supervises his daily care. This involves preparation in intravenous techniques since the infusion may need to be restarted.

Supportive care is important in helping the patient to overcome the infection. Usually, bed rest is ordered at first. When the patient begins to improve, he is permitted gradually to go to the bathroom and later to be up and about. While the patient is on bed rest, everything possible should be done to spare him exertion and to make him as comfortable as possible. Extra blankets should be provided if he has a chill; they should be removed when the chill is over. Usually, at this time his temperature will have risen, and he will feel too warm with more than a light blanket or two. Bedding that becomes damp from perspiration, as it often does when the patient's fever abates, should be changed promptly. The patient should be encouraged to eat, and particularly to drink fluids; fluids are especially important because of the fever and the sweating.

The patient is observed carefully. Fluctuations in temperature are noted. The temperature usually is taken rectally every four hours. It is important to be alert for changes in the rate and the quality of the pulse and for the appearance of any new symptoms, such as petechiae. Observation for signs and symptoms of embolization is necessary.

Without drugs, patients with bacterial endocarditis almost surely die. Nursing intervention, too, helps him through the attack. As his symptoms subside, gradually he will be allowed increased activity. The nurse observes that he does not overdo, and that new activities are stopped short of fatigue. When the antibiotic treatment is discontinued, any recurrence of the symptoms is noted. Sometimes,

although the infection seems to be conquered, it flares up again after the drugs have been discontinued. Then the treatment has to be resumed and continued until the infection has been eradicated.

No drug, however dramatic in its effect, renders skilled nursing care unnecessary. Nowhere is this need more evident than in the care of patients with bacterial endocarditis, who are seriously ill and subject to a variety of complications that may appear without warning.

### Prognosis

It has been estimated that about 90 per cent of patients with bacterial endocarditis can recover from the infection. Much depends on the sensitivity of the organism to available drugs. Some resistant strains make therapy more difficult and the outcome more uncertain. The amount of heart damage that existed before the attack, as well as that which may result from the endocarditis, also affects the prognosis. Some patients have the infection controlled by drugs, but not before heart damage or embolization has occurred. These patients may be incapacitated by or succumb to congestive heart failure or damage inflicted on the vital organs by the emboli.

### Prevention

Any patient with damaged heart valves should have antibiotics just before and for a short time after any event that might cause bacteremia, whether it be a tooth extraction or childbirth. The patient must understand that this precaution is a lifelong necessity. Unfortunately, bacterial endocarditis does not provide immunity to further attacks. The patients who develop the condition are usually those whose previous valvular damage predisposes them to it. They will continue to be vulnerable to this disease as long as they live.

## PERICARDITIS

The heart wall is composed of three distinct layers of tissue. The bulk of the heart is muscle tissue (myocardium). The delicate layer of endothelial tissue lining the interior of the heart which the circulating blood directly contacts is the endocardium. Covering the myocardium on the outside is a loose-fitting inelastic sac known as the *pericardium*. The outermost layer is the fibrous pericardium. The serous pericardium lies beneath the fibrous pericardium and consists of two layers. The innermost layer, or that adhering to the myocardium, is the visceral layer or epicardium. The parietal layer of the serous pericardium lies between the fibrous pericardium and the epicardium. Between the parietal and visceral layers is a potential space known as the pericardial space which contains a few drops of pericardial fluid. This fluid lessens the friction between the myocardium and the pericardium. Since the pericardium does not stretch, overdilatation of the heart during diastole cannot take place.

Inflammation of the pericardium (pericarditis) can result from infection, trauma, or neoplasms. Blood, excess fluid, or pus can accumulate in the pericardial space and produce partial or complete cardiac tamponade with fall in cardiac output or death. Sections of the two linings (epicardium and pericardium) can adhere and cause chronic constrictive pericarditis (Fig. 35-3).

## Acute Pericarditis

Pericarditis can be caused by an infection with any organism. For example, tubercle bacilli and streptococci can cause a purulent pericardial exudate. Infection from a virus or pneumonia or a lung abscess can spread to the pericardium. Myxedema and uremia can produce a nonbacterial, serofibrinous pericarditis. In acute pericarditis there may be sharp pain aggravated by moving and breathing due to the rubbing together of the two inflamed surfaces. A pericardial friction rub can usually be heard with a stethoscope and is the most striking sign.

The pain of acute pericarditis is very similar to the pain of acute myocardial infarction—sudden, severe, beginning over the sternum and radiating to the neck and left arm. However, the pain of the patient with pericarditis is usually increased by rotating the chest or deep breathing and is relieved by sitting up and leaning forward. In contrast, the pain of acute myocardial infarction is not usually influenced by position, movement, or breathing. Acute pericarditis is a disease of the younger age group (15 to 35 years) and is generally preceded by an upper respiratory infection or hay fever. There are characteristic changes in the S-T segments of the ECG. X-ray may show dilatation of the heart with pericardial effusion. Serum enzyme changes are confusing in that they are similar to those of acute myocardial infarction. If there is

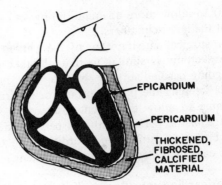

EPICARDIUM

PERICARDIUM

THICKENED, FIBROSED, CALCIFIED MATERIAL

**Figure 35-3.** Pericarditis. Normally, the epicardium and the pericardium slide over each other easily. They are lubricated by a small amount of fluid, which in pericarditis is replaced by thicker material that can cause the surfaces to adhere.

sufficient fluid in the pericardial space to compress the heart (*tamponade*), there may be signs of congestive heart failure and a pulse that is weaker on deep inspiration (*paradoxical pulse*).

The patient with acute pericarditis is generally treated with coronary precautions until myocardial infarction is ruled out.

Treatment depends on the underlying cause. Rest, analgesia, antipyretics, and other supportive treatment is given. Antibiotics and steroids may be ordered.

## Chronic Constrictive Pericarditis

Patients may have no symptoms and no disability, even when there is some adherence of the two linings. However, as scar tissue forms in chronic constrictive pericarditis, there is compression of the heart (as there is when fluid is present in the pericardial sac) that prevents the ventricle from filling fully. The cardiac output of blood is decreased, even though the heart rate increases to compensate. The patient tires easily and eventually shows such signs of cardiac failure as hepatomegaly, dyspnea, edema, and distention of the superficial veins, especially of the neck.

**Treatment.** When there is fluid in the pericardial sac, the surgeon may aspirate it (pericardial paracentesis), or if there is pus in the sac, he may incise the pericardium and insert a drain. A chronic accumulation of fluid may be treated by making a pericardial opening (window), thus allowing the fluid to drain into the pleural space. Constrictive pericarditis is treated surgically by removing the binding pericardium (pericardectomy or decortication) to allow more adequate filling and contraction of the heart chambers.

The surgical nursing care of the patient having pericardectomy is similar to that of other patients undergoing cardiac surgery. Nursing care may also include keeping the patient prone for several hours at a time to allow dependent drainage if surgical drainage of the pericardium was performed for the management of purulent pericarditis. (See Chapter 63 for care of the cardiac surgical patient.)

## Postpericardiotomy (Postcardiotomy) Syndrome

A febrile illness with symptoms and signs characteristic of acute pericarditis may develop one to three weeks after the pericardium has been surgically opened. It is thought to be due to reaction to the presence of fibrin and blood in the pericardial sac. In most patients the episode resolves spontaneously in one to three weeks. Analgesics and antipyretics may be ordered as well as steroid therapy.

## REFERENCES AND BIBLIOGRAPHY

Ad Hoc Committee of the Council on Rheumatic Fever and Congenital Heart Disease: Jones criteria (revised) for guidance in the diagnosis of rheumatic fever, *Circulation* 32:664, 1965.

BAILEY, C. (ed.): *Rheumatic and Coronary Heart Disease,* Philadelphia, Lippincott, 1967.

BEESON, P. B., and McDERMOTT, W. (eds.): *Cecil-Loeb Textbook of Medicine,* ed. 13, Philadelphia, Saunders, 1971.

BISHOP, L. F.: Pericarditis vs. myocardial infarction, *Hosp. Med.* 3:9, 1967.

BRETT, B.: The prevention of rheumatic fever, *Canad. J. Publ. Health* 63:486, November-December 1972.

CREIGHTON, H.: The saving grace of saving face, *ANA Clin. Sess. 1970,* 175.

ERB, B., and WILSON, G.: Rheumatic heart disease, *Cardiovasc. Nurs.* 4:1, January-February 1968.

FEENEY, R.: Preventing rheumatic fever in schoolchildren, *Am. J. Nurs.* 73:265, February 1973.

FOX, E. N., et al.: Antigenicity of the M proteins of group A hemolytic streptococci: III Antibody responses and cutaneous hypersensitivity in humans, *J. Exp. Med.* 124:1135, 1966.

HARRISON, T., and REEVES, T.: *Principles and Problems of Ischemic Heart Disease,* Chicago, Yearbook Publishers, 1968.

Inter-Society Commission for Heart Disease Resources: Community resources for the diagnosis and acute care of patients with rheumatic fever, *Circulation* 44:A-197, July 1971.

——: Community resources for the management of patients with rheumatic heart disease, *Circulation* 44:A-273, December 1971.

——: Prevention of rheumatic fever and rheumatic heart disease, *Circulation* 43:A-1, May 1970.

MANDELL, G.: Enterococcal endocarditis, *Arch. Int. Med.* 125:258, February 1970.

MARKOWITZ, M.: Eradication of rheumatic fever—an unfulfilled hope, *Circulation* 41:1077, June 1970.

McINTYRE, H. M., and MASON, D. T.: The prevention of heart disease: A greater challenge, *Cardiovasc. Nurs.* 7:77, September-October 1971.

MICHAELSON, M.: Wyoming's war on deadly strep, *Today's Health* 49:40, March 1971.

MOTOCK, E.: A patient with sarcoma of the pericardium, *Nurs. Clin. N. Am.* 1:15, March 1966.

National Health Education Committee: *Facts on the Major Killing and Crippling Diseases in the United States Today,* New York, 1966.

QUINN, R. W., et al.: Mortality rates for rheumatic fever and rheumatic heart disease, 1940-65, *Pub. Health Rep.* 85:1091, December 1970.

RABINOVICH, S., et al.: The changing pattern of bacterial endocarditis, *Med. Clin. N. Am.* 52:1091, September 1968.

STAMLER, J.: *Lectures on Preventive Cardiology,* New York, Grune, 1967.

STITT, A.: The rheumatic heart in pregnancy, *Emerg. Med.* 3:122, July 1971.

STOLLERMAN, G. H., et al.: Relationship of immune response to group A streptococci to the cause of acute, chronic, and recurrent rheumatic fever, *Am. J. Med.* 20:163, 1956.

TARANTA, A.: Rheumatic fever, in *Current Therapy, 1971,* H. F. Conn (ed.), Philadelphia, Saunders, 1971.

——: Prevention of bacterial endocarditis, *Circulation* 31:953, 1965.

——, and MOODY, M. D.: Diagnosis of streptococcal pharyngitis and rheumatic fever (Symposium on Laboratory Diagnosis), *Ped. Clin. N. Am.* 18:125, 1971.

WATSON, H. T.: The role of the school nurse in the support of children with certain cardiovascular disorders, *Nurs. Clin. N. Am.* 1:35, March 1966.

WOOD, P.: *Diseases of the Heart and Circulation,* ed. 3, Philadelphia, Lippincott, 1968.

WANNAMAKER, L. W., et al.: Prevention of rheumatic fever, *Circulation* 31:948, 1965.

# The Patient with Coronary Heart Disease; Functional Heart Disease

## CHAPTER 36

## CORONARY CIRCULATION

Contrary to what might be expected, blood does not pass directly from the chambers of the heart into the heart muscle. Rather, the myocardium has its own blood supply through a system of coronary arteries. Blood flows through these vessels and through branches over the outer surface of the heart, then into smaller arteries and capillaries in the cardiac muscle and finally back to the systemic circulation through the coronary veins which empty via the coronary sinus in the right atrium (Fig. 36-1).

There is considerable variation among individuals in the anatomic pattern of their coronary arteries. This variability accounts for some of the diversity in the responses of patients to similar forms of heart disease. Genetic factors are probably important in determining the pattern of coronary arteries possessed by any one individual.

Usually there are two main coronary arteries, a right and left, and these originate from the aorta immediately above the aortic valve. Thus the coronary arteries get the first supply of the rich, oxygenated blood leaving the left ventricle. Four per cent of the cardiac output goes to the coronary circulation and of this, 80 to 85 per cent goes to the left coronary artery.

The main left coronary artery branches 4 to 5 cm. after its origin into both a left circumflex and a left anterior descending branch. The left circumflex courses anteriorly at first in the groove between the left atrium and left ventricle, giving off branches to the left atrium and the lateral aspect of the left ventricle. The left

637

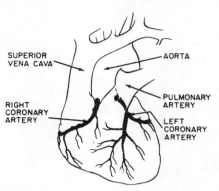

**Figure 36-1.** Anterior view of the heart, showing the right and the left coronary arteries that supply the myocardium with blood.

anterior descending coronary artery runs inferiorly along the anterior surface of the heart in the groove between the right and left ventricles. The branches of the left coronary artery supply most of the anterior surface of the left ventricle and also the anterior portion of the intraventricular septum. The left anterior descending artery has traditionally been called the artery of sudden death.

The right coronary artery passes at first anteriorly and then around to the posterior aspect of the heart in the groove between the right atrium and right ventricle. Its branches supply most of the right ventricle, a variable portion of the left ventricle posteriorly, the right atrium, and the tissues of the atrioventricular (A-V) node. The sinoatrial (S-A) node is supplied by an artery which also originates from the right coronary artery in about 60 per cent of people. Generally an uncomplicated inferior (or posterior) wall infarction has a less serious immediate prognosis than infarction resulting from occlusion of the left coronary artery (anterior wall infarction).

Coronary arteries have very few functional, interconnecting (anastomotic) channels in health. The myocardium is nourished with very little overlap of vessels from one region to another. Thus, if a coronary artery is acutely blocked, few other vessels can take over the blood supply to the area served by the blocked artery and the viability of the myocardial tissue is threatened. During the course of slowly advancing atherosclerotic disease of the coronary arteries, or with time, after an acute coronary occlusion, pre-existing anastomotic channels open up and grow into the involved area. In the person with coronary heart disease the rate

of development and the extent of this new collateral circulation is of critical importance in the survival and viability of myocardial tissue.

Hypoxia, or diminished oxygen supply to cells, is a stimulant to myocardial blood supply. In addition, the pressure gradient between the area supplied by an atherosclerotic artery and the surrounding normal areas is thought to stimulate the development of collateral circulation.

Thus the person with slowly progressive coronary atherosclerosis may have developed some collateral vessels over the course of time which may stand him in good stead in the event of a sudden occlusion of a major vessel. However, the young man who never had the need or opportunity to develop collaterals has a greater chance of dying instantly following a coronary occlusion due to the sequelae of overwhelming oxygen lack to a critical portion of the myocardium.

## INCREASING BLOOD FLOW TO THE MYOCARDIUM

Since almost all cellular processes ultimately require oxygen for the sustained production of energy, the delivery of oxygen to the tissue across the capillary membrane is vitally important. Normally, oxygenated arterial blood contains about 19 ml. of oxygen per 100 ml. of blood. In health this arterial oxygen concentration is fairly constant. At any instant it is exactly the same in all the arteries supplying the many tissues of the body. Thus every 100 ml. of arterial blood flow to an organ (whether to liver, kidney, or brain) can potentially supply that organ with 19 ml. of oxygen. However, no organ uses all the oxygen presented to it, and the draining venous blood usually contains a certain quantity of oxygen that is not used during its passage through the organ. Thus, the draining venous blood has a certain oxygen content. This varies from organ to organ depending on the rate at which the organ uses oxygen and on the rate of blood flow through it. The difference between the arterial and venous oxygen concentrations is called the arteriovenous difference (A-V difference). In an organ such as the kidney where the rate of blood flow is high and the oxygen utilization fairly low, the venous oxygen content is high and therefore the A-V difference for oxygen is very small. The heart muscle (myocardium), on the other hand, uses large quantities of oxygen during its rhythmic contractions, has a low venous oxygen content, and therefore a very large A-V difference.

If a muscle begins to perform increased work as it does during exercise, its needs and demands for oxygen increase.

How can the oxygen supply keep up with the increased needs for oxygen? There are generally three ways:

1. A-V extraction can be increased, that is, the muscle may increase the amount of oxygen it extracts from the inflowing arterial blood.

   As noted, however, the myocardium at rest (supplied by the coronary arteries) extracts near maximal amounts of oxygen. Its venous oxygen content is the lowest of any vein draining any organ of the body. Thus unlike skeletal muscle, during periods of increased work by the heart, the increased need for oxygen *cannot* be adequately achieved by increasing the oxygen extraction.

2. Certain tissues such as skeletal muscle can employ another mechanism to compensate for increased oxygen demands. They can incur an "oxygen debt."

   When the demands for oxygen exceed the supply of oxygen, a tissue may switch its metabolism from oxygen-consuming (aerobic) to nonoxygen-consuming (anaerobic) pathways. Thus during exercise (or shock when little blood is brought to an organ) when a muscle is called upon to perform short periods of strenuous exercise, glycogen is broken down in organs such as skeletal muscle or liver and, after a series of reactions in which no oxygen is used, lactic acid begins to accumulate. This series of reactions, however, produces only small amounts of energy, and after a while, the muscle involved in exercise fatigues. After the increased activity ceases or the low blood flow becomes corrected, oxygen is then required for a prolonged period of time to metabolize the large amount of lactic acid which has accumulated. This quantity is known as the oxygen debt.

   As an example, an athlete who strenuously overexercises his skeletal muscles in fast, hard running develops an oxygen debt and accumulates lactic acid. At the end of the race, with his muscles exhausted, he uses oxygen to pay back his oxygen debt, so to speak, and he recovers after the lactic acid is metabolized.

   Although contractions of skeletal muscle can be maintained temporarily by anaerobic metabolism, the mechanical contractions of heart muscle cannot be maintained by anaerobic metabolism. Thus, the myocardium is unable to build up an oxygen debt and this mechanism for increasing oxygen supply *is not* available to the heart.

3. If the extraction of oxygen remains the same in an organ but blood flow doubles to it, then the oxygen delivery will be effectively doubled. Like skeletal muscle and other organs, the myocardium *can* employ this compensatory mechanism to increase its oxygen supply.

To summarize, then, of the three methods for increasing oxygen supply to an organ, that is, (1) increasing arteriovenous oxygen extraction, (2) accumulating an oxygen debt, or (3) increasing blood flow, the heart can use only one of the three —that of increasing blood flow through the coronary arteries. Thus we can appreciate how critical an adequate coronary blood flow is to the viability of cardiac tissue.

The massaging action of the cardiac contraction itself can become more active and be utilized to increase coronary blood flow. This action can result from stimulation of the sympathetic nervous system which can also result in dilation of the coronary vessels, thus bringing more blood to the myocardium.

If blood flow cannot be increased through the use of drugs or sympathetic stimulation, or surgery, because of atherosclerosis of the coronary arteries, then the only resort is to lessen the demands made on the heart through rest.

## CORONARY ARTERY DISEASE

Like other arteries in the body, the coronary arteries may develop degenerative changes or disease. The pathologic change most responsible for coronary artery disease is atherosclerosis—the gradual deposition of substances, such as lipids and calcium, within the walls of the arteries, making them narrower. Cholesterol is one of the lipid substances believed to be implicated. The lipid deposits are often called *plaques*. Coronary artery disease is more common among people over 50, but it may occur in younger people. A familial tendency toward early development of the condition has been noted. During early middle life men are affected much more frequently than women.

Atherosclerosis usually is not recognized until it interferes sufficiently with the blood supply to cause symptoms. Coronary artery disease is primarily responsible for sudden deaths attributed to heart disease. Sometimes neither the patient nor his physician has any warning that serious and possibly fatal illness is imminent. It is not unusual to hear that a man who was apparently in robust health and had recently passed his physical examination with flying colors had suddenly dropped dead from a "heart attack." Most such attacks are due to the sudden occlusion of an already narrowed coronary artery.

Most of the atherosclerotic lesions are located in the first 4 cm. of the major coronary arteries near the surface of the heart. Rarely are lesions found in the smaller branches which penetrate deep within the myocardial walls. The presence of atherosclerotic plaques and narrowed segments of coronary artery does not necessarily signify a reduction of myocardial blood flow. Usually the lumen of the artery has to be reduced about 35 to 40 per cent of its original diameter before a significant reduction of flow occurs. In a man at rest, a normal myocardial blood flow may be maintained despite considerable coronary artery narrowing; however the ability to increase this flow sufficiently during exercise in order to meet the increased metabolic needs of the heart may be markedly impaired. Beyond the narrowed segment, the vessels supplied by the artery dilate (due probably to local accumulation of metabolites and a pressure gradient between normal and ischemic tissue). This dilation decreases the resistance to blood flow, which can then be maintained at normal levels. Because of this vasodilation and the development of a good collateral circulation, patients with significant coronary atherosclerosis may be fairly asymptomatic and their disease may go unrecognized during their lifetime particularly if they lead a sedentary existence. During exercise or emotional stress with increased cardiac workload, however, the normal coronary arterial vasodilation which usually allows myocardial blood flow to increase proportionately can no longer occur since the local capillary bed is already in a maximally dilated state. Under these circumstances the myocardial demand for oxygen and metabolic nutrients exceeds the ability of the coronary circulation to supply them and clinical manifestations of coronary heart disease such as chest pain of cardiac origin (angina pectoris) may then ensue. Pain results when nerve endings are stimulated by acid metabolites which accumulate in ischemic tissue.

## Epidemiology

Coronary heart disease (CHD) in epidemic proportions continues to rage in this country. Approximately 600,000 people die each year from this, the leading cause of American deaths. Many of these deaths are premature in the sense that the victims are young adults or those in middle life with basically sound myocardiums. Sudden death accounts for more than half of all coronary fatalities under age 65. For each fatality, there are two nonfatal but disabling events. The disease is most serious because its ravages affect the prime productive years of life. The patient, his family, and society as a whole all suffer from this loss of productivity.

The nature of CHD is indeed grim. One study showed that 48.6 per cent of all CHD deaths were sudden, occurring out of the hospital, without medical assistance in most cases. Of these sudden deaths, more than one-half were completely unexpected in that the persons had never had an episode of clinical CHD (Stamler, et al., 1969). Relatives, friends, employers, and other associates of these people must cope with the reality of sudden death with all its ramifications.

CHD is recognized as a disease of mature, industrial societies; American society has been negligent in dealing with it. As yet, there has been no concerted effort to deal with CHD as an epidemic such as has been employed in the past with communicable disease epidemics like tuberculosis and poliomyelitis. Unlike these epidemics, CHD doesn't appear as a plague and wipe out large populations who live in close proximity. Though just as destructive, the gradualness of its increase and the spottiness of its incidence have probably contributed to its being relatively ignored. Though there has been considerable effort expended in recent years to improve the treatment of patients hospitalized for acute myocardial infarction through the coronary care concept (see Chap. 62), the statistics on the nature of the disease point out that if it is to be conquered, it must be prevented. Lown (1968) notes that close to two-thirds of the victims die before reaching a hospital. Of the one-third who reach the hospital, mortality has been reduced from about 30 to 20 per cent in coronary care units, which is conceded to be about the maximum contribution that inhospital care can make to reduction in CHD mortality for the foreseeable future. Thus, the data compel the conclusion that *prevention* of CHD should be a primary national goal.

As with other epidemic diseases, coronary artery disease is considered to be due to multiple causative factors rather than to a single cause. Considerable study is being directed toward the discovery of measures to diagnose coronary artery disease before an acute myocardial infarction occurs and to develop ways of decreasing, or at least arresting, the process of atherosclerosis before damage occurs to the muscle of the heart.

Coronary risk factors are those traits, abnormalities, or habits which, when present in an individual, subject him to a sizable increase in risk of the disease in middle age or young adulthood as compared with persons lacking such factors. A coronary risk factor is defined by The American Heart Association as a finding associated with at least a doubling of the risk, that is when its presence increases the chance of disease by at least 100 per cent. When multiple risk factors are present, studies have shown that their effects are additive.

Factors which when present are thought to increase the risk of coronary artery disease are:

- Age
- Sex
- Family history of coronary disease (heredity)
- Hypertension
- Blood lipid abnormalities, i.e., elevated serum cholesterol and triglycerides
- Lack of regular physical activity
- Electrocardiographic abnormalities
- Cigarette smoking
- Other diseases, such as gout and diabetes mellitus
- Glucose intolerance
- Obesity
- Personality-behavior patterns
- Emotionally stressful situations

Three factors, hypertension, hypercholesterolemia, and cigarette smoking are considered *major* risk factors for premature atherosclerotic disease, especially of the coronary circulation (Fig. 36-2).

## Prevention: Eliminating or Modifying Risk Factors

**Assessment.** Most of the risk factors can be readily measured by a nurse without trauma or risk to the patient. The nurse can assist with the prevention of coronary heart disease through education of the public regarding risk factors and through encouraging individual adults to be tested for coronary proneness. Another aspect of care is to prompt individuals with one or more risk factors to seek early remedial help.

Such risk factors as age, sex, body build (mesomorphs, or those with a muscular body build, show increased risk), and family history cannot be changed, but modifications can be made to reduce the risk. Although people in late middle life and old age are the most likely to show symptoms of the condition, it is believed that atherosclerosis

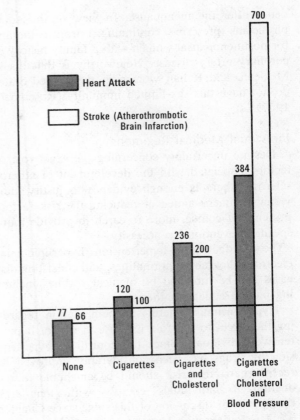

Source: *The Framingham Heart Study: Habits and Coronary Heart Disease,* Bethesda, Md., National Heart Institute

**Figure 36-2.** The danger of heart attack and stroke increases with the number of risk factors present. Example: A 45-year-old male with an abnormal blood pressure level of 180 systolic, and a cholesterol level of 310. (Reprinted from "Heart Facts 1974" with permission of The American Heart Association)

develops gradually over many years; therefore whatever preventive measures may be found to be useful will have to be begun early in life. The need for preventive measures is especially apparent among those who seem predisposed to the condition—for example, those who have a family history of coronary artery disease occurring early in life.

An autopsy study showed that 77 per cent of American soldiers with an average age of 22 killed in action in the Korean war had significant coronary atherosclerosis. The incidence of coronary artery disease in women rises after the menopause and becomes similar to that among men. It has been suggested that estrogens may protect younger women from coronary artery disease, and that lack of this protection may account for the rise in incidence after the menopause. In view of this some physicians prescribe continuing estrogen therapy for postmenopausal women with a family history of coronary artery disease. Noteworthy is that black, Mexican, and Italian women in the United States do not have this sex-limited immunity (Rosenman, 1967).

### Individual Medical Regimens

Despite uncertainty concerning the exact role of factors associated with the development of atherosclerosis, there is enough evidence to justify individual regimens aimed at reducing the risk factors present. Of course, more research to provide more specific prevention is a necessity.

The risk factors of hypertension, hyperlipidemia, electrocardiogram abnormalities, and coexisting diseases can be modified by medical regimes including patient education therapy.

**Hypertension.** There is documentation regarding the three- to fourfold increase in risk of hypertensive individuals. Since the control of hypertension by drugs has been considerably improved in recent years, this risk should be amenable to reduction if individuals comply with long-term therapy. (For discussion of this subject see Chapter 37, The Patient with Hypertension.)

**Hyperlipidemia.** Blood (serum) lipids include cholesterol, triglycerides, and phospholipids. There is evidence that elevation of serum lipids is related to the atherosclerotic process. The cholesterol and triglyceride concentrations determine whether hyperlipidemia is present in the patient. Extensive research related to atherosclerosis has concentrated on the role of serum cholesterol, but recent research studies suggest that elevated serum triglycerides may also increase the risk of coronary artery disease. Frederickson (1972) states that hyperlipidemia deserving some attention exists when cholesterol exceeds 220 mg. per 100 ml. or the triglyceride concentration exceeds 140 mg. per 100 ml. in all patients under the age of 55.

Secondary hyperlipidemia can exist in association with other diseases such as hypothyroidism, nephrotic syndrome, obstructive jaundice, multiple myeloma, lupus erythematosus, and poorly controlled diabetes mellitus. Secondary hyperlipidemia is not treated as such; if the underlying disorder is treated, hyperlipidemia is reduced or eliminated.

Primary hyperlipidemia is that which exists with no other associated disease. The cholesterol and triglyceride elevations can then be localized to one or more of the specific groups of lipoproteins that carry the fats in plasma. The hyperlipidemias are then classified into five major types of hyperlipoproteinemias, some of which lead to the diagnosis of a specific inherited disease. A person with normal cholesterol but elevated triglyceride would suggest the more common Type 4. Determining the type helps put therapy on a more rational basis.

Diet is the keystone of therapy for all hyperlipidemia (hyerlipoproteinemia). The basic components of the diet are reduction of calories to maintain ideal body weight and reduction of cholesterol and saturated fats; and in some cases primarily a reduction of simple carbohydrates (sugars as found in candy, soft drinks, syrups, table sugar). However, the dietary prescription varies according to the specific type of hyperlipoproteinemia (Frederickson, 1972; Cox and Wear, 1972).

When dietary treatment is unsuccessful in reducing elevated lipids, the physician may order drug therapy, the particular drug depending on the age of the patient, the type of hyperlipoproteinemia, and determination of drug effectiveness by monitoring cholesterol and triglyceride values during a trial period. Two such drugs are clofibrate (Atromid-S) and cholestyramine (Questran). Drugs are prescribed with caution because neither the mechanism of action nor all the possible side effects of most hypolipidemic agents are known. In addition, the benefit of treatment in terms of reducing coronary risk is still unproved.

The nurse who participates in coronary risk factor screening programs has an opportunity to explain to the public and the individual about risk factors and the reasons for tests, such as why a blood specimen is taken for cholesterol and triglycerides. Another important role of the nurse is the education and support of the patient on a dietary regime in order to secure his compliance with long-term, but as yet unproved, therapy.

The American Heart Association through its local chapters has a great deal of helpful literature for the lay public on risk factor reduction, including dietary treatment. For example, *Planning Fat-Controlled Meals for 1,200 and 1,800 Calories* (Revised), is available, as is information on meals of 2,000 to 2,600 calories. More stringent dietary recommendations are found in the professional series, *A Maximal Approach to the Dietary Treatment of the Hyperlipidemias.*

**Electrocardiographic Abnormalities.** There is evidence that electrocardiographic abnormalities, such as intraventricular block, left ventricular hypertrophy, abnormal S-T segment displacement, and T wave abnormalities at rest or ischemic S-T and T wave abnormalities after exercise testing, or unexplained arrhythmias are indicators of increased risk, and that the patient should be referred for medical care.

**Coexisting Diseases.** Every effort should be made to assist persons with contributing disease states such as gout, diabetes, anemia, or thyroid disease to seek and maintain long-term medical care.

Other Risk Factors

The following risk factors can be modified by the person at risk, given appropriate nursing, medical, psychological, and sociocultural support:

**Cigarette Smoking.** There is evidence that cigarette smoking increases atherogenesis as well as vascular clotting. Many studies show an increase in coronary heart disease and myocardial infarction in cigarette smokers. Notably, however, this risk is reversible in that once smoking is discontinued, the person's risk reverts to that of a nonsmoker. Nurses can emphasize this point in their teaching.

**Physical Activity.** Regular exercise apparently stimulates collateral circulation. Sports and other activities begun in youth such as skating, dancing, hiking, or swimming are beneficial when continued into middle life. Sudden vigorous exercise such as playing tennis once yearly during a vacation, running for a train, or shoveling snow can overstress myocardial reserve.

Much of the U.S. population is sedentary at work and at leisure activities. Physical exercise programs have been shown to be beneficial in increasing myocardial performance when they are individually prescribed, undertaken regularly, and medically approved.

Jogging or other exercise programs should not be engaged in by middle- or older-aged persons without a physical examination including an exercise electrocardiogram. Myocardial reserve decreases as age increases and individual exercise tolerance varies.

**Obesity.** Studies have shown that while there is only a slight increase in the incidence of coronary artery disease in the obese, the risk of sudden death as well as angina pectoris is considerably elevated. The obese person frequently has other characteristics which increase his risk. Hypertension, hyperlipidemia, diabetes mellitus, and gout are more frequently present in the obese person. A diet designed to reduce weight can have indirect beneficial effects on these other factors as well.

Obesity is defined by some as an increase in body weight of 30 per cent or more above that recommended in standard tables of desirable weight.

**Personality.** Studies have identified a personality type described as the Type A—aggressive, hard-driving, time-pressured, deadline-oriented—individual as being more prone to CHD. Rise in serum cholesterol and acceleration of blood clotting were noted in men subjected to a sense of time urgency (Rosenman, 1967; Freidman and Rosenman, 1974).

A five-year prospective survey of the relation between occupation, education, and coronary heart disease revealed that men who had high levels of responsibility or who were promoted rapidly did not have any added risk of CHD compared with men who remain at lower levels. The data suggested, on the other hand, that there are important determinants of the risk of CHD already in existence before men reach adulthood and that the period of early growth and development may be the important one in the development of CHD (Hinkle, et al., 1968).

Since personality classification is not precise, the relationship between personality and risk cannot be exactly defined. Should an individual's personality and behavior pattern seem to constitute a risk, special attention should be paid to minimizing all other risk factors.

In addition, the clinical nurse specialist can participate in programs which help Type A individuals alter excessive responses, such as time urgency and accompanying impatience, and develop more appropriate responses.

**Acute Emotional Stress.** Intense emotional states such as anger or sudden shock can precipitate myocardial ischemia. This can have the same effect on the heart as unaccustomed physical exertion. One cannot always avoid such intense emotional states. They are part of life and learning to deal with one's emotions is a lifelong task. A person can be assisted to express emotion in a reasonably acceptable manner and thus avoid becoming consumed with pent-up rage, for example. If, however, a person is unable to modify repetitive overwhelming response to a situation or doesn't have the assistance available to him to help him change his response, then the situation itself may have to be avoided or changed.

## Pathophysiology

The symptoms of coronary heart disease result from an insufficient supply of blood to the myocardium. Like other muscles, the myocardium requires more blood when it works hardest—as is the case during physical exertion or emotional stress. Blood supply through narrowed arteries may be sufficient for a body that is at rest, but not adequate for some of the more strenuous activities of daily living.

If the normal vessels or collateral circulation are not adequate for the needs of the heart during exertion, symptoms of *myocardial ischemia* develop.

*Coronary occlusion*, or the closing of an already narrowed coronary artery, can occur from a variety of mechanisms. Usually a clot lodges in the vessel (coronary thrombosis). Occlusion can also result from subintimal hemorrhage of a coronary artery or from a gradually increasing buildup of atheromata. A sudden loss of blood supply to a portion of the myocardium from an occluded coronary artery often leads to necrosis (death) of that portion of the muscle of the heart. The area of necrotic tissue is called a *myocardial infarction*. This condition is usually accompanied by persistent, severe pain and clinical evidence of dead heart tissue. *Coronary insufficiency* is a term used to describe a clinical condition in which cardiac pain is frequently more severe than typical *angina pectoris,* but death of heart muscle does not take place. This condition may also be termed "preinfarction angina" or "crescendo angina."

Coronary occlusion does not necessarily result in myocardial infarction. A small coronary vessel may be occluded, but collateral circulation may be adequate to prevent infarction. On the other hand, myocardial infarction may occur in conditions other than coronary occlusion; for example, drastic curtailment of the blood supply to the myocardium during shock or general anesthesia can result in myocardial infarction.

## ANGINA PECTORIS

The chief symptom of myocardial ischemia is pain. When ischemia and the resulting pain are fleeting, as is often the case during periods of stress when the blood supply is briefly inadequate for the heart's increased needs, the condition is called *angina pectoris*. It is not clear whether the coronary arteries also undergo spasm during attacks of angina pectoris, thus further diminishing blood supply to the myocardium.

**Assessment Factors.** Attacks of angina pectoris are characterized by sudden chest pain or pressure, which may be most severe over the heart under the sternum (substernal). Sometimes, the pain radiates to the shoulders and the arms, especially on the left side, or to the jaw, neck, or teeth. Some patients may deny that they have "pain," but will describe other sensations such as tightening in the chest, a squeezing, choking feeling in the upper chest or throat, indigestion, or burning in the epigastric region.

The patient may experience dyspnea, pallor, sweating, and faintness. Although the intensity of the pain and the apprehension that it arouses may make minutes seem to be hours, the attack usually lasts less than five minutes. Sometimes, the patient seems to "freeze"—the pain makes him suddenly stop whatever he is doing, and he waits, tense and motionless, for it to subside. The attacks characteristically occur during periods of physical or emotional stress. Sometimes, a particular activity almost invariably brings on an attack. For one patient this might be the morning walk to his train; for another, an argument with his wife.

In some patients the severe pain comes without any apparent relation to meals, activity, rest, excitement, or anything that is under the patient's control. These patients are prone to a particularly helpless feeling, because there seems to be little that they can do to lessen the frequency of the attacks.

For the patient whose attacks are more predictable there is the problem of continuous decision making. One man who was able to continue in his work as a shoe salesman found that the day was filled with asking himself, "Will this bring on an attack?" He had to hesitate before climbing up the ladder to reach for a pair of shoes, before bending over to lace a customer's shoe, and before many other regular activities in his workday. Another problem common with other long-term illnesses is that because the pain is exquisite and repetitive, it can all too easily exceed the patient's ability to tolerate it gracefully. It can exceed also the ability of family and friends to empathize with the patient's distress. Whether the patient complains or not, it is obvious to all who are with him that he is in pain when he has an attack, and it is not unusual for people to try to spare themselves the distress of being with the patient. This uncomfortable situation is more conducive to resentment and avoidance than a helpful attitude. Anxiety can cause chest pain similar to that of angina, and it also can make the pain of angina more severe and of longer duration. It is often difficult, and sometimes impossible, for the physician to differentiate functional chest pain and angina pectoris (Master, 1964). Very careful study is required. Angina sufferers frequently delay their entry into the hospital coronary care unit (CCU) with an infarction because they are accustomed to the pain.

**Nursing Intervention.** The pain usually subsides as soon as the patient rests, thus lessening the need of the heart for blood. Most patients quickly discover this, and they need no further urging to stop their activity. Occasionally, a patient may feel that if he just ignores it and refuses to "give in to it," the pain will disappear. The pain is a warning that the heart is not receiving enough oxygen.

Heeding the warning may help the patient to avoid serious illness or even sudden death. The possibility of the sudden death of patients who have angina pectoris is very real. The underlying problem of atherosclerosis and diminished circulation makes the heart especially vulnerable to serious arrhythmias and myocardial infarction (see Chaps. 61 and 62), which may cause sudden death.

The patient need not lie down to rest. In fact, having him lie down often increases his sensations of breathlessness. Merely stopping the activity and standing or, if it is possible, sitting quietly for a few minutes usually suffices. Some patients with angina learn to cease their activity quite inconspicuously—for example, by pausing in a walk and appearing to look in a store window or by merely sitting down quietly and waiting for the attack to subside.

The flustered ministrations of a person who does not understand his condition can be very upsetting to the patient, especially if he knows what is wrong and what to do. A nurse with a patient who often has had attacks in the past should take her cues from him. He should be helped to find a place to rest, and to locate and take any medication that the physician has prescribed. Staying quietly and calmly with the patient and assuring him by one's presence and manner that the attack soon will be over are helpful. If the pain does not subside within 10 to 15 minutes, the patient should be kept at rest and his physician notified. If his physician is not imme-

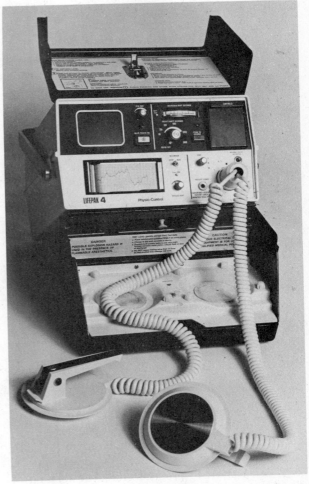

**Figure 36-3.** Lifepak 4, a portable cardioscope-recorder-defibrillator. (Courtesy of Physico-Control)

diately available, the patient should be transported to a hospital with cardiac monitoring facilities.

**Drug Therapy.** Nitroglycerin often is used to relieve attacks that do not disappear quickly with rest and also to prevent attacks. Nitroglycerin is thought to act by relieving spasm of the coronary arterioles, thus permitting vasodilation. Another theory is that nitroglycerin causes peripheral vasodilation, thus reducing the amount of blood returning to the heart and, in effect, temporarily reducing the cardiac workload so that the heart has a chance to rest.

Nitroglycerin is given sublingually in doses of 0.3 to 0.6 mg. (gr. 1/200 to 1/100). Nitroglycerin tablets are prepared in such a way as to dissolve quickly under the patient's tongue. Nitroglycerin relieves the pain within two or three minutes. The duration of its effect is also brief, lasting only about half an hour. Sometimes nitroglycerin causes throbbing headache, flushing, and nausea; usually these side effects can be minimized by decreasing the dose. A patient who is not accustomed to taking nitroglycerin should remain seated for a few minutes after taking the medication since some people experience a feeling of faintness. If they take the drug while they are seated, fainting and injury due to falls can be prevented.

When a patient is about to undertake an activity that usually causes anginal pain, such as sexual intercourse, taking a nitroglycerin tablet a few minutes beforehand often will prevent the attack. Nitroglycerin is a safe drug; many patients take it for years without ill effect. If the drug has been taken repeatedly for a prolonged period, it may lose its effectiveness temporarily, but cases of this sort are rare. Stopping the use of the drug for a short time usually restores the patient's susceptibility to its effects.

Amyl nitrite works faster and has a similar action, but it is used much less commonly than nitroglycerin. It comes in ampuls that are broken into a handkerchief and inhaled. Most patients find the nitroglycerin more convenient, less conspicuous, and cheaper than the amyl nitrite.

Drugs such as aminophylline and pentaerythritol-tetranitrate (Peritrate), isosorbide dinitrate (Isordil), or erythrityltetranitrate (Cardilate) sometimes are given in an effort to produce prolonged dilation of the coronary arteries, thereby preventing attacks of angina. Aminophylline may be given orally in doses of 0.1 to 0.2 Gm. or in rectal suppositories. Peritrate is given in doses of 10 to 20 mg. several times daily. Side effects of Peritrate include weakness, palpitation, flushing, and headache. Some patients find these drugs helpful; others experience little relief from their use.

A newer drug, the beta-adrenergic blocking agent propranolol (Inderal) has been found effective in the treatment of angina. Reflex coronary vasoconstriction may be blocked with this drug. Also cardiac energy requirements and therefore coronary blood flow need are reduced. A dose of 40 to 400 mg. per day is ordered to achieve a resting heart rate of 55 to 60 beats per minute. The drug is contraindicated in congestive heart failure.

Treatment of angina with narcotics is not considered advisable. The pain is likely to recur over a period of years, and the danger of narcotic addiction is considerable. Some physicians apply this restriction to tranquilizers as well.

For an extensive review of drugs used in coronary artery disease, see Chapters 30 and 31 in Rodman, M., and Smith, D.: *Clinical Pharmacology in Nursing*, Philadelphia, Lippincott, 1974.

**Surgery.** Surgical attempts to correct the pathology caused by the diseases of the blood vessels that serve the muscle of the heart have been directed mainly toward improving vascularization, because the basic problem of coronary artery disease is insufficient blood supply to the muscle of the heart. There are several approaches (see Chap. 63).

**Other Treatment.** Occasionally, the nerves over which the pain sensation passes are cut or injected with alcohol, so that the patient no longer will feel the pain. Patients who have this type of treatment must learn to rest, even when they experience very slight discomfort, since they no longer have the warning of severe pain.

Cervicodorsal sympathectomy may help some patients by relieving pain but has little effect on the continuing disease process. Also, the pain of angina may spontaneously improve if the patient sustains a myocardial infarction. (Necrotic tissue loses its pain fibers.)

Sometimes the patient's metabolism is slowed by decreasing the activity of his thyroid gland, thus decreasing the work of the heart and its need for blood. Radioactive iodine and propylthiouracil have been used for this purpose.

External counterpulsation (a modality of noninvasive assisted circulation) has been used recently in some patients with angina pectoris to augment diastolic pressure. It is reported to produce significant subjective and objective improvement in some patients with angina pectoris, possibly by enhancing collateral circulation (Banas, et al., 1973).

**Patient Education.** The patient is advised to stop smoking, because of the association of smoking with the increased risk of coronary artery disease.

Patients with angina are advised to eat small meals rather than large ones, as large meals increase cardiac output and so may precipitate attacks of angina. Regular exercise, such as walking out of doors, often is beneficial in promoting collateral coronary circulation, thus lessening the frequency and the severity of attacks. Overweight patients in most instances benefit from weight reduction.

Many patients continue to live active, productive lives despite attacks of angina pectoris. Vasodilators and careful regulation of activity may decrease the frequency and the severity of the attacks. For instance, the patient who has attacks of angina every morning while he is walking to the railroad station may find that leaving the house earlier, walking more slowly, and taking a nitroglycerin tablet will prevent the attack.

**Activity Prescription.** The amount of activity permitted in work and leisure is best determined by the physician's interpretation of data obtained from evaluation of the patient's performance in a series of tests administered at a cardiac work evaluation clinic. (See Chapter 39, Rehabilitation of Patients with Heart Disease.) The nurse can assist the patient to plan his daily activities in accordance with his activity prescription.

Some patients find that their symptoms remain the same for years. In others the atherosclerosis advances rapidly, and anginal attacks become more frequent and severe despite treatment. These patients are crippled by such severe interference with blood supply to the heart that everyday activities must be curtailed.

The patient with angina faces the problem of finding what his level of tolerance for activity is and then learning to live within that level. He also has to learn to live with the ever-present possibility of an attack. For some patients the fear aroused by the attack is worse than the pain. Some feel each time that an attack comes, "Well, this is it." Some patients react to this illness by being more angry at the necessary curtailment of their activity than by being afraid. All who care for the patient must strive to relieve and, if it is possible, to prevent the symptoms. They will need to help the patient to strike a reasonable compromise with his condition: to avoid the one extreme of giving up all activity and allowing his entire life to revolve around the possibility of an attack and to avoid the other extreme of refusing to acknowledge that his heart places some definite restrictions on the amount of exertion that he can undertake safely. Because the prognosis is so variable—the patient may live for years, or he may die suddenly because of the poor circulation to his heart—he is encouraged to live each day as it comes, to take reasonable precautions, and to continue with his prescribed activities, provided that they do not precipitate attacks of angina pectoris.

## MYOCARDIAL INFARCTION

For a presentation of the care of the patient with acute myocardial infarction, see Chapter 62.

## FUNCTIONAL HEART DISEASE

Anxiety can produce a variety of physical discomforts—headache, diarrhea, nausea, to name just a few common ones (see Chap. 7). Symptoms associated with heart disease also can be produced by anxiety, and they are referred to as functional heart disease. Other terms sometimes used to describe the condition are neurocirculatory asthenia, soldier's heart, and effort syndrome.

Careful examination of the patient is essential to rule out organic heart disease and to assure the patient that his heart is normal. Regular, complete physical examinations are especially important for any patient who has functional disturbances, because organic disease can develop in this patient just as it can in anyone else. Because the patient is known to have had a functional disturbance, early symptoms of organic disease may be ignored or attributed to the functional disorder.

Symptoms of functional heart disease can include any symptom referable to heart function. Pain over the heart, dyspnea, palpitation, and exhaustion are common.

The treatment of functional heart disease is similar to that of any other functional disorder:

- Carefully evaluating the factors, both in the patient's personality and in the environment, that seem to be related to the attacks.
- Providing symptomatic relief while the underlying causes of the condition are investigated. In functional heart disease, relief might be obtained by a vacation or by the use of sedatives or tranquilizers.
- Gradually helping the patient to understand that his symptoms may be due to anxiety, and that treatment involves helping him to recognize and to deal with his emotional problems, and sometimes modifying his environment.

Often the treatment of functional heart disease must continue throughout life. New and taxing situations often provoke symptoms, such as dyspnea, fatigue, and chest pain. Treatment involves a gradual and lifelong process of re-education, in which the patient is helped by his physician and, hopefully, by his family, his employer, and his friends. Psychotherapy with a psychiatrist, psychologist, or clinical nurse specialist, individually or with a group, may be beneficial.

## REFERENCES AND BIBLIOGRAPHY

American Heart Association: *Coronary Risk Handbook. Estimating Risk of Coronary Heart Disease in Daily Practice,* New York, 1973.

————: *A Maximal Approach to the Dietary Treatment of the Hyperlipidemias. Physician's Handbook,* New York, 1973.

Banas, J., et al.: Evaluation of counterpulsation for the treatment of angina pectoris, *Circulation* 46: supplement II-74, October 1972.

Cox, M., and Wear, R.: Campbell Soup's program to prevent atherosclerosis, *Am. J. Nurs.* 72:253, February 1972.

Elek, S.: Emotional tension as a factor in coronary disease, *Hosp. Med.* 6:15, February 1970.

Fox, S., et al.: Physical activity and cardiovascular health: I. Potential for prevention of coronary heart disease and possible mechanisms, *Mod. Conc. Cardiovasc. Dis.* 41:17, April 1972.

Fredrickson, D.: A physician's guide to hyperlipidemia, *Mod. Conc. Cardiovasc. Dis.* 41:31, July 1972.

Freidman, M., and Rosenman, R.: *Type A Behavior and Your Heart,* New York, Knopf, 1974.

Germain, C. P., and Minogue, W.: Precoronary care: Nursing considerations, *Cardiovasc. Nurs.* 8:1, May-June 1972.

Gotto, A. M.: Recognition and management of the hyperlipoproteinemias, *Heart Lung* 1:508, July-August 1972.

Grollman, A.: How drugs work in atherosclerosis, *Consultant* 13:99, March 1973.

Harrison, T., and Reeves, T.: *Principles and Problems of Ischemic Heart Disease,* Chicago, Year Book, 1968.

Hinkle, L., et al.: Occupation, education, and coronary heart disease, *Science* 161:238, July 1968.

Inter-Society Commission for Heart Disease Resources: Primary prevention of the atherosclerotic diseases, *Circulation* 43:A-55, 1970.

Kagan, A., et al.: The Framingham study: A prospective study of coronary heart disease, *Fed. Proc.* 21: 52, 1962.

Kannel, W.: The disease of living, *Nutrition Today* 6:2, May-June 1971. Condensed and reprinted in *Nurs. Digest* 2:67, May 1974.

————, et al.: Relative importance of factors of risk in the pathogenesis of coronary heart disease: The Framingham study, in Russek, H., and Zohman, B. (eds.): *Coronary Heart Disease.* A Medical-Surgical Symposium sponsored by the American College of Cardiology and St. Barnabas Hospital, Philadelphia, Lippincott, 1971.

Kershbaum, A., and Bellet, S.: Cigarette, cigar, and pipe smoking; some differences in biochemical effects, *Geriatrics* 23:126, March 1968.

Kratz, A. M.: Cardiac drugs today: Antilipemic agents. Part 5, *Nurs. '73* 3:53, September 1973.

Lown, B.: Intensive heart care, *Sci. Am.* 219:19, July 1968.

Master, A. M.: The spectrum of anginal and noncardiac chest pain, *JAMA* 187:894, March 1964.

Rockwell, S.: Low-cholesterol meals for cardiologists —and for you, *RN* 35:72, May 1972.

Rosenman, R.: Emotional factors in coronary heart disease, *Postgrad. Med.* 42:165, September 1967.

Shapiro, S., et al.: The H.I.P. study of incidence and prognosis of coronary heart disease. Preliminary findings of incidence of myocardial infarction and angina, *J. Chron. Dis.* 18:527, June 1965.

Stamler, J.: The primary prevention of coronary heart disease, *Hosp. Pract.* 6:49, September 1971.

————, et al.: Detection of susceptibility to coronary disease, *Conference on Automated Multiphasic Health Screening,* New York, New York Heart Association, 1970. Reprinted from *Bull. N.Y. Acad. Med.* 45:1257, December 1969.

What happens in practice. Treating the cardiac neurosis, *Roche Image Med. Res.* 14:24, November 1972.

# The Patient with Hypertension

With the development of newer, more effective anti-hypertensive agents, patients may expect longer life with fewer complications. Between 1951 and 1965, the death rate from *hypertensive heart disease* decreased 49 per cent. This was largely due to the development of antihypertension drugs. In the Veterans Administration Cooperative Study a significant decrease in morbidity and mortality associated with elevated blood pressure was reported for male patients receiving drug treatment when compared with placebo-treated control subjects with similar degrees of hypertension (Freis, 1971; U. S. Veterans Administration, 1967, 1970, 1972). When untreated or ineffectively managed, however, hypertension is still a dangerous ailment, significantly impairing prognosis for health and longevity. It is said to be more prevalent and more destructive than cancer, tuberculosis, and pneumonia combined (Thomas, 1969). It is estimated that from 20 to 30 per cent of adults in the United States have blood pressures at the level of or greater than 160 mm. Hg systolic and 95 mm. Hg diastolic (Aagaard, 1973). The incidence of high blood pressure, as well as its complications, is significantly higher among the black race.

Untreated hypertension contributes to cardiovascular diseases such as myocardial infarction and congestive heart failure; cerebrovascular disease, mainly stroke; and progressive renal failure. To reap the benefits of improved therapy, the patient and his family may need nursing help in living each day as fully and as hopefully as possible, avoiding the pitfalls of ignoring the illness and failing to follow medical treatment, yet escaping the potential anxiety neurosis generated by excessive attention to the disease.

The term *hypertension* refers to a disease entity characterized by sustained elevation of arterial pressure. The systolic, diastolic, and mean arterial pressure may be elevated.

## ARTERIAL BLOOD PRESSURE

*Systolic blood pressure* is determined by the rate and volume of ventricular ejection and the distensibility of the aorta. Normally the walls of the aorta are elastic and yield to the volume of blood which bursts into it on ventricular contraction. In older persons with a rigid, atherosclerotic aorta, however, systolic blood pressure may be quite elevated due to loss of this elasticity. Systolic hypertension is a response to change in central hemodynamics.

*Diastolic blood pressure* is the pressure recorded during the period of ventricular relaxation. It depends on the peripheral resistance and the diastolic filling interval. The rate of outflow or runoff from the systemic arterial system depends on the state of the peripheral resistance through which the blood flows. If arterioles are constricted, blood will have to flow under an increased pressure to overcome the increased resistance which is a factor in raising the diastolic pressure. If the arterioles are dilated there will be less impedance to blood flow and diastolic pressure will fall rapidly. The slower the heart rate, the longer is the diastolic interval during which aortic pressure continues to fall and the lower is the final end diastolic pressure. This low diastolic blood pressure may occur with marked sinus bradycardia and complete heart block. Diastolic hypertension is a response to change in peripheral hemodynamics.

The *mean arterial pressure* is the average pressure tending to push blood through the system's circulation and is measured as the diastolic pressure plus one-third of the pulse pressure. It is usually slightly less than the average of the systolic and diastolic pressures, however, since arterial pressure is nearer to diastolic level during the greater portion of the pulse cycle. Mean arterial pressure is important since it takes into account systemic resistance, blood flow, and blood pressure. A high mean arterial pressure can be produced by a high systolic pressure and a normal diastolic pressure, or a normal systolic pressure and an elevated diastolic pressure, or when both pressures are elevated. It is sometimes said that of the two, the high diastolic pressure is more significant, because it has been associated with more vascular complications of high blood pressures. Another view holds that a rise in mean arterial pressure is of greatest importance.

*Pulse pressure* is the difference between the systolic and diastolic pressures. The magnitude of the pulse pressure largely determines the forcefulness and the volume of the radial pulse. Factors which *increase* the systolic pressure, such as a rigid, atherosclerotic aorta, or factors which decrease the diastolic pressure, such as a slow heart rate, will increase the pulse pressure. A strong bounding pulse reflects a wide pulse pressure.

Factors which *decrease* the systolic pressure and increase the diastolic pressure will decrease the pulse pressure. A rapid, weak, and thready pulse reflects a decreased or narrowed pulse pressure. This is the case in shock.

Normal blood pressure for adults ranges from about 100/60 to 140/90. Although a progressive increase in blood pressure with age has been frequently noted in the United States, this is not invariably true. The reasons for the changes in blood pressure in advancing age are not fully understood.

Blood pressure normally fluctuates with changes in posture, exercise, and emotion. It is lowest when an individual is sleeping, slightly higher when he is awake but lying down, higher still when he is sitting up, and elevated even further when he is standing. Exercise and emotional stress cause elevation of blood pressure. These normal fluctuations show the importance of measuring blood pressure under constant conditions. For example, the patient's blood pressure should not be taken before he has been out of bed one morning, and the next morning while he is sitting in a chair immediately after he has taken a shower. The designated circumstances for taking the patient's blood pressure so that conditions are most nearly duplicated should be recorded on the nursing care plan.

### Physiologic Control of Arterial Pressure

The system for the control of arterial pressure is multifaceted. Arterial pressure is regulated by the autonomic nervous system, the kidneys, and the endocrine glands.

Nervous Control (Acute or Short-Term)

**Sympathetic Nervous Control During Exercise.** When the motor area of the cerebral cortex becomes active during exercise, nerve impulses excite sympathetic vasoconstrictor fibers throughout the body, elevating the blood pressure. During exercise the vessels in active muscles dilate. Without the sympathetic regulatory mechanism, which also prevents a decrease in arterial pressure during exercise, blood pressure would fall drastically.

**Baroreceptors.** These bodies are located mainly in the carotid sinuses and the arch of the aorta. When arterial pressure rises, they are stimulated and transmit signals to the vasomotor centers of the brain to cause reflex vasodilation throughout the body and reflex decrease in heart rate. If an extraneous factor, such as a sudden infusion of fluid, increases blood pressure above normal, functioning baroreceptors will decrease the amount of potential rise in pressure. Baroreceptors, however, adapt quickly to continued stimulation and over a period of time their output may no longer be effective in blood pressure regulation.

**Ischemia.** Nerve cells in the vasomotor center of the medulla are themselves sensitive to ischemia. When arterial pressure falls to shock levels and blood flow is reduced to the vasomotor center, they will increase heart rate and peripheral vasoconstriction, thus elevating the blood pressure. This activity occurs mainly at the lethal level of arterial pressure and can be termed a "last ditch stand" in an attempt to maintain life (Guyton, et al., 1969).

## Capillary Fluid Shift Mechanism

Movement of fluid through the capillary membrane helps to moderate changes in blood pressure. Following severe hemorrhage, fluid is absorbed from the tissue spaces into the bloodstream increasing the circulating volume toward normal and raising the blood pressure. Overinfusion is followed by loss of much of the excess fluid into the tissue spaces with lowering of the blood pressure.

## Stress Relaxation and Reverse Stress Relaxation

Excess pressure from an overload of blood causes a slow stretch of all vessels of the body, but especially of the veins and venous reservoirs such as the liver and spleen. Thus the circulatory system effectively enlarges to accommodate the increased blood volume. When hemorrhage occurs, venous reservoirs diminish in size so that the circulatory system more nearly fits the volume of blood.

Blood volume eventually adjusts itself to the capacity of the circulatory system.

## Long-Term Regulation of Blood Pressure

Present experimental evidence and clinical experience point to the kidney as the organ probably vested with long-term control of arterial pressure. This mechanism is the subject of much present study and debate. Some prevalent theories are:

**Humoral Theories.** The renin-angiotensin or vasoconstrictor theory holds that low blood pressure causes the juxtaglomerulus apparatus of the kidney to secrete renin. In turn, renin catalyzes the conversion of a plasma protein, angiotensinogen, into a substance called angiotensin I, which is converted in the lung by another enzyme into angiotensin II. Angiotensin causes constriction of systemic arterioles throughout the body, thereby raising arterial pressure. Angiotensin also stimulates the adrenal cortex to secrete aldosterone, which causes the kidneys to retain sodium and water resulting in increased blood pressure.

**Body Fluid and Electrolyte Theories.** Excess sodium in the vessel wall results in increased arteriolar vasoconstriction. Retention of water and electrolytes by the kidneys causes an increase in arterial pressure. Initially the pressure increase results from an increase in cardiac output. This causes increased total peripheral resistance by the mechanism of reflex autoregulation. (Autoregulation means the capacity of each local tissue to control its own blood flow.) This phenomenon of autoregulation secondarily increases the total peripheral resistance while cardiac output returns to its original mean level. The further increased peripheral resistance causes greater increase in arterial pressure with only a slight decrease in blood flow through the tissues.

## HYPERTENSIVE DISEASE

A person having a sustained blood pressure of greater than 140/90 is usually considered to be hypertensive. This is a potentially serious condition because it causes increased work by the heart and damage to the arteries. Congestive heart failure, myocardial infarction, stroke, and renal failure are serious sequelae of hypertension.

When cardiac abnormalities (such as electrocardiographic or x-ray evidence of enlargement of the left ventricle) are present with the elevated blood pressure, the term *hypertensive heart disease* is used. When extracardiac vascular damage is present without heart involvement, the term *hypertensive vascular disease* is used. When both heart and extracardiac pathology are present with hypertension, the appropriate term is *hypertensive cardiovascular disease* (Stamler, et al., 1967).

Hypertension is divided into two main categories: primary (essential) and secondary. The cause of primary hypertension is unknown although heredity seems to play a major role. About 90 per cent of hypertensive patients have the primary or essential type.

Secondary hypertension is a term used to describe a variety of conditions in which elevation of blood pressure is secondary to some known cause. Pheochromocytoma (a tumor of the adrenal gland) is an example of a condition causing secondary hypertension which is curable by the removal of the tumor. Determination of catecholamines and/or VMA (vanillylmandelic acid) in a 24-hour urine collection is a reliable screening procedure for pheochromocytoma.

Secondary hypertension is also associated with such conditions as toxemia of pregnancy, increased intracranial pressure, congenital blood vessel and heart malformations, and diseases of the kidney such as glomerulonephritis, pyelonephritis, and polycystic disease. Rarely, tumors of the adrenal cortex may cause high blood pressure by excess production of cortisol (Cushing's syndrome) or aldosterone (Conn's syndrome). Only 10 per cent of persons with hypertension are estimated to have the secondary type. Treatment is directed at relief of the underlying cause.

## PRIMARY (ESSENTIAL) HYPERTENSION

Primary hypertension is characterized by sustained elevation of the diastolic pressure. A diastolic pressure of 95 mm. Hg or greater is generally accepted as abnormally elevated (Stamler, et al., 1967). Most physicians believe that sustained diastolic pressure over 90 mm. Hg requires treatment.

### Theories About Etiology

Among the many theories concerning the cause of primary hypertension are these:

- Heredity. Many investigators have noted a strong familial tendency toward the development of primary hypertension; there is also a relationship between hypertension and a family and/or personal history of diabetes mellitus (Stamler, et al., 1967).
- Fluid-electrolyte metabolism. A disturbed relationship among salt intake, body fluid-electrolyte metabolism, and renal-adrenal function has been observed in many studies, but the results are inconclusive.
- Emotional stress. Patients with hypertension may have difficulty expressing and dealing with their aggressive impulses. Although outwardly calm and composed, inwardly they may be in a turmoil.
- Obesity. Overweight persons have a higher incidence of hypertension, but obesity may not of itself cause high blood pressure.
- Bacteruria. Higher prevalence rates of bacteria in the urine have been found in hypertensive persons (Stamler, et al., 1967).

### Epidemiology

Hypertension is presently estimated to affect approximately 23 million Americans (National Institute of Health, 1973). Only half are aware that they have the disease and only one-eighth are aware and have adequate blood pressure control (American Heart Association, *1974 Heart Facts*) (Fig. 37-1). In 1960 to 1962 the National Health Survey estimated that over 1,000,000 Americans in the age group 35 to 44, of a total population of about 24,000,000 in this age range, had definite *hypertensive heart disease*. Almost 170,000 were black men and 170,000 black women, showing a markedly higher proportionate incidence among

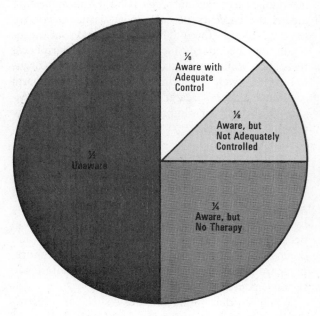

Source: National Heart and Lung Institute

**Figure 37-1.** Awareness and therapy of 22 million persons in the United States with high blood pressure. (Reprinted from "Heart Facts 1974" with permission of The American Heart Association)

blacks than among whites. Hypertensive heart disease is the major health problem of black Americans today; the mortality rate among blacks is three and one-half times greater than in the white population. The reason for this excessive difference in mortality is not known. It may reflect basic biological differences in the natural history of the disease between the two races, or it may reflect accessibility and patterns of usage of medical care resources (Finnerty, *Circulation* 47:73).

Sporadic elevated blood pressure readings in young adulthood often indicate increased risk for later development of sustained hypertension (Stamler, et al., 1967).

Among women, the incidence of high blood pressure rises at middle age to equal that of men. The potential for complications is of equal magnitude for males and females and is related to the height of the pressure elevation (Fig. 37-2).

### Prevention

Despite the lack of knowledge concerning the etiology of primary (essential) hypertension, the information available from current epidemiologic studies affords a useful basis for prevention of its complications.

Measures to decrease the risk in susceptible populations may help to forestall the development of symptoms or curtail advancement of the disease.

People with a family history of hypertension or those who have shown transient elevations of blood pressure may be helped by:

- Having a periodic health examination at least annually. For the poor population this necessitates major changes in our health care delivery system.
- The correction of obesity and the direction of efforts to remain lean and trim through a nutritious diet and physical exercise.
- Moderation in salt intake—about 5 Gm. per day instead of 15 to 20 Gm.
- Routine midstream urine cultures for the early detection and treatment of urinary tract infections.
- Learning to deal more effectively with problems at work, home, or in other circumstances. Some people may need professional assistance. If, for some reason, the patient doesn't learn to cope more effectively, it may become necessary for him to avoid certain stress-producing situations.
- Improving general health habits. Adequate sleep, rest, and relaxation may prove to be helpful in controlling high blood pressure.

As noted above, studies indicate that only a fraction of the hypertensive population is identified and

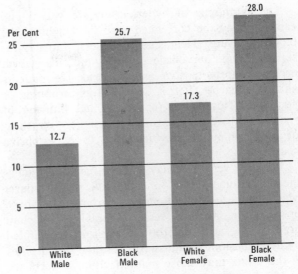

Source: National Health Examination Survey

**Figure 37-2.** Hypertension prevalence by sex and race in adults age 20 and over, United States, 1971 estimate. (Reprinted from "Heart Facts 1974 with permission of The American Heart Association)

receiving adequate treatment. Detection of those people affected is a needed public health measure. The nurse can help by participating in screening programs in industrial clinics, community centers, and student health centers, and by referring those people with elevated blood pressure for medical care. The physician can then evaluate key target organs by history, physical exam, and appropriate laboratory investigation. The encouragement of periodic health examinations of adults in colleges, offices, and industry would constitute a major detection effort. Particular attention needs to be given to mass screening and medical followup of inner-city black populations in view of their marked susceptibility to the complications of high blood pressure as well as their experience with the social problems of discrimination and poverty and the inaccessibility of preventive health care.

### Symptoms

The onset is insidious; usually, hypertension is first discovered during a routine physical examination.

A sustained elevation in blood pressure may occur without any symptoms. High blood pressure may be present for 10 or 15 years before the patient experiences symptoms of target organ disease.

The symptoms of hypertension are varied and cannot always be correlated with the height of the blood pressure. Headache, dizziness, fatigue, insomnia, and nervousness are symptoms which occur in normotensive and hypertensive patients alike. Headache often is described as throbbing or pounding. Nosebleeds (epistaxis) and blurring of vision may occur. Angina pectoris or shortness of breath may be the first clue to hypertensive heart disease.

The left ventricle may enlarge, and eventually the patient may develop congestive heart failure. Many of the complications arise from hemorrhage or occlusion of blood vessels supplying important organs. The atherosclerotic process is accelerated by hypertension. Hemorrhage from the tiny arteries in the retina may cause marked visual disturbance or blindness. Cerebrovascular accident may result from hemorrhage or occlusion of a blood vessel in the brain. Myocardial infarction may result from occlusion of a branch of a coronary artery. Impaired circulation to the kidney is believed to be related to the frequency of degenerative kidney disease among hypertensive patients.

The clinical symptoms may be an indication of the stage of the disease. Progression from the asymptomatic stage to that of symptoms of target organ involvement and target organ failure is usually slow and fortunately can be delayed by appropriate therapy. The earlier treatment is instituted, the more effective it is likely to be.

The term *malignant hypertension* refers to an abrupt onset of accelerated high blood pressure associated with severe symptoms of vascular disease. The prognosis without treatment is poor. Untreated patients usually live only a few months to one or two years. Death frequently is caused by damage to heart, brain, or kidneys.

## Diagnostic Assessment

Five to 10 percent of patients with high blood pressure have an underlying cause such as renal artery stenosis, coarctation of the aorta, or pheochromocytoma, or they develop hypertension as a result of the ingestion of drugs such as oral contraceptives or menopausal estrogen therapy. A careful medical history is taken, and information related to the patient's psychosocial functioning and life style is also obtained.

If secondary causes are ruled out, further diagnostic tests are ordered to determine whether target organ disease is present before treatment is begun. Treatment for primary hypertension is most successful in preventing complications when it is initiated before target organ damage has occurred.

## Treatment

Although it has not been possible to develop a cure for primary hypertension, many forms of treatment are available which control high blood pressure quite well. The objective of the health care team is to secure the patient's compliance with lifelong dietary, hygienic, pharmacologic, and education therapies in order to prevent the major cardiovascular and renal complications of hypertension.

Securing compliance in a program of lifelong treatment which sometimes causes side effects for an often symptomless disease involves many cognitive, affective, and cultural dimensions, and can best be achieved by the gradual building of a trusting relationship between patient and health care team. The primary relationship may be with a physician or a nurse specialist working in collaboration with the physician. The nurse as primary therapist works with hypertensive patients in such facilities as hospital or industrial clinics, neighborhood storefront health centers, or mobile health units in rural areas.

Many patients adhere to a treatment program only until blood pressure returns to normal or symptoms are relieved. Others drop out of treatment programs due to factors such as family crises, cost of care, long waiting times in offices or clinics, interference with working hours, transportation difficulties, drug-induced side effects, or failure to understand the treatment program. For the poor, the constant struggle to acquire the barest necessities for survival on a day-to-day basis may result in the patient's assigning the lowest priority to treatment of an asymptomatic chronic disease.

Federally funded programs are seeking more effective methods for administering antihypertensive treatment to a wide spectrum of persons in large communities. In addition to participating in mass screening efforts in these locales, nurse specialists in charge of *Stepped Care* clinics are attempting to make treatment more accessible, convenient, and compatible with the patient's priority system at little or no cost. The nurse, aware of noncompliance factors, may need to become involved in getting more welfare money for a client, or better housing, or medical care for a sick child through referral to appropriate agencies. Vigorous followup of individuals who miss appointments is carried out by an "outreach" worker. *Stepped Care* treatment involves the use of a protocol which begins a treatment program with the mildest standard antihypertensive medications and after careful evaluation of the patient adds more potent standard drugs as necessary to control the blood pressure (National Institute of Health, 1973).

**Dietary Treatment.** Weight reduction and moderate salt restriction may help lower blood pressure in a number of patients with mild labile high blood pressure. Shaker salt and grossly salty foods such as pretzels, potato chips, anchovies, and herring should be eliminated. The physician may recommend that no salt be added in food preparation in the home. Some patients may find salt restriction unpalatable; salt substitutes may be utilized with the physician's approval or oral diuretics prescribed.

Control of lipid abnormalities in cholesterol and triglycerides may be accomplished by appropriate diet with adjunctive drug therapy, such as Atromid-S.

**Physical Activity.** Where cardiovascular stress testing techniques are available, physical activity can be prescribed on an individual basis. A progressive program of physical fitness exercises compatible with the patient's capacity is recommended and may include tennis, swimming, and skiing.

**Sexual Function.** There appears to be little increased risk of heart attack or stroke with sexual intercourse (Howard, 1973). It is recommended that patients with angina use appropriate treatment such as nitroglycerin in advance. In the male, antihypertensive drugs such as reserpine and methyldopa (Aldomet) may interfere with sexual potency and libido; guanethidine may cause retrograde ejaculation into the urinary bladder. Such sexual considerations are an important part of individual patient management and play a major role in compliance with therapy.

**Psychosocial Factors.** The personality of the patient is an important factor in his reaction to stress and, therefore, an important consideration in the overall plan of high blood pressure management. Helping the patient to understand his problems, the role of his life style, and his emotional reactions may help in the treatment of his disease. The patient who rushes at the last minute to meet scheduled activities may be helped to see the wisdom of conducting his daily activities at a less frenzied, more leisurely pace. Techniques which encourage muscular relaxation such as yoga exercises are helpful for the tense, hyper-reactive, hypertensive individual (Aagaard, 1973).

Individual or group counseling with a clinical nurse specialist or other counselor may be necessary to help the patient (and family) deal more effectively with aggravating interpersonal situations arising in the home or school, or on the job.

## Drug Therapy

Several drugs are used to lower blood pressure. The principal ones in current use are the oral diuretics, reserpine, alpha-methyldopa, hydralazine, guanethidine, and diazoxide. They vary in their mechanisms of action. None of them is considered ideal in always producing the desired results without unpleasant or dangerous side effects. Many, however, particularly the newer agents, have proven extremely effective.

There is wide variation in the response of hypertensive patients to individual drugs. The physician seeks a regimen which provides the most effective blood pressure control with the fewest side effects. Compliance often is increased by simplifying the treatment, such as by prescribing one pill (or as few pills as possible) per day.

Most hypertensive patients are treated as outpatients. Patients are hospitalized for drug therapy of malignant high blood pressure or where the physician suspects a secondary cause.

**Oral Diuretics.** These can be classified as (1) thiazides and related diuretics, (2) loop diuretics—furosemide and ethacrynic acid, and (3) potassium-sparing diuretics.

Thiazides such as chlorothiazide (Diuril) and hydrochlorothiazide (HydroDiuril) as well as the related compounds chlorthalidone and quinethazone are considered the cornerstone of an antihypertensive regimen. Although the mode of action is not entirely understood, it is believed to be related to the reduction of sodium in the arterial wall as well as depletion of plasma volume and direct vasodilating effect on arteriolar smooth muscle (Fig. 37-3).

Therapy with chlorothiazide may be continued for many years. Side effects are infrequent but fatigue, weakness, and gastrointestinal upsets occur. Hypokalemia (hypopotassemia) is a complication

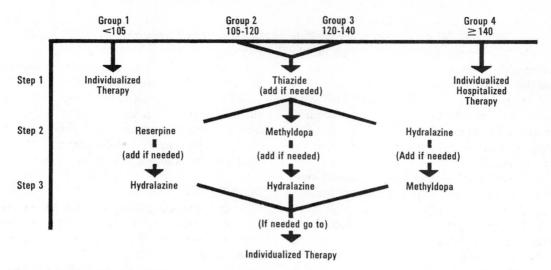

Therapeutic objective: Diastolic pressure under 90 mm. Hg, or, if untoward effects cannot be tolerated, under 100 mm. Hg. "All hypertensives should have treatment for any lipid disorder and obesity and should be instructed to stop smoking cigarettes and to engage in appropriate regular exercise." Report of Inter-Society Commission for Heart Disease Resources, Circ. Vol. XLIV, November 1971.

**Figure 37-3.** Outline of recommended antihypertensive regimens for groups with varyingly severe hypertension as indicated by diastolic pressure (in mm. Hg). (Adapted from National High Blood Pressure Education Program, Task Force 1, September 1973. By permission of The American Heart Association)

of prolonged therapy with chlorothiazide. It can be prevented by administration of supplementary potassium in the form of KCl or by additional dietary intake of potassium such as in fruits or juices. The patient may be instructed to drink a large glass of orange juice every morning or to eat a banana every day. Chlorothiazide alone may be given to patients with mild hypertension, and in severe cases it may be given in conjunction with other antihypertensive agents. The dose ranges from 250 mg. to 500 mg., orally one to three times daily. Chlorothiazide and other oral diuretics of the thiazide type potentiate the action of the stronger antihypertensive drugs. Combined therapy with chlorothiazide and one of the more potent drugs permits a smaller dose of the latter and thus reduces the likelihood of toxic effects.

LOOP DIURETICS. Furosemide (Lasix) and etha-crynic acid (Edecrin) are potent diuretics employed to counteract marked excesses of extracellular volume which are not controlled with conventional diuretics and sodium restriction. Potassium loss may be great, and hyperuricemia is common with prolonged daily administration. Doses of 40 to 200 mg. orally of furosemide or 25 to 200 mg. of ethacrynic acid daily may be effective. A precipi-

tous fall in arterial pressure may be due to volume depletion and can be treated by volume expansion. Deafness has been reported following treatment with ethacrynic acid. These diuretics are particularly useful in hypertensive patients with renal insufficiency.

POTASSIUM-SPARING DIURETICS produce sodium diuresis without potassium loss. Spironolactone (Aldactone) is a steroidlike compound and an aldosterone inhibitor. It is given in a dose of 50 to 100 mg. per day in divided doses. Triamterene (Dyrenium) is a pteridine derivative which acts on the distal tubule independently of aldosterone. A usual dose is 100 mg. twice daily after meals. Both these drugs are contraindicated in patients with renal insufficiency in whom potassium retention is a therapeutic problem.

**Rauwolfia alkaloids** such as reserpine are effective in the treatment of mild hypertension. The primary action is to impair the intracellular storage of norepinephrine.

Local vasodilation may result in nasal congestion. Additional side effects include diarrhea, gastro-intestinal bleeding, lethargy, drowsiness, nightmares, and decreased libido. The most serious side effect is mental depression. Reserpine is contraindicated in patients with a history of depression or psychosis and should be used with caution in patients with obesity or peptic ulcer. The average dose is 0.25 mg. one to two times daily.

**Methyldopa (Aldomet)** acts as a false neurotransmitter displacing norepinephrine, the major vasoconstrictor to the blood vessels. Side effects include postural hypotension, drowsiness, depression, decreased libido, arthralgias, myalgias, and drug fever. A daily dose of 250 mg. two times daily to 500 mg. four times daily may be prescribed, titrated according to the individual patient's response. This drug can be used in patients with chronic renal insufficiency but is contraindicated in patients with liver disease. Drowsiness and dry mouth are bothersome side effects. A rare serious toxic effect is hemolytic anemia occurring during the first six weeks of therapy.

**Guanethidine (Ismelin).** This most potent of all antihypertensive drugs exerts its effect by depletion of tissue levels of norepinephrine. Hypotension is most marked when the patient stands, especially in the morning or after exercise. Guanethidine may produce unfavorable effects on renal function and should be used with caution in patients with renal insufficiency. Diarrhea, nasal stuffiness, impotence, failure of ejaculation, peptic ulcer, and muscular weakness are other side effects. Guanethidine is prescribed in the smallest effective dose, such as 10 to 25 mg. once daily; dosage can be increased by 12.5 to 25 mg. increments to 100 mg. per day if necessary.

**Hydralazine (Apresoline)** is a moderately powerful antihypertensive drug. Side effects include tachycardia, palpitation, headache, anxiety, and nausea. Edema, fever, and psychoses may occur. The dosage varies from 10 to 100 mg. four times daily. Small doses (10 mg. three times daily) are given at first to minimize the side effects, and the dose is gradually increased. Although usually given orally, hydralazine also may be prescribed intravenously. A lupuslike syndrome may be associated with doses larger than 400 mg. per day. The drug can be prescribed when renal insufficiency exists.

**Table 37-1.** Contraindications, Side Effects, and Treatment for Side Effects of Antihypertensive Drugs

| DRUG | CONTRAINDICATIONS | SIDE EFFECTS | TREATMENT OF SIDE EFFECTS |
|---|---|---|---|
| *Oral Diuretics*<br>Thiazides and related diuretics | *Absolute*—acute gout<br>*Potential*—azotemia, hypokalemia | Hypokalemia, muscle cramps, gastrointestinal distress | 1. Monitor plasma K bimonthly<br>2. Supplemental K routine only when patient taking digitalis<br>3. K 3.2—liquid K<br>K 2.5—liquid K and omit drug<br>4. K-sparing drugs |
| | | Hyperuricemia (uric acid 10) | 1. Monitor uric acid every 3 to 4 months. Probenecid 250–500 mg b.i.d., or allopurinol 100 mg. b.i.d. or t.i.d.<br>2. Acute gouty arthritis: colchicine |
| | | Hyperglycemia | 1. Monitor blood glucose every 3 to 4 months; not necessary to discontinue drug |
| | | Hypotension | 1. Decrease frequency and dose; restore to maintain volume |
| | | Generalized aching | No good treatment |
| *Loop Diuretics*<br>Furosemide (Lasix)<br>Ethacrynic acid (Edecrin) | *Potential*—acute gout<br>*Potential*—acute gout | Same as thiazide<br>Same as thiazide | Same as thiazide } with emphasis<br>Same as thiazide } on volume replacement |
| *Potassium-sparing Diuretics*<br>Spironolactone (Aldactone) | *Absolute*—renal insufficiency; azotemia of any consequence | Nausea, vomiting<br>Weakness, headache<br>Drug rash<br>Gynecomastia | 1. Give drug after meals<br>1. Decrease dosage<br>1. Decrease dosage<br>1. Discontinue drug |

**Table 37-1.   (Continued)**

| DRUG | CONTRAINDICATIONS | SIDE EFFECTS | TREATMENT OF SIDE EFFECTS |
|---|---|---|---|
| Triamterene (Dyrenium) | *Absolute*—azotemia; severe hepatic disease | Same as spironolactone except for gynecomastia | |
| *Rauwolfia serpentina* Reserpine | *Absolute*— depression, psychoses | Nasal congestion | 1. Nasal vasoconstrictor; omit during respiratory infection |
| | *Potential*—peptic ulcer, chronic sinusitis, obesity | Weight gain | 1. Diuretics and stricter diet |
| | | Gastrointestinal bleeding | 1. Omit drug, substitute methyldopa |
| | | Lethargy, sluggishness | Omit drug |
| | | Depression (frequently preceded by changes in sleeping habits) | Omit drug |
| | | Nightmares | Omit drug |
| | | Decreased libido | Prayer |
| *Methyldopa* (Aldomet) | *Potential*—liver disease | Drowsiness and dryness of mouth | 1. Common during first weeks; tends to diminish later |
| | | Mood disturbances | 1. Discontinue drug |
| | | Bradycardia | 1. Decrease dosage |
| | | Hemolytic anemia | 1. Monitor hematocrit every 3 or 4 months; a positive Coombs' test is not an indication for discontinuation of drug |
| *Hydralazine* (Apresoline) | *Potential* 1. Arteriosclerotic heart disease with angina | Headaches | 1. Pretreatment with reserpine 2. Antihistamine drugs |
| | | Angina, tachycardia, palpitations | 1. Pretreatment with reserpine 2. Gradually increasing dosage |
| *Hydralazine* (Apresoline) | 2. Congestive heart failure | Peripheral edema | 1. Diuretics |
| | | General myalgia | 1. Usually remits spontaneously; if not, discontinue drug |
| | | Lupus erythematosus–like reaction | 1. Discontinue drug |
| *Guanethidine* (Ismelin) | *Absolute*— pheochromocytoma *Potential*—azotemia | Postural syncope; dizziness | 1. Patients must be trained to protect themselves from fainting: (a) Good support stockings (b) Should never get out of bed quickly (c) Should never stand quietly for more than a few minutes (d) Be warned of existence of hypotension (e) Enhancement of antihypertensive effects with diuretics plus dose reduction |
| | | Diarrhea | 1. Parasympathetic blocking drugs, e.g., atropine or oxyphenonium (Antrenyl) |
| | | Fluid retention | 1. Diuretics |
| | | Failure of ejaculation | Prayer |

From Finnerty, F.: Critical considerations in the treatment of arterial hypertension, *Mod. Conc. Cardiovasc. Dis.* 42:37, August 1973. By permission of The American Heart Association and the author.

## Patient Education

The patient must adhere to a program of long-term therapy to prevent target organ complications. Instruction and support of the patient sustain his motivation and improve cooperation with a treatment program. Group teaching affords the opportunity for sharing his concerns, needs, understanding, or misunderstanding with others who share a similar diagnosis. The nurse-teacher recognizes that giving information is not equivalent to patient education. She capitalizes on patients' contributions to improve knowledge and change misconceptions as well as to promote positive attitudes and a higher level of motivation for members of the group. An education program for the hypertensive patient as well as his family or others responsible for his care should include the following points geared to the cognitive capacities, affective responses, and psychomotor abilities of the persons involved:

- **Facts regarding sodium restrictions in the diet, weight and blood lipid control, exercise, relaxation techniques and cessation of smoking.**
- **Facts about blood pressure elevation, e.g., that it is a chronic condition which can be controlled but which can worsen without treatment and cause stroke, heart failure, kidney and eye disease.**
- **Specific drug actions, side effects, and toxic effects of the patient's regime and what to do when these occur.**
- **The importance of lifelong regular blood pressure checks and compliance with a therapeutic regimen. Some patients or a family member may be taught to use the sphygmomanometer and stethoscope and record blood pressures at home; the physician will direct some in self-regulation of medication dosage according to pressure levels.**
- **The importance of continuing treatment even though symptoms are relieved, a sense of well-being is achieved, and blood pressure returns to normal.**
- **The importance of not increasing medication dosage without medical advice when symptoms worsen, and explanation of the system for obtaining such advice.**
- **The necessity of informing additional medical therapists such as a surgeon, psychiatrist, or dentist of the hypertensive condition and its treatment regimen in view of the possibilities of drug interactions.**

### Nursing Assessment and Intervention

Most patients with hypertension are first seen by the physician and nurse as outpatients. However, patients can be hospitalized for diagnostic assessment, establishment of a treatment regimen, or for hypertensive crisis.

## The Hospitalized Patient

When antihypertensive drugs are administered, the patient should be observed carefully for side effects, which should be promptly reported. Since some of these drugs may cause orthostatic hypotension, the patient must be instructed to get up slowly to avoid weakness or fainting. When he arises in the morning, he first should sit on the edge of the bed a few moments and then stand. He should be told to sit or, preferably, to lie down promptly if he feels faint. Blood pressure must be taken carefully at the intervals ordered by the physician and additionally upon the judgment of the nurse. The patient must be in the desired position when the blood pressure is taken; the position should be recorded with the blood pressure. Some physicians will order blood pressure to be checked each morning before the patient arises; others will order it to be taken with the patient standing as well as sitting or recumbent. At this time, the patient may be taught how to take his own blood pressure. Then therapy after hospital discharge can be planned and adjusted according to multiple blood pressure recordings made in the patient's usual surroundings. The patient is encouraged to participate in his own care.

Often the patient seeks repeated reassurance and explanation which the nurse may provide. The nurse should know what the physician has told the patient about his particular problem, so that he does not become confused by variance in explanations. The pitfalls of giving the patient information for which he is not prepared or of withholding information that he has long considered necessary for self-care must be avoided.

For example, a patient who has been admitted for diagnosis, and who asks his blood pressure, should not be told blithely, "It's 160/120." Such information, in the absence of a definite diagnosis and an explanation of his problem, could be very upsetting to him. On the other hand, a patient who has had high blood pressure for years, and who has been taking and recording his own blood pressure at home, may be justifiably irritated if he is refused his blood pressure reading.

When the patient learns that he has hypertension, he needs a great deal of explanation and reassurance concerning its possible consequences. Almost everyone has heard of people who have had strokes or heart attacks that were attributed to high blood pressure. Often the patient's first thought is that such a catastrophe is about to befall him. The physician and nurse help the patient to understand the course of the disease, and explain how the patient can help himself.

### Hypertensive Crisis

Acute severe elevation of diastolic blood pressure above 140 mm. Hg is a life-threatening crisis which may rapidly produce congestive heart failure with pulmonary edema, hypertensive encephalopathy, intracranial hemorrhage, or aortic dissection because of the high degree of stress placed on the heart and arterial vessels. Blood pressure must be rapidly reduced without producing renal, cerebral, or myocardial ischemia and disabling hypotension. The physician selects the appropriate antihypertensive drug such as hydralazine (Apresoline), trimethaphan (Arfonad), reserpine, or methyldopa (Aldomet), which is usually given parenterally to reduce the diastolic pressure to 100 to 110 mm. Hg. A new very effective antihypertensive drug, diazoxide (Hyperstat), is administered by the physician using rapid IV injection technique (Diazoxide, *Nursing '73*).

Aspects of nursing assessment and intervention include:

- **Blood pressure measurement at times as often as every 30 seconds. Physicians' orders regarding drug dosage, flow rates, and blood pressure range must be clearly understood and accurately followed.**
- **Observation for signs of central nervous system complications, heart failure, cardiac arrhythmias, fluid intake and output, patient's appearance, behavior, and comments. He should not be left alone until out of crisis.**
- **Protection of the patient from injury during convulsions. A padded tongue depressor should be at the bedside with side rails up. Anticonvulsant drugs (such as Dilantin or sodium amobarbital) should be readily available.**
- **Vasopressor agents (such as Levophed) should be readily available should there be a precipitous drop in blood pressure, shock, and ischemia of vital organs. Physicians' orders for the drug, dosage, flow rate, and range of blood pressure should be clearly written and understood.**

### The Ambulatory Outpatient

Nursing assessment often begins with participation in screening programs involving entire communities, random populations who congregate in large public facilities such as shopping centers, or selected groups such as those taking pre-employment physicals. Such screening programs are ineffectual however without a built-in referral system for diagnostic assessment and treatment.

Nursing specialists in hypertension can be responsible for groups of hypertensive patients, helping them to achieve blood pressure control through maintenance of a treatment program as well as through teaching, counseling, and referral to appropriate agencies. In clinics using a *Stepped Care* plan the nurse follows a medical protocol established by the physician, starting with the mildest standard antihypertensive medications. She may, through continuous assessment of blood pressure response, add more potent drugs as necessary to control blood pressure, conferring with the physician when she or the patient finds it necessary. Compliance with long-term therapy will be enhanced if the nurse recognizes the importance of listening to the patient, respecting his priorities, and referring him for financial or other kinds of help. Counseling, guiding, and teaching, in addition to an expanded role in treatment, are major components of the nursing role in the hypertension clinic. Cardiovascular physical assessment, including funduscopic examination of the retina, is also part of the role of the nurse who is primary therapist for patients with hypertension.

Further informational material on high blood pressure is obtainable from High Blood Pressure Information Center, 120/80 National Institute of Health, Bethesda, Maryland 20014, and from local chapters of the American Heart Association.

### REFERENCES AND BIBLIOGRAPHY

AAGAARD, G.: Treatment of hypertension, *Am. J. Nurs.* 73:621, April 1973.

American Heart Association: *1974 Heart Facts,* New York, 1974.

BAINE, R., and SHERMAN, W.: Arterial hypertension, Chap. 15 in MacBryde, C., and Blacklow, R. (eds.): *Signs and Symptoms,* ed. 5, Philadelphia, Lippincott, 1970.

BEESON, P. B., and McDERMOTT, W. (eds.): *Cecil-Loeb Textbook of Medicine,* ed. 13, Philadelphia, Saunders, 1971.

BREST, A.: Preoperative and postoperative considerations in the hypertensive patient, *Hosp. Med.* 6:59, September 1970.

———, and MOYER, J.: *Cardiovascular Disorders,* Philadelphia, Davis, 1968.

Byrom, F.: *The Hypertensive Vascular Crisis: An Experimental Study,* New York, Grune, 1969.

Caldwell, J., et al.: The dropout problem in antihypertensive treatment, *J. Chron. Dis.* 22:579, February 1970.

Carr, A. A.: Identifying endocrine hypertension, *Consultant* 12:25, June 1972.

Del Greco, F., et al.: Malignant hypertension, *Hosp. Med.* 9:8, July 1973.

Diazoxide. Report on rapid reducer of hypertension. Drug update, *Nurs. '73* 3:13, June 1973.

Eliot, R. S.: Cri de coeur, *Emerg. Med.* 4:21, May 1972.

Finnerty, F., Jr.: Critical considerations in the treatment of arterial hypertension, *Mod. Conc. Cardiovasc. Dis.* 42:37, August 1973.

————: Drugs used in the treatment of hypertension, *Mod. Conc. Cardiovasc. Dis.* 42:33, July 1973.

————: Hypertension is different in blacks, *JAMA* 216:1634, June 7, 1971.

————, et al.: Hypertension in the inner city. I. Analysis of clinic dropouts, *Circulation* 47:73, 1973; II. Detection and follow-up, *Circulation* 47:76, 1973.

Freis, E.: Medical treatment of chronic hypertension, *Mod. Conc. Cardiovasc. Dis.* 40:17, April 1971.

Genest, J. (ed.): *Hypertension—1972,* New York, Springer, 1972.

Griffith, E., and Madero, B.: Primary hypertension: Patient's learning needs, *Am. J. Nurs.* 73:624, April 1973.

Grollman, A.: Hypertension: What does it really mean? *Consultant* 13:26, August 1973.

Guyton, A. C.: *Textbook of Medical Physiology,* ed. 4, Philadelphia, Saunders, 1971.

————, et al.: Physiological control of arterial pressure, *Bull. N.Y. Acad. Med.* 45:811, September 1969.

The heart and the whole body. Steps to understanding hypertension. Part 2, *Emerg. Med.* 4:128, January 1972.

The heart and the whole body. Drugs for the patient as well as the disease (hypertension). Part 3, *Emerg. Med.* 4:140, January 1972.

Howard, E.: Sexual expenditure in patients with hypertensive disease, *Med. Asp. Human Sexuality* 7:82, October 1973.

*The Hypertension Handbook,* Rahway, N.J., Merck, 1974.

Inter-Society Commission on Heart Disease Resources: Part 1. Cardiovascular disease—primary prevention. Primary prevention of hypertension, *Circulation* 42(suppl.):A-39, July 1970.

Kimball, J. T., et al.: Circulatory emergencies, Part III. Hypertensive crisis, in Meltzer, L., et al.: *Concepts and Practices of Intensive Care for Nurse Specialists,* Philadelphia, Charles Press, 1969.

Kirkendall, W. M.: What's with hypertension these days? *Consultant* 11:13, January 1971.

Lancour, J.: The nurse and cardiovascular drug therapy, *Cardiovasc. Nurs.* 9:19, July-August 1973.

Lewis, C. E., et al.: Nurse clinics and progressive ambulatory patient care, *New Eng. J. Med.* 277:1236, December 1967.

Marston, M. V.: Compliance with medical regimens: A review of the literature, *Nurs. Res.* 19:312, July-August 1970.

Mayer, J.: Don't salt it, season it, *Family Health* 3:34, December 1971.

McCombs, N., et al.: *The Atlanta Community High Blood Pressure Program Treatment Center,* Supplement Number IV to *Circulation,* Vols. VII and VIII, AHA Abstracts, IV-235, October 1973.

National Health Education Committee: *Facts on the Major Crippling Diseases in the United States Today,* New York, 1966.

National Institute of Health: *Hypertension Detection and Follow-Up Program of the National Heart and Lung Institute* (pamphlet), Bethesda, Md., 1973.

Page, L., and Sidd, J.: *Medical Management of Primary Hypertension,* Boston, Little, Brown, 1973.

Redman, B.: Patient education as a function of nursing practice, *Nurs. Clin. N. Am.* 6:573, December 1971.

Rodman, M.: Drugs used in cardiovascular disease. Treating hypertension. Part 2, *RN* 36:41, April 1973.

Schoenberger, J. A., et al.: Current states of hypertension control in an industrial population, *JAMA* 222:559, October 30, 1972.

Stamler, J.: *Lectures on Preventive Cardiology,* New York, Grune, 1967.

————, et al.: *The Epidemiology of Hypertension,* New York, Grune, 1967.

Stewart, R., and Cluff, L.: A review of medication errors and compliance in ambulant patients, *Clin. Pharmacol. Ther.* 13:463, 1972.

Thomas, C. B.: Developmental patterns in hypertensive cardiovascular disease: fact or fiction? *Bull. N.Y. Acad. Med.* 45:831, September 1969.

Tracht, M. E.: The laboratory evaluation of hypertension, *Consultant* 13:79, January 1973.

U. S. Veterans Administration, Cooperative Study Group on Antihypertensive Agents: *Effects of Treatment on Morbidity in Hypertension.* Results in patients with diastolic blood pressure averaging 115 through 129 mm. Hg., *JAMA* 202:1028, December 11, 1967; Results in patients with diastolic blood pressure averaging 90 through 114 mm. Hg., *JAMA* 213:1143, August 17, 1970; Influence of age, diastolic pressure, and prior cardiovascular disease, further analysis of side effects, *Circulation* 45:991, May 1972.

Wilber, J., and Barrow, J.: Hypertension: A community problem, *Am. J. Med.* 52:653, May 1972.

Wilkins, R. W., et al.: Evaluation of hypertensive patients, *Clin. Symp.* 24:5, 1972.

# The Patient with Peripheral Vascular Disease: Thrombosis and Embolism

## CHAPTER 38

The term peripheral vascular disease (PVD) refers to diseases of the blood vessels that supply the extremities. The disease may involve the veins, arteries, or lymphatics, or all of these.

The long-term nature of peripheral vascular diseases is discouraging. Treatment is often painful, and healing is slow. A small ulceration that may be looked upon by the hospital staff as relatively "minor" compared with more dramatic patient conditions is a tragedy to the patient if he loses his ability to walk. It may require months of treatment for healing to take place. Worry about finances, loss of job, and suspension of family and civic responsibilities compound the patient's burden.

The number of patients with peripheral arterial disease is growing due to the lengthening of the life span. The elderly are especially vulnerable to peripheral vascular disease. They frequently suffer also from coexisting medical conditions such as diabetes and hypertension. The possibility of recurrence of the condition after a long treatment process, increasing incapacitation, and dependence on others are formidable problems.

Caring for these patients often does not provide opportunity to see rapid, dramatic recovery. Instead, it involves working patiently and painstakingly with persons whose illnesses can sometimes be ameliorated but seldom cured. In spite of advances in surgical treatment, a large group of these patients can be helped at present only by symptomatic treatment. The importance of expert nursing care cannot be overemphasized, because this care and the education of the patients and their families can in some instances prevent invalidism.

An important part of the nursing role is to teach the patient and family methods of prevention of tissue breakdown. There is a precarious balance between the blood flow to ischemic tissues and the metabolic needs of the tissues. The slightest chemical, mechanical, or thermal injury, or local bacterial infection of the tissues, can upset the balance and lead to ulceration or gangrene. The patient needs to understand those measures which can limit the progress of his underlying disease and prevent complications so that he can live in relative good health and comfort.

In some instances severe disability results in spite of the most meticulous and thoughtful care because the disease process has outstripped current knowledge of treatment.

## ANATOMY AND PHYSIOLOGY

All body tissues depend on efficient functioning of arteries, veins, and lymphatics—arteries to bring blood rich with oxygen and nutrients, veins to remove blood that has given up its oxygen and taken on waste products, and lymphatics to transport tissue fluids. Diseases of the blood vessels, unless promptly controlled, lead to damage of the tissues that are supplied by the vessels.

Arteries have thicker, more muscular walls than veins. The walls have a great deal of elasticity, enabling them to pulsate or "give" with each gush of blood pushed through by the heart, as well as to dilate and to constrict, so that the amount of blood flowing to any part of the body can be regulated according to the varying metabolic needs of the tissues.

When the circulation is impaired, the body compensates by developing collateral circulation, so that tissues still can receive blood. Collateral circulation is effected by the greater utilization and dilation of existing vessels to carry more blood, as well as by the development of new vessels to carry blood to the deprived tissues. Collateral circulation has more opportunity to develop if the circulatory impairment develops slowly. Sudden occlusion of an artery does not allow time for collateral circulation to develop, and if the artery is a major one, serious damage to the tissues results unless the obstruction in the artery can be removed quickly. The body's ability to develop collateral circulation is greatly diminished in peripheral vascular disease.

## Factors Affecting the Tissues' Need for Blood

What increases the need of a part of the body for blood? Exercise, added warmth, and infection all increase the metabolism of the tissues and, therefore, their need for blood. For example, vigorous exercise of the leg causes vasodilation and increased blood supply to the leg muscles. Placing the hands in hot water causes the superficial blood vessels to dilate, making the hands look red. More blood is needed during infection, because blood carries leukocytes and antibodies to combat the infection. If infection occurs near the surface of the body, redness and swelling caused by the dilation of superficial blood vessels can be observed readily. Dilation and constriction of blood vessels helps to regulate body heat. When the surface of the body is cold, superficial blood vessels constrict in order to conserve heat. When the part is warmed, blood vessels dilate in order to dissipate heat. The body thus is capable of maintaining its optimum temperature despite changes in the temperature of the environment.

The blood supply is adjusted automatically to meet the varying needs in all parts of the body. Activity of the sympathetic nervous system causes vasoconstriction. Removal of sympathetic activity by surgery or drugs causes vasodilation.

Decreased metabolism lessens the need of the part for blood. Rest and chilling slow the metabolism of the tissues and decrease their need for blood. Chilling also induces vasoconstriction, thus reducing the blood supply to the region.

## CIRCULATORY ASSESSMENT

*Ischemia* is the term used to describe a lack of blood supply to meet the needs of the tissues. At one time or another almost everyone has had the experience of "pins and needles" in the foot or leg, perhaps from sitting on the leg or with the legs crossed for a long time, causing pressure that interferes with blood supply. When the leg is first moved, it feels heavy, numb and awkward. However, these sensations quickly vanish when change of position and exercise improve the circulation to the leg.

What would happen to the leg if circulation were impaired for a long time? What kinds of pathologic change can cause diminished blood supply? A blood clot (embolus) can lodge in an artery, quickly occluding it and preventing the blood from reaching its destination. Excessive vasoconstriction can result in diminished flow of blood. Gradual occlusion of the lumen of the artery by fatty deposits (atherosclerosis) can slowly and inexorably reduce the amount of blood that the arteries can deliver. Such occlusion may be speeded by formation of a blood clot at the atherosclerotic site (thrombosis). Regardless of the particular pathology responsible for the decreased blood flow, certain changes in the affected part will occur if the diminished blood supply is severe and persistent.

## Signs and Symptoms of Ischemia

- Coldness. Ordinarily, the body feels warm to touch, because of the presence of warm blood. When the blood supply is markedly decreased, the part is cold to touch and also feels uncomfortably cold to the patient. The body normally becomes chilled when it is exposed to cold. However, warmth usually returns quickly when one is in a warm environment. The patient with diminished blood supply to an extremity has coldness of the extremity even in a warm environment. If only one extremity is affected, its temperature may readily be contrasted with that of the opposite hand or foot.
- Pallor. The normal pink hue of the skin is due to the blood in superficial vessels. Diminished arterial blood supply causes pallor. Blanching is noted particularly when the part is elevated above the level of the heart, since this elevation further diminishes arterial blood flow to the region.
- Rubor (redness). Redness—usually a reddish-blue color—results when the superficial blood vessels have been injured by anoxia or coldness and remain dilated. The color is different from that of the normal rosy-pink and indicates impaired rather than improved circulation. The extremity is both blue-red and cold, rather than pink and warm, as it normally should be. Although blood remains in the tiny superficial vessels, circulation to the part as a whole is impaired.
- Cyanosis (blueness). Cyanosis indicates that the blood in the part contains less than the normal amount of oxygen. Cyanosis usually results from a blood supply that is diminished and yet not diminished sufficiently to cause blanching.
- Pain. Pain is characteristic when the blood supply is not adequate for the requirements of the tissues. Pain that occurs only after a certain amount of exercise is called *intermittent claudication*. The patient may walk a block and then have to stop because of severe aching in his calf muscles. His arteries are not able to deliver the amount of blood required by his legs during this exercise. The pain disappears when the patient rests, but it promptly returns when he repeats the same amount of exercise. Pain occurs even at rest (rest pain) when sudden occlusion of an artery by an embolus occurs,

because there is not sufficient blood supply to sustain the tissues even when no exercise is undertaken. Rest pain also occurs when the patient has severe circulatory impairment from any cause, and particularly when an ulcer has formed on the part, or gangrene is imminent.
- Trophic changes. This term refers to abnormal changes in the skin and the nails due to impaired circulation. The skin becomes smooth, shiny, taut, dry, and hairless. It has very little resistance to infection. Tiny injuries, like stubbing the toe or scratching the skin, can lead to infection. Because of poor blood supply, the body's ability to fight the infection and to heal the lesion are diminished, and an ulcer is likely to form. Gangrene may follow. The nails become thickened, brittle, and deformed.
- Pulsation (see Fig. 38-10 for major arteries of the lower extremities that can be palpated for pulsation). There may be abnormal pulsations or the presence of bruits. Arterial pulsation (for instance, that normally felt at the wrist or the ankle) may be diminished or absent.

## Diagnostic Tests for Determining Adequacy of Blood Supply

- Oscillometry. The oscillometer is an instrument used to measure the volume of blood delivered to the extremity with each heartbeat. A cuff attached to the oscillometer is wrapped around the limb. The fluctuations in blood volume caused by pulsation are transmitted by the cuff to the oscillometer and are indicated by a needle that moves across a dial.
- Testing skin temperature. The skin temperature of an affected limb is an important diagnostic sign. The examiner feels and notes the temperature of the extremity, and then contrasts it with that of the limb on the opposite side. Sometimes, a hot-water bottle or an electric heating pad is placed on the patient's abdomen, and the response of each extremity is noted. Normally, the extremities grow warmer because of reflex vasodilation. However, if the arteries of one limb are diseased, that limb may remain cool while the others become warmer. Changes in skin temperature when the part is placed in a warm or cold environment may be noted. For instance, the extremity may be placed in warm or cool water. The patient should be as relaxed as possible when skin temperature is tested, because the temperature of the extremities is affected by emotional states as well as by organic disease. Most clinicians who treat patients with peripheral vascular disease become very skillful at judging whether skin temperature is normal just by feeling the extremity. Skin temperature may be taken readily with direct-reading skin temperature thermometers, but the use of these thermometers ordinarily is not necessary in the usual clinical examinations.
- Angiography may be performed (see Chap. 23).
- Testing the response to deprivation of arterial circulation. After constriction has caused a tempo-

rary lack of blood supply, blood normally rushes back to the part. The skin quickly becomes warm and flushed. Patients with diminished circulation do not have a prompt, full flushing of the skin. Their response often is slow, with a faint flush that may not extend to all the areas that have been deprived of blood. To test this response a blood-pressure cuff is applied and inflated for approximately three minutes. The pressure is then released. Observation is made of how fully, quickly, and completely the skin flushes in the area below the cuff and whether or not there is capillary bleeding.

- Exercise tests. The amount of exercise that the patient can perform without experiencing pain is another indication of the adequacy of circulation. The patient is asked how far he can walk before experiencing pain. The patient may be asked to perform a simple exercise in the office or clinic to note whether he experiences pain in the extremity, and if so, how soon the pain occurs after the exercise is begun.
- Doppler flowmeter. A commercially available transcutaneous blood flow velocity meter utilizing ultrasound and the Doppler effect may be used to indicate blood flow through arteries over which the transducer is placed. It is more sensitive in detecting evidence of pulsatile flow than digital palpation, and its use is innocuous to the patient.
- Phlebography. Radiopaque dye is injected into a foot vein and the veins most likely to produce large emboli are displayed. This is useful in depicting the exact site, extent, and nature of a thrombus.

## Measures to Increase Blood Supply

In what general ways can the blood supply to an extremity be increased? How may these measures be utilized in the care of patients with diminished blood supply to an extremity?

- Position. The flow of arterial blood to the limb is improved when the part is dependent (lower than the heart) or at least flat, rather than raised. Raising the limb will further diminish the amount of blood reaching the part. Patients with lessened circulation to the feet are advised to keep the legs flat on the bed or to sit in a chair with their feet on the floor. Elevating the legs on pillows or with a gatch bed is contraindicated, except when the legs are briefly elevated during prescribed exercises. Sometimes the head of the bed is elevated on 6-inch blocks, so that the legs will be lower than the rest of the body.
- Warmth. At first glance, added warmth might seem the ideal solution to diminished circulation in the extremities. But heat must be used with caution, because the tissues are unusually susceptible to burns. Often, the patient has diminished sensation in the part, making him less able to note when excessive heat is applied and therefore placing him in even greater danger of being burned. The benefits of applying heat are greatly limited by the fact that increased heat speeds up tissue metabolism. Arteries

unable or barely able to deliver sufficient blood to meet minimal metabolic needs cannot supply the part adequately when metabolism is increased. In persons with normal arteries, increased heat causes vasodilation and increased blood supply. But if the vessel has lost its elasticity (arteriosclerosis) and is unable to dilate, the discrepancy between supply and demand for blood will be increased, leading to greater ischemia. Gangrene may be precipitated by the ill-advised use of a heating pad or hot-water foot bath.

The kind of warmth that merely insulates the extremity from a cold environment may be safely used. Warm gloves and socks are examples. Extra heat provided by hot-water bottles, hot foot soaks or heating pads never should be used. Heat sometimes is applied to the abdomen to cause reflex dilation of the blood vessels in the extremities. Warm (95 degrees F ) baths or thermoregulated cradles are sometimes recommended. The question may be asked, "Why not use cold applications to decrease the metabolism, so that the extremity won't need so much blood?" Although cold applications are used occasionally to decrease metabolic needs of the tissues, thus helping to relieve rest pain, they also induce vasoconstriction, and therefore they may lessen the blood supply further.

- Interrupting sympathetic stimuli. Interruption of sympathetic stimuli to the extremity prevents vasoconstriction. If the vessels have enough elasticity to enable them to dilate, and if the disease process has not occluded the lumen (for example, by a clot), cutting off sympathetic innervation may result in vasodilation and improved blood supply. This may be accomplished by the use of sympatholytic drugs, such as tolazoline (Priscoline) and phenoxybenzamine (Dibenzyline), or by sympathectomy. Sympathetic stimuli may be removed temporarily by injecting the vertebral sympathetic ganglia with lidocaine (Xylocaine), thus temporarily preventing the transmission of sympathetic impulses to the extremity.

Permanent interruption of sympathetic stimulation is achieved by cutting the nerve. Usually, Xylocaine injections are carried out before surgery is done, to determine whether the arteries are still capable of dilating when sympathetic stimuli are removed. Many authorities believe that sympathectomy increases blood supply primarily to the skin rather than to the deeper tissues. Therefore, sympathectomy is performed less frequently now in the treatment of impaired deep circulation resulting from organic occlusive vascular disease, but it may be done in the treatment of Raynaud's phenomenon.

- Vasodilators. In order to be effective, vasodilators must have more than a fleeting action. Alcohol and papaverine are examples of drugs used to cause vasodilation. The usefulness of vasodilators is limited by the fact that organic changes, such as arteriosclerosis, often make the vessels incapable of dilating. Thus, diseases characterized by spasm of vessels or vasoconstriction respond best to vasodilators.

- Dissolving and/or preventing clot formation. If clots are impeding circulation, such anticoagulants as heparin and dicumarol may be given to prevent further clot formation. Enzymes, such as streptokinase and thrombolysin, are sometimes used to dissolve clots. Their usefulness in the treatment of vascular disease is being studied.

- Avoidance of vasoconstriction. Nicotine leads to vasoconstriction; therefore, smoking or the use of tobacco in any form is contraindicated in any patient with diminished arterial circulation. Exposure to cold causes vasoconstriction and should be avoided whenever possible. The constriction of vessels by pressure also must be avoided. For instance, sitting with the knees crossed causes pressure on popliteal vessels and lessens further the blood supply to the legs.

- Exercise. If exercise does not cause greater demand for blood than the body can supply to the extremity, it is beneficial. Mild exercise with frequent rest periods is usually recommended. Pain is a warning that the patient has exercised more than his blood supply will allow; he should stop and rest. No exercise is permitted when the circulation is impaired drastically. For example, when a clot occludes an artery, the part is kept at complete rest until adequate circulation can be restored.

- Replacement or bypass of diseased arteries using synthetic vessels or veins (grafts). When successful, surgery of this type produces the most rapid and dramatic improvement possible.

## GENERAL NURSING CONSIDERATIONS IN THE CARE OF PATIENTS WITH PVD

In addition to nursing assessment and intervention aimed at increasing blood supply and in specific clinical conditions, there are important general nursing considerations for patients with peripheral vascular disease.

**Socioeconomic.** Peripheral vascular disease is especially common among older people. Many of the disorders are chronic and tend to be progressive with advancing age. Often, only palliative treatment is possible. Care consists of a multitude of detailed measures to control the disease, to halt its progress, and to prevent complications.

Patients with peripheral vascular disease often are obliged to change the type of work they do. Among the types usually contraindicated are those involving considerable outdoor exposure to cold or prolonged standing or repeated trauma to the feet. Indoor, sedentary occupations are the most suitable. However, a change of job is frequently difficult or impossible for the older person. Often, illness carries the threat of prolonged disability, loss of earning power and, as a consequence, lessened personal independence. Retirement from active work may be necessary earlier than had been anticipated.

**Coexisting Conditions.** Many of these patients have multiple diagnoses. Peripheral vascular disease is often only one manifestation of a widespread vascular disorder affecting many different organs. For instance, the patient may have suffered myocardial infarction due to atherosclerosis of coronary vessels, and he may have failing vision due to vascular changes in the tiny blood vessels of the retina. Diabetics are especially prone to arteriosclerosis and atherosclerosis. Plans for the nursing care must encompass not only the peripheral vascular disease, but also any other conditions for which the patient requires nursing assistance.

**Chronicity.** The nurse must have a great deal of patience and willingness to carry out the detailed care that can mean the difference between invalidism or continued ability to carry out daily activities. Often, the patient requires treatment for the rest of his life. He is faced with the management of a condition that usually necessitates changes in his mode of living for years, not merely for weeks or months.

**Position.** Understanding the factors that may hamper or facilitate peripheral circulation is essential in caring for patients with peripheral vascular disease. It is important to know whether the arteries, veins, lymphatics or all three are involved in the disease process, and what pathologic changes are responsible for the symptoms. For instance, the idea that elevating the legs always improves circulation is erroneous. Elevating the legs promotes venous and lymphatic return; it does not improve—it actually reduces—the blood supplied by the arteries.

Errors in positioning the patient can be avoided by:

- **Basic understanding of the dynamics of circulation to the extremities**
- **Understanding the patient's particular disease**
- **Frequent conferences with the patient's physician so that specific procedures concerning important details, such as positioning the patient, can be fully discussed**

If there is doubt about positioning the patient, it is best to have him keep his legs flat rather than elevated or dependent until the opportunity for discussion is available.

## Leg Ulcers

Ulcers often complicate peripheral vascular disease, and they require a great deal of care (Fig. 38-1). Because the ulcers tend to heal very slowly, the patient and those who care for him may become discouraged. Meticulous technique is especially important when carrying out prescribed care, such as the application of ointments and dressings. Sometimes, the patient (and, occasionally the staff, too) grow so accustomed to the lesion that they use technique that would be considered unthinkable in the care of a surgical incision; for example, the patient may apply ointment with his fingers instead of as he was taught.

Patients with peripheral vascular disease are especially vulnerable to infection. They develop infection readily, and their ability to control it and to heal wounds is so lessened by poor circulation that gangrene and amputation are not unusual. The most careful technique possible must be used by staff and patient. Washing the hands thoroughly before starting to care for the lesion, applying prescribed medication with a sterile tongue blade to sterile gauze, and then laying the gauze and medication against the ulcer are examples of simple techniques that can lessen the incidence of infection. The patient is taught not to touch the side of the gauze that he places next to the ulcer.

When the patient has a leg ulcer, he often must stay off his feet for weeks or even months. Part or all of this time may be spent in the hospital. Diversion is very important. Hours and weeks pass slowly, and the patient often worries about his finances, his family, and his job. The nurse must take time to listen when the patient expresses some of his worries and fears—perhaps of amputation or of losing his job—and refer the patient to other sources of help such as the social service department if indicated.

## Foot Care

If the patient is feeble, has poor vision, or has an unsteady hand, someone else must assume the responsibility for inspecting his feet regularly, bathing them, and trimming the nails. A member of the family may give this care, or, if the patient lives alone, a weekly visit from the community health nurse can provide this important care, as well as continued instruction and encouragement in the care that the patient can still perform himself.

The services of a podiatrist are valuable in managing such problems as the cutting of thickened, brittle nails. The patient should explain that he has peripheral vascular disease and give the name of his physician. These measures enable the podiatrist to carry out treatment with consideration of the patient's impaired circulation, as well as to confer with the patient's physician concerning particular needs and problems.

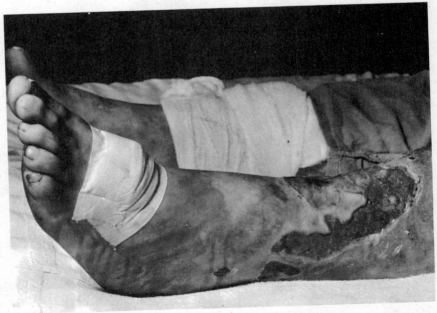

**Figure 38-1.** Ulcers on the legs of a patient who has peripheral vascular disease.

## Pain and Discomfort

Pain is common, but the kind of pain may vary. For example, the patient with an ulceration often experiences constant and severe pain, which interferes with his ability to sleep as well as to carry on his usual activities. While the pain of varicosities may not be as acutely intense, nevertheless, the heaviness and burning interfere with the patient's ability to concentrate, and restrict his activities. Constant pain undermines morale and affects the patient's response to his surroundings, his associates, and his medical treatment.

Chronic pain occurs with special severity at certain times of the day. The relief of pain presents a difficult challenge. Ideally, the pain is treated by employing measures that improve circulation, thus relieving ischemia and healing ulcers. Sometimes the realization of this goal is impossible, or it can be achieved only to a limited degree. Narcotics usually are avoided, if possible, because of the long-term nature of the condition and the consequent danger of addiction. Salicylates may give relief, particularly when they are used in combination with measures to improve circulation, such as position, exercise, warmth, and vasodilators. Sometimes, codeine is given with the salicylates.

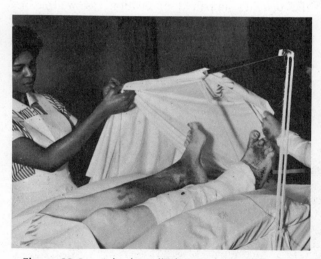

**Figure 38-2.** A bed cradle keeps the weight of the covers off the patient's feet. Note the discoloration of the skin and the thickening of the nails that occur typically in patients with peripheral vascular disease. The pillows under the patient's legs have been protected with plastic covers. The dressing is being kept wet with enzymes used to dissolve clots and fibrinous exudates. The enzymes pass through the tubing to the dressing.

The reluctance to use narcotics stems from the danger of addiction; it does not mean that the pain is trivial. As much concern and zeal to relieve pain are required for these patients as for any others. All too often the patient senses a slackening of interest, and he may have the impression that his pain is not so dramatic or given as careful consideration as that of a postoperative patient, for example. Its chronicity makes the pain harder to bear rather than easier. The pain itself is added to the fatigue from many sleepless nights and the uncertainty about when the symptoms will abate. Prolonged pain can set nerves on edge and make the patient seem to be cranky or demanding.

What can the nurse do to help to lessen the patient's pain?

- **Measures that improve circulation can be used. For example, placing the legs of a patient with arterial insufficiency in a dependent position often helps. The patient can put his legs over the side of the bed but must be careful that this position does not also cause pressure from the edge of the bed against the popliteal space, since this pressure could further impair circulation. A stool or a chair can be used to support the feet, so that the pressure behind the knees is relieved.**

- **The feet should not become chilled. If a patient gets up at night to put his legs over the edge of the bed or to sit in a chair, he should wear warm socks and have a blanket over his legs and his feet.**

- **P.r.n. analgesics must be given promptly when they are needed. A dose given about one-half hour before a dressing change or soak may make the pain of the treatment easier to bear.**

The patient sees concern for his welfare reflected in promptness, in measures concerning warmth and position, and in the nurse's manner, if it conveys a feeling of caring.

Flexibility in carrying out the care is important in promoting comfort. A patient who is awake most of the night should not be wakened for a bath just because it is 8 A.M. If a patient is restless at night, he should be placed where he will be least likely to disturb others. The emphasis should be on helping him to rest rather than on chiding him to consider the needs of other patients.

A foam rubber pad should be positioned so that the heels are off the bed to help to prevent necrosis, a frequent complication in patients with peripheral vascular disease. A bed cradle or a footboard may be used to keep the weight of the bedclothes off the feet (Fig. 38-2).

## Burns

Nurses carry major responsibility for the patient's safety as well as his comfort. Patients with peripheral vascular disease are especially prone to burns. The temperature in thermoregulated cradles is set according to the physician's directions (95 degrees F is usual), and it can be maintained constant as long as desired.

The Aquamatic pad is another example of a device that can be used to apply heat safely. Heat provided by an ordinary light bulb is difficult to regulate and can result in burns.

The temperature of bath water should be tested with a bath thermometer before the patient places his feet in the basin or bathtub (95 degrees F is a safe temperature); he is instructed to do the same when he is without supervision. For the patient with peripheral vascular disease, bath water that is too hot may result in a severe burn or even the loss of a leg.

External heat is used with approval of the physician.

## Patient and Family Education

Although the patient may require hospitalization for acute exacerbations of his illness or for complications arising from the condition, the bulk of his care usually is carried out at home. Therefore, the teaching of self-care and the arranging for continued medical and nursing supervision through the physician or nurse specialist and the community health nurse are of special significance.

The following instructions are applicable to most patients with peripheral vascular disease. Teaching can be done by the nurse with groups of patients who can also benefit from the peer support and sharing of ideas and affective responses afforded by the group interaction.

These general instructions are modified and supplemented in the light of each patient's particular program of treatment. Many are on special diets, such as reducing diets, low-cholesterol diets (in atherosclerosis), or diabetic diets. Instruction concerning diet forms an important part of the teaching program for such patients.

- **The feet must be kept clean by bathing daily. They should be inspected regularly for cuts or bruises. Socks or stockings should be changed daily.**
- **The feet should be kept dry because constant moistness predisposes to infections, like athlete's foot. Skin between the toes should be dried well after bathing. Excessively warm socks or shoes should not** be worn in a warm environment, because overly warm footwear can lead to profuse perspiration. Shoes should be aired after each wearing.
- **Toenails should be trimmed regularly, at least once a week. Nail clippers and an emery board are safer to use than pointed scissors. A razor blade should never be used for this purpose. Nails are cut straight across, and not too short. If vision is not good another person or a podiatrist should cut the nails.**
- **Cuts, corns, or calluses should be treated only after medical advice. An accidental cut on the foot should be cleansed with 70 per cent alcohol; a dry sterile dressing should be applied and the physician or nurse notified. Medication, such as corn plasters, should not be applied to feet without medical advice.**
- **Lotion or cream should be applied to dry feet after bathing. Prolonged soaking increases dryness and should be avoided.**
- **Shoes should fit comfortably. Heels that are too high cause pressure on the toes. Sneakers make the feet perspire and are not advisable. A comfortable shoe with good support and a leather sole is preferable. Shoes made of soft leather with rounded rather than pointed toes help to prevent pressure and friction.**
- **Socks and stockings should be large enough to avoid any tightness or pressure. Bulky darns that could cause pressure and irritation of the foot are hazardous.**
- **Circular garters should never be worn. A girdle or a garter belt should be used to hold up stockings. If circular garters are tight enough to hold up stockings, they are tight enough to impair circulation. This rule applies also to hose with elasticized tops that are tight enough to stay up without garters and to panty girdles and other garments that cause constriction around the thigh.**
- **Going barefoot, even at home, affords too great a chance of cutting or bruising the feet. "Thong" sandals do not give adequate protection to the feet.**
- **Positions that cause pressure on the legs must be avoided. The legs should not be curled under the body when the patient is sitting and the knees should not be crossed. The edge of the chair should not come right behind the knees.**
- **The exercise prescription should be followed. If walking causes pain, the patient is advised to learn to judge distances, so that he can stop and rest before pain occurs. Walking slowly often enables the person to walk farther without experiencing pain.**
- **Prolonged standing must be avoided. Unless prescribed otherwise, rest should be alternated with mild exercise, such as walking.**
- **The feet should be kept warm, but excessive heat avoided; it may make the condition worse. External heat can cause burns. An extra blanket at the foot of the bed, warm socks, and fleece-lined boots are examples of safe ways to keep the feet and legs warm. Bath water (95 degrees F) should be tested with a thermometer. An electric heating pad, hot-water bottle, or hot foot soak should never be used without medical advice.**

- **Smoking must be stopped. (See Chapter 11 regarding helping the patient stop smoking.)**
- **If job or travel requires sitting for long periods, plans should be made to walk around for five minutes each hour.**

## RAYNAUD'S DISEASE

Raynaud's disease is characterized by periodic constriction of the arteries that supply the extremities. The digital arteries of the hands and the feet commonly are affected. Other extremities, such as nose, ears, and chin, are involved less commonly. In many instances, the symptoms are confined to the hands.

The underlying cause of Raynaud's disease is not entirely clear; however, it is believed to be related to emotional stress and exposure to cold. (Vasoconstriction on exposure to cold and emotional stress can be symptomatic of other underlying constitutional diseases such as scleroderma.) The condition is much more common among women than men, and it usually occurs in young adults. Familial predisposition may play a part in causing the disease.

**Symptoms.** The attacks occur intermittently and with varying frequency, but especially with exposure to cold. The hands become cold, blanched, wet with perspiration; they feel numb and prickly. Awkwardness and fumbling are noted, especially when fine movements are attempted. After the initial pallor, the hands, and especially the fingers, become deeply cyanotic. The cyanosis often is accompanied by aching pain. Usually, the patient learns that the attack can be relieved by placing the hands in warm water or by going indoors, where it is warm. The warmth relieves the vasospasm, and blood rushes to the part. The skin in the deprived areas becomes flushed and warm, and the patient has a sensation of throbbing.

In the early stages of the disease, the hands usually appear perfectly normal between attacks. However, when the disease is severe and of long duration, cyanosis of the fingers may persist between the attacks, and trophic changes gradually may occur. Ulcers and superficial gangrene may appear at the fingertips and are exquisitely painful. The fingers may become thin, and the skin white, shiny, taut, and smooth. The nails may be deformed. The fingers are especially vulnerable to infection. Healing of even minor lesions is often slow and uncertain. The disease does not necessarily progress to cause severe disability. In many instances the symptoms are mild, and they may even improve spontaneously.

**Treatment.** The treatment of Raynaud's disease involves avoidance of the factors that precipitate attacks. The patient is instructed to avoid chilling. Electric blankets are helpful. Warm gloves and footwear should be worn outdoors in the winter. Today with lightweight clothing items such as leotards which can be removed upon going indoors, as well as high fleece-lined boots and fur-lined gloves, it is possible for patients to dress warmly without compromising style.

The patient also should be helped to recognize situations that cause emotional upset. Often, counseling is effective in helping the patient to change her environment and/or her ways of reacting to it, in order to minimize stress. One woman's attacks disappeared entirely when she established her own home and no longer had to live with her mother-in-law. Smoking is contraindicated, since it causes vasoconstriction. Some patients are helped by moving to a warmer climate.

Sympatholytic drugs, such as tolazoline and phenoxybenzamine, often are prescribed. Intra-arterial injection of reserpine is under investigation.

These drugs are particularly valuable in the treatment of Raynaud's disease, because they help to relieve spasm of the arteries, thus providing greater blood supply to the tissues. Vasodilators, such as alcohol or papaverine, are also useful in preventing or relieving the attacks. Nylidrin (Arlidin), cyclandelate (Cyclospasmol), or nicotinyl alcohol (Roniacol) may also be prescribed.

Sympathectomy is performed occasionally when the disease is severe and progressive, and when medical treatment fails to relieve the condition. Sympathetic stimuli to the affected extremities are abolished permanently by this operation, and the resulting vasodilation relieves the condition. The areas from which sympathetic stimuli have been removed will no longer perspire. However, this is a relatively minor consideration. The patient is instructed to apply cream daily to prevent excessive dryness of the skin.

## THROMBOANGIITIS OBLITERANS (BUERGER'S DISEASE)

The name of this disease describes the pathology —inflammation of blood vessels associated with formation of clots and with fibrosis of arteries. This condition leads to the obstruction of the blood vessels. The disease affects primarily the arteries and the veins of the lower extremities. The upper extremities occasionally are involved.

The cause of thromboangiitis obliterans is not established definitely; however, some believe it to be an allergic response to tobacco. It is far more common among men than women, and it usually has its onset during young adulthood.

**Symptoms.** The patient notes that one foot or both feet are always cold. *Intermittent claudication* is a common symptom. The patient has aching in his calf muscles after a certain amount of exercise; the aching is relieved when he rests, but it promptly recurs when he does similar exercise. Usually, the symptoms fluctuate in severity. Attacks of acute distress often are followed by remissions, during which the disease is quiescent.

Cyanosis and redness of the feet and legs are noted often. Frequently, the color is a mottled purplish-red. Ulcers that heal slowly or progress to the development of gangrene may occur, particularly at the toes and the heel (Fig. 38-3). Trophic changes in the skin and the nails are characteristic when circulation has been impaired for a considerable period. Phlebitis is common. Rest pain occurs when circulation has been impaired seriously, and particularly when ulcers have formed. Although the disease usually is most pronounced in one leg and foot, both legs usually are affected to some degree.

**Treatment.** Much of the treatment is directed toward eliminating the factors known to aggravate the condition. The use of tobacco in any form is contraindicated, and it never should be resumed, even if the symptoms of the disease abate. The resumption of smoking leads to an exacerbation of the disease. The patient is instructed to avoid chilling and to be especially careful to keep his extremities warm. Warm socks, boots, and gloves are essential in cold weather. Prolonged standing should be avoided. Exercise within the limits of the patient's tolerance is beneficial, but he should rest if he experiences pain when he is exercising. Sometimes, these requirements mean that the patient must change his job. The prevention of injury and of infection of the extremities is very important.

Exercise is helpful in stimulating circulation, provided it is not excessive and does not cause pain. *Buerger-Allen exercises* involve elevating the feet and the legs until the feet blanch, lowering them until they appear red, and then resting with the legs and the feet in a horizontal position. The patient performs the exercises while he is lying on a bed or a sofa, first raising the legs, then dangling them over the side of the bed, and finally resting with his legs flat on the bed. The patient is instructed regarding the length of time that he is to spend in each position and the number of times the exercise is to be repeated. He is taught to watch the color of his legs and feet and to lower them as soon as they turn white. Blanching indicates an inadequate blood supply. The maintenance of this position could harm the tissues.

*Walking and active foot exercises* may be prescribed instead of Buerger-Allen exercises.

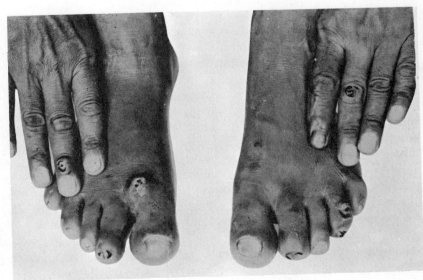

**Figure 38-3.** Thromboangiitis obliterans, with gangrenous ulcers. (Vakil, R. J., and Golwalla, A.: *Clinical Diagnosis,* Bombay, Asia Publishing House)

The *oscillating bed* stimulates circulation by providing a frequent change of position. The bed is operated electrically. The amount of position change can be adjusted according to the needs of the patient. The bed provides a smooth, continuous, seesaw motion. The head is raised, and the feet are lowered; then the feet are raised, and the head is lowered. Many patients who have pain at night find the oscillating bed especially helpful in relieving pain and promoting sleep. Although some patients say that the constant motion makes them feel "seasick" at first, most become quite accustomed to the movement and do not find it uncomfortable. The patient feels more secure if he is given the switch and shown how to stop the movement of the bed when he wishes (for example, during meals or for use of the bedpan).

The patient's legs are kept horizontal or slightly dependent, except during Buerger-Allen exercises, if these have been prescribed. Elevating the legs increases the ischemia, and therefore it causes or increases pain.

The vasodilating effect of heat may be utilized, provided that the heat is properly applied. The heat is not set above body temperature, and no appliance should be used in which the amount of heat cannot be reliably regulated. (The optimum temperature is 95 degrees F.) An electric blanket may be used provided that it is in good condition and the temperature can be regulated safely. Thermoregulated heat cradles also may be used, if they are kept at body temperature or slightly below it.

Sympatholytic drugs such as tolazoline (Priscoline) and phenoxybenzamine (Dibenzyline) may be ordered, but these may not be successful. Analgesics often are required to lessen pain. The aim is to control the pain without resorting to narcotics. Because thromboangiitis obliterans is a chronic illness, the danger of addiction from the use of narcotics is great.

Sympathectomy is performed sometimes to relieve vasospasm. If lesions occur on the extremity and become infected, antibiotics are ordered to help to control the infection. Enzymes, such as streptokinase-streptodornase, are ordered sometimes to debride the lesion. If the circulation becomes so impaired that gangrene results, amputation may be necessary. The site of the amputation is determined by the area of the limb in which satisfactory blood supply has been maintained. The stump must have a good blood supply so that it

can heal, and further necrosis of tissue will not occur. (The care of patients after amputation is discussed in Chapter 21.)

## ARTERIOSCLEROSIS AND ATHEROSCLEROSIS

Arteriosclerosis and atherosclerosis commonly accompany the aging process. *Arteriosclerosis* refers to the hardening and the loss of elasticity of the arteries. *Atherosclerosis* refers to the deposition of fatty plaques (composed chiefly of cholesterol) inside the artery and is the most common cause of peripheral arterial disease. These calcified plaques can ulcerate and cause thrombosis, gradually reducing the size of the lumen, resulting in partial or complete obstruction of the artery and in impairment of the blood supply to the part of the body served by the artery. Narrowing and roughening of the lumen of the artery make obstruction of the vessel by clots a particular hazard. The discovery of the location of the site of the occlusion is aided by an arteriogram or an aortogram. Usually, both arteriosclerosis and atherosclerosis exist in aging arteries. It is the atherosclerotic process that is primarily responsible for the reduction of the blood supply to the part. However, the entire process often is described by the single term *arteriosclerosis*.

Arteriosclerosis and atherosclerosis affect many different parts of the body. Heart, brain, and kidneys, as well as extremities, frequently are involved. Diseases caused by arteriosclerosis and atherosclerosis are discussed in many different sections of this book. For example, angina pectoris is brought about by atherosclerosis of coronary arteries; this condition is discussed in Chapter 36. The discussion in this chapter will be limited to the effects of arteriosclerosis and atherosclerosis on the extremities.

Legs and feet are affected most often. Frequently, one extremity is affected more severely than the other, although the circulation to both legs and both feet usually is impaired. The condition frequently does not manifest itself until the patient is over 50. It is believed that the loss of elasticity and the deposition of fatty substances occur gradually over many years. The process usually is not advanced enough to cause symptoms until late middle life or old age.

The rate at which the changes occur varies in different persons. Patients with diabetes mellitus suffer these changes quite early in life. Other factors that may influence the age of onset and the severity of the condition are hypertension, smoking, heredity, and diet. Some authorities assert that a diet high in fat, and particularly in cholesterol, may contribute to the occurrence of atherosclerosis. Patients with a family history of vascular disease may be especially prone to develop the condition.

**Symptoms.** The symptoms are those of ischemia of the feet and the legs. These symptoms have already been discussed and can be briefly summarized as follows:

- Color changes (pallor, rubor, cyanosis)
- Coldness
- Absent or diminished pulses
- Trophic changes in skin and nails
- Susceptibility to infection, lessened ability to fight infection, tendency to develop ulcers and gangrene.
- Pain—intermittent claudication and rest pain. Cramping pain may occur at night, particularly in the calf muscles.
- Numbness and tingling

**Treatment.** A large component of treatment is patient education, as well as symptomatic treatment which may be summarized as follows:

- Keeping the parts warm, such as by wearing warm clothing, but avoiding excessive warmth and taking special precautions to avoid burns and other trauma.
- Cleanliness. A warm tub bath at a temperature of 95 to 100 degrees (a bath thermometer must be used) or a foot bath in water of the same temperature can be used if the skin is intact. No friction should be used when drying the skin. Lanolin can be applied gently to dry skin. Socks or stockings should be loose-fitting and soft and changed daily.
- Prompt medical care of even minor cuts or infections. Toenail care by a podiatrist if necessary.
- Prevention of athlete's foot (fungus infection) by drying feet well, especially between the toes, and using a nonmedicated powder such as cornstarch. Medicated antifungicidals should be prescribed by the physician.
- Avoiding factors, such as exposure to cold and smoking, that cause vasoconstriction.
- Moderate exercise, provided that it does not exceed the patient's tolerance.
- Avoidance of prolonged standing or sitting in a position that places pressure on the legs, particularly pressure in the popliteal space. Avoiding all constricting clothing.
- Resting with the legs somewhat lower than the rest of the body. Elevating the head of the bed on shock blocks accomplishes this and facilitates the flow of blood to the legs.
- Measures to lessen vasoconstriction. Because vasoconstriction often is not a prominent factor in causing the symptoms, the use of these measures

frequently gives disappointing results. However, sympatholytic drugs like tolazoline (Priscoline) and vasodilators such as cyclandelate, nylidrin, alcohol, and nicotinyl alcohol may be prescribed. The patient requires instruction in their use. Sympathectomy may also be tried.
- Treatment of ulcers and infections by cleansing, use of antibiotics, and all the measures previously mentioned to improve circulation.

The patient, family, community health nurse, and physician collaborate in the treatment process.

There is no cure for arteriosclerosis. Such measures as meticulous attention to personal cleanliness and avoidance of injury and exposure often can preserve the limb, as well as lessen the patient's discomfort.

Surgical procedures, such as endarterectomy (removal of an atherosclerotic plaque from the lumen), bypass operations, shunts, and the replacement of diseased vessels with prostheses made from such materials as nylon are sometimes effective in increasing the blood supply to the part (see p. 683).

If gangrene occurs, amputation may become necessary.

## VARICOSE VEINS

Veins serving the extremities have valves that keep the blood flowing in one direction only. The closure of successive sets of valves along the veins keeps the blood moving up toward the heart and prevents it from seeping down toward the feet (Fig. 38-4).

Varicose veins are dilated, tortuous veins. Blood collects in these veins and cannot be returned efficiently to the heart. The valves of the veins are incompetent. They close incompletely or not at all, and blood is permitted to reflux backward, rather than being propelled always onward toward the heart. This reflux causes further congestion of the part with venous blood and further distention of the veins. The saphenous veins of the legs commonly are affected (Fig. 38-5).

Some people have a familial tendency toward varicose veins. The valves of the veins become incompetent early in life, resulting in the development of varicosities. Men as well as women suffer from varicose veins—a point sometimes overlooked because men's trousers conceal their legs. Often, the condition first manifests itself when other factors impair venous return. For example, pelvic tumors or pregnancy may exert pressure on the veins,

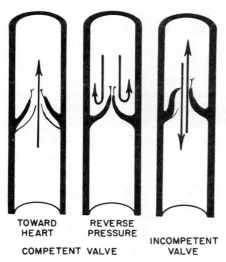

TOWARD HEART
REVERSE PRESSURE
COMPETENT VALVE
INCOMPETENT VALVE

**Figure 38-4.** Competent valves in the veins permit the blood to flow toward the heart and prevent the flow of the blood in the opposite direction. Incompetent valves, by failing to close tightly, permit the blood to flow in both directions.

causing interference with venous return. Prolonged standing aggravates the condition, because the venous return is impaired further by the force of gravity. The action of the leg muscles during exercise, such as vigorous walking, aids venous return. Anything that causes constriction or pressure on the legs makes varicosities worse. Circular garters and panty girdles are familiar examples. Obesity contributes to inefficient venous return by placing excess weight on the legs. Thrombophlebitis (discussed later in this chapter) sometimes leads to the development of varicose veins, because the valves of the veins may be damaged during the inflammatory process. Often several of these factors combine to produce varicose veins.

**Symptoms.** When blood is not returned efficiently from the legs, it tends to collect in the saphenous veins. Because these veins are superficial and less well supported by surrounding tissues, they are especially prone to distention. (The deeper veins of the legs are better supported by muscles.) The veins become swollen and tortuous. They can be seen under the skin as dark blue or purplish swellings. The patient's legs feel heavy and tired and often become edematous, particularly after prolonged standing. There may be cramping pains. Inefficient venous return causes congestion of the tissues of the leg and the foot. This congestion leads to diminished arterial blood supply and results in impaired nutrition of the tissues with

consequent reduction in their ability to resist infection and to allow wounds to heal. Minor injuries readily become infected and ulcerated. The healing of such lesions is slow and uncertain.

Varicose ulcers usually appear on the lower leg over a vein. It is believed that the ulcer is usually caused by inflammation of the vein and the surrounding tissues. This inflammatory process impairs the blood supply to the overlying skin and leads to the development of an ulcer. Varicose ulcers are painful and disabling, since elevation of the leg usually must be maintained in order to facilitate venous repair and promote healing.

**Diagnosis.** Ordinarily, the clinician needs only to examine the extremity, noting distended, tortuous veins, sometimes edema and possibly ulcers. Sometimes, *Trendelenburg's test* is done. The leg is elevated above the level of the pelvis, so that the veins empty by gravity. Digital pressure is applied over the saphenofemoral junction in the groin. The patient then is asked to stand, and the examiner notes the filling of the veins. The manner in which

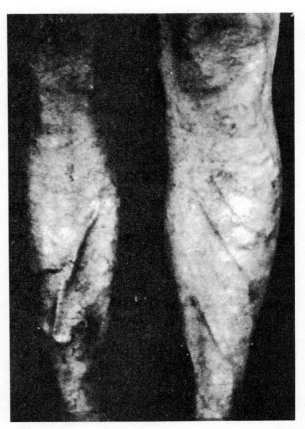

**Figure 38-5.** Varicose veins. (Medichrome–Clay-Adams, Inc., New York, N.Y.)

the veins fill (how rapidly, and whether from above or below) helps to determine which veins are incompetent. If the veins fill rapidly from above downward when digital pressure is removed at the saphenofemoral junction, the valve there is incompetent. Normally, the blood should be held back by the valve; however, if the valve is incompetent, blood will surge down into the legs when the pressure is released. If the veins fill from below while pressure is still being applied, the lesser saphenous or communicating veins are incompetent.

**Treatment.** Small varicose veins are treated sometimes by the injection of sclerosing solutions, such as sodium morrhuate or sodium tetradecyl sulfate. These drugs cause an inflammation of the vein and the formation of a thrombus. The injection is made into the vein usually with the patient in a standing position. The lumen of the vein is obliterated by this process, and blood can no longer pass through the vein. The injection of veins very rarely causes embolism by the release of the clot into the bloodstream. Some patients have severe allergic reactions to certain sclerosing agents; the treatment is similar to that of any severe allergic response (see Chap. 9). While the injection is being done, it is important to ensure that the patient can hold on to something, because undergoing this treatment while he is standing may make him feel faint. After the injection the site is covered with a small sterile dressing. The patient should remain in the office or clinic for fifteen minutes so that he can be observed for allergic response.

The treatment of varicose veins usually is surgical. One frequently used procedure is called *ligation and stripping*. The affected veins are ligated, severed from their connections, and removed. The entire great saphenous vein, which extends from the groin to the ankle, usually must be removed. In the course of stripping, numerous small incisions are made on the leg. These incisions are covered with sterile dressings, and then elastic bandages are applied firmly from the foot to the groin. The operation may be performed under local or general anesthesia.

### Nursing Assessment and Intervention

The patient returns from the operating room with the elastic bandages in place. The foot of his bed usually is elevated in the immediate postoperative period to aid venous return. Elevation can be accomplished by using shock blocks or, with some of the newer beds, by merely turning a crank or pushing a foot pedal. The standard knee gatch is not satisfactory for this purpose, because it causes a bend in the knee and pressure behind the knee. The operative sites are observed for bleeding. If any is noted, manual pressure is applied over the bleeding area, the limb is elevated, and the surgeon is notified.

The patient's legs are painful and stiff after surgery. Analgesics are frequently necessary during the first day or two after the operation.

Early ambulation is an important aspect of postoperative treatment. It stimulates circulation and helps to prevent venous thrombosis. If the patient asks how the blood will be returned from the leg "now that my veins have been removed," he can be told that the blood will be returned by the deep veins of his leg, which are still working efficiently.

The patient must be helped to understand that walking is a part of his postoperative treatment. Often, he is startled to learn that he is expected to take a walk shortly after he recovers from anesthesia. Unless he understands the reason, this treatment may seem like unmitigated cruelty to him. He must have assistance the first few times that he gets up. His legs will feel clumsy and painful. This, plus the effect of preoperative medications and anesthesia, makes it especially important to protect the patient from falls. If the patient is elderly or unusually weak, it is wise to ask a male nurse or a nursing assistant to help the first time that the patient is out of bed.

As a rule, the patient remains in the hospital only two or three days. After the immediate postoperative period, nursing care involves helping the patient to plan his activities so that he takes frequent short walks, alternating with periods of rest in bed and in the chair. Often, the patient is instructed to elevate his legs when he is sitting in a chair. However, the foot of the bed usually is elevated only during the immediate postoperative period. Elastic bandages must be checked regularly and reapplied as it is necessary, because they tend to become loose when the patient walks about. These bandages may be initially changed and reapplied by the surgeon; later they are changed by the nurse. Before his discharge from the hospital the patient is instructed in the correct procedure for applying the bandages, because he ordinarily is advised by the physician to continue their use at home; the patient also is told if and when to begin to wear elastic hosiery.

The postoperative period provides an excellent opportunity to teach the patient how to minimize the possibility of the recurrence of varicosities or (if only one leg was affected) their development in the other leg. The patient has already found that he has a tendency to varicose veins and therefore must make every effort to control and, if it is possible, to prevent them in the future. Unfortunately, many patients cherish the belief that the operation will make further precautions unnecessary.

The importance of follow-up care must be emphasized (Fig. 38-6). General instructions include:

- Whenever possible, the patient should elevate the legs when he is sitting.
- He should avoid prolonged standing. For example, it is better to walk about at a bus stop than to stand still.

# BE GOOD TO YOUR VEINS
## DO          DON'T

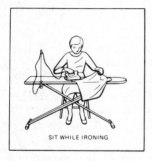
SIT WHILE IRONING

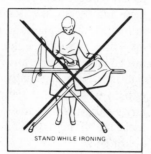
STAND WHILE IRONING

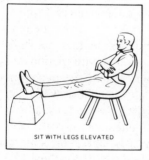
SIT WITH LEGS ELEVATED

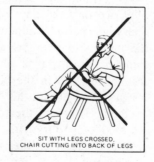
SIT WITH LEGS CROSSED,
CHAIR CUTTING INTO BACK OF LEGS

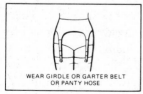
WEAR GIRDLE OR GARTER BELT
OR PANTY HOSE

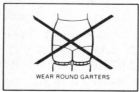
WEAR ROUND GARTERS

**Figure 38-6.** Posters like this are useful in teaching patients. This one was designed for the waiting room of a peripheral vascular disease clinic.

- An elastic stocking should be washed daily and replaced when it becomes worn or loose.
- On long rides such as in a plane, the patient should walk for at least five minutes every hour. The same applies if work involves sitting at a desk or bench.
- The skin must be kept clean by daily bathing. Lanolin can be used at bedtime if the skin is dry.
- Fungal infection of the toes should be prevented by drying well and by powdering between them.
- Bumping, cutting, bruising, or scratching the legs must be avoided.
- Circular garters or tight girdles should not be worn.
- Weight reduction to normal range may be indicated.
- Some patients may be directed by the physician to keep the foot of the bed elevated on six-inch blocks to aid venous return.

**Treatment of Varicose Ulcers (Stasis Ulcers).** This treatment involves primarily the treatment of the varicose veins that have led to the formation of ulcers. Every effort should be made to persuade patients to have treatment before ulcers develop. The ulcers are slow to heal and have a tendency to recur. They cause considerable pain and disability. Elevation of the leg is often necessary to promote venous return, thus helping to restore more normal circulation and permitting the healing of the ulcer. Sometimes a gelatin paste boot (Unna's paste boot) is applied, and the patient is permitted to walk about. The principle is similar to that of an elastic bandage or stocking. The boot, which consists of a circular gauze bandage and a special paste, is applied while the patient's foot is elevated. It dries and "sets" after about 20 minutes, and it provides firm support, compressing the superficial varicose veins and facilitating the return of the venous blood through the deeper veins of the leg.

Careful technique is important in the application of dressings or local medications, because the tissues have poor ability to combat infection. Antibiotics often are ordered to treat infection locally if it occurs. Such enzymes as streptokinase-streptodornase may be used to remove clots and dead tissue.

(Care of leg ulcers is discussed above.)

## THROMBOPHLEBITIS AND PHLEBOTHROMBOSIS

*Thrombophlebitis* means inflammation of a vein accompanied by clot formation. *Phlebothrombosis* refers to the presence of clots in a vein that has little or no inflammation.

**Avoiding Venous Stasis.** Venous stasis predisposes to the development of both conditions. The factors contributing to venous stasis are inactivity after surgery or any illness, heart failure, and pressure on the veins in the pelvis or legs.

Unless leg exercises are contraindicated by the patient's condition, all patients who are unable to walk about should do leg exercises while they are in bed. Preferable are active exercises, such as bending the knee, rotating the foot at the ankle, and wiggling the toes. However, if the patient is unable to carry out these active exercises, passive exercise should be given by the nurse.

Pressure should not be applied to the legs. For example, pillows and blanket rolls should not be placed behind the knees, and the knee gatch should not be elevated for prolonged periods. Prolonged sitting is inadvisable, because the chair may cause pressure behind the knees. Convalescent patients should alternate sitting with walking about the room or lying on the bed. The vague instruction, "Move your legs often," or "Don't sit in the chair too long" is not effective in motivating patients who are in particular danger of developing thrombophlebitis—for example, fresh postoperative or aged patients. Giving specific instructions, which should include a demonstration of the exercise and an indication of how many times and how often it is to be done, is far more likely to result in the patient's actually performing the exercise.

The patient must be encouraged in his exercise throughout his period of inactivity and observed to see that his performance is adequate as often as necessary. Instruction is easily overlooked or forgotten, especially when a patient is tired or in pain. The activity prescription should be written in the nursing care plan so that all who care for the patient will carry it through.

Elderly patients and those with heart disease, infections, or dehydration are susceptible to thrombophlebitis. And it does not occur only in hospitals. Prolonged sitting on airplane flights, on bus rides, or in front of TV has led to thrombophlebitis. The importance of changing position frequently and of exercising the legs at intervals cannot be overemphasized.

Wrapping the legs with elastic bandages or wearing elastic stockings or support hose may help to prevent thrombophlebitis in susceptible persons by giving added support to the veins and facilitating venous return from the legs. Sometimes, anticoagulants are given to patients who are especially susceptible to thrombophlebitis in an effort to prevent the development of thrombi. Elevating the foot of the bed on 6-inch blocks aids venous return, and this measure is sometimes used to help to prevent thrombophlebitis when illness necessitates bed rest.

**Symptoms.** The symptoms of *thrombophlebitis* include pain, heat, redness, and swelling in the affected region. Usually, the legs are involved. If there is marked interference with deep venous return, the leg becomes markedly swollen and may have a mottled bluish color. Often, the patient has systemic symptoms of fever, malaise, fatigue, and anorexia.

*Phlebothrombosis* produces few if any symptoms, since inflammation is slight or absent. Sometimes, the limb suddenly becomes swollen and cyanotic, calling attention to the condition. The patient may experience pain in the calf on dorsiflexion of the foot (Homans' sign).

**Treatment.** The treatment of thrombophlebitis usually includes complete rest of the limb and promotion of venous return by elevating the foot of the bed on 6-inch blocks. Keeping the leg at rest and avoiding massage help to prevent clots from being dislodged and traveling in the bloodstream. The affected part *never* is rubbed since rubbing might dislodge a clot and result in embolism. Because clots may form without producing symptoms, as happens in phlebothrombosis, a patient's legs are never massaged as a comfort measure. Any patient who shows symptoms or signs that might indicate thrombophlebitis should be kept at rest until the physician has had an opportunity to examine him.

Some difference of opinion exists among physicians concerning the advisability of elevating the leg and keeping it at complete rest. Some permit the patient to exercise the affected leg, in the belief that exercise facilitates circulation and lessens the likelihood of further extension of the disease. These physicians believe that the likelihood of causing emboli by exercising the limb is not great. Specific orders concerning the position of the part and the amount of activity permitted should be obtained.

Some physicians order warm wet packs to lessen pain and to decrease inflammation. Others do not think this helps. Since the area to which heat is applied is usually extensive, bath towels or large flannel cloths are used. Petrolatum is applied to the skin to lessen the danger of burning and maceration. The warm towels are wrung out as dry as possible. The foundation of the bed should be covered with plastic material, so that it does not become wet. The pack should be kept warm (usually with an Aquamatic pad) during the entire time ordered for its application. The foot should be incorporated in the pack. The extremity and pack are covered with a dry bath blanket.

Dry heat using a thermoregulated cradle or pad such as the Aquamatic pad, which provides accurate and constant temperature control, is used sometimes instead of warm wet packs to apply heat to the limb (Fig. 38-7).

Anticoagulants are ordered to prevent further clot formation. Dosage is ordered on a daily basis according to laboratory prothrombin levels.

Enzymes such as fibrinolysin and streptokinase may be used to dissolve clots that have already formed. However, the use of such drugs to dissolve clots is relatively new and is still being studied. Sometimes, the clot is removed surgically, or the vein is ligated in order to prevent embolism. Analgesics may be ordered for the relief of pain.

When symptoms have subsided, the patient gradually is permitted more activity. The limb is elevated for only part of the day, and the patient is

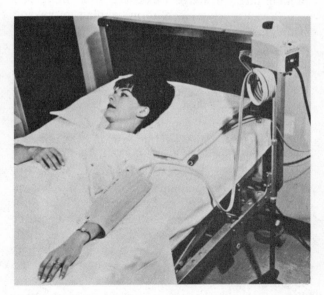

**Figure 38-7.** The Aquamatic K-pad is an example of equipment which is used to apply heat to a part. It permits the maintenance of a constant temperature at the level prescribed by the physician. Therefore, it is both safer and more effective than a hot water bottle or an electric heating pad. (Gorman-Rupp Industries, Inc., Bellville, Ohio)

allowed to walk about. Usually, elastic bandages or elastic stockings are advised at first to give support and to promote venous return. The condition frequently subsides completely, and the patient may resume his accustomed activities. The illness and the convalescent period often last several weeks or even several months, The patient requires encouragement to continue his treatment, including anticoagulant therapy, as long as it is necessary. Diversion helps the time to pass more quickly and lessens the restlessness and the impatience that so often accompany restricted physical activity.

## LYMPHEDEMA

Lymph is similar in composition to tissue fluid and plasma. A system of vessels called *lymphatics* carries tissue fluid from the body tissues to the veins. The lymph becomes mixed with venous blood and is returned to the right side of the heart. Lymph channels, like veins and arteries, serve nearly all parts of the body, nails and hair excepted. Obstruction to lymph vessels causes accumulation of tissue fluid in the affected part. Edema (often massive) occurs, resulting in deformity and poor nutrition of the tissues. This condition is called *lymphedema.*

Lymphedema occurs usually in the legs and the genitalia. It also occurs quite frequently in the arms, particularly in patients who have had radical mastectomy.

Lymph vessels can be damaged in a variety of ways. For example, filarial worms may invade lymph channels, causing a condition known as *elephantiasis.* The legs and often the genitalia become tremendously edematous and deformed.

Burns and excessive radiation can damage the lymphatics and cause lymphedema. Some children are born with inadequate lymph channels, although the edema may not manifest itself until puberty. Carcinoma often spreads by way of the lymph channels. Often, the lymphatics are damaged, either by the malignancy or by the extensive surgery required to cure it. The infection of lymph channels by such organisms as the streptococcus also can lead to lymphedema. Lymphedema can also follow repeated bouts of phlebitis and supervening streptococcal (erysipeloid) infection. With each attack more permanent scar accumulates and edema fluid becomes trapped in small "fibrous" lakes (Oschner, 1969).

**Symptoms.** The symptoms of lymphedema include enlargement due to edema of the limb and tight, shiny skin. Sometimes, the skin becomes thickened, rough, and discolored. Because nutrition of the tissues is impaired, ulcers and infection are common.

**Treatment.** The treatment of lymphedema consists of removing the cause, if it is possible. Rest, prevention of reinfection, and a drug such as diethylcarbamazine citrate (Hetrazan) are used to combat filarial worms. An antibiotic such as penicillin may be given to treat streptococcal infections of the lymphatics. The obstruction of lymphatics caused by injuries, such as burns, can be corrected sometimes by surgery. The Kondoleon operation, a radical excision of involved tissue, is occasionally performed for severe, disabling lymphedema.

Mild cases of lymphedema may respond to symptomatic treatment. The limb is elevated at intervals to promote lymphatic drainage. Elastic bandages or an elastic stocking is worn when the part is dependent. Massage starting at the toes or the fingers and moving up toward the body may be helpful (see Fig. 54-5).

## THROMBOSIS AND EMBOLISM

When an embolus reaches a blood vessel that is too small to permit its passage, the vessel is occluded, and blood is prevented from flowing through the rest of the vessel. The tissues lying beyond the obstruction are deprived of their blood supply. Thrombosis of a blood vessel means that a clot has formed within the vessel. Often, the clot enlarges, causing partial or complete obstruction of the vessel. Clots form relatively easily in arteries whose lining has become roughened and narrowed from the deposition of fatty plaques (atherosclerosis). The occlusion of a vessel by an embolus usually is followed by thrombosis of the portion of the vessel distal to the obstruction. The speed with which thrombosis occurs varies; sometimes it occurs within a few hours after the embolus has become lodged in the vessel. One of the main objectives of therapy is to remove the embolus and to re-establish normal circulation before the distal part of the blood vessel becomes obstructed by clots.

**Symptoms.** The symptoms of an embolism affecting the extremities are due to ischemia of the tissues that depend on the obstructed vessel for their blood supply. If the occluded vessel is a large one, the blood supply to the extremity may be completely and suddenly cut off below the level of the obstruction. If the vessel is a small one, the blood supply, though diminished, may be sufficient to keep the tissues alive. Sometimes, the obstruction of the vessel is not complete. The small amount of blood that reaches the part through the vessel, aided by the collateral circulation developed in the body's effort to supply the deprived tissues with blood, may suffice to prevent necrosis of tissue.

If the curtailment of blood supply is drastic, the extremity suddenly becomes white, cold, and excruciatingly painful. Normal arterial pulse is absent below the area of the obstruction. The patient may feel numbness, tingling, or cramps. Surrounding vessels go into spasm. These symptoms are followed by a loss of sensation in the affected area of the limb and a loss of the ability to move the part. Unless the obstruction is promptly relieved, necrosis of tissue occurs and necessitates amputation. Symptoms of shock frequently occur if a large vessel has been obstructed. When a small vessel is occluded, symptoms of ischemia, such as pallor and coldness, occur, but they are less severe.

**Initial Care.** To save the limb, the treatment must be immediate. Patients who already are hospitalized have a better chance for cure, since treatment is available immediately. The symptoms usually occur suddenly. The nurse may be the only person with the patient at the time, particularly if the embolism occurs during the evening or the night. *The physician is notified immediately* upon the nurse's suspicion of embolism, and the signs and symptoms are described accurately and concisely. The patient is told that the physician is coming and the nurse remains with the patient. The extremity is placed in a dependent position to facilitate some possible blood flow to the part, and the part is kept at complete rest. The patient is kept warm, since chilling may lead to further vasospasm, thus further decreasing the blood supply to the extremity. The extremity is wrapped in cotton to prevent radiation of heat and pressure necrosis. Direct heat never is applied to ischemic tissues, because it may burn the skin and accelerate the development of gangrene.

As emergency treatment the physician may order an immediate injection of heparin to help to prevent the development of further clots or the extension of those already present. An attempt may be made to improve the circulation by relaxing the vasospasm. Such drugs as papaverine may be used for this purpose. A block of the sympathetic nerves, usually by injecting procaine into the sympathetic ganglia, may relieve vasospasm. A narcotic, such as meperidine (Demerol), may be ordered to relieve the pain and to lessen the patient's apprehension.

**Surgery.** If, as a result of this treatment, the limb does not regain normal color and warmth, surgery is performed. The patient must be prepared for the operating room as quickly as possible. However, giving him the feeling of disorganization or confusion must be avoided.

Surgery may be done under local anesthesia, though this may not be the case when a clot has become stuck at the bifurcation of the aorta into the iliac arteries (saddle embolism). In an embolectomy the vessel is cut above the clot, the clot is suctioned out, grasped with a forceps, or eased out digitally, and the vessel is sutured together (arteriorrhaphy). A Fogarty balloon catheter can be pushed through a thrombus so that it does not break up or detach from the vessel wall (Browse, 1974). When the tip passes beyond the end of the thrombis, its balloon is inflated and the clot withdrawn gently with the catheter.

### Nursing Assessment and Intervention

Both preoperatively and postoperatively, the patient with an acutely occluded vessel needs to be constantly attended. The pain is severe, and the patient is apprehensive. Postoperative observations include blood pressure readings and continued checking of the extremity. The blood pressure should not vary widely, as fluctuation tends to increase clotting. The extremity is checked for temperature, sensation, color, return of pulses, or for increasing ischemia. The vessel that was operated on may become plugged again due to clot formation from surgical trauma. When normal circulation has been re-established, the part becomes warm and normal in color and sensation. It is no longer paralyzed. The pulses can be felt again.

The patient is observed for bleeding on the dressing as well as a drop in blood pressure and a rapid pulse. The patient may have been given anticoagulants, such as heparin or warfarin (Coumadin). Hemorrhage, if it occurs, may be severe. While waiting for the physician to arrive, the limb is elevated and pressure is applied at the nearest pressure point or directly over the wound. Supportive treatment, such as keeping the patient flat and warm and giving as much assurance as possible, is impor-

tant. The patient may have to be returned to the operating room in order to stop the bleeding. Transfusions are given to replace lost blood.

Exercise of the affected limb is not given postoperatively without the direction of the surgeon. The knee gatch should not be elevated; pillows should not be placed under the knees unless the surgeon specifically orders them, because pressure on the legs may impair circulation and lead to thrombosis.

### Pulmonary Embolism

An embolus is any foreign substance, such as a particle of fat or a clot, that travels in the bloodstream. A clot can become dislodged from a vein and is carried back toward the heart and the lungs. Often, the clot occludes one of the pulmonary vessels, causing infarction. If the blood vessel is large and the area of infarction is extensive, the patient may go into acute cor pulmonale (right heart failure). Complete cardiovascular collapse (cardiac arrest) may follow and the patient may die despite resuscitative attempts.

Pulmonary embolism is a dreaded complication of thrombophlebitis and phlebothrombosis, but previous thrombosis or thrombophlebitis is found in only 20 to 50 per cent of patients with pulmonary embolism. Pulmonary embolism is identified as the sole cause of 47,000 deaths per year and a contributory cause in 150,000 other deaths (Silver et al., 1970). It is one of the most frequent causes of death in the hospital population. The postmortem incidence is found to be in excess of 25 per cent but a correct diagnosis is made before death in only half of the cases (Dalen and Dexter, 1969).

Predisposing conditions to pulmonary embolism, in addition to thrombophlebitis and phlebothrombosis, are recent surgery, confinement to bed rest, fracture or trauma of the lower extremities, the postpartum state, and debilitating diseases. Studies are presently being conducted to determine the relationship between thromboembolic disorders and the use of oral contraceptives.

If the occluded blood vessel is small, the patient may experience chest pain, dyspnea, wheezing, tachypnea and tachycardia, cough, hemoptysis, and cyanosis.

An ECG and chest x-ray may be ordered. Their results are suggestive but not specifically diagnostic. They are used in conjunction with the results of a lung scan and angiogram. A pulmonary radioisotope scan would show an area of hypoperfusion, but the physician needs to distinguish this from other causes such as tumor or pneumonitis.

The patient is treated with heparin and other measures such as complete rest, oxygen, and analgesia. Heparin prevents the extension of the thrombus in the pulmonary artery and prevents the development of additional thrombi in the veins from which the embolus arose. Heparin is preferably given intravenously, initially in higher doses than usually recommended for anticoagulation since there is evidence that high initial dosage decreases mortality. For example, the physician can give 35,000 to 40,000 U.S.P. units of heparin as an initial rapid IV and then 7,500 to 15,000 units every four hours for the first 24 hours. The dosage may then be reduced and gradually tapered. One guide used by the physician for ordering dosage is to maintain the patient's clotting time at 30 minutes. Warfarin (Coumadin) may be used after six to seven days of heparin therapy (Silver et al., 1970).

Oxygen is given to treat hypoxia, which is a usual response to acute pulmonary embolism, and the patient is kept at complete rest.

Other forms of therapy include the use of fibrinolytic agents such as urokinase. For massive embolus, embolectomy may be performed using cardiopulmonary bypass to support the circulation while the embolus is being removed. However, the mortality rate is about 50 per cent.

Since the embolus to the lungs passes through the inferior vena cava, it can be interrupted by various means if pulmonary embolus is recurrent. Because of the problem of severe venostasis and edema in the lower extremities following ligation of the inferior vena cava, methods which attempt to stop large emboli without blocking blood flow have been devised. These include plication of the inferior vena cava (stitching folds between the walls), creation of a suture filter, application of a smooth or serrated plastic clip around the vessel, or use of an intracaval "umbrella."

Pulmonary embolism is a greater danger in phlebothrombosis than in thrombophlebitis, because the absence of inflammation makes clots less likely to adhere to the vein and more likely to be dislodged and to travel in the bloodstream.

Because of the ever-present danger of pulmonary embolism, thrombophlebitis and phlebothrombosis can cause serious and even fatal consequences, which are made all the more tragic if they appear when the patient is recovering from the illness or the operation that initially caused his inactivity. At best, the period of illness and disability is prolonged. At worst, the patient suddenly loses his life. Therefore, every possible effort must be made to prevent thrombophlebitis and phlebothrombosis.

## SURGICAL CONDITIONS OF THE OTHER BLOOD VESSELS

It is a good rule to assume that the patient with a vascular disease has other circulatory problems. A thrombus in the leg may precede a coronary occlusion. Anything that affects one blood vessel may have repercussions throughout the entire cardiovascular system, and patients should be cared for with this in mind. Observations of the blood pressure and of the rate and the quality of the pulse may give important clues to pathology elsewhere in the system.

The preoperative and postoperative care of a patient undergoing vascular surgery is similar to that of a patient who has heart surgery. When the surgery involves opening the thoracic cavity, preoperative and postoperative care are similar to the nursing care of any patient who has chest surgery. Points of nursing for specific conditions are given below.

### Aneurysms

The middle layer, or *media*, of the walls of arteries is elastic, allowing for pulsation with every heartbeat. When the elasticity is weakened by disease or trauma, an outpouching, called an *aneurysm*, of the wall is created. The aneurysm grows progressively larger under the pressure of the blood. Some aneurysms become very large, and they exert relentless pressure on surrounding structures. Untreated, some few aneurysms lay down layer on layer of clots, but the overwhelming majority become larger and larger until they burst, and then the patient bleeds to death.

Arteriosclerosis is the commonest cause of aneurysms. Also, syphilitic changes in the wall of an artery can so weaken the media that an aneurysm is produced. Bacterial infection, trauma, and congenital weakness also can cause aneurysms. Trauma can create an aneurysm either directly, such as in a gunshot or stab wound, or indirectly, as in an automobile accident in which a sudden stop at high speed causes tears in the media and the intima. The aorta is the most common site of aneurysms (Fig. 38-8).

A *fusiform* aneurysm affects the entire circumference of the involved artery. A *sacciform* aneurysm involves only a portion of the wall. A *dissecting* aneurysm occurs when blood dissects between the layers of the vessel wall. As the blood progresses inside the wall, it cuts off circulation to the branches coming off that vessel.

When the walls of the aneurysm contain deposits of calcium, the exact location of the outpouching can be seen on a roentgenogram. Aortography may be done.

Aneurysms may cause pain. Other symptoms may be related to pressure or nearby structures. For example, a thoracic aortic aneurysm can cause bronchial obstruction, dysphagia, or dyspnea. An abdominal aortic aneurysm can produce nausea and vomiting from pressure exerted on the intestines, or it may cause back pain from pressure on the vertebrae. Sometimes it can be felt as a pulsating mass. Sometimes an aneurysm of a superficial vessel can be seen as a pulsating bulge. Sometimes aneurysms go undetected, producing no symptoms until the patient has a massive hemorrhage.

Aneurysms are treated surgically whenever it is possible; there is no other cure. A fusiform aneurysm is excised and replaced with a graft. Portions of blood vessels can be replaced by grafts of human vascular tissue or by such synthetic fibers as Dacron and Teflon woven or formed into appropriate shapes (Fig. 38-9). A sacciform aneurysm may be cut off at its base, and the vessel sutured (aneurysmorrhaphy). A dissecting aneurysm may be treated by excision of the diseased segment of the vessel, or by recreating a passageway between the false lumen in the wall and the true lumen of the vessel and eliminating the false lumen by suturing the inner and the outer walls together.

Heparin is used during these procedures to control the formation of thrombi. The diseased vessel is clamped off above and below the aneurysm while surgical repair is in progress. If the heart or the aortic arch is involved, the situation may call for, or the surgeon may elect, diversion of the bloodstream from the work site temporarily by the use of a heart-lung machine. Bypass also may be used when the surgery would interrupt the circulation to important organs, especially the kidneys.

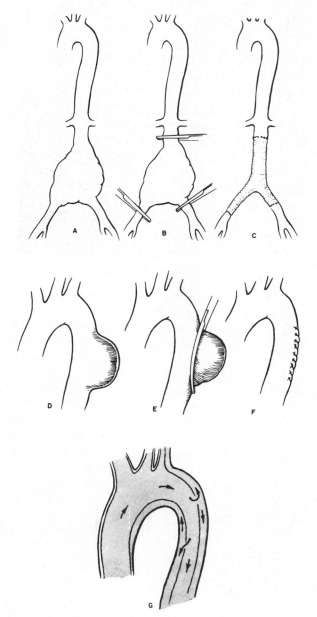

**Figure 38-8.** Aneurysms. (A) A fusiform aneurysm of the abdominal aorta. (B) It is clamped off before removal. (C) Replacement with a graft. (D) Sacciform aneurysm. (E) Clamping before suturing. (F) The sutured vessel. (G) Dissecting aneurysm. In this instance blood is seeping between the layers of the vessel wall through two holes.

### Arteriovenous Fistula

Fistulas may be congenital or caused by trauma. Because arterial blood goes directly into the vein without passing first through the capillary bed, the tissues ordinarily supplied by that artery are deprived of oxygen and nutrients. The vein may become distended, and an aneurysm may form. It may pulsate. The parts distal to the fistula may have color change. A fistula can lead to cardiac failure by returning abnormally large amounts of blood to the heart. The symptoms of arteriovenous fistula are highly variable, depending on the size and the location of the communication between the artery and the vein. An arteriogram enables the physician to visualize the abnormality. A common surgical treatment is excision of the fistula along with the affected portions of the artery and the vein. If collateral circulation is poor and the artery is important to the nutrition of a part, it is reconstructed by the insertion of a graft or by reanastomosing it.

### Trauma

The surgical treatment of direct trauma to a blood vessel includes simple closure of the laceration, resection and closure, and graft replacement. A patient entering the hospital with vessel damage—for example, after he has been injured in an automobile accident, or after he has been shot—usually will have multiple injuries that will complicate both his treatment and his nursing care.

Nursing Care Following Revascularization Procedures

The correction of an aneurysm or other reconstructive vascular procedure frequently necessitates a long incision. The abdominal aorta is reached through a midline abdominal incision, and the intestines are retracted to one side. To reach the thoracic aorta, the chest cavity must be entered. The aneurysm may not have been easily accessible, and the surgery may have been long and taxing. Consequently, the patient can be expected to have considerable incisional pain, which may interfere with his willingness to turn from side to side and to cough. The incisional area should be supported with the palms of the nurse's hands while the patient coughs. An abdominal binder can be applied when ordered for an incision in that area.

Postoperatively, the nurse should maintain careful observation of the pulses, especially during the first 24 hours, including the apical-radial pulse as well as the pulses distal to and fed by the vessel operated on (Fig. 38-10). If the pulse cannot be detected, the surgeon should be informed. A thrombus may have formed. Sometimes a reflex

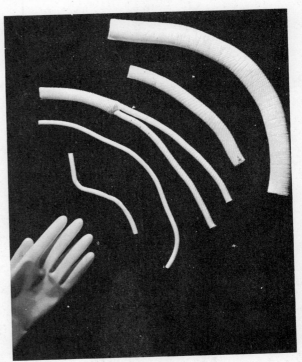

**Figure 38-9.** Synthetic blood vessel grafts. (National Heart and Lung Institute)

spasm will prevent pulsation. The area where the pulse can be felt may be marked with ink preoperatively. Overvigorous palpation of a distal pulse can obliterate it. It is possible to be feeling one's own pulse rather than the patient's. When the nurse is in doubt, another person can count the radial or precordial pulse, or the cardiac monitor pulse meter simultaneously with the uncertain observer. Following revascularization surgery, distal pulses may not return for 6 to 12 hours but this is not prognostically significant if replacement transfusion has been adequate (Breslau, 1968). Following thrombectomy, endarterectomy, or vessel replacement with a synthetic graft, the physician may order the patient's systolic blood pressure to be maintained approximately 20 mm. Hg above his unpremedicated preoperative pressure for about 12 hours. The suture line is "stented" internally by a high pressure column of blood flowing through it. One of the reasons for this is to promote adherence of a smooth thin layer of fibrin and platelets on the internal suture line to make the suture line resistant to clot formation. Renal function is monitored by intake and output and laboratory data.

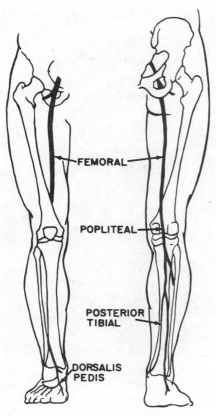

**Figure 38-10.** Major arteries of the leg that can be palpated for pulsation where they come close to the surface, such as in the popliteal area and immediately below the ankle.

The patient is positioned flat in bed or with his head elevated, or the revascularized part may be ordered to be positioned above the level of the heart (perhaps 15 degrees) in order to improve venous and lymphatic drainage, reduce the formation of edema, and facilitate fresh arterial blood flow. This elevation prevents engorgement of the previously ischemic part so new arterial blood flows in. The patient's body should not be jack-knifed, as this position impedes the free flow of blood. The knee gatch is not raised nor pillows placed under the knees, because pressure on the popliteal vessels is not desirable. The patient's position is changed at least every two hours, and he is encouraged to move his legs frequently. Any pain or cramping in the leg should be reported immediately, as it may indicate the occlusion of an artery or a thrombosis in a vein.

When an abdominal aortic aneurysm has been repaired, the appearance of back pain may be serious. It may indicate a hemorrhage or a thrombosis at the graft site. Abdominal distention may be an uncomfortable complication, but it is less serious. Distention may occur because the intestines were handled during surgery. A Levin tube may be passed and attached to suction apparatus.

(See Chapter 63 for further nursing care of the patient after cardiopulmonary bypass and Chapter 59 for care of the patient in shock.)

Patients who have had successful surgery may look forward to complete or partial relief from symptoms. The activity prescription is gradually increased to the patient's optimal level of functioning. The nursing measures for the protection of the extremity from tissue damage, including teaching the patient and family, are continued.

### Frostbite

Frostbite, largely a peripheral vascular disorder, is discussed in Chapter 13.

### REFERENCES AND BIBLIOGRAPHY

ABBOT, W. M.: Leg ulcers: Ways of healing, *Consultant* 13:97, February 1973.

ADAMS, J., and DeWEESE, J.: Partial interruption of the inferior vena cava with a new plastic clip, *Surg. Gynec. Obstet.* 123:1087, November 1966.

AJEMIAN, S.: Bypass grafting for femoral artery occlusion, *Am. J. Nurs.* 67:565, March 1967.

BEESON, P. B., and McDERMOTT, W. (eds.): *Cecil-Loeb Textbook of Medicine,* ed. 13, Philadelphia, Saunders, 1971.

BERGAN, J., and YAO, J.: Modern management of abdominal aortic aneurysm, *Surg. Clin. N. Am.* 54:175, February 1974.

BRAK, M. J.: Help for the patient with problem veins, *Patient Care* 8:158, March 1974.

————: Leg pain. Dealing with arterial insufficiency (pictorial), *Patient Care* 8:124, March 1974.

BRESLAU, R.: Intensive care following vascular surgery, *Am. J. Nurs.* 68:1670, August 1968.

BROWSE, N. L.: Current thoughts on thromboembolism, *Surg. Clin. N. Am.* 54:229, February 1974.

CALINOG, J., et al.: Newer approaches in the bedside diagnosis of massive pulmonary embolism, *Thorac. Cardiovasc. Surg.* 63:300, 1972.

COBEY, J. C., et al.: Chronic leg ulcers . . . ongoing treatment (pictorial), *Am. J. Nurs.* 74:258, February 1974.

CONN, J.: Thoracic outlet syndromes, *Surg. Clin. N. Am.* 54:155, February 1974.

CROW, T., and BRAK, M.: Aortic aneurysm: A patient study, *Nurs. Clin. N. Am.* 4:131, March 1969.

DALE, W. A.: Ligation, stripping and excision of varicose veins, *Surgery* 67:389, February 1970.

DALEN, J., and DEXTER, L.: Pulmonary embolism, *JAMA* 207:1505, February 1969.

DAVIS, R. W.: The intracaval umbrella, *AORN* 13:234, February 1971.

DE WEESE, M., and HUNTER, D.: A vena cava filter for the prevention of pulmonary embolism, *Arch. Surg.* 86:852, 1963.

EASTCOTT, H.: *Arterial Surgery,* Philadelphia, Lippincott, 1969.

ELIZABETH, SR. M.: Occlusion of the peripheral arteries: Nursing observations and symptomatic care, *Am. J. Nurs.* 67:562, March 1967.

FAIRBAIRN, J. F., II, et al.: Allen-Baker-Hines *Peripheral Vascular Diseases,* ed. 4, Philadelphia, Saunders, 1972.

FITZMAURICE, J., and SASAHARA, A.: Current concepts of pulmonary embolism, *Heart Lung* 3:209, March-April 1974.

Frostbite. New approaches plus the best of the old, *Patient Care* 5:66, November 15, 1971.

GAUL, A.: Hyperbaric oxygen therapy, *Am. J. Nurs.* 72:892, May 1972.

HILLIER, E. M.: Elephantiasis (Care St.), *Dist. Nurs.* 15:275, March 1973.

HOUGIE, C.: Thromboembolism and oral contraceptives, *Am. Heart J.* 85:538, April 1973.

JACKSON, B. S.: Chronic peripheral arterial disease, *Am. J. Nurs.* 72:928, May 1972.

MILES, R., et al.: A partial occluding vena caval clip for prevention of pulmonary embolism, *Am. Surg.* 30:40, 1964.

MILLER, V. M.: Femoropopliteal bypass graft with the saphenous vein: Nursing care, *RN* (OR-1), November 1972.

MOSER, K., and STEIN, M.: *Pulmonary Thromboembolism,* Chicago, Year Book, 1973.

O'BRIEN, J.: The mechanisms of venous thrombosis, *Mod. Conc. Cardiovasc. Dis.* 42:11, March 1973.

OSCHNER, A.: The sequelae of phlebitis, *Postgrad. Med.* 45:103, April 1969.

POWERS, M.: Emotional aspects of cardiovascular surgery, *Cardiovasc. Nurs.* 4:7, March-April 1968.

Proposed vascular surgical guidelines for screening, *Bull. Am. Coll. Surgeons* 59:6, June 1974.

RODBARD, S.: The clinical utility of the arterial pulses and sounds, *Heart Lung* 1:776, November-December 1972.

RODMAN, M., and SMITH, D.: *Clinical Pharmacology in Nursing,* Philadelphia, Lippincott, 1974.

ROSE, M. A.: Home care after peripheral vascular surgery, *Am. J. Nurs.* 74:260, February 1974.

ROSE, O.: Thrombophlebitis, *Hosp. Med.* 5:6, May 1969.

SABISTON, D., and WAGNER, H., JR.: The diagnosis of pulmonary embolism by radioisotope scanning, *Ann. Surg.* 160:575, 1964.

SASAHARA, A., and FOSTER, V.: Pulmonary embolism: recognition and treatment, *Am. J. Nurs.* 67:1634, August 1967.

SILVER, D., et al.: Management of pulmonary embolism, *Med. Clin. N. Am.* 54:361, March 1970.

The threat of thrombophlebitis, *Nurs. '73* 3:38, November 1973.

VERSTRAETE, M.: The present state of thrombolytic agents, *Drugs* 5:353, 1973.

WOOD, J. E.: The cardiovascular effects of oral contraceptives, *Mod. Conc. Cardiovasc. Dis.* 41:37, August 1972.

# Rehabilitation of Patients with Heart Disease

CHAPTER **39**

Physical activity is a reassurance of vitality and an affirmation of life. Decreased capacity to perform self-care activities and the other ordinary physical activities of daily living reduces self-esteem. The "homecoming" depression following myocardial infarction has been found to be directly related to physical weakness resulting from the deconditioning effects of enforced rest during the hospitalization period (Cassem and Hackett, 1973). A similar concern may be noted among patients with other diagnoses who are weak due to illness and inactivity.

In recent years technological advances such as telemetry, measurement of oxygen consumption and energy expenditure, the findings of basic research in myocardial ischemia and exercise physiology, and the development of sophisticated and safe methods of cardiac stress testing have contributed to a more scientific approach to activity prescription for the cardiac patient.

Studies have indicated that the prescription of bed rest has not been scientifically based (Browse, 1965; Duke, 1971). Gradually, the pattern of prolonged restriction of activity after acute myocardial infarction has been changing. For example, prior to World War II the average hospital stay for patients without complications was 42 days; today it is 21 days, and the trend is toward a shorter hospital stay. Formerly, return to work followed a convalescent period of six months; today many patients return to their former work in two to four months.

In the past, views concerning the rehabilitation of cardiac patients were so nebulous that there was a tendency for it to be overlooked. If the goal of maximal

**Overall Points in Rehabilitation**

**Cardiac Physical Rehabilitation**

**Rehabilitation of the Wage Earner**

**Functional and Therapeutic Classification**

686

functional capacity for each patient with heart disease is to be achieved, all who care for the patient must give specific well-coordinated instruction and guidance to the patient and family. No longer is it sufficient to advise, "Take it easy," "Do not do too much," or "Don't overdo it." Vague instructions such as these are not helpful to the patient in learning to live as fully as possible despite the cardiac condition. Such vague instructions lead to confusion and contribute to the depression that many cardiac patients experience. In addition, other negative behavioral responses are fostered since the patient may fear sudden death or invalidism if he exceeds these nebulous limits. Then inactivity leads to further deterioration of physical fitness which, in turn, may make the heart less able to tolerate the numerous stressors encountered in the activities of daily living. One study demonstrated that in all of the families or couples interviewed, a steady eroding conflict had developed which 75 per cent of the time was focused on disputes about instructions for convalescence (Cassem, 1973).

Specific, knowledgeable advice helps the patient guide himself back to health in an orderly fashion. To return to his job and recreation successfully, he and the physician, nurse, family, employer, and other team members need to know what the goals are each step of the way. If the patient understands the goals, and they are his goals, and if he receives guidance in achieving them, he is likely to have a high level of motivation. When family and health team members are more certain about the plan of rehabilitation, they are less apt to advise the patient to restrict his activities unnecessarily. This lessens the tension and worry which sometimes can be far worse than the sickness and it also can help promote more positive relationships among the patient, the family, and the health care team. Thus, patient and family education and counseling are essential components of cardiac rehabilitation programs.

Rehabilitation includes measures to halt or delay progression of the disease and to educate the patient about his condition so that he can participate knowledgeably in his care program. Part of the nurse's role in cardiac rehabilitation is to teach the patient about coronary risk factor reduction.

For many cardiacs, especially those men with atherosclerotic coronary artery disease, the concept of cardiac rehabilitation—returning to as near normal as possible—may well mean doing more physically after a "heart attack" than before. Lack of regular physical exercise could have been one of the major factors leading to the illness. Exercise is of extreme importance in reconditioning the heart muscle. Its efficiency improves just as any other muscle which is made to work harder. Exercise is prescribed on a regular basis with gradually increasing loads. The danger is to move ahead too rapidly with the possibility of overload. Thus, specific graded programs are essential for safety.

Though patients with compensated congestive failure and those following myocardial revascularization require rehabilitation, the vast majority of patients today requiring conditioning programs are those with coronary artery insufficiency or myocardial infarction. Recent medical opinion holds that these conditions can be grouped into the category of anoxic cardiomyopathy. This essentially means that the heart muscle cannot get the amount of oxygen needed to perform efficiently at various levels of effort. The rehabilitation process is an attempt to change this relationship. In addition to a prescribed physical conditioning program, the patient is strongly urged to cease smoking since smoking results in increased catecholamine secretion (epinephrine and norepinephrine) which causes the myocardium to use more oxygen. Many studies have indicated that smoking is associated with increased pulse rate and some deviation of blood pressure.

Avoiding or correcting obesity is important, since overweight can increase strain on an already damaged heart. Dietary restriction of calories, concentrated sugars, and foods high in saturated fat to reduce elevated triglycerides and cholesterol, as well as treatment to control hypertension, may be part of the overall program.

Rehabilitation also involves learning how to minimize emotional tension, or if the kind of assistance needed for the patient to learn this is lacking, then it may be necessary for him to avoid certain stress situations. Emotional tension leads to catecholamine excretion, which is oxygen wasting and can result in serious cardiac dysrhythmias. (See Chapter 36 for further discussion of risk factors in coronary artery disease.)

## OVERALL POINTS IN REHABILITATION

The concept of rehabilitation is to help the patient to return as soon as possible to a life that is as nearly normal as possible. However, the rehabilitation of the cardiac patient presents some particular problems and challenges. Heart disease is not an obvious disability. In some ways this aspect helps the patient to resume his previous relationships and activities; on the other hand, it may make it harder for others to recognize his limitations.

The rehabilitation benefits may seem less visible than, say, those in the rehabilitation of patients with neuromuscular disorders. Helping a patient to learn to walk with crutches or to feed himself again is a concrete goal toward which the patient and those who care for him can strive.

All who care for the patient—physicians and nurses, as well as family members—must guard against the insidious temptation to protect themselves by overprotecting the patient. (It is so easy to think: "If I don't let him do anything, it won't be my fault if something happens to him.") They may have a tendency to assume total responsibility for anything that may happen to the patient, forgetting that there are many unpredictable events over which human beings have no control. For the cardiac patient, rehabilitation means evaluating how much and what kind of activity the patient's heart will allow him to do and helping him to live as fully and contentedly as possible within these limitations.

The goal of rehabilitation of a cardiac patient is to increase the quality of life potentially available by minimizing or eliminating the disabling consequences of heart disease. Cardiac disability involves physical, psychological, and social dimensions.

Physical disability can result from the inefficiency of the heart as a pump to maintain normal circulation; or from myocardial ischemia as a result of coronary artery disease which limits the heart's capacity to perform work; or from both.

Psychological disability in the cardiac patient can result from the patient's emotional and behavioral response to the illness. His response, in part, depends on his pre-illness personality and how he has coped with stressors in the past. However, impressions or appraisals given the patient, consciously or unconsciously by members of his family, employers, physicians, nurses, and others in his environment, can contribute to a negative behavioral response if others view the patient as inadequate to perform various roles. For example, the patient may be more likely to develop feelings of inadequacy as a spouse, a sexual partner, a parent, or a worker as a result of being a cardiac.

Unnecessary disability can result if the family, employer, or community at large have uninformed or inaccurate attitudes and beliefs concerning heart disease. For example, negative attitudes or misinformation about heart disease can be reflected in the failure to employ or to re-employ the cardiac patient who is able to continue his accustomed work. The lack of a suitable job opportunity in work for which the cardiac patient is prepared and which he can do is socially and economically disabling.

Helping the cardiac patient extend his physical independence benefits him emotionally and socially as well. The earlier physical rehabilitation is initiated, the less likely is the patient to develop satisfaction in the secondary gains of illness such as overdependence or disability income benefits, or to develop cardiac neurosis.

## CARDIAC PHYSICAL REHABILITATION

Guidelines for cardiac physical rehabilitation programs have largely been prepared with emphasis on the patient with clinical evidence of coronary (ischemic) heart disease, especially as manifested by acute myocardial infarction. Though comparable principles and resources are required for the rehabilitation of patients with other types of cardiovascular disorders, coronary heart disease receives emphasis because of its increased prevalence and increasing incidence at lower ages and because of concern that newer medical and surgical techniques which increase survival should enhance optimal function as well.

About 600,000 patients are hospitalized annually in the United States for an acute coronary episode, and approximately two-thirds survive. The annual cost for medical care, lost income, and taxes is estimated to be ten billion dollars. A further estimate indicates a national annual savings of forty million dollars if hospital medical care for each surviving patient were reduced by one day (Wenger, 1973). This is a realizable goal if greater emphasis is put on therapy which prevents deconditioning and furthers early reconditioning with the aim of self-care by the patient at the time of discharge. Indeed there is growing realization that the third week of hospitalization adds no benefit to the recovery of the uncomplicated AMI (acute myocardial infarction) patient (Cassem and Hackett, 1973). This supports the view that this time period is best spent in specific programs of patient and family education and other aspects of rehabilitation rather than in simply "resting" with consequent furtherance of deconditioning and increased physical weakness.

Because of the degree of cardiac damage from repetitive insults, self-care is an unrealistic goal for some patients. But helping the patient assess strengths as well as limitations can point out the direction for more meaningful participation in activities within his functional capacity. (See below for further information on functional capacity.)

Increasing emphasis on physical assessment for the cardiac does not decrease the need for nursing assessment of the patient's emotional responses (such as anxiety, denial, depression, regression) and their manifestations as well as for the appropriate nursing intervention. But the gradual and early return to physical activity to the extent possible enhances the patient's ability to cope with his situation.

Physical rehabilitation of the cardiac is concerned with:

- Assessing functional capacity at each phase of illness. Factors which influence function include the severity of the disease, complications, emotional response, age, response to therapies, and coexisting conditions.

- Establishing goals for each phase.
- Giving the patient an exercise prescription for each phase of illness which includes the activities that can be performed, the duration, the intensity, and the frequency (type, duration, intensity, frequency).
- Monitoring certain parameters appropriate to each phase during and after exercise to determine "strain" or disproportionate responses to the degree of effort.
- Helping the patient achieve maximal physical capacity through performance.
- Educating the patient regarding his role at various phases.
- Teaching and counseling patient and family regarding their emotional responses and risk factor reduction.
- Advising regarding energy conservation or avoidance of strain through physical rearrangements of the working environment or adjustment of schedule.
- Periodically reassessing function and represcription, usually increasing the exercise load to a point of maximal functional load without hazard.

To translate his exercise prescription into activities of daily living, the patient is taught to use charts which give approximate energy requirements for common self-care, occupational, housework, and recreational activities. Such charts may be expressed in calories per minute (see Table 39-1) or more commonly today as METs (see Table 39-2). A

**Table 39-1. Approximate Energy Requirements of Common Activities in Calories per Minute**

| PERSONAL AND SELF-CARE | | OCCUPATIONS | |
|---|---|---|---|
| Resting, supine | 1.0 cal./min. | Typing | 1.8 cal./min. |
| Feeding self, sitting | 1.4 cal./min. | Using hand tools | 2.5 cal./min. |
| Conversation | 1.4 cal./min. | Saw, power hand | 3.1 cal./min. |
| Washing face, hands, brushing teeth | 1.8 cal./min. | Plastering; brick laying | 4.0 cal./min. |
| Changing hospital gown | 2.3 cal./min. | Assembly line work | 4.5 cal./min. |
| Bedside commode | 3.6 cal./min. | Carpentry | 6.8 cal./min. |
| Dressing, washing, shaving | 3.8 cal./min. | Shoveling earth | 8.5 cal./min |
| Showering | 4.2 cal./min. | Ascending stairs with 17 lb. load | 9.0 cal./min. |
| Using bedpan | 4.7 cal./min. | Tending furnace | 10.2 cal./min |

| EXERCISES | | RECREATION | |
|---|---|---|---|
| Passive range of motion, lower extremities | 1.4 cal./min. | Knitting | 1.5 cal./min. |
| Deep breathing, active exercises of wrists and ankles, isometrics of quadriceps and buttocks | 2.0 cal./min. | Driving car | 2.8 cal./min. |
| Walking slowly, 1 mile in 24 min. | 3.5 cal./min. | Bowling | 4.4 cal./min |
| Cycling 5.5 m.p.h., 1 mile in 11 min. | 4.5 cal./min. | Dancing fox-trot | 5.5 cal./min. |
| Swimming 20 yds./min. | 5.0 cal./min. | Gardening, moderate | 5.6 cal./min. |
| Walking downstairs | 5.2 cal./min. | Golf, pulling cart or carrying bag | 7.0 cal./min. |
| Climbing, descending 2 flights stairs/min. | 8.5 cal./min. | Tennis doubles | 7.1 cal./min. |
| Running 1 mile in 11 min. | 11.0 cal./min. | Skiing, tow, down-hill | 9.9 cal./min. |
| Walking uphill, 10% slope | 13.0 cal./min. | | |

| HOUSEWORK ACTIVITIES | | OCCUPATIONAL THERAPY | |
|---|---|---|---|
| Cooking, standing | 1.6 cal./min. | Leather tooling, reclining | 1.2 cal./min |
| Light ironing, standing | 2.7 cal./min. | Rug hooking, sitting | 1.3 cal./min. |
| Hand washing small clothes | 3.0 cal./min. | Hand sewing | 1.4 cal./min. |
| Vacuum cleaning | 3.2 cal./min. | Leather carving, sitting | 1.8 cal./min. |
| Scrubbing floors | 3.6 cal./min. | Weaving, floor loom | 2.0 cal./min. |
| Mowing lawn, power | 3.8 cal./min. | Light gardening | 2.1 cal./min. |
| Making beds | 4.1 cal./min. | Power sanding | 2.2 cal./min. |
| Carrying 50 lbs. | 6.7 cal./min. | Playing piano | 2.5 cal./min. |
| Shoveling snow moderately wet, 10 lb./min. | 11.4 cal./min. | Sawing soft wood | 6.3 cal./min |

**Table 39-2. Approximate Metabolic Cost of Activities***

| | OCCUPATIONAL | RECREATIONAL |
|---|---|---|
| 1½–2 METs†<br>4–7 ml. O$_2$/min./kg.<br>2–2½ kcal./min.<br>(70 kg. person) | Desk work<br>Auto driving‡<br>Typing<br>Electric calculating<br>   machine operation | Standing<br>Walking (strolling 1.6 km. or 1 mile/hr.)<br>Flying,‡ motorcycling‡<br>Playing cards‡<br>Sewing, knitting |
| 2–3 METs<br>7–11 ml. O$_2$/min./kg.<br>2½–4 kcal./min.<br>(70 kg. person) | Auto repair<br>Radio, TV repair<br>Janitorial work<br>Typing, manual<br>Bartending | Level walking (3¼ km. or 2 miles/hr.)<br>Level bicycling (8 km. or 5 miles/hr.)<br>Riding lawn mower<br>Billiards, bowling<br>Skeet,‡ shuffleboard<br>Woodworking (light)<br>Powerboat driving‡<br>Golf (power cart)<br>Canoeing (4 km. or 2½ miles/hr.)<br>Horseback riding (walk)<br>Playing piano and many musical instruments |
| 3–4 METs<br>11–14 ml. O$_2$/min./kg.<br>4–5 kcal./min.<br>(70 kg. person) | Brick laying, plastering<br>Wheelbarrow (45 kg. or<br>   100 lb. load)<br>Machine assembly<br>Trailer-truck in traffic<br>Welding (moderate load)<br>Cleaning windows | Walking (5 km. or 3 miles/hr.)<br>Cycling (10 km. or 6 miles/hr.)<br>Horseshoe pitching<br>Volleyball (6-man noncompetitive)<br>Golf (pulling bag cart)<br>Archery<br>Sailing (handling small boat)<br>Fly fishing (standing with waders)<br>Horseback (sitting to trot)<br>Badminton (social doubles)<br>Pushing light power mower<br>Energetic musician |
| 4–5 METs<br>14–18 ml. O$_2$/min./kg.<br>5–6 kcal./min.<br>(70 kg. person) | Painting, masonry<br>Paperhanging<br>Light carpentry | Walking (5½ km. or 3½ miles/hr.)<br>Cycling (13 km. or 8 miles/hr.)<br>Table tennis<br>Golf (carrying clubs)<br>Dancing (fox-trot)<br>Badminton (singles)<br>Tennis (doubles)<br>Raking leaves<br>Hoeing<br>Many calisthenics |
| 5–6 METs<br>18–21 ml. O$_2$/min./kg.<br>6–7 kcal./min.<br>(70 kg. person) | Digging garden<br>Shoveling light earth | Walking (6½ km. or 4 miles/hr.)<br>Cycling (16 km. or 10 miles/hr.)<br>Canoeing (6½ km. or 4 miles/hr.)<br>Horseback ("posting" to trot)<br>Stream fishing (walking in light current<br>   in waders)<br>Ice or roller skating (15 km. or 9 miles/hr.) |
| 6–7 METs<br>21–25 ml. O$_2$/min./kg.<br>7–8 kcal./min.<br>(70 kg. person) | Shoveling 10/min.<br>   (4½ kg. or 10 lbs.) | Walking (8 km. or 5 miles/hr.)<br>Cycling (17½ km. or 11 miles/hr.)<br>Badminton (competitive)<br>Tennis (singles)<br>Splitting wood<br>Snow shoveling<br>Hand lawn-mowing<br>Folk (square) dancing<br>Light downhill skiing<br>Ski touring (4 km. or 2½ miles/hr.)<br>   (loose snow)<br>Water skiing |
| 7–8 METs<br>25–28 ml. O$_2$/min./kg.<br>8–10 kcal./min.<br>(70 kg. person) | Digging ditches<br>Carrying 36 kg. or 80 lbs.<br>Sawing hardwood | Jogging (8 km. or 5 miles/hr.)<br>Cycling (19 km. or 12 miles/hr.)<br>Horseback (gallop)<br>Vigorous downhill skiing<br>Basketball<br>Mountain climbing<br>Ice hockey<br>Canoeing (8 km. or 5 miles/hr.)<br>Touch football<br>Paddleball |

| | OCCUPATIONAL | RECREATIONAL |
|---|---|---|
| 8–9 METs<br>28–32 ml. O$_2$/min./kg.<br>10–11 kcal./min.<br>(70 kg. person) | Shoveling 10/min.<br>(5½ kg. or 14 lbs.) | Running (9 km. or 5½ miles/hr.)<br>Cycling (21 km. or 13 miles/hr.)<br>Ski touring (6½ km. or 4 miles/hr.)<br>(loose snow)<br>Squash racquets (social)<br>Handball (social)<br>Fencing<br>Basketball (vigorous) |
| 10 plus METs<br>32 plus ml. O$_2$/min./kg.<br>11 plus kcal./min.<br>(70 kg. person) | Shoveling 10/min.<br>(7½ kg. or 16 lbs.) | Running:  6 mph = 10 METs<br>7 mph = 11½ METs<br>8 mph = 13½ METs<br>9 mph = 15 METs<br>10 mph = 17 METs<br>Ski touring (8+ km. or 5+ miles/hr.)<br>(loose snow)<br>Handball (competitive)<br>Squash (competitive) |

\* Includes resting metabolic needs.
† 1 MET is the energy expenditure at rest, equivalent to approximat ely 3.5 ml. O$_2$/kg. body weight/minute.
‡ A major excess metabolic increase may occur due to excitement, anxiety, or impatience in some of these activities, and a physician must assess his patient's psychological reactivity.
From Fox, S., Naughton, J., and Gorman, P.: Physical activity and cardiovascular health, *Mod. Conc. Cardiovasc. Dis.* 41:27, June 1972. Reproduced with the permission of the authors and The American Heart Association.

MET is a metabolic equivalent which relates physical energy to basal energy requirements. One MET is the basal energy requirement of an individual at rest; it is roughly equivalent to 1.3 to 1.5 calories per minute depending on the individual or 3.5 to 4.0 ml. oxygen per kilogram of body weight per minute. METs are approximate equivalents since the values have usually been determined on normal subjects and do not account for the effects of psychological factors which increase intensity and energy costs, such as competitiveness, impatience, or excitement, as noted in Table 39-2.

### Rehabilitation Programs

There are several types of rehabilitation programs for persons with coronary heart disease. All include patient and family teaching and counseling as well as physical reconditioning. The roles of team members (nurse, physician, dietitian, psychiatrist, vocational counselor, physical education instructor, social worker) vary according to the phase of illness and the needs of the patient. Programs include:

- A precoronary phase program of graded exercises for those with high-risk coronary profiles or controlled angina pectoris.
- Inpatient programs for the clinically stable AMI patient starting with the first day after admission (Phases I and II).
- Posthospital convalescent phase programs for the recovering patient (Phase III).

- Work evaluation and reconditioning programs for the recovered AMI patient (Phase IV).

**Angina Pectoris Program.** The principles are the same as for Phase IV post-AMI reconditioning programs and are discussed later in this section.

**Inpatient Program.** Phases I and II of the rehabilitation program involve the acute illness period, which is usually 21 days in uncomplicated cases; these are discussed in Chapter 62, The Patient with Acute Myocardial Infarction.

**Convalescence After Discharge.** Phase III takes place after discharge from the hospital and is generally spent at home. It is usually two to eight weeks in duration. At the time of homecoming a patient who has met the usual goals of Phases I and II has reached the activity level for self-care at home, including most usual light household activities and climbing stairs. Making beds, scrubbing floors, and washing and hanging heavy clothes are to be avoided. One exercise that may be given prior to hospital discharge is the rapid ascent of two flights of stairs. This "two-flight" test is considered comparable in terms of physical demand to the energy expenditure during sexual intercourse. The affective response to return to sexual activity should be dealt with explicitly, and preferably with both patient and spouse.

Although able to care for themselves, patients should be told that they can anticipate some degree of weakness on homecoming, which is related to the degree of deconditioning involved in the hospitalization phase.

Activities in Phase III are in the range of 3 to 5 METs. Walking is the primary activity, progressively increased in speed and distance. At the end of the sixth week the patient may walk one to two miles per day divided into two or three activity periods. At the end of Phase III (up to eleven weeks post-AMI) the patient who has progressed on schedule can walk at a speed of three miles in one hour, an energy expenditure level of four to five METs, which is higher than that required for most desk or bench jobs in our society.

Support during this phase is provided by the community health nurse, office or clinic nurse, occupational health nurse, nurse in private practice, physician, family, friends, and employer.

**Recovery-Maintenance and Return to Work Program.** Today multi-stage exercise testing is recommended as a guide for prescription for higher levels of physical activity which promote maximum function (Phase IV). Exercises may be begun three to six months postinfarction for uncomplicated cases or after a similar period of stability for the patient

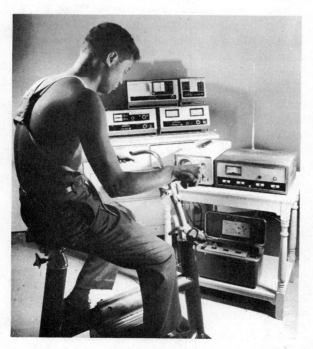

**Figure 39-1.** Exercise test using ergometer with controls and radio receiver. (Hackensack Hospital, Hackensack, New Jersey)

with angina pectoris or myocardial revascularization surgery.

Where there is no local or regional facility for newer modes of exercise testing, the physician can use a standardized test in the office, such as the "Master Two-Step" test to give the patient a definite amount of exercise and evaluate his response. The test involves a specified number of trips up and down two steps, each 9 inches high, within a definite time interval.

This test requires approximately 8.5 calories (6 METs) per minute, which is higher than almost all kinds of work except extremely heavy work. The pulse and blood pressure response of the patient, as well as the ECG, can allow the physician to estimate what the heart might do under actual work conditions.

Cardiac work evaluation units or commercial cardiac rehabilitation centers have specialized equipment and staff to perform stress tests consisting of increasing levels of work on a treadmill or bicycle ergometer (Fig. 39-1). Heart rate, ECG, and blood pressure are continuously monitored. The goal is to raise the pulse rate high enough to gain a stressful enough response to help strengthen the myocardium. This will vary according to age, with younger people able to attain higher rates. The fact that maximum heart rate declines with age is very important. This is often overlooked by potential cardiacs who self-prescribe their physical conditioning program (such as jogging) without benefit of a physical examination and stress ECG (see Tables 39-3 and 39-4).

Patients are generally tested to 70 to 85 per cent of maximal pulse rate for age. If during stress testing (or increase in activity at any phase) evidence of myocardial hypoxia appears, such as chest pain

**Table 39-3. Relationship of Pulse to Degree of Work**

| AGE | 100% (CAPACITY) | 50% (HEAVY) | 30% (MODERATE) | 10% (LIGHT) |
|---|---|---|---|---|
| 20 Yrs. | 198 | 130 | 102 | 70 |
| 30 Yrs. | 188 | 125 | 98 | 70 |
| 40 Yrs. | 180 | 120 | 96 | 70 |
| 50 Yrs. | 170 | 116 | 92 | 70 |
| 60 Yrs. | 160 | 110 | 90 | 70 |
| 70 Yrs. | 152 | 108 | 86 | 70 |

Derived from Communications from the Testing and Observation Institute of the Danish National Association for Infantile Paralysis, Hellerup, Denmark, 1959.

**Table 39-4. Classification of Work by Energy Required**

| DEGREE OF WORK | ENERGY REQUIRED |
| --- | --- |
| Light | Up to 4.9 cal./min. |
| Moderate | 5.0 to 7.5 cal./min. |
| Heavy | Over 7.5 cal./min. |

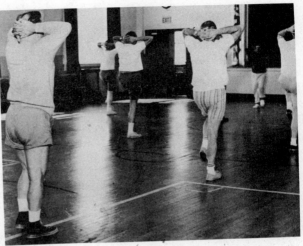

**Figure 39-2.** Exercise class for cardiac patients. (Hackensack, N.J.)

or dyspnea, or ECG evidence of dysrhythmia or S-T displacement, or if there is a fall in blood pressure or rapid progression of fatigue, the effort is considered to be excessive and the exercise prescription would be for activities of lesser output.

Because of the potential for cardiac emergencies to occur if the patient is inadvertently overstressed, each cardiac evaluation unit is equipped with a "crash cart" containing cardiac emergency drugs and equipment to be used by prepared personnel.

Patients are referred to these units by their own physician or by their employers. Often, the staff consists of a physician, nurse, and technician. Evaluation and consultation services are available on a part- or full-time basis with other team members such as a psychologist, psychiatrist, social worker, or vocational counselor. Each state in the United States has a Rehabilitation Commission which can provide such specialized services. The patient's capacity for work is evaluated and recommendations made concerning his employment and physical conditioning program. These units help to educate patients, physicians, and employers concerning heart disease and the employment of patients with heart disease, to evaluate workers' capacity for specific kinds of jobs; unit staff members work with sponsors of conditioning programs or plan, direct, and supervise such programs themselves for individuals and groups (Fig. 39-2).

Exercise tests are not done on patients with such conditions as manifest congestive heart failure, rapidly increasing angina pectoris, thrombophlebitis, or active myocarditis, or usually within three months of acute myocardial infarction. Other conditions are considered relative contraindications, and special precautions are utilized if stress testing is performed (Fox, et al., 1972).

An exercise prescription takes into consideration the patient's job, recreation, and home life. He is helped to understand the concept of calorie or MET expenditures that can be "spent" in accordance with his prescription. He is also taught to count his own pulse rate since heart rate is a determining factor of myocardial oxygen demand. Today the concept is to work at 40 to 50 per cent of maximal capacity and exercise at 70 per cent using the pulse as a guideline.

A trial work situation in the actual or an equivalent setting often is used to determine how well the worker can tolerate a certain type of activity. Knowing this is of great value, because the ability to perform a certain task comfortably depends on many factors other than sheer physical exertion. Some of these factors are:

Temperature
Humidity
Oxygen content of air
Toxic exposures
Rate of work
Skill and coordination
Self confidence
Rest periods—length and environment
Shift changes (biologic rhythms)
Anxiety over type of work, quality of work, effects of work on self and others
Interpersonal relations with supervisors and coworkers
Physical condition
Food habits
Smoking

Recently it has become possible to monitor a person's electrocardiogram throughout his daily activities by use of a portable, magnetic tape recorder (Holter monitor, Fig. 39-3). Electrodes are placed on the chest and connected to a recorder contained in a small bag carried over the shoulder or attached to the belt. The patient carries out his usual daily

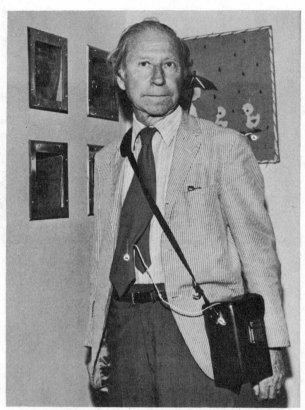

**Figure 39-3.** Patient wearing the Holter cardiac monitor.

functions and keeps a diary of his activities and his subjective response to them. The physician replays the ECG tape and notes the effects of various activities such as work, recreation, sexual intercourse, or emotional stress on heart rate, rhythm, and metabolism as denoted in any S-T-T wave ischemic changes. A special rapid scanning device enables the physician to review an entire ten-hour ECG record in ten minutes and to stop it when necessary to study irregularities.

Another type of physiologic monitoring is through a biotelemetry system. This is being used more and more frequently as the patient increases his physical activity in the hospital, or performs in a mock work situation. The patient goes through his usual activities with chest electrodes connected to a small radio transmitter attached to his belt. This sends his ECG to a radio receiver not more than 1,500 feet away. The physician or nurse views the transmitted radio signal (ECG) directly on an oscilloscope screen, or it can be printed on standard ECG equipment for study at a later time.

## Physical Conditioning Programs

These usually start about three or four months after infarction. Generally patients have been in a Phase III walking program and can tolerate three or four miles every other day at a moderate pace. Aerobic exercises (physical activities characterized by a steady supply of oxygen being delivered through the cardiopulmonary system to active muscle cells as opposed to anaerobic exercises, in which oxygen debt is incurred) are performed to promote cardiovascular endurance. Classes of beginners meet in a community center two or three times a week. Sessions consist of a *warm-up* period, the *training-stimulus* period during which time activities are designed to increase the pulse rate to the prescribed target rate, and a *cool-down* period followed by a warm shower. Hot shower and sauna baths following exercise are contraindicated because they impose added vasodilation due to heat stress.

A physician and, at times, a nurse are available to answer questions. Resuscitation equipment and drugs are present at all beginners' sessions, which are generally led by a physical educator.

The patient is taught to monitor his body's response to physical stress and stops every few minutes during the training-stimulus period to check his pulse. As endurance increases, higher level activities can be performed for longer periods. Periods of relative inactivity such as those due to illness necessitate starting out again at a lower level.

The process of defining the patient's capacities and limitations is a continuous cooperative effort of the patient and the rehabilitation team—a process of learning gradually how the patient responds in a variety of situations rather than a matter of dictating a list of permitted and forbidden items. Actually, physical activity prescription emphasizes what the patient can do, as opposed to so many other dictums that say what he can't do.

The patient's intelligence and emotional balance in relation to the stability of his home life and his job play a large part in determining the success of rehabilitation. The person who has developed valuable skills through education and experience, one whose work is valued at his place of employment, has a firm foundation for vocational rehabilitation. The patient who has a loyal family to help and to support him in his efforts toward recovery has an extra measure of strength in coping with stress, including that of illness.

694

Modern technology has much to contribute, too. Air conditioning at home or at work lessens strain in warm weather. The heart works harder and less efficiently when temperature and humidity are high—a point that takes on great importance when the patient has heart disease. The machines that now do much of what used to constitute heavy physical labor, both at home and at work, have been a particular boon to the disabled.

## REHABILITATION OF THE WAGE EARNER

In the American culture, work occupies the major part of life. Not only is it necessary to obtain money to live, but it provides contact with other people and, for most people, feelings of usefulness and satisfaction. Attitudes toward work vary, however. Some few may consider it a necessary evil and welcome the chance to be relieved of responsibility. Attitudes toward work influence the success of rehabilitation. The diagnosis of heart disease used to be considered to be a sufficient reason for the cessation of employment. "He has a bad heart, and so he can't work anymore," was a familiar attitude. Nowadays there is a growing tendency to ask such questions as these before advising the patient about his ability to work:

- How much and what kind of work can the patient do without experiencing symptoms?
- What kind of activity and how much activity are compatible with his total program of treatment?
- What kind of work was the patient doing before the illness? How much exertion and what kind of exertion did this work entail, in relation to physical exercise, degree of responsibility, emotional strain?
- What is the before and after work energy expenditure? For many patients the energy cost of traveling to and from work on public transportation or by driving on crowded expressways is far greater than that of the actual job requirements.
- What kinds of rest facilities are available?
- What does work mean to the patient?
- What are his attitudes toward his job, coworkers, employer?
- How does his job influence his relationships with his family, his friends, his community?

The question is not the simple one, "Can he work?" The requirements of each job situation must be evaluated as carefully as possible. No one merely "works." We do a certain kind of job that presents its own assortment of physical and emotional demands and rewards. The same principles apply for the cardiac homemaker. Tasks around the home can be viewed as a form of exercise, and doing routine things may serve as a tension reliever. Most household tasks are not too heavy in terms of caloric or MET expenditure, and the problem is lessened if labor-saving devices such as a clothes washer and dryer and power lawn mower are available. The American Heart Association has several pamphlets depicting energy costs of household activities and methods of conserving energy expenditures. Advice regarding community resources for homemaker services for the cardiac is also available.

It is the specific job situation, in relation to a particular patient and his physical, emotional, and intellectual abilities, that must be evaluated. The final test is how well the worker performs in the actual job situation, and how the work affects his health status.

Recent data indicate that over 85 per cent of patients under age 65 had returned to work within two to four months after an uncomplicated myocardial infarction; over three-fourths resumed their preinfarction level of physical activity (Wenger, et al., 1973).

For some patients, the degree of cardiac involvement will necessitate a change in job. This may be dictated by the strenuousness of the work, coexisting health conditions, the exposure to environmental hazards such as heat and humidity, or the potential risk to others by such employees as airline pilots or truck drivers. Vocational guidance needs to be given early because the difficulty of returning the cardiac patient to work increases with his length of separation from it.

Some patients can return to their former job but with modification. The occupational health or community health nurse can assist in the planning whenever possible. Some ways of modifying a job to allow for decreased cardiac reserve are:

- Initially working a part-time day
- Working four days a week instead of five
- Sitting, whenever possible, rather than standing
- Traveling at off-hours to avoid rush-hour congestion and confusion
- Taking more frequent rest periods
- Utilizing air-cooled rest facilities, which should be provided for patients who work in hot environments
- Rearranging work space
- Planning work to avoid sudden and excessive spurts of energy expenditure

When the job can be modified, the employer benefits from the continued contribution of an experienced, skilled worker. The cardiac benefits from continued income, social contact with coworkers, and feelings of usefulness and satisfaction. The economy as a whole benefits because the worker continues to pay taxes, has income to purchase goods and services, and is not the recipient of disability income.

Unfortunately, some have difficulty finding employment or returning to their former jobs. Many employers refuse to hire people with heart disease. This reluctance to hire cardiacs has been attributed partly to Workmen's Compensation laws. For example, if the worker has a myocardial infarction on the job, the illness often is considered compensable, even though no unusual situation occurred at work, and although it might be argued that the attack might have been as likely to occur while the worker was at home. There has been much discussion of the ways in which such laws could be changed to lessen the financial problem for the employer and thus to encourage the employment of cardiacs who are able to work, and who want to work. Fear that the worker will have "attacks" while he is at work, which might upset others or damage property, or a conviction that people with heart disease do not belong at work also may contribute to the reluctance to hire people with heart disease. Absentee rates of cardiac patients who return to their former jobs were found to be significantly lower than the general absentee rate of the company (Feldman, 1968).

The need for a broader viewpoint in relation to the employment of cardiacs has been highlighted by the more widespread use of careful physical examinations, x-ray examinations, and even electrocardiograms before employment. Many persons who have slight cardiac abnormalities and few, if any, symptoms are being discovered. This is a good trend, since treatment can be initiated in the early stages of heart disease, with the possibility of preventing serious illness. However, this trend could work a hardship for some people, if employment is denied or discontinued without considering the worker's capabilities.

The person with heart disease who lives and works within the limits of his capacity is usually healthier and happier than is the person who gives up his accustomed pursuits. Idleness is no guarantee of long life, and, in fact, may hasten the person's death.

## FUNCTIONAL AND THERAPEUTIC CLASSIFICATION

The functional and the therapeutic classifications developed by the New York Heart Association have helped to establish a precise definition of what the patient is physically able to do (functional classification) and what he should do as part of his treatment (therapeutic classification). These two are not always the same in degree of restriction. For example, a patient with active rheumatic fever may be physically able, so far as cardiac function is concerned, to be up and about. However, to derive maximum value from treatment, it may be necessary for him to remain on bed rest to protect his heart. Such a patient might be classified IIE (see Table 39-5).

### THE CLASSIFICATION OF PATIENTS WITH DISEASES OF THE HEART*

#### Functional Capacity

CLASS I. Patients with cardiac disease but without resulting limitation of physical activity. Ordinary physical activity does not cause undue fatigue, palpitation, dyspnea, or anginal pain.

CLASS II. Patients with cardiac disease resulting in slight limitation of physical activity. They are comfortable at rest. Ordinary physical activity results in fatigue, palpitation, dyspnea, or anginal pain.

CLASS III. Patients with cardiac disease resulting in marked limitation of physical activity. They are comfortable at rest. Less than ordinary activity causes fatigue, palpitation, dyspnea, or anginal pain.

CLASS IV. Patients with cardiac disease resulting in inability to carry on any physical activity without discomfort. Symptoms of cardiac insufficiency or of the anginal syndrome are present even at rest. If any physical activity is undertaken, discomfort is increased.

#### Therapeutic Classification

CLASS A. Patients with cardiac disease whose ordinary physical activity need not be restricted.

CLASS B. Patients with cardiac disease whose ordinary physical activity need not be restricted, but who should be advised against severe or competitive physical efforts.

CLASS C. Patients with cardiac disease whose ordinary physical activity should be moderately restricted, and whose more strenuous efforts should be discontinued.

---

*This classification was developed by the New York Heart Association and is used here with permission.

**Table 39-5. Classes of Organic Heart Disease: Guide for Evaluating Impairment of the Whole Person**

| CLASS I (MINIMAL) | CLASS II (MODERATE) | CLASS III (SEVERE) | CLASS IV (VERY SEVERE) |
|---|---|---|---|
| Energy expenditure continuous up to 5 calories/min., intermittent to 6.6 calories/min. | Energy expenditure continuous up to 2.5 calories/min., intermittent to 4 calories/min. | Energy expenditure continuous up to 2 calories/min., intermittent to 2.7 calories/min. | Energy expenditure up to 1.5 calories/min. |
| No symptoms with ordinary activity | Slight symptoms with ordinary activity; none at rest | Less than ordinary activity causes symptoms; none at rest | Symptoms even at rest |
| Walking, climbing stairs, and usual activities of daily living do not produce symptoms | Walking on level, climbing one flight of stairs (average pace), and usual activities of living do not produce symptoms | Walking more than one block on level or climbing one flight of stairs (average pace) or usual activities of daily living produce symptoms | Performance of any of activities of daily living beyond personal toilet or its equivalent produce increased discomfort |
| Intermittent (2 min. or less), severe physical exertion, hurrying, hill-climbing, active recreation, and marked emotional stress do not produce symptoms | Emotional stress, hurrying, hill-climbing, active recreation, or similar physical activity produce slight symptoms | Emotional stress, hurrying, hill-climbing, active recreation, or similar activities produce marked symptoms | Symptoms increase with emotional reaction; any physical activity increases discomfort |
| Signs of congestive heart failure are not present | Signs of congestive heart failure are not present | Signs of congestive heart failure may be present, and if so, are usually relieved by therapy | Signs of congestive heart failure, if present, are usually resistant to therapy |

Adopted with revisions from The American Heart Association (New York Heart Association) and American Medical Association (Committee on Medical Rating of Physical Impairment).

CLASS D. Patients with cardiac disease whose ordinary physical activity should be markedly restricted.

CLASS E. Patients with cardiac disease who should be at complete rest, confined to bed or chair.

By using the functional classification of heart disease along with the energy expenditure of common activities expressed in calories per minute or METs, the physician can initiate a progressive energy-expenditure prescription for the patient. The final plan would depend on a real or simulated work trial.

For example, from a physical rehabilitative standpoint the patient with a myocardial infarction who has an uncomplicated course of healing may have the following level of energy expenditure:

- In the coronary care unit (one to three days), from 1 gradually up to 2 calories per minute (1 to 2 METs).
- During remainder of hospital stay (about two weeks), up to 3 calories per minute (2 to 3 METs).
- During convalescence at home (eight to twelve weeks) up to 4 to 5 calories per minute (3 to 5 METs).
- After recovery (twelve weeks), dependent upon the functional classification of the patient (see Table 39-5).

- After twelve weeks and indefinitely, a program of graded activities under medical supervision merged into a regimen of physical conditioning that becomes a lifetime program of regular exercise as strenuous as the patient is able to perform with safety. According to the functional classification of the patient, energy expenditure would be prescribed for:

Class I patients—eventually from 6.6 to 11 to 12 calories per minute or higher (6 to 10+ METs).

Class II patients—eventually from 4 to 6 to 7 calories per minute (5 to 6 METs).

Class III patients—possibly only a slight increase, up to 3 to 3.5 calories per minute (3 to 4 METs).

Class IV patients—probably no practical physical rehabilitation possible.

When the level of permitted energy expenditure is established, the patient can be assisted by the physician, nurse, and other team members to live within his limits by using a table of approximate energy requirements of common activities. (See Tables 39-1 and 39-2.)

## Nursing Assessment and Intervention

Nurses in many practice settings such as community health agencies, hospital outpatient departments, occupational health departments, and in private practice can assist in the cardiac's rehabilitation program throughout its phases by:

- **Expecting a specific activity prescription from the physician for the patient rather than vague suggestions.**
- **Assessing patient response to increased activity by observing for danger signals such as anginal pain, palpitation, dyspnea, dizziness, undue fatigue, dysrhythmias, increase in S-T-T displacement, precordial bulge, appearance of S-3, S-4 gallops, decrease in blood pressure, or increase in pulse rate above 120 per minute or above target rate. Discussing these with the physician before the patient repeats the activity is necessary (see Table 39-6).**
- **Listening to the patient as he talks about his illness—what led up to it, what the illness means to him, and what he thinks about the future. Helping the patient to establish realistic goals and to assess his strengths and assets as well as his losses and liabilities can assist him in a realistic way to make the most of what he has.**
- **Counseling the patient and family regarding adjustments to be anticipated during the convalescent phase.**
- **Teaching regarding risk factor reduction.**
- **Knowing how to respond in a cardiac emergency.**
- **Using a positive though realistic approach to the patient. For example, when the hospitalized patient is asked to move his legs and feet, the need should be emphasized to maintain the muscles in good condition since these will have to carry him when he starts to walk again, rather than placing emphasis on the prevention of venous thrombosis and emboli. The physical activities the patient can do rather than the don'ts should be stressed.**

- **Working with the vocational counselor, psychologist, physicians, nurses, and other team members in various settings so that the best program for the individual cardiac patient can be achieved.**
- **Being aware of the facilities available in the community for stress testing, physical conditioning, vocational evaluation, and job retraining and placement, such as the State Rehabilitation Commission.**
- **Realistically appraising work and home situations whenever possible. For example, the occupational health nurse should test the assembly line worker's pulse response at his place of work, not after he has walked to the dispensary. The visiting nurse can assist the homemaker to evaluate the home situation in terms of energy expenditure and make recommendations for conserving energy.**
- **Helping those who cannot resume their former occupation or any job at all to find meaningful pursuits within their limitations.**
- **Recognizing that the patient is the driving force for his own rehabilitation. The team makes his potential evident and provides encouragement and continued support.**

## REFERENCES AND BIBLIOGRAPHY

BARRY, E., et al.: Hospital program for cardiac rehabilitation, *Am. J. Nurs.* 72:2174, December 1972.

BROWSE, N. L.: *Physiology and Pathology of Bed Rest,* Springfield, Ill., Thomas, 1965.

BUGG, R.: They're mending hearts with exercise, *Today's Health* 45:50, October 1967.

CASSEM, N., and HACKETT, N.: Psychological rehabilitation of myocardial infarction patients in the acute phase, *Heart Lung* 2:382, May-June 1973.

DUKE, M.: Bed rest in acute myocardial infarction: A study of physician practices, *Am. Heart J.* 82:486, October 1971.

ELIOT, R., and MILES, R.: What to tell the cardiac patient about sexual intercourse, *Resident Intern Consult.* 2:14, October 1973.

FELDMAN, D.: Rehabilitation of the cardiac patient, *Mod. Treatm.* 5:93, September 1968.

FOX, S., et al.: Physical activity and cardiovascular health: I. Potential for prevention of coronary heart disease and possible mechanisms. II. The exercise prescription: Intensity and duration. III. The exercise prescription: Frequency and type of activity, *Mod. Conc. Cardiovasc. Dis.* 41:17, April 1972; 41:21, May 1972; 41:25, June 1972.

FRASHER, W., et al.: Office procedures as aids to work prescription for cardiac patients (Parts I and II), *Mod. Conc. Cardiovasc. Dis.* 32:769, 32:776, January and February, 1963.

GERMAIN, C. P.: Exercise makes the heart grow stronger, *Am. J. Nurs.* 72:2169, December 1972.

HELLERSTEIN, H.: Exercise therapy in coronary disease, *Bull. N.Y. Acad. Med.* 44:1028, August 1968.

———: Sexual activity and the post-coronary patient, *Med. Asp. Human Sexuality* 3:70, March 1969.

**Table 39-6.** "Target" Heart Rates for Subjects without Signs or Symptoms Suggesting Circulatory Insufficiency*

| AGE (YEARS) | SCANDINAVIAN AND MYRTLE BEACH CRITERIA | SHEFFIELD ET AL. (90%) |
|---|---|---|
| 20–29 | 170 | 175 |
| 30–39 | 160 | 172 |
| 40–49 | 150 | 168 |
| 50–59 | 140 | 164 |
| 60–69 | 130 | 160 |

*A subject should neither be permitted nor encouraged to press on to any such arbitrary intensities if signs or symptoms suggest significant or impending problems. Approximate maximum heart rates for "normals" adjusted for age can be calculated by either of the following formulae:

High estimate: Maximum predicted heart rate = 210 minus ½ age (in years)

Low estimate: Maximum predicted heart rate = 220 minus age (in years)

From Fox, S., Naughton, J., and Gorman, P.: Physical activity and cardiovascular health, *Mod. Conc. Cardiovasc. Dis.* 41:23, May 1972. Reproduced with the permission of the authors and The American Heart Association.

———: Rehabilitation of the postinfarction patient, *Hosp. Prac.* 7:45, July 1972.

HOUSER, D.: Outside the coronary care unit, *Nurs. Forum* 12:96, #1, 1973.

KOHN, R. M.: Physical reconditioning after myocardial infarction, *N.Y. Med. J.* 70:516, 1970.

KOS, B.: The nurse's role in rehabilitation of the cardiac patient, *Nurs. Clin. N. Am.* 4:513, December 1969.

LARSEN, O. A., and MALMBORG, R. O. (eds.): *Coronary Heart Disease and Physical Fitness,* Baltimore, University Park Press, 1971.

LAVIN, M. A.: Bed exercises for acute cardiac patients, *Am. J. Nurs.* 73:1226, July 1973.

LESHER, S.: There comes a time to live—well, *The New York Times Magazine,* January 27, 1974, p. 9.

LEVITAS, I.: The prescription of exercise, Chap. 15 in Zohman, L., and Phillips, R. (eds.): *Medical Aspects of Exercise Testing and Training,* New York, Intercontinental Medical Book Corp., 1973.

ROBINSON, A.: Stress-testing: Key to activity for the heart patient, *RN* 36:ICU-1, December 1973.

SCALZI, C.: Nursing management of behavioral responses following acute myocardial infarction, *Heart Lung* 2:62, January-February 1973.

WEINBLATT, E., et al.: Return to work and work status following first myocardial infarction, *Am. J. Pub. Health* 56:169, February 1966.

WENGER, N. K.: Medical data: Background for nursing assessment. In Papers Presented (at) National Nursing Conference (on) Posthospital Care of Coronary Patients, held at Richmond, Va., Feb. 25-26, 1970.

Rockville, Md., Office of Communications and Public Information, Heart Disease and Stroke Control Program, U.S. Regional Medical Programs Service, 1971, pp. 13-15.

———: *Rehabilitation After Myocardial Infarction,* New York, American Heart Association, 1973.

———, et al.: Uncomplicated myocardial infarction. Current physician practice in patient management, *JAMA* 224:511, 1973.

When should your coronary patients return to work? *Patient Care* 4:82, August 15, 1970.

WISHNIE, H., et al.: Psychological hazards of convalescence following myocardial infarction, *JAMA* 215:1291, 1971.

ZOHMAN, L.: New methods of work prescription for the coronary patient, in Russek, H. I., and Zohman, B. L. (eds.): *Coronary Heart Disease,* Proceedings, American College of Cardiology Symposium, New York, 1971, Philadelphia, Lippincott, 1971.

———, and PHILLIPS, R. (eds.): *Medical Aspects of Exercise Testing and Training,* New York, Intercontinental Medical Book Corp., 1973.

———, and TOBIAS, J. S.: *Cardiac Rehabilitation,* New York, Grune, 1970.

**Films**

Available through the local Heart Association

*Gotta Lotta Living to Do*
*It's Your Heart*

# UNIT
# EIGHT

## Disturbances of Ingestion, Digestion, Absorption, and Elimination

# Assessment of the Patient with Gastrointestinal Disorders

## CHAPTER 40

Disorders of gastrointestinal function are associated with a wide variety of health problems. Symptoms common to all of these disorders are disturbances in ingesting, digesting, and absorbing nutrients, and eliminating waste products from the gastrointestinal tract.

The patient's condition may be caused predominantly by emotional or physical factors. Dysphagia (difficulty in swallowing) due to a life situation the patient "cannot swallow" is an example of the former. Dysphagia caused by swallowing a harmful chemical is an example of the latter, if damage to the esophagus was accidental. On the other hand, if the harmful substance was swallowed in an attempt at suicide, the underlying cause of the problem is psychological rather than physiologic, even though damage to the esophagus is clearly physical.

There are many patients with gastrointestinal disturbances whose conditions cannot be classified as emotional or physical in origin; their illnesses seem to be both psychological and physiologic malfunction, with each of these spheres constantly interacting with the other. Thus a patient with constipation may find her condition is aggravated by an argument with her domineering husband, or by lack of exercise. The patient recovering from peptic ulcer may suffer a relapse when his daughter goes away to college, or when he overworks or eats unwisely. The cause of many gastrointestinal disturbances is debated by those who specialize in this field. The nurse must recognize that among many patients, particularly those with a gastrointestinal disorder, psychological as well as physiologic factors are etiologically significant.

**Functional Disorders: Interaction of Psychological and Physical Factors**

**Nursing Care of Patients with Gastrointestinal Tubes**

**Alternative Feeding Methods**

703

## FUNCTIONAL DISORDERS: INTERACTION OF PSYCHOLOGICAL AND PHYSICAL FACTORS

Of patients who consult a physician for gastrointestinal disturbances, those with a functional disorder far outnumber all others. The processes of eating and eliminating have many psychologic implications. Many important needs and satisfactions revolve around them, beginning in infancy and continuing throughout life. Food and love become associated, because the mother brings both to her infant as she nurses him. Dining is one way in which ties with other people are established and maintained. Mealtime is usually a time of being with friends and family, of talking and of sharing. In addition to satisfying physical hunger, eating a meal with others helps to fill the need for companionship and belonging.

The young child learns to modify his habits of elimination to conform to those of adults. This process, too, has many psychological meanings to the child as he strives to please his parents and in the process submits to rules and restrictions concerning habits of elimination and personal cleanliness. Some of these concerns persist throughout life, and they may contribute to disturbances of bowel function. The physical processes of taking in (eating) and eliminating sometimes have important, though unconscious, meanings to the individual. For example, vomiting may occur when the patient is rejecting some aspect of his life that has become intolerable to him.

Functioning of the gastrointestinal tract is affected greatly by the autonomic nervous system, which in turn is affected by the patient's emotions. For instance, it has been demonstrated that frustration and repressed anger are associated with hyperemia and with increased secretion and motility of the stomach. A variety of social, psychological, and physiologic factors cause the gastrointestinal tract to be a common area for functional disturbances. These disturbances can cause distressing symptoms, and yet they may not be accompanied by permanent pathologic changes in the affected organs.

Almost everyone at one time or another has experienced some of these functional disorders.

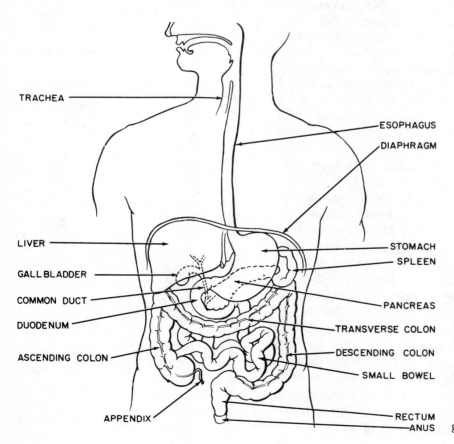

TRACHEA

ESOPHAGUS
DIAPHRAGM

LIVER

GALL BLADDER

COMMON DUCT

DUODENUM

ASCENDING COLON

STOMACH
SPLEEN

PANCREAS

TRANSVERSE COLON

DESCENDING COLON

SMALL BOWEL

APPENDIX

RECTUM
ANUS

**Figure 40-1.** Diagram of the gastrointestinal tract.

Commonplace are an attack of indigestion before an examination, a sudden loss of appetite before an important date, constipation or diarrhea during the first day or two at a new job. Usually these disorders disappear promptly when the tension and the anxiety are relieved. Some people are chronically anxious, or they become involved in situations that make excessive demands on their emotional resources so that their symptoms continue unabated. These individuals need help in differentiating the condition from organic disease, in providing symptomatic relief, and in coping with their tensions.

This section presents a systematic approach to the assessment of patients with a gastrointestinal disorder. The nurse may or may not perform all of the activities discussed, depending upon where and when she has contact with a patient and upon her role and her skill.

For example, in a health maintenance organization or other neighborhood clinic the nurse may examine patients to detect possible pathology, thus initiating the process of health care.

## Taking the Health-Illness History

History taking is a valuable tool. In many cases the information gained during an interview will form the basis for identifying the problem(s) and for guiding proper management.

Utilization of these data presumes knowledge of the disease processes; it is difficult to know which questions are pertinent, without this knowledge. However, techniques of history taking can be learned, practiced, and perfected as the knowledge of disease processes increases.

**Rapport.** It is essential that the nurse gain the patient's confidence and trust to get his cooperation and to facilitate communication. By demonstrating her sincerity, concern, integrity, and warmth, the nurse shows that she accepts the patient. These qualities are difficult to quantify and define; basically they are conveyed by a willingness to listen, avoiding value judgments about the patient's symptoms or illness. Etiology will determine management, but vomiting, regardless of its cause, will lead to the same fluid and electrolyte disturbances. Also, continued vomiting from any cause will lead to anxiety and emotional tension.

**Setting.** If possible, privacy should be provided during the interview. Some patients are reluctant to talk about their feelings, family problems, or bowel habits in the presence of other patients or of visitors. A lack of privacy may lead to questionable responses.

**Skill.** Certain skills are necessary to obtain a complete and accurate account from the patient. The manner in which questions are phrased may influence the response. Some questions such as "Tell me more . . ." and "What happened next?" require more verbalization than a direct question. "How are you?" may elicit a polite "fine," and "When did that happen?" may reap only "1939." If details are needed, direct questions to elicit details are useful.

The nurse should avoid "putting words in the patient's mouth" by describing a symptom for him. However, if he is having difficulty describing his symptoms, she can offer a selection of terms from which he may choose.

The nurse should avoid assuming that failure to state something means nonoccurrence; he may have forgotten it or dismissed it as not meaningful.

The patient should be encouraged to tell his story in his own words. However, the nurse must help make his terms precise and check statements with him to be sure they are clear and accurate. To one person "constipation" means not having a bowel movement one day; to another it may mean a hard, dry stool is passed two times a day.

### Biographic Data

Name, age, sex, race, occupation, marital status, family composition, and habits form a biographic sketch of the patient and provide important information. Some races are prone to certain diseases; some conditions occur more frequently in specific age groups; some occupations are more hazardous than others. That a patient appears older than his stated age, has just been through his fourth divorce, or one of his children has just had a serious accident, is significant.

### Presenting Problem

A statement of why the patient is seeking help or of his primary concern constitutes the presenting problem or chief complaint. This statement, in the patient's own words, provides the basis for the rest of the investigation. Sometimes no particular problem is stated. The patient may feel vaguely ill, and describes multiple symptoms and concerns.

### History of Present Illness

To elicit a history of the patient's present illness requires skill, patience, and understanding as well as the ability to help the patient focus on relevant information. He should be encouraged to relate his story in his own words, interrupted only when unavoidable. When he has finished, it is necessary to return to specific symptoms so as to describe them fully, according to the following.

Quantity. How severe is the symptom? Just annoying, or does it interfere with normal activities? Severe, moderate, mild?

Quality. Is it sharp, dull, burning, itching, throbbing, heavy, aching, and so on?

Location. Where specifically in the body does it occur? Does it radiate? Is it localized?

Duration. How long has it been experienced? How long does it last? Is it intermittent or constant? When was it last experienced?

Setting. Where does it usually occur?

Aggravating or alleviating conditions. Is there anything which usually brings it on? Anything that usually relieves it?

Associated manifestations. Are there other symptoms or alterations in body functions associated with it?

## Previous Health-Illness History

The patient's previous illnesses and injuries as well as his past hospitalizations and medical care may provide significant information. Some of his present complaints may be exacerbations of a pre-existing condition, or may be related to past injuries or surgical operations. Dates, name of hospital, and/or physician are requested so that records may be obtained to substantiate or clarify the patient's statements. Some of this information may have been acquired during the review of the patient's present illness.

Medications the patient is taking, whether by prescription or "over-the-counter," are important. Some people neglect to state that they are taking aspirin or vitamin pills, for example, because they believe these medications are not drugs. Allergies to foods, drugs, pollen, or other substances are determined.

**Social History.** In addition to biographical data, further information about the habits and life situation of an individual is helpful in understanding his problem or how he reacts to it. In some instances the patient may withhold certain facts until a future session, when rapport with the examiner has improved.

Sleeping and eating habits, the use of alcohol and tobacco, and recreational or exercise activities should be recorded. Ask about such symptoms as periods of anxiety, depression, anger and its fre-

quency, and measures used to relieve stress. Many factors influence responses. The patient may not remember exact dates or his memory, in general, may be poor; there may be a language barrier; the patient may be ill-at-ease or unable to describe his symptoms accurately. Some people try to please and may say what they think the nurse wants to hear. Or, they may say "yes" or "no" to all questions.

These factors must be kept in mind when evaluating and correlating the data. Perhaps the presence of a family member or an interpreter will be necessary to complete the history.

Interviewing a patient for history taking requires skill, patience, understanding, and the ability to develop rapport with him to elicit valid and useful information.

## Nursing History

The patient is asked about matters that bear directly on the present plan for nursing care. Significant are such matters as the response to previous illness and hospitalization, physical or emotional considerations that require adaptation in nursing care (such as fear of anesthesia, or use of a prosthesis that complicates postoperative ambulation). Personal habits that must be considered while the patient is hospitalized are also important, such as his preferred routine for personal hygiene. Attitudes toward visitors (or the fact that he is far from home and has no visitors) are important. Are there people the patient especially wishes to contact? What is his response to shared living accommodations with other patients, if his is a multiple bed unit? Does he wish to see a clergyman? If the patient is being treated on an outpatient basis, it is essential to inquire carefully about his living situation, his coworkers, and whether his home and work environments interfere with his treatment.

In addition to asking specific questions to acquire data, the nurse should allow the patient time to freely express concerns he may have, and allow him to select those he wishes to discuss. At this time patients often bring up concerns that are especially significant but not elicited during specific questioning to elicit factual data.

## Physical Assessment

### Mouth

As the orifice through which foods and liquids are ingested, the mouth is considered part of the gastrointestinal tract and is examined by inspection and palpation. A tongue depressor allows unobstructed views of all areas of the mouth. Good lighting is essential during the examination so that the posterior portion of the oral cavity can be inspected. The examiner should note abnormal breath odors, since these may accompany infection of the mouth and conditions of maldigestion. A foul odor may indicate oral or sinus infections or putrefaction of food in the stomach due to stasis from obstruction. Acetone breath is found with diabetic or starvation acidosis. Severe liver disease imparts a musty odor to the breath. Drugs such as paraldehyde and chloroform, as well as alcohol, can be detected in the breath.

**Lips.** The general appearance, color, and skin integrity of the lips should be inspected. Note old scars and check them against the patient's history. Further information concerning them may be sought during the examination. Lesions, especially those of the lower lip where carcinoma is most common, should be investigated.

**Teeth and Gingiva.** Disorders of the teeth and gingiva may cause or reflect systemic changes; caries may be associated with systemic manifestations and malocclusion may hamper the ingestion of food, leading to malnutrition.

If the patient wears dentures, these should be removed before the gingiva are inspected. Bleeding from the gingiva is common and may represent the only source of blood expectorated.

*Gingivitis* is infection of the gums and, if untreated, may lead to *pyorrhea*. In adults the gingiva naturally recede. When gingivitis is accompanied by pyorrhea, the gums may recede to the extent the teeth fall out.

**Tongue.** The dorsum of the tongue is inspected first. The color and size of the papillae are noted. The tongue may be coated, but this is usually due to diet and habits, such as smoking or poor oral hygiene, rather than to disease. Be aware of the range of appearance of normal tongues.

The ventral surface is inspected for lesions or tumors, as most tongue malignancies originate here and then invade the dorsum.

The tongue is then gently palpated for tumors not apparent on inspection.

**Buccal Mucosa and Palate.** The oral mucosa and the soft and hard palates are inspected. Ulcerative lesions and fungal infections of these structures are common and will be discussed in Chapter 41.

## Abdomen

The abdomen is examined by inspection, auscultation, palpation, and percussion. It is useful to divide the abdomen into topographical areas to gain a picture of underlying structures. Usually the abdomen is divided into quadrants by a vertical line

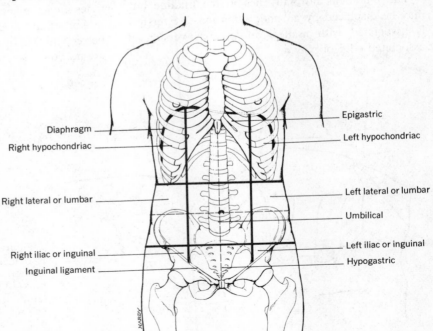

**Figure 40-2.** The four quadrants (dotted lines) and the nine regions (solid lines) of the abdomen with underlying structures.

Diaphragm
Right hypochondriac
Right lateral or lumbar
Right iliac or inguinal
Inguinal ligament

Epigastric
Left hypochondriac
Left lateral or lumbar
Umbilical
Left iliac or inguinal
Hypogastric

that extends from the xiphoid process to the symphysis pubis and a horizontal line that bisects the umbilicus. To achieve greater accuracy the abdomen is further divided into nine areas. Visualize underlying structures while examining the abdomen (Fig. 40-2).

**Inspection.** To inspect the patient's abdomen have him lie supine with his arms in a comfortable position but away from his abdomen. Raise his head on a small pillow and have him flex his knees to relax, so that the abdominal muscles are not contracted and rigid. Draping the patient adds to his comfort and preserves his modesty. The abdomen is exposed from the sternum to the pubis, leaving the breasts and pelvic area covered. Good lighting is essential for the examination. A movable light source provides oblique views that emphasize minimal changes in contour and is preferred. The light should shine across and level with the abdomen. Symmetry and contour of the abdomen are noted. Masses or hernias may be visible, if the abdomen is inspected from the sides as well as from above, and are explored further by palpation. The abdomen may be flat, depressed, or distended and may reflect the patient's nutritional state.

Visible peristaltic contractions are associated with obstruction of the bowel in the presence of a distended abdomen.

The umbilicus normally lies in the midline but may be displaced by an underlying mass. Eversion is associated with ascites, and deep inversion is associated with obesity.

Distended veins are present when liver disease is accompanied by obstruction of the portal circulation.

Changes in hair distribution may reflect disorders of the liver or endocrine glands.

The skin should be similar to that elsewhere on the body. Some conditions that may be observed and should be noted include: striae, visible streaks caused by rapid weight gain or endocrine disorders; rashes and petechiae; spider nevi associated with liver disease; abnormal pigmentation, as in jaundice or hemorrhage into the tissues; and scars, indicative of previous operations. The skin may be taut and glistening in ascites.

**Auscultation.** Auscultation should be performed before the abdomen is manipulated. If manipulation is performed first, the examiner should wait at least ten minutes before auscultating. Use the diaphragm of the stethoscope, applying only light pressure, to avoid compression and friction.

Normal bowel sounds reflect normal peristaltic activity at least every ten seconds. To appreciate the wide range of normal bowel sounds, it is helpful to listen to as many normal bowels as possible. A thorough knowledge of normal bowel sounds is imperative before abnormalities can be detected or defined. Increased bowel sounds normally occur postprandially or in anticipation of food. Borborygmus is a loud gurgling or rumbling sound produced by the propulsion of gas in the intestines. Sometimes it can be heard at a distance.

Abnormal bowel sounds are pathologic and must be recognized. In paralytic ileus or peritonitis there are no bowel sounds. One must auscultate all quad-

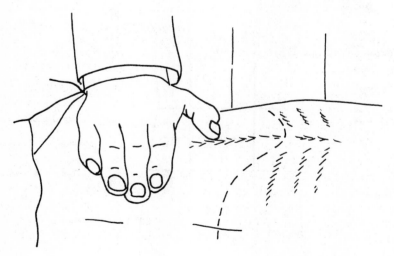

**Figure 40-3.** Light palpation. The palm is placed lightly but firmly upon the abdomen, and the fingertips are lightly pressed into the abdominal wall. The hand indents the abdomen, and care should be taken that the fingertips do not "dig in."

rants for several minutes before stating that bowel sounds are absent. *Tinkles* are high-pitched sounds associated with increased bowel activity and indicate bowel obstruction. A succussion splash is created by the movement of fluid or air in a hollow organ. This may be caused by an obstruction of the pylorus or a portion of intestine. This sound can be produced by jiggling or rocking the patient's abdomen.

Friction rubs are created by an inflamed or enlarged liver or spleen. They are soft sounds and must be distinguished from breath sounds or the friction rub of the stethoscope against the skin.

Bruits in blood vessels are also heard when the abdomen is auscultated.

**Palpation.** Palpation is probably the most important maneuver in the abdominal examination. The patient must be supine and relaxed, and the examiner should warm his hands so that the patient will not become tense. Assure the patient that discomfort will be minimized. If a painful area has been noted, avoid it until the end of the examination. Conversing with the patient helps him to relax and may elicit further information.

*Light palpation* with the tips of the fingers, barely indenting the abdomen, is performed first (Fig. 40-3). The entire abdomen is palpated in this manner, as the patient breathes normally and as he takes deep breaths. Areas of tenderness, distended hollow organs, and muscle rigidity are noted. Tenderness related to anxiety may cause the muscles to become rigid and this cause must be distinguished from involuntary rigidity due to irritation of underlying organs. To do so the examiner palpates lightly with the diaphragm of the stethoscope. As patients do not equate the stethoscope with pain, they will be more relaxed. To accentuate the rectus muscles and distinguish them from organs or masses, the examiner should have the patient raise his head.

*Deeper palpation* then follows (Fig. 40-4). This maneuver detects deeper tenderness or pain, masses, and organs not felt on light palpation. The palm and distal portion of the fingers of one hand or one hand placed on top of the other is used for deeper palpation.

**Organs and Masses.** An enlarged spleen or liver may be palpated. The examiner should stand to the patient's right to palpate these organs.

The liver is examined by placing the right hand on the right upper quadrant, and the spleen by

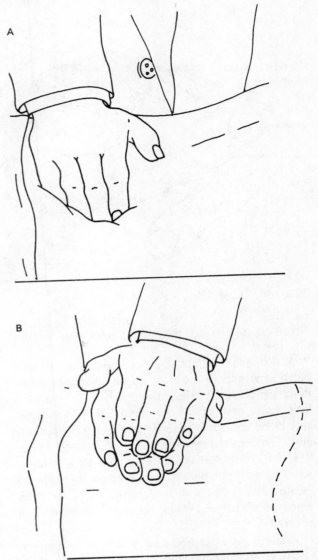

**Figure 40-4.** Deeper palpation. (A) Single-handed method in which the entire palmar surface of the hand and the fingers is pressed into the abdomen. (B) Reinforced method in which the right hand is placed as in the single-handed method, but the pressure is exerted by the tips of the left fingers on the terminal, interphalangeal joints of the right.

placing the left hand on the left upper quadrant and the right hand under the patient's left side. The patient is instructed to take a deep breath. If the spleen is enlarged, it will be displaced by the examiner's left hand and felt with his right hand. The enlarged liver will slide over the examiner's fingers when the patient breathes in deeply. Caution must

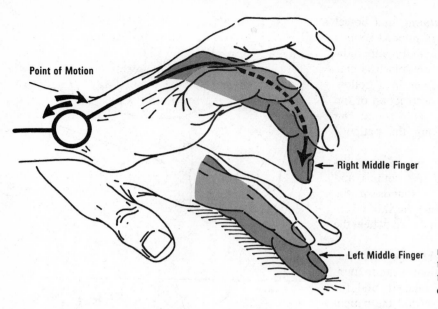

Point of Motion

Right Middle Finger

Left Middle Finger

**Figure 40-5.** Percussion. The middle finger of one hand strikes the middle phalanx of the middle finger of the other hand, using only wrist motion.

be taken not to overlook an organ that is so enlarged as to extend below the umbilicus or the iliac crest.

A distended gallbladder can sometimes be palpated as a mass in the right upper quadrant; stones in the gallbladder prevent distention.

A mass that cannot be identified as an organ should be recorded as to its location, size, tenderness, and consistency.

LOCALIZING AREAS OF PAIN OR TENDERNESS. After general palpation, an attempt is made to localize areas of pain or tenderness. There are three types of abdominal pain: visceral, somatic, and referred.

*Visceral pain* is produced when an abdominal viscus is affected by noxious stimuli. The pain is characterized as dull, poorly localized, and difficult to describe by the patient.

*Somatic pain* is produced by noxious stimulation of the peritoneum. The pain is usually more intense and is localized at the site of the lesion, as in appendicitis.

*Referred pain* is felt in areas thought to be supplied by the same neural pathway but remote from the affected organ.

REBOUND TENDERNESS. This maneuver confirms the presence of peritonitis underlying a tender or painful area located by palpation. The pain is felt after the examiner applies pressure over an affected area, then relaxes that pressure suddenly.

The patient's facial expression as well as his verbal remarks will confirm the pain.

**Percussion.** Percussion is performed by striking the middle finger of the dominant hand against the middle phalanx of the middle finger of the other hand which is placed over the part to be examined (Fig. 40-5). The sound thus produced travels into the abdomen and is reflected back to the examiner's ears and fingers. This procedure is less valuable and requires much more practice and experience than does palpation, but it does provide useful information. It is used to detect hollow air-filled or fluid-filled organs and to delineate borders of solid organs. A pattern for percussion should be established so that areas are not missed and comparisons can be made.

Air-filled organs are tympanic and resonant; fluid-filled and solid organs are dull. To assess the presence of free fluid a test for shifting dullness is used. The patient lies supine, the abdomen is percussed, and the area of dullness is marked on each side. The patient is then asked to lie first on one side and then on the other, and the area is percussed again. Any shift in dullness indicates intraperitoneal fluid.

Rectal Examination

External and internal examinations of the rectum provide important information about the patient and are too often overlooked or deferred. The examination can be performed with the patient in one of several positions:

Left lateral, with knees drawn up to the abdomen.
Standing, bending over a table or bed, feet slightly apart, toes pointing in.
Knee-chest, resting on knees and chest, not elbows, head turned to one side.
Supine, with knees spread apart.

As the patient cannot see the examiner and is usually apprehensive, he must be told before the examination that his rectum will be examined.

**External Inspection.** This is accomplished by spreading the buttocks and asking the patient to "bear down." The area is inspected for external hemorrhoids; fissures, a slit-like tear; and lesions secondary to scratching or rubbing due to pruritus ani.

**Internal Palpation.** A gloved, liberally lubricated index finger is inserted into the rectum. The patient should try to relax during the insertion; gentle pressure on the anal sphincter may help. Sphincter tone and strictures should be noted.

The examining finger moves in a circle, palpating the area. The normal prostate is firm on palpation. To palpate the rectum for tumors and polyps, ask the patient to bear down so that structures located higher up in the rectum become more accessible. Fecal material adhering to the examining glove is tested for occult blood.

## Diagnostic Tests

The need for specific diagnostic tests is determined from the patient's history and the findings of the physical examination. The purpose and performance of various tests and the role of the nurse relative to each will be described.

### Specimens

Samples of gastric contents and secretions, stool, tissue, or fluid from the gastrointestinal tract as well as blood or serum are collected and submitted for analysis.

**Gastrointestinal Analysis.** A nasogastric or orogastric tube is inserted to collect gastric or intestinal contents for analysis. (Further details are given on pp. 716 to 718.) There are various types of tubes available that can be used for this purpose.

TYPES OF TUBES. A Levin tube is used most often for gastric analysis (Fig. 40-6). It is a rubber or plastic tube that has holes or "eyes" in several locations near its tip to permit aspiration of gastric contents.

A sump tube, which is a two-lumen tube, has holes in its proximal tip. The other lumen is open to the atmosphere. The sump tube has an advantage in that it prevents the buildup of negative pressure in the stomach so that the gastric mucosa is not injured by the suction.

An Ewald tube, or stomach pump, is similar to the Levin tube in that it has a single lumen with several openings at the proximal end. It is unique in that its diameter is large and it has a bulb on its distal portion to provide suction. The Ewald tube is passed through the mouth and used to quickly withdraw large volumes of gastric contents, for example, when the patient has swallowed a harmful substance.

A Dreiling tube is a double lumen tube that is used for pancreatic function tests. One lumen is placed in the stomach and connected to a suction

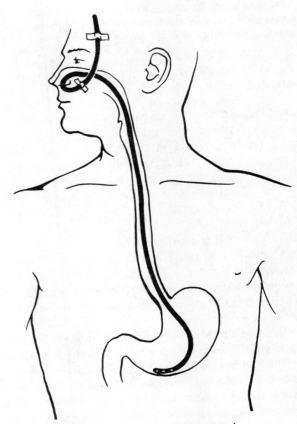

**Figure 40-6.** A Levin tube in place.

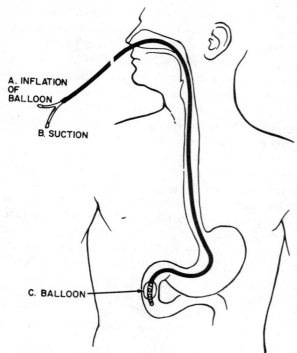

A. INFLATION OF BALLOON

B. SUCTION

C. BALLOON

**Figure 40-7.** A Miller-Abbott tube in place. It is advanced through the intestines to the prescribed point. The Miller-Abbott tube has a double lumen. (A) Portion of the metal tip leading to the balloon. (B) Portion of the metal tip leading to the lumen that can be suctioned. (C) Balloon inflated with air.

machine; the other is advanced into the duodenum where samples are also aspirated.

A Rehfuss tube is a single lumen tube which terminates in a small metal bulb with vertical slits. It is used for gastric or duodenal aspiration.

The Miller-Abbott and Cantor tubes are long tubes for intestinal use (Figs. 40-7 and 40-8). The Miller-Abbott tube has two lumina, one of which ends in a small collapsible balloon. The other lumen has "eyes" at its tip. When the balloon has passed through the pylorus, it is inflated with air, and then propelled along the intestinal tract by peristalsis. The intestinal contents are aspirated through the holes.

Because the Miller-Abbott tube has two lumina, each with a separate opening, it is very important to differentiate between them. The adapter at the end of the tube has two openings, one marked "suction" and the other leading to the balloon. The balloon should never be connected to suction or used for irrigation. Labeling the lumina with tape helps to distinguish between them.

The Cantor tube has one lumen with a sealed rubber bag, into which mercury is injected with a needle and syringe before the tube is inserted. The weight of the mercury helps to propel the tube along the intestinal tract. The bag is elongated when the tube is inserted so that it can be passed more easily and with little discomfort.

PROCEDURES FOR GASTRIC ANALYSES. There are many procedures for removing samples for gastric analysis. These are performed after the patient has fasted for 10 to 12 hours to be sure his stomach is empty. All medications affecting gastric secretions are withheld for at least 24 hours before the test. Basal secretion of gastric acid is assessed from specimens collected at 15-minute intervals for at least one hour, after the stomach has been completely emptied. The volume of this aspirate is noted. At times the nurse will be responsible for collecting these specimens. They are aspirated with a syringe and all gastric juice that can be obtained is deposited in appropriately labeled containers, after the volume of each is recorded.

The aspirate should be examined for bile or blood. If bile is noted, the tube may have entered the duodenum and should be readjusted. If bile is still obtained, the location of the tube is checked by fluoroscopy. The presence of a small amount of blood may be due to the trauma of insertion. If the bleeding persists, the test is postponed and the site of bleeding determined. Basal secretion tests are replacing the once popular 12-hour or overnight fast.

Stimulants that induce maximal gastric acid secretion are used. Histamine and betazole are the two stimulants used most widely in this country. Both have potentially serious side effects and the nurse must be knowledgeable about them and their use in treatment. Sometimes the nurse gives the prescribed dose and carries out the test; at other times the stimulant is administered by the physician but the nurse collects the specimens and terminates the test.

Histamine and betazole may cause hypotension, shock, pain at the injection site, dizziness, nausea, flushing, and headaches. Antihistamines are usually given prior to these drugs to decrease the severity of their side effects without decreasing their stimulant effect. Gastric secretions are collected every 15 minutes for two hours after injection and the patient must be observed frequently for side effects. The nurse must be prepared to administer epinephrine and intravenous fluids, should hypotension occur. New stimulant drugs, such as gastrin, tetragastrin, and pantagastrin, which produce fewer side effects, have been synthesized but have not yet been approved for use by the U.S. Food and Drug Administration. Since insulin can produce hypoglycemia, which induces vagal stimulation of gastric acid secretions, it is used to test the completeness of vagotomy.

The main hazard is hypoglycemic coma. The patient must be under constant observation and 50 per cent glucose must be available for intravenous use. Specimens are collected at 15-minute intervals for two hours.

The volume of gastric aspirate is recorded and aliquots are analyzed for gastric acid, electrolytes, occult blood, pepsin, bacteria, mucus, or intrinsic factor.

Secretin, given intravenously, stimulates pancreatic secretions. Samples are collected through a Dreiling or a Rehfuss tube from the duodenum.

**Gastrointestinal Analysis without Tubes.** Diagnex Blue, an exchange resin, is taken orally and, in the presence of acid in the stomach, dissociates, is absorbed, and then is excreted in the urine, coloring it blue. This test cannot be quantified and is mainly used as a screening test for achlorhydria.

Stool samples are frequently examined and tested as an aid to diagnosis or to evaluate the effects of therapy. The nurse is responsible for collecting the fecal samples and must instruct ambulatory patients to use a bedpan or stool container when a specimen is required. Usually, only a small portion of stool is needed. Therefore, a tongue blade can be used to place it in a disposable waxed container, which is then labeled and sent to the laboratory. If the stool is to be examined for ova and parasites, or cultured, it should be taken to the laboratory while it is still warm and fresh so that the motion of living parasites can be seen through a microscope and bacteria are not killed. A hot-water bottle is often placed around the specimen box to keep the material warm until it reaches the laboratory. Samples or 24-hour specimens may also be examined in the laboratory for fat, their volume and weight measured and, rarely, their electrolyte content determined.

Stool is frequently tested for occult blood, using Hematest tablets or guaiac reagent. Directions for the test are available with the tablets or reagent. In many hospitals the laboratory technician

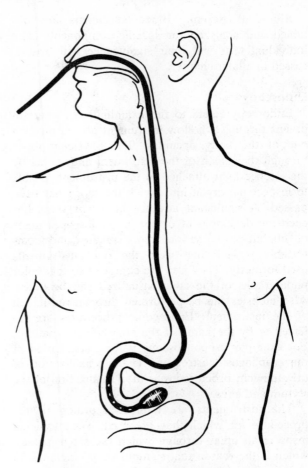

**Figure 40-8.** A Cantor tube in place.

performs these tests, although sometimes the nurse is required to do so.

The nurse must observe the stools and report any change in consistency, contents, or color. She should not hesitate to order or to perform a test for occult blood when she suspects blood in the stool and when the stool is free of contamination from gross vaginal or hemorrhoidal bleeding.

**Biopsies.** A sample of tissue from various organs of the gastrointestinal system and peritoneum is obtained for histologic examination.

A flexible tube with a light source and biopsy forceps, (see below) is inserted perorally or perrectally, advanced to the desired area, and a sample of tissue is obtained.

Biopsies of the liver, spleen, or peritoneum can be obtained subcutaneously with a needle.

Nursing care involves preparing the patient both physically and emotionally for the procedures.

**Blood or Serum.** Blood specimens are obtained and analyzed for specific components. The individual tests and their significance will be discussed in a later chapter.

### Endoscopy

Endoscopy refers to the examination of certain organs through a hollow instrument passed through one of the body openings. The physician looks through the lumen of the instrument and, aided by the electric light attached to the instrument, is able to inspect the organ into which the scope has been passed. A significant advance in recent years has been the development of flexible endoscopes made of fiberglass. These are more readily and comfortably passed than were the rigid instruments used formerly. They also are equipped so that color photographs of the areas visualized can be taken. Also biopsies can be performed through the lumen of the instrument. Endoscopic procedures are referred to by the name of the area being visualized. For example: esophagoscopy is the visualization of the esophagus; gastroscopy is the visualization of the stomach; proctoscopy is the visualization of the rectum and anus.

The instruments are named according to the procedure for which they are used. The physician inspects all areas through which the scope passes, which is the reason that sigmoidoscopy includes an examination of the anus, the rectum, and the sigmoid. The area of the gastrointestinal tract to be examined must be as empty as possible to permit effective visualization of the tissues.

**Helping with Endoscopy.** Passing a scope into any body cavity is uncomfortable and, sometimes, quite painful. Usually, it causes apprehension; tension and fear tend to increase the discomfort associated with the examination. Not only are these reactions distressing to the patient, but they make it more difficult to complete the examination quickly and successfully. After the purpose of the examination has been discussed with the patient, the nurse can help to allay his fears by explaining what is required of him.

### Esophagoscopy, Gastroscopy, and Jejunoscopy

Nothing is given by mouth eight hours before esophagoscopy and gastroscopy so that visualization of organs will not be obscured by food and the patient will not regurgitate as the gastroscope is passed down the esophagus. Usually, this procedure

is carried out in the operating room, and the patient is prepared in a manner similar to that of any other who is going to the operating room. For example:

- Personal hygiene is completed before the patient leaves the ward.
- Dentures, jewelry, and hairpins are removed.
- Patients usually wear turbans; hospital clothing is worn. Since the examination entails only the upper part of the body, male patients are permitted to wear a shirt and trousers.
- The patient is given the opportunity to void just before going to the operating room, so that he will not be uncomfortable or embarrassed by this need during the procedure.
- The patient signs written permission for the examination.
- Sedation is given as ordered by the physician.

A barbiturate, such as phenobarbital, and meperidine (Demerol), are often ordered one hour before the patient leaves the ward.

Usually, sedatives are sufficient for adults. Occasionally, if the patient is very apprehensive and unable to hold still, general anesthesia may be required.

After the patient arrives in the operating room, his posterior pharynx is sprayed with cocaine or tetracaine (Pontocaine) by the physician. This suppresses the gag reflex and lessens discomfort when the gastroscope is introduced. Five or ten minutes must be allowed for the local anesthetic to take effect. During this period the nurse can quietly explain further details of the procedure by staying with the patient and by conveying her concern gently. An emesis basin and tissues are provided so that the patient can spit out mucus and saliva.

When the physician notes that the gag reflex has disappeared, the patient is positioned on the table, and the scope is passed. The nurse helps the patient to maintain the position requested by the physician, so that the examination can be carried out quickly and successfully and the esophagus will not be injured by any sudden movement while the scope is in place. For esophagoscopy, the patient's head and shoulders extend over the end of the table; for gastroscopy, the patient lies on his side.

Brief explanations and encouragement are given by both the physician and the nurse throughout the examination. Physician and nurse should impart a real feeling of support throughout the unpleasant procedures. The patient should be given the impression that the procedure will be carried out as quickly and as painlessly as possible, and that any fear or discomfort he may show will be accepted, not condemned.

When the patient returns to the ward, he is permitted nothing by mouth until the gag reflex returns. Return of this reflex, which may take three or four hours, can be tested by touching the back of the patient's throat with a tongue blade. Usually, the patient is very tired and needs an opportunity to rest. Note any expectoration or vomiting of blood, since this may indicate injury to the esophagus. However, expectoration of a small amount of blood-tinged mucus is not unusual. When local anesthesia wears off, the patient's throat will feel sore. Assure him that this soreness will disappear gradually over a period of several days. Severe pain should be reported to the physician.

## Colonoscopy, Sigmoidoscopy, Proctoscopy, and Anoscopy

These procedures usually are performed in the ward treatment room, the clinic, or the physician's office. Enemas are given before the examination, since feces in the lower bowel prevent adequate visualization during the examination. If the enemas are not effective or all solution is not expelled, the physician should be notified before the examination is begun. Disposable, commercial enemas are used often in cleansing the lower bowel. Sometimes, the patient is instructed to limit his supper on the evening before the test to foods low in residue; for example, raw fruits and vegetables and whole-grain cereals would be excluded. Usually, the patient is permitted a light breakfast on the morning of the examination.

Of course, explanation before and support during the test are indicated.

Placed in the knee-chest position on the treatment table, the patient is draped with a fenestrated sheet. Show the patient how to assume this position before the test is started since it is awkward and some patients make the mistake of resting on their elbows instead of their chest. Some physicians prefer that the patient lie on his left side, with the head of the table elevated approximately 15 degrees; the thighs are flexed on the abdomen and the legs are extended. As the scope is advanced, the patient is asked to extend his thighs and legs so that they are almost straight. It has been claimed that this position facilitates visualization of the

rectum and low sigmoid and is more comfortable for the patient.

The physician performs a digital examination of the anus and the rectum first, using rubber gloves and a lubricant. The scope is then lubricated and inserted. To facilitate examination with the lighted instrument, the lights in the room are turned off and the shades drawn. While the sigmoidoscope is in place, the physician uses long, cotton-tipped swabs to remove particles of feces or mucus that interfere with visualization. The swabs are passed through the scope and discarded immediately after use in a waste container. Also, since a suction tip may be inserted through the scope to remove fluid, a suction machine should be available.

The nurse's role in these tests involves the following preparative and supportive measures:

- **Preparation of the patient—giving the enemas, explaining the procedure, and showing him how to assume the knee-chest position.**
- **Positioning and draping the patient for the test; observing and encouraging him during it.**
- **Preparing the equipment and assisting the physician (for example, turning the lights on and off, handing him swabs).**
- **Cleansing the anal region after the test is completed, and assisting the patient back to bed. Many patients can cleanse the area themselves when provided with tissues.**
- **Caring for used equipment; discarding waste, sending specimens to the laboratory, as ordered.**

*Peritoneoscopy* is a procedure in which the contents of the peritoneum are examined through a lighted instrument inserted through a small abdominal incision. A local anesthetic is usually all that is required. The procedure causes little discomfort and it may provide enough diagnostic information to eliminate the need for surgical exploration.

### Roentgenography and Fluoroscopy

Roentgenograms and fluoroscopy are very valuable aids to diagnosis, because with them the entire gastrointestinal and biliary tract can be visualized.

With an upper GI series or barium swallow and with a barium enema the upper and lower gastrointestinal tract are examined by fluoroscope and roentgenograms taken. Barium is a radiopaque, nonabsorbable, contrast medium. In studies of the upper GI tract, the patient swallows barium and its passage is followed fluoroscopically and by x-ray films. The speed with which the barium passes

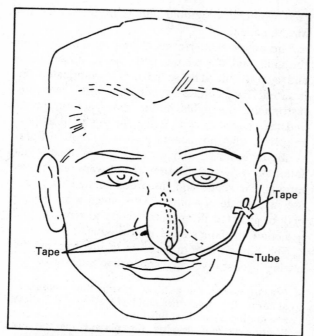

**Figure 40-9.** Preferred method of taping gastrointestinal tubes. The tape is split in two halfway up; the wide portion is secured to the patient's nose and the two split ends wrapped in opposite directions around the tube. The tape suspends the tube so it does not touch the skin of the nares opening. Thus there is no tension on the nares, and ischemia does not develop. The tube is then taped horizontally on the patient's cheek to promote drainage and to prevent obstruction of vision.

through the tract, the appearance of the organs themselves, and tumors or ulcers are noted.

The patient usually fasts after midnight, omits breakfast, and has a late lunch. The nurse checks with the x-ray department to find out whether the series has been completed before giving the patient anything to eat. Sometimes, he must return to the radiology department for additional films. The nurse must be sure that his meal is palatable because barium has a chalky taste which is sometimes somewhat lessened by flavorings.

*Cholecystography* and *cholangiography* are contrast x-ray studies of the gallbladder and common bile duct, respectively. The contrast medium for a cholecystogram is a radiopaque dye taken orally in tablet form. The patient then fasts until studies are completed. After ingestion, the dye takes about 13 hours to reach the liver, is excreted into the bile, and passes into the gallbladder, making it visible radiographically. If on two occasions, the gall-

bladder cannot be demonstrated, this is presumptive evidence of stones and/or inflammation. It is important to explain to the patient that this test is sometimes repeated, so he does not become needlessly alarmed.

Cholangiograms also utilize a radiopaque dye. The dye may be injected intravenously (intravenous cholangiogram or IVC), through a T-tube or by the percutaneous transhepatic approach (percutaneous transhepatic cholangiogram or PTC). IVC or T-tube cholangiography may be done during the operation to be sure that stones, which may be missed visually, are removed completely. PTC involves the insertion of a long needle through the abdominal wall into the liver. The needle is slowly withdrawn until bile is obtained, the radiopaque substance is injected into the bile duct, and filling of the biliary hepatic trees is monitored by fluoroscopy.

An abdominal plain film will expose calcium deposits in the form of stones or concentrated bile. The plain film alone usually is not diagnostic, and contrast films are used.

## Isotope Studies

Isotope studies involve the ingestion or injection of a radioactive substance specific to an organ, which picks it up. The organ is then "scanned" by an isotope sensitive machine (scintiscanner) and areas of activity and inactivity are mapped out. This technique is used most often for liver function studies and helps to determine nonfunctional areas and the site from which a biopsy should be taken. Pancreatic scanning does not provide the information gained by hepatic scans.

For the procedure, the patient is required to lie still on an x-ray table for one to two hours. He is usually not anesthetized for this procedure but must lie flat and still. To gain his cooperation and relieve his anxiety the nurse should instruct him about his role in this test and assure him that it is not painful.

### Inserting a Gastric or Intestinal Tube
#### EQUIPMENT
*Tube*

The intestinal tube is usually inserted by the physician. Its purpose will determine the kind of tube selected, its size, and length. The more viscous the material to be introduced or removed, the larger the diameter of the tube should be. If a tube smaller than that required is used greater pressure must be exerted to remove the desired volume. However, the size of the tube is also limited by the portal of insertion (nose; mouth) and the discomfort to the patient.

### Lubricant

Friction is created at the interface between the tube and the gastrointestinal mucosa. Lubricating the tube before it is inserted will reduce the amount of friction. A water-soluble lubricant should be used to prevent lipid pneumonia, should tracheal intubation and/or aspiration occur.

### Emesis Basin and Towel

Coughing and/or gagging may occur because the tube stimulates reflexes in the nasopharynx. An emesis basin and towel should be readily available to prevent the patient from soiling himself.

### Glass of Water

If allowed, the patient is given water to drink as the tube is being inserted to help reduce friction and propel the tube by the peristaltic action of the esophagus.

## SECURING THE TUBE

### Tape

The tube is secured to the patient with paper tape or adhesive tape. Gastric tubes are secured immediately after they reach the stomach. Intestinal tubes are only loosely attached until they have been completely advanced into the desired area. (See Figure 40-9 for the desired method of securing nasal tubes.)

### Rubber Band and Safety Pin

These are used to secure the distal end of the tubing to the patient's gown. Sufficient length of tubing is left to prevent the tube from being pulled as the patient moves or turns.

## DETERMINING PROPER PLACEMENT OF THE TUBE

### Catheter Tip Syringe and Stethoscope

Determining the location of the tube can be accomplished by quickly injecting 10 to 20 cc. of air through the tube while listening with a stethoscope at the cardia of the stomach. A "pop" or gurgling is heard with proper placement. This procedure is repeated if there is any question about the location of the tube.

### Catheter Tip Syringe

Another alternative is to aspirate for return of gastric contents. If gastric contents do not return on aspiration, it is impossible to determine the location of the tube by this method.

### Glass of Water

A third alternative is to place the distal end of the tube in a glass of water and observe for air bubbles at regular intervals. The relationship of the bubbles to respiration should be observed because gastric gas may mimic this. If the bubbling is continuous, the tube is in the trachea and must be withdrawn. If bubbling occurs in short spurts and is not related to respiration, gas is moving from the stomach.

## ESTABLISHING FUNCTIONING OF THE TUBE

### Infusing Apparatus

If the purpose is gastric gavage, a drip apparatus, infusion pump, or syringe will be needed to introduce the formula.

### Suction Apparatus

If the purpose of the tube is to remove material, a suction apparatus will be connected. The usual methods utilize a thermotic drainage pump or wall suction, which is continuous and should be used only with single lumen tubes.

### Clamp or Plug

If the tube functions intermittently, as with periodic collections of specimens or periodic tube feedings, it must be clamped or plugged to prevent aspiration of air into the stomach.

## PROCEDURE FOR INSERTION

### Explanation to the Patient

Explain the tube and the procedure for insertion. Explanation increases control and reduces fear of the unknown.

### Patient Position

The patient is then positioned so as to minimize friction in the nares and nasopharynx. Because of the structure of the nares, friction is inherent in passing the tube. If the patient is positioned so that the tube follows the floor of the nose, friction is minimal. The best nostril into which the tube should be inserted is determined by asking the patient about nasal injuries or by observing for septal deviation. The patient can be in any relaxed position, but sitting at a 45-degree angle with the head slightly backward facilitates movement along the floor of the nares. If this position is impossible, Sims' position is acceptable.

### Distance to Insert Gastric Tube

The distance a tube must be passed to reach its destination must be measured before insertion begins. Gastric tube length is measured by placing the distal tip of the tube at the xiphoid process, then extending the tube to the earlobe and across to the nose. This distance is marked with tape or with the fingers (Fig. 40-10).

### Insertion

Drape the patient's chest with the towel. The tube is lubricated and inserted into the nares,* passing it along the floor of the sphenoid. From the time the tube is in the nasopharynx until it reaches its destination, the patient is asked to take some water into his mouth and swallow it when requested. Advancement of the tube and the patient's swallowing are timed to occur

*The mouth may be the portal of entry for larger bore tubes or those used for only a short period of time.

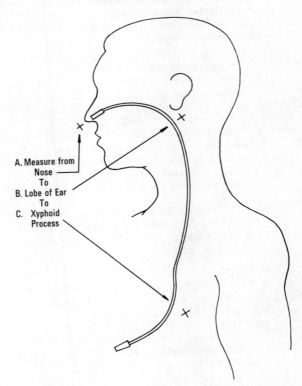

A. Measure from
   Nose
   To
B. Lobe of Ear
   To
C. Xyphoid
   Process

**Figure 40-10.** Proper measurement of gastric tube length.

simultaneously. The glottis closes and the trachea is covered so that aspiration is prevented. Also, swallowing is part of the first -phase of digestion, and stimulates peristalsis.

*Test for Proper Placement*

The tube is tested for proper placement, gastric tubes are secured with tape, and the distal end of the tube is attached to the type of equipment needed to accomplish the purpose of intubation.

## NURSING CARE OF PATIENTS WITH GASTROINTESTINAL TUBES

### MOUTH CARE

Since the nasogastric tube forces mouth breathing and the patient is usually allowed nothing by mouth, mouth care is particularly important (see Chap. 41).

### MAINTAINING PATENCY

Each time the nurse enters the patient's room she should note whether the suction is working. Intermittent Gomco suction machines are difficult to assess but aspirate should be visible in the tube and as it drips into the bottle. In a sump tube the aspirate will move constantly at the connection, and a glance can ascertain the patency of the tube. If it is not functioning, the following may be tried:

**CAUTION: On any patient with gastric surgery, esophageal stricture, or whose tube was positioned during surgery or who was difficult to intubate—Do Not Touch or Irrigate without a Physician's Order.**

1. If a sump tube, inject about 10 cc. of air through the airway.
2. If the above is not successful or the tube does not have an airway, disconnect and irrigate with normal saline. (Tubes can also be irrigated with air in this manner.)
3. Note amount and type of returns. If returns equal irrigating fluid, no notations are needed. If either input or aspirate is in excess of the other, it is charted as intake or output. (Of course if air is used, notations are not necessary.)
4. If irrigations do not re-establish function or irrigation fluid does not return, the tube may be lying against the gastric mucosa or it may be coiled up.

### ACTION

Loosen the tape and adjust the position of the tube (still connected to suction). A slight pull on the tube may dislodge it from the mucosa, and returns will be seen. Occasionally the tube must be manipulated further if it is coiled inside the stomach. If necessary, remove the old tape and resecure the tube.

### RECORDING

Accurate measurement of all intake and output of patients with gastrointestinal decompression is essential. Often the amount of gastric aspirate is replaced by intravenous infusion of replacement solutions. If regular irrigations or instillations are ordered, check with colleagues, so that a mutually understood policy is established. Some write each irrigation on the intake and output sheet, while others keep notes on a slip of paper at the bedside and the data are either totaled and transferred to the sheet or subtracted from the total amount of fluid in the drainage bottle.

### REMOVAL

When the tube is no longer needed, it is gently withdrawn. Keep the tube attached to suction while withdrawing, to prevent aspiration of gastric contents.

The nasogastric tube can be withdrawn quickly. However, intestinal tubes are removed gradually, several inches at a time. Some resistance to the removal of the tube usually is felt; the tube should never be forced. When the end of the tube reaches the pharynx, the balloon or the bag of mercury is removed through the patient's mouth. The remainder of the tube is then withdrawn through the nose.

Usually, a great deal of mucus is secreted, due to irritation caused by the tube. Be sure that tissues are handy, so the patient can blow his nose and expectorate. Mouth care is given after the tube has been removed. Soreness of the throat may persist for several days, but this gradually abates once the tube has been removed.

## ALTERNATIVE FEEDING METHODS

### GAVAGE

Gavage is the instillation of liquids (nourishment or medications) through a tube into the gastrointestinal tract. The tube may be passed through the nose or mouth into the stomach or it may be inserted through a surgically created opening into the stomach (gastrostomy), duodenum (duodenostomy), or jejunum (jejunostomy).

Introduction of fluids into the gastrointestinal tract involves moving the fluids from an area of greater pressure to an area of lesser pressure. The pressure gradient depends on the size of the tubing, the viscosity of the fluid, and the height of the column of fluid. The higher the column of fluid from the source to the intended site, the greater the pressure exerted. This pressure is due to gravity, and gravity is often used to insert fluid into the gastrointestinal tract. If the fluid cannot be administered by gravity, additional pressure may have to be exerted. This pressure may be manual, as with a syringe, or it may be created with an infusion pump.

*Preparation of formula or medication.* Depending upon the type of feeding being used, it might be necessary to refrigerate the nutrients prior to use. The newer canned, sterilized, formulas may be kept at room temperature. Formulas prepared by the dietary department usually require refrigeration to prevent spoilage.

Although some authorities recommend heating the formula before administering it, there is no evidence to support this recommendation. As heating is time consuming and can destroy vitamins and proteins, it is recommended that this step be omitted.

*Intermittent feeding.* Nutrients can be administered by attaching a syringe (without the plunger) to the distal end of the tube and slowly pouring the measured amount of food into the barrel of the syringe. The rate of flow is regulated by raising or lowering the syringe. The higher the syringe, the faster the flow. Continue to pour the feeding slowly into the barrel. Do not allow the barrel to empty. If it does, an air pocket will form in the tubing and air will be introduced. Flush the tubing with water and clamp the tube before all of the water flows through. Remove the syringe and wash out all equipment.

*Continuous drip feeding.* The formula is measured and placed in a disposable feeding bag or an intravenous bottle and tubing. The rate of flow is regulated with a clamp placed on the tubing (not the feeding tube), and must be monitored regularly as changes in the patient's position or settling of the formula may alter the rate. The formula and apparatus should be changed every four hours to prevent spoilage and bacterial overgrowth.

*Infusion pump.* If gravity is not sufficient to move the solution (i.e., the formula is too viscous or the tube is too small), an infusion pump may be used. The advantages of an infusion pump are that it provides a slow constant rate of delivery regardless of the patient's position when the patient cannot absorb larger amounts of feedings, and a smaller feeding tube, which decreases irritation of the gastrointestinal mucosa, can be used. The most commonly used is the Barron food pump.

One end of the tubing is inserted into a container of formula (this container may be placed in an ice solution to retard spoilage), the tubing threaded through the rollers of the pump, and the free end connected to the feeding tube. The rate of flow with this pump may be adjusted from 43 to 200 ml. per hour.

Dry medications can be crushed and mixed with a small amount of water; oil-based solutions flow better if warmed. It is preferable to administer medications separately, just before the tube feedings, rather than pour them into the bulk of the tube feeding.

*Patient position.* The patient should be in a sitting position or on his left side, with head elevated during the feeding and for at least 30 minutes after the feeding, to prevent aspiration and to aid in the gravity flow.

**It is imperative to determine the position of the tube before administration.**

*Administration.* Initially, tube feedings are small and frequent, with gradually increasing amounts and decreasing frequency. The amount of each feeding will depend upon the composition of the formula and the ability of the patient to digest and absorb the feeding.

Aspiration of all gastric contents before instilling the feeding determines how well the patient has absorbed the previous feeding. A syringe is used to aspirate the contents, which are placed in a graduated container to measure the amount of residual. Depending upon such factors as the amount of the previous feeding and the time lapse since the previous feeding, the next feeding may be postponed if the residual is above a certain specified amount. The aspirate is replaced through the tube to prevent loss of gastric juices and electrolytes.

Dehydration may accompany high-solute tube feedings with insufficient water. This can be prevented with adequate amounts of water in the tube feeding or by administering water after the feeding. The tube is rinsed with water after feedings to clear it, thereby reducing the medium for bacterial growth between feedings, but the recommended 30 ml. usually is not sufficient to prevent dehydration. It is the nurse's responsibility to assure that the patient is receiving sufficient amounts of water along with the formula.

HYPERALIMENTATION

Hyperalimentation is total parenteral nutrition. The solution, infused into the subclavian vein, contains glucose, vitamins, electrolytes and amino acids sufficient to promote anabolism and tissue synthesis.

This method of nutrition is indicated when oral or intestinal alimentation is not feasible for long periods or when the gastrointestinal absorption of protein or other nutrients is impaired.

Specific conditions found to benefit from hyperalimentation are: gastrointestinal fistula, chronic pancreatitis, dumping syndrome, intestinal obstruction, malnutrition due to cancer, peritonitis, ulcerative colitis, regional enteritis, intractable vomiting and diarrhea, gastrointestinal resection, anorexia nervosa, severe malnutrition, and paralytic ileus.

Since hyperalimentation fluid is high in glucose, sufficient time must be allowed for the patient's pancreatic function to adjust to this increased load. Therefore it is started slowly; the dose is built up while blood and urine sugar are monitored. Urine sugar and acetone tests are performed routinely, usually every four hours, while the patient is on hyperalimentation.

Septicemia is a potential and serious complication of hyperalimentation. Since the catheter is in place for up to 30 days and the solution is an excellent medium for the growth of organisms, strict aseptic care of the insertion site, tubing solution, and container must be maintained. The following is an example of an accepted procedure:

I. Change subclavian dressing every day.
   1. Remove old dressing.
   2. Cleanse area around insertion site with acetone for defatting.
   3. Apply an iodine solution for its antibacterial action.
   4. Apply an antibiotic ointment.
   5. Apply an occlusive dressing.

II. Change tubing and filter at least every 48 hours.

III. Do not use the line for anything other than hyperalimentation. (Do not draw blood from or give other medications through the line.)

Hyperalimentation infusions are discontinued gradually since rebound hypoglycemia may occur if the pancreas has been stimulated maximally. A 5 per cent dextrose solution is then given to allow insulin production to return to normal.

Similarly, it is possible for a patient to become hyperglycemic from a too rapid infusion.

Hyperalimentation is a lifesaving but potentially hazardous measure. It is becoming a common procedure in some hospitals.

Adapted from the Gastrointestinal Intubation Module by Nancy Hutchings and Wanda Avery, School of Nursing, University of California Medical Center, San Francisco. (Unpublished, used with permission of the authors.)

## REFERENCES AND BIBLIOGRAPHY

BELINSKY, I., SHINYA, H., and WOLFF, W. I.: Colonofiberoscopy: Technique in colon examination, *Am. J. Nurs.* 73:306, February 1973.

BUCKINGHAM, W., SPARBERG, M., and BRANDFONBRENER, M.: *A Primer of Clinical Diagnosis,* San Francisco, Harper and Row, 1971.

COLLEY, R., and PHILLIPS, K.: Helping with hyperalimentation, *Nurs. '73* 6:17, July 1973.

DAVENPORT, H.: *Physiology of the Digestive Tract,* ed. 3, Chicago, Yearbook Medical Publishers, 1971.

FOWKES, W., and HUNN, V.: *Clinical Assessment for the Nurse Practitioner,* St. Louis, Mosby, 1973.

PRIOR, J., and SILBERSTEIN, J.: *Physical Diagnosis,* St. Louis, Mosby, 1973.

SLEISENGER, M., and FORDTRAN, J.: *Gastrointestinal Disease: Pathophysiology, Diagnosis, Management,* Philadelphia, Saunders, 1973.

SMITH, J., JR.: *Essentials of Gastroenterology,* St. Louis, Mosby, 1969.

SPIRO, H. M.: *Clinical Gastroenterology,* New York, Macmillan, 1970.

WILLACKER, J.: Bowel sounds, *Am. J. Nurs.* 73:2100, December 1973.

# Patients with Disorders of the Mouth

## CHAPTER 41

## THE TEETH AND THE MOUTH

Some adults lavish dental care on their children, yet neglect their own teeth. Perhaps they believe that such care becomes less important when adulthood is reached, or possibly they feel that resources for health care should be expended primarily on the young. Although proper care of the mouth and teeth should be taught during childhood so that the individual can carry out similar care throughout life, many people have grown up without the benefit of such instruction.

Knowledge concerning care of the teeth has changed too, with the result that the instruction received by many adults when they were children is now outmoded. For example, plaque production is known to cause caries and chronic periodontal disease. Refined carbohydrates contribute to tooth decay by favoring the production of plaques, which must be removed daily to prevent caries and periodontal disease.

### Nursing Responsibilities

All too often, the patient's mouth is neglected in favor of other, more exciting or more obvious aspects of care. However, if the dangers and complications that arise from inadequate mouth care are recognized, proper care of the mouth will be given priority.

A painful mouth can lead to anorexia, which can lead to poor nutrition and fluid intake. All patients must be assessed for their ability to perform their own oral hygiene and be given instructions if it is not done properly.

Those patients needing particular attention and assistance with oral hygiene include:

1. Those with xerostomia (dryness of the mouth) which may be due to a number of causes: mouth breathing; anxiety; drugs, such as atropine, chlorpromazine, and propantheline; systemic dehydration, which may be caused by prolonged diarrhea or high fever; systemic diseases such as diabetes, connective tissue diseases (Sjögren's syndrome), chronic granulomas; therapeutic radiation to the head; and aging. Short-term xerostomia leads to oral discomfort, problems associated with wearing dentures, dysphagia, reduction in or loss of the sense of taste and, often, voice changes. Chronic xerostomia can lead to mucosal changes and dental caries, in addition to the effects of short-term xerostomia.

2. Those who are unable to care for themselves, including: those with neuromuscular or joint diseases that make it difficult or impossible for the patient to manage a toothbrush or to realize that mouth care is needed; patients who are confused or disoriented.

3. Those with mandibular or maxillary fractures, or with extensive oral surgery requiring specialized mouth care.

4. Heavy smokers are subject to oral irritation and discomfort and unpleasant mouth odors, and have increased susceptibility to oral cancer. These problems tend to be exacerbated by illness.

### Techniques of Good Mouth Care

The classic lemon and glycerin swabs and mouth washes are inadequate. The teeth must be brushed with a toothbrush in an up-and-down rather than a back-and-forth motion. Care should be taken to reach all accessible surfaces so that food particles do not collect and promote dental caries and periodontal disease. It is sometimes helpful to ask the patient to demonstrate the way he brushes his teeth and, if necessary, to show him how to do it more thoroughly. Dental tape or floss is used to clean between the teeth. A length of floss is held between both hands and drawn up between the teeth to dislodge food particles and plaque.

Next, the mouth is rinsed with plain water to wash out the debris. If the patient is unable to expectorate, his head is turned to the side and his mouth irrigated with water, by means of a large syringe, while a suction apparatus is used to remove the fluid. A waterpick, used with caution on alert patients, may be helpful for patients whose jaws are wired or those whose teeth are hard to reach.

### Dentures and Partial Plates

Dentures present a problem to many people. Often the necessary tooth extraction and the fitting of dentures are delayed, causing a severe emotional impact. The same reaction may be found in patients whose dentures have to be removed for a surgical procedure. Many people are embarrassed and distressed to be seen without their teeth. The nurse must use tact and understanding when working with these patients.

Usually, dentures are uncomfortable at first. However, if the patient persists in their use, he usually becomes accustomed to them, and they then cause him little discomfort. The cosmetic effect as well as the fit of modern dentures usually is excellent. Too often people remember the discomfort that their parents and grandparents had with dentures, without realizing that improvements have been made in their construction. The patient should report to his dentist any persistent discomfort that he experiences. Poorly-fitting dentures can cause ulceration and infection, leading to decreased food intake. It has been suggested that ill-fitting dentures may predispose the patient to cancer. There is little evidence to support this notion, but rare cases have been reported.

Dentures should remain in place by proper fitting and contact with the gums. Some patients prefer using denture adhesive for an increased feeling of security, but should adhesives be necessary to keep the denture in place, the patient should see his dentist.

Dentures and partial dentures should be scrubbed with a toothbrush. They should be removed periodically (some authorities recommend daily) to aerate the gums and wash out any debris that collects between the appliances and the gums or palate. When the dentures or partial dentures are removed they should be placed in water for protection.

### Gingivitis

Gingivitis means inflammation of the gums, which may be caused by inadequate toothbrushing, resulting in the buildup of plaque and calculus, ill-fitting dental appliances, or spaces between teeth allowing food impaction. Poor general nutrition causes decreased resistance and reparative ability. Gingivitis is first manifested by bleeding upon even gentle brushing or probing. It is treated by removal of all plaque and irritating factors.

### Periodontitis

Periodontitis is inflammation of the soft tissue and the bone surrounding the teeth. It usually starts

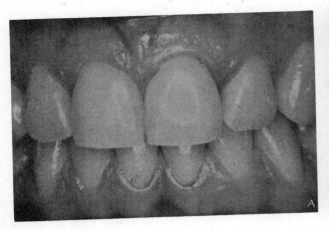
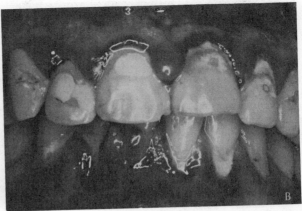
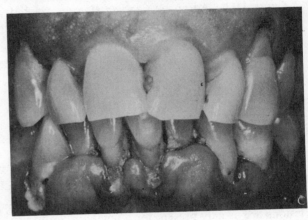

**Figure 41-1.** Progression of periodontitis. (A) Normal teeth. (B) Heavy calculus, edematous, and inflamed gingiva. (C) Retraction of the gums and further plaque buildup. (Courtesy, Gary Armitage, D.D.S.)

as gingivitis and, in a susceptible host, progresses along the roots of the affected teeth. It is characterized by retraction of the gums from the teeth, exposing the roots, and eventual loss of teeth (Fig. 41-1). It is diagnosed by thorough clinical and roentgenographic dental examinations.

The treatment of early periodontitis is the same as for gingivitis; in later stages or more involved cases, surgery may be required. If there is extensive involvement, teeth may be lost. In the United States this condition is responsible for the loss of more adult teeth than all other causes combined.

### Parotitis

Parotitis is inflammation of the parotid gland(s). There is one parotid gland on each side of the lower jaw just below the ear. Their function is to produce saliva. When parotitis occurs, it usually is caused by bacteria normally present in the mouth. Parotitis is especially likely to occur postoperatively and in debilitated patients. Eating stimulates salivation and helps to keep the mouth moist and in

good condition. However, when the patient's resistance is poor, when normal eating is impossible, or when oral hygiene is neglected, the parotid gland is more likely to become infected. Parotid enlargement is seen in the following: Sjörgren's syndrome and other forms of chronic sialadenitis, acute sialadenitis, virus infections, chronic granulomas, allergic reactions, diabetes mellitus, alcoholism with liver disease, malnutrition, hyperlipoproteinemia, lymphoma, and glandular neoplasms.

The patient with parotitis has pain and swelling on one or both sides of his face, over the parotid gland. Saliva does not flow from the affected gland, and often purulent exudate seeps from its duct. The treatment includes careful oral hygiene and antibiotics. If an abscess forms, incision and drainage may be necessary. Some physicians advise those patients who are not permitted oral feedings to chew gum in order to stimulate the flow of saliva.

Stones sometimes form in the ducts of salivary glands, preventing the flow of saliva. The gland enlarges and becomes tender. Sometimes, the stone

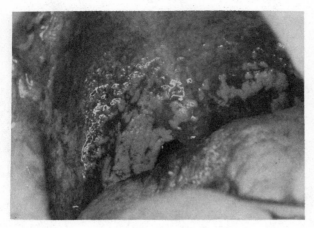

**Figure 41-2.** Advanced *Candida albicans*. Candida begins with one or two small white patches and is often missed at the beginning stages unless the nurse routinely and specifically observes for this condition. (Courtesy, Troy E. Daniels, D.D.S.)

can be removed with a fine probe; in other instances, an operation must be performed. It is sometimes necessary to remove the entire parotid gland if it is filled with stones, or if an infection persists.

*Aphthous ulcers* are small, white, painful lesions commonly known as canker sores. Their cause is unknown. However, emotional stress has been found to be closely associated with their formation. The lesions are usually present for a few days, up to two weeks, and regress spontaneously. No known cure exists and susceptible people usually have recurrences for years.

*Recurrent herpes simplex* is characterized by vesicular eruptions that become ulcerated, infected, and encrusted. It is commonly referred to as cold sore, fever, or sun blister. The herpes simplex virus lies dormant until activated by sunburn, trauma, gastrointestinal disturbances, or the common cold. No cure is known. Bland and protective ointments may help relieve the discomfort. The lesions usually heal in one to two weeks.

## IATROGENIC DISEASE

Iatrogenic disease is defined as that caused by medical therapy, and, in this context, medications. In some cases the offending drug may be discontinued. In many cases, such as epilepsy, that is not feasible and the iatrogenic condition itself must be treated and controlled. Nursing interventions include observing for and reporting the diseases and educating the patient.

Antibiotics used for a period of time will alter the normal flora of the mouth and may cause oral moniliasis, an overgrowth of *Candida albicans*, a fungus normally found in the oral cavity (Fig. 41-2). This condition is treated with a topical antifungal agent such as nystatin (Mycostatin). Mycostatin vaginal suppositories are effective. The patient should be instructed to allow the suppository to slowly and completely dissolve in his mouth; it is not effective systemically. (It is probably best not to tell the patient exactly what he is receiving as it may alter his acceptance of it.)

Aspirin, placed on the gum of an aching tooth, and *anesthetic lozenges* can cause marked irritation and inflammation of the oral mucosa. Patients should be warned against such practices and encouraged to seek treatment for the underlying cause.

Diphenylhydantoin (Dilantin sodium), in some cases, causes gingival hyperplasia. The patient is encouraged to practice meticulous oral hygiene and to seek regular dental care. Once the hyperplasia forms it usually must be removed surgically. In most patients it can be prevented from occurring or returning by the maintenance of careful oral hygiene.

## TRAUMA

Injuries to the oral cavity vary in their severity from a tongue or cheek bite to severe lacerations and fractures caused by falls, automobile accidents, gunshot, and so on. A blow against the teeth frequently cuts the mouth and lip and may break or knock out teeth. Trauma can also be caused by chemical burns, such as the ingestion of lye in an attempt at suicide.

Fortunately, tissues of the mouth heal quickly and are relatively resistant to infection. Whether this resistance is acquired because the mouth normally is in contact with infectious material, or because saliva has antibacterial properties is being debated.

Minor injuries, such as those caused by biting the cheek while eating, usually heal promptly without treatment other than good oral hygiene and the prevention of further injury. Frequent rinses with normal saline help to keep the area clean and reduce discomfort.

Larger wounds are gently debrided and closed with fine sutures. Every effort is made to prevent or to minimize facial disfigurement by carefully preserving all viable tissue and by avoiding marks from sutures. Infection and any interference with the blood supply are avoided, since these conditions impair healing and, in addition, could lead to a poor cosmetic result. For instance, dressings should not be so tight that they interfere with circulation. Usually, the patient is more comfortable with his head elevated, since the elevation minimizes edema and helps to prevent the dressings from becoming too tight. His dressings are observed for any evidence of bleeding or purulent drainage.

Fractures of the mandible are treated frequently with wires that splint the lower jaw to the upper jaw (Fig. 41-3). Wire cutters should be at the bedside and the nurse and the patient should know which wires to cut to prevent aspiration should the patient vomit. While edema of the surrounding tissues is present, the patient may not be able to swallow his secretions, so oral suctioning should be done at regular intervals to prevent aspiration. Alert patients are often taught to suction themselves. Elevation of the head of the bed promotes drainage.

Because the patient cannot chew, he is on a high calorie, nutritious, liquid diet, which he either sips or drinks through a straw. If he cannot sip through a straw, he may be fed parenterally or by nasogastric tube until he is able to take oral feedings.

Oral hygiene must be done thoroughly every two hours and after every meal. Often, the mouth is rinsed with normal saline to keep the area clean and to prevent unpleasant odors. If the patient is discharged while his jaws are still wired, he is given wire cutters and instructions on their use. Often, plastic and reparative dental work may be necessary after the patient has recovered sufficiently from the initial injury.

## MALIGNANT ORAL TUMORS

Five per cent of all cancers are found in the mouth. Yet, the cancer is frequently missed until it has become large or metastasized, because oral tumors often are asymptomatic early in their course. Numerous tumors are found in the mouth, most of which are benign. *However, only a biopsy can confirm or dismiss a diagnosis of malignancy.* The nurse should report any abnormality to the physician or dentist.

Malignancies can occur in any area of the mouth, the most common sites being the lip, tongue, floor of the mouth, and oropharynx.

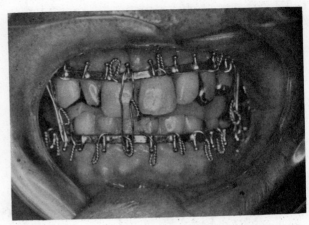

**Figure 41-3.** Jaw wiring. One method of mandibular fixation. The vertical wires hold the maxilla and the mandible together. They are the wires to cut if the patient vomits, to prevent aspiration. (Courtesy, Raymond Huebsch, D.D.S.)

The *etiology* of oral cancer is unknown but certain predisposing factors have been identified: the use of tobacco, alcoholic cirrhosis, jagged teeth, and, rarely, ill-fitting dentures. Those persons who overuse alcohol and who smoke excessively are at particularly high risk.

### Medical Treatment

Radiation is the treatment of choice for many oral carcinomas. Teeth may be extracted to expose the site. In some cases, chemotherapy and radiotherapy are combined.

### Surgical Treatment

The surgical excision of malignant tissue in the mouth may result in complete cure, provided it is performed early. Sometimes, surgery is so extensive that it is not only mutilating but may interfere with normal breathing and swallowing. For instance, considerable edema may occur postoperatively, leading to the obstruction of respiratory passages. A tracheostomy may be necessary during the postoperative period until edema subsides. (Care of patients with a tracheostomy is discussed in Chapter 28.) The patient may have to be fed through a nasogastric tube until healing is sufficient to allow him to swallow.

### Common Types of Operations

*Maxillectomy* is performed to excise cancer of the hard palate or lower maxilla. A silicone obtura-

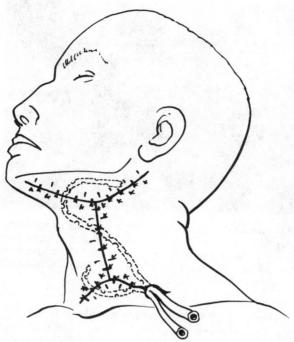

**Figure 41-4.** Diagram showing radical neck dissection. Note placement of drains under surgical flap. These are connected to suction.

tor combined with a maxillary denture is used to seal off the defect in the palate.

*Mandibular resection* is performed for cancer of the tongue or floor of the mouth. Prostheses and appliances are difficult to construct for repair of the numerous defects left by this procedure. Speech is altered, the patient may drool constantly, and severe facial deformity may result. Bone and skin grafts and plastic reconstruction, along with newer prosthetic techniques are improving the outlook for these patients. A therapist can help the patient to improve the intelligibility of his speech.

*Radical neck dissection* eradicates the cervical lymphatic network, thereby eliminating routes for the metastasis of oral cancer, and the primary site is excised. This operation is less mutilating than it used to be, due to advances in surgical technique. It may be combined with the removal of oral structures and the mandible in a procedure called a "combined resection."

A tracheostomy is usually not necessary, unless a bilateral neck dissection is done, but is always performed with a combined resection. Usually, drains are placed under the surgical flap and con-

nected to suction to prevent the accumulation of fluids (Fig. 41-4).

### Postoperative Care

When the patient returns from the operating room, ordinarily he is positioned flat, either on his abdomen or on his side, with his head turned to the side to facilitate drainage from the mouth. Suction is carried out to prevent aspiration of secretions postoperatively.

When the patient recovers from the effects of anesthesia, he is often more comfortable if the head of his bed is elevated. This position usually makes it easier for him to breathe deeply, to cough up secretions, and to help control edema. Coughing and deep breathing prevent postoperative pneumonia and atelectasis. Firm support of the patient's head and neck helps to lessen pain when he coughs. At first the nurse provides this support for the patient; by placing her hands gently but firmly on either side of the patient's head, supporting it to prevent excessive movement when he coughs. Later the patient is taught to support his head without help.

Bleeding on dressings, rapid pulse, fall in blood pressure, or coughing up of bright red blood should be reported. Expectoration of some dark blood is to be expected during the immediate postoperative period. The patient's breathing should be noted. The physician should be called immediately if the patient experiences respiratory difficulty or cyanosis. Equipment for suction, administration of oxygen, and the care or performance of a tracheostomy should be kept at the bedside during the immediate postoperative period.

A great deal of care and judgment is necessary in the administration of narcotics postoperatively, since these drugs can cause respiratory depression. Usually, the physician orders them in relatively small doses, and he requests that they be given only when they are essential for the relief of pain.

Old blood and mucus tend to collect in the mouth during the postoperative period. Unless the mouth is kept scrupulously clean, infection is likely to occur. Very unpleasant odors and an offensive taste in the mouth are distressing to the patient and those near him. Cleansing must be done frequently and with great care so as not to cause trauma or introduce infection. Sterile technique is used in some hospitals. In others, clean technique is practiced, based on the theory that sterile technique is not necessary because the mouth normally harbors bacteria and cannot be kept sterile.

Usually the mouth is irrigated gently to keep it clean. The frequency of irrigations and the type of solution to be used are ordered by the physician. Often normal saline is used as the irrigant.

To irrigate the mouth, turn the patient's head to the side and allow the solution to run in gently and to flow out into the emesis basin. A soft rubber catheter is useful for this purpose, because it does not cause trauma. The mouth should not be irrigated until the patient regains consciousness after surgery, otherwise he might aspirate the solution. Care should be taken to avoid wetting the dressings or the patient's bed or gown during irrigations. Place the emesis basin carefully in position to catch the return; do not allow too much solution to run in at one time and use plastic material to protect dressings and linen.

In most cases extensive pressure dressings have been applied immediately after surgery to lessen edema and to provide firm support, thus lessening pain. These dressings are bulky and cumbersome, and the patient often is greatly relieved when the dressing is changed and a smaller one applied by the surgeon, usually about a week after surgery.

Because the postoperative patient often is unable to swallow, he is given parenteral fluids immediately, followed by feedings through the nasogastric tube. When able to swallow, he is given small amounts of liquid at first, and gradually progresses from liquids to soft foods, as they are tolerated. The patient should be observed carefully when he first attempts to swallow small amounts of liquid. If he coughs and has difficulty swallowing, he should be suctioned immediately. Further oral feedings should not be given without checking with the physician. Some patients have had such extensive surgery that they continue to require tube feedings, and learn to carry out the feeding themselves.

## Problems

Communication with others presents a real problem to patients who have had extensive oral surgery. The patient's ability to tell others about his discomfort, to express his fears, to ask questions, or to call for help is impaired at the very time he needs to communicate with others. The Magic Slate is so useful that many nurses consider it standard equipment at the bedside of a patient who is unable to speak but can write. Merely lifting the plastic cover erases the writing and the slate is ready for reuse. Special care should be taken that the call bell is within reach at all times and that the call light is answered promptly. When surgery has been extensive, speech therapy may be necessary to help the patient learn to speak as normally as possible.

Changes in appearance often present extremely difficult problems for the patient and his family. Facial disfigurement and the use of plastic surgery are discussed in Chapters 56 and 57.

Specific points that may help minimize the patient's distress over his appearance after oral surgery are:

- **Providing privacy during his first attempts to swallow and to eat.**
- **Helping the patient to minimize the problem of drooling. See that he has plenty of tissues and tilts his head at intervals so that the saliva is directed back, where it can be swallowed. Sometimes a small catheter attached to low-pressure suction is used to remove excess saliva from the mouth.**
- **Helping him to pay extra attention to personal cleanliness and grooming. Clean pajamas, neatly combed hair, and a shave, as soon as the doctor permits, all help the patient to feel more presentable.**
- **Allowing dressings to be left in place longer than is absolutely necessary to cover gross defects until they can be corrected by plastic surgery. (This is sometimes done; often the decision to do so is reached after consultation between the doctor and the nurse concerning the patient's reaction.)**

## Complications

**Hemorrhage.** Large blood vessels, such as the carotid arteries, are located near the operative area. Serious hemorrhage may result when an artery is invaded by cancer and perforates or when necrosis follows radiotherapy. Discussion between physician and nurse is important in identifying which patients are most likely to hemorrhage. These patients should be placed near the nurse's station so they can be observed frequently.

If hemorrhage should occur, the nurse applies direct digital pressure over the bleeding point until the physician arrives. Another nurse, or even another patient, should be asked to report the emergency immediately.

The physician usually orders a narcotic to relieve apprehension. Transfusions are administered to replace lost blood. Often it is necessary to ligate bleeding vessels. The nurse's role involves assisting the physician to control bleeding rapidly and assuring the patient, by her swift, calm, competent care, that everything possible is being done to control the bleeding. After the bleeding has stopped, the patient is not only exhausted but also very apprehensive that it may recur. Visiting and observing him frequently are important to detect further bleeding and to assure him that his condition is being checked carefully. Pulse rate and blood pressure must be checked frequently.

**Respiratory Obstruction.** If respiratory obstruction should occur, an emergency tracheostomy may be necessary. Labored breathing and cyanosis should be noted and reported promptly. Pneumonia and atelectasis may be caused by aspirated secretions or blood. Suction, avoiding oversedation and depression of the cough reflex, and encouraging the patient to cough up secretions are important to prevent pneumonia and atelectasis.

## REFERENCES AND BIBLIOGRAPHY

DAVENPORT, H. W.: *Physiology of the Digestive Tract,* ed. 3, Chicago, Yearbook Medical Publishers, 1971.

NIEBEL, H. H., and KEOUGH, G.: Oral cancer detection, *Am. J. Nurs.* 73:684, April 1973.

REITZ, M., and POPE, W.: Mouth care, *Am. J. Nurs.* 73:1728, October 1973.

ROBINSON, C.: *Robinson's Normal and Therapeutic Nutrition,* ed. 14, New York, Macmillan, 1972.

SCHWARTZ, S., et al.: *Principles of Surgery,* ed. 2, San Francisco, McGraw-Hill, 1974.

SCOPP, I.: *Oral Medicine,* St. Louis, Mosby, 1973.

SMITH, J. N., JR.: *Essentials of Gastroenterology,* St. Louis, Mosby, 1969.

SPIRO, H. M.: *Clinical Gastroenterology,* New York, Macmillan, 1970.

# Patients with Disorders of the Esophagus

Disorders of the esophagus are characterized by a variety of symptoms and may be caused by, or may be the cause of, various conditions. For example, esophageal varices are associated with portal hypertension (see Chap. 46), while an inability to swallow leads to malnutrition.

## SYMPTOMS AND DEFINITIONS

### Dysphagia

Dysphagia is defined as difficulty in swallowing and may be physiologic or psychogenic. The usual description given by the patient is that something has lodged in his throat. When dysphagia is associated with actual food swallowing, it must be investigated. A similar complaint in the absence of food swallowing is termed *globus hystericus.*

Dysphagia may be caused by a motor dysfunction, abnormalities in the sphincter, or the presence of a stricture or tumor. The way in which the patient relieves his dysphagia is of diagnostic importance. For example, does he throw his head back, drink water, or eat alone?

### Heartburn

Heartburn is a word used to describe indigestion or discomfort in the abdomen or chest. It usually follows overeating, the ingestion of highly seasoned or rich foods, or lying down too soon after a large meal has been eaten. Patients seek to relieve the discomfort by assuming various positions or by taking antacids.

729

## Belching

Belching, the expulsion of air via the esophagus, is considered an esophageal symptom, but it is usually due to excessive gas or air in the stomach.

## Reflux

Reflux or regurgitation is the return of solids or liquids from the stomach into the esophagus or mouth, without belching or vomiting. All of the above symptoms (dysphagia, heartburn, belching, and reflux) are common and are pathologic only when they are excessive or interfere with the activities of daily living.

## HIATAL HERNIA (DIAPHRAGMATIC HERNIA)

The esophagus and vagus nerves pass through a small opening (hiatus) in the diaphragm. When there is an alteration in the hiatus, the stomach and lower portion of the esophagus protrude through into the thoracic cavity (Fig. 42-1).

A sliding hiatal hernia is one that occurs while the patient is recumbent but disappears when the patient stands upright because gravity pulls the stomach downward.

## Etiology

It is believed that congenital or acquired shortening of the esophagus "pulls" the gastric cardia up through the diaphragm. Also implicated are muscle weakening, increased abdominal pressure from straining, obesity, vomiting, and trauma to the diaphragm.

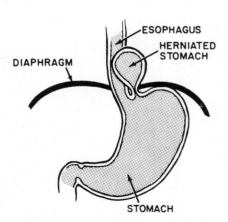

**Figure 42-1.** Esophageal hiatal hernia–paraesophageal (sliding) type. The herniated portion of the stomach protrudes through the diaphragm into the chest cavity.

## Diagnosis

Signs and symptoms include pain or heartburn when recumbent, which is relieved by an upright position; reflux causing sternal pain that may radiate to the shoulders and arms and may be confused with angina; dysphagia when the hernia is accompanied by esophagitis.

Diagnostic studies include a barium swallow with the patient in an upright and Trendelenburg position, and esophagoscopy.

## Treatment and Nursing Care

Medical treatment consists of relieving the symptoms and conditions causing the hiatal hernia to give it time to heal. The nurse instructs the patient in methods to alleviate or prevent symptoms. The patient should avoid activities that increase abdominal pressure, such as coughing, straining, bending. Medications may be given to control coughing and vomiting and stool softeners are given to prevent straining. Obese patients should lose weight. Diets are usually bland, with small frequent feedings and antacids to control ulceration. Meals are taken in an upright position to prevent reflux. The recumbent position is avoided; the patient may use two to three pillows at night; the hospital bed is in the reverse Trendelenburg; and the head of the bed at home can be placed on 6-inch blocks.

Patients who do not respond to a rigid medical regimen are treated surgically.

Surgical treatment involves replacing the hernia into the abdominal cavity and repairing the hiatus. An abdominal or thoracic approach may be used; the postoperative nursing care depends upon the approach used.

## ACHALASIA

Achalasia is characterized by a double defect in esophageal function: 1) the esophagogastric sphincter fails to relax, and 2) normal esophageal peristalsis is absent.

## Etiology

The cause of achalasia is unknown but is associated with disintegration of ganglion cells of the myenteric plexus or the absence of sympathetic receptors in the sphincter. Psychogenic factors have been considered because the condition sometimes follows severe emotional trauma or illness.

## Diagnosis

Signs and symptoms include dysphagia of both solids and liquids, substernal pain, and regurgitation. The patient may throw his neck and shoulders back to help food pass through the esophagus.

Diagnostic tests include barium swallow, esophagoscopy, and manometric pressure studies.

## Treatment and Nursing Care

The patient is encouraged to chew food thoroughly. The environment should be as calm as possible while the patient is eating. Some patients find that drinking liquids with food helps to increase pressure above the sphincter, forcing it open. Mild sedation about a half hour before meals helps to relax the patient.

**Medical Treatment.** Medical treatment includes dilatation of the lower esophageal sphincter with a hydrostatic or pneumatic dilator (Fig. 42-2). The patient is placed on a liquid diet the night before the procedure and given sedation before dilation is done. The dilator is inserted and positioned under fluoroscopy; the bag is inflated and left in position for 10 to 15 seconds.

When the patient returns to his room after the procedure, he will usually complain of some pain. If the pain is severe, the physician should be notified. The patient is allowed nothing by mouth for six to eight hours and vital signs are taken hourly during this time. Any temperature elevation or signs of esophageal perforation (sudden dyspnea, diaphoresis, tachycardia, severe pain) are reported immediately. If no complications occur, the patient is given clear liquids and gradually placed on a regular diet. If dilation is successful, the patient will be able to eat without dysphagia. Occasionally, a subsequent dilation may be necessary.

**Surgical Intervention.** Surgical intervention is performed if bag dilation is unsuccessful or if cancer is suspected. An esophagomyotomy, a sphincter-weakening procedure, is used most often. Slight pressure then pushes the food into the stomach. This may also be accomplished by a thoracotomy or a laparotomy. Nursing care depends upon which approach is used.

## INTERRUPTIONS TO ESOPHAGEAL WALL INTEGRITY

### Lacerations, Perforations, and Ruptures

*Lacerations* of the esophagus may result from forceful vomiting, particularly in alcoholics (Mallory-Weiss syndrome). Symptoms include hematemesis; epigastric and back pain may or may not be present. Diagnosis is confirmed by esophagoscopy.

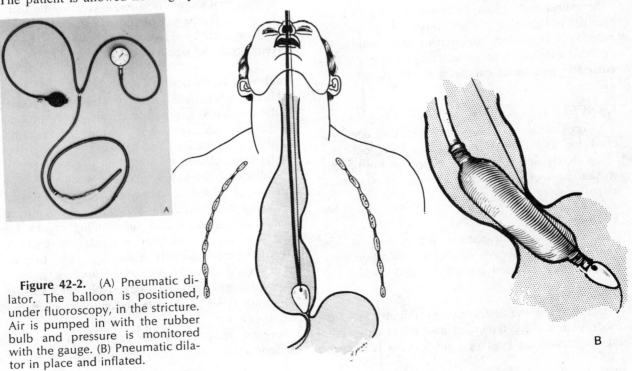

**Figure 42-2.** (A) Pneumatic dilator. The balloon is positioned, under fluoroscopy, in the stricture. Air is pumped in with the rubber bulb and pressure is monitored with the gauge. (B) Pneumatic dilator in place and inflated.

*Perforations and ruptures* may also be caused by forceful vomiting (Boerhaave's syndrome); by instrumentation, esophagoscopy, or forceful dilation; by automobile accidents; or by the ingestion of corrosive chemicals, such as lye or cleaning agents, either by accident or in a suicide attempt. Symptoms include those discussed above in relation to esophageal perforation. The patient may be in shock. Diagnosis is confirmed by esophagoscopy, x-ray films, and/or barium swallow, and must be distinguished from a perforation due to peptic ulcer.

### Treatment and Nursing Care

Most lacerations, when not very severe, will heal spontaneously. The patient is advised not to drink alcohol and to avoid foods or activities that precipitate vomiting.

Arterial bleeding and perforations are treated surgically. The bleeding site is oversewn and the perforation or rupture is closed. Postoperative care after a perforation or rupture is identical to that after a thoracotomy or laparotomy. In addition, antibiotics are given to control the pneumonitis or peritonitis that occurs with perforation.

Damage caused by ingesting caustic substances may lead to perforations or may heal spontaneously, depending on the length of exposure to, and the concentration of, the substance.

Strictures may result from the healing and are treated by dilation. When most or all of the esophagus is eroded, the patient may require an artificial esophagus or gastrostomy. These are discussed in relation to cancer of the esophagus.

## CANCER

Cancer of the esophagus is a relatively common condition and a discouraging one. Symptoms develop slowly and may be dismissed by the patient so that he seeks care when the cancer is already extensive.

### Etiology

As with cancer in general, the etiology is unknown. Smoking, heavy alcohol consumption, and familial predisposition have been implicated.

### Clinical Picture

Dysphagia is the first symptom, initially to solid foods, with a vague feeling of discomfort, progressing to intolerance even of liquids. Pain is a later symptom and usually indicates extension of the carcinoma. Weight loss, anorexia, and an inability to swallow even saliva are late but predominant signs and symptoms. Pain usually is not present but may be if the tumor has extended beyond the esophageal wall.

### Complications

The tumor may completely obstruct the lumen of the esophagus, leading to aspiration pneumonia. It may erode into the trachea, creating a tracheoesophageal fistula or it may involve the laryngeal nerve, producing hoarseness or muteness.

### Diagnosis

Radiologic studies are used and include a routine barium swallow. The patient may also be asked to swallow a barium-impregnated bolus, such as a piece of bread, and observed for specific areas of narrowing or strictures.

Cytologic studies are performed by inserting a gastric tube into the esophagus just above the lesion, washing the area with saline, and aspirating the material. This procedure is repeated in the stomach. If a barium test was done first, the cytologic test should be delayed a few days because barium abrades the tissues and might affect test results.

By esophagoscopy the lesion is visualized directly and a portal for biopsy provided. The bronchi may also be viewed by endoscopy to evaluate any involvement of the trachea and/or bronchi.

### Treatment and Nursing Care

Unfortunately, most of the treatments for cancer of the esophagus are palliative and rarely prolong the patient's life. However, the relief of suffering, dysphagia, aspiration, and choking is a goal and can be accomplished.

**Radiation.** Radiation may be performed as a curative or palliative procedure. The position of the lesion determines the feasibility of irradiation because the stomach and surrounding organs are very sensitive to radiation, whereas the thoracic structures are relatively resistant. This therapy results in a decrease of edema and swelling, relieves dysphagia, and provides marked although usually temporary relief. Even a five-year cure rate by irradiation is rare.

**Surgical Resection.** Surgical resection of the carcinoma is usually reserved for patients whose overall condition is good and in whom metastasis has not occurred. The lower third of the esophagus responds best to surgical intervention. Surgery involving the upper two-thirds is difficult to perform, and anastomotic leaks are common. These sites are usually treated with radiation therapy.

**Palliative Surgery.** Palliative surgery is sometimes performed to improve patient comfort. Rarely, the esophagus may be removed and replaced by a segment of colon; more frequently, a Mackler tube may be inserted. This procedure necessitates a laparotomy. The tube is inserted through a gastrotomy incision and passed up the esophagus until the funnel reaches the site of the stricture.

Semisolid food can be eaten but more solid food or large pills may block the tube. Patients are advised to chew food thoroughly or to grind or strain it before eating. They must remain upright, as there is no sphincter, and reflux is likely. When other methods are not successful, a gastrostomy is performed to provide a portal through which food can be ingested.

Gastrostomy is a relatively minor procedure. It can be performed under local anesthesia and can be done even if the patient is very weak and debilitated. During the procedure a catheter is inserted into the opening and secured to the abdominal wall by either a suture or adhesive tape. To prevent gastric contents from leaking, the end of the catheter is clamped except during the time the patient is fed. Leakage around the tube is extremely troublesome because gastric contents are very irritating to the skin. Dressings are applied to absorb any drainage around the tube, and must be changed frequently. The skin must be washed often with mild soap and water to prevent excoriation. Ointments, such as zinc oxide or petrolatum, may be applied to the skin to help prevent irritation.

Initial feedings through the tube usually consist of small amounts of tap water, with gradual increase to larger amounts, as tolerated. The amount of fluid and the frequency with which it is administered are specified by the surgeon. Once clear liquids can be ingested through the tube, feedings are started. The principles and technique are the same as those used with tube feeding through a nasogastric tube.

As soon as the patient is able, he is taught to feed himself through the tube. Problems of instructing the patient whose normal body functions have been modified by surgery are similar to those of any patient who has a stoma, and they are discussed in relation to the care of patients with an ileostomy or colostomy.

When sufficient healing has taken place, the gastrostomy tube is removed and inserted only for feedings. The patient learns to insert the catheter approximately 4 inches into the gastrostomy and to pour the feedings into a funnel attached to the end of the catheter. Usually, about 300 to 500 ml. is given at one time. Some patients feel uncomfortably full and even nauseated, unless the feedings are small. They must take their feedings more frequently to receive the total amount ordered by the physician. The tube and funnel are washed and rinsed thoroughly after each use. A permanent plastic "button," with a screw-in plug, is sutured to the abdominal wall to keep the stoma closed between feedings.

Many physicians recommend that the normal diet be converted in a food blender to a form suitable for tube feeding. Both liquids and solids are mixed together, forming a thick liquid; this is strained and then introduced through the gastrostomy tube. This method is considered desirable if tube feedings must be continued for a long period so that the patient's normal nutrition can be maintained, and his meals can readily be prepared at home. Sometimes it is recommended that the patient chew his food, just as he normally would, and then place it in the funnel so that it will pass into his stomach. In this way the patient may enjoy the taste of food, and his mouth and his teeth remain in better condition because he is chewing normally. Because this method of eating can be quite offensive to others and embarrassing to the patient, privacy is especially important.

It is very difficult for most patients to face the prospect of gastrostomy. Eating is one of the basic pleasures of life. Although nutrition can be maintained by gastrostomy, the person with one is denied the physical satisfaction of taste and the emotional satisfaction of companionship. It is the unusual patient who does not prefer privacy during this procedure.

## ESOPHAGITIS

Inflammation of the esophagus is usually caused by reflux of the acidic gastric contents of the stomach, but may be due to reflux of bile or pancreatic juice.

## Etiology

A hiatal hernia, carcinoma, prolonged use of a nasogastric tube, or any condition causing reflux may lead to esophagitis.

## Clinical Picture

Esophagitis is manifested by dysphagia; heartburn, which may radiate to the arm, simulating angina; vomiting; and, rarely, bleeding. These signs and symptoms are aggravated by lying down, bending, or stooping, and are usually alleviated by the upright position or ingestion of antacids.

## Diagnosis

Esophagitis may be a separate entity, or a symptom of a variety of conditions. Barium studies, esophagoscopy, and manometric studies are used to determine the underlying cause.

## Treatment and Nursing Care

Treatment is directed to the underlying cause. Nursing care is directed toward preventing the gastric contents from contacting the esophagus so as to diminish esophageal irritation. The patient is positioned to keep the esophagus above the level of the stomach at all times, even during sleep. This may be accomplished as discussed in the section on hiatal hernia. The nurse encourages the patient to avoid extremely hot, cold, or spicy foods, tobacco, and aspirin. Food should be chewed thoroughly to prevent mechanical irritation. Antacids are given to reduce gastric acidity in case of regurgitation.

## REFERENCES AND BIBLIOGRAPHY

DAVENPORT, H. W.: *Physiology of the Digestive Tract,* ed. 3, Chicago, Yearbook Medical Publishers, 1971.

ROBINSON, C.: *Normal and Therapeutic Nutrition,* ed. 14, New York, Macmillan, 1972.

SCHWARTZ, S., et al.: *Principles of Surgery,* ed. 2, San Francisco, McGraw-Hill, 1974.

SLEISENGER, M., and FORDTRAN, J.: *Gastrointestinal Disease: Pathophysiology, Diagnosis, Management,* Philadelphia, Saunders, 1973.

SMITH, J. N., JR.: *Essentials of Gastroenterology,* St. Louis, Mosby, 1969.

SPIRO, H. M.: *Clinical Gastroenterology,* New York, Macmillan, 1970.

# Patients with Disorders of the Stomach and Duodenum

The stomach and duodenum are considered together because of their close proximity, duodenal control of gastric secretion and motility, and common conditions affecting both.

## SYMPTOMS, DEFINITIONS, AND CARE

### Nausea and Vomiting

Nausea is a feeling of wanting to vomit. It is accompanied by increased salivation, perspiration, and tearing of the eyes. It may be produced by psychogenic responses to unpleasant or disgusting experiences or by thoughts of them. Noxious smells or sights may also cause nausea. It is stimulated by many drugs, diseases of the gastrointestinal tract, and some systemic diseases.

Vomiting often closely follows nausea. It is the forceful expulsion of gastric (and sometimes duodenal) contents through the mouth. Vomiting is accompanied by an increase in abdominal pressure, which may lead to wound dehiscence and, as mentioned before, lacerations of the esophagus; bradycardia, due to vagal stimulation; and, if prolonged, to fluid and electrolyte disturbances. Aspiration of the vomitus can also occur.

Vomiting is also a valuable diagnostic aid that should be observed and reported, utilizing the seven characteristics of a symptom, as outlined in the section on assessment of the patient. Vomiting may be a transient act or a manifestation of a serious underlying condition.

Nursing care centers on preventing vomiting by removing the stimulus, administering antiemetics, evaluating fluid and electrolyte loss, preventing aspiration, providing oral hygiene, and cleaning the area.

The nurse's actions, such as holding the patient's head, can convey support at a time when lack of control and acute discomfort are experienced. Vomiting may be accompanied by other distressing symptoms, such as diarrhea and syncope. Severe or repeated attacks of vomiting can lead the patient to feel helpless and anxious.

### Anorexia

Anorexia is the lack of desire to eat foods not previously disliked. It may be transient. Almost everyone has had a sudden loss of appetite before an important appointment, or when he has a cold. Anorexia may also be the cause of more serious underlying pathology and if food intake is reduced, will ultimately lead to weakness, weight loss, and nutritional deficiency.

Some patients have difficulty swallowing food; they may feel that food sticks in the throat and will not go down. Frequently, no structural abnormality of the esophagus is found; however, it is noted that the patient has severe emotional problems. He may gradually eliminate most solid foods from the diet and may become malnourished.

Some patients constantly feel as though a lump was in the throat, which may make them feel continually uncomfortable, particularly at mealtime. When the condition is psychogenic, it is called *globus hystericus*. The sensation is similar to that of a lump in the throat.

Anorexia nervosa is a severe disorder in which the patient has a true aversion to food. The condition is most often found in women, and usually begins during young adulthood. Anorexia nervosa is related to profound emotional problems. There are many theories concerning causation, one of which is that it may be related to difficulties associated with assuming the adult role. Emaciation often is extreme and is accompanied by a variety of symptoms, such as nausea, abdominal pain, and amenorrhea. Treatment includes psychotherapy and painstaking help in restoring normal nutrition. It often takes years and is not always successful. Sometimes, the person is ill for a long time, and may be hospitalized periodically. Nursing care requires much tact and patience. Although the nurse's first impulse might be to try to force the patient to eat in order to "put some meat on the bones," this method often succeeds only in making the patient vomit. It also leads to antagonism and distrust between nurse and patient. For example, pressuring the patient to eat may cause her to dispose of the food down the toilet when the nurse is not looking.

### Nursing Care

The following suggestions may be practiced when dealing with patients who have functional anorexia, nausea, or vomiting:

- **Help the patient to avoid emotional upsets at mealtime. Make a special effort to avoid scheduling painful or upsetting procedures at this time.**
- **Avoid focusing constant attention on how much the patient eats. Observe unobtrusively what he eats so that you can keep informed, and yet avoid making the patient feel that someone is counting every mouthful.**
- **If the situation permits, arrange for the patient to eat with others who are up and about, perhaps by setting a table in the solarium. Ambulatory patients may take their meals in the dining room. Pleasant conversation with others, and cheerful surroundings that do not remind the patient constantly of illness, are often very effective. A friendly chat with the nurse at mealtime may put the patient at ease.**
- **Avoid blaming the patient for not eating. When he is having particular difficulty with meals, make a special effort to spend time with him and let him express some of his feelings. Diversion is important too—a trip to the lounge for a game of cards or to watch television. Notice fluctuations in the patient's appetite and any situations that seem to precipitate them.**
- **Work with the dietitian to see that the patient is served the foods that tempt his appetite. Be sure they are served attractively and in very small portions.**
- **If you know that a particular food or meal may be especially difficult for the patient (for example, a patient who has difficulty swallowing and is trying to eat solid food for the first time in days), remain nearby, so that he knows you are ready to help.**
- **Avoid suggesting to the patient that any particular kind of food makes him sick. In most cases it is not the food, but the patient's reaction to it that is causing the difficulty. Some are very likely to blame the last food eaten for their symptoms and gradually restrict their diets to very few foods. Encourage the patient (without pressuring) to try new things served to him.**

## GASTRITIS

Gastritis is an inflammation of the gastric mucosa. It is caused by anything that irritates the mucosa and is defined as acute or chronic, depending upon the etiologic agent and the time it takes for the symptoms to occur.

## Acute Gastritis

### Etiology

There are numerous drugs, substances, and conditions associated with acute gastritis. Most people are familiar with the nausea, vomiting, and pain associated with excessive alcohol ingestion. This is caused by the direct effect of alcohol on the mucosa. Aspirin and phenylbutazone (Butazolidin) are well-documented causes of gastritis. The ingestion of hot liquids has been implicated. Emotional stress that increases gastric acidity and bile reflux damages the gastric mucosa.

### Clinical Features

Acute gastritis may be asymptomatic or it may cause epigastric pain, nausea, and vomiting. The damaged mucosa may bleed.

Diagnosis is based on symptoms and gastroscopic findings. The mucosa is edematous and hyperemic, with erosions; hemorrhagic spots may be visible.

### Treatment and Nursing Care

Acute gastritis usually subsides spontaneously. Food and fluids are withheld until the acute symptoms have subsided. Bleeding may be stopped by an iced saline lavage. The iced normal saline is injected through a nasogastric tube and then aspirated. The returns become progressively more clear as the bleeding is controlled. If control is not established, surgery may be necessary. Vagotomy and pyloroplasty or gastroenterostomy are usually performed. These are discussed below.

Medications may be given to control the vomiting. Intravenous infusions may be administered to correct fluid and electrolyte imbalances.

After the acute episode, the patient may resume oral intake. Frequent bland meals should be given initially, with the patient progressively resuming a normal diet, as tolerated. He is taught to avoid aspirin, alcohol, phenylbutazone, and other agents or activities that may cause acute gastritis.

## Chronic Gastritis

### Etiology

There is no evidence that chronic gastritis arises from the same factors as acute gastritis, or that chronic gastritis arises from acute gastritis. Endocrine disorders, such as diabetes mellitus, thyroid disease, and Addison's disease; nutritional disorders, such as ulcerative colitis; chronic infection; and rheumatoid arthritis have been implicated. Chronic superficial gastritis, characterized by involvement of the superficial epithelium, has no clinical significance other than that some believe it progresses to atrophic gastritis. This condition is significant in that the functioning cells progressively atrophy and cease to produce secretions and mucus. There may be a vitamin $B_{12}$ deficiency due to lack of intrinsic factor.

Diagnosis is reached by gastroscopy and microscopic examination of the mucosa. Carcinoma must be ruled out.

### Treatment

Treatment is symptomatic, eliminating factors that seem to precipitate attacks, and, if a specific etiologic factor is discovered, such as vitamin $B_{12}$ deficiency, specific therapy is instituted.

## PEPTIC ULCER

A peptic ulcer is a circumscribed loss of tissue in the gastrointestinal tract due to contact with hydrochloric acid and pepsin (see Plate 2). Most peptic ulcers occur in the duodenum (duodenal ulcers). However, they may occur at the lower end of the esophagus, the stomach (gastric ulcer), or in the jejunum, after the patient has had an anastomosis between stomach and jejunum.

### Etiology

Peptic ulcer formation is dependent upon two conditions that occur simultaneously: (1) the presence of gastric acid and pepsin, and (2) decreased mucosal resistance to the acid and pepsin. Various conditions, drugs, or situations cause either an increase in gastric acid production or a decrease in mucosal resistance. The most commonly accepted factors in the formation of a peptic ulcer are discussed below.

### Psychogenic

Emotional tension, particularly repressed anger, frustration, and aggression, has been cited as predisposing to peptic ulcers. Whether this leads to an increased acid-pepsin secretion or reduction in mucosal resistance, or both, is not clear. Some say that insomnia, fatigue, and increased smoking caused by emotional stress are the etiologic factors, rather than the emotional tension itself. Increased emotional stress is known to aggravate a pre-existing peptic ulcer.

## Stress

Patients with severe stress, such as that caused by a serious illness, burns, extensive fractures, sepsis, or neurological disorders, are especially prone to stress ulcers. That associated with central nervous system stress is called *Cushing's ulcer,* while that caused by burns is referred to as *Curling's ulcer.* The mechanism producing these ulcers is unknown.

The nurse must be sure that each seriously ill patient receives frequent antacid therapy to prevent the formation of stress ulcers, and test stools and gastric secretions for occult blood, which would suggest bleeding ulcers.

## Drugs

Certain medications have been found to cause or aggravate peptic ulcers. It is important for the nurse to know the medications that do to institute preventive therapy, observe for ulcer formation, and teach patients about them.

Corticosteroids and salicylates are the main drugs implicated, especially in patients with rheumatoid arthritis whose medical treatment includes both drugs. These patients should be made aware of the hazards of these drugs so they can take preventive measures or seek immediate medical care should an ulcer develop. Also, many people take large amounts of salicylates, such as aspirin, APC, Excedrin, or Alka Seltzer, unaware of the hazards and sometimes unaware that the preparation contains salicylate. Salicylates also increase clotting time and should be strictly avoided in the presence of a peptic ulcer. Patients with ulcers are advised to read all labels closely to avoid medications containing salicylates.

Caffeine and nicotine are also thought to provoke or aggravate ulcers.

## Heredity

Genetic makeup influences susceptibility to peptic ulcers. Which factors of heredity are responsible is not known.

## Zollinger-Ellison Syndrome

This syndrome, produced by a tumor of the non-beta cells of the pancreas, is more prevalent than previously thought. The tumor stimulates excessive secretion of gastric acid.

**Symptoms.** The symptoms are due largely to irritation of the ulcer by hydrochloric acid. Pain, which may be described as burning or gnawing, occurs in the epigastric region, and bears a definite relationship to eating. It usually occurs one to several hours after meals, and is often relieved by ingesting protein foods, such as milk. Sometimes the pain is accompanied by nausea, and the patient may find that vomiting relieves the pain. Those who are severe hypersecretors of acid may experience night pain, disturbing their sleep, and back pain, indicating pancreatic irritation by the ulcer. In about 20 per cent of patients, bleeding, hematemesis, and melena may be the first signs of an ulcer. Protracted vomiting, secondary to scarring, and resultant obstruction are also seen as the first symptoms in those who have ignored their "indigestion."

**Diagnosis.** Diagnosis is usually suggested by history and confirmed in most patients by a GI series. In some, x-ray studies are not helpful, and a trial of therapy may suggest the diagnosis. Duodenal ulcers are always benign, but gastric ulcers may be either benign or malignant. To differentiate between benign and malignant ulcers the combined use of roentgenography, gastric analysis, gastric washing for cytologic examination, and gastroscopy is required. Even if all these studies indicate benignity, a trial of therapy, in the hospital, must be the next step. Failure to show significant healing by x-ray examination and gastroscopy after three weeks is usually reason to operate for suspected malignancy, as is healing followed by a recurrence a few months after therapy.

## Complications

**Bleeding.** As stated earlier hematemesis or melena may be the first sign as well as a complication of peptic ulcer. Depending upon the amount and rate of blood loss, the patient may show signs of shock. Hyperperistalsis is associated with upper gastrointestinal bleeding, and the nurse should listen for increased bowel sounds when bleeding ulcers are suspected.

The site and magnitude of the bleeding and often the decision to operate are determined by endoscopy.

TREATMENT. Treatment consists of an intravenous infusion to maintain blood volume. It is desirable to measure central venous pressure. Blood is drawn for type and crossmatch. A nasogastric tube is inserted and continuous iced-saline lavages are administered. The nurse must maintain a constant record of serial vital signs, state of consciousness, urinary output, and laboratory test results. The hematocrit and red blood count are not reliable indices of the initial blood loss because of hemodilution. However, they do provide a guide to effective replacement therapy. Blood urea nitrogen, which rises with the digestion and absorption of blood, and the white blood count, which rises with gastrointestinal bleeding, provide the most accurate laboratory guides. A drop in blood pressure, urine output, hematocrit, or red blood count and a clouding sensorium associated with a rising pulse rate, blood urea nitrogen, and white blood count indicate increased bleeding, and the physician must be notified. Transfusions are begun and the lavage is continued. If the bleeding is not controlled medically, surgical intervention is required.

**Perforation.** The ulcer may penetrate the tissues so deeply that perforation occurs, allowing the contents of the gastrointestinal tract to seep out and cause peritonitis.

Symptoms of perforation and ensuing peritonitis usually are dramatic; once seen, they are unforgettable. The patient experiences sudden, excruciating abdominal pain, his face becomes ashen and drawn, and he perspires profusely. Body temperature at this time may be normal or subnormal. The abdomen becomes as hard as a stone, it is extremely painful and tender, and there is resistance to having it touched, no matter how gently. Usually the patient lies with his knees flexed to lessen the pain. The extreme hardness of the abdomen, often described as boardlike, is due to rigidity of the abdominal muscles. Breathing is rapid and shallow. After an hour or two, the patient's face becomes flushed, and fever develops. The abdomen becomes very distended and less rigid; bowel sounds are absent. Respirations become even more rapid and shallow; pulse becomes rapid and weak; the patient will die unless treatment is given promptly.

Perforation is an emergency situation. Treatment includes immediate surgical closure of the perforation so that no further leakage can occur; suction during surgery to remove the gastric contents from the peritoneal cavity; and the administration of large doses of antibiotics. Every moment counts. The longer the perforation goes untreated, the less likely is the patient's recovery.

The nurse has an important role. Sometimes, she is the one who first observes the symptoms, perhaps during the night, when she is the only one to see the patient. Immediate recognition of the significance of the symptoms and prompt, accurate reporting to the physician can save the patient's life. Never assume that sudden, severe pain is just a flare-up from the ulcer and delay calling the physician; never try to provide relief with antacids that may have been ordered for treatment of the ulcer.

When the physician arrives, he usually performs a physical examination to validate the nurse's assessment and orders a roentgenogram to determine the cause of the symptoms. If he finds that perforation has occurred treatment is instituted promptly, with nurse and physician working quickly together. Although he is very ill, the patient is often aware of what is going on around him, and he is usually very frightened. The nurse should briefly explain what she is doing as she proceeds, and avoid any comments in his presence that might add to his apprehension.

Despite the need for speed in preparing the patient for the operating room, the nurse should not forget to give him a word of encouragement as he is taken there. She could say, "I'll be here to take care of you when you get back from surgery."

When the patient returns from the operating room, a Levin tube will be in place, connected to suction. After he has reacted from anesthesia, he is placed in a low sitting position. Nothing is given by mouth, and parenteral fluids are administered. Antibiotics are given to combat infection in the peritoneal cavity, and the patient is observed carefully. Usually, his fever subsides, his abdomen becomes less distended, he breathes more easily and deeply, and his pulse is stronger and slower. Continued elevation of temperature, distention, weak rapid pulse, and shallow rapid breathing should be reported to the physician, since they may indicate that peritonitis is not responding to treatment or that an abscess has developed. The patient should also be observed for signs and symptoms of paralytic ileus, such as distention, failure to pass flatus or stool, and absence of bowel sounds. When the patient recovers from surgery, treatment of the underlying condition, the peptic ulcer, is continued.

Occasionally, a small perforation that is diagnosed promptly is treated medically. Continuous suction is used to keep the stomach empty, and intravenous fluids and electrolytes are administered. Antibiotics are used to combat infection. The purpose of therapy is to facilitate healing of the perforation and to prevent and treat infection.

**Obstruction.** Edema, spasm, inflammation, and scar tissue surrounding the ulcer may interfere with the passage of food, so that food is retained in the stomach for abnormally long periods. Obstruction commonly occurs in the pyloric region. The degree to which the normal flow of gastric contents is impeded varies. If it is slight, the patient may notice that after eating he has a feeling of fullness, distention, and nausea. If the obstruction is severe, the patient is nauseous, vomits, has pain, and is distended.

Physical examination, x-ray study of the gastrointestinal tract, and aspiration of the stomach contents help determine the location and the severity of the obstruction. If there is an obstruction, large amounts of food and secretion are obtained when a gastric tube is passed and the contents of the stomach are withdrawn.

Obstruction due to edema and inflammation often subsides when the ulcer is treated medically.

If retention is still present, as evidenced by the aspiration of more than 200 ml. of gastric contents after an overnight fast, the gastric tube is connected to continuous suction and parenteral fluid therapy is instituted. The physician then determines the cause of the obstruction. Medications, cancer, fibrosis, and spasm can all cause obstruction and when it is due to a chronic ulcer associated with scarring and deformity, a gastroenterostomy, a subtotal gastric resection, or a pyloroplasty may be performed to bypass the obstruction. These operations are discussed below.

### Medical Treatment and Nursing Care

Medical treatment of peptic ulcer is designed to provide optimum conditions for healing the lesion. Neutralization of acid, so that it does not further irritate the ulcer, and the reduction of hypermotility and secretions are objectives of therapy. This is accomplished by diet, antacids, and physical and emotional rest.

### Diet

There is no evidence to support the hourly "milk and cream" therapy of yore or a bland diet. On the contrary, milk has been shown to *cause* a higher gastric acidity than a normal meal (Fordtran, 1973). The notion of giving small frequent meals is also being challenged. There has been little research done on the reduction of gastric acidity. From what is known, most clinicians recommend a normal diet for patients with an ulcer, excluding caffeine and alcohol (Walker and Richardson, 1973), which have been proven to damage the gastric mucosa. As these patients seem to have increased secretory responses to meals, and as the acid stays in the stomach longer, the patients are advised not to eat anything close to bedtime (when they will not be taking antacids).

### Antacids

There are many antacid preparations on the market, and their effectiveness in ulcer therapy is also being challenged. Until conclusive evidence has been presented proving them ineffective, and because clinical trials with animals demonstrate their efficacy, they will continue to be used in the treatment of ulcers. One study in humans has shown that antacids given one hour after meals significantly reduces gastric acidity (Fordtran).

For active ulcers, antacids are given one hour after meals and then hourly or half-hourly if severe pain is present. While the ulcer is healing, antacids are taken one and three hours after meals. After the ulcer has healed, antacids are recommended one hour after meals and at bedtime, if there is a tendency toward recurrence.

For severe ulceration, antacids may be given by continuous drip through a nasogastric tube.

Antacids containing magnesium tend to cause diarrhea, while those containing aluminum hydroxide tend to cause constipation. The patient may take these antacids alternately to avoid these complications.

Some antacids contain sodium, and should not be given to patients with cardiac problems. Other antacids have other side effects, as described in textbooks of pharmacology.

### Reduction of Hypermotility and Secretions

Antispasmodics, such as tincture of belladonna and atropine, often are given to decrease gastric motility and acid secretion. Tincture of belladonna is given in doses of 0.6 ml. (10 drops); atropine, in doses of 0.4 to 0.6 mg. The side reactions include dryness of the mouth, dilatation of the pupils, blurring of vision, and difficulties in voiding. Methantheline (Banthine) and propantheline (Pro-Banthine) are newer preparations with effects similar to those of atropine and belladonna. The side effects are also similar but may not be as marked. Banthine is given in tablets of 50 mg., and Pro-Banthine in tablets of 15 mg., several times daily. Diphemanil

(Prantal) has similar actions and side effects; it is given in doses of 100 mg. several times daily. Other drugs that reduce motility and secretion include: methscopolamine bromide (Pamine Bromide, Lescopine Bromide), 2.5 mg. to 5 mg.; methscopolamine nitrate (Skopolate Nitrate), 2 mg. to 4 mg.; and hexocyclium methylsulfate (Tral), 25 mg. These drugs are given orally and parenterally. Side effects are similar to those of atropine. These drugs are usually given 30 minutes before meals to suppress the increased acid secretion that follows food ingestion; they are usually also administered at bedtime. These drugs are contraindicated in patients with partial obstruction since they further decrease the motility of an atonic stomach and add to obstructive symptoms.

Rest and relaxation are of prime importance in the treatment of peptic ulcer. In the absence of complications this aspect of treatment may not necessarily entail rest in bed. In most instances the patient may be permitted bathroom privileges and may relax in a chair as he reads or watches television. Sedatives may be prescribed to promote rest. It is sometimes desirable for the patient to be in the hospital when treatment is started, so that the entire program of diet, medications, and rest can be carried out exactly as it was prescribed. Later, when the patient's condition improves, a restful vacation may be advised. If situations that cause a great deal of stress exist either at home or at work, the patient is helped to modify them, so that as far as possible he can avoid emotional upsets. For instance, if he characteristically becomes worried and tense over everyday affairs, or if he has difficulty in his relationships with others, considerable personal counseling may be needed to help him cope more effectively.

The long-term management of peptic ulcer involves avoidance of fatigue and stress; sometimes a diet must be maintained in which substances that might cause irritation and excess secretion of hydrochloric acid are eliminated. Patients are advised to avoid smoking; to avoid drinking alcoholic beverages, coffee, and tea; and to take medications as they are ordered. Decaffeinated coffee is permitted. Peptic ulcer tends to recur, and each recurrence carries the possibility of complications. Every effort is made to help the patient regulate his life in such a way that the possibility of a recurrence is minimized. With proper medical treatment and re-education of the patient, 85 per cent of peptic ulcers can be healed. Recognizing sources of stress and learning to deal with them without somatizing is of great importance.

Irradiation of the stomach occasionally is used to decrease the secretion of hydrochloric acid. Its use is limited largely to older persons with gastric ulcers who have not benefited from medical treatment and for whom surgical treatment is contraindicated.

### Surgical Treatment

Peptic ulcers that do not respond to medical treatment, that recur frequently, or that are associated with complications may require surgery. Various surgical procedures are used, depending on the location of the ulcer and the degree and location of deformity caused by the ulcer.

**Subtotal Gastrectomy; Gastrectomy; Vagotomy.** In subtotal gastrectomy with gastroenterostomy the lower one-half to two-thirds of the stomach is removed, and the remaining portion is joined to the jejunum. The surgical procedures in which the stomach and small bowel are joined (anastomosis) is called gastroenterostomy. The operation removes the ulcer and that portion of the stomach that stimulates the secretion of acid; the food passes directly from the upper portion of the stomach to the jejunum. (Sometimes the terms subtotal gastric resection and hemigastrectomy are used rather than subtotal gastrectomy.) The stomach may be joined to the duodenum (Billroth I) or to the jejunum (Billroth II). If the duodenum is deformed by an ulcer, the remainder of the stomach may have to be joined to the duodenum.

Sometimes, in patients who are too infirm to tolerate such extensive surgery, a gastroenterostomy alone without gastrectomy is performed. The jejunum is drawn up close to the stomach and an opening made between the stomach and jejunum. This opening allows the food to pass directly from the stomach into the jejunum, bypassing the duodenum which may be obstructed.

*Vagotomy* (division of the vagus nerves) is frequently performed in the treatment of peptic ulcer. When impulses traveling down the vagus are prevented from reaching the stomach, both the secretion of hydrochloric acid and gastric motility are lessened.

As motility lessens, gastric secretions may accumulate, leading to stasis and distention. Therefore, along with a vagotomy, a drainage procedure is performed.

*Antrectomy* is preferable because it also removes the main gastric secretory cells. This procedure has a higher mortality rate and causes more side effects than does a pyloroplasty.

*Pyloroplasty* is a surgical enlargement of the pylorus done because vagal stimulation for sphincter control has been removed. It is followed by a Billroth I or II reconstruction (Fig. 43-1).

**Preoperative and Postoperative Nursing Care.** Nursing care of the patient whose peptic ulcer has been treated surgically involves all of the general principles required for any surgical patient, as well as the care required for gastric intubation and suction.

Preoperatively, careful attention is given to water and electrolyte regulation. Whether fluids are given orally or parenterally, care is taken that the patient

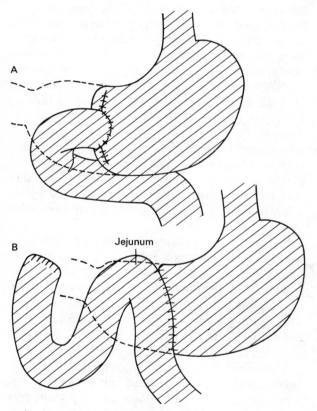

**Figure 43-1.** Partial gastrectomies. Dotted lines show portion of stomach removed. (A) Billroth I, which preserves the normal pathway for food. The remaining stomach is anastomosed to the duodenum (gastroduodenostomy). (B) Billroth II, which bypasses the duodenum in cases of duodenal alterations. The remaining stomach is anastomosed to the jejunum (gastrojejunostomy).

is well hydrated. Usually a Levin tube is inserted and connected to suction before surgery, to empty the stomach of food and secretions.

The patient is usually anxious about his condition and treatment and the nurse should reassure him as much as possible, explaining the equipment and why it is needed. In an emergency there may not be time, but the nurse can still reassure him by her manner and air of confidence.

The patient returns from the operating room with the Levin tube in place. It is attached to suction, as ordered by the physician, and left in place as long as necessary—usually two or three days. Its purpose is to promote healing by keeping the operative area clean and free of pressure. Although at first a small amount of bright red blood may be mixed with drainage, this promptly disappears. If large amounts appear, or if the drainage should continue to be streaked with blood, the doctor should be notified immediately. Drainage usually is dark red or brownish at first, indicating the presence of old blood, but then changes to the normal greenish-yellow color of gastric secretion plus bile. The amount, as well as the color of the drainage, is carefully noted. Usually, the physician orders irrigation of the Levin tube, so that it will remain clean and patent. It is important to use only the amount and the type of solution specified by the physician, since it is being introduced into the operative area. Too much fluid could cause strain and pressure, and might injure the incision.

Nothing is given by mouth for one or two days. Mouth care greatly relieves the discomforts of dryness, unpleasant taste, and odor from anesthesia; the inability to take oral fluids; and the presence of the Levin tube. Usually, the patient is given 30 ml. of water orally, starting on the second day. If this is well tolerated, the amount is increased, first to 60 ml. and then to 90 ml. The patient gradually progresses to a soft diet and then, in most instances, to a normal diet. However, feedings are small and frequent.

The patient is observed carefully for any sensation of fullness or distention and for vomiting. Repeated vomiting of small amounts of food usually indicates that the feedings are not progressing normally through the gastrointestinal tract. Sometimes this condition is due to edema near the incision. The Levin tube may have to be reinserted for one or two days, and the oral feedings may be temporarily reduced or discontinued.

The patient is encouraged to breathe deeply and to cough up mucus. Both are especially important, because the incision is high in the abdomen, and the patient tends to take shallow breaths to avoid pain. In most cases he is allowed to take a few steps and to sit in a chair for a short period on the day after surgery. This change in position can be achieved without dislodging either the infusion needle or the Levin tube (both of which may still be in place), provided that the tubing is long enough and the patient is helped slowly and carefully. When these treatments have been discontinued and the patient feels stronger, he is helped to walk about and encouraged to carry out more of his own personal hygiene.

Hemorrhage may occur postoperatively. Any changes in vital signs or laboratory results indicating blood loss should be reported immediately. Often, by the time the patient returns home he is able to eat six small meals daily. Most patients who have had a subtotal gastrectomy are gradually able to eat larger meals and to eat less frequently, because their bodies slowly adjust to the loss of a large portion of the stomach.

## Complications of Surgery and Nursing Care

**Dumping Syndrome.** A few patients experience the dumping syndrome, a complication of gastric surgery, that is characterized by a sensation of weakness and faintness, frequently accompanied by profuse perspiration and palpitations. It is believed that these symptoms may be due to rapid emptying of large amounts of food and fluid through the gastroenterostomy into the jejunum. (Normally, the food would pass through the entire stomach and duodenum before reaching the jejunum.) The presence of this hypertonic solution in the gut draws fluid from the circulating blood volume into the intestine, thereby reducing the effective blood volume and producing a syncopelike syndrome.

Patients who experience the dumping syndrome are instructed to:

1. Eat small, frequent meals.
2. Avoid drinking fluids with meals. Fluids are taken later.
3. Follow a low carbohydrate, high protein, moderate fat diet.
4. Lie down for about a half-hour after eating.

**Retention and Gastric Atony.** Gastric distention and vomiting in a postoperative gastric patient indicate atony; gastric decompression must be instituted before gastric dilation and fluid and electrolyte imbalances occur. Gastric suction, and intravenous infusions are restarted and the patient is given nothing by mouth. Sometimes the patient is maintained on hyperalimentation until the condition is relieved.

Any postoperative vomiting and distention should be reported immediately and oral feedings and liquids withheld. These symptoms may be due to obstruction by adhesions, herniations, intussusception, or paralytic ileus.

**Duodenal Stump Dehiscence.** After a Billroth II gastrectomy, the remaining duodenal stump may distend due to obstruction, edema, or infection and abscess, causing a "blow-out" of the stump. The patient manifests symptoms of peritonitis and acute pain. This is a serious complication that requires immediate surgical intervention.

**Infection and Abscesses.** The possibility and incidence of postoperative infections and abscesses are high with gastrointestinal surgery. The nurse should carefully inspect all incisions for signs of infection and maintain strict aseptic technique during dressing changes. Any signs of infection are reported. The surgeon usually opens the wound and packs it with saline-soaked gauze. Antibiotic therapy is started.

## CANCER OF THE STOMACH

The number of cases of gastric cancer in the United States is decreasing, for reasons not understood. Unfortunately, by the time most people seek medical care the cancer is already advanced, and the cure rate for advanced carcinoma of the stomach is extremely low.

### Etiology

As with most cancers, the cause is unknown, but certain factors have been found to influence the development of stomach cancer. Gastric *ulcers, atrophy,* and *polyps* may be precursors. A familial tendency has also been noted. Persons in these categories should be examined regularly to detect the cancer early. Tobacco and alcohol have not been found to be associated with stomach cancer.

### Diagnosis

Signs and symptoms include early changes in bowel or eating habits. These are gradual and progressive, and the patient may not even be aware of them. He usually decreases food intake because

743

of dysphagia or anorexia, with resultant weight loss and anemia. The anemia is further aggravated by the gastric bleeding that occurs. The bleeding is occult so the patient is usually not aware of it. Most often, the resultant weakness, dizziness, and dyspnea are the reasons the patient seeks medical attention. The American Cancer Society encourages everyone who experiences a change in bowel or eating habits to receive a medical examination. The nurse is responsible for educating patients to follow this suggestion.

Diagnostic tests include tests for stool occult blood, anemia, and the presence of the carcino-embryonic antigen in the serum which is present in 50 per cent of patients with stomach cancer. Barium studies, gastroscopy, and cytology confirm the diagnosis.

### Treatment and Nursing Care

Surgical excision is the only curative therapy for stomach cancer. The type and extent of excision depends upon the location and extent of the malignancy.

Treatment often involves total gastrectomy. The entire stomach is removed, and the continuity of the gastrointestinal tract is restored by joining the jejunum and the esophagus (Fig. 43-2). Depending on the location and the size of the tumor, it may be possible to perform a subtotal rather than a total gastrectomy, thus preserving a more normal digestive function. The spleen is also removed, since metastasis to the splenic lymph nodes is common.

Care of the patient after total gastrectomy differs from that after subtotal gastrectomy in that:

- The thoracic cavity, as well as the abdominal cavity, must be entered to remove the entire stomach. The patient therefore requires care similar to that of any patient who has had chest surgery.

- Very little drainage returns through the nasogastric tube because the stomach, which normally forms the secretions, has been removed.

- Oral feedings are started several days postoperatively, with small amounts of tap water given at frequent intervals. Gradually, the patient progresses to frequent small feedings of bland foods.

- The patient continues to eat small meals very frequently. Because his entire stomach has been removed, he is unable to tolerate large meals and often has difficulty digesting his food. He should be given easily digested foods, should eat slowly, and chew his food thoroughly. If he cannot tolerate oral feedings, jejunostomy tube feeding or hyperalimentation is indicated.

- Injections of vitamin $B_{12}$ are sometimes necessary for the rest of the patient's life, because once the stomach has been removed, the intrinsic factor, necessary for the absorption of vitamin $B_{12}$, is no longer produced. If therapy with vitamin $B_{12}$ is not administered, the patient will have symptoms of pernicious anemia. Unfortunately, most patients do not live long enough following gastrectomy for carcinoma to use up the body stores of $B_{12}$, and clinical pernicious anemia rarely develops.

- Prognosis depends on whether the disease has metastasized. Unfortunately, metastases usually have developed before symptoms are so marked that the patient seeks medical attention. Thus treatment is seriously delayed. Surgery for these patients is often palliative rather than curative. Although the mortality remains high, advances in surgical management and earlier diagnoses are permitting survivals of five years or longer.

## REFERENCES AND BIBLIOGRAPHY

DAVENPORT, H. W.: *Physiology of the Digestive Tract,* ed. 3, Chicago, Yearbook Medical Publishers, 1971.

ROBINSON, C.: *Normal and Therapeutic Nutrition,* ed. 14, New York, Macmillan, 1972.

SCHWARTZ, S., et al.: *Principles of Surgery,* ed. 2, San Francisco, McGraw-Hill, 1974.

SLEISENGER, M., and FORDTRAN, J. S.: *Gastrointestinal Disease,* Philadelphia, Saunders, 1973.

SMITH, J. N., JR.: *Essentials of Gastroenterology,* St. Louis, Mosby, 1969.

SPIRO, H. M.: *Clinical Gastroenterology,* New York, Macmillan, 1970.

WALKER, CHARLES O.: Chronic duodenal ulcers, and RICHARDSON, CHARLES T.: Reduction of acidity, in Sleisenger, M., and Fordtran, J. S.: *Gastrointestinal Disease,* Philadelphia, Saunders, 1973.

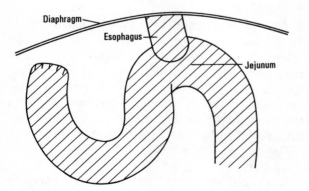

**Figure 43-2.** Total gastrectomy. The entire stomach is removed and the esophagus is anastomosed to the jejunum.

# Patients with Disorders of the Intestines

## CHAPTER 44

Disorders of the intestines are caused by inflammation, obstruction, disorders of absorption and motility, and anatomical abnormalities. The two main symptoms of intestinal disorders are alterations in normal elimination, i.e., diarrhea and constipation.

## DIARRHEA

Diarrhea is defined as loose, watery stools, usually occurring frequently. If prolonged, it can lead to extracellular fluid volume deficit (dehydration), hypokalemia, and acidosis.

Osmotic diarrhea, as in the dumping syndrome, occurs when the volume of solutes in the intestines increases above that of plasma, drawing fluid into the intestine. This may also occur with the administration of high-solute tube feeding without adequate water.

Increased intestinal motility due to psychogenic causes, irritation of the intestines, or excessive use of laxatives propels the contents along the intestinal tract too rapidly for water absorption.

Altered intestinal bacteria caused by antibiotic therapy or intestinal infections may cause diarrhea.

### Treatment and Nursing Care

Even before the cause of diarrhea has been determined, it must be controlled to prevent fluid imbalances. Medications such as diphenoxylate (Lomotil) or Kaopectate, antispasmodics, a change in diet or more effective coping with stress are generally recommended. Sedatives or tranquilizers are sometimes prescribed. Many times diarrhea cannot be controlled until the underlying cause is determined and corrected.

Diarrhea

Constipation

Inflammatory Diseases

Malabsorption

Intestinal Obstruction

Diverticulosis and Diverticulitis

Appendicitis

Peritonitis

Hernia

Cancer

Urgency with diarrhea and perhaps fecal incontinence, are embarrassing to patients. Keep the bedpan within reach at all times (two may be needed so that one is available while the other is being cleaned). The perianal area needs special care, as diarrhea causes skin excoriation. After the area is thoroughly washed and dried, a protective ointment, such as zinc oxide or A & D ointment, is applied liberally and frequently to avoid skin breakdown.

## CONSTIPATION

Constipation is defined as hard, dry stools, usually occurring infrequently. Prolonged constipation can lead to impaction of fecal matter in the intestine (liquid feces is usually passed around this bolus and it is usually palpable), and hemorrhoids from the increased pressure required to defecate.

Constipation results from decreased intestinal motility so that more water is absorbed, thus leading to hard, difficult to expel, stools. Emotional stress, poor diet, or repeatedly ignoring the urge to defecate are examples of some common causes of constipation. The busy person may not "have time," some people need complete privacy, and others cannot defecate when they must assume an unusual position, such as when using a bedpan or a higher or lower stool than they are used to. Frequently the patient is not actually constipated; he just defecates less frequently than he believes is normal. Too much emphasis on the importance of moving the bowels once daily can lead the patient to depend on laxatives. Instead of a normal movement every other day, he may induce a very loose stool with a cathartic, then have no movement the next day; this leads him to take another dose of cathartic. These patients need to be assured that a daily evacuation is not necessary provided that the stool is not very hard and dry, and that avoiding laxatives will allow the bowels to function normally again.

Enemas, too, unless carried out with careful technique and on the advice of the physician, can disturb normal bowel function and even lead to injury. Under normal circumstances the bowel does not require cleansing or washing. Some people routinely take enemas once or twice weekly to be sure they "have a good cleaning out." It is not unknown for a patient to fasten the tubing directly to a faucet, so that the pressure and the temperature of the solution are not controlled. Hanging an enema can or bag on a hook at the top of the bathroom door, rather than at a height of about 18 inches above the patient's rectum, is another common mistake. Introducing the fluid under high pressure can cause severe cramping, and it may, by causing too rapid dilatation of the colon, result in injury. The rectal tube should be inserted only 3 to 4 inches; hard rubber tips should be avoided, as they can injure the rectum.

If the physician advises the patient to take enemas, help the patient to understand just what solution to use and how to carry out the procedure safely. Some patients find it most convenient to lie in the bathtub; thus bedding is not soiled and they are near the toilet when the treatment is over. The patient should lie down while the solution is running in, so that the abdomen will be relaxed and the enema can be given with as little discomfort as possible. Small, commercially prepared enemas packaged in disposable units are now recommended frequently for home use. They insure that the correct amount and the correct type of solution are given with clean equipment and without excess pressure.

The regular use of cathartics is avoided whenever possible. If the patient needs medication to help him gradually reestablish normal function, a bulk-producing laxative, such as agar or some commonly used commercial preparations, such as senna (Senokot), a vegetable product that stimulates bowel function, or bisacodyl (Dulcolax), which acts directly on the colonic mucosa to stimulate peristaltic waves, may be used. A glycerin or a Dulcolax suppository often effectively stimulates evacuation. Stool softeners such as colace are commonly recommended.

Major emphasis is placed on helping the patient to maintain habits that foster normal elimination. Eating plenty of raw fruits and vegetables and whole grain bread and cereal, maintaining a high fluid intake, and getting regular rest and exercise are important. Allowing sufficient time for evacuation at a definite time each day is also very helpful in restoring normal function. The program of therapy is designed to help the patient return to a normal pattern of elimination with the least possible use of enemas and cathartics.

## INFLAMMATORY DISEASES

### Crohn's Disease (Regional Enteritis)

Regional enteritis was previously thought to occur only in the terminal ileum. It has now been described in the stomach, duodenum, jejunum, small and large intestine, and rectum. It is an inflammatory condition that involves all layers of the mucosa and thus thickens the wall. It is characterized by epithelial nodules, called granulomas, and skip lesions (the process is not continuous; there are segments of healthy tissue separating the affected tissue). The etiology is unknown.

## Diagnosis

Signs and symptoms vary from patient to patient but include diarrhea, fever, right lower quadrant pain, and cramping. Anorexia and vomiting are sometimes present. The symptoms of Crohn's disease are so similar to those of appendicitis that many cases are diagnosed only at laparotomy.

Diagnostic studies include barium x-ray studies, endoscopies, and biopsies. A thickened wall on x-ray films and microscopic examinations confirms the diagnosis.

## Treatment and Nursing Care

There is no known cure for regional enteritis. Therapy is mainly supportive and directed toward preventing complications. The patient is placed on bedrest, and medication, such as paregoric and codeine, is given to control diarrhea. If vomiting continues, gastric decompression may be necessary and intravenous infusions may be given. Steroids may be required for stubborn cases to reduce inflammation. Diet has no known influence unless there is an associated obstruction.

The nurse can provide much needed psychologic support to the patient by listening to him and being available when needed. She should help him maintain good nutrition.

Surgical treatment is indicated only if intensive medical therapy has not helped, or to relieve complications. Some complications include obstruction, fistulas, and major bleeding. The operative therapy consists of a colectomy, bypassing the diseased portion. There is a high recurrence rate.

## Ulcerative Colitis

The term *ulcerative colitis* refers to inflammation and ulceration of the colon. The mucosa of the colon becomes hyperemic, thickened, and edematous. The ulceration is sometimes so extensive that large areas of the colon are denuded of mucosa.

**Etiology.** The cause is obscure. Many who have studied this disease comment that the illness seems more prevalent in those who have certain kinds of emotional problems. Patients who develop the disease are sometimes described as inwardly hostile

yet outwardly submissive, and have strong needs for dependence. Patients with this disease often exhibit a hopeless, helpless attitude. It has been suggested that an altered blood supply to the mucosa of the colon may occur in response to emotional influences and may eventually lead to ulceration of the mucosa. Others point out that functional disorders, such as attacks of diarrhea when the person is frightened, rarely progress to ulcerative colitis, and that emotional factors may have little to do with the disease. Usually, no pathogenic organisms or parasites can be demonstrated. The possibility that symptoms are caused by infection seems slight, although it has been suggested that organisms are present that cannot be demonstrated. Ulcerative colitis may be a disease caused by multiple factors that may include infection, allergy, autoimmunity, and emotional stress. The term *idiopathic* (no known cause) often is used to describe ulcerative colitis.

**Frequency.** Ulcerative colitis is most common during young adulthood and middle life, but it can occur at any age. Both men and women are affected.

**Symptoms.** The condition may have an abrupt or a gradual onset. The patient experiences severe diarrhea (12 to 20 bowel movements per day) and expels blood and mucus along with fecal matter. Weight loss, fever, severe electrolyte imbalance and dehydration, anemia, and cachexia may follow. Often diarrhea is accompanied by cramps, and the patient may experience anorexia, nausea, and vomiting, as well as extreme weakness. The urge to defecate may come so suddenly and with such urgency that the patient is incontinent of feces. Some patients have particular problems with incontinence while they are asleep; they are unaware that defecation has taken place until they awaken.

The condition may continue in fairly mild form for years, or it may run a rapid, fulminating course, causing death from hemorrhage, peritonitis, or profound debility. Some patients recover suddenly and dramatically. They may remain free of the disease for years, or their illness may recur.

**Complications.** Cancer of the colon is much more frequent among patients with ulcerative colitis than among the general population. Patients who are chronically ill with colitis must be examined frequently for malignant tumors. X-ray films of the colon, proctoscopy, and sigmoidoscopy may be ordered by the physician at regular intervals. Severe hemorrhage may occur if the ulcerative process affects blood vessels. Perforation of the colon is another serious complication and leads to peritonitis. Among patients with ulcerative colitis the incidence of arthritis is high. The relationship between the two diseases is unclear yet the clinical picture resembles rheumatoid arthritis, which is thought, by some investigators, to support the autoimmune theory of etiology. Other serious complications are fistulas between the rectum and vagina or bladder.

**Diagnosis.** In addition to the history and the physical examination, x-ray examination, proctoscopy, sigmoidoscopy, and stool examination are used to diagnose the disease. A careful search is made for another condition that could be responsible for the symptoms, such as cancer, amebic dysentery, or diverticulitis.

Cathartics are contraindicated when preparing the patient with colitis for a barium enema if the disease is at all acute. They may cause severe exacerbation of the disease, and have been implicated as a cause of toxic megacolon—a marked dilation of the colon sometimes leading to perforation and death. The physician may postpone the barium enema until the more acute phase is passed and, in the more acute phase, employ such diagnostic measures as sigmoidoscopy. Even then he may elect to have the patient on a liquid diet for a few days before, and give some gentle tap water enemas the morning of the x-ray examination.

## Treatment

Medical treatment is supportive, and it is designed to provide rest for the bowel, opportunity for healing, and correction of anemia and malnutrition. About three-fourths of patients can be managed medically and helped into remission. The remainder usually come to a total colectomy and permanent ileostomy when medical treatment fails or an acute complication occurs, such as perforation or severe hemorrhage.

**Diet and Supplements.** The patient usually is given a bland diet. Any substances that might further irritate the bowel, such as raw fruits and vegetables or highly seasoned foods, usually are eliminated. The patient is encouraged to eat as nourishing a diet as is possible. Protein foods, such as meat and eggs, are important. Often, small frequent meals are necessary because the patient feels too ill to eat large meals. The quantity and type of food the patient eats are carefully noted, as are fluid intake and output as well as the number and character of bowel movements. Some physicians advocate greater flexibility in the diet prescribed for the patient who is not acutely ill, advising restriction only of those foods that increase the patient's symptoms. The rationale behind this approach to diet therapy is that at present there is no clear evidence that certain categories of food make the condition worse. Foods that are well tolerated are permitted, and as the condition improves, the patient is encouraged to vary his diet as much as possible. During periods of acute illness it may be necessary to discontinue all oral intake and begin intravenous feedings. These seriously ill patients are returned to a varied diet gradually commencing with liquids and very bland, easily digested foods.

Transfusions and iron are given to correct anemia. Parenteral fluids and electrolytes may be needed. Because the patient's diet often lacks essential nutrients, such as vitamin C which is found in raw fruits and vegetables, and because the disease itself may interfere with the absorption of nutrients, supplementary vitamins are often given.

Rest in bed is important during the acute phases of the illness and is continued until severe symptoms subside and the patient begins to gain weight and to feel stronger. Pressure sores must be prevented, particularly if the patient is very thin.

**Drugs.** A variety of drugs may be given. Although they do not cure the disease, they may lessen the symptoms and promote healing of the diseased bowel. The effectiveness of the various treatments is difficult to evaluate, because the course of the illness is characteristically variable.

Sedatives and tranquilizers often help the patient to relax and to rest. Drugs that slow peristalsis, such as atropine or tincture of belladonna, or drugs used to coat and to soothe the mucosa, such as kaolin and pectin, may be ordered. Antispasmodics must be given with great caution as they may be factors in precipitating toxic megacolon. Any rather sudden onset of abdominal distention in a patient with acute ulcerative colitis is an ominous sign and should be reported at once.

ACTH and cortisone may be given when the disease does not respond to other measures. A dramatic relief of symptoms often follows their use. In the acutely ill patient with severe diarrhea, fever, and abdominal pain, these steroids are often given intravenously for a few days until they can be taken orally. To maintain remission, the drug may be continued for weeks or months in as low a dose as possible. Use of these potent drugs is not without hazard; they may mask symptoms of peritonitis and produce other undesirable reactions, such as moon face and edema. Although potentially dangerous, corticosteroids have helped many patients with this disease, as well as other diseases, for which no certain cure is available, to live longer and more comfortably. They have also helped some to recover who otherwise might have succumbed. Corticosteroids have probably played a major role in reducing the operative mortality of elective colectomy by providing a patient who is a better operative risk and who is not as debilitated by his disease as was the case in the presteroid era. If a patient does not appreciate the drug's toxicity, he may not understand why he should not take a larger dose than the physician has prescribed, because the drug usually imparts a feeling of well-being. The patient should be given ample opportunity to discuss therapy with his physician. Because corticosteroids are not curative, they should be viewed as one aspect of treatment rather than as a replacement for other types of therapy.

Antibiotics, especially nonabsorbable sulfonamides, penicillin, or streptomycin, may be given. Antibiotics are particularly used to prepare the patient for surgery. These drugs decrease the number of bacteria in the bowel and thus lessen the possibility that infection will complicate surgery on the bowel.

**Psychotherapy.** When the illness is a manifestation of emotional problems, psychotherapy may be helpful. The patient is gradually assisted, through individual or group therapy, to understand and to cope more effectively with stress. Often it is necessary for close associates, too, to learn how their responses to the patient affect him. The process of reeducation may benefit not only the patient but others as well, as the patient and those close to him learn to relate to one another in ways which promote health.

Surgery is sometimes necessary when the disease does not respond to other treatment, or when complications occur. For example, perforation of the colon is an acute, surgical emergency, because it promptly leads to peritonitis. Surgical treatment of severe, intractable ulcerative colitis usually includes total colectomy (removal of the entire colon and rectum) and a permanent ileostomy (opening the ileum onto the abdomen for the passage of fecal matter). Many patients adjust well, once the diseased colon has been removed. Others have considerable difficulty in adjusting to the ileostomy. Fecal matter is very liquid because it does not go through the colon where water normally is absorbed; it is discharged immediately from the ileum. Therefore, ileostomy is more difficult to care for than colostomy. If the patient is one who has had severe emotional problems, management of a permanent ileostomy may exceed his emotional resources. Both he and his family often realize that surgery offers a hope of cure or improvement, whereas lack of response to medical treatment threatens survival. If time permits, it is sometimes of great value for the patient to be visited by someone who has had a similar procedure and made a good adjustment. There are "ostomy" clubs throughout the country whose members are glad to perform this service.

## Nursing Care

The care of patients with ulcerative colitis is a challenge to the most skillful nurse. Supportive care, both physical and emotional, can do a great deal to lessen symptoms and to assist the patient in overcoming the disease.

Any illness associated with fecal incontinence is physically and emotionally distressing. Our culture emphasizes cleanliness in habits of elimination. The importance of not soiling oneself is stressed from earliest childhood, and finding that he has soiled his bedding or his clothing can embarrass the patient profoundly. The problem is quite different from that of the unconscious or stuporous person who is not aware that he has defecated involuntarily. Patients with ulcerative colitis are usually painfully aware of the situation.

The patient should be helped to minimize soiling by keeping a clean bedpan within easy reach, so that it is available if he needs it in a hurry. He should be assisted to clean himself and to wash his hands after he has used the bedpan. This care is important, not only for aesthetic reasons, but because the skin around the rectum becomes easily excoriated. Applying petrolatum after the area has been cleansed helps to prevent irritation of the skin. If incontinence cannot be controlled (for example, the patient defecates while asleep), perineal pads and disposable bed pads placed under the buttocks help to control the extent of soiling and make it easier to cleanse the patient.

When the patient is allowed up and about, he may at first need the extra protection and assurance provided by his wearing a disposable pad; otherwise, he may be so afraid of having an accident that he will refuse to go more than a few yards away from his bathroom. Any type of disposable pad is usually better accepted by women than men, because men so often associate these with femininity.

Helping maintain an adequate dietary and fluid intake is essential. Serve small portions of food the patient enjoys in an environment that is clean and odor free. Appetite often improves as morale does. Moving his bed so that he can look out the window, giving extra attention to personal grooming, or having a visit from a friend may help the patient to feel more like eating.

Some patients with ulcerative colitis appear to be both emotionally and physically ill. They may show this state by being excessively dependent on the nurse, by seeming apathetic, or by constantly criticizing whatever is done for them. They may become extremely frightened by symptoms that seem commonplace to the nurse. Emotional problems do not rule out physical illness. The patient has a serious, possibly a fatal illness that may or may not be related to emotional disturbances.

One patient who had an ileostomy saw a tiny spot of blood on her dressing, which had been caused by the excoriation of skin around the ileostomy. She became pale, trembled, and cried, "I'm bleeding." Previously, various members of the nursing staff had changed the dressing for her ileostomy; after this incident she insisted that one particular nurse do this for her. She refused to allow the others to change the dressing, saying, "They're rough," or "They haven't had enough experience."

How could the nursing staff help this patient? They helped, not by dismissing the drop of blood as nothing to worry about, because to the patient it meant a great deal. Instead, extra care and gentleness were taken with the dressing, and the patient was shown just how the excoriated skin would be treated so that it would heal. When at first the patient wanted only one nurse to change her dressing, that nurse did so. After two or three day, when the patient's skin had improved and the slight bleeding had stopped, that nurse and another worked together on the dressing. The next day the new nurse carried out the care alone, and shortly afterward all members of the staff participated in the patient's care, exactly as they formerly had done.

**Table 44-1. Regional Enteritis Contrasted with Ulcerative Colitis**

| PARAMETER | REGIONAL ENTERITIS | ULCERATIVE COLITIS |
|---|---|---|
| Incidence | Familial tendency; common in young children | Less familial tendency; common in young children |
| Etiology | Less psychogenic | Psychogenic |
| Location and extent | Anywhere along gastrointestinal tract | Starts distally, moves proximally |
| Cancer | Rarely | Frequently |
| Malabsorption | Usually | Rarely |
| Surgical response | High recurrence rate | Low to no recurrence rate |

The nurses in this situation recognized that the patient should not be pushed. When she was very upset, she was given the extra care and the support that she needed. They recognized, too, that the patient could readily become too dependent on one member of the staff, and that this nurse could not always be available to change the dressing.

The period of acute illness is not the time to expect the patient to conquer his emotional problems —even those that seem extreme, or those that present difficulties in relationships with the staff. Later, with physical improvement, the combined efforts of the physician, the nurse, and the family may help the patient to deal more effectively with his emotional problems.

## MALABSORPTION

Many conditions interfere with normal intestinal absorption of nutrients, water, and vitamins. Malabsorption results in general symptoms of weight loss, weakness, wasting, and the passage of abnormal stools. The stools are usually quite bulky, frothy, pale in color, and foul smelling due to the high content of fat, i.e., steatorrhea. The cause of malabsorption may reside in the wall of the small intestine itself, as in adult celiac disease, or it may be secondary to a deficiency of digestive enzymes, as in pancreatic disease, e.g., chronic pancreatitis. A bowel resection or bypass reduces the surface area for absorption. Symptoms are related to the particular type of malabsorption experienced. For example, deficient absorption of vitamin B complex can cause glossitis, muscle tenderness, dermatitis, and peripheral neuritis. Vitamin K loss leads to hypoprothrombinemia and easy bleeding; loss of calcium causes tetany and bone demineralization.

Patients with adult celiac disease are unable to metabolize gluten, a protein contained in wheat, rye, and barley. In some way not fully understood, ingestion of gluten damages the intestinal mucosa, thus interfering with the absorption of nutrients, vitamins, and water. Symptoms improve dramatically with the administration of a gluten-free diet, which must be continued indefinitely because symptoms recur if the diet is discontinued. A marked familial tendency toward this disease has been noted.

Pancreatic insufficiency with secondary malabsorption is treated by ingestion of pancreatic extract with meals. Pancrelipase (Cotazyme) is one of the newer pancreatic extracts.

The diagnosis of malabsorption is not always apparent in patients who do not have a severe form and are not malnourished. Therefore, the nurse's accurate description of the character of the stool seen in a patient with diarrhea may be critical in establishing a diagnosis of malabsorption.

A quantitative determination of fat in the stool will confirm the presence or absence of steatorrhea and then additional tests may elucidate the specific cause. For example, in adult celiac disease, the urinary excretion of D-xylose administered by mouth is low, while in pancreatic disease it is normal.

## INTESTINAL OBSTRUCTION

In intestinal obstruction, neither gas nor intestinal contents are passed through the bowel.

Common causes of intestinal obstruction are mechanical or neurogenic. Tumors are an example of the former. In neurogenic obstructions, interference with intestinal innervation inhibits peristalsis. This condition is often called paralytic ileus. An intestinal obstruction may be complete or partial, and it may occur in either the small or the large intestine. In paralytic ileus, failure of peristalsis usually is generalized throughout the intestine.

### Paralytic Ileus

In this condition the nerve impulses required to maintain normal peristalsis may be inhibited by infections, such as peritonitis, by the handling of viscera during surgery, and by such systemic diseases as pneumonia.

Because peristalsis is inhibited, secretions and gas collect in the intestine, leading to severe abdominal distention. Vomiting may ensue, and there is failure to pass feces and flatus. If the condition persists, the patient becomes very weak and dehydrated; marked abdominal distention interferes with breathing. Death may occur if normal peristalsis does not return.

In contrast with the treatment of mechanical obstruction, surgery usually is not indicated for paralytic ileus. Intestinal decompression and parenteral therapy are used supportively and to relieve symptoms. Supportive therapy helps to maintain the patient in the best possible condition to promote normal peristalsis. Neostigmine (Prostigmin) sometimes is given intramuscularly in an effort to stimulate peristalsis. A rectal tube and heat can be used to help the patient pass flatus.

Paralytic ileus is prevented by promptly treating conditions that may cause peritonitis, such as perforation of the intestine; care and gentleness in handling the intestines during surgery; and routine use, after major abdominal operations, of gastric intubation to help prevent the accumulation of secretions and flatus.

### Mechanical Obstruction

Cancer is the most common cause of intestinal obstruction, particularly in older persons. The tumor gradually becomes larger until it completely obstructs the bowel. The patient may note changes in bowel habits if the obstruction is partial. Often, he has alternating constipation and diarrhea. The diarrhea results from very forceful peristalsis, which is the body's way of pushing the intestinal contents through the narrowed lumen of the bowel. If the patient receives treatment promptly, complete obstruction may be averted.

Volvulus, twisting or kinking of a portion of the intestines, can cause sudden obstruction of the intestines (Fig. 44-1). Strangulated hernia is a third common cause of acute intestinal obstruction.

#### Symptoms

Symptoms of a severe intestinal obstruction may arise suddenly in a previously healthy individual. When the bowel is obstructed, the portion proximal to the obstruction becomes distended with intestinal contents, while the portion distal to the obstruction is empty. If the obstruction is complete, neither gas nor feces is expelled rectally. However, one or two

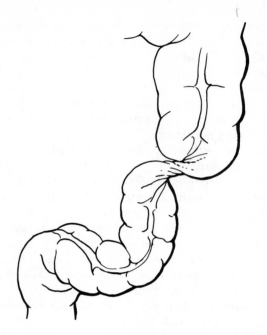

**Figure 44-1.** Volvulus of the colon. The twisting can cause complete obstruction.

bowel movements may occur soon after obstruction has developed because the material already past the obstruction can be expelled normally.

Peristalsis becomes very forceful in the proximal portion, as the body attempts to propel the material beyond the point of the obstruction. These forceful peristaltic waves cause severe cramps, which tend to occur intermittently. Very forceful peristalsis often causes bubbling and gurgling sounds, which are audible even without the use of a stethoscope. When the examiner listens to bowel sounds with a stethoscope, he finds that the gurgling is occurring in that portion of the intestine proximal to the obstruction; the distal portion is quiet.

Digestive fluids are constantly secreted into the intestinal tract. However, with bowel distention, normal reabsorption by the intestinal mucosa is impaired. Even though the patient stops eating, that portion of bowel proximal to the obstruction becomes more and more distended with accumulated secretions as well as with gas. The problem is aggravated by the patient's tendency to swallow air when he feels nauseated and apprehensive.

When an obstruction occurs high in the gastrointestinal tract, the patient usually vomits whatever contents are in the stomach and in the small bowel. Vomiting often is severe and continued. After the stomach is emptied, the vomiting is brought about by reverse peristalsis, which pushes the material up through the mouth, since the obstruction prevents its passage downward through the normal route. The vomitus initially contains the food and gastric secretions present in the stomach. Later, the vomitus resulting from reverse peristalsis is dark, thick, and foul-smelling, because the material has been stagnant in the gastrointestinal tract, and the bacteria normally present have multiplied. On the other hand, if the obstruction is low—for example, in the colon—vomiting usually does not occur at all.

The patient becomes very dehydrated, is unable to take oral fluids, and loses water and electrolytes through vomiting. Failure of the mucosa to reabsorb secretions poured into the intestine contributes to the water and electrolyte imbalance.

Increasing pressure on the bowel, due to severe distention and edema, often impairs circulation and leads to gangrene of a portion of the bowel. If the gangrenous bowel perforates from pressure against weakened tissue, the intestinal contents seep into the peritoneal cavity, causing peritonitis. Intestinal obstruction is extremely dangerous and can be rapidly fatal if not treated promptly.

### Diagnosis

The physician studies the patient's history and performs a careful physical examination. Roentgenography of the intestinal tract is usually necessary.

### Treatment

Mechanical obstruction usually must be relieved surgically. Sometimes, especially if the patient's general health has been poor (as is often true among older persons with cancer), definitive surgical treatment must be delayed until the patient can withstand extensive surgery. Obstruction is relieved by a relatively minor surgical procedure, such as a temporary colostomy or cecostomy. Once the obstruction has been relieved, supportive therapy, described later in this section, is given; and once the patient's condition has improved, more extensive surgery may be undertaken. For example, a portion of bowel containing a malignant tumor may be excised and the remaining portions anastomosed. Sometimes, because of the location and the extent of the malignant process, a permanent colostomy is necessary.

Intestinal decompression, parenteral therapy, and antibiotics are used preoperatively to help improve the patient's condition so that he can withstand surgery better and make more rapid progress during the postoperative period. For intestinal decompression, a long tube, such as the Miller-Abbott tube, is passed into the intestine. Large amounts of accumulated secretions and gas are drawn out through the tube by gentle suction, greatly relieving distention and vomiting. Parenteral fluids and electrolytes are administered to correct fluid and electrolyte imbalance. Antibiotics may be ordered to combat infection.

## Cecostomy

A cecostomy is an artificial and temporary drainage opening used to decompress the distended bowel. The cecum and transverse colon bear the brunt of intestinal obstruction, since they are the most distensible part of the colon. A catheter is placed in the cecum and attached to gravity drainage.

The drainage will be liquid stool and, if leakage occurs, will irritate the skin. A collection bag (such as that used for a colostomy or ileostomy) may be used to trap the drainage and prevent it from remaining on the skin. The tube may be irrigated periodically to prevent blockage. After the tube is removed, the wound may still ooze, requiring frequent skin care.

## Nursing Care of a Patient with an Intestinal Obstruction

The nursing care involves assessment of pertinent data, such as the amount and type of vomitus and drainage obtained from intestinal intubation; the degree of abdominal distention; the location and intensity of abdominal pain; and whether gas or feces is being passed rectally. Accurate measurement of intake and output is needed to determine the need for and response to parenteral therapy. Any urinary retention is noted.

Mouth care, changing the patient's position, and the care of equipment for intubation and parenteral therapy all play a part. Keeping the patient and his surroundings clean and neat and ventilating his room will lessen his distress at the sight and smell of vomitus and drainage. Often the patient whose abdomen is markedly distended can breathe more comfortably if the head of his bed is elevated slightly.

If enemas are ordered, they should be given with extreme care and gentleness. To make certain that little pressure is exerted as the solution flows in, place the reservoir of fluid no higher than 18 in. above the patient. If he complains of discomfort,

or if the solution does not flow in readily, discontinue the treatment and notify the physician. Returns from the enema should be noted and reported carefully.

Sometimes heat is applied to the abdomen to relieve distention. A hot-water bottle or electric heating pad may be used. An electrically operated heating pad, in which the temperature can be set and maintained constantly at the same level (e.g., the Aquamatic pad), is safer than the conventional type in which heat regulation is only approximate. A rectal tube also may be ordered to facilitate the expulsion of flatus.

The patient's pain often is severe. Nursing measures are discussed in Chapter 10.

## DIVERTICULOSIS AND DIVERTICULITIS

Diverticula are sacs or pouches caused by herniation of the mucosa through a weakened portion of the muscular coat of the intestine or other structure (Fig. 44-2). They are common in the colon and are especially likely to occur in the sigmoid.

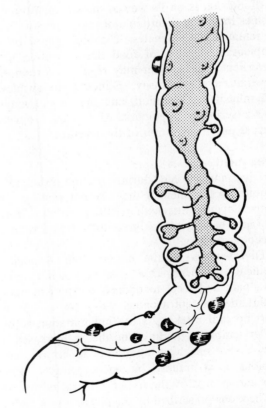

**Figure 44-2.** Diverticulitis. Note the numerous small out-pouchings of the intestinal wall.

The cause of diverticula is unknown. It is believed that some diverticula are congenital, though most are thought to be due to weakness in the muscular coat, associated with aging. They are most common in persons over 50 years of age. The term diverticulosis refers to the presence of multiple diverticula; diverticulitis means inflammation or infection of the diverticula.

### Symptoms

Diverticulosis is often asymptomatic and may be noted only when x-ray films are taken for some other condition, or at autopsy. However, the contents of the gastrointestinal tract often become trapped in these pouches, causing irritation and leading to inflammation and infection. For example, fecal material may accumulate in the pouches of the sigmoid, leading to irritation and infection of the diverticula. There may be constipation, diarrhea, or flatulence, pain and tenderness in the left lower quadrant, fever, leukocytosis, and rectal bleeding may occur. Intestinal obstruction or a perforation leading to peritonitis occasionally results from the inflammatory process.

Food that is on its way to the stomach often becomes lodged in diverticula of the esophagus, where it remains and stagnates. The breath may be very unpleasant because of food decomposition in the diverticula; the patient may regurgitate food eaten several days previously. Difficulty in swallowing (dysphagia) is common, and the patient may become seriously malnourished. Cough sometimes occurs due to irritation of the trachea.

### Treatment

Diverticula noted during routine examinations require no treatment if they are not causing symptoms. Diverticulitis with resultant stricture formation may be difficult to differentiate from carcinoma, except at surgery.

Diverticulitis of the colon often responds to medical treatment. During a very acute episode with pain and local tenderness the patient may be maintained on intravenous fluids for a few days, with no oral intake. As the inflammation subsides under antibiotic therapy, the diet is increased to a low-residue one. Constipation is to be avoided by copious fluid intake, by encouraging a regular evacuation, and by the use of mineral oil (or other medications prescribed by the physician) at bedtime. If the condition does not respond to medical treat-

ment, or if such complications as perforation, intestinal obstruction, or severe bleeding occur, surgery is necessary. The portion of colon containing the diverticula is removed, and bowel continuity is reestablished by joining the remaining portions. Depending on the location and the extent of the disease and on the presence of intestinal obstruction, a temporary colostomy sometimes must be performed. Bowel continuity is restored at a later operation, and the colostomy is closed.

Diverticula of the esophagus usually are excised, if they are symptomatic. The resulting opening in the esophagus is closed, thus restoring normal function and giving complete relief of symptoms. If a diverticulum is located in the upper portion of the esophagus, the postoperative patient may take a liquid diet, followed by a bland diet, soon after surgery. General postoperative nursing is required. If a diverticulum is lower in the esophagus, the operation must be performed through an incision into the thoracic cavity.

## APPENDICITIS

Appendicitis is one of the most common surgical emergencies. The appendix—a narrow, blind tube located at the tip of the cecum—may become inflamed, for reasons that are not entirely clear. It is believed that obstruction occurs, making it difficult or impossible for the contents of the appendix to empty normally. Since the intestinal contents are laden with bacteria, an injury to tissues in contact with the contents will often result in an infection. A hard mass of feces, called a fecalith, may obstruct and mechanically irritate the appendix. Inflammation and infection may follow quickly. Pressure from the fecalith and the edema of tissues that occurs with inflammation may interfere with the blood supply, making the tissues more vulnerable to infection, and sometimes leading to gangrene and perforation. Perforation is a dreaded complication, because if the intestinal contents flow into the peritoneal cavity, generalized peritonitis or, in localized peritonitis, an abscess will follow (Fig. 44-3).

### Incidence and Symptoms

Appendicitis can occur at any age. However, it seems to be more common among adolescents and young adults. An attack of severe abdominal pain is the most common symptom. Often, the pain is

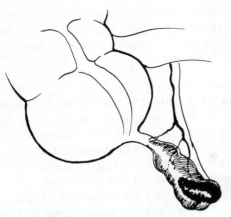

**Figure 44-3.** Appendicitis. The entire appendix is red and swollen, and the tip is gangrenous. The gangrenous portion is likely to rupture, spilling its contents into the peritoneal cavity.

generalized throughout the abdomen at first, or it is localized around the umbilicus. Later in the attack, the pain typically occurs in the lower right quadrant of the abdomen. McBurney's point, midway between the umbilicus and the right iliac crest, is usually the site of the most severe pain. Rebound tenderness is present; slight or moderate fever and moderate leukocytosis often occur; and nausea and vomiting may be present. Symptoms among the very young and the very aged are often atypical.

## Diagnosis

A physical examination is done, noting especially the location of the pain and tenderness in the abdomen. A white blood count is usually taken, and additional tests and examinations may be ordered, as required, to rule out other possible causes.

## Treatment

The appendix is removed surgically, and cure is complete. The appendix has no known function within the body, so its removal causes no change in body function. Parenteral fluids may be administered preoperatively or postoperatively. On the day after surgery the patient usually is permitted food and fluids as tolerated, and is usually allowed out of bed. Convalescence is rapid, but it depends on the patient's age and general physical condition. A healthy young adult is usually able to return to his regular activities within two to four weeks. He is advised to avoid heavy lifting or unusual exertion for several months.

## Nursing Care

The nurse's role involves reporting symptoms that may indicate appendicitis, preparation of the patient for emergency surgery, and postoperative nursing care required by any patient who has had abdominal surgery. Preparation for emergency surgery is discussed in Chapter 14, and postoperative care in Chapter 16.

**Preventing Complications.** Early diagnosis and modern surgical treatment have made death from appendicitis a rarity in our country. Nevertheless, death can and does occur. Severe illness and death result all too often from a delay in seeking medical attention and from attempts to relieve the symptoms with home remedies.

Who has not at some time suffered pain in the abdomen or nausea and vomiting? It is easy to understand why self-medication and a delay in seeking treatment occur.

The nurse can help to reduce complications and death from appendicitis by instructing families in what to do (and especially what *not* to do) when abdominal pain occurs:

- **Consult a physician for any abdominal pain that is severe, or that does not disappear promptly.**
- **Do not take a cathartic or an enema. Either of these increases peristalsis, which may result in perforation of the inflamed appendix and in peritonitis.**
- **Take nothing by mouth. Eating may aggravate the condition, and if surgery should be necessary, it is best that the stomach be empty.**
- **Lie quietly in the position that is most comfortable until the physician arrives.**

A nurse is often the first person to see the patient, in a health office, in industry or school, or as an independent practitioner in the community. The nurse assesses the patient's condition carefully, noting such factors as location and duration of pain, fever, nausea, and rebound tenderness. She refers the patient to the physician as necessary. One nurse, when referring a patient, used this description:

"Ms. Burns has severe pain in the right lower quadrant of her abdomen. She says she vomited her lunch, and that the pain has been getting worse since then. Her temperature is 101°."

The physician planned to see Ms. Burns in a few minutes. Meanwhile, the nurse had the patient lie down on a cot, and made her as comfortable as possible by covering her with a blanket, and letting her lie on her side, with her right knee drawn up. This position seemed to lessen the pain. Ms. Burns said that her mouth was dry, and she asked for water. The nurse allowed her to rinse her mouth but advised her not to drink anything.

Ms. Burns asked whether she could have something to relieve the pain, and the nurse explained gently that the physician would first have to examine her and determine what was wrong before ordering any treatment. She assured the patient that the physician was on his way and stayed with her until he arrived, about 20 minutes later. After initial examination he arranged for Ms. Burns to be admitted to the hospital.

The nurse in this situation contributed to Ms. Burns' care by:

- **Carefully assessing important symptoms.**
- **Promptly referring the patient.**
- **Doing nothing that might make the condition worse. (She kept the patient at rest and gave her nothing by mouth.)**
- **Staying with the patient, assuring her and observing any further symptoms, until the physician arrived.**

It is very important to avoid masking any of the patient's symptoms before the physician has made the diagnosis. The severity and the location of pain are important clues to its cause. Therefore, analgesics are not given until the diagnosis is certain. Relieving the pain without treating the underlying condition could result in perforation and peritonitis. Patients have developed appendicitis while they have been hospitalized for some other condition. Hence, when the patient complains of a new or different type of pain, never administer a narcotic previously ordered for some other condition. Refer the patient to the physician for further assessment.

## PERITONITIS

The term *peritonitis* means inflammation of the *peritoneum,* a serous sac lining the abdominal cavity. The intestines, normally filled with bacteria, are among the organs enclosed in the peritoneum. Any break in the continuity of the intestines that causes a leakage of the intestinal contents can lead to inflammation and infection of the peritoneum. Two of the most common causes of peritonitis are perforation of the appendix and perforation of a duodenal ulcer. In both instances the intestinal contents escape into the peritoneal cavity, causing peritonitis. The infection may be widespread within the peritoneum (generalized peritonitis), or it may be localized and lead to abscess formation. Initial

chemical inflammation of the peritoneum often follows the rupture of various organs; however, chemical inflammation is usually followed promptly by bacterial invasion.

### Symptoms

Symptoms of peritonitis include severe abdominal pain and tenderness, nausea and vomiting. Fever may be absent initially, but the temperature rises as the infection becomes established. The pulse becomes rapid and weak, and respirations are shallow. The patient avoids movement of the abdomen when he breathes, because such movement increases his pain. He often lies with his knees drawn up toward his abdomen, because this position seems to lessen the pain. *Paralytic ileus* (paralysis of intestines), a condition in which peristalsis fails, and flatus and intestinal contents accumulate in the bowel, typically accompanies peritonitis. The patient's abdomen is rigid and boardlike at the onset of peritonitis. As the condition progresses, the abdomen becomes somewhat softer and very distended with the gas and intestinal contents that cannot pass normally through the tract. Marked leukocytosis commonly occurs in peritonitis.

If the infection is uncontrolled, the patient becomes very weak; his pulse becomes even more rapid and thready; his abdomen is distended further, leading to even more shallow breathing; and his temperature falls. The patient is moribund.

### Diagnosis

The most severe pain and tenderness usually occur over the area of the greatest peritoneal inflammation. The location of the pain helps the physician to determine, for example, whether the peritonitis is due to a perforation of the appendix or of the duodenum. A leukocyte count and a roentgenogram of the abdomen are other important aids in diagnosis.

### Prevention and Treatment

Modern treatment has saved many patients who would have died from peritonitis in years past and has prevented its occurrence in many other patients. Early diagnosis and treatment of such conditions as appendicitis have decreased the incidence of peritonitis. Strict surgical asepsis and the use of antibiotics before performing surgery on the intestines have reduced cases of peritonitis as a complication of surgery.

Preventing further leakage of intestinal contents into the peritoneal cavity is an important measure in treatment. If the duodenum has perforated due to peptic ulcer, the area of perforation is closed surgically, so that no further escape of intestinal contents can take place. If the intestinal contents are leaking from a ruptured appendix, the appendix is removed. Gastrointestinal decompression is used to drain accumulated gas and intestinal contents that are prevented, by intestinal paralysis, from passing normally through the tract.

Fluids and electrolytes must be replaced. The patient can take nothing by mouth, and water and electrolytes are being lost in vomitus and drainage from gastrointestinal intubation. Large quantities of body fluids and electrolytes collect in the peritoneal cavity instead of circulating normally throughout the body, thus increasing the problem of water and electrolyte imbalance.

Large doses of antibiotics are given to combat infection. Analgesics, such as meperidine (Demerol), are often necessary to relieve pain and to promote rest. The head of the patient's bed is elevated to allow drainage to settle in the pelvic region, where, if abscesses occur, they can be drained more readily.

All these measures are designed to aid the body in its fight against the infection, and provide favorable conditions for healing.

### Nursing Care

The patient with peritonitis is very ill and requires detailed care and observation. His symptoms often change rapidly, and the nurse must assess such factors as:

- **Is his abdomen more distended? Is it softer, or more rigid?**
- **Is the pain diminishing? Where is it most severe?**
- **Are bowel sounds present?**
- **Is gas being passed rectally? Has the patient had a bowel movement?**
- **Is he vomiting? What is the character of the vomitus?**
- **Is the pulse weaker, or more rapid? Is his temperature rising?**
- **How much has he voided? How much drainage has been returned through the tube? How much parenteral fluid has he received?**

The patient is usually in great pain. Make him as comfortable as possible. Usually, the head of the bed is kept elevated, and a footboard, against which the patient can brace his feet, helps to keep him from sliding down in bed. Administer analgesics as prescribed.

Mouth care is very important. Often the patient is vomiting. The inability to take anything by mouth, the presence of a gastrointestinal tube, and fever make the patient's mouth feel dry and parched, causing an unpleasant taste and odor.

Cleanliness and an orderly environment help the patient to rest. Linen that has become wet with perspiration or soiled by vomitus should be changed. Bedside equipment, such as infusion poles and drainage bottles, should be arranged neatly.

Sometimes the patient becomes disoriented. Siderails on the bed are needed to prevent him from harming himself, and he should be observed frequently.

The patient requires gentleness above all else. Every movement causes him added pain. Every unnecessary jolt of his bed or stretcher adds to his agony. If he must be moved from his bed to a stretcher for roentgenography or for surgery, have ample assistance and lift him as gently and as smoothly as possible. Guard carefully against accidentally placing pressure on the fiercely tender abdomen.

## HERNIA

Although the term hernia may be used in relation to the protrusion of any organ from the cavity that normally confines it, it is used most often to describe the protrusion of intestines through a defect in the abdominal wall. The word rupture is used sometimes by lay persons to describe this condition. When a hernia occurs, a lump or swelling appears on the abdomen underneath the skin (Fig. 44-4). The swelling may be large or small, depending on how much of the viscera has protruded. Because hernia occurs frequently and sometimes causes no symptoms other than a swelling, its potential seriousness is often overlooked.

### Types of Hernia

The most common types of abdominal hernia are the inguinal, the umbilical, the femoral, and the incisional. Certain points on the abdominal wall are normally weaker than others, and they are more vulnerable to the development of a hernia. These points are the inguinal ring, the point on the abdominal wall where the inguinal canal begins; the femoral ring located at the abdominal opening of the femoral canal; and the umbilicus.

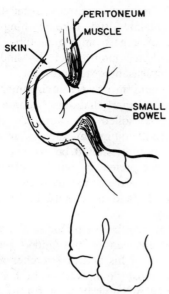

**Figure 44-4.** Inguinal hernia, demonstrating how the small bowel can become caught in the herniated sac.

Incisional hernias occur through the scar of a surgical incision when healing has been impaired. They often can be prevented by careful surgical technique, with particular emphasis given to preventing wound infection. Obese or elderly patients and those who suffer from malnutrition are especially prone to an incisional hernia.

If the protruding structures can be replaced in the abdominal cavity, the hernia is said to be reducible. Having the patient lie down and applying manual pressure over the area often reduces the hernia. An irreducible hernia is one that cannot be replaced in the abdominal cavity. The protruding structures become edematous and the opening through which they have emerged constricts, making it impossible for them to return to the abdominal cavity. This condition is called incarceration. If the process continues without treatment, the blood supply to the trapped viscera can be cut off, leading to gangrene of the trapped tissues. This condition is called a strangulated hernia and is an emergency.

### Etiology

Congenital defects account for a large number of hernias, including those that appear after childhood. The hernia may be apparent in infancy, or it may appear in young adulthood in response to increased intra-abdominal pressure, as occurs with heavy lifting, sneezing, or coughing, or during pregnancy. Obesity and muscle weakening may give rise to hernia in later middle life and old age.

### Frequency

Inguinal hernias, the most common type, are more likely to develop in men; women are more likely to experience umbilical and femoral hernias.

Diagnosis usually can be made by physical examination. Occasionally, x-ray films of the intestinal tract are ordered.

### Symptoms

Often, the hernia causes no symptoms other than a swelling on the abdomen when the patient coughs, stands, or lifts something heavy. Sometimes the swelling is painful; the pain disappears when the hernia is reduced. Incarcerated hernias cause severe pain. If they are not treated, they may become strangulated. (Symptoms of strangulated hernia are discussed under complications.)

### Complications

When a hernia first occurs, the defect in the abdominal wall is usually small. However, as the hernia persists and the organs continue to protrude, the defect grows larger, making surgical repair more difficult. The hernia may become incarcerated or even strangulated. Strangulation is an acute emergency characterized by extreme abdominal pain and severe pressure on the loop of intestine protruding outside the abdominal cavity and causing intestinal obstruction. Unless surgery is performed promptly, the patient may die. If a portion of the bowel has become gangrenous because its blood supply has been curtailed, that part of the intestine must be excised and the remaining portions of the intestine anastomosed.

When a hernia has been neglected for many years, the tissues in the area become weakened and do not heal as readily. Obese persons who have put off surgical repair of the hernia for years are especially likely to have a recurrence. Usually, the physician advises the obese patient to lose weight before the surgery is undertaken, to lessen the possibility of recurrence.

### Treatment

Herniorrhaphy is surgical repair of a hernia. The protruding structures are replaced into the abdominal cavity, and the defect in the abdominal wall is repaired. Herniorrhaphy may be performed under spinal or general anesthesia.

**Importance of Early Treatment.** The nurse can help patients to understand the importance of seeking medical care for hernias that are not painful. It is very hard to seek care (especially when one is quite sure an operation is needed) for something that causes little discomfort. By the time the hernia causes discomfort, an operation that might have been relatively simple may be complicated by the poor condition of the patient's tissues or even by strangulation. Therefore, most physicians advise hernia repair promptly to avoid years of possible discomfort and the threat of complications.

Increasing recognition of possible complications of hernia and the importance of prompt repair to prevent these complications—as well as the fact that the appearance of a hernia after employment is compensable—has caused some employers to delay hiring until the hernia has been corrected, particularly if the work is strenuous. Industrial nurses have a role in explaining the need for treatment to employees or prospective employees who have a hernia.

## Nursing Care

Before and after herniorrhaphy nursing care usually presents no special difficulties. Usually, the patient is permitted out of bed the day after the operation. If he has difficulty voiding, he may be permitted to stand at the bedside with assistance, while he uses the urinal. If possible, an orderly or a male nurse should stay with the patient who must stand to void on the day of surgery. If this help is not available, evaluate the patient by noting his color and pulse, whether or not he feels dizzy or faint, and whether it is safe to step outside the curtain for a moment to give the patient some privacy.

Usually, food and fluids can be tolerated the day after surgery. However, some patients, either because of the type and the extent of the necessary surgery or because complications such as strangulation exist, are permitted nothing by mouth for several days postoperatively. These patients receive parenteral fluids, and a nasogastric tube, connected to gentle suction, frequently is used to prevent postoperative distention and vomiting.

Every effort is made to prevent conditions that might impair healing, since this could cause the hernia to recur. Strict aseptic technique is required

to prevent infection. An increase in intra-abdominal pressure, as occurs when the patient is lifting or coughing, must be avoided. If he has a chronic cough, its cause is investigated, and treatment is given to relieve it before the herniorrhaphy is performed. The patient is observed carefully after surgery to be sure he does not experience sneezing or coughing. These symptoms, if they occur, are reported promptly to the physician. The patient is instructed to splint the incision with his hand if he coughs or sneezes.

Walking about and breathing deeply help prevent postoperative complications. The patient is encouraged to move, provided that he does not strain the operative area. Some patients are afraid to move or walk lest the hernia reappear. If the height of the bed is adjustable, a footstool will help the patient to easily step from the high bed to the floor. He is instructed not to lift heavy objects.

After repair of an inguinal hernia, male patients sometimes have scrotal pain and swelling due to inflammation and edema. Ice bags may be ordered to relieve the pain and swelling, and the scrotum often is supported with a suspensory.

If the patient seems to be having severe pain, is reluctant to move after the first 24 to 48 hours postoperatively (when the most severe pain near the incision has usually subsided), and has painful swelling of the scrotum, the physician should be notified.

Because the operation is usually performed in the inguinal region, a male patient may be embarrassed when the nurse checks the dressing postoperatively. By carefully arranging the bedding, or giving the patient a towel to use as a drape, he need not be exposed.

## Restriction of Activities

Postoperative recovery is usually rapid. Those who had been in good health preoperatively often go home within a week. Once home, the patient is instructed to avoid strenuous exertion or heavy lifting until his physician feels this can be undertaken safely. Many factors are considered in determining how much and for how long activities must be restricted, such as the location and size of the repair, the condition of the patient's tissues, his age, and whether or not he is obese. Those who always have performed heavy physical labor may have to do some other kind of work, whereas those who perform sedentary or light physical work usu-

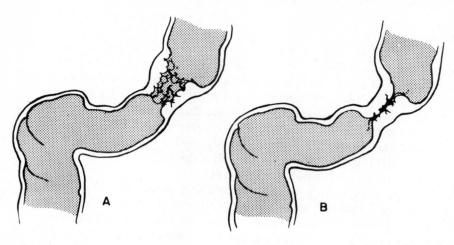

**Figure 44-5.** Cancer of the colon. (A) The new growth proliferates. (B) As the malignancy grows, it can occlude the lumen of the colon and cause obstruction.

ally can return to full employment within a few weeks. Healthy young persons in whom an uncomplicated hernia was repaired often have no restrictions on their later activity.

## CANCER

Cancer of the intestines causes the same symptoms and is diagnosed in the same way as is cancer elsewhere along the gastrointestinal tract (Fig. 44-5).

Treatment of cancer of the colon is primarily surgical, although a combination of surgery and radiotherapy may be utilized. Depending on the location of the tumor and the time treatment is instituted, it may be possible to completely remove the malignant tissue of the affected section of bowel and to restore normal continuity of the tract by joining the remaining segments. If this treatment is not possible because of the size and spread of the tumor or because of the patient's general condition, a temporary or a permanent colostomy may have to be performed to relieve the obstruction. Sometimes, a temporary colostomy is carried out to relieve obstruction, and more radical surgery is performed to remove the malignant growth and to reestablish the continuity of the bowel when the patient's physical condition has improved.

## REFERENCES AND BIBLIOGRAPHY

DAVENPORT, H. W.: *Physiology of the Digestive Tract*, ed. 3, Chicago, Yearbook Medical Publishers, 1971.

HEYDMAN, A. H.: Intestinal bypass for obesity, *Am. J. Nurs.* 74:1102, June 1974.

JACKSON, B.: Ulcerative colitis from an etiological perspective, *Am. J. Nurs.* 73:258, February 1973.

ROBINSON, C.: *Proudfit—Robinson's Normal and Therapeutic Nutrition*, London, Macmillan, 1971.

SCHWARTZ, S., et al.: *Principles of Surgery*, ed. 3, San Francisco, McGraw-Hill, 1974.

SLEISENGER, M., and FORDTRAN, J.: *Gastrointestinal Disease: Pathophysiology, Diagnosis, Management*, Philadelphia, Saunders, 1973.

SMITH, J. N., JR.: *Essentials of Gastroenterology*, St. Louis, Mosby, 1969.

SPIRO, H. M.: *Clinical Gastroenterology*, New York, Macmillan, 1970.

# Patients with Disorders of the Rectum and Anus

The afternoon report was in progress, and the nurse was discussing several patients who had had surgery that day. Considerable detail was mentioned concerning Ms. Ryan, who had had a cholecystectomy, and Mr. Cohen, who had had an appendectomy. Then the nurse said, "Oh, yes, and Mr. Ross went to surgery today, too. He only had a hemorrhoidectomy, though. He's all right."

How often and how glibly we say this of patients who undergo rectal surgery! The operation seems so minor compared with those in which the abdominal or the thoracic cavity is entered. However, the needs of the patient for nursing care are not necessarily minor, even if his operation is not classified as major surgery.

## HEMORRHOIDS

Hemorrhoids are varicose veins of the anus and the rectum. They may occur outside the anal sphincter (external hemorrhoids) or inside the sphincter (internal hemorrhoids) (Fig. 45-1). These sphincters keep the orifice closed except during defecation. External hemorrhoids appear as small, reddish-blue lumps at the edge of the anus.

**Etiology.** The contact of anal and rectal tissues with feces often leads to infection, which in turn may cause dilation and thinning of the walls of the veins. Pregnancy, intra-abdominal tumors, chronic constipation, and hereditary factors also are believed to be responsible for fostering hemorrhoids.

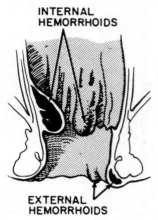

INTERNAL
HEMORRHOIDS

EXTERNAL
HEMORRHOIDS

**Figure 45-1.** Internal and external hemorrhoids.

**Symptoms.** Thrombosed external hemorrhoids are painful lumps appearing near the anus. One or two such swellings may appear and disappear spontaneously within a few days. The pain and swelling are caused by clotting of blood within the vein. Thrombosed external hemorrhoids rarely cause bleeding. However, they may become large and numerous, causing a great deal of pain as well as embarrassing itching. The pain is especially severe when the patient has a bowel movement, so he puts off defecation as long as possible. Constipation results, or if it is already present, is aggravated. Constipation and straining at stool make the hemorrhoids worse.

Internal hemorrhoids often cause bleeding, but they are less likely to cause pain unless they protrude through the anus. The bleeding may vary from an occasional drop or two of blood on toilet

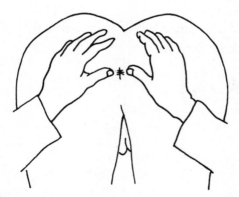

**Figure 45-2.** External inspection of the anus. The buttocks are spread by the examiner to detect external lesions. The patient is asked to "bear down," which accentuates the area and may prolapse internal hemorrhoids.

tissue or underwear to a chronic loss of blood that leads to anemia. Internal hemorrhoids usually protrude each time the patient defecates. At first, he is able to push them back inside the sphincter with his finger. Gradually, as the masses grow larger, they remain permanently outside the sphincter and often cause a chronic discharge of blood and mucus.

**Diagnosis.** External hemorrhoids are noted on inspection. Unless internal hemorrhoids protrude through the anus, an anoscope or proctoscope must be used to visualize them. Since the symptoms may be similar to those of cancer, a thorough examination of the anal and rectal areas is necessary. The patient who experiences rectal bleeding may have hemorrhoids, cancer, or both.

Anyone who experiences pain, bleeding, or swelling in the anal region should have a medical examination promptly so that the cause of the condition can be determined.

The nurse who functions as a primary care agent has responsibility to inquire about symptoms, such as rectal bleeding, pain upon defecation, and the sensation of a mass being present (or actually feeling a mass) in the rectum. Visual inspection of the anus (see Fig. 45-2) and digital examination are carried out by the nurse to detect such conditions as hemorrhoids. If the findings are abnormal, referral for therapy is made. Such examinations are especially important in long-term settings like nursing homes and mental hospitals, where patients' physical needs frequently receive inadequate attention from physicians. The nurse in the community can assist in bringing people to treatment. Older people living alone constitute a group among whom concerns about elimination are common, and who frequently have anal fissures and hemorrhoids. The nurse can offer instruction about bowel hygiene which can alleviate these problems, and can provide postoperative instruction to patients after procedures like hemorrhoidectomy.

### Treatment and Nursing Care

A small external hemorrhoid often disappears without treatment, or it may be relieved by warm sitz baths. Ointments containing local anesthetics may be recommended by the physician for the relief of discomfort. Ointments containing dibucaine (Nupercaine) frequently are used for this purpose. Correction of constipation is important both in relieving the condition and in preventing its recurrence. Often, mineral oil is recommended to soften the stool.

Surgical excision of dilated veins (*hemorrhoidectomy*) frequently is necessary for cure; it is the most common type of rectal surgery among adults. Occasionally, sclerosing solutions are injected into the dilated veins.

What are the patient's particular needs for nursing care? How can the nursing staff help the patient?

- The location of the operative area causes embarrassment; hence the patient should be draped and a screen should be used during treatments and examinations.
- The patient, and sometimes the staff as well, may assume that pain and discomfort will be minimal, since the operation itself is not considered a major procedure; however, the pain after a hemorrhoidectomy is likely to be severe at first. Narcotics, careful positioning, and explanation concerning what to expect, all help to lessen the discomfort.
- Although cleanliness of the operative area is essential, the anal region cannot be kept sterile. For instance, although the tub used for the sitz bath must be kept very clean, the procedure itself is not sterile.
- Gentleness is as important as cleanliness. A rubber ring should be provided for the patient to sit on, and local cleaning should be done gently.
- Some patients have difficulty voiding following hemorrhoidectomy. Often, with the physician's permission, the male patient is permitted to stand at the bedside to void. Women may find it easier to void if they use a commode, or if a bedpan is placed on the seat of a chair next to the bed.
- The sitz bath provides considerable relief from pain and also cleans the area. It is a good idea to give the sitz bath when the patient is especially likely to experience pain—for example, after bowel movements.
- The first bowel movement is dreaded by most patients who have had rectal surgery. He needs an explanation of how he is being prepared for the bowel movement (for example, by the use of mineral oil). When the movement occurs, he needs the assurance that someone is nearby to help him if he needs assistance with cleaning and measures for the relief of pain afterward.
- Plans must be made for continued care when the patient returns home. He is shown how to take sitz baths and instructed in the use of medications, such as mineral oil, to soften the stool. Any problems that predisposed to the hemorrhoids must be corrected if possible. For instance, treatment and instruction may be necessary to overcome constipation.

Principles in the care of any patient after rectal surgery are similar, regardless of the type of surgery performed. The following conditions are also encountered frequently among adults.

## ANAL FISSURE

Anal fissure may be described by the patient as a crack that does not heal. Actually, it is an ulcer involving the skin of the anal wall. Severe pain is caused when the patient defecates, and the pain usually persists for some time afterward. Slight bleeding often accompanies defecation. Constipation frequently results from delaying painful bowel movements. The ulcer is caused by an infection that localizes in the anal skin.

Sitz baths and local anesthetic ointments give symptomatic relief. Mineral oil may lessen the constipation and minimize the pain caused by passing hard feces; however, surgery is almost always necessary to cure the condition. The ulcer is excised, and the remaining healthy tissue is then able to heal.

## ANAL ABSCESS AND ANAL FISTULA

Anal abscess is caused by an infection of the tissues near the anus. The infection localizes, forming an abscess. Rupture of the abscess leads to the formation of an anal fistula—an abnormal tunnel or passageway within the tissues. The fistula may have several openings onto the skin, each of which periodically exudes pus, causing irritation and soiling the skin and clothing. The abscess causes severe throbbing pain, which may be accompanied by chills and fever. The spontaneous discharge of pus often temporarily relieves the acute pain.

Anal abscess is treated by incision and drainage. However, treatment often results in the formation of a fistula. Surgical treatment of the fistula is then carried out approximately one week after the abscess has been incised and drained.

Anal fistula is treated by *fistulotomy*, a surgical procedure that opens the entire fistulous tract, thus allowing healthy tissues to heal and to obliterate the fistula. Recurrent fistulas should alert one to the possibility of an underlying disease of the intestinal tract, and appropriate studies should be done to look for regional enteritis or ulcerative colitis. Such patients may not have diarrhea as a prominent symptom and may seek medical treatment initially with a history of repeated rectal fistulas. Local surgery in these instances usually makes a bad situation worse, until the underlying disease is recognized and treated.

### Nursing Care

This is similar to that of any patient who has rectal surgery. However, the following additional points must be considered:

- **There usually is a gauze packing in the wound, to keep the wound edges apart. This prevents more superficial tissues from closing over before the deeper tissues have had an opportunity to heal. The nurse may be asked to change the packing, as well as the outer dressing covering the wound, at intervals specified by the physician. Sometimes the gauze packing is moistened with normal saline. The packing must be placed deeply into the wound, making sure that all spaces are filled with gauze. Several thicknesses of gauze should be used for the outer dressing, since profuse purulent drainage is likely to occur. If the packing has been moistened with normal saline, plastic material is placed over the dressing to keep the bedding dry.**
- **Women must have special care during and after voiding, to prevent soiling dressings in the anal region. The patient lies on her abdomen and voids into an emesis basin that has been placed in position to catch the urine. The area is carefully dried by the nurse after each voiding.**
- **Bowel movements may be delayed until healing has progressed sufficiently. Liquid or low-residue diets may be ordered for several days. Drugs, such as camphorated tincture of opium (paregoric), usually are given to lessen peristalsis. After several days of this treatment, a regular diet is resumed, and mineral-oil or oil-retention enemas may be ordered to help stimulate regular elimination and decrease the pain associated with the first few bowel movements.**

### PILONIDAL SINUS

*Pilonidal* means "a nest of hair." The words *sinus* and *cyst* are both used to describe the condition, although the lesion is not a cyst but a sinus. The condition typically occurs after puberty, when the hair in the anogenital region becomes thick and stiff. The skin deep in the cleft in the sacrococcygeal region becomes macerated. Predisposed are persons with a deep cleft in this region and those who are hirsute. Inadequate personal hygiene, obesity, and trauma to the area are other predisposing factors. Stiff hairs in the sacrococcygeal region irritate and pierce the soft macerated skin, becoming imbedded in it. The hairs then become foreign bodies, causing the tissues to become inflamed. Infection readily follows, due to the break in the skin which permits microorganisms to enter. Several channels lead from the sinus to the skin; their openings on the skin are called *pilonidal openings*. Often, hair protrudes from them.

Usually, the patient is unaware that he has a pilonidal sinus until it becomes infected. The patient experiences pain and swelling at the base of his spine, and he may note purulent drainage on his clothing.

Treatment involves an operation in which the sinus and all its connecting channels are laid open; drainage of purulent material, removal of the hair, and cleaning facilitate healing with normal, healthy tissue. Antibiotics may be administered.

### Nursing Care

Particular points in nursing care after surgery include:

- **Care must be taken not to soil the dressings. Women void while lying on the abdomen.**
- **Moving the bowels is avoided for the first few days. Mineral-oil and oil-retention enemas may be used before the first bowel movement.**
- **After the first few postoperative days the nurse may be asked to change the dressing.**

During the immediate postoperative period the patient lies on his abdomen. The length of time that he is kept in bed varies from one to several days. When he is first permitted out of bed, he is instructed to take short steps and to avoid prolonged sitting, so that strain will not be placed on the incision. The height of the bed should be adjusted, or a footstool should be used, when the patient gets in and out of bed to prevent strain on the operative area.

### CANCER OF THE RECTUM

The role of the nurse in detecting warning symptoms of rectal cancer cannot be overemphasized. Skilled observation for signs and symptoms is particularly essential in older age groups. Note any masses or bleeding; be alert for the patient's complaints of obstruction to passing his stool. Patients with any suspicious symptoms should be promptly referred for evaluation by a physician.

The location of the tumor will help the surgeon to decide whether to utilize an abdominoperineal resection or a "pull-through" operation that removes the diseased area of the rectum but preserves the anus. In some instances it is beneficial to give radiotherapy before undertaking surgical treatment.

## Surgical Treatment

In an abdominoperineal resection, the anus, the rectum, and part of the sigmoid colon are removed. The operation is a major, lengthy procedure. First, an abdominal incision is made; through it the sigmoid is divided and its proximal portion brought out onto the abdomen to form a permanent colostomy. The patient is then placed in the lithotomy position, and the anus, the rectum, and the lower portion of the sigmoid are removed through the perineal incision. The operation actually involves two major procedures, and in some instances it is performed by two teams of surgeons working simultaneously. One team performs the abdominal operation; the other, the perineal operation. Abdominoperineal resection is necessary when the malignant tumor is located in the lower section of the rectum near the anus.

When the tumor is located higher in the rectum near the sigmoid, it is sometimes possible to remove the tumor and the involved portion of the rectum, to leave the anal sphincter intact, and to pull the sigmoid colon down to the anus, thus enabling the patient to continue to evacuate through the anus.

Because abdominoperineal resection involves such extensive surgery, it is especially important to observe the patient for shock after he returns from the operating room. Observation of pulse, respirations, and blood pressure are made carefully; an increased pulse rate and a fall in blood pressure are reported immediately.

## Nursing Care

Nursing care involves the preparation for, and the care following, a permanent colostomy. In addition to having an abdominal incision and colostomy, the patient returns from the operating room with a perineal wound. Dressings over the wound must be checked carefully for bleeding. Usually, there is profuse serosanguineous drainage, and sometimes the dressings must be reinforced a short time after surgery to prevent soiling. Placing small disposable bedpads under the patient's buttocks helps to protect the bedding. The pads can be changed easily and quickly whenever they become soiled. When sufficient healing has taken place, the entire rectal dressing is changed by the nurse whenever it becomes soiled.

These patients usually are acutely uncomfortable during the first few days after surgery. Most surgical patients have one operative area that causes pain; these patients have two—one on the abdomen and one in the perineal region. Thus narcotics may be required more frequently than after less extensive surgery, but the patient should not be so heavily sedated that he cannot move, exercise his legs, or breathe deeply.

Measures that help to prevent respiratory complications and thrombophlebitis are essential, because after abdominoperineal resection patients usually are kept in bed longer than most other surgical patients to permit the extensive perineal wound to heal. If the patient stands and walks about before the pelvic floor has healed sufficiently, a hernia may develop in the perineal region.

Careful positioning helps to minimize pain. The patient often is most comfortable on his side, a position that avoids pressure on either of the operative areas. During the early postoperative period, he is turned frequently from one side to the other and is encouraged to breathe deeply, to cough, and to exercise his legs. When the most acute discomfort has subsided, the patient frequently finds that he can lie on his back as well as on either side. Supporting the perineal dressings firmly with a T-binder encourages the patient to move about in bed. Unless the dressings are held snugly in place, he often is reluctant to turn and to move his legs for fear of dislodging the dressing.

Because a distended bladder is more subject to injury during operation, an indwelling catheter (Foley) is usually inserted just prior to surgery to keep the bladder empty. It is left in place for several days after the operation, because most patients have difficulty voiding immediately after abdominoperineal resection. The catheter also helps to prevent urine from soiling perineal dressings during the immediate postoperative period. When the catheter has been removed, the time and the amount of each voiding are carefully noted to determine whether the patient is able to empty his bladder satisfactorily. If the perineal dressings become soiled with urine, they should be changed promptly. Female patients are most likely to soil their dressings. A carefully positioned female urinal often helps to prevent soiling during urination.

Gastrointestinal decompression ordinarily is carried out for several days postoperatively. Intravenous fluids and transfusions are given as necessary during this period. The patient then begins taking oral fluids, and he progresses gradually to a regular diet. The patient is usually given antibiotics to prevent infection.

The length of time the patient must remain in bed varies. Because of the extensive surgery and the longer period of bed rest, he is usually quite weak and needs considerable assistance. Placing a rubber ring or foam rubber pad on the seat of his chair helps to lessen discomfort while sitting.

The surgeon sometimes packs the perineal wound to promote healing from the inside out (rather than healing of superficial tissues before deeper tissues have healed). The packing is removed gradually as the wound heals. Irrigation of the wound may be ordered. The surgeon will specify the type of solution to be used and the frequency of irrigations.

When the patient is allowed out of bed, sitz baths often are ordered to promote perineal wound healing. Because the patient is weak and may become faint, he must not be left alone while in the sitz bath for the first few times. Depending on the patient's condition and the distance between his bed and the sitz bath, it is often advisable to take him to the bathroom in a wheelchair. A rubber ring is placed in the bottom of the tub to lessen the discomfort caused by sitting in the hard tub and to allow warm water to circulate freely around the operative area. Most patients find the sitz baths a great help in relieving their discomfort and in promoting healing of the wound.

Dressings are worn over the perineal wound until healing occurs, and drainage ceases. Later, when healing has progressed and the patient is stronger, he learns to change the perineal dressings as well as the colostomy dressings or appliance. During convalescence, perineal pads often are used instead of perineal dressings. The patient is taught to continue taking sitz baths at home, using either the bathtub or a large basin.

Gradually, the patient regains his strength after the operation provided that all malignant tissue has been removed. He must learn to live with a permanent colostomy (see Chap. 47).

Convalescence is usually lengthy due to the magnitude of surgery and its inevitable physical and emotional effects.

## REFERENCES AND BIBLIOGRAPHY

DAVENPORT, H. W.: *Physiology of the Digestive Tract,* ed. 3, Chicago, Yearbook Medical Publishers, 1971.

ROBINSON, C.: *Proudfit—Robinson's Normal and Therapeutic Nutrition,* London, Macmillan, 1971.

SCHWARTZ, S., et al.: *Principles of Surgery,* ed. 2, San Francisco, McGraw-Hill, 1974.

SLEISENGER, M., and FORDTRAN, J.: *Gastrointestinal Disease: Pathophysiology, Diagnosis, Management,* Philadelphia, Saunders, 1973.

SMITH, J. N., JR.: *Essentials of Gastroenterology,* St. Louis, Mosby, 1969.

SPIRO, H. M.: *Clinical Gastroenterology,* New York, Macmillan, 1970.

# Patients with Disorders of the Liver, Gallbladder, or Pancreas

## CHAPTER 46

## THE PATIENT WITH LIVER DISEASE

Care of patients with liver disease presents nursing challenges. Two common liver diseases are emphasized in this chapter—cirrhosis and hepatitis. Care of patients with these conditions involves particular concern for nutrition, for health teaching over an extended period, and for meticulous physical care during acute illness. Although some work is being done in liver transplants, it is still in the very early stages. Emphasis in nursing care of patients with liver disease, therefore, is on measures to support the patient physiologically so that his liver will have the best possible chance to regain adequate function, and to support the patient emotionally during a lengthy and often discouraging period of illness.

### Anatomy and Physiology

The liver is the largest glandular organ in the body, weighing between 1.0 and 1.5 kg. It is located in the right upper abdomen, just under the right diaphragm, which separates it from the right lung. The liver has two major lobes, right and left, and two small lobes located on the undersurface, the caudate and quadrate lobes. The liver is supported in place by intra-abdominal pressure, and by ligaments or mesenteries. These attachments connect the liver to adjacent intestines, abdominal wall, and diaphragm.

A liver of normal size usually is not palpable. It may be felt in tall, thin persons or in those with low diaphragms, such as a patient with chronic lung disease. The liver receives arterial blood from the hepatic artery, an indirect branch of the aorta. The portal vein transports blood from the intestinal tract to the liver. After it has traversed vascular pathways inside the liver, the blood is collected by the hepatic veins, transported to the inferior vena cava, and then returns to the heart for further circulation.

Microscopically, the internal structure of the liver includes smaller ramifications of the hepatic artery, the hepatic and portal vein, lymphatics, and bile ducts. The cellular constituents of the liver are the hepatic parenchymal cells, which carry out most of the liver's metabolic functions, and the Kupffer's or reticuloendothelial cells, which carry on the immunologic, detoxifying, and blood-filtering actions of the liver.

The liver is involved in several vital, complex metabolic activities. Among the most important functions are the formation and excretion of bile; the utilization, transformation, and distribution of vitamins, proteins, fats, and carbohydrates; the storage of energy-yielding glycogen; the synthesis of factors needed for blood coagulation, including prothrombin and fibrinogen; the detoxification of endogenous and exogenous chemicals, bacteria, and foreign elements which may be harmful; and the formation of antibody substances.

## Diagnosis of Liver Disease, and Related Nursing Care

Because an understanding of diagnostic measures is important to the nurse when explaining these measures to the patient and preparing him for the tests, some of the factors considered in the diagnosis of liver disease will be briefly discussed, as well as nursing measures that can help the patient as he experiences various diagnostic tests.

Different liver diseases require different kinds of treatment, so great care by the physician is required in making the medical diagnosis, and many tests are often necessary.

Jaundice may be due to parenchymal liver disease, biliary tract obstruction, or both. Treatment may include numerous medical or surgical measures. The nurse who understands the basis of disease as well as its treatment can help the patient to appreciate the importance of undergoing necessary diagnostic tests.

The importance of an accurate diagnosis accents the necessity for nursing intervention, stressing emotional support during diagnostic tests and an explanation of procedures. Nursing measures can

diminish the patient's discomfort. For example, he is often kept fasting in the morning until blood samples are drawn. Promptly serving his tray as soon as the blood specimens have been taken and making sure that the food served is hot can lessen discouragement and promote adequate nutrition. The patient frequently must have many venipunctures, and may become very tense about this procedure. While in most hospitals a technician draws the blood, it is essential for the nurse to remain with the patient during the procedure if he is frightened. Diverting attention from the venipuncture by asking him to look at you and to concentrate on squeezing your hand is a useful nursing measure that will help him tolerate the venipuncture, make it easier for the technician to draw the blood, lessen discomfort, and minimize trauma to the veins.

Tests of liver function are done. In addition, of course, a physical examination is performed and the patient's history is taken. The patient is observed, especially for signs and symptoms of liver disease, which will be discussed in relation to specific illnesses. Function tests are employed to detect liver disease and in evaluating the extent of liver damage and the prognosis. When these tests are repeated at appropriate intervals during the course of illness, they indicate the effectiveness of therapy.

**Liver Function Tests.** Most tests of liver function require samples of blood drawn while the patient is fasting. Ordinarily the blood specimens are taken in the morning, and breakfast is omitted until after the blood has been drawn. A laboratory technician usually is assigned to see that specimen bottles are accurately labeled, and carefully transported to the chemistry laboratory, and that tubes containing special additives are used when required (for prothrombin determination, for example, to avoid clot formation). In tests that employ a dye, such as the BSP test, the dose of dye must be calculated, based upon the patient's weight, as well as accurate timing of the period between the injection of dye and the collection of blood. In most hospitals the physician injects the dye, such as for a BSP test, and specimens are collected at carefully timed intervals after the dye is administered. It is important to have an understanding ahead of time about which physician will administer the dye and when the dye will be given. Similar planning should occur with personnel from the laboratory. If telephone reminders are necessary during the test, give the ward secretary the names of persons to be called and the times when the calls should be made.

TOTAL SERUM BILIRUBIN. The level is elevated in jaundice from bile duct obstruction, diseases of the liver, and certain forms of anemia (see section on jaundice).

URINE BILIRUBIN, URINE UROBILINOGEN, FECAL UROBILINOGEN are other pigment tests to assist in confirming findings indicated by serum bilirubin testing.

ALKALINE PHOSPHATASE, SERUM GLUTAMIC OXALOACETIC TRANSAMINASE AND GLUTAMIC PYRUVIC TRANSAMINASE (SGOT AND SGPT), AND LACTIC DEHYDROGENASE (LDH) are liver enzymes, blood levels of which help to identify hepatic neoplasms, obstruction, or infection. Liver cells are rich in enzymes, such as transaminase. When the cells are damaged by viruses (as in hepatitis) or by alcohol (as in Laennec's cirrhosis), the enzyme is released into the bloodstream and is readily measured.

Both albumin and cholesterol are synthesized in the liver. In major liver dysfunction, blood levels of both may be depressed. In obstruction of bile ducts, blood cholesterol may be elevated.

Alkaline phosphatase of liver origin is elevated in obstructive jaundice whether of intra- or extra-hepatic origin.

PROTHROMBIN TIME measures the level of coagulation factors, synthesized by the liver.

SULFOBROMOPHTHALEIN SODIUM TIME. This test is generally called BSP, or Bromsulphalein time. It is a dye-excretion test that determines liver damage. Because BSP is excreted by the liver in the same fashion as bilirubin, the BSP test has been used as a fine measure of excretory function when the level of serum bilirubin is still normal. Whenever a patient is to receive a dye or medicine, especially if intravenously, a history of possible allergy should be ascertained.

SERUM ALBUMIN AND GLOBULIN LEVEL, THYMOL TURBIDITY, AND CEPHALIN FLOCCULATION are tests of liver proteins and may reflect the nature and degree of hepatic disease.

SERUM CHOLESTEROL level is reduced in severe liver damage, but is usually elevated with biliary obstruction and liver cancers.

SERUM AMMONIA level may be increased when a failing liver cannot detoxify this endogenous waste product of protein metabolism.

More complex tests to define hepatic disorders include liver biopsy for direct, microscopic analysis of liver tissue. This may be done percutaneously, by passing a special biopsy needle through the skin into the liver, or through a small abdominal incision, under general or local anesthesia. Percutaneous needle biopsy is not performed by the physician if there is a bleeding tendency, if there is obstructive jaundice which may result in bile leakage from the biopsy site, or if there is fluid in the abdomen which can mask hemorrhage.

The patient is asked to sign an operative permit before the biopsy is performed. Preoperative prothrombin time, platelet counts, and, often, partial thromboplastin times are determined. Sedatives are administered, as ordered, before the procedure, and the patient is kept fasting. Blood for transfusion may be ordered and kept in readiness. Postoperatively the patient is maintained at rest; vital signs and the condition of the dressing are observed every 15 minutes for the first 4 hours, every 30 minutes for the next 4 hours, every hour for the next 4 hours, and every 4 hours thereafter. Fall in blood pressure, tachycardia, shoulder pain, abdominal pain or distention, and staining of dressing with excessive blood or bile are indications of complications, and should be immediately reported to the physician.

ESOPHAGOSCOPY, BARIUM ESOPHAGOGRAM AND UPPER GASTROINTESTINAL X-RAY STUDIES (GI SERIES) may be ordered to help the physician assess the status of the esophagus and other parts of the upper gastrointestinal tract, because these organs are often affected by liver disease.

PORTAL VENOGRAPHY AND HEPATIC ARTERIOGRAPHY SPLENOGRAM, AND CELIAC-HEPATIC ARTERIOGRAPHY are methods by which contrast material is introduced into the hepatic circulation. Appropriate x-ray films will then define the character of the blood vessels and outline defects within the liver substance. Pressure in the portal venous system can also be determined in portal hypertension and cirrhosis.

Liver scan following intravenous administration of radioactive substances, such as iodine ($^{131}$I), labeled albumin, technetium and colloidal gold can give a picture of liver size, shape, and effect due to space-occupying lesions, such as tumors (primary or metastatic) or abscess. The pattern of radioisotope uptake may yield information as to the extent of liver damage and help to differentiate various diseases. No special precautions are required in relation to radioactivity when the patient has received substances such as $^{131}$I intravenously.

## SPECIFIC LIVER DISORDERS

### Jaundice (Icterus)

Jaundice is a greenish yellow discoloration of tissue due to staining by an abnormally high concentration of the pigment bilirubin in the blood. Normally, total bilirubin concentration is less than 1.2 mg. per 100 ml. of blood. If this reaches over 3 mg. per 100 ml. of blood, jaundice is visible. The skin, mucous membrane of the mouth, and especially the sclera (white portion of eye) are sites to observe for jaundice.

Jaundice occurs in numerous diseases which directly or indirectly affect the liver. It is probably the most common sign of liver disorder. Important to the understanding of jaundice is a knowledge of bile formation and excretion (Fig. 46-1).

When red blood cells are old or injured, they are picked up by the spleen and bone marrow where they are broken down by reticuloendothelial cells. Hemoglobin released from these red blood cells is then reduced to the compound known as "unconjugated" or "indirect" bilirubin. This bilirubin is then carried by the blood to the liver where further chemical processes transform it into "conjugated" or "direct" bilirubin. These two forms of bilirubin are distinct, can be differentiated chemically, and are important in the clinical discrimination of diseases producing jaundice.

The "conjugated" bilirubin enters the bile ducts, reaches the intestine, and is there transformed into urobilinogen. Urobilinogen is then changed into urobilin, the brown pigment of stool. Urobilinogen enters the bloodstream and is carried back to the liver, where it is changed into bilirubin for re-excretion in the bile. Another portion of urobilinogen is carried from the intestine to the kidney and is excreted in the urine.

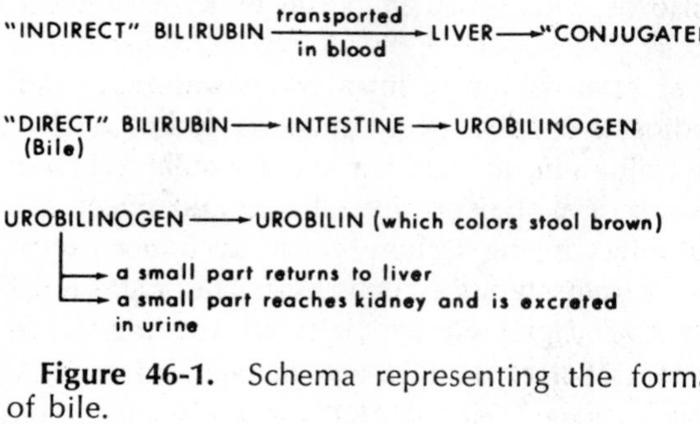

In diseases causing jaundice, laboratory determination of the type of pigments in blood, urine, and stool allows the physician to arrive at a more accurate diagnosis, and thus the appropriate therapy.

For purposes of discussion, jaundice may be classified into three forms: (1) hemolytic jaundice (due to the overabundance of breakdown products of blood); (2) hepatocellular jaundice (due to internal liver disease preventing normal transformation of bile by the liver cells); and (3) obstructive jaundice (due to the inability of normally formed liver bile to be passed into the intestine because of duct blockage).

### Some Conditions Causing Jaundice

#### HEMOLYTIC JAUNDICE

Congenital hemolytic anemias (sickle cell; thalassemia; spherocytic)

Acquired hemolytic anemias (sepsis; chemical or drug induced; mismatched blood transfusion; hemolysin from snake and other poisons; severe burns)

#### HEPATOCELLULAR JAUNDICE

Physiologic jaundice of newborn; cirrhosis; liver cancer; hepatitis (parasitic, bacterial, or viral; chemical-toxic)

#### OBSTRUCTIVE JAUNDICE

Extrahepatic (bile duct blockage due to congenital atresia, or acquired stones, stricture, or tumor)

Intrahepatic (blockage of fine bile structures induced by infection, drugs, or no known cause)

### Companion Signs and Symptoms

Jaundice is both a sign and a symptom; it is not a separate disease. The patient's other signs and symptoms are those of the underlying disease.

Pruritus may be an extremely disquieting feature of obstructive jaundice and difficult to control. Soda or starch baths, calamine, and other soothing lotions may be helpful. Drugs, including antihistamines, cholestyramine, sedatives, and tranquilizers are sometimes ordered, but are used with extreme care to avoid further possible liver damage.

In addition to the morning bath, sponge bathing with tepid water, several times a day, may help to lessen itching. Explain to the patient that scratch-

RBC $\xrightarrow[\text{MARROW}]{\text{SPLEEN}}$ HEMOGLOBIN $\longrightarrow$ "UNCONJUGATED" or

"INDIRECT" BILIRUBIN $\xrightarrow[\text{in blood}]{\text{transported}}$ LIVER $\longrightarrow$ "CONJUGATED" or

"DIRECT" BILIRUBIN $\longrightarrow$ INTESTINE $\longrightarrow$ UROBILINOGEN
(Bile)

UROBILINOGEN $\longrightarrow$ UROBILIN (which colors stool brown)

　　└→ a small part returns to liver
　　└→ a small part reaches kidney and is excreted in urine

**Figure 46-1.** Schema representing the formation of bile.

ing can lead to infection of his skin, and help him avoid scratching and skin infections by such measures as:

- **Keeping his nails short and clean.**
- **Avoiding too-warm bed clothes.**
- **Assisting the patient to find diversion, because concentrating on itching makes it worse.**
- **Giving the patient a supply of calamine lotion (if ordered) and cotton swabs with instruction to apply it to particularly itchy spots.**
- **Making special efforts to promote comfort when the patient is prepared for his night's sleep by such methods as soothing backrubs, a starch bath (if ordered), and an evening snack. Itching tends to be worse at night, when the patient's attention is not diverted. If he scratches while asleep, have him wear white cotton gloves or mittens while sleeping.**

The jaundiced patient often is embarrassed because of his appearance. There are measures which the staff can take to lessen the patient's embarrassment, such as:

- **Make sure his bed is not opposite a mirror.**
- **Avoid remarks or facial expressions that convey that his appearance is odd or unattractive.**
- **Explain to visitors before they enter the room that the patient is jaundiced and help them find ways of controlling their responses to the patient's changed appearance so that the patient's embarrassment is not heightened by his visitors' reactions.**
- **Listen when the patient wishes to discuss his jaundice, and avoid pretending that the jaundice does not exist.**
- **Encourage the patient to ask questions about the jaundice, if he seems puzzled. The condition can seem mysterious to the patient, and often he is helped by understanding what it is, such as that the yellow color is due to excessive bile pigment in the blood.**

Because of associated blood coagulation defects, jaundiced patients may have bleeding tendencies, such as rectal bleeding, tarry stool, blood in urine, bleeding gums, and black and blue marks (ecchymosis) from minor skin trauma. Observe for bleeding and perform procedures in a way that lessens the likelihood of bleeding. For example, intramuscular medicines should be given with small-gauge needles and the injection site should be firmly pressed and observed for hematoma formation. After removal of an intravenous catheter, immediate and prolonged pressure should be applied to prevent seepage which allows hematomas to form making the vein unusable. These patients may require frequent blood tests or intravenous therapy; therefore every effort should be made in order to preserve venous integrity.

Specific care of jaundiced patients will be discussed in relation to the underlying disease.

## Cirrhosis

### Pathology

There are several types of hepatic cirrhosis, depending on etiology, pathology, and clinical manifestations. Basically, liver damage is followed by scarring with development of excessive fibrous connective tissue. This occurs as the liver attempts to repair itself and leads to considerable anatomical distortion, including partial or complete occlusion of blood channels within the liver.

### Etiology

Conditions leading to cirrhotic scarring are listed below. Of these, Laennec's portal cirrhosis is most common in the United States. It is associated with a heavy, chronic alcohol intake, usually coincident with poor nutrition. In the Orient, parasitic disease is a more common etiologic agent. Laennec-type cirrhosis can also follow chronic poisoning with carbon tetrachloride, a cleaning agent.

> TYPES OF CIRRHOSIS
> Laennec's portal cirrhosis (alcoholic; nutritional; toxic)
> Postnecrotic cirrhosis (posthepatitis)
> Parasitic (following schistosomiasis, malaria, etc.)
> Biliary cirrhosis (primary-idiopathic; obstructive)
> Congestive (cardiac cirrhosis)
> Wilson's disease

### Frequency of Laennec's Cirrhosis

This type of cirrhosis is seen most often in males between the ages of 45 and 65 years with a history of alcoholism. Men are affected two to three times more often than women.

### Signs and Symptoms

In addition to signs and symptoms of the underlying disease, general manifestations of liver damage occur. There are disorders of protein, fat, carbohydrate, and vitamin metabolism as well as defects of blood coagulation, fluid and electrolyte balance, and ability to combat infections and toxins.

Clinically, advanced findings include poor nutrition with tissue wasting; poor hemostasis and easy bleeding; vitamin deficiencies; water retention; decreased sodium concentration in the blood (but increased total body sodium); weight loss; weakness, mental dullness; anorexia, nausea, vomiting; intra-abdominal fluid (ascites), low blood sugar (hypoglycemia), and low blood protein (hypoproteinemia). The skin is thin, with dilated veins especially noted over the abdomen. Nosebleed (epistaxis), jaundice, ecchymosis, scant body hair, palmar erythema (bright pink palms), and cutaneous spider angiomata (tiny pulsatile skin vessels of face and chest) also occur. Testicular atrophy is common and is probably due to the inability of the damaged liver to metabolize estrogenic factors produced by organs such as the adrenal gland.

A most important factor secondary to hepatic scarring in Laennec's cirrhosis is portal hypertension. Intrahepatic obstruction to the return of portal blood from the intestines leads to backup and diversion of blood through venous pathways in the stomach and esophagus. These engorged collateral vessels are called esophageal or gastric varices. As this obstructed back-flow increases, pressure within the portal system also increases (portal hypertension). Gastric and esophageal veins distend and are then apt to rupture. Subsequent bleeding into the stomach and esophagus may be slow, with melena, but is often rapid and may result in massive hematemesis with exsanguination and death. Bleeding is aggravated by clotting disorders common in liver damage.

Another serious complication of advanced cirrhosis is infection due to reduced natural resistance as liver function is reduced. Cirrhotic patients are to be protected from others with infection, colds, or other contagious disease. The patient should be instructed in basic principles of hygiene, such as avoiding scratching and obtaining rest and nutrients, to help his body fight infection. Nurses and physicians should wash their hands before caring for the decompensated cirrhotic patient. Established infection is treated by appropriate antibiotics, surgery, or both.

Hepatic coma may occur in any form of liver failure; it frequently follows a bleeding episode, paracentesis, infection, surgery, or other stress. The patient becomes lethargic, drowsy, confused, irritable, and eventually stuporous, drifting into coma. Delirium tremens (DT's) may occur early in the development of hepatic coma. Elevated serum ammonia may be a contributing toxic factor.

Renal failure may occur at the same time as liver failure and add to existing fluid and electrolyte problems. It may be related to pre-existing kidney dysfunction or disturbed blood supply to the kidney. Combined hepatorenal failure has an extremely poor prognosis.

The cirrhotic process may be so minimal that there may be no obvious signs or symptoms of liver dysfunction on clinical or laboratory analysis.

In some patients the disease process gradually advances, especially if therapeutic precautions are not taken. Initially the patient may feel absolutely well or have only minor discomfort. Subtle changes occur with gradual progression through a range of symptomatic intensity, leading eventually to the full-blown manifestations of advanced disease. Hepatic coma is a toxic encephalopathy. The mechanism is not completely understood. It is based on the inability of the diseased liver to metabolize protein adequately. These metabolites adversely affect cerebral function. At first the changes in mentation may be very subtle and go unrecognized for months, e.g., mild lethargy, memory defects, and disordered thinking. Later there may be a flapping tremor of the outstretched hands (asterixis), and finally coma, jaundice, and renal failure. At any point in the progression of these symptoms the level of serum ammonia may be elevated, but this is not a constant finding. Characteristic changes are seen in the electroencephalogram.

## Diagnosis

Diagnosis involves analysis of history, physical examination, and the various laboratory, blood, and radiographic tests mentioned previously. Other diseases with similar findings are ruled out, the diagnosis is established, and therapy is instituted. Biopsy is essential to a definitive diagnosis.

## Care of the Patient

There is no specific cure or medicine for hepatic cirrhosis. The aim of therapy is to prevent further deterioration by abolishing underlying causes and to apply supportive measures while the liver attempts to re-establish its functional integrity.

If treatment begins early when signs and symptoms are few and mild, satisfactory recuperation is frequent and long-term prognosis is good. To rescue patients with advanced disease who are jaundiced, who are hypoproteinemic, and who have ascites as well as other manifestations of severe injury is considerably more difficult to do.

**General Supportive Measures.** Encouraging the patient to eat is a major nursing task. Sustained, adequate nutrition is extremely important. The physician will usually prescribe a diet high in carbohydrates, proteins, and vitamins in the form of meat, fish, eggs, milk, fruit, and vegetables. Fats are sometimes omitted, or included in amounts less than ordinary daily requirements. Tobacco and especially alcohol are prohibited because of the damage alcohol inflicts on the liver. If a high blood level of ammonia is present and impending liver coma is suspected, proteins (which are ammonia precursors) are omitted from the diet. When improvement occurs, proteins are added to the diet. The anorexia of severe cirrhosis may require frequent, small, semisolid or liquid meals rather than three full meals a day. Nausea and vomiting may require parenteral feedings. Vitamin B complex, especially folic acid, vitamins $B_{12}$, K, and C and iron may be prescribed. Intravenous albumin may be given in severe hypoproteinemia, and blood transfusions may be necessary for anemia. Because of the tendency toward salt and water retention (which can lead to edema, circulatory congestion, and heart failure), the intake of these substances is carefully regulated and often restricted. Salt makes food more palatable, so restriction of it poses a challenge to find other seasonings the patient enjoys and is permitted to have. Consult the dietitian, who can help the patient learn to follow his prescribed diet in as palatable a form as possible. The dietitian also sees to it that the patient receives the prescribed amount of protein, fat, carbohydrate, and total calories, and in collaboration with nurse and physician, teaches the patient how to make these calculations himself when he goes home.

Observation of daily weight, intake and output, vital signs, and the color, number, and consistency of bowel movements are important to the care of the cirrhotic patient. Changes in any of these indicators of the patient's condition should be reported to the physician.

Bed rest is ordered should signs of liver failure, such as mental or neurologic disturbance, ascites, jaundice, and weakness arise. Thoughtful, attentive nursing care can make the difference between a relatively comfortable, really rested patient and an exceedingly uncomfortable, restless one. Helping the patient with bed baths and mouth care, applications of soothing lotions or powders, frequent turning to avoid pressure sores, and keeping the urinal and bedpan accessible are examples of measures that can increase comfort during the period of acute illness.

As the patient's condition improves, help him to walk and to find quiet diversion. Teaching the patient and his family assumes increasing importance as he recovers; it is a collaborative effort of physician, nurse, and dietitian. Emotional support is particularly important. Sensitivity to his concerns and a willingness to listen can help him assess his own motivation and goals. Cirrhosis requires long-term therapy and usually re-education. Its success depends considerably on the patient's ability to change his pattern of living—for example, avoiding alcohol if it is a factor in his illness. Often he feels guilt and remorse, and blame from his family, over habits which have contributed to his illness, such as dietary neglect and heavy drinking. Condemnation by others does little to help and can lead the patient to further self-neglect. Setting limits is often necessary and useful, however. For instance, the nurse may matter-of-factly enforce the rule that no alcohol is to be brought to the patient, and encourage visitors to bring, instead, some of the patient's favorite food, provided it is allowed on his diet.

Because immoderate use of alcohol is a significant factor in causing cirrhosis, the assumption is sometimes mistakenly made that cirrhotic patients are necessarily alcoholics. Some cirrhotic patients whose illness is not related to alcohol consumption are burdened by these assumptions of others, and by rejection which, regardless of the etiologic factors in the patient's illness, interferes with treatment and rehabilitation.

The nurse who believes that the patient can follow and benefit from prescribed treatment can often help him begin to believe this too, thus helping him combat discouragement and commence rehabilitation. Several weeks of treatment may be necessary before improvement is obvious. The improvement itself can be a powerful motivating force for the patient as he begins to experience signs of well-being, such as improved appetite, greater mental alertness, and increased strength.

**Increased Fluid Retention.** This condition is manifested as ascitic intra-abdominal fluid and tissue edema and involves factors that are not entirely clear. Overproduction of the hormone aldosterone by the adrenal glands probably occurs in cirrhosis, causing intense sodium and water retention, combined with potassium excretion. This, in addition to associated protein deficiency and factors affecting kidney function, causes fluid to accumulate.

Ascites and edema may be partially alleviated by restricting sodium intake to 1.0 Gm. or less per day and giving a diet rich in protein. The drug spironolactone (Aldactone) specifically antagonizes aldosterone, reversing its effects so that sodium and water are excreted and potassium is retained. The physician looks for acute hyponatremia (low serum sodium) and hyperkalemia (high serum potassium) when this drug is used. Other diuretic agents, including furosemide (Lasix), ammonium chloride, mercuhydrin, hydrochlorothiazide (Hydro-Diuril), and acetozolamide (Diamox), are sometimes prescribed, but with extreme care. Injudicious use of these drugs may aggravate an existing fluid and electrolyte disorder, intensify neurologic defects, and precipitate coma.

Usually ascites can be relieved by severe sodium restriction and diuretic therapy. However, when the abdomen is tense with fluid and kidney function is impaired, a paracentesis may be required. Even then, no more than 1 to 2 liters of fluid is removed, because removal of large quantities of fluid at once can cause drastic shifts between vascular and extravascular compartments and resultant circulatory collapse.

The rapid removal of abdominal fluid by paracentesis is achieved by carefully introducing a needle through the abdominal wall and allowing the ascites to drain. This may quickly relieve the severe discomfort of distention and difficulty in breathing due to the large volume of abdominal fluid pressing upon the diaphragm and lungs. Circulatory collapse (shock) can occur immediately after the tap from acute fluid, mineral, and protein shifts acting to replace the lost ascitic fluid. Other complications of paracentesis include perforation of intestine or bladder with peritonitis, and leakage of fluid from the needle site. To avoid perforation of the bladder, the patient must void before paracentesis. Prior to paracentesis an infusion is usually ordered and plasma is made available for rapid administration if necessary. Pulse, blood pressure, and breathing should be carefully observed after this procedure. Any changes in vital signs or abdominal pain should be reported.

As in patients with decompensated heart and kidney disease, fluid and electrolyte levels in patients with liver damage should be carefully monitored by frequent determinations of serum levels of Na, K, Cl, $CO_2$, and BUN. Clinical features that can confirm and help differentiate such disorders as low sodium, dehydration, overhydration, urinary failure, and high potassium include the character of the skin (dry or moist); level of thirst; blood pressure; volume and specific gravity of urine; pulse rate; state of mentation; and the presence of muscular cramps and weakness. These indicators must be monitored carefully both by physicians and nurses.

## Care of the Cirrhotic Patient with Severe Complications

**Hepatic Coma.** Coma may occur in any form of hepatic failure. Signs and symptoms have been described. Increased serum ammonia level seems to be related to the development or aggravation of hepatic coma, but is not the absolute cause. Therapy to reduce the blood ammonia level seems to ameliorate the comatose state. Ammonia formed in the intestine by bacterial action on ingested proteins is normally detoxified in the liver by conversion to urea, which is then excreted by the kidneys. A failing liver, as in advanced cirrhosis, can no longer break down ammonia and allows it to accumulate in the blood. Also, with portal venous obstruction, ammonia-rich intestinal blood may be diverted from the liver, further reducing detoxification.

Therapy of coma includes reducing protein intake to zero; avoiding drugs or stress; and removing residual protein or blood (if there has been recent hemorrhage) from the intestine by cathartics and enemas. Broad-spectrum antibiotics, such as neomycin, may be ordered in the presence of hepatic encephalopathy. Because it is only poorly absorbed from the gastrointestinal tract, neomycin is used frequently to disinfect the bowel, thereby lessening the production of ammonia by intestinal flora. Cleansing enemas are often ordered to reduce the fecal bacterial substrate in the colon. Careful medical support of the comatose patient involves maintaining fluid and electrolyte balance with parenteral nutrition. Multivitamins are often added to infusions.

Nursing care involves the management of a semicomatose or fully unresponsive patient. Observation of vital signs, frequent turning to avoid pressure sores, mouth care, endotracheal suction to prevent aspiration pneumonia, use of side rails and frequent observation to prevent falling, and similar common-sense measures are essential. When it is impossible to reverse the pathologic process, hepatic coma is a terminal state. In other instances, medical and nursing measures succeed and the patient recovers from coma.

In certain instances of severe hepatic coma, treatment has been by "washout" of toxic blood and reinfusion of fresh blood. When this new investigational technique has been used, the blood has sometimes been perfused through a human cadaver liver or the liver of a pig or baboon. By this cross-circulation system, an attempt is made to achieve detoxification as well as perhaps replenishment of needed liver factors.

**Portal Hypertension and Bleeding Esophageal Varices.** As noted previously, in the scarred cirrhotic liver the intrahepatic veins may be squeezed shut so that blood backs up into the portal vein and on into diverting channels around the esophagus and stomach. If the portal vein itself is obstructed (by tumor, clot, infection or by unknown cause),

similar collateral diversion occurs. The buildup of pressure in the portal system (portal hypertension) can be measured by manometry, and an x-ray film taken of the portal vascular system by arteriography of the celiac, splenic, or superior mesenteric arteries.

Before this test is ordered the physician evaluates the patient's bleeding tendency, because a severe bleeding tendency would make the test very hazardous to the patient. It is necessary for the patient to sign an operative permit. Sedation is ordered prior to the test, which is performed in the x-ray department. Under sterile conditions a needle is introduced through the skin into the spleen. Since the venous drainage of the spleen is into the portal vein, the pressure in the spleen will be a good reflection of portal pressure. This is recorded. If it is over 25 cm. of water (18 mm. Hg), it is diagnostic of portal hypertension and indicates the patient is a potential bleeder from esophageal varices. The most life-threatening complication for the cirrhotic patient is hemorrhage from esophageal varices. These patients have a high incidence of duodenal

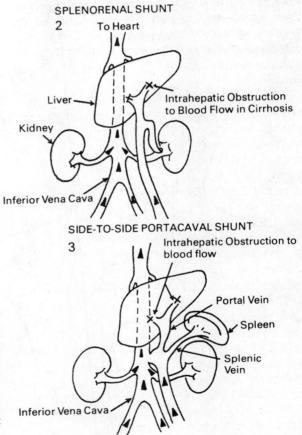

**Figure 46-2.** (1) Normal anatomy showing blood flow back to the heart. Note that major systemic veins pass through the liver. (2) Splenorenal shunt. The spleen has been removed and the splenic vein connected to the left renal vein. Now some portal blood can flow into the inferior vena cava by thus passing the liver. (3) Side-to-side portacaval shunt. The side of the portal vein is anastomosed to the side of the inferior vena cava. Now blood can flow from the portal circulation into the systemic circulation if there is significant intrahepatic obstruction.

ulcers, which may be another cause of gastro-intestinal bleeding.

Contrast dye may be introduced through the needle in the spleen and, as it circulates in the portal system, the character of the portal vein (its size and patency) and the nature of the collateral diverting veins can be evaluated from the x-ray films.

As after liver biopsy, vital signs and evidences of bleeding should be looked for after these procedures.

In some instances emergency esophagoscopy may be carried out to verify bleeding from the esopha-gus. Another test to evaluate possible bleeding sites is the arteriogram. In this procedure radiopaque dye is injected into the circulation. If a significant leak has occurred, x-ray films may define its loca-tion in the gastrointestinal tract.

TREATMENT. Portal hypertension can be re-lieved by surgically draining blood from the portal vein into an adjacent systemic vein. As less blood goes through the portal system, the pressure drops and there is less chance of a burst collateral vessel with resultant hemorrhage.

The portal vein lies just next to the inferior vena cava. A connection can be made surgically between these vessels so that portal blood is released into the vena cava, reducing hypertension. This is called a *portacaval shunt*. Sometimes a similar beneficial effect is achieved by connecting the splenic vein (a tributary of the portal vein) to the renal vein (a tributary of the vena cava). This is called a *spleno-renal shunt* (see Fig. 46-2, p. 175).

These are major operations. If done electively or prophylactically to prevent future hemorrhage, the patient should be in the best possible preoperative condition. The jaundiced, hypoproteinemic patient with electrolyte disorders and ascites is a poor risk and frequently will not tolerate this surgery. Such complications should be rectified before surgery.

Often a portacaval or splenorenal shunt must be done as an emergency operation in a patient with high portal pressure and with massively bleeding esophagogastric varices. In these cases conserva-tive measures to stop bleeding have failed, and an attempt to rapidly lower portal pressure and shunt blood away from the engorged bleeding site is necessary to save life.

Other emergency operations to stop bleeding from varices include direct division and ligation of varices in the stomach and esophagus. Both before and after surgery, physicians and nurses work as a team to carry out the intensive program of care and observation needed to pull these critically ill people through.

The stress of surgery usually produces further

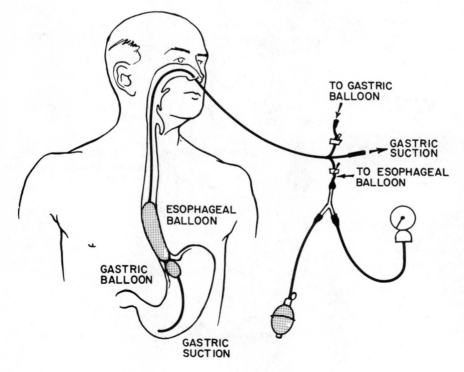

**Figure 46-3.** A Sengstaken-Blakemore tube in place. The clamp on the tube that leads to the esophageal balloon is kept tightly closed to maintain the inflated balloon at the pre-scribed pressure. The clamp is loosened to check the pressure with the manometer. The gas-tric suction tube is attached to continuous suction to keep the patient's stomach empty and to prevent vomiting, which would dislodge the esophageal balloon. Irrigations of the gas-tric suction tube may be or-dered to prevent clogging with blood.

transient liver impairment or frank failure with coma. Associated problems may include kidney failure, further hemorrhage, and electrolyte imbalance. After surgery, coma may be additionally aggravated by the fact that intestinal blood, rich in ammonia, is now being directly shunted into the systemic circulation. This is not an infrequent postoperative complication, even when all else is going well, and must be treated aggressively. (Treatment to reduce ammonia levels has already been discussed.)

Both pre- and postoperative blood volumes must be maintained by transfusion; measures are taken to avoid hepatic coma; vitamins (especially K, B, and C) and glucose are given parenterally; vital signs, intake, and output are constantly monitored; oversedation is avoided; urine catheter and nasogastric drainage tubes are checked frequently for patency; blood counts and chemistries are followed carefully.

As the patient improves after surgery, the supportive measures previously outlined for the therapy of patients with cirrhosis and liver impairment are carried out. Before major surgery, conservative measures are carried out in the hope of slowing bleeding down enough to better prepare for emergency surgery. If bleeding stops, surgery may be postponed to an elective date.

SENGSTAKEN-BLAKEMORE ESOPHAGEAL-GASTRIC BALLOON TUBE. In addition to the supportive measures mentioned, a most useful device to stop bleeding from esophageal varices is the Sengstaken-Blakemore esophageal-gastric balloon tube (illustrated in Figure 46-3).

Use of this tube can be hazardous and requires *constant vigil by both physicians and nurses* to get the best effect. It has three separate openings: one inflates the esophageal balloon, another inflates the gastric balloon, and the third aspirates the stomach. The distended, bleeding varices of portal hypertension are in the lower esophagus and upper stomach. As the gastric balloon is inflated to the prescribed pressure, it is gently pulled up. In this way constant application of this balloon to the upper stomach wall squeezes any bleeding vessels shut. Similarly, as the esophageal balloon is inflated, it expands against the esophageal wall and ruptured bleeding varices are pressed closed. In this way bleeding can be controlled. Through the tube opening into the stomach, clots can be irrigated out (reducing protein by-products of digested blood,

leading to the production of ammonia and possible hepatic coma). Later, small liquid tube feedings may be given; however, it is usually wiser to keep the patient fasting as long as the tube is in place. This reduces the possibility of gastric distention or retching, with regurgitation of the balloon.

Constant nursing care and observation are needed, so the patient is usually placed in the intensive care unit. These problems should be anticipated: too much pressure in the balloons can cause necrosis of the esophageal or gastric wall; the balloons can be pulled up into the oropharynx, interfere with breathing, and cause asphyxia; with the balloons inflated, saliva cannot be swallowed and must be suctioned away to prevent aspiration into the trachea.

The most common iatrogenic cause of death associated with the tube is asphyxiation. If the patient shows signs of respiratory distress, the tubes leading to both balloons should be cut at once, thereby deflating them and letting the patient breathe. Since the tube is introduced through the nose and traction is applied to the exposed ends coming from the nose, care must be taken to avoid pressure to the nasal walls causing necrosis and loss of a portion of nose.

As the patient's condition stabilizes, the tube may be deflated 24 to 48 hours later. It is hoped that bleeding will not recur. The tube is not removed yet, but kept loosely in place so that rapid reinflation can be carried out if necessary. During this period the patient is observed for melena, further hematemesis, fall in blood pressure, fall in hematocrit, and tachycardia, which indicate further bleeding. If bleeding occurs or is uncontrolled, emergency shunt or ligation operation may be necessary.

With this tube in place the patient may be restless, apprehensive, and uncomfortable. Simple sedatives, such as antihistamines, may be useful. Barbiturates that are usually metabolized in the liver should not be used.

Vasopressin (Pitressin), a pituitary extract with strong vasoconstrictive action, is often added in the medical attempt to temporarily control bleeding varices. It is injected directly into the arteries drained by the bleeding varices.

Gastric lavage with iced saline and methods to indirectly cool the stomach and esophageal walls are usually not effective and if used alone may cause loss of precious time.

## Viral Hepatitis (Infectious or Serum Hepatitis)

### Pathology

Hepatitis is an infectious, contagious disease caused by a virus. The infection may cause simultaneous damage to the intestine and other organs, but the most significant damage is to liver cells, which become necrotic and die. In fatal cases parenchymal damage is severe. Internal damage to the liver may prevent normal bile secretion or excretion, causing jaundice in addition to the metabolic dysfunction of parenchymal injury.

### Etiology and Frequency

There are two types of hepatitis, both caused by viruses which, although similar in nature, produce slightly different clinical diseases. Infectious hepatitis is caused by the IH virus, or virus A; serum hepatitis is caused by the SH virus, or virus B.

Both of these viruses resist drying, freezing, heating, and other physical and chemical treatments. They can be destroyed by heating at 60 degrees C for ten hours. Albumin may be made virus-free, whereas whole blood and pooled plasma cannot be decontaminated and are frequent transmitters of the virus.

Infectious hepatitis is usually disseminated by contact with contagious virus in the stool of infected people. The virus may be transmitted by close contact with carriers, contaminated food, water, or other items apt to be taken orally. Contaminated rectal thermometers, bedpans, and linen harbor the virus, which then reaches the fingers and may be subsequently ingested. Diseased food handlers, cooks, or waiters may create an epidemic especially in the army, schools, or similar close community environment. Virus A also occurs in the bloodstream of infected people, so that it can also be transmitted by this route. The virus may be in the blood before, during, and after the period of infectivity. Duration of infectivity may be difficult to determine, and the patient should be assumed to be infectious for several weeks after the onset of the jaundice.

Serum hepatitis, virus B, is usually found only in blood and is transmitted by transfusions of blood or plasma and inoculation via contaminated syringes, needles, surgical and dental equipment. More recently, there is evidence that virus B may be passed in the saliva and urine, and via sexual intercourse. Carriers are asymptomatic and may be infective for long periods. This condition has increased in areas where drug abuse is widespread. Drug addicts often use unsterile syringes, and by so doing, contract the disease.

Many people probably have subclinical infectious hepatitis some time in life, presenting as a very mild illness, without jaundice or significant liver damage. Following a bout of infectious hepatitis, immunity built up to that causative virus will not protect the patient from a subsequent attack of serum hepatitis.

### Signs and Symptoms

Serum hepatitis and infectious hepatitis are not clinically distinguishable. The incubation period of infectious hepatitis is from 6 days to 6 weeks, whereas serum hepatitis takes 60 to 120 days to develop after infection occurs.

The disease pattern, except for the difference in incubation period, is basically the same. In the preicteric (early or prejaundice) phase, manifestations include fever, rash, joint pain, lymph-node enlargement, anorexia, nausea, vomiting, weakness, pain over the liver, and diarrhea. The liver may be enlarged and tender to percussion; there is often a distaste for smoking tobacco; fatigue may be profound. The spleen is occasionally palpably enlarged.

All these manifestations may occur with varying speed of onset before jaundice is seen. Icterus may be evident from one to three weeks after the onset of symptoms. Occasionally, a patient will die of massive liver failure even before becoming jaundiced. As jaundice appears, patients usually improve clinically, with better appetite, less pain, and increased strength. Jaundice usually persists for one or two weeks. An important concern of the physician is to differentiate between jaundice due to hepatitis and jaundice due to obstruction.

### Laboratory Tests

The earliest indication of parenchymal damage is an elevation in transaminase. This usually precedes the rise in bilirubin and alkaline phosphatase. Alteration in proteins leads to a positive cephalin flocculation and thymol turbidity. Transaminase levels may not return to normal for as long as 12 to 36 months although the patient is clinically well.

### Prognosis

A small number (less than 1 per cent) of patients will proceed to hepatic coma and death. Most will recover, but they will be forever barred from being blood donors. A few patients will suffer from chronic active hepatitis. These patients usually go on to cirrhosis and death unless corticosteroid treatment slows the active and inflammatory process.

### Prevention

Gamma globulin has been used as a preventive against hepatitis, with some small success. It may make the attack of hepatitis less severe. It does not give 100 per cent protection; it probably gives no protection against serum hepatitis and it is of no help if the patient already has contracted the disease.

Blood is screened for a hepatitis associated antigen (HAA or Australia antigen), which is found in serum hepatitis, and rejected if the antigen is discovered. Recently the test for SH antigen by radioimmunoassay or electrophoresis has become a popular method to determine possible exposure to or presence of the hepatitis virus. Although the test is not 100 per cent accurate in all cases, it is a valuable new device.

Patients scheduled for elective surgery, who may require blood transfusions, are requested to donate their own blood a few weeks in advance of surgery. This eliminates the possibility that the patient will contract hepatitis from a blood donor and it also minimizes transfusion reactions.

Cardiac and vascular surgery, organ transplantation, and renal dialysis in which repeated infusions and transfusions are likely have also added to the patient, nurse, and physician population at risk. Physicians and nurses can contact hepatitis from patients, for example, by pricking a finger with a contaminated needle.

With both types of hepatitis, extreme caution is required to avoid direct contact with the patient's blood, stool or other drainage. The nurse should use great care to see that she is not pricked accidentally by the needle that has been used to withdraw blood from a hepatitis patient. Disposable syringes and needles should be used. In the unusual situation in which none is available, the needle and the syringe should be rinsed with water and placed in a rack or boat containing solvent or soap solution. If the needles are cared for immediately after use, the chance of anyone's pricking himself with them is lessened. Should it occur, however, injections of gamma globulin should be given.

Needles and syringes should not be used again for a patient until they have been autoclaved at 15 pounds of pressure for a minimum of 20 minutes. If boiling is the only method of sterilization available, the equipment should be completely covered by bubbling water for no less than 30 minutes. However, boiling is not considered to be as sure a method of killing the virus as is autoclaving, and should be used only in emergencies. There is no antiseptic known that kills the viruses, and placing equipment in alcohol or other antiseptic solutions does not sterilize it against these stubborn organisms. Therefore, this practice is discouraged in any setting, even when there is no known patient with hepatitis. Also, to be absolutely condemned is the practice of using the same syringe for more than one patient without sterilizing between uses. When the plunger is pulled back, a small amount of serum enters the syringe. Changing the needle, but using the same syringe, does not prevent the injection of that serum into the next patient, and hepatitis can be readily spread from "healthy" carriers in this way.

### Treatment

As there is no known drug or medical therapy that directly affects the viruses of hepatitis, treatment is directed at strengthening the patient's body to withstand the insult of the infection. Rest is the cornerstone of treatment.

Bed rest and a nourishing diet, often one higher in protein than carbohydrate, are offered. Although the patient probably will be grateful for the rest, his poor appetite will make it difficult for him to accept the diet. Some physicians have allowed patients to regulate their own activity—staying on complete bed rest if they feel that ill, or, gradually, going to the bathroom and staying up in their rooms if they feel equal to more exertion. When the illness is severe, corticosteroids may be used but their effectiveness has not been proven.

### Nursing Care

Because the treatment is concerned mainly with improving resistance so he can fight the virus, nursing care is of paramount importance. Bed rest should not be a mere twisting and turning in an uncomfortable tangle of sheets. Comfortably positioning the patient, with pillows and changes of position, may help him to rest. The nurse also protects her patient from disturbances by maintaining quiet in the halls, explaining the need for rest to visitors, and doing as much as is necessary for the patient at one time so that he need not be bothered at frequent intervals.

His interest in food may be enlivened by an attractively served tray. A small quantity of food does not look as discouraging to the anorectic patient as does a full tray. Hot drinks that are really hot, and cold drinks that are iced are more tempting than those that are lukewarm. Any patient with jaundice (unless the presence of edema or another disease contraindicates the rule) should drink a hearty quantity of fluid each day: 3,000 ml. is a desirable goal. Dehydration can lead to hepatic coma. Color of skin, stool, and urine should be observed.

Although the mode of transmission of serum hepatitis and infectious hepatitis is different, differential diagnosis between the two diseases may be difficult. Therefore all patients with hepatitis are usually placed in isolation. Linen is handled separately, and dishes and eating utensils are sterilized. When paper plates are used, they should be heat-retaining and able to contain food without becoming soaked. It is understandable that patients resent being served meals that arrive cold and on soggy plates. Patients may view paper plates as further evidence of rejection, especially because they are told that a good diet is important and they observe that other patients are served hot food on china plates. The patient should be provided with his own glass and straw.

Since the virus of infectious hepatitis lives in the gastrointestinal tract, stool precautions are required. The patient has his own thermometer, and, if it is a rectal thermometer, the nurse is especially careful to scrub her hands after handling it. Thermometers resist autoclaving, so it is good economy to throw them away after the patient's discharge from the hospital. This practice is less expensive than trying to sterilize them and possibly infecting another patient with hepatitis. The bedpan is kept for the hepatitis patient's sole use, and it is autoclaved or boiled for an hour when he leaves the hospital. The disposal of feces is carried out according to the hospital rules for stool precautions, with strict attention to technique. The nurse washes her hands well after handling the bedpan. Rubber gloves should be used when giving the patient a rectal treatment, such as an enema. Some recommend that all staff wear gloves whenever handling stool or blood and when bathing the patient.

Visitors should be given enough instruction in isolation precautions to enable them to protect themselves. Warn them against close contact with the patient, sharing his food, or giving him the bedpan.

Viral hepatitis lowers resistance to secondary infection. Hand washing on entering the patient's unit protects him. No effort should be spared to separate the patient from infective organisms.

Patients generally are kept in isolation until the fever has subsided and the jaundice begins to fade, usually for one or two weeks after the onset of symptoms. As the patient begins to feel well, he may have a tendency to overexert and cause his symptoms to recur. The nurse should encourage a return to bed, if he seems to be a person who drives himself. The medical regimen may require that the patient remain on bed rest for a month or more. This may be a good time for him to catch up on reading, to follow baseball on television, or to start a handicraft project. An inquiry into previous interests may give a clue as to the kind of activity that will hold his enthusiasm.

Part of the nurse's role is the interpretation of the physician's orders and, with the patient and his family, helping to establish a convalescent regimen that will be feasible within the framework of the physician's prescription.

## Noninfectious Hepatitis (Toxic or Chemical)

Exposure to cleaning solutions with carbon tetrachloride, insecticides, cinchophen (a drug used in arthritis), and some other drugs and chemicals can cause severe liver derangement. Degree of damage and signs and symptoms will vary with the amount of poisoning as well as associated damage to kidneys and other organs. The clinical picture may evolve gradually or abruptly and be indistinguishable from viral hepatitis. History of exposure, high WBC count, acute onset of jaundice, and hepatic failure, with a rapidly enlarging tender liver usually is more indicative of toxic hepatitis.

Therapy involves removal of the toxic agent, a diet high in carbohydrates, proteins, and vitamins, and rest in bed. General supportive and convalescent care is similar to that prescribed for viral hepatitis.

Prophylaxis of this form of disease requires education of children, parents, industrial workers, and others by nurses, physicians and public health-minded individuals. Advise the public to read labels carefully and observe precautions in use of cleaning solutions, insecticides, and other chemicals; provide adequate ventilation when using volatile chemicals; keep chemicals away from children; take no medicines unless specifically prescribed by the physician. Often patients will save the unused portion of a prescribed medicine, then pass it on to a friend or relative, or even use it for a different condition, without medical consultation, to avoid expense.

### Pyogenic Liver Abscess

Pyogenic liver abscess is a localized bacterial infection of the liver resulting in a pus-filled abscess cavity. Bacteria reach the liver from nearby or distant sources by way of the biliary tract, the hepatic artery, or portal vein inflow into the liver. In this way conditions such as cholangitis, appendicitis, diverticulitis, peritonitis, kidney infection, pneumonia, cholecystitis, and bacterial endocarditis may be responsible for one or multiple abscesses. Any organism may be the offending agent, but *E. coli* and *S. aureus* are the most common.

Clinically, fever, chills, right upper abdominal pain, weight loss, anorexia, jaundice, and right pleural fluid accumulation may be seen in any combination. Liver function tests usually show abnormalities, as may roentgenograms of the abdomen, a liver scan, and an hepatic arteriogram. Treatment is by surgical drainage and appropriate antibiotics. Rupture of the abscess with peritonitis is a serious, often fatal, complication.

### Parasitic Diseases

Parasitic diseases of the liver include amebic abscess due to *Entamoeba histolytica* and hydatid cyst due to the echinococcus tapeworm. These conditions, though uncommon, are occasionally seen and diagnosed by history, laboratory, and radiographic studies. Their treatment involves surgical drainage and the use of amebicidal drug therapy for the one and excision of the echinococcus cyst for the other.

Nursing care in these infectious conditions is supportive as in any liver disease or following major surgery. Additionally, especially where drainage has been instituted, instruments, equipment, and dressings must always be carefully handled in order to avoid reinfection of patients, as well as physicians, nurses, aides, and technicians.

### Trauma

Trauma to the liver can be by direct penetration (knife or sharp object) or by blunt injury, fracturing the liver (automobile or similar forceful accidents). Other organs may be simultaneously damaged. Immediate mortality is high because of bleeding and associated injuries. If the abdomen has not been perforated, there may be no early external evidence of injury. If the patient is conscious, pain may be present. Shock with pallor, hypotension, and tachycardia develop, according to the rate of bleeding. The abdomen may fill with blood as the hematocrit drops. Careful tap of the abdominal cavity by needle aspiration may disclose blood. Initial treatment includes blood volume replacement. Emergency surgery includes hemostasis, removal of necrotic liver tissue, and drainage of bile that leaks from the bare liver surfaces. In certain situations the common bile duct may be drained with a tube to decompress the biliary system and liver of bile.

Abscesses may occur within or around the liver, requiring further surgery at a later date.

### Tumors of the Liver

Neoplasms of the liver can be benign or malignant. Benign tumors include hemangiomas (a collection of blood vessels), rare adenomas, cysts, and hamartomas. These may pose problems in differentiation from malignant tumors or may enlarge enough to become symptomatic. On this basis surgical intervention may be required for biopsy or removal.

Malignant tumors include the rare primary liver cell carcinoma (hepatoma) and bile duct carcinoma (cholangiocarcinoma). When diagnosed, these tumors are usually fatal within one year without treatment or if treated by simple excision. Radical resection by removal of an entire lobe of the liver is occasionally feasible and permits longer survivals. Primary carcinoma of the liver (hepatoma) occurs more often in patients with underlying cirrhosis.

More commonly, the liver is afflicted with metastatic cancer from other organs, such as the breast, lung, stomach, or colon. On occasion, a single metastatic implant may be excised. Systemic chemotherapy by anticancer drugs is occasionally valuable in the treatment of liver cancers that cannot be removed surgically. The administration of cytotoxic chemicals directly into the liver through a catheter placed in the hepatic artery may produce temporary remission. Radiotherapy by external x-ray or radioisotopes is not used routinely in the management of liver cancers.

The presence of primary or secondary malignancy in the liver usually signifies a fatal outcome in the near future. Supportive measures include diet and vitamins as for other forms of hepatic insufficiency. When pain is a major factor, analgesics should be used to provide relief.

### Liver Transplantation

In cases where an otherwise incurable destructive benign or malignant liver disease is present, it has recently become technically feasible to totally replace the damaged liver with a normal liver from a donor, or place the donor liver in another region of the abdomen to augment the activity of the patient's own failing liver. In addition to the operative mortality inherent in this highly complex procedure, graft rejection and infection are later complications. A very few patients have lived as long as a year. This procedure is still in the investigational stage. The aftercare of these patients requires a highly specialized and individualized program utilizing all of the principles of nursing and medical therapy discussed previously.

## DISEASES OF THE BILIARY SYSTEM

### Anatomy and Function

The gallbladder is attached to the midportion of the undersurface of the liver. Normally it has a thin wall and a capacity of about 60 ml. of bile. Bile formed in the liver enters the intrahepatic bile ducts and travels to the common hepatic duct. It usually then passes into the cystic duct and is stored in the gallbladder. When required, the gallbladder empties its bile, which now goes out of the cystic duct, into the common bile duct, and on into the duodenum. Stones can be found in any portion of this bile system, most frequently in the gallbladder. Arteries, veins, and lymphatics are associated with all sections of the biliary tree, and along with the ducts themselves are subject to considerable variation.

The liver forms up to 1 liter of bile per day. Upon reaching the gallbladder, bile is altered by the absorption of water and minerals to form a more concentrated product. Upon reaching the intestine after gallbladder contraction (stimulated by ingested food, especially fats), this bile functions in the absorption of fats, fat-soluble vitamins, iron, and calcium. Bile also activates the pancreas to release its digestive enzymes as well as an alkaline fluid, which may neutralize stomach acids reaching the duodenum.

### Cholecystitis and Cholelithiasis

These terms signify gallbladder inflammation and stones within the gallbladder. Gallstones represent the most common abnormality of the biliary system, occurring in about 20 per cent of people over 40 years. There is a progressively increased incidence with aging. They occur in women about four times more often than in men, particularly in women with a history of pregnancies, diabetes, and obesity. The etiology of gallbladder stones has not been definitely established. Bile stasis and infection have been generally implicated. Hemolytic anemia associated with excessive bilirubin is associated with development of pigment stones; hypercholesterolemia is associated with the accumulation of cholesterol stones.

Chronic cholecystitis is rarely present without stones. Stones and infections are intimately related. Symptoms in this condition are probably secondary to transient blockage of the outflow of bile due to stones or spasm of the ductal system. Most usually, after a meal containing fried, greasy, spicy, or fatty foods, the patient experiences belching, nausea, and right upper abdominal discomfort, with pain or cramps. When pain is very severe it is called "biliary colic." Pain may radiate around the right to the back and shoulder. Vomiting may occur.

In simple, uncomplicated colic of chronic cholecystitis with stones, there is no jaundice, fever, chills, liver damage, leukocytosis, or evidence of peritonitis on abdominal examination. Many patients with stones in the gallbladder may never have significant symptomatology.

### Diagnosis

In addition to suggestive signs and symptoms, definitive demonstration of cholelithiasis is by the cholecystogram (gallbladder series). The evening before roentgenography a special dye-containing tablet is given the patient, after which he should fast until the time of testing. The nurse should be sure he gets and takes the tablet and remains fasting during the night.

Giving cathartics or enemas simultaneously or shortly after the dye tablets should be avoided. These may cause increased intestinal motility and evacuation of the dye before it can reach the liver and gallbladder. The dye tablets themselves may cause diarrhea, so may be prematurely lost from the intestine. Under such circumstances, when x-ray films are taken the following day nonvisualization of the gallbladder will perhaps be due to lack of dye rather than disease. Thus, if diarrhea has occurred, the nurse must record this and inform the physician. After ingestion, this dye reaches the liver, is excreted into the bile, and passes into the gallbladder, making it visible radiographically. Preliminary films are taken. Then, following a small fatty meal (such as olive oil, butter, or egg yolk), another film is taken to determine whether or not the gallbladder contracts normally.

This series of x-ray films can show a normal gallbladder, a nonfunctional gallbladder, or stones in the gallbladder. If there is obstructive jaundice or hepatocellular disease preventing normal bile flow, this test is not used because it will not demonstrate the gallbladder. If the gallbladder is not visualized, the test is repeated. If on two occasions there is failure to demonstrate the gallbladder, this is presumptive evidence of stones or inflammation. It is important to explain to the patient that this test is sometimes repeated, so that he does not become needlessly alarmed.

## Treatment

Because of the distress associated with this condition, removal of the gallbladder (cholecystectomy) is usually advised. Even in mild cases, because of the possibility of future distress and the complications of acute cholecystitis, cholecystectomy is still advised by many surgeons who prefer to operate electively rather than anticipate a more urgent situation.

**Medical.** Patients known to have gallbladder stones should be advised to avoid fried, greasy, spicy, and high-cholesterol foods. These include eggs, pork products, rich dressings, cheese, cream, and whole milk. A dietitian should instruct the patient and outline a palatable, wholesome diet also aimed at maintaining a reasonable body weight.

During an attack of colic, therapy usually involves rest, a bland liquid diet, and sedation. If vomiting is a feature, hospitalization, nasogastric suction, and parenteral fluids may be needed. Meperidine (Demerol) and morphine may be used to reduce severe pain or colic. These drugs should be used sparingly and only, if necessary, because they are known to cause spasm of portions of the common duct. Nitroglycerine and aminophylline may be used to try to relieve spasm; however, many doctors believe these drugs are not often required.

General nursing care is supportive, to create as comfortable an environment as possible for the patient until the attack passes. Because the pain during an acute attack can be extremely severe, it is important to observe the patient carefully and to make sure his call light is answered promptly. The severity of the pain can cause fear, which in turn causes more severe pain. Assure the patient that you are nearby and visit him frequently. Administer sedatives and analgesics promptly when they are ordered, and note the patient's response to medication. Mouth care and prompt emptying of the emesis basin can lessen distress due to vomiting.

**Surgical.** Patients whose attacks continue or grow worse are usually treated surgically. Cholecystectomy is planned under general anesthesia. The day before surgery a liquid diet helps to keep the bowel clean; after midnight the patient is given nothing by mouth; the morning of operation a nasogastric tube is usually put in place so that postoperative secretions and swallowed air can be removed from the stomach. The chart should be checked for a signed operative permit; physicians will have reviewed the cardiogram, chest roentgenograms, complete blood count, urine analysis, and liver chemistries to be sure they are satisfactory.

Following cholecystectomy, and after a period in the recovery room, the patient is returned to the floor, where special measures for care after general anesthesia should be observed. Side rails should be up; the nasogastric tube should be checked for patency and irrigated if necessary; infusions should be observed and vital signs monitored. The patient must be encouraged to cough to prevent postoperative stasis pneumonia. Limited ambulation and frequent turning during the first day improve venous circulation, prevent phlebitis, and help keep the lungs clear of secretion. (For details of postoperative nursing care, see Chapter 16.)

Of particular importance in postoperative care are:

- **Emphasis on deep breathing and coughing. Because the incision is high on the abdomen, these patients find full expansion of the chest more painful than with a lower incision. Because of this, they are prone to shallow breathing and avoidance of coughing, which predisposes them to respiratory complications.**

Show the patient how to splint the incision with his hands to lessen the pain when coughing and taking deep breaths. Sometimes a folded draw sheet drawn tightly about the incision when the patient is in sitting position helps lessen pain by splinting the incision and helps the patient carry out the necessary coughing and deep breathing. The patient should be taught preoperatively this aspect of what is expected of him and he should practice the exercises before his operation.

- Medication for relief of pain must be administered frequently so the patient can rest and carry out his postoperative exercises, yet not so frequently that his activity is diminished and his respirations become shallow or even depressed.

- Measures to help the patient void are discussed in Chapter 16. It is preferable to begin using these measures before the patient becomes uncomfortable from bladder distention. Thus, attention to positioning, privacy, lack of haste, and an attitude of calmness can help the patient void before the bladder becomes distressingly distended. Otherwise his tension, physical discomfort, and preoccupation with voiding militate against spontaneous voiding; and catheterization, which might have been avoided, becomes necessary. If the patient is unable to void after eight to ten hours, notify the physician, who usually will order catheterization. However, use nursing measures to promote spontaneous voiding thereafter, so that further catheterizations do not become necessary.

For a simple cholecystectomy, one or two soft rubber drains are usually placed in the area of the excised gallbladder to remove blood and bile which may accumulate after surgery. If the dressing is stained excessively with blood or bile, the doctor should be immediately informed.

With a smooth course, the nasogastric tube is usually removed in 24 to 48 hours. Liquid feedings are started and gradually progressed to a general low-fat diet. The rubber drain is usually taken out by the third to the fifth day. Patients are usually told to keep to a low-fat diet indefinitely.

**Acute Cholecystitis** is a progression of chronic cholecystitis in which a stone completely blocks off flow of bile from the gallbladder. If the stone impacted in the cystic duct is not dislodged spontaneously, the walls of the distended gallbladder may become gangrenous, causing rupture and subsequent peritonitis. These patients are usually very sick, with fever, vomiting, severe abdominal pain, and tenderness over the liver. The gallbladder may be so swollen that it becomes palpable; the white blood count is high; jaundice may be slightly evident due to associated hepatic inflammation.

Medical management, including antibiotics, parenteral fluids, and nasogastric suction, fails to relieve a significant number of patients. In these cases surgery may be lifesaving and consists either of cholecystectomy or cholecystostomy (opening the gallbladder, removing stones and placing a tube for bile drainage to the exterior). If medical therapy is successful, cholecystectomy is carried out two to three months after inflammation has subsided.

**Choledocholithiasis** means the presence of stones anywhere in the ducts of the biliary system. The usual origin is the gallbladder. However, a small number of people form stones within the ductal system even after the gallbladder is removed.

Signs and symptoms are those of cholecystitis and cholelithiasis, but in addition jaundice is typical. If stones completely block the common duct, the stools will be clay colored because no bilirubin reaches the intestine. The urine will darken with bilirubin, as this pigment backs up into the blood and reaches the kidney.

If the ducts become infected, fever and chills mark the onset of cholangitis or infection of the bile ducts. This may progress to septicemia and shock. Parenteral antibiotics will be required.

The presence of common duct stones is suggested by history and the physical finding of jaundice. Liver chemistries will show elevated bilirubin, cholesterol, and alkaline phosphatase, suggesting obstructive disease. Unless long-standing obstruction with infection has been present, there should be no chemical indication of hepatocellular damage. This testing usually differentiates the jaundice of hepatitis from that due to other diseases. If the patient is only slightly jaundiced (less than 2 or 3 mg. of bilirubin per 100 ml. of blood), an intravenous cholangiogram will define the common duct radiographically and show stones within it. This test involves the use of an intravenous dye that is quickly absorbed by the liver and excreted in the bile so that the duct can be visualized within one hour. Query the patient to find out if he is sensitive to iodine.

If obstruction and jaundice have been present, the prothrombin time may be elevated, indicating a deficit in coagulation. This will occur because vitamin K is used in the manufacture of prothrombin by the liver. Vitamin K is fat soluble and poorly absorbed from the intestine, if bile is absent. Vitamin K is prescribed for these patients and, if it is at all possible, surgery is deferred until the prothrombin time is normal.

784

Treatment of choledocholithiasis is surgical exploration of the common duct, removal of stones, and cholecystectomy if the gallbladder is present. At the end of this operation, a small T-shaped tube is placed into the common duct. The small end is placed in the duct lumen aligned lengthwise; the long end comes out through the skin (Fig. 46-4). If bile flow is temporarily obstructed because of postsurgical spasm of the duct, this tube will allow decompression by releasing bile externally. Before the operation is terminated, dye may be introduced into the T-tube to visualize the ductal tree, insuring that all stones have been removed.

The postoperative care is similar to that following cholecystectomy, except that in this case there is a T-tube to be observed. This is connected to straight gravity drainage. The collection bag, or bottle, is attached to the bed below the level of the operation site, to prevent reflux of bile into the duct and avoid an excessive height against which bile would have to "climb" in order to drain. The receptacle must have a vent opening to prevent pressure build-up, which would hinder bile drainage.

Particular care is taken to avoid dislodging the tube by a sudden stress or yank. It should be firmly secured to the abdominal wall; the collection tubing should not be allowed to tangle and should have sufficient slack to allow some freedom of movement. Care should be taken when turning the patient; when conscious, he should be alerted to the presence of this tube.

The tube is usually left constantly open. Kinking or allowing the patient to roll over and occlude the lumen must be avoided. It should not be clamped without a physician's order. Drainage usually amounts to a few hundred milliliters of bile per day, since most of the bile is expected to pass on into the intestine. However, if total obstruction is present in the common duct, up to 1 liter of bile may drain and the stool will be light colored. If such significant bile loss is expected for more than a week, the bile may be mixed with chilled fruit juice and fed to the patient in small quantities during the day. Thus, he does not lose the benefit of bile constituents necessary for proper digestion.

The T-tube is usually removed after the tenth postoperative day. Frequently a T-tube cholangiogram (in which dye is introduced into the tube and an x-ray picture is taken), is done before the tube is removed in order to make certain that there is no residual obstruction.

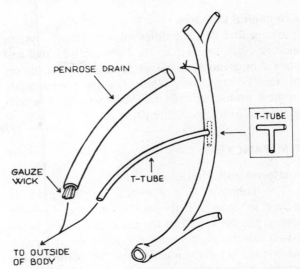

**Figure 46-4.** After cholecystectomy the Penrose drain helps to remove exudate from the area formerly occupied by the gallbladder. The T-tube diverts bile to the outside.

When the patient returns from the radiology department, be sure that unless physicians have indicated otherwise, the tube is unclamped and draining freely. This is done to avoid prolonged contact of residual dye within the bile duct, which may be irritating. Following the T-tube cholangiogram there may be transient temperature elevation, nausea, and vomiting. The patient should be carefully observed and the physician notified. Persistent fever, especially if with chills, may signal inflammation of the bile ducts or pancreatic duct. This may develop into a full-blown cholangitis or pancreatitis requiring antibiotics, intravenous fluids, and other measures.

The usual postoperative measures include early ambulation, nasogastric tube aspiration, observation of vital signs, and wound drainage for blood or bile.

## Carcinoma

Carcinoma of the gallbladder and bile duct is infrequent and has an extremely poor prognosis. Surgery, often involving partial hepatectomy, is the only curative method at present. Perfusion with cytotoxic agents is only palliative; liver transplantation is being investigated.

It should be noted that up to 90 per cent of patients with cancer of the gallbladder have associated stones, further supporting the argument for removing all gallbladders with stones.

## Congenital Diseases

Congenital abnormalities of the biliary system include cystic swelling of the common bile duct and atresia or stenosis of all or some of the segments of the biliary tree. When feasible, appropriate surgical procedures can relieve the pathologic consequences of these conditions.

## THE PANCREAS

### Anatomy and Physiology

The pancreas is a glandular organ about 10 inches in length that lies behind the stomach, against the back wall of the upper abdomen. It has a rich arterial supply with correspondingly numerous veins that drain mainly into the portal venous system. Lymphatic vessels also provide drainage from the pancreas into adjacent lymph nodes. Sympathetic and parasympathetic nerve fibers pass to and from the pancreas, carrying pain impulses and stimuli for the secretory and excretory activities of the pancreas. A main pancreatic duct collects enzymes and other solutions formed by the pancreas and carries these directly into the duodenum, or more often into the terminal portion of the common bile duct, just before it enters the duodenum.

Microscopically, it is possible to differentiate at least two major cellular components in the pancreas. One group, the acinar cells, are involved in the exocrine functions, forming the digestive enzymes. The other group consists of cells of the islands of Langerhans, which control the endocrine function of the pancreas, and the secretion of insulin.

The pancreas has two major functions. As an endocrine organ it produces insulin and glucagon. These hormones maintain the blood sugar level and are secreted directly into the blood. As an exocrine organ it produces protein, fat, and carbohydrate digesting enzymes. These do not enter the bloodstream directly, but instead enter the ducts of the pancreas and eventually are released into the lumen of the duodenum, where they act directly on arriving food. By a complex interplay of chemical and nervous stimuli, the pancreas is activated by ingested foods to release its enzymes at the appropriate time for most efficient digestion.

### Acute Pancreatitis

The exact etiology of pancreatitis is unknown. In simplest terms pancreatitis may be defined as an inflammatory disease characterized by the destruction of pancreatic tissue as well as functional capability. Pancreatitis may be acute and mild, or may occur abruptly with a fulminant, often quickly fatal course. Later it may occur as a chronic disease, with a long history of relapse and recurrent attacks. Mortality in acute cases may reach as high as 20 per cent.

Pancreatitis is often noted to develop in people with a history of biliary tract disease, and high alcohol intake. However, many persons with pancreatitis have no other illness. In those situations where the common bile duct and the pancreatic duct release their contents into the duodenum via a common channel, it has been theorized that when the single opening is obstructed by a gallstone or inflammatory edema, stricture or spasm, enzyme-rich juice cannot escape from the pancreas. With increasing back pressure, this solution, which is concentrated with potent digestive agents, may then actually digest and destroy surrounding pancreatic tissues. Certain drugs, including certain diuretic and corticosteroid agents, have been implicated in the etiology of pancreatitis. Coincident with mumps pancreatitis is felt to be induced by the same virus that affects the parotid or other salivary glands. Whatever the cause, once underway pancreatitis may proceed to cause a variable degree of insufficiency and disorder.

### Signs and Symptoms

In acute pancreatitis, the most common complaint is severe middle-upper abdominal pain, which may radiate to both sides and straight through to the back. Usually, nausea and vomiting are present. If the pancreatic inflammation is intense, with necrosis and hemorrhage of the gland, peritonitis, severe fluid and electrolyte imbalance, and shock may ensue. In fulminant cases the fatty tissue around the pancreas is digested by lipase, a fat-digesting enzyme. Calcium binds with the released fatty acids. In rare cases, this reduces circulating calcium to dangerously low levels, resulting in tetany and convulsions. Also, in the more advanced circumstances of hemorrhagic pancreatitis, released blood may discolor the skin of the lateral abdominal wall.

In addition to radiologic and blood tests that may be carried out in diagnosis, a test of serum amylase and lipase level is usually ordered. These two enzymes, normal secretions of the pancreas, will appear in elevated quantities in the bloodstream of most patients with significant pancreatitis. They may subsequently be detected in peritoneal fluid and the urine. This determination aids the physician in establishing a correct diagnosis. Serum amylase may also be elevated in other conditions causing abdominal pain, but it is not usually as high as in acute pancreatitis. Urine amylase may continue to be high after serum amylase has returned to normal, enabling the diagnosis to be made even several days into the attack.

### Recurrent (Relapsing) and Chronic Pancreatitis

Recurrent pancreatitis is the reappearance of intermittent attacks of pancreatic inflammation after an initial attack earlier in life. With chronicity, there may be partial to ultimate complete loss of function as pancreatic tissue is progressively destroyed.

With the late development of chronic recurrent pancreatitis, stones and strictures may obstruct the pancreatic ducts. Areas of pancreatic breakdown may disrupt to form pseudocysts, which are fluid-filled pouches budding from the diseased pancreas. These cause symptoms by putting pressure upon adjacent organs or by rupturing, bleeding, or becoming infected. With the development of chronic pancreatitis, pain, weight loss, digestive disturbances, diabetes, malnutrition, and steatorrhea occur, in addition to the usual signs and symptoms of acute pancreatitis. These problems are caused by the progressive loss of exocrine and endocrine actions of the gland.

### Treatment

In acute pancreatitis measures are taken to relieve pain, reduce pancreatic secretion, restore fluid and electrolyte losses, and combat infection. The patient usually receives nothing by mouth, and continuous nasogastric aspiration is applied. This will relieve nausea, distention, and vomiting as well as reduce stimulation of the pancreas by gastric contents entering the duodenum. Atropine or other anticholinergic drugs may be administered to reduce the activity of the vagus nerve, because this nerve stimulates the pancreas. Drugs to decrease the activity of proteolytic enzymes released from the pancreas may be given to reduce their autodigestive action. Meperidine is the analgesic of choice, being less likely to cause spasm of the sphincter at the entrance of the common duct into the duodenum. Shock with acute pancreatitis is combatted with solutions of blood plasma, albumin, and electrolytes in appropriate quantities to avoid deficits secondary

to hemorrhage, peritonitis, and protein and mineral loss. The management program usually also includes antibiotics, a cooling blanket for extremely high temperature, accurate measure of intake and output, frequent checking of vital signs, and repeated clinical and laboratory examinations.

Improvement usually occurs in about a week. The diet initially prescribed is extremely bland, with slow progress to a low-fat diet. Alcohol, coffee, tea, and other irritants or rich foods are withheld. Prolonged use of narcotic pain relievers may lead to addiction, a common complication of pancreatitis in its chronic or recurrent stages. Care and thought in the prescription and administration of narcotics is therefore essential. The use of alcohol for its pain-killing effect establishes a vicious circle in which alcohol precipitates further attacks and more pain. The alcoholic patient needs assistance to overcome his dependence on alcohol (see Chap. 11).

There is no direct surgical therapy for acute pancreatitis. However, if pancreatic abscess is suspected, this must be drained surgically. Also, if acute cholecystitis or obstruction of the common duct is felt to be a coincident or inciting factor, drainage and simple stone removal may be necessary. Simple bile diversion by cholecystostomy or choledochostomy is believed to give relief and hasten healing.

A few weeks after the acute attack subsides, roentgenograms of the upper gastrointestinal tract, including the biliary tree, are done. If surgically treatable disease, such as stones in the gallbladder or common duct, is demonstrated, the operation is delayed for several months until pancreatic healing is complete.

The treatment of chronic, recurrent pancreatitis depends on the etiology and whether or not the pancreatic duct is obstructed. If pancreatic duct obstruction is not yet present, abstinence from alcohol, a bland fat-free diet, and correction of associated biliary tract disease or hyperparathyroidism may give good results. If there is scarring with stricture and stenosis of portions of the pancreatic duct, surgical measures are carried out to attempt reconstitution of an unobstructed flow into the intestine.

Pseudocysts of the diseased pancreas can be removed, but often are simply drained directly into the intestinal tract. Chronic pain may be relieved by surgically removing nerve fibers supplying the pancreas as well as part or all of the pancreas. Diabetes and digestive enzyme deficiency seen with advanced pancreatic destruction may be treated with insulin and exocrine enzyme replacement.

### Nursing Care

Because severe pain is the outstanding symptom of pancreatitis, nursing intervention involves relieving pain by carefully administering prescribed analgesics and by other measures, such as changes of position. The patient usually will show the nurse the position in which he is most comfortable, or at least the position in which he is the least uncomfortable. Supportive pillows may help.

During the acute attack the patient will need mouth care, as does any patient with continuous nasogastric suction. His nasal passage also may feel dry and sore from the tube, and a small amount of glycerine may help. However, be sure that it is only a tiny amount that cannot be aspirated. Care can be arranged so that he is not disturbed when dozing. Do what needs to be done when he is awake, and avoid interrupting his sleep. Make certain that the suction device is working satisfactorily.

During the weeks and months of convalescence the nurse can help the patient to establish a routine for eating and living that he will find possible to maintain and that will not violate the physician's prescriptions. Taking a full measure of exercise and avoiding rich meals, alcohol, and fatty foods can be a very difficult regimen for the patient to maintain.

Learning to cope with emotional stress is another important phase of treatment. During the acute phase of illness, the nurse conveys emotional support by reliably using all possible measures to relieve the patient's pain and to help him rest. As the patient recovers, she can spend time listening to his concerns and helping him find ways to cope with emotional stress.

### Trauma

Since the pancreas lies in a relatively fixed, deep position in the posterior midabdomen, it is well protected. However, deeply penetrating stab or gunshot wounds may injure the pancreas. Injuries to adjacent organs, such as the liver or intestines, may be more obvious, obscuring the pancreatic damage. Principles of therapy are those for any penetrating abdominal wound and usually involve exploring the abdomen, controlling the bleeding, removing necrotic tissue, suturing lacerations, and draining the pancreatic leakage.

Blunt trauma to the abdomen may injure the pancreas without penetrating the abdominal wall. This type of crushing accident may cause extravasation of pancreatic enzymes and subsequent acute pancreatitis. Operation may become indicated if bleeding or leakage from damaged portions of the pancreas is suspected.

### Tumors

Pancreatic tumors can arise from the ductal or acinar cells; they may be benign adenomas or malignant adenocarcinomas. Rarely, tumors arise from the island cells. These tumors may be benign or malignant and can produce excessive insulinlike and other humoral agents.

Cancer of the pancreas often cannot be removed by surgery because adjacent vital structures may have been invaded by the time the condition is diagnosed. Cancer in the most proximal portion of the pancreas (head of the pancreas) is most common. It produces pain, digestive disturbance, weight loss, and jaundice by blocking the end of the common bile duct. Less commonly, the tumor appears further distally (in the body and tail of the pancreas), and signs and symptoms appear later, when metastases have already occurred. Laboratory tests and x-ray studies are usually not specifically diagnostic, and exploratory laparotomy is often necessary to clarify the diagnosis.

In those few patients in whom the tumor is resectable, surgery is the only chance for cure. Removing the diseased portion or the entire pancreas along with the adjacent duodenum, common duct, distal stomach, and regional lymph nodes is an extensive operation with significant postoperative mortality and morbidity. Of those surviving surgery, only about 5 to 10 per cent will survive for 5 years. When the cancer is not resectable, palliation may be achieved by diverting bile from the obstructed biliary tree into a portion of intestine away from the blockage. Chemotherapeutic drugs such as 5-fluorouracil have given occasional transient palliation.

Recurrent phlebitis and venous thrombosis in the arms and legs are often seen in advanced pancreatic malignancy and are indicative of a poor prognosis.

### Nursing Care

As soon as the diagnosis is made and operation has been decided on, every effort is made to increase the patient's vitality before surgery. He may be given vitamin K. Extra carbohydrate may be administered intravenously. The diet is high in protein and carbohydrate and low in fat. As the patient lacks appetite, and eating is an important aspect of his preoperative treatment, this situation offers a real challenge to the ingenuity of the nurse. Nausea is especially brought on by the smell and taste of food.

Postoperatively, the dressings should be watched for drainage. The patient will have nasogastric suction. Complications can occur. Bleeding, wound infection, and skin breakdown around drain sites may be problems in the early postoperative course. Vitamin deficiencies of fat-soluble A, D, and K are guarded against by appropriate supplementation. Meticulous care is required for support following such major surgery in a patient already stressed by an intra-abdominal cancer.

## REFERENCES AND BIBLIOGRAPHY

*BELINSKY, I., SHINYA, H., and WOLFF, W.: Colorofiberoscopy: Technique in colon examination, *Am. J. Nurs.* 2:306-308, February 1973.

*BUCKINGHAM, W., SPARBERG, M., and BRANDFONBRENER, M.: *A Primer of Clinical Diagnosis,* San Francisco, Harper and Row, 1971.

*COLLEY, R., and PHILLIPS, K.: Helping with hyperalimentation, *Nurs. '73* 6:17, July 1973.

DAVENPORT, H. W.: *Physiology of the Digestive Tract,* ed. 3, Chicago, Yearbook Medical Publishers, 1971.

FOWKES, W., and HUNN, V.: *Clinical Assessment for the Nurse Practitioner,* St. Louis, Mosby, 1973.

GAMBILL, E. E.: *Pancreatitis,* St. Louis, Mosby, 1973.

JACKSON, B.: Ulcerative colitis from an etiological perspective, *Am. J. Nurs.* 2:258-264, February 1973.

PRIOR, J., and SILBERSTEIN, J.: *Physical Diagnosis,* St. Louis, Mosby, 1973.

*REITZ, M., and POPE, W.: Mouth care, *Am. J. Nurs.* 10:1728-1730, October 1973.

ROBINSON, C.: *Proudfit—Robinson's Normal and Therapeutic Nutrition,* London, Macmillan, 1971.

SCHIFF, L.: *Diseases of the Liver,* ed. 3, Philadelphia, Lippincott, 1969.

SCHWARTZ, S., et al.: *Principles of Surgery,* ed. 2, San Francisco, McGraw-Hill, 1974.

SCOPP, I.: *Oral Medicine,* St. Louis, Mosby, 1973.

SHERLOCK, S.: *Diseases of the Liver and Biliary System,* ed. 4, Springfield, Illinois, Thomas, 1968.

SILVERMAN, S., JR., and GALANTE, M.: *Oral Cancer,* San Francisco, University of California, 1972.

SLEISENGER, M., and FORDTRAN, J.: *Gastro-intestinal Disease,* Philadelphia, Saunders, 1973.

SMITH, J. N., JR.: *Essentials of Gastroenterology,* St. Louis, Mosby, 1969.

SPIRO, H. M.: *Clinical Gastroenterology,* Macmillan, 1970.

*WILLACKER, J.: Bowel sounds, *Am. J. Nurs.* 12:2100-2101, December 1973.

*Especially recommended for students.

# The Patient with an
# Ileostomy or a Colostomy

## CHAPTER 47

## WHAT IS AN OSTOMY?

*Ostomy* is a suffix that means "formation of an open-ing or outlet." Recently it has come to be used as a noun to refer to individuals in whom an opening (stoma) has been artificially created to provide an outlet for intestinal waste products or excretions. The words ostomy and stoma are frequently used inter-changeably. As used here, ostomy refers to intestinal stomas; both ileostomy and colostomy will be dis-cussed. Although the terms sound much alike and both operations involve an opening into the intestine, *expec-tations in care do differ and should not be confused by patients or personnel.*

An ostomy is created for both benign and malignant disorders. The site of the problem indicates the type of procedure performed and thus the type of ostomy assumes the name of the body area in which the open-ing is created. Ostomies may be temporary or perma-nent depending upon the pathology of the disorder. Various types of ostomies and a description of as well as implications of each are given in Table 47-1.

## WHO HAS AN OSTOMY?

Anyone at any age can have an ostomy. Individuals both young and old are subject to conditions that require an ostomy. Infants have colostomies for im-perforate anus or anomalies of the bowel; teenagers, young adults, and persons under 50 years of age gener-ally have ileostomies, whereas those 50 to 90 years of age have colostomies more frequently, chiefly because of bowel malignancy.

**Table 47-1. Classification of Various Types of Ostomies Giving Definition, Indication for, Anatomical Changes and Implications**

| CLASSIFICATION | DEFINITION | INDICATIONS | ANATOMICAL CHANGES | IMPLICATIONS |
|---|---|---|---|---|
| Ileostomy Permanent | A surgically created opening between the ileum and the outside of the abdomen. | Chiefly for ulcerative colitis, (cause unknown) birth defects, Crohn's disease, familial polyposis, diverticulitis, injury (and rarely cancer). | Removal of the entire colon and rectum, or the entire colon but not the rectum, or part of the colon only, leaving lower portion of the colon and rectum.<br><br>The end portion of the ileum is brought through the abdominal wall and forms the stoma. Ileal discharge is excreted through the stoma. | Ileal discharge is usually liquid or semisolid and contains proteolytic enzymes which may digest the skin around the stoma therefore a collecting device must be worn at all times. Meticulous skin care is essential.<br><br>There is no control over the drainage—drainage may occur at any time. (Usually within $1/2$-2 hrs. of eating.) Removal or bypass of the large colon will interfere with fluid absorption.<br><br>Electrolyte imbalance may occur from loss of large amounts of fluid. Replacement of fluid loss is essential. |
| Loop Ileostomy Temporary | | In very ill patients with inflammatory disease as a temporary measure before bowel is removed. | Where part of the colon remains there may be a second stoma to the left of the ileostomy stoma. This is called a mucus fistula. | Mucus is secreted from this second stoma and only a gauze pad may be needed to cover the second stoma. |
| Colostomy | A surgically created opening between some part of the colon and the outside of the abdominal wall. A colostomy may be formed in any one of the divisions of the colon—ascending colon, transverse colon, descending colon or sigmoid colon. It may be temporary or permanent. | Chiefly disease—such as cancer of the colon or rectum, diverticulitis, sigmoid volvulus, familial polyposis, birth defects, and trauma. | Diseased portion of bowel and rectum removed or diseased portion of the bowel removed without rectum. | The water absorption takes place in the colon. Interruption of this function depends upon the location of the colostomy. Management of the colostomy is by irrigation and/or diet.<br><br>After continence is achieved a stomal cap, 4 x 4 pad or close-ended pouch may be used. |
| End colostomy or Single-barreled end colostomy | Part of the colon and rectum removed. | As above—usually cancer. | Removal of part of the colon and rectum. The end portion of the remaining colon is brought through the abdominal wall to form a stoma (one stoma only). | Mucus discharge varies with individuals but some type of stomal covering is required to prevent soiling of clothing. Usually stool is firm and dry. |
| Transverse colostomy May be loop or double-barreled | A surgically created opening between the transverse colon and the abdominal wall. | As above—usually diverticulitis, cancer, inflammatory condition or perforation. | The stoma is located on the upper abdomen, middle or to the right. | Irrigation helps to decrease number of movements — a pouch is usually worn. Digestive enzymes in stool will cause skin breakdown. |
| Loop colostomy | A surgically created opening into a loop of the transverse colon. A glass rod may be placed underneath for support for a week to ten days. | Usually temporary as above. | A loop of bowel is brought through a hole in the abdominal wall. The outside of the loop is slit laterally and a single stoma is created with openings to the right and to the left. | Fecal discharge may be liquid—semisoft from one stoma—the other stoma and the rectum drain mucus. A double-barreled pouch, Hollester loop or Marsans Loop-Loc can be used.<br><br>Irrigation helps decrease number of movements. |

**Table 47-1.** (Continued)

| CLASSIFICATION | DEFINITION | INDICATIONS | ANATOMICAL CHANGES | IMPLICATIONS |
|---|---|---|---|---|
| Double-barreled colostomy | The transverse colon is divided and two separate openings made into the colon. They may or may not be separated by skin. The stomas may be constructed side by side or above and below each other. | As above — may be temporary or permanent — is usually temporary. | The end portion of the divided colon is brought out to the abdominal wall. The rectum is not removed. If a portion of the colon is removed the stomas may be distant from each other. | One drains fecal matter, the other and the rectum drain mucus. Consistency of drainage varies from soft to firm. May be controlled by irrigation. |
| Sigmoid colostomy | A surgically created opening made in the sigmoid colon and the abdominal wall. | As above — may be temporary or permanent—is usually permanent. | The end portion of the sigmoid colon is brought to abdominal wall. Rectum may or may not be removed. (Rectum is removed if end colostomy is constructed). | Simplest to manage. Can be managed by irrigation or diet. After regulated, may only require gauze pad, or stoma cap. Stool is firm and dry, usually. |
| Descending colostomy | A surgically created opening between the descending colon and abdominal wall. | May be temporary or permanent—is usually permanent. | The end portion of the descending colon is brought to the abdominal wall—the rectum may or may not be removed. (Rectum is removed if it is an end colostomy.) | Can be managed by irrigation or diet. Functions similarly to sigmoid colostomy. May require use of a disposable pouch. |
| Cecostomy | A surgically created opening between the cecum and right lower side of abdomen. | Usually temporary to rest the colon or bypass an obstruction of the colon. | An opening is made into the cecum—stoma may be flush with the skin. Tube may be inserted during surgery, if it slips out, only the surgeon should replace it. | Drainage is liquid and contains digestive enzymes that irritate the skin. A collecting pouch is necessary—special attention must be given to protect skin. Karaya or cement-on type of pouch is useful.<br><br>Irrigation usually is not carried out.<br><br>If tube used, connect to drainage bottle or pouch. Protect skin as above from leakage around tube. |
| Wet colostomy | A colostomy in which the distal end of one or both ureters has been transplanted into the colon. | Diseased state—usually cancer. | An opening usually is made in the descending or sigmoid colon and a stoma is constructed as described above. One or both ureters are placed into the colon. Urinary bladder and rectum may or may not be removed. | Stoma drains both urine and fecal matter.<br><br>A collection pouch is necessary—bowel control usually is not achieved.<br><br>Infection is potentially great. |

The very young have the fewest problems and learn to adjust more readily than young adults. Young adults have many developmental problems, are struggling with identity, forming their life style of dating and mating, and establishing personal relationships; the stoma makes it difficult for them to accept and adjust to their body changes. The older married individual who frequently has raised a family, is entrenched in his life work, and has established a life style, may therefore adjust more easily than the younger person.

## ACCEPTANCE OF THE OSTOMY

Degree of illness, disability, and emotional resources are factors that influence the degree to which the patient accepts the need for the procedure. Those with long periods of weakness, frequent episodes of diarrhea, repeated hospitalizations necessitating painful tests, may welcome the relief surgery provides. Those with short periods of illness, few or no troublesome symptoms, and an unexpected diagnosis and surgery, often question the need for so drastic a procedure. They frequently complain that their physicians used them as guinea pigs, and they have great difficulty accepting the ostomy, even if they are having no problems with its control (Katona, 1967).

## Attitudes and Reactions

The ostomate is conditioned by the attitude of individuals responsible for his care—the medical and nursing staff; members of his immediate family, his relatives, his friends, his peers, and all others significant in his life, such as his employers and business associates. Factors that influence the acceptance of and adjustment to having an ostomy are:

1. Time (length of illness or incapacitation due to illness)
2. Life style and interruption or changes in it
3. Acuteness or chronicity of condition
4. Age—adjustment capacities
5. Stage of maturation
6. Pain—discomfort—control
7. Other events occurring around or at time of surgery
8. Past experiences with other ostomates
9. Kind and amount of information individual has about ostomies
10. Physical conditions *unrelated* to the ostomy (arthritis, stroke)
11. Attitude and manner of the professionals caring for him
12. Extent of care achieved
13. The relationships of significant others with whom he interacts—degree of support he obtains
14. Resocialization skills
15. Coping abilities

The patient perceives the behavior of caring persons as a reflection of the world at large. Therefore, it is extremely important that the nurse be aware of her own reactions to fecal incontinence and not withdraw from or reject the patient because of them. The patient who is unable to control his bowel movements experiences great anxiety about possible rejection by the nursing staff, his family, visitors, and other patients. He may soil himself or his clothing, there may be an odor, he suffers loss of self-esteem, and lack of control makes him insecure. He has to spend more time in the bathroom to take care of himself. He lives in dreaded fear of having an accident. He is acutely aware of odor and noises that emanate from the stoma. He is sure the appliance will bulge and be obvious to all. He worries about his ability to do his work, to engage in recreational activities, and to perform sexually. Time alone will help resolve some of these fears, but a visit from a recovered ostomate will help immeasurably to dispel fears and doubts in a much shorter time and enable him to resume his previous life style with confidence.

## Psychologic Implications of and Adjustment to an Ostomy

Ostomy surgery, which represents a severe blow to an individual's self-esteem and to the intactness of his body, produces profound emotional reactions that are normal and common.

Each patient's reactions depend on his own ego-strength; most people experience shock and anger, then depression and shame about this mutilating procedure, and, perhaps, withdrawal from family and friends.

Often patients must make a transition from a status and life style of sickness to newly gained health. It is a difficult transition, often accompanied by depression.

There are many vital factors to be considered if the patient is to be restored to emotional health. For example:

1. Careful preparation for surgery
2. Careful management of the stoma
3. Time—helping the patient through stages of grief, loss, and accepting change
4. Family adjustment and support
5. Overall understanding and thoughtful support of physicians, nurses, families, and other ostomates
6. Assistance with resumption of usual role and activities, at home and at work

## Handicap of Having a Stoma

Most ostomates do not consider the presence of a stoma a handicap. The healthy stoma does not interfere with physical activity of any kind. The only physical limitation is that the patient should not lift heavy objects because of the danger of herniation around the stoma. Emotionally, it is difficult for most persons to accept a stoma. A well-integrated individual can survive the experience, while a fragile ego may be devastated.

A handicap may result from a poorly fashioned or incorrectly placed stoma; rejection by employers and insurance companies; inadequate information and instruction about essential equipment; and a lack of ready sources of supply of ostomy care products and appropriate follow-up programs (Lenneberg, et al., 1972).

## STANDARDS OF CARE

Some medical and hospital practices and routines applicable to nonostomates do not apply to the ostomate. The ostomate's comfort, well-being, and personal safety may depend upon his knowing the need to be treated differently, with consideration for his stoma. This information must be communicated appropriately to physicians and other personnel when necessary. This is especially important when the patient with an ostomy is being treated for a nonostomy ailment.

### Appliances and Accessories for Care

Manufacturers of ostomy equipment and supplies have concentrated on developing a wider variety of more durable and streamlined products for ostomy care than were previously available. These include appliances and accessories for conduits, irrigating equipment, drainage collection pouches, skin protection and odor control products which provide greater personal comfort and security, and ease in their use. Nevertheless, the search for new and better methods to meet and satisfy individual preferences continues.

Some companies provide small kits with samples of their products for use in teaching and demonstration programs for patients and staff. These are available at nominal cost or on an extended loan basis.

These advances enable the patient to resume his previous life style more quickly and to simplify the task of learning to live with the ileostomy or colostomy. The patient must learn to manage and regulate his own ostomy.

### Knowledgable and Skillful Health Workers

There are a great number of well-informed, skillful persons to assist in caring for the stoma and to aid in the rehabilitation process, and the number of enterostomal therapists, enterostomal technicians, or ostomy specialists is increasing rapidly. Educational committees of ostomy groups provide teaching sessions for nursing and medical students and for nursing personnel through hospital inservice education programs.

### Patient Education

A wide variety of teaching aids, charts, models, diagrams, and printed materials are available to aid in instructing the patient and the family about the ostomy.

Patient education programs are being planned to improve patient teaching pre- and postoperatively. Many hospitals employ an enterostomal therapist or arrange for a member of the nursing staff to obtain appropriate enterostomal instruction in care and product information. Meyers (1974) states that hospitals are placing ostomy products in the Central Service or Pharmacy Department for more efficient economic management of ostomy appliances and supplies. The hospital enterostomal therapist assists by identifying the types of items needed in the selection of ostomy equipment for specific situations. Having adequate supplies and equipment on hand is a problem especially in smaller hospitals. Some of these have made arrangements with surgical supply dealers in the community to obtain the needed items rather than stock a large number of different items that may deteriorate from disuse. These same resources then are used when the patient is discharged. It helps to eliminate a major problem for the ostomate as he can then see other types of ostomy equipment from a variety of suppliers when he needs to consider changing the type of equipment he is currently using.

## VISITORS

Assessment of when to have a visitor, preoperatively, postoperatively, or not at all, is also part of the plan of care and the decision is made on an individual basis. It is often beneficial to have a member of the visiting committee of the local ostomy group or a selected former patient visit the patient. The visitor is visible proof that care of the stoma and management of the ostomy can be successfully mastered. It conveys to the patient a sense that it is possible to be well-groomed, attractive, and successful despite an ostomy.

Ostomy groups require that the patient's physician agree to the visit before sending a visitor. It is desirable to educate ostomy groups in the role of the professional nurse practitioner, to encourage their contact with the person responsible for nursing care. An attempt is made to match the visitor in sex, age, occupation, language, physical handicaps, or other pertinent factors significant to rehabilitation. Members of the ostomy visitor program are carefully selected, screened, and trained in visiting etiquette either by the Visitors Advisory Committee of the local ostomy association or the Ostomy Rehabilitation Program of the local cancer unit. It is essential, if the ostomate visitor has not made contact with the nurse, for the latter to initiate this contact and to communicate with the visitor so that a collaborative approach to the patient can be made.

## Stoma Rehabilitation

The ostomy patient needs someone thoroughly versed in ostomy care and rehabilitation available to him at the time of hospitalization.

Ostomy associations are of vital help in rehabilitation, but they cannot meet the need alone. They serve largely in the resocialization of the person and as a source of information and reassurance after surgery.

Enterostomal therapists have been added to the staffs at hospitals in many states. Their services have been expanded to outpatient followup through stoma clinics, which indicates a breakthrough in rehabilitation of the ostomate.

In addition to established stoma clinics the number of enterostomal therapy training programs in the United States and Europe has increased. Certified enterostomal therapist schools have been established to provide skilled personnel trained in the care and rehabilitation of the ostomy patient. Initially many of the applicants to these programs were ostomates. Many nurses have been trained and current requirements indicate preference for either the licensed practical or registered nurse background. Therapists work with nurses, physicians, family, and patients pre- and postoperatively to facilitate the patients' care and adjustment.

## Assessment

People involved in care of the ostomy, regardless of their role, know that effective communication is essential for the continuity of care. Each patient requires an individual plan of care based upon a careful assessment of the problem and adapted to his individual needs.

The assessment should contain a profile of the patient's life style, age, occupation, personality, and physical state, the meaning of the illness to him and his family—how illness affects life style, antici-

pated problems or necessary alterations; previous methods of coping with stressful situations; the role of the patient in the family, at work, and in the community; strengths; weaknesses; significant others at home or at work and the patient's relationship to them. In particular, previous bowel habits, frequency of movements, consistency of stool, use of laxatives, enemas, or other difficulties should be noted.

**Physical Assessment.** The patient's physical state is also assessed. Particular attention should be given to nutrition, the condition and integrity of the skin, and general physical build, together with other physical disabilities. It is important to note any disability which may interfere with care of the stoma, such as arthritis of the hands or blindness (see Chap. 40).

## PLANNING FOR NURSING INTERVENTION

Each patient requires a care plan that is adapted to his individual requirements and that considers not only his surgical experience but his preparation for surgery, his recovery from it, and his learning to live with the ostomy.

The patient may be given instruction about the ostomy, and about equipment and general principles of care prior to surgery. Some patients are taught to apply the device even before surgery. Others, too ill or too bewildered to learn, are taught later.

The overall plan of care is adapted to each patient's needs. For example: the plan includes instruction; but just how this instruction is carried out varies according to such factors as the patient's previous knowledge about ostomies and his emotional reaction.

The patient with a stoma has no sphincter, and thus no sphincter control; he is left with a problem of incontinence for the rest of his life. Therefore, efforts to assist him to regain the continent state are imperative. Every effort is made to help the patient reach the stage of recovery in which he feels he has mastery over the stoma.

The patient should be allowed to express his feelings about the stoma. It is not unusual for a patient who appeared very brave and eager to learn before surgery to become depressed and withdrawn after the operation. Usually, however, if those who care for him show patience and support, the patient soon begins to look at the stoma and to develop interest in its care. Sometimes a casual and yet factual comment like, "The drainage is more formed today," helps. If he continues avoidance, however, members of the health team should discuss and plan together so that further help with the patient's emotional reaction can be given. Sometimes the nurse's attention is focused quite narrowly on the stoma and its care. It is important for her to spend some time with the patient when she is not busy with his dressing—time when she can listen and show her concern for the patient, without the stress (for the patient) engendered by the care of the stoma. Particularly if the patient is experiencing difficulty accepting his stoma, such periods can be of special importance in helping him to cope with his feelings.

As soon as the patient begins to observe and demonstrate interest in caring for his stoma, the nurse should explain each step as she proceeds. After several periods of observation, he should be encouraged to help. The nurse should ask him to hold the equipment and hand her supplies as she needs them. The patient should be allowed to wash his hands after he has helped with his bag or dressing change. Too often this important detail is forgotten, even though it is taken for granted that the nurse will wash her hands.

Every patient needs to know that his nurse cares about him and understands some of his problems, *and also that she has the knowledge and the ability to help him resolve these problems.* The nurse demonstrates this concern and knowledge by her manner, her skill, and by her attitude with which care is given. Choice of words and tone of voice are important when the nurse discusses the ostomy with the patient. For example the nurse who gushingly refers to the ostomy as a "rosebud," may impress the patient as insincere and unrealistic; this approach may interfere with the patient's ability to express his feelings (especially negative ones) concerning the ostomy. It is preferable for the nurse to use terms that are neutral, and that are not laden with her own emotional reactions or with efforts to cover up her reactions.

When the patient has help with his stoma care a few times and is regaining his strength, he is usually ready to begin to carry out the procedure himself. The nurse should stay with him the first few times, and help when needed. Sometimes she may think that the patient who carries out the procedure correctly for the first or second time needs no further help. This often gives the patient the feeling that the nurse is eager to be rid of the task of caring for his ostomy. Even though the patient can carry out the technique of his stoma care adequately, the nurse should arrange to be with him sometimes when he changes the dressing. This will enable her to observe how he is applying what he has learned. It will also give her an opportunity to note the condition of the skin, and the type and the amount of fecal drainage, and it will convey to the patient her continued interest and willingness to help.

For most patients this change in body function constitutes a loss. The nurse can help by exploring with the patient what the loss means to him. For example, one patient described it as loss of a diseased body part that endangered his health and even his life. By losing the diseased part, he gained freedom from disease, an opportunity to regain his normal health, and a chance to return to living a useful, productive life.

Because the surgery involves loss and a change in body image, patients go through a grieving process. This cannot be hurried. It takes time and patience and a sincere sustained concern and interest for the patient in order to help him at this time. The patient may experience a period of disbelief, denial, anger, discouragement, or despair before he finally accepts the situation.

He may even be suicidal. The nurse's and physician's presence, their concern and their helpfulness are essential not only in accepting the patient in his grief but in helping him to see the progress he has made (however slight).

The nurse and the physician should discuss each patient and his care as it evolves. The nurse and physician should collaborate in teaching the patient. *Decisions about who will teach the patient various aspects of his care must be made promptly and definitely lest the patient be discharged before he is able to care for himself.* The physician informs the patient what surgery is required and why and explains the pathology to the patient. The nurse reviews this with the patient as necessary. *The plan of who teaches what must be definite and agreed upon by the nurse and physician.* The nurse teaches what is necessary for self care, appliance, skin care, as detailed elsewhere in this chapter. The patient should *receive the equipment and instruction in its use and care while hospitalized, and should have an opportunity to demonstrate his ability to manage the ostomy prior to discharge.* Referral to the visiting nurse service or a stoma clinic for nursing care should be made upon discharge.

*Follow-up care after discharge is an essential aspect of the plan of care even when the patient seemingly has demonstrated the ability to perform the self-care activities.*

*The patient and his family* are to be actively involved in the care and management of the ostomy.

## THE PATIENT WITH AN ILEOSTOMY

An ileostomy is a surgically formed opening into the ileum for the drainage of fecal matter. A loop of ileum is brought out onto the lower right quadrant of the abdomen, slightly below the umbilicus, near the outer border of the rectus muscle, and a stoma is formed. The stoma is "matured" at the time of surgery by everting the bowel and suturing the cut end of the ileum to the skin. The rationale for maturing the stoma is that it provides a seal at the base of the stoma. This technique promotes healing and provides a smooth peristomal area, thus permitting the application of the permanent appliance much sooner than is permissible in the non-matured stoma. Serositis is prevented from developing as this technique eliminates the ileal flow over the serosal surface.

Fecal drainage from the ileostomy is of a liquid consistency at first since it is discharged before it passes through the colon where water absorption normally takes place. Therefore, *an ileostomy requires the immediate application of a collecting appliance over the stoma to collect this fecal matter.* The surgeon applies a temporary disposable plastic pouch to the skin over the stoma at the time of the operation. This pouch should be of the *drainable type* and may have an adhesive facing or a karaya gum seal with or without an adhesive facing.

**Indications for Ileostomy.** Ulcerative colitis is a common indication for ileostomy. When a temporary ileostomy is performed, the disease process in the colon persists despite the diversion of the fecal stream. Removal of the diseased colon (colectomy) is necessary to halt the disease. When the colon has been removed the ileostomy is permanent. The procedure may be done in one, two, or three stages.

### Immediate Postoperative Care

The principles of postoperative care are the same as those for any patient who has had surgery on the gastrointestinal tract. The use of a Levin tube and suction and the administration of parenteral fluids are usual in the immediate postoperative period. Within several days these treatments usually are discontinued, and oral feedings of easily digested foods are begun. The patient is encouraged to gradually resume a normal diet, excluding only those foods that he has found cause him to have gas or diarrhea.

Electrolyte imbalance due to a large output of fluid through the ileum is a *particular* problem for the patient with an ileostomy. The nurse observes for weakness, trembling, and confusion, especially when the ileal output is profuse and intravenous fluids for fluid electrolyte replacement may be required. Therefore, these symptoms should be reported to the physician when they occur. The nurse should have a *thorough understanding* of fluid requirements and fluid therapy replacement within the context of the nursing role.

Nursing measures for deep breathing, coughing, turning, and exercising the toes and legs are carried out as for other surgical patients. Medication for relief of pain and discomfort should be given as required. Nursing care should be planned to provide the patient with adequate time to rest.

Some surgeons advocate the use of elastic stockings to both legs for several days until the patient

**Table 47-2.  Factors Considered in Planning Location and Construction of Stoma and Selection of a Permanent Pouch**

| LOCATION OF STOMA | CHARACTERISTICS OF ABDOMINAL CONTOUR AND TEXTURE | CHARACTERISTICS OF STOMA |
|---|---|---|
| Distance from hip bone navel, waistline, incision, pubic bone, groin | Muscular, fleshy, soft, firm<br>Scars within disk area<br>Other depressions or bumps near the stoma | Flush<br>Short, 1½ in. or longer<br>Proud flesh tabs surrounding stoma or irregularly shaped stoma |

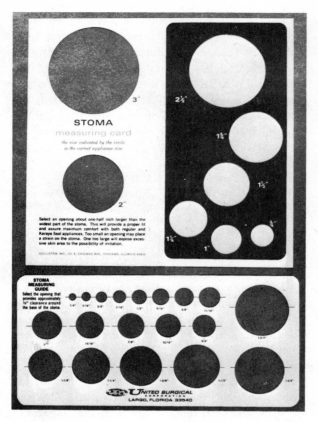

**Figure 47-1.** Examples of colostomy and ileostomy stoma measuring guides. (Hollister Inc. and United Surgical Corp.)

is ambulating well (to prevent thrombophlebitis). If used they should be removed at least once in each eight-hour period.

The patient returns from the operating room with a stoma and a surgical incision through which the operation has been performed. The stoma is usually covered with a plastic disposable pouch. Sometimes the close proximity of the stoma to the surgical incision makes it especially difficult to avoid fecal contamination of the surgical incision. The plastic pouch, which can be fitted snugly around the stoma and secured with adhesive, helps to prevent fecal drainage from seeping into the surgical incision. Wide strips of adhesive may be applied tightly over the entire dressing, covering the incision to protect it from fecal drainage.

**Colostomy.** Often when a colostomy is performed, the stoma is matured at surgery. That is, the stoma is everted and sutured down, and thus is open. If the stoma is not matured at surgery, a loop of bowel is brought out onto the abdomen. About

24 to 36 hours after the operation, the loop of bowel is opened by cutting or cautery to form the stoma. In this way initial healing of the incision takes place without danger of contamination. The latter procedure is not physically painful, since the bowel is not as sensitive to pain as the skin is. The opening of the colostomy usually is carried out at the patient's bedside or in the treatment room. The bed should be well protected, and a temporary ostomy pouch rather than a basin, is used to receive the initial flow of liquid feces. The initial gush of fecal material from the stoma can be upsetting to the patient even when he understands what to expect. The patient should be prepared for the pungent odor of the cauterized tissue, which will disappear shortly.

Dressings may still be used over the stoma initially after the operation. Fluffed, clean gauze is shaped into rings or doughnuts, and several of these are placed around the stoma. The stoma itself is then covered with several gauze fluffs. A similar result may be achieved by cutting holes the size of the stoma in several cellulose pads and placing them, one by one, over the stoma; several pads, left whole, are placed over the top of the stoma. This method of applying the dressing helps to absorb and control leakage around the stoma. Depending on the amount of drainage, the entire dressing may be covered with several combination or "abd" pads. Montgomery straps are used to hold the dressings in place. Their use makes the application and removal of adhesive less frequent, and thus irritation of the skin is lessened.

Moving about in bed, coughing, and early ambulation may be made more difficult by the patient's fear of soiling his clothing and his bedding. Apply the dressing snugly, and change it frequently enough, so that the patient is more willing to move about. Above all, give him the feeling that some soiling is inevitable in the immediate postoperative period, and that the dressing and even bedding changes are accepted and expected by the nursing staff. Promptness in changing the soiled dressings and proceeding in a matter-of-fact manner with a sure touch do more than words to assure the patient that his condition is accepted.

Temporary Pouches

A temporary disposable pouch usually is placed over the stoma during the immediate postoperative period. The stoma is measured and a hole is cut in

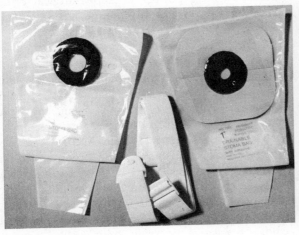
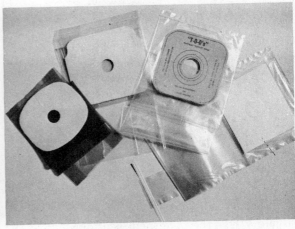

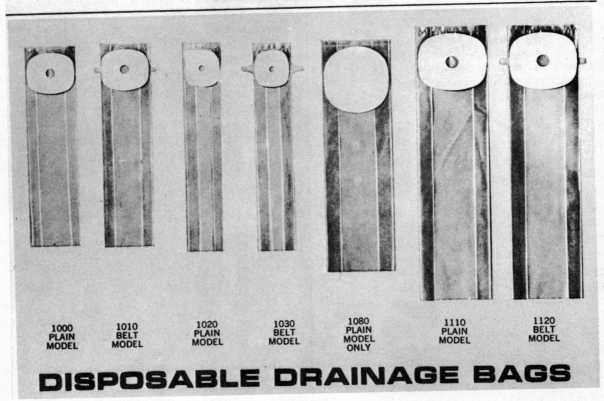

**OSTOMY ACCESSORIES**

| 1000 PLAIN MODEL | 1010 BELT MODEL | 1020 PLAIN MODEL | 1030 BELT MODEL | 1080 PLAIN MODEL ONLY | 1110 PLAIN MODEL | 1120 BELT MODEL |

**DISPOSABLE DRAINAGE BAGS**

**Figure 47-2.** Temporary ostomy drainable bags for postoperative use. Temporary ostomy bags are available in various sizes, widths, and lengths. (*Top, left*) Karaya seal bag with adhesive facing and bag with karaya seal. (Hollister Inc.) (*Top, right*) Examples of adhesive type bags, T-O-D (temporary ostomy drain) and coloplast with closure attachment. (United Surgical Corp. and Atlantic Surgical Co.) (*Bottom*) Temporary bags are available with precut openings or uncut so opening can be fashioned by user. Some temporary bags also have belt attachments. (United Surgical Corp.)

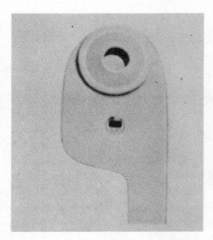

**Figure 47-3.** The permanent ileostomy appliance. A variety of permanent ileostomy appliances are available from the manufacturer. The features of these appliances vary as to pouch size, pouch length, pouch shape and faceplate (disk) design. (United Surgical Corp.)

the top of the pouch with a ⅛-inch clearance around the stoma (Fig. 47-1, p. 798). Some pouches have a precut opening at the top, however, this hole often has to be enlarged so that it will fit over the stoma. A commonly used type of pouch is made of plastic and has a square of double-faced adhesive at the top (Fig. 47-2, p. 799). One side of the adhesive sticks to the skin around the stoma; the other adheres to the plastic material (or may be plastic with a karaya ring). The lower end of the plastic pouch is folded securely and held closed with elastic bands. When the pouch is emptied, a large emesis basin is placed to catch the return and the elastic bands are removed, allowing the drainage to flow out the bottom of the pouch into the emesis basin. The entire appliance is disposable, and a fresh one used if *leakage* occurs.

The disposable plastic pouch is used for a variety of conditions in which drainage occurs from a stoma. Because of edema, the stoma is larger immediately after surgery than it will be later. Thus, the temporary appliance is especially useful because fresh ones can be cut to fit the stoma as often as they are necessary. After healing has occurred and the stoma has reached its permanent size and shape, a permanent appliance is fitted.

**Application of the Temporary Postoperative Appliance.** ADHESIVE TYPE. Prepare the skin by cleansing with soap and water. Pat dry. Apply one or two coats of tincture of benzoin on wet skin and dust on karaya powder or apply surgical cement. Permit cement to dry five minutes if used. Tincture of benzoin should be tacky and dry before applying the appliance. If the temporary bag does not have the exact size opening, measure the stoma and add ⅛-inch clearance around stoma to allow for stomal size change. A karaya ring can be placed around the base of the stoma before applying bag. Secure end of bag with bands or barrette-type clamp.

KARAYA GUM RING WITH ADHESIVE FACING. Prepare skin as above. Peel off protective backing from adhesive facing and align carefully to guide over stoma evenly. Karaya gum ring should fit snugly around stoma. Secure closure as above.

KARAYA GUM RING. Prepare skin as above. Remove protective covering from karaya ring and guide over stoma. Secure closure as above. The karaya ring can fit snugly around the base of stoma without injuring stoma. Care should be taken not to use hard surface rings close to stoma to avoid injury to stoma.

Permanent Appliances

The three basic features of the permanent appliance are:

1. A *disk* (faceplate) surrounds the stoma and usually is adherent to the body.
2. A *pouch* for collecting the feces, usually oblong with a spout for emptying.
3. *Accessories* such as a belt, belt attachments, spout closures, bands, or clips.

The permanent appliance may be made adherent with surgical cement, a karaya gum ring or a double faced adhesive disk.

Considerations for choosing a permanent appliance are concerned with the disk and its design (Fig. 47-3). Therefore, the location of the stoma, the characteristics of abdominal contour and texture, and the characteristics of the stoma must be analyzed for each individual. The material and size of the disk will depend upon individual specifications and patient preferences (Fig. 47-4).

The pouch is that part of the appliance which collects the feces. If there is no fitting problem, pouch size may be the deciding factor in choosing the appliance. There is a wide variety of types of plastic and quality of rubber used with respect to odor permeability. This may be the decisive factor for some patients. Allergy to rubber or other materials may be a factor.

**Allergy to Rubber and Liquid or Creams.** For

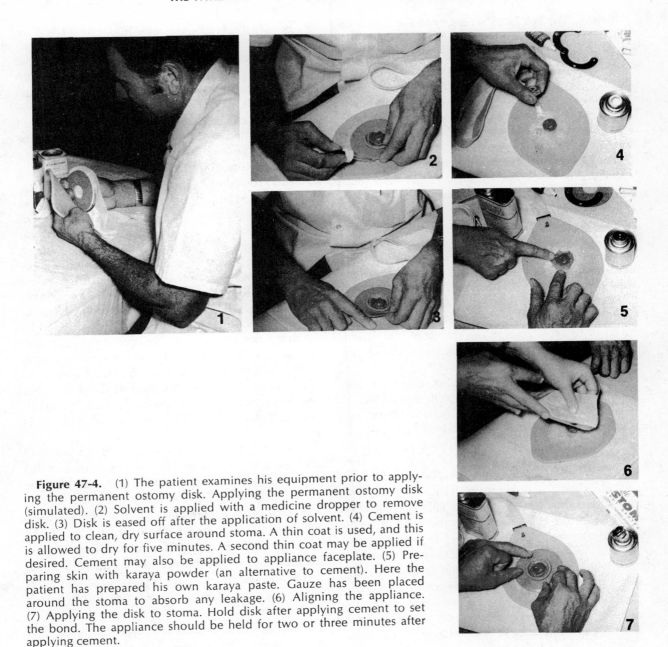

**Figure 47-4.** (1) The patient examines his equipment prior to applying the permanent ostomy disk. Applying the permanent ostomy disk (simulated). (2) Solvent is applied with a medicine dropper to remove disk. (3) Disk is eased off after the application of solvent. (4) Cement is applied to clean, dry surface around stoma. A thin coat is used, and this is allowed to dry for five minutes. A second thin coat may be applied if desired. Cement may also be applied to appliance faceplate. (5) Preparing skin with karaya powder (an alternative to cement). Here the patient has prepared his own karaya paste. Gauze has been placed around the stoma to absorb any leakage. (6) Aligning the appliance. (7) Applying the disk to stoma. Hold disk after applying cement to set the bond. The appliance should be held for two or three minutes after applying cement.

those individuals allergic to rubber, patch-testing can be done with small bits of rubber (worn on the skin for 24 hours) obtained from the manufacturers of rubber appliances. A simpler solution would be for them to wear an all-plastic appliance or a two-piece appliance with plastic disk and synthetic rubber pouch or rubber pouch with a cloth cover in order to avoid irritating contact.

To test for allergy to liquid, saturate ½-inch square of gauze (Band-Aid) with liquid or cream to be tested. Apply to inner surface of arm or leg and leave in place for 24 hours. A positive reaction (sensitivity) to the material is signified by a burning sensation. Remove test material immediately and clean with soap, water, or alcohol. The absence of redness after 24 hours usually indicates no sensitivity. Delayed reaction may occur even after periods of a week in some individuals.

**Belts.** The belt is an accessory to the appliance. However, it is usually worn for 24 hours just as is the appliance; bathing and sleeping are no exceptions. It may occasionally be omitted when a snugly fitted girdle is worn or if disk edge is reinforced with Micropore tape (3M) or reinforcement crescents (Nu Hope). A rubber belt can be used while bathing or swimming, as the elastic tends to stretch when wet.

The belt is used for several reasons: it holds the appliance in place when cement is not used, or it provides pressure for a good bond when cement is used. It may be used to support the weight of the appliance and filled pouch and thus prevent the disk from being pulled away from the abdomen by the weight of the liquid fecal material. It provides the new ostomate with the assurance that the appliance will not fall off.

Reston, gauze, or flannel padding can be used under a belt which cuts into the flesh. Care should be taken to avoid upward or downward pull on the stoma, or double belts can be used to equalize pull on the top and bottom of the disk.

Cement is a combination of latex, a hydrocarbon solvent, and usually some prophylactic additives. It is used to stick the appliance onto the body and it must be applied to a clean, dry surface. Always *apply cement in thin coats* and *permit each coat to dry thoroughly before applying the next one.* This technique permits adequate evaporation of the solvent. Allow five minutes for drying of the cement and evaporation of the solvent. This prevents excoriation of the skin and permits the bond to form. Two thin coats of cement applied to the appliance and the skin will insure a complete covering of the area without excess cement building up. Finding the right cement is a trial-and-error procedure. The skin should be tested for sensitivity before a cement is used because sensitivity is common. It is not necessary to remove all paste from the disk each time the appliance is changed. Slight paste buildup provides for better adherence. However, the skin beneath the disk must be left as clean as possible.

Cement can be rolled off the skin and appliance after several days of wearing. If it does not roll off, a little solvent applied with a medicine dropper can be used *gently* with a gauze pad to rub off traces of cement. A *little* solvent is all that is necessary; wipe off the area with water after solvent has been used.

Solvent is a hydrocarbon which is highly inflammable. It is also very irritating and therefore should be applied sparingly between the body and the bag, with a medicine dropper. *Excessive* rubbing will cause skin irritation. *Never* use carbon tetrachloride in place of ileostomy solvent. Carbon tetrachloride is the most toxic of all commonly used solvents and is highly dangerous. *Benzine* can be used in an emergency but *not benzene*, which is a hydrocarbon and also hazardous.

**Skin Protection Agents.** KARAYA GUM POWDER, KARAYA GUM RINGS, AND NEO-KARAYA. Karaya gum powder is made from the resin of the *Sterculia urens* tree in India. It is a useful product in that it protects the skin while is permits healing underneath and it also serves as an adherent for the ostomy appliance. Karaya gum is used by many in place of cement. Karaya gum powder becomes gelatinous when brought in contact with moisture and can be used in this gummy state.* It can be resealed by applying pressure. Rings of karaya gum are also available commercially. These rings can be cut, pulled, or pushed into any shape desired and therefore can be used as a protection at the base of the stoma to correct the problems created by an ill-fitting appliance. Karaya paste is also available in a tube.

Neo-karaya is karaya gum powder mixed with aluminum hydroxide gel. The watery portion of the aluminum hydroxide gel is poured off and only the thick part is used. This mixture reduces the burning sensation of an excoriation and increases the healing power of the karaya. However, it is not tacky but leathery and when pulled off it will not restick on itself under renewed pressure as do karaya and water. In severe cases of skin breakdown, alternating layers of aluminum hydroxide and karaya is recommended.

Although karaya rings are readily available and less expensive in managing problems related to stoma size changes, scar tissue, proud flesh tags and fistula problems, the overall problem must be assessed in terms of adequacy of protection of skin, and promotion of healing of excoriated areas or prevention of excoriation. The use of either Marsan's new formula skin barrier seal (Mason's) Colby

---

*To prepare karaya gum paste: for each one level teaspoonful of karaya add two teaspoonfuls of water. Stir until smooth and tacky and apply to skin. Increase proportions according to amount needed.

Seel, and Squibbs Stomahesive or Davol ReliaSeal (if allergic to karaya), is recommended for greater protection and greater economy since the appliance may need to be changed less frequently.

## Changing the Appliance

The important factors with regard to changing the appliance are *time* and *frequency*.

**Time.** There are two points to remember. The *first* and the cardinal rule for changing the appliance is that when there is burning or itching underneath the disk or pain around the stoma the appliance should be removed immediately. This should be done regardless of whether the appliance has been on one hour or several days. The stoma and skin should be examined carefully to determine the cause of the difficulty. Excoriation of the skin is to be avoided at all costs. Resorting to the use of a temporary postoperative appliance may be advisable until the cause is identified and eliminated. The most frequent cause is leakage of fecal drainage or reaction to solvent or cement. (Stinging, tingling or itching may be experienced immediately after an appliance change, and will subside quickly. If the sensation is prolonged or intensified, remove the appliance.)

*Second,* the appliance should be changed at a time when the bowel is relatively quiet. For most ostomates this time is early in the morning, before eating or two to three hours after mealtime. However, it is best to check the patient by listening for bowel sounds to note the times of least bowel activity. A record of these times should be made on the patient's chart in order to coordinate plans for the patient's care. The patient will be very much aware and even concerned about the frequency of bowel activity in the beginning. However, he should be assured that as the bowel adjusts to its new state, the activity lessens. Usually, it is most active after he has eaten and relatively quiet at other times. The patient should have quiet and privacy when making the appliance change.

**Frequency.** A few surgeons believe that the first appliance change should be made in 24 hours. Most other surgeons think that the first change should be made in 48 hours unless there is evidence of difficulty such as burning, itching, pain, or a tendency for the patient's skin to become irritated. In this case, the appliance is removed so the skin and stoma may be inspected. Too-frequent changes are thought to be inadvisable, because, in removing

the appliance one may remove the protective layers of epithelium and cause it to become raw and excoriated. However, if the skin and stoma appear intact, wearing time can gradually be increased to a week or longer. The two-piece appliances permit inspection of the stoma by removing only the pouch while the disk remains cemented to the body.

## Care of the Skin

It is imperative that meticulous care be given the circumstomal area to prevent excoriation and skin breakdown. Time and expense should not be spared, because ileal discharge contains digestive enzymes and acids which undermine the skin; the resulting excoriation may take weeks to heal. The nurse should be aware of such problems so that they may be prevented or treated early should they occur. She should be especially careful to protect the circumstomal area from ileal drainage by placing a tissue cuff around the stoma or using a small receptacle to collect the drainage (a paper cup) while caring for the skin.

## Control of Odor and Gas

Odor is an individual matter. There are two kinds of odor that the ostomy patient is concerned about: the odor present when emptying the ileostomy pouch, and the odor which occasionally envelops an ileostomate and follows him about. Personal cleanliness is essential; however, the ostomate must cope with special problems, such as care of his pouch, to lessen odors.

The really serious odor problem is the particularly identifying smell that occasionally clings to the person. Leakage, the pouch, inadequate changing of the pouch, certain foods, or an impending complication may be responsible. Try to ascertain the cause so it can be remedied.

There are many deodorants and deodorizers on the market. These include tablets to be taken orally, such as charcoal, chlorophyll, bismuth subcarbonate, and Derifil (these must be prescribed by the doctor). There are tablets which are inserted in the pouch after each emptying, such as charcoal, chlorophyll, ordinary aspirin, oxychinol or Dis-Pel, and Odo-Way tablets. Others are in liquid form. These include Nilodor (only one drop is needed), Deo-Drops, Banish, and isopropyl alcohol. A paper tissue sprayed or saturated with alcohol can be placed in the pouch. There are also aerosol deodorant sprays, such as Turgasept, Ozone, and Lysol. In an emergency, aerosol underarm deodorant sprays can be used to clear the odor from the room.

To reduce odor in warm weather, try slipping a plastic bag or plastic wrap over the appliance. Keep the appliance clean.

To control odor at its source, a restricted diet of tea, toast, and marmalade and the addition of one food at a time may be tried. Foods containing condiments, fish, eggs, onions, and cheese should be omitted. These frequently cause odors that linger. However, the patient must do this under medical supervision and progress to an adequate diet.

Medications, especially antibiotics and antituberculosis drugs, may cause particularly strong odors that cling to the appliance. An old pouch or disposable pouches used while taking these medications is helpful.

Intestinal gas is often as much as 85 per cent swallowed air. Sighing, chewing, gulping down food, and breathing with the mouth open all contribute to gas formation. Eating slowly and chewing food well with the mouth closed help to reduce gas formation.

Some foods are gas-producing and should be avoided temporarily, such as cabbage, onions, pork, beans, and peppers. Later some individuals find they can add small amounts of these foods to the diet.

Both charcoal tablets and Mylicon tablets or Mylicon liquid are prescribed sometimes to relieve distress due to gas. They break up the gas bubble at its source and reduce the discomfort of bloating.

## Complications

**Blockage.** A blockage is a serious complication. It may be due to a twisted, strangulated, or incarcerated bowel, an internal hernia, or a bolus of food caused by poorly chewed, inadequately digested, stringy, pasty, or fibrous foods. A liquid or no ileal flow will signify an obstruction. *The physician should be consulted.*

*The permanent appliance should be removed and a temporary postoperative appliance with a larger disk opening than that normally worn should be used to allow for stoma swelling and to permit observation of the stoma.* The stoma may become edematous and cyanotic.

Careful lavage by the physician may relieve the obstruction, if it is due to food blockage. The patient may need surgical intervention if the bowel is twisted or strangulated.

Stenosis, tightening, and narrowing of the stoma may eventually require surgical revision. The surgeon may wish to have the patient dilate the stoma daily for a while to prevent further difficulty. The patient inserts a well-lubricated index finger into the stoma for a few minutes. This should be done only on the surgeon's advice. The nail should be cut short to prevent injury to the bowel.

**Prolapse** or protrusion of the ileostomy is fairly common, and if it is of moderate degree (2 to 3 inches) it can be disregarded. Even longer prolapses might be symptomless and harmless. A truss can be worn on the advice of the patient's physician. *However, should there be a sudden prolapse of the stoma, the permanent appliance should be removed immediately, a temporary appliance applied, and the physician notified.* A prolapse should be replaced by the physician as soon as possible. Edema may occur and lead to obstruction, with restriction of blood supply. Necrosis may result if the prolapse is not promptly and skillfully managed. Once prolapse of the stoma has occurred, its recurrence is more likely. Occasionally the prolapse occurs when the patient is far from medical help. In this instance either the patient or a companion replaces the prolapse and medical care is sought as quickly as possible.

**Retraction** of the ileostomy is also common, and is often related to or alternates with prolapse, both being due to a stretched opening in the abdominal wall. It usually is harmless, except for the control of discharge, which is more difficult and may require modification of the appliance or revision of the ileostomy on this basis.

**Hernia** (bulging) around the ileostomy is due to a weakening of the muscles and ligaments at that point. It may be controlled by the ring of the appliance itself and it is left alone. If it is very large, an operation may be necessary.

**Fistula** is an opening in the side of the stoma, and may drain fecal contents through its opening. Its presence makes control of discharge more difficult. Surgery is sometimes necessary. Frequently, injury to the stoma from an improperly applied or too-small bag opening may be the cause.

## THE PATIENT WITH A COLOSTOMY

A colostomy is an artificial opening of the large bowel brought out to the abdomen and fashioned into a stoma. The stoma is a small round structure, pink in color and moist and velvety smooth

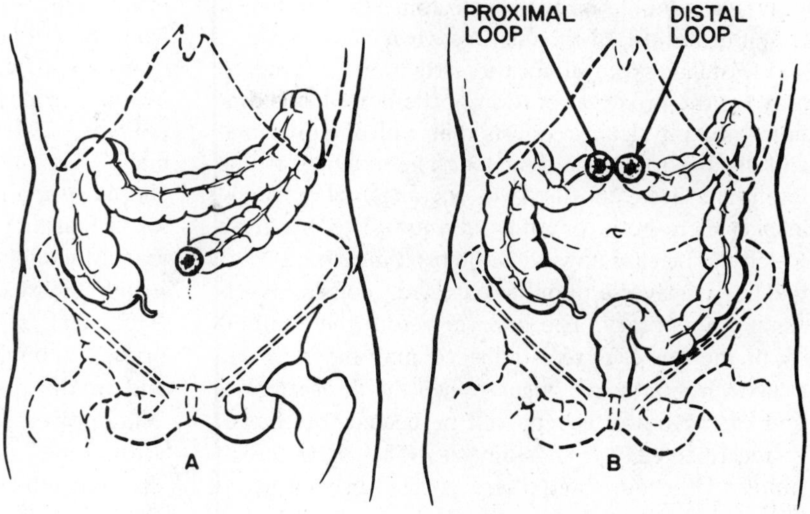

**Figure 47-5.** Single- and double-barreled colostomy. (A) One type of single-barreled colostomy. The distal portion of the bowel has been removed, and the colostomy is permanent. (B) One type of double-barreled colostomy, showing proximal and distal loops. This type of colostomy may or may not be permanent.

in texture. Changes in size and color of the stoma vary with activity and emotional status. Anger or extreme annoyance may produce a very red or purplish color. Small beads of blood may ooze from the surface. Fright may cause the stoma to blanch. These are normal reactions and are significant in that the tissues will revert to their normal state when the cause is alleviated. The nurse must explain to the patient that these are normal reactions.

A cancerous lesion, an ulcerative inflammatory process, multiple polyposis, and injury are indications for a colostomy.

## Types of Colostomies

A colostomy may be described in a number of ways depending upon its purpose, duration, or location. It may be temporary or permanent. If described by location, it may be ascending, transverse, descending, or sigmoid. It may have a single loop or a double loop (double-barreled). It may be described in terms of its therapeutic effect on the patient and be either curative or palliative.

The type of colostomy will not only tell the location of the stoma but will also help the nurse to anticipate the patient's needs. When a colostomy is spoken of in general terms, it usually relates to a sigmoid location. Problems experienced by patients who have this procedure depend to a large extent upon the type of colostomy created.

**Single- and Double-barreled Colostomies.** Colostomies may be double-barreled or single-barreled (Fig. 47-5). A double-barreled colostomy connects with both the proximal and the distal portions of

the bowel. The portion of the bowel leading from the small intestine to the stoma, through which the feces passes to the outside, is called the *proximal portion,* and its opening is called the *proximal opening* or *loop* of the colostomy. The *distal portion* of the bowel leads from the stoma to the anus. Because fecal drainage has been diverted, the distal portion of the bowel does not pass feces by way of the anus. However, mucus often collects in this portion of bowel. Sometimes, the double-barreled colostomy is a temporary procedure and, after disease or injury in the distal portion has been treated, the continuity of the bowel is restored.

A single-barreled colostomy consists of one opening through which fecal matter is passed. The opening is that of the proximal portion of the bowel. The distal portion of the bowel usually has been surgically removed, and the colostomy is permanent.

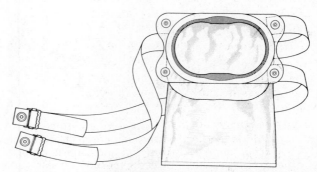

**Figure 47-6.** Disposable bag for double-barreled colostomy. Note size and shape of hole. (Courtesy, Atlantic Surgical Company, Merrick, N.Y.)

When a double-barreled colostomy is irrigated, it is important to distinguish between the proximal and distal loops. Often the irrigation is ordered only for the proximal portion of the bowel. At other times, the physician requests that both the proximal and distal portions be irrigated. The nurse must differentiate between the two openings. She should inspect them both for a few minutes. The one from which the feces is flowing is the proximal loop.

The transverse double-barreled colostomy is usually temporary. The interval before the continuity of the bowel is re-established may be from one to sixteen months or longer. When the diseased portion of the bowel is removed or healed, the bowel is reconnected by anastomosis. This is a much simpler procedure and there is less discomfort to the patient than from the original procedure. Most physicians will insert a nasogastric tube and give intravenous fluids for a few days. As soon as bowel function returns, these measures are discontinued. The patient occasionally will experience some distress with gas-producing foods, for the bowel may narrow at the anastomotic site. Rarely is it necessary to hospitalize the patient for this distress.

**Loop Colostomy.** The loop colostomy is a temporary procedure for diverting the fecal stream in obstruction of the colon. This procedure is being done more frequently in the aged, especially for diverticular conditions. The surgical technique most commonly used in the past was to pass a glass, rubber, or plastic rod through the mesentery of the colon to support the loop on the abdominal wall. Distinct disadvantages to this technique are: (1) the rod may become displaced, allowing the exposed loop to retract, and (2) fitting a leakproof appliance, while the rod is in place, is difficult and

troublesome, resulting usually in skin excoriation from the fecal drainage.

A breakthrough in management of the loop colostomy is now benefiting professionals as well as patients. Two new appliances available commercially eliminate the problems while utilizing the simple support technique. The appliances are similar in that they constitute (1) a support, (2) a gasket assembly, and (3) use a disposable, drainable stoma pouch that can be applied to the gasket. In one (Hollister), a flat, butterfly-shaped polyethylene bridge, 1 mm. thick, is used in place of the rod, and in the other (Marsan), a plastic rod is used. The appliances are available in sets, and are used at the time of surgery. The prime advantage is that they keep the skin free from fecal soilage and at the same time the surgeon and the nurse can view the stoma, and the staff can provide care by removing the drainable pouch attached to the gasket, leaving the rod and protective agent in place (Figs. 47-7 and 47-8). If the surgeon, either by preference or necessity, uses the traditional glass rod technique, management can be simplified with an oversized drainable pouch for the double-barreled or loop colostomy. These pouches are completely disposable, are made of leakproof, odorproof polyethylene materials, and can remain in place for several days. Adjustments can be made for very troublesome situations by altering the placement of the adhesive facing on the pouch, or they can be made to order. The savings in cost of dressings, soiled clothing, and soiled linen, in addition to the self-esteem of the patient, and the nurse's time and effort that is saved far exceeds the additional cost of the pouch. A plan should be made with the surgeon to coordinate the time for inspection of the stoma with the

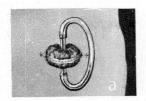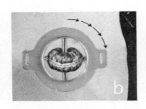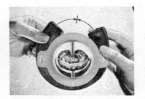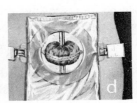

**Figure 47-7.** Marsan loop colostomy method. (A) Flexible tubing is placed over one end of plexiglas rod. Rod is then passed through a defect in the mesocolon at the apex of the loop. Other end of tubing is placed over free end of rod and loop is brought to surface. (B) Tubing is removed and rod is left in place. Gasket is then placed over loop on skin surface; rod is fitted into slots on inner rim of gasket and rotated to lock in place. (C) To help prevent excoriation, a karaya gum washer is applied under gasket and around stoma. (D) A drain is fitted to gasket when colostomy is opened and secured over stoma by an adjustable belt. (Courtesy, Marsan Manufacturing Co., Inc., Wausau, Wis.)

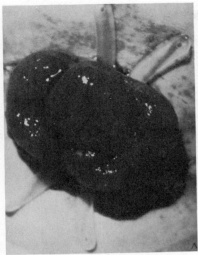 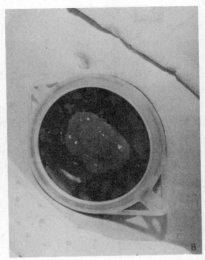 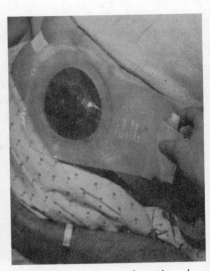

**Figure 47-8.** Hollister loop colostomy appliances. (A) Polyethylene bridge in place. (B) Gasket placed over loop on skin surface. (C) Drain is fitted to gasket and secured over stoma. (Courtesy, Hollister, Incorporated, Chicago, Ill.)

need for pouch change so that time and equipment are not wasted.

### Keeping the Patient Clean

The contents of the large bowel are liquid in the ascending colon, semiliquid to pasty in the transverse colon, semisolid in the descending, and solid in the sigmoid colon. Functions of the large bowel are to reabsorb water and to store feces until evacuated.

Control of fecal evacuation, therefore, is based upon the location of the stoma and the function of

that portion of the bowel. An ascending colostomy will need a carefully applied temporary appliance or an ileostomy type permanent pouch (Fig. 47-9).

The appliance will have to be emptied more frequently. This should be done promptly to maintain the seal and to protect the patient from soiling. Observe the patient to determine the frequency with which the appliance must be emptied.

At first, the stoma constantly exudes soft and liquid feces, and the plastic pouch must be emptied frequently day and night to keep the patient as clean as possible, to control odors, and to prevent

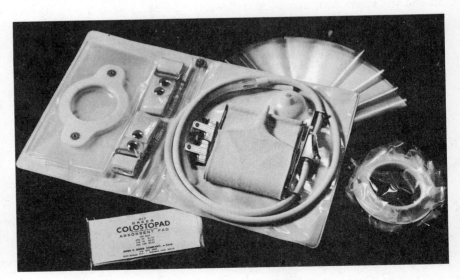

**Figure 47-9.** An example of appliances available for care of colostomy: colostomy shields and belts, and irrigation equipment. (John F. Greer Co.)

excoriation of the skin around the stoma which results from leakage.

The transverse colostomy will be more manageable if irrigated daily to reduce the number of movements and to help eliminate odor (although some surgeons do not consider its irrigation strictly necessary). Discuss the need for irrigation with the surgeon. A temporary ostomy bag will protect the skin and prevent contamination of the surgical wound. The descending and sigmoid colostomies are easier to manage because the content of the bowel is semisolid to solid. Scheduled daily irrigation to establish regularity will help the patient achieve control more rapidly. When control is obtained on a once-a-day basis, the patient is ready to try an every-other-day schedule of irrigations.

Clean rather than sterile technique is used because the opening is into the bowel, which normally contains many bacteria, and because the fecal drainage is laden with bacteria. Wash your hands carefully before and after caring for the stoma. Collect all needed equipment first so that you will not have to obtain supplies from cupboards or supply cart while the dressing change is in progress. If you should require additional supplies, wash your hands thoroughly before leaving the patient's unit.

It is convenient to keep all necessary supplies at the patient's bedside, replenishing them as needed. The supplies include newspapers or paper bags for wrapping soiled dressings, extra dressings or plastic pouches, and any medication that has been ordered for the patient's skin.

Remove the plastic pouch, empty it if necessary, and wrap it in newspaper. Gently wash the skin around the stoma with mild soap and water. Gauze fluffs or disposable washcloths usually are used for cleansing. If the skin is inflamed, use only water, no soap. Wash gently and yet thoroughly; avoid rubbing because the skin is very easily irritated.

Work neatly. Avoid leaving soiled articles within the patient's view. Wrapping the soiled dressings in newspaper as soon as they are removed helps to control odor and make the entire procedure more acceptable to the patient. Provide adequate ventilation, but do not chill the patient. Room deodorizers may be helpful or an aerosol deodorant spray may be used.

Various preparations may be ordered by the physician to treat or to prevent excoriation of the skin. Whatever preparation is used, it is important to remove it periodically and to observe the condition of the skin underneath. Apply the dressings or the plastic pouch snugly to minimize leakage. The adhesive that holds the plastic pouch against the skin will not stick unless the skin is clean and dry. (If ointment is used it is used sparingly and the excess is wiped off.) Apply the bag smoothly to avoid wrinkles.

Change everything that is soiled, including gowns or bedding as necessary.

Try to empty the pouch at least a half-hour or so before meals. Changing it close to mealtime or during the serving of trays interferes with the patient's appetite.

## Methods of Colostomy Management

There are three popular methods of colostomy management—irrigation by the standard method, irrigation by bulb syringe, and nonirrigation.

The first and most widely advocated method for irrigation is the standard method in which the colostomy is irrigated daily, as scheduled, with 1,000 to 2,000 ml. of normal saline or tap water. The schedule gradually progresses to every other day, every third day, or even twice a week. Equipment used is the standard irrigation setup: receptacle for solution (can or bag) attached to tubing and catheter, and irrigation sleeve or sheath for the fecal return. The amount of fluid instilled varies from 500 to 2,000 ml. The patient may be free of spillage from one to three days with effective results.

The second method employs a bulb syringe [Postel, et al., and Still] of soft rubber and a short rubber catheter. The equipment consists of the bulb syringe, a container for the solution, and a plastic sheath. This method calls for several instillations of 50 to 100 ml. of solution at a time. Few patients have found this method effective for freedom of spillage for 24 hours or more. Some patients use two instillations a day. It may be an alternate choice when the standard method cannot be used for irrigation.

The nonirrigation or natural method is the third method. With this method, the patient may use a variety of devices to stimulate an evacuation. Prune or orange juice on arising or before bedtime, liquid breakfast, coffee, mild exercises, a mild laxative, or lemon juice in warm water may be effective. The patient usually does not know when the evacuation will occur.

Another device used by nonirrigators is the suppository (glycerine or Dulcolax). Seven days elapse before a pattern begins to be established. Movements occur three to four times daily. Each day the movements decrease and the time lapse is greater until the patient has two movements a day—one in the morning and one in the evening, but neither at a scheduled time (Katona).

Some patients use the suppository in addition to the irrigation method.

### The Irrigation Procedure

It is essential that the colostomy patient be assisted with the irrigation procedure, because the effectiveness of the irrigation is the basis for establishing control. It can be easily and simply taught so that the patient can begin to do his own irrigation after it has been demonstrated by the nurse (Fig. 47-10).

Once the equipment is assembled, the irrigation solution prepared, and air removed from the tubing, the patient is seated on the toilet seat or on a chair in front of the toilet with the irrigation sheath directed into the toilet bowl. He is then ready to begin the irrigation. The bottom of the bag containing the irrigating solution is hung approximately at shoulder height. (The size of the catheter lumen and height of the bag determine the rate of flow. The catheter size may vary from size 18 to 28 Fr.)

The catheter is inserted through the plastic cup or through the irrigation sleeve, lubricated, and then inserted into the stomal opening. The belt can then be secured after the catheter is inserted into the stoma. The catheter or irrigation tube should be inserted *slowly* and *gently* 2 to 3 inches by rotating the catheter. Difficulty inserting the catheter may be due to a hard piece of stool or to a fold of tissue. If there is difficulty inserting the catheter, withdraw the catheter and reinsert or permit water to flow during insertion. *Never* force the catheter. Once the catheter is in place it can be advanced 4 to 10 inches as desired. However, it is necessary only that the catheter be introduced far enough for water to be retained in the bowel. Allow the water to enter the bowel slowly and gently because too rapid an instillation of fluid will result in painful cramping and an ineffective irrigation. If water returns as it is being introduced, clamp off the tubing until the flow ceases. Do not remove the catheter because the return will flow around the catheter; also, difficulty may be encountered during reinsertion. Then release clamp and continue irrigation until desired amount of solution has been used. Remove the

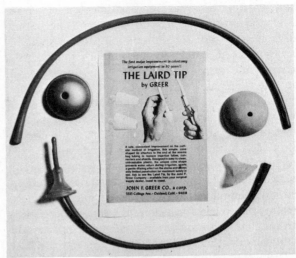

**Figure 47-10.** Items used to prevent backflow during water insertion for irrigation. Items include half of a rubber ball (*upper right*) and a similar device made of metal. (United Surgical Corp.) A baby's bottle nipple may also be used. The Laird Tip is shown on the bottom of the picture. (John F. Greer Co.)

catheter and permit the return to flow into the irrigation sleeve. The patient may remain seated on the toilet or may close off the edge of the sleeve and walk about to help stimulate an evacuation. Shaving or other personal care can be done while awaiting a fecal return.

It requires 20 to 30 minutes for the return to be completed. This time varies from individual to individual and even in the same person at first. The patient will get to know when the irrigation is sufficiently effective and the bowel is clean of feces by a spurt of gas or just a sensation which, he has learned, indicates that sufficient evacuation has occurred. *A clue to the effectiveness of the irrigation can be made by observing the returns. If the return is watery and slightly colored and contains no stool, the bowel is probably clean. If the return is heavy with stool or thick, the bowel is not clean and an additional instillation of 500 or 1,000 ml. of fluid may be necessary.* Use as a guide the amount of water which returns. If what is instilled is returned, you can safely put in more. If what is instilled is not returned, you may need to siphon back the fluid or discontinue the irrigation at that point. Fluid which is not returned at time of irrigation is absorbed by the bloodstream and is later voided. Patients should be discouraged from using more than two quarts of water at a time lest water intoxication result. Soap is not recommended. Some surgeons may advise addition of salt or soda bicarbonate to the water for individual patients. As a general rule this is not necessary. Ordinary tepid tap water will suffice (105 degrees F).

Cramping may be a problem during the irrigation. A slight cramp may simply be a signal that the bowel is ready to empty. Water which is too cold or introduced too rapidly or failure to release air from tubing before inserting the fluid may cause cramping. If cramping occurs, merely pinch off the tubing, and have the patient sit up straight, take a few deep breaths, and relax. Cramping usually will last about a minute. When the cramp is gone, release the tubing and continue the irrigation.

The water may fail to return on occasion, even in experienced individuals, because the catheter was inserted too far and the water remained in the bowel temporarily, or the water may be trapped behind a hard stool. To encourage the return of fluid material more promptly, one or several of the following activities is suggested to the patient: gentle massage of the lower abdomen, tightening the abdominal muscles, taking several deep breaths and relaxing, gently twisting the body (at waist) from side to side, standing up or sitting more erect. If these measures are not effective and the patient is uncomfortable or distressed, notify the physician.

Flushing the bag from below or through a small opening made near the top of the bag will help to eliminate odors from drainage. The irrigation set can be used to flush the bag. The opening at the top of the bag should be covered with a small piece of adhesive tape to prevent leakage.

After the irrigation is completed, remove the irrigation sheath. Rinse it in cool water to reduce odor and discard, or clean it in warm soapy water if it is to be reused.

Irrigation of the proximal loop has been discussed. If the distal loop is to be irrigated, the patient should sit on a bedpan or on the toilet seat because the solution will be expelled through the rectum. Usually mucus and, sometimes, necrotic tissue are expelled along with the solution. Examine the return carefully before discarding it. Sometimes, to decrease the number of bacteria in the bowel, an order is given for one of the sulfonamide drugs or neomycin to be instilled into the distal loop after the irrigation has been completed. The drug is dissolved in water and is instilled through the catheter into the distal loop of the bowel. Ask the patient to retain this solution as long as possible. Having him lie down while the medication is inserted helps him to retain it. Make sure that the bedding is well protected, and that a bedpan is handy.

## Stomal Covering

The stoma may be covered with a gauze pad or temporary postoperative ostomy bag. If a gauze pad is worn, apply a small amount of lubricating jelly over the area which will come in contact with the stoma to prevent irritation of the stoma. Stomal caps are also available. An adhesive drainable bag or a karaya seal drainable bag is recommended for those individuals who continue to have drainage problems between irrigations. A permanent bag is not recommended.

## Scheduling of Irrigations

There should be uninterrupted use of the bathroom for at least one hour for the irrigation. Select a time convenient to the patient according to his schedule of activities. Other members of the household should be considered when setting the time for irrigation.

A regularly scheduled time for the irrigation should be adhered to in the beginning. Later, when control is established, the time can be varied, and the following schedule is recommended: a daily irrigation at first until control is established for 24 hours; then observe the patterning of bowel activity (Katona). When there is little or no fecal return at the time of irrigation, the irrigation can be done every other day; by observing the same pattern, it can be extended to every third day. Some patients who have a tendency to have gas prefer to irrigate daily. This is a personal preference rather than a necessity.

## Diet

Occasionally the physician may prescribe a special diet if there are irregular bowel movements or excessive gas. Otherwise a regular diet (unless there is a particular problem) can be taken with special attention to avoiding gas-forming foods, such as dry beans, cabbage, uncooked onions, cheese, and fish. When trying new foods, introduce one new food at a time to determine if it can be tolerated. Allow at least one day to lapse between adding new foods.

The diet can be adjusted if diarrhea or constipation is a problem. Elimination of distressing food items will help to control diarrhea. Increasing the amount of bulk and water in the diet will help to correct constipation. The physician should be consulted on these problems should they persist after temporary measures have been used. Attention to eating slowly with mouth closed and chewing food well will reduce gas which is caused chiefly by swallowing air rather than by processes of digestion.

## Clothing

With the exception of tight-fitting items, no adjustment needs to be made regarding type of clothing worn. Women are advised to wear girdles without bones or stays, lest the stoma be injured. Those of lightweight expandable material such as Lycra or Spandex are suggested. It is *not* advisable to cut a hole in the garment to allow the stoma to protrude as this defeats the purpose of the garment. Those individuals who require a firm support (such as patients who have back disorders and who wear braces) may find a stoma shield helpful in preventing undue pressure or irritation of the stoma.

## Travel

Travel can be undertaken as the patient's physical state improves or with his physician's permission if physical circumstances require caution. Upsets can be avoided by planning in advance and by having an established routine. There are three things the ostomate should consider in traveling: (1) what equipment to take along and how to carry it, (2) what to do in case of medical emergencies, (3) where to obtain additional ostomy supplies.

Always, whether on a short or a long trip, the ostomate should carry *with him* the minimum equipment to remedy a leak or make a quick change. If travel is at a distance or the trip extended, more than bare essentials should be taken, with thought given to purchasing readily available items at one's destination. Practical, dual-purpose containers and items are preferable. It is wise to plan a short stay away from home purposely, in order to gain experience, especially if one is contemplating a lengthy trip.

A few travel pointers for the patient to keep in mind are:

- **Water which is not safe to drink is not desirable for irrigation either. Boiled or bottled water can be used.**
- **Changes in climate and temperature can interfere with the efficiency of established practices. Example**
—items that are pressurized or liquids in plastic containers should be avoided.
- **Experiment with substitutes at home to test their efficiency and adequacy.**
- **Use caution in trying new or exotic foods. Be prepared for sudden intestinal upsets, which may occur if you want to be adventuresome.**
- **Make a list of essential items to take along, and refer to it when packing.**

What to do should a medical emergency arise will depend upon the distance and the patient's location. A call to a physician may be sufficient or the proximity to a medical facility will have a bearing on the decision. In any event, be prepared with names, addresses, phone numbers of possible sources of help, such as physicians, ostomy associations, and supply houses. The *Ostomy Quarterly* carries lists of both suppliers and ostomy associations.

## THE PERINEAL WOUND

The perineal wound, the space left after the rectum has been removed, may constitute a greater problem than the ostomy to some people with a total colectomy. The blood supply (necessary for satisfactory healing) is not really adequate, and thus fistulas and abscesses may form here. The perineal wound usually is left to granulate rather than close completely to lessen the possibility of infection from poor healing.

When the skin surface of the perineal wound closes before the rest of the opening, matter accumulates and will eventually drain to the outside, often in a rush of liquid. If it is infected, there will be pain and swelling. It is a frightening event to the ostomate.

The time for complete healing of the perineal wound varies widely from several months to many years. Often a stitch or exudate within the wound itself prevents healing. Once the cause has been removed, healing will take place rapidly.

The perineal wound is kept clean by sitz baths (immersion of the buttocks and perineum in 5 to 6 inches of very warm water, usually for 20 minutes.

Sitz baths are ordered three to four times daily for proper cleansing of the tissues. The persistent discharge will be quickly reduced in volume and thickness to a thin watery discharge after several treatments.

The wound may be irrigated with a solution of 50 per cent normal saline and 50 per cent peroxide or povidone-iodine (Betadine) solution. The physician determines the depth and the direction the catheter should be inserted to irrigate the perineal defect.

In perineal resection for a malignancy, a larger area is excised, more tissue is removed, and healing is delayed. In perineal resection for ulcerative colitis, a smaller area is excised and less tissue is removed. Therefore, healing is more rapid and fewer problems occur in perineal resection of the ileostomate.

### New Surgical Technique

The creation of an ileostomy alone is a satisfactory substitute for bowel evacuation when proctocolectomy is necessary. This procedure, however, does require a "stick on" pouch, *an absolute necessity* to protect the skin from excoriation due to fecal drainage. Most patients with an ileostomy may soon have a choice of a traditional stoma or the newer version of ileostomy with an ileal reservoir. On the basis of the work done by Koch, Beahrs, and others, some surgeons in the United States and Europe are offering selected ileostomy patients a choice of the ileal reservoir over the traditional ileostomy.

Most American surgeons view the procedure with caution. The advantages of a continent ileostomy and freedom from leakage, gas, and time-consuming rituals are primary, but the disadvantages are still a matter of great concern to most surgeons. The potential is great for breakdown of the suture line as a consequence of the method of constructing the pouch thus dumping the fecal contents into the peritoneum, as is the potential for perforation during catheterization of the internal pouch to evacuate the reservoir. As the technique for constructing the ileal reservoir and the effect of changes within the ileal pouch itself become better understood, it may become the procedure of choice. Since the procedure is not standardized, and the technique continues to be refined, the reader is referred to recent publications in the surgical journals for details about the construction of the ileal reservoir.

### CECOSTOMY

An opening made in the cecum for the drainage of intestinal contents is called a cecostomy. Usually, this is a temporary measure performed to relieve intestinal obstruction. When the patient's physical condition has improved, further surgery may be carried out. It is a relatively minor procedure, usually done under local anesthesia. An opening is made into the cecum through a small incision in the lower abdomen, and a large catheter is placed in the cecostomy to drain feces. The catheter is connected to a drainage bottle that collects the liquid feces, and it is sutured to the skin to prevent displacement.

Although the fecal material draining from the cecum is usually liquid, small clumps of formed stool also may be present and may clog the catheter. Irrigations of the catheter usually are ordered to prevent clogging. The frequency of irrigations and the amount and type of solution to be used are ordered by the physician. Normal saline is commonly used. It is allowed to run into the cecostomy tube by gravity, through an Asepto syringe. The glass portion of the syringe without the rubber bulb is used as a funnel through which the normal saline flows into the cecostomy tube. It is important not to exert pressure (as by using the rubber bulb) when you are doing the irrigation, because this might injure the bowel. If the fluid will not run into the tube by gravity, the physician should be consulted. The tube may be obstructed, and another may need to be inserted.

Fecal material may leak around the tube onto the skin. Dressings, if used, are applied to absorb the drainage and are changed frequently to control soiling, odor, and to prevent excoriation of the skin.* Principles of caring for a patient who has an opening of his bowel onto the skin are similar to those for a patient with a colostomy or an ileostomy.

### REFERENCES AND BIBLIOGRAPHY

ALEXANDER, E. L., BURLEY, W., ELLISON, D., and VALLERI, R.: *Care of the Patient in Surgery Including Techniques,* St. Louis, Mosby, 1967, pp. 642-663.
BACON, H. E.: *Cancer of the Colon, Rectum, and Anal Canal,* Philadelphia, Lippincott, 1964, p. 498.
———, and OCHSNER, A.: *Ulcerative Colitis,* Philadelphia, Lippincott, 1958.
BEAHRS, O. H., KELLY, K. A., ADSON, M. A., and CHONG, G. C.: Ileostomy with ileal reservoir rather than ileostomy alone, *Ann. Surg.* 179:634, May 1974.

---

*Temporary postoperative bags are preferred to dressings.

BEHNKE, H. D. (ed.): *Guidelines for Comprehensive Nursing Care in Cancer,* Springer, New York, 1973, p. 391.

BELAND, I. L.: *Clinical Nursing,* ed. 2, New York, Macmillan, 1970, pp. 920-1004.

BROOKE, B. N.: *Ulcerative Colitis and Its Surgical Treatment,* Chap. 6, Edinburgh, Livingstone, 1954.

CHUGHTAI, S. Q., and ACKERMAN, N. B.: Perforated Diverticulum of the Transverse Colon, *Am. J. Surg.* 127:508-510, May 1974.

DAVIS, F., and EARDLEY, A.: Coping with a colostomy—the importance of the nurse, *Nurs. Times* 70:580-2, April 1974.

DAVIS, L.: *Christopher's Textbook of Surgery,* ed. 9, Philadelphia, Saunders, 1968.

DENNIS, C., and KARLSON, K. E.: Cancer risk in ulcerative colitis; formidability per year in late disease, *Surgery* 50:568, 1961.

DERRICKS, V. C.: Rehabilitation of patients with ileostomy, *Am. J. Nurs.* 61:48, May 1961.

DEVLIN, H. B.: Stoma care: A surgeon's viewpoint, *Nurs. Times* 70:576, April 1974.

DISON, N. G.: *American Atlas of Nursing Techniques,* St. Louis, Mosby, 1967, pp. 165-174.

ELLISON, E. H., FRIESEN, S. R., and MULHOLLAND, J. H.: *Current Surgical Management, III,* Philadelphia, Saunders, 1956, pp. 409-424.

FINN, B.: Training the stoma care nurse, *Nurs. Times* 70:579, April 1974.

GALLAGHER, A. M.: Body image changes in the patient with a colostomy, *Nurs. Clin. N. Am.* 7:699, December 1972.

GIVEN, B. A., and SIMMONS, S. J.: *Nursing Care of the Patient with Gastrointestinal Disorders,* St. Louis, Mosby, 1970, pp. 263-264.

GUTOWSKI, F.: Ostomy procedure: Nursing care before and after, *Am. J. Nurs.* 72:262, February 1972.

HILL, L. D., STONE, C. S., and BAKER, J. W.: One-stage abdominoproctocolectomy and ileostomy, *AMA Arch. Surg.* 83:98, 1961.

———, STONE, C. S., and PEARSON, C. C.: Surgical aspects of ulcerative colitis, *AMA Arch. Surg.* 72:968, 1956.

INGLES, T., and CAMPBELL, E.: The patient with a colostomy, *Am. J. Nurs.* 58:1546, 1958.

KATONA, E. A.: Learning colostomy control, *Am. J. Nurs.* 67:3, 1967.

———: Patient centered living oriented approach to the patient with artificial anus or bladder, *Nurs. Clin. N. Am.* 2:623, December 1967.

LENNEBERG, E. S., et al.: Modern concepts in the management of patients with intestinal and urinary stomas, *Clin. Obstet. Gynecol.* 15:542, June 1972.

LINDER, J.: Inexpensive colostomy irrigation equipment, *Am. J. Nurs.* 58:1544, 1958.

POSTEL, A. H., GRIER, W. R., and LOCALIO, S. A.: A simplified method of irrigation of the colonic stoma, *Surg. Gynec. Obstet.* 121:595, 1965.

SAUNDERS, H. B.: Stoma care nurse—a new role, *Nurs. Times* 70:578, April 1974.

SIEGEL, R., and PAPUSH, H.: *The ABC of Ileostomy,* Jamaica, N.Y., Custom Service, 1963, p. 90.

SUTTON, A. L.: *Bedside Nursing Techniques in Medicine and Surgery,* ed. 2, Philadelphia, Saunders, 1969.

TURNBULL, R. B., JR.: Management of the ileostomy, *Am. J. Surg.* 86:617, 1953.

VUKOVICH, V. C., and GRUBB, R. D.: *Care of the Colostomy Patient,* St. Louis, Mosby, 1973, p. 138.

WHELTON, M. J., FINDLEY, J. M., MACDONALD, M. A.: Ileostomy and colostomy care, *Br. J. Hosp. Med.* 6:315, September 1971.

*Your Ileostomy: A Guide for the New Patient,* Q.T. Inc. (c/o The Medical Foundation, Inc., 29 Commonwealth Ave., Boston, Mass. 02116), 1962.

ZIMMERMAN, I. M., and LEVINE, R.: *Physiologic Principles of Surgery,* ed. 2, Chap. 22, Philadelphia, Saunders, 1964.

ZOPF, D.: How could Patti, 20 and newly married, ever face a colostomy? (care st) *Nurs. '73* 3:14, October 1973.

## SUPPLEMENTARY BIBLIOGRAPHY

Abdominoperineal resection of the rectum, *Nurs. Times* 68:186, February 1972.

BACON, H. E., et al.: Is colostomy a necessary complement to elective left colonic resection?, *Dis. Colon Rectum* 16:29, January-February 1973.

BARCKLEY, V.: A visiting nurse specializes in cancer nursing, *Am. J. Nurs.* 70:1680, 1970.

BEAHRS, O. H., et al.: Ileal pouch with ileostomy rather than ileostomy alone, *Am. J. Surg.* 125:154, February 1973.

BODE, H., and HENDREN, W. H.: Healing of fecal fistulas initiated by synthetic low-residue diet, *Lancet* 1:954, 1970.

BRANDBERG, A., et al.: Bacterial flora in intraabdominal reservoir. A study of 23 patients provided with "continent ileostomy," *Gastroenterology* 63:413, September 1972.

BROOKE, B. N., et al.: Further experience with azathioprine for Crohn's disease, *Lancet* 2:1050, 1970.

BURMAN, J. H., et al.: The effects of diversion of intestinal contents on the progress of Crohn's disease of the large bowel, *Gut* 12:11, 1971.

BURY, K. R., STEPHENS, R. V., and RANDALL, H. T.: Use of chemically defined liquid elemental diet for nutritional management of fistulas of the alimentary tract, *Am. J. Surg.* 121:174, 1971.

CASE, T. C.: Simple technic for transverse colostomy, *J. Am. Geriat. Soc.* 21:333, July 1973.

CIHLAR, J., et al.: Courage with a colostomy, *Am. J. Nurs.* 67:1050, May 1967.

CROMAR, C. D. L.: The evolution of colostomy, *Dis. Colon Rectum* 11:256, 1968; 11:367, 1968; 11:423, 1968.

DAILEY, T. H.: Office management of common intestinal stoma problems, *Dis. Colon Rectum* 13:401, 1970.

DAVIS, L. P.: The "average" ostomy patient, *J. Med. Assoc. Ga.* 62:314, September 1973.

DERRICKS, V. C.: *Booklet of Instructions for Persons with a Colostomy,* 1966, The New York Hospital, 525 East 68th Street, New York.

DEVLIN, H. B.: Colostomy. Indications, management and complications, *Ann. R. Coll. Surg. Engl.* 52:392, June 1973.

———, and PLANT, J. A.: Colostomy and its management, *Nurs. Times* 65:231, February 20, 1969.

DLIN, B., et al.: Psychosexual response to ileostomy and colostomy, *Ostomy Quarterly,* Winter, 1969, pp. 4-5, 16-24.

DRUSS, R. G., O'CONNOR, J. F., and STERN, L. O.: Psychological response to colectomy, *Arch. Gen. Psych.* 18:53, 1968.

EIN, S. H., et al.: Ulcerative colitis in children under one year: A twenty-year review, *J. Pediat. Surg.* 6:264, 1971.

FINCH, H. M.: Enterostomal therapy—a new approach to ostomy care, *J. Med. Assoc. Ga.* 59:299, 1970.

FOLEY, W. J., et al.: Toxic megacolon in acute fulminant ulcerative colitis, *Am. J. Surg.* 120:769, 1970.

FRENAY, SISTER MARY A. C.: Dynamic approach to the ileal conduit patient, *Am. J. Nurs.* 64:80, January 1964.

GIBBS, G., and WHITE, M.: Stomal care, *Am. J. Nurs.* 72:268, 1972.

GILL, N. N., and MILLER, D.: The care of ileostomies, *Mich. Nurse,* January 1971.

GIVEN, B. A., and SIMMONS, S. J.: *Nursing Care of the Gastrointestinal Disorders,* St. Louis, Mosby, 1971.

GOODARD, G. M.: The patient with a colostomy, Part 3, *Nurs. Mirror* 134:43, March 31, 1972.

GRIFFIN, M.: Survey of the incapacity of patients with permanent colostomy, *Proc. R. Soc. Med.* 66:204, February 1972.

GROSS, G. F., et al.: Perforations of the colon from barium enema, *Am. Surg.* 38:583, November 1972.

GUTOWSKI, F.: Ostomy procedure: Nursing care, *Am. J. Nurs.* 72:262, 1972.

HALLBURG, J. C.: Patient with surgery of the colon, *Am. J. Nurs.* 61:64, March 1961.

HANEY, M. J., and McGARITY, W. C.: Ureterosigmoidostomy and neoplasms of the colon, *Arch. Surg.* 103:69, 1971.

Helping your ostomy patient cope. *Nurs. Update* 3:1, October 1972.

HUDSON, C. N.: Ileostomy in pregnancy, *Proc. R. Soc. Med.* 65:281, March 1972.

HUGHES, E. S.: Ileostomy care, *Med. J. Aust.* 2:110, July 8, 1972.

Human problems in nursing . . . helping patients live with colostomy, *Nurs. '72* 2:4, July 1972.

HUNGELMANN, J., and KOLBA, SISTER M. T.: Bridging the gap between hospital and home, *RN* 32:56, June 1969.

JAVETT, S. L., and BROOKE, B. N.: Reversed ileal segment for ileostomy diarrhea, *Lancet* 1:291, 1971.

JETER, K.: Count your blessings, 1969, Columbia-Presbyterian Medical Center, 622 West 168th St., New York.

———, and BLOOM, S.: Management of stomal complications following ileal or colonic conduit operations in children, *J. Urol.* 106:425, 1971.

JOHNSON, W. C.: Large para-ileal conduit hernia, treated with the aid of preoperative progressive pneumoperitoneum: a case report, *J. Urol.* 108:863, December 1972.

KAFETSIOULIS, A., and SWINNEY, J.: A study of ileal conduits, *Br. J. Urol.* 42:33-36, 1970.

KATONA, E. A.: Nurse initiated and conducted clinic for colostomy patients, in *Maintaining the Integrity of the Individual; a Nursing Responsibility* (Convention Clinical Sessions, 1964, No. 6), New York, Am. Nurses' Assoc. 1964, p. 22.

———: Learning colostomy control, *Am. J. Nurs.* 67:534, 1967.

KEE, J.: Fluid and electrolyte imbalances, *Nurs. '72,* January 1972.

KORELITZ, B. I., et al.: Controversy on recurrent ileitis after ileostomy: background and speculation, *Gastroenterology* 65:498, September 1973.

KRAMER, P., and LEVITAN, R.: Effect of 9-0 fluorohydrocortisone on the ileal excreta of ileostomized subjects, *Gastroenterology* 62:235, 1972.

LAPIDES, J., and TANK, E. S.: Urinary complications following abdominal perineal resection, presented at the National Conference of the Colon and Rectum, San Diego, California, January 1971.

LENNEBERG, E., and ROWBOTHAM, J. L.: *The Ileostomy Patient,* Springfield, Ill., Thomas, 1970.

———, et al.: Modern concepts in the management of patients with intestinal and urinary stomas, *Clin. Obstet. Gynecol.* 15:542, June 1972.

LETTON, A. H., et al.: Rehabilitation of the patient with colostomy, *Cancer* 28:219, 1971.

MacLEOD, J. H.: Colostomy irrigation—a transatlantic controversy, *Dis. Colon Rectum* 15:357-360, September-October 1972.

McCONNELL, E.: Enterostomal therapy in the community hospital, *AORN* 10:44, December 1969.

McGARITY, W. C.: Colostomy—to irrigate or not to irrigate, *J. Med. Assoc. Ga.* 62:93, March 1973.

MEYERS, B.: Some psychological aspects of the colostomy. Paper presented at a meeting of the Colostomy Society of New York, Martinique Hotel, October 4, 1963.

NEWTON, C. R.: The effect of codeine phosphate, lomotil, and isogel on ileostomy function, *Gut* 14:424, May 1973.

———: Comparison of bowel function after colectomy and ileostomy or ileorectal anastomosis for inflammatory bowel disease, *Gut* 13:855, October 1972.

O'BRIEN, P. H.: The colostomy rehabilitation program, *J. SC. Med. Assoc.* 68:394, October 1972.

ORBACH, C. E., and TALLANT, N.: Modification of perceived body and of body concepts, *Arch. Gen. Psychiat.* 12:126, 1965.

ORR, K. B.: Closure of colostomy, *British Med. J.* 4:552, December 2, 1972.

PELOK, L. R., et al.: Colostomy in the trauma patient, *Dis. Colon Rectum* 16:290, July-August 1973.

PEMBERTON, L. B.: Immediate mucocutaneous suture for loop colostomy, *Surg. Gynec. Obstet.* 135:793, November 1972.

Psychiatric nursing intervention with a colostomy patient, *Perspect. Psychiat. Care* 10, 2:69-71, 1972.

ROSS, F. B.: Opening a loop colostomy by a simple method, *Surg. Gynec. Obstet.* 136:446, March 1973.

ROWBOTHAM, J. L.: Stomal care, *New Eng. J. Med.* 279:90, July 1969.

————: Colostomy problems—dietary and colostomy management, presented at the National Conference on Cancer of the Colon and Rectum, San Diego, California, January 7-9, 1971.

————, et al.: Helping your ostomate patient cope, *Patient Care* 6:46, 1972.

SANCHEZ, E.: How well do we know our patients? *Am. J. Nurs.* 9:1263, June 1969.

SECOR, S. M.: Colostomy care—1964, *Am. J. Nurs.* 64:127, September 1964.

SHAW, B. L.: Current concepts of stomal care, *RN* 32:52, 1969.

SILL, A. R.: Bulb syringe technique for colonic stoma irrigation, *Am. J. Nurs.* 70:536, March 1970.

SINGER, A. M., et al.: Blood and urinary changes in patients with ileostomies and ileorectal anastomoses, *British Med. J.* 3:141, July 21, 1973.

A slightly neglected area? *Nurs. Times* 69:126, January 1973.

SPARBERG, M., et al.: Solid state karaya gum ring for use in disposable and permanent ileostomy appliances, *Am. J. Surg.* 111:610, April 1966.

STERLING, W. A., and MCHEATH, D.: A normal life with a colostomy, *Postgrad. Med.* 47:80, 1970.

STITT, A.: When the problem is ileostomy, *Emergency Med.* 2:107, 1970.

————: Coping with a colostomy, *Emergency Med.* 2:85, 1970.

THOMPSON, W. R., et al.: Use of the "space diet" in the management of a patient with extreme short bowel syndrome, *Am. J. Surg.* 117:449, 1969.

THOMSON, J. P.: Results of closure of loop transverse colostomies, *British Med. J.* 3:459, August 19, 1972.

TRUNKEY, D., et al.: Management of Rectal Trauma, *J. Trauma* 13:411, May 1973.

TURNBULL, R. B., et al.: Choice of operation for the toxic megacolon phase of nonspecific ulcerative colitis, *Surg. Clin. N. Am.* 50:1151, 1970.

————, and WEAKLEY, F.: Atlas of intestinal stomas, St. Louis, Mosby, 1967.

WILSON, E.: A place for colostomy in treatment of ulcerative colitis, *Dis. Colon Rectum* 16:98, March-April 1973.

WRIGHT, H. K., and TILSON, M. D.: A method for testing the functional significance of tight ileostomy stomas, *Am. J. Surg.* 123:147, 1972.

# The Urologic Patient

Both male and female patients with disorders of the urinary tract not only suffer from the accompanying physical discomfort, but often from embarrassment and anxiety as well. Because genitourinary difficulties often involve sharing very personal information and the experience of an extensive physical inspection and examination of this part of the body, patients tend to delay seeking medical help. The sex organs and urinary tract are in close physical proximity so that disturbances of urinary elimination may pose threats to usual sexual functioning. Every effort should be made to protect the patient's modesty and privacy and to deal matter-of-factly with problems. It may be necessary for the nurse, for example, to help the patient translate his complaints from the vernacular to more scientific language. This may be somewhat difficult for the nurse to do. It requires a sensitivity to the patient's cultural and emotional patterns with recognition that effective understanding of what is happening to him may involve some instruction in normal anatomy and physiology. Diagrams may be useful. Knowing the customary anatomic terms may make the patient less hesitant to ask questions (see Figs. 48-1 to 48-4).

Urologic patients, like others, can express their anxiety in a variety of ways. The threatened male patient, for example, may become immodest and aggressive toward the female nurse. The nurse should try to understand the reason for the patient's behavior. However, she need not tolerate this behavior. Instead, it is necessary to set limits to behavior and to listen and talk with the patient about his concerns. Overt sexual behavior of this type may be anxiety producing for the nurse and she may react by withdrawing from the patient. The patient, in turn, becomes more threatened and his self-esteem is lowered even more. Asking the patient to behave more appropriately shows a response to his overt behavior and respect for his capacity to change it, and paves the way for more culturally appropriate anxiety-relief mechanisms, such as talking with the nurse or physician about what is bothering him.

## THE URINARY TRACT

The urinary tract is one of several waste disposal systems by which the body rids itself of the by-products of metabolism. This system is also essential to regulation of body fluids and their electrolyte content. When the kidneys are diseased or injured, and their function is impaired, or when there is an obstruction to the free flow of urine to the outside, serious illness is present or imminent. Often, conditions develop that require long-term care and treatment.

Certain problems that occur with advancing age, such as benign prostatic hypertrophy, are seen more frequently today since people live longer.

The urinary tract consists of the *kidneys,* which manufacture urine, and the various tubes and reservoirs necessary to discharge this fluid from the body. The kidneys have at least three known functions: (1) they excrete excess water and the nitrogenous waste products of protein metabolism; (2) they play a significant role in maintaining the acid-base balance of the body and the equilibrium of plasma electrolytes; and (3) they produce enzymes, such as

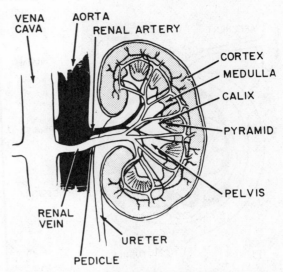

**Figure 48-2.** Interior of kidney.

renin, which act on certain plasma constituents to form a compound that raises blood pressure. The kidneys selectively filter over 50 gallons of plasma daily. All but a quart or so of this volume is reabsorbed into the circulation every 24 hours.

The formed urine is excreted into the renal *pelves* and carried down the *ureters* to the *bladder.* Here the urine is stored until bladder fullness is reached, at which time the patient voids the urine to the out-

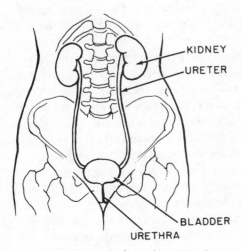

**Figure 48-1.** The urinary tract.

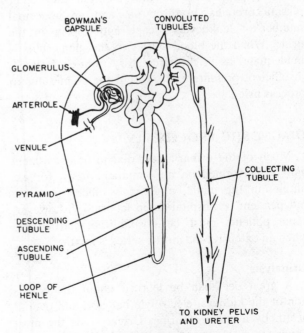

**Figure 48-3.** A nephron.

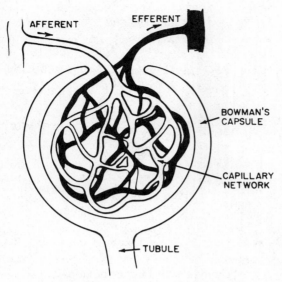

**Figure 48-4.** Bowman's capsule.

side through the *urethra*. Any disorder that interferes with this process is likely to cause serious repercussions unless it can be corrected. These disorders include interference with circulation to the kidney, disease of the kidney itself, and obstruction to drainage of the urinary tract.

In some diseases, such as chronic glomerulonephritis, the permeability of the filtering membranes is increased, so that albumin and other plasma proteins, erythrocytes, and an abnormal number of leukocytes escape and appear in the urine. When the blood supply to the glomerulus is inadequate, as in the circulatory failure of shock, insufficient pressure exists within the glomerulus to process urine.

## DIAGNOSTIC PROCEDURES

Much of the urinary tract diagnostic assessment can be performed on an outpatient basis, for example, in the clinic, physician's office, or in an independent or hospital-based laboratory; however, some patients must be hospitalized, particularly when an extensive diagnostic series is required.

### Urinalysis

A great deal can be learned about the condition of the kidneys, electrolyte balance, and overall health by a study of urine. Urinalysis is the most important diagnostic study of the urinary tract.

The characteristics of normal urine are:

| | |
|---|---|
| Specific gravity | 1.005 to 1.025 |
| Color | Pale yellow to dark amber |
| Turbidity | Usually clear (cloudiness not always abnormal) |
| Acidity | pH 4.8 to 7.5 |
| Protein | None to trace |
| Glucose | None to trace |
| Red blood cells | 0 to 3 per high power field |
| White blood cells | 0 to 4 per high power field |
| Casts | Rare per high power field |

A red color of the urine may mean that blood is present, but must be proved by microscopic examination of the sediment. Certain metabolic disturbances, ingested dyes, or foodstuffs may impart a red color that is not blood. One-fifth of the patients admitted to the hospital with gross blood in the urine (hematuria) have cancer in the urinary tract and this finding requires a complete urologic investigation. Cloudiness of the urine may be due to phosphates (a normal finding) or to white cells, suggesting an infection or irritation of the tract. Proteinuria (usually albumin) may occasionally be normal. More often it implies disease of the system. Little of this material filters through the pores of the normal glomeruli. Casts are molds of the renal tubules, and their size will vary with the size of the portion of the nephron whence they originate. They may be constituted of red cells, of white cells, or of precipitated protein.

The container in which the urine specimen is collected should be clean and dry; it should be sterile if a culture is to be taken. It is preferable to have the patient void directly into the container that is sent to the laboratory. Taking a urine specimen from a bedpan or a urinal that contains sediment from previous use may lead to inaccurate results.

When infection is suspected, a specimen may be taken for culture. It is usually sufficient to have the male patient cleanse the glans penis with soap and water, after which he voids about 60 ml., which is discarded, and then voids into a sterile specimen bottle (clean-catch specimen). The bottle is capped in such a way that it is not contaminated.

Because there is always the danger of introducing infection into the urinary tract with a catheter, the sterile-voided or clean-catch procedure is used for women also. The labia are held apart, and the vulva and urethral meatus are cleansed. While the labia are held open so that the orifice of the urethra is exposed, the client voids into a sterile container after the initial 60 ml. is discarded (midstream collection). The nurse gives instructions to the client and provides for physical assistance if necessary.

Catheterization may be necessary for a specimen for culture. Since bacteria multiply in urine and its contents decompose on standing, the specimen is delivered immediately to the laboratory or promptly refrigerated on the ward.

Fractionated urine specimens may be required to determine where a urinary abnormality, such as pus, originates. One method used is the three-glass test. The first 60 ml. voided represents urethral washings. A second, similar volume is from the bladder and kidneys. A third specimen, obtained after the physician performs prostatic massage, includes secretions from that organ. Papanicolaou smears of urine may identify cancer cells arising from the lining of the kidney, ureter, and bladder. Specimens are secured in the same manner as described for suspected infection.

Sometimes a specimen of all urine excreted over a period of time, such as 24 hours, may be needed for examination of such constituents as tubercle bacilli and 17-ketosteroids. The patient empties his bladder immediately prior to the start of the time period and this urine is discarded. The entire specimen is refrigerated to prevent bacterial growth. To prevent any part of the specimen from being lost or contaminated, the patient is instructed to use separate receptacles for voiding and defecation.

## Blood Chemistry

Several blood tests are useful in evaluating the patient with a urologic problem.

When the nephrons fail to remove waste products efficiently, the composition of the blood is altered. Deterioration in renal function is manifested chemically by a rise in blood urea nitrogen (BUN) and creatinine values, both of which are protein breakdown products. However, there must be a decrease of 50 to 75 per cent in function before these values rise. The normal BUN is 8 to 18 mg. per cent, and creatinine 0.5 to 1.0 mg. per cent. High blood levels of urea nitrogen can be accompanied by disorientation and convulsions.

This information can serve as one guide to planning nursing care. For example, if the patient's BUN is high, he should be observed particularly for disorientation and convulsions and the necessary protective equipment must be kept in readiness, such as side rails and a padded tongue blade.

Serum electrolytes may be altered with the onset of acidosis. Other useful determinations are acid phosphatase, an enzyme produced by the prostate. In 75 per cent of patients with prostatic cancer extending beyond the prostatic capsule, acid phosphatase is elevated. Alkaline phosphatase may be elevated with spread of cancer to the bones, although other disorders may cause a rise in this value.

Blood calcium, phosphorus, and uric acid studies may be ordered to evaluate metabolic causes for certain types of urinary calculi (stones).

## Renal Function Studies

Renal function studies are used to evaluate damage to the kidney. In general, these tests require that the patient be well hydrated and that specimens be obtained on time, in clean containers which are carefully labeled. A close working relationship between the nurse and laboratory personnel who may draw blood specimens is essential so that timing is accurate and repetition of the tests is avoided.

**Concentration and Dilution Tests.** Specific gravity shows the concentration of particles, such as electrolytes, in water. The specific gravity of distilled water is 1.000. Normally, the specific gravity of urine is responsive to the water and electrolyte situation in the body. On a hot day a person who is perspiring profusely and taking little fluid will have urine with a high specific gravity. Much of the water passing into the glomerular filtrate will be reabsorbed in the tubule. Conversely, a person who has a high fluid intake and who is not losing excessive water from perspiration, diarrhea, or vomiting will have copious urine with a low specific gravity.

When the kidneys are damaged, this ability to concentrate or produce dilute urine is impaired: the specific gravity remains relatively constant, no matter what the water needs of the body are or how much the patient drinks. It is often fixed between 1.010 and 1.015. To test for the capacity to adjust the specific gravity of urine, the patient may be dehydrated by restricting fluids, and a specimen taken; then he is well hydrated by giving him a large amount to drink in a short time, and another specimen is taken. The specific gravity of each specimen is tested.

**Urea Clearance Test.** The ability of the kidneys

to remove various substances from the plasma is termed plasma clearance. The clearance of various substances as a measure of kidney function can be determined by analyzing the concentrations of substances simultaneously in plasma and urine. Normal urea clearance is 60 to 90 ml. of plasma per minute. A value below 60 ml. indicates decreased renal function. A fasting blood specimen is taken, and the patient voids. The patient drinks several glasses of water and, one hour later, voids again. The exact time between the two urine specimens is recorded on the label of the second specimen. The urea contents of blood and urine are compared. Urine flow per minute is calculated on the basis of the volume of the second specimen and the time between specimens. In some kidney diseases an elevated urea level in blood and a decreased urea level in urine are expected.

**Creatinine Clearance.** Creatinine is a breakdown product of muscle metabolism. It is excreted by glomerular filtration and by the tubules, so the value is slightly greater than the true glomerular filtration rate. Since creatinine excretion is not particularly influenced by diet or hydration, sources of error are few if specimen collection and laboratory technique are adequate. Normal creatinine clearance is between 130 and 140 ml. per minute.

**Phenolsulfonphthalein (PSP) Test.** Phenolsulfonphthalein (PSP) is a red dye that the kidneys excrete after IV injection. The amount of dye excreted by the patient is compared with that excreted by a person with normal kidney function. In renal disease, particularly when the tubules are involved, there is a delay in excretion.

The procedure varies slightly from hospital to hospital. It is important that the directions be followed exactly. A few drops of urine lost or a specimen collected four minutes late may mean that test results are inaccurate, with resultant misleading diagnostic data. These are the steps, as followed in one hospital:

1. The procedure is explained to the patient.
2. The patient drinks about 400 ml. of water.
3. Twenty minutes later the patient voids. This urine is discarded.
4. The physician injects exactly 1 ml. (6 mg.) of PSP intravenously. The time of the injection is recorded.
5. A series of specimens is collected at these intervals after the injection: fifteen minutes; thirty minutes; one hour; two hours. The patient must void as fully as he can for each specimen.

The bottles are labeled with the exact time of voiding. The time of the injection is included on the label of the first bottle. Normally 15 to 35 per cent of the dye injected appears in the first specimen, and 80 per cent by the last specimen. If all the urine is not collected, or if the bottles are not labeled accurately, the test results will be inaccurate. If the patient is unable to void at the stated times, catheterization may be ordered or a catheter may be inserted for the duration of the study. Patients who are not acutely ill and who are able to assume responsibility for the procedure may be provided with a watch, labeled specimen bottles, and written instructions, and asked to collect their own specimens. PSP dye becomes colorless in acid urine and red only if the urine is alkaline. The patient should be forewarned that a red color to his urine during the test does not indicate that he is bleeding.

**Intravenous Pyelogram (IVP).** This x-ray study is based on the ability of the kidneys to excrete a radiopaque contrast medium, such as Conray, in the urine. Injected intravenously, the contrast medium reveals the outlines of the kidney pelvis, the ureters, and the bladder on x-ray film as it moves along the urinary tract.

These media contain iodine, to which the patient may be allergic. Reactions of a mild allergic nature, such as hives, are rather common. Serious reactions, such as angioedema and vascular collapse, are infrequent. However, the physician cannot detect potential allergic reactions because skin testing for allergy to these substances is unreliable and ocular testing is dangerous. If there is a history of allergy, he may inject a minute amount of medium intravenously and observe the patient for five or ten minutes.

Whenever these dyes are used, the nurse carefully observes the patient's response and promptly reports to the physician any untoward effect, such as increasing anxiety, restlessness, wheezing, tachycardia, or signs of cardiovascular collapse. Oxygen, antihistamines, epinephrine (Adrenalin), steroids, and vasoconstrictor agents such as metaraminol (Aramine), as well as resuscitation equipment should be readily available in the department where the test is done, such as the x-ray or the cystoscopy room, as well as on the ward to which the patient is returned.

If the patient is undergoing an extensive diagnostic workup, barium studies of the gastrointestinal tract are delayed until urologic studies are completed. It may take several days for barium to be removed from the gastrointestinal tract and its presence in the gastrointestinal tract can distort IVP findings. Orders before the procedure usually include nothing by mouth for 12 hours before the pyelogram is scheduled. This fasting dehydrates the patient so that the urine (and therefore the contrast medium) will be at maximum concentration.

Cleansing the bowel is necessary so that its contents do not interfere with visualization of the kidneys. Usually, a cathartic is ordered the evening before the test and a rectal suppository or enema may be ordered early on the morning of the pyelogram. Because poor cleansing of the bowel may require that the test be repeated, it is a nursing responsibility to check that the bowel preparation has been effective, even if given by someone else. The thoroughness of the bowel cleansing is tiring, especially to older or debilitated patients. After the cathartic has been given, the patient's call bell is kept near him so that he may ask for assistance if he needs it. The bedpan is kept close by and a night light kept on to guide him to the bathroom if he is ambulatory.

Some patients have other conditions that make the usual preparation inadvisable. For example, in diverticulitis there is the danger of intestinal perforation, and therefore the bowel-cleansing procedure must be modified.

On the day of the test, a plain x-ray film (KUB —kidneys, ureter, bladder) is taken of the abdomen. This film will show the presence of any radiopaque stones in the urinary tract, and it can be used as a control when it is compared with the subsequent x-ray films. The contrast medium is injected intravenously. The patient may experience a salty bitter or metallic taste, flushing of the face, a surge of warmth and nausea. These sensations should pass away in a few moments. The patient is instructed to breathe deeply and slowly. He is observed for signs of allergic response. He should be made comfortable while he waits in the x-ray department. Postinjection films are taken at 7-, 15-, and 25-minute intervals. They not only reveal abnormalities of the outline of the urinary tract, but also indicate the level of kidney functioning as they excrete the dye. A postvoiding film may be ordered to estimate the efficiency of bladder emptying. The pyelogram is monitored by the physician who then may order subsequent films to visualize a kidney with delayed function, such as in hydronephrosis. After the test, the patient is encouraged to rest and to take fluids liberally to overcome any dehydration and to flush any remaining dye from the urinary tract. Films may be taken as long as 24 hours later, to obtain additional information.

**Nephrotomogram.** This is a variation of intravenous pyelogram. A larger dosage of contrast medium is used in combination with body section radiography (laminography). The latter technique utilizes "cuts" wherein only a certain plane of the body is in focus, many cuts being taken at various levels. The aim is to better delineate the nature of a mass lesion of the kidney, primarily to differentiate a malignant tumor from a benign cyst. The preparation and observation of the patient is the same as for intravenous pyelography.

**Cystourethrography.** For this x-ray study, contrast material is instilled into the bladder through a urethral catheter. Following an initial plain film, the physician fills the bladder by gravity with an Asepto syringe held 15 cm. above the bladder neck (intra-abdominal resting pressure) and a film is exposed. The bladder is filled further and a picture taken while the patient is voiding and another after it is empty. The cystogram may outline filling defects, such as tumors within the cavity, or delineate a smooth or trabeculated bladder wall, diverticula, or other abnormality. The urethra will be outlined on the voiding film. Particularly in children, the physician will note whether or not there is reflux of material up into the ureters and kidneys and under what pressures it may occur. This vesicoureteral reflux is abnormal and, if not corrected surgically, results in permanent and severe damage to the urinary tract.

**Arteriography.** Renal arteriograms are used to evaluate blood vessels to the kidneys and delineate the nature of mass lesions. For example, cancer of the kidney often takes on a characteristic vascular blush, whereas a benign cyst will be an empty avascular area.

Accurate information as to the location and number of renal arteries can be obtained, especially since multiple vessels to the kidney are not unusual. The commonly used method is the percutaneous catheter technique. A catheter is passed up the femoral artery into the aorta to the level of the renal vessels. At this point, contrast material is injected directly to produce an aortogram, or the

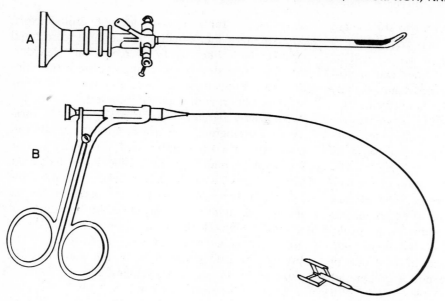

**Figure 48-5.** (A) A cystoscope. (B) A ureteral dilator. Opening and closing of the dilating end are controlled by the handle.

catheter may be manipulated into separate arteries individually.

After the examination, a pressure dressing is applied to the femoral area for four hours and the pulses in the legs and feet are palpated for signs of interference with the circulation. The femoral area is observed for bleeding. Because of these considerations, arteriography is best done as an inpatient hospital procedure. Preparation is the same as for pyelography.

**Ultrasonography.** The application of ultrasonics in urology is rapidly becoming a practical reality. This risk-free study is a measurement of sound echo patterns from various parts of the body using high frequency sound waves close to the wavelength of light. The echo pattern thus obtained is recorded on film using an electronic scanner. The experienced interpreter can outline the size of a lesion and determine whether it is solid or cystic. The technique is particularly useful and complementary to other radiographic procedures in evaluating mass lesions of the kidney.

## Cystoscopy and Retrograde Pyelography

Cystoscopy is the visual examination of the inside of the bladder, by the urologist, using a metal instrument known as a cystoscope (Fig. 48-5). It consists of a sheath with a light source at its tip, either an incandescent bulb or a fiberoptic bundle. A telescope containing numerous prisms, an objective, and an ocular lens, is inserted into the sheath for visualization. The cystoscope enables the examiner to see the interior of the bladder clearly magnified. Inflow and outflow valves allow for irrigation. The valve mechanism permits the bladder to be filled with clear sterile solution, which is retained in the bladder until it is released through the outflow tap. The size of the cystoscope is graded in the French (F.) scale; usually, 20 to 24 F. is used in adults.

Cystoscopy may be done for the following three purposes:

- Inspection. Prostate, urethra, bladder (dilated with transparent fluid), and ureteral orifices can be seen. Cystoscopy usually is done in instances of bleeding of the urinary tract, since the bleeding may be a symptom of cancer. A catheter may be threaded into each ureter to gather separate specimens of urine from each kidney to indicate which one is affected by pus, cancer cells, tubercle bacilli, or other evidence of disease. A contrast medium (about 3 to 5 ml.) can be injected into the catheters to outline the upper urinary tract and a retrograde pyelogram is thus obtained. An alternate method is the use of specially designed catheters with widened tips. These tips are inserted much like a cork into the ureteral orifice, and the entire ureter and renal pelvis are filled. Although historically antedating intravenous methods, retrograde pyelograms are usually ordered only when visualization by intravenous pyelography has been inadequate or when a history of serious allergy to the intravenous media is obtained.
- Biopsy. Specimens of tissue may be taken from the bladder or urethra through the cystoscope.
- Treatment. Tumors of the urethra or bladder can be treated by electrosurgery (fulguration). Electrodes

are passed through the cystoscope tube. Small stones and other foreign bodies can be removed through the cystoscope. Sometimes, larger stones are crushed and then removed. Stenosed ureteral orifices can be incised, ureters dilated, the kidney pelves drained and irrigated, and radon seeds implanted.

## Nursing Intervention

Nursing care before and during cystoscopy can lessen the patient's discomfort and embarrassment and contribute to the success of the examination. The procedure must be explained to him, including what he will actually experience, in accordance with his level of understanding as well as his level of anxiety.

Cystoscopy can be very frightening to the patient. The more tense he becomes, the more chance there is of increased pain due to spasm of the vesical sphincters.

When the cystoscope passes the internal sphincter at the bladder neck and the bladder is filled, the patient will feel the urge to void.

The nurse can help the patient by explaining what is happening, by encouraging him throughout the procedure, and by helping him to relax his abdominal muscles. Because the physician must concentrate on the procedure, it is essential that a nurse place her major attention on assisting the patient. In some instances, one nurse can perform both the functions of assisting the urologist and of comforting the patient. If this is not possible, it is desirable to have two nurses present, especially if the patient is awake throughout the examination.

Additional preparation includes encouraging fluid intake so that adequate urine will be in the ureters for specimens. The patient should drink at least 400 ml. about one hour before the examination, or fluids may be given intravenously, if general anesthesia is to be used. Usually, food is withheld because the discomfort of the procedure may cause nausea. If x-ray films are to be taken during cystoscopy, the bowel is cleansed as for an intravenous pyelogram to remove gas and stool, which may throw confusing shadows on the x-ray film. A sedative and a narcotic may be given before cystoscopy. Signed permission must be obtained for this procedure. The examination can be performed without anesthesia or with local, spinal, or general anesthesia.

The patient is placed on the examination table in the lithotomy position. A sandbag or firm pillow may be placed under his buttocks to raise them about 4 inches. The stirrups should be padded for the patient's comfort and to decrease pressure on the common peroneal nerves and on blood vessels behind the knees. At best this is an uncomfortable position, especially so for an older patient or one with arthritis, for example. When an interval in the examination allows for it, the nurse should remove the patient's feet from the stirrups and flex and extend the legs.

With the patient in position, the external genitalia are cleansed with surgical soap and water and then with an antiseptic solution. A woman may be given an antiseptic douche. Procaine may be instilled into the urethra and bladder for local anesthesia. Legs and lower abdomen are then covered with sterile drapes, leaving the genitalia exposed. Strict aseptic technique is maintained throughout the examination, since the grave danger of infection exists whenever anything foreign is introduced into the urinary tract. Antibiotics may be given prophylactically.

## Procedure

Before the instrument is inserted, the urologist hands one end of the light cord to the assistant who attaches it to the power source. The other end is connected to the rotating electrical contact attached to the instrument and the lamp and intensity of illumination are tested. The well-lubricated sheath with an obturator in it is inserted through the urethra into the bladder and urine is evacuated. The obturator is removed, the telescope is then inserted, and the bladder filled with warm irrigating solution, and observations begun.

The examiner estimates the size of the bladder and evenness of expansion. He will inspect the bladder wall for signs of inflammation, neoplasia, and changes (trabeculation, cellules, and diverticula) seen with such conditions as obstruction at the bladder neck.

A blockage to the bladder outlet causes characteristic changes. Because of the increased resistance resulting from the impediment to flow, the three-layered smooth muscle of the bladder (detrusor) becomes thickened and hypertrophied. The intervening areas of the bladder with less muscle become pitted and the wall assumes a honeycombed or trabeculated appearance. When the pits deepen, they are identified as cellules. When the cellules bulge beyond the general contour of the bladder, they are known as diverticula.

During cystoscopy, the size, shape, and location of the ureteral orifices and the nature of urinary outflow from either kidney are observed. To test kidney function the examiner may observe the length of time until intravenously injected colored materials, such as indigo carmine, are excreted from either ureteral orifice. A biopsy of a suspicious lesion may be taken, ureteral catheterization or a retrograde pyelogram performed, or cultures taken.

If ureteral catheterization is performed, for easy differentiation, the catheter going into the right kidney is sometimes a different color, has different markings, or its end is cut at a different angle from the catheter going into the left kidney. Urine specimens from the kidney pelvis may also be examined for their urea content, and for blood or pus, or for cancer cells.

Ureteral catheters may be left in place after the cystoscope is removed, especially before surgery in this region, to aid in identifying the ureters, thus preventing cutting of them.

The cystoscope is constructed to visualize the interior of a sphere, such as the urinary bladder. To view a tubular structure, such as the urethra, the urologist uses a similar but straight tubular instrument, the panendoscope. The latter is more suitable for examining the prostate gland (see Chap. 53). This endoscopy may be performed prior to or subsequent to cystoscopy. At the conclusion of cystoscopy the sequence is reversed. The bladder is emptied, the telescope is removed, and the obturator is inserted, following which the intact instrument is removed.

## Postcystoscopy Care

When the examination is over, the patient's external genitalia are cleansed and he is helped to descend from the lithotomy position slowly. He is observed for dizziness and permitted to rest for a few minutes before proceeding back to his hospital room (via wheelchair or stretcher) or before getting dressed, if he is an outpatient.

The decision whether to perform these examinations on an ambulatory or inpatient basis and the type of anesthesia to be used will depend on an individual assessment of the patient, including emotional as well as physical considerations. Outpatients should rest for a half-hour before going home, and they should not travel unaccompanied. Not only has the patient just been through an uncomfortable procedure, but he may have had sedation. He should

not plan to drive a car. Patients who have had spinal anesthesia are hospitalized at least overnight, and they are kept flat in bed for six hours or more after the procedure.

Fluids should be encouraged liberally to dilute the urine and to lessen irritation of the lining of the urinary tract. The patient should be told that voiding will be painful for about a day. Mild hematuria is not unusual. Discoloration of the urine may be expected if dyes were used. Analgesics, several warm sitz baths, and explaining beforehand what to expect are ways that the patient's discomfort can be alleviated.

Underlying pathology may be aggravated by the instrumentation. For example, significant prostatic obstruction may culminate in complete urinary retention. If there is precedent urinary infection, instrumentation may be followed by chills, fever, and possibly serious septicemia. The patient is observed for these symptoms and they are promptly reported to the physician, who may order antibiotics. There may have been damage to the walls of the tract, even perforation (anuria and sharp abdominal pain often accompany perforation).

Ureteral colic occasionally occurs and may be treated with atropine or related drugs. Many patients have a dull ache caused by distention of the renal pelvis with dye. The pain may be relieved by a hot bath or codeine. Outpatients should be instructed to contact the urologist promptly if there is frank bleeding, anuria, pain, or fever.

## Technical Considerations

Since electrical currents are involved for fulguration, the irrigating solutions must be of a nonelectrolyte nature (sterile distilled water); otherwise, currents will be dispersed throughout the bladder and rendered ineffectual. Also, electricity is involved for light source connections and x-ray films. Consequently, if a general anesthetic is administered, only nonexplosive agents are used. All electrical equipment must be adequately grounded.

The cystoscope is delicate in construction, but will last indefinitely if given proper care and gentle handling. Cystoscopic equipment is *never* sterilized by boiling or autoclaving. Gas sterilization is a lengthy but safe method. If technicians care for equipment or assist in the cystoscopy room, the nurse instructs and supervises them in aseptic techniques and the care of delicate instruments.

## GENERAL NURSING CARE OF THE UROLOGIC PATIENT

Nursing care common to many urologic patients is considered in this section. For special points of nursing care, the learner should refer to the specific disease entities (for example, observation for stones is discussed under "Calculi"; for care of the patient in renal failure, see Chapter 64).

### Assessment

In order to plan nursing care, the patient is questioned about his urinary pattern and habits, aids to elimination, or urinary diversion. In the nursing history particular note is made regarding frequency, dribbling (retention with overflow), dysuria, polyuria, oliguria, urgency, hesitation, nocturia, hematuria, pyuria, urethral discharge, or incontinence. Significant information for planning nursing care may be obtained from the female patient's menstrual and obstetric history and the male patient's history of testicular pain or swelling. Further pertinent aspects of the urologic patient's history may include sexual problems, stone formation, and venereal disease.

A distended bladder is manifested by swelling of the abdomen, and a tense highly sensitive area determined by palpation. Percussion over the swollen area may yield a "kettledrum" sound.

The urine should be observed for amount, color, odor, degree of opacity, sediment, mucus, clots, shreds of material, or other unusual constituents. If the patient has an indwelling catheter the specimen for examination is collected from the catheter, not from the drainage container.

Because the function of the urinary tract is the elimination of metabolic products and electrolytes, and because it uses water as the vehicle for the movement of these substances, the nurse, in observing any patient with a disorder of the urinary tract, is constantly alert for symptoms of electrolyte and water imbalance. For instance, in greeting the patient in the morning she looks at his lips to see if they are dry. While she bathes him, she inspects his skin. Is it edematous or dehydrated? Does the pressure of a finger leave a mark in the skin, indicating pitting edema? Edema may first become obvious as puffiness around the eyes (periorbital edema). With dependent edema, the sacral area, lower extremities, or hands would swell if they remained in a dependent position. Patients who have had swollen ankles when they were ambulatory may be pleased to discover that the condition disappears once they are on bed rest, not realizing that now their buttocks are edematous.

Laboratory reports should be reviewed as they are received. They give clues to the progress of the patient's illness and the symptoms to observe.

For example, if calcium is low, the patient is observed for signs of tetany, and ampules of calcium gluconate or calcium chloride are kept available. If the calcium level is so low that the patient has had convulsions or is in such danger, side rails are padded and kept up and a padded tongue blade is taped to the head of his bed. High or low potassium levels are a cue that the nurse must be especially alert to the rate, quality, and regularity of the patient's pulse. Whenever there is edema, the patient usually is weighed every day to keep track of possible loss or gain of fluids. The lungs are auscultated for rales. Intake and output are also measured.

Anemia and other blood changes may lead to a hemorrhagic disorder. The stool is observed for unusual blackness, which may indicate the presence of old blood from gastrointestinal hemorrhage, and bleeding from other sites is reported promptly. The daily amount of urine is an important indication of the adequacy of renal function. Less than 500 ml. a day when the intake has been adequate means that there is serious trouble in the urinary tract that should be promptly discussed with the physician, as should a wide discrepancy between intake and output. The total intake and output for the 24- or 8-hour period should be checked to see whether the figures are approximately equal. Here is an example of one patient's intake and output:

| | MONDAY | TUESDAY | WEDNESDAY | THURSDAY |
|---|---|---|---|---|
| Intake | 950 ml. | 1,300 ml. | 1,670 ml. | 1,950 ml. |
| Output | 840 ml. | 6,680 ml. | 3,640 ml. | 1,730 ml. |

In this hypothetic example, note that on Monday and Tuesday the patient was on restricted intake. On Tuesday diuresis occurred, and it continued to a lesser extent into Wednesday. As the output improved, the patient was allowed more to drink. By Thursday the relationship between intake and output was more normal. When insensible loss (perspiration, breathing) is taken into account, output approximates intake.

When the BUN is extraordinarily high, and when

there is cerebral edema, the patient may become disoriented, apathetic, stuporous, or completely comatose. A patient who spoke sensibly one day and by the next is confused or drowsy is exhibiting a symptom of progressive pathology. Conversely, a patient who has been unaware of his surroundings and who becomes alert shows an important step toward recovery. Such observations should be discussed with the physician. When cerebral edema is present or imminent, ampules of hypertonic intravenous solutions are kept readily available.

Blood pressure is another index. The patient's usual blood pressure, if he knows what it usually is, and what it was on admission, should be recorded. These will give a standard against which to judge pressure readings. Blood pressure usually is taken every four hours on patients with nephritis, all those with active kidney pathology, and those with uremia. If the blood pressure is not stable, it is taken more frequently. If the patient seems sluggish or complains of headache, the blood pressure should be taken even more often. A progressive rise should be called to the physician's attention. A danger of hypertension is cerebral vascular accident.

Any patient with a disorder of the urinary tract can develop renal failure. The earlier renal failure is recognized, the earlier treatment can start, before there is severe damage to electrolyte regulation. The nurse remains alert for any symptoms that may indicate early or advanced renal failure (see Chap. 64).

## Fluids

Each day, the specific fluid-intake goal for each patient should be known. As a general rule, fluids are encouraged to keep the urine dilute. Dilute urine does not crystallize and form calculi as easily as does concentrated urine; in cystitis it burns less on urination; it rids the kidney quickly of noxious substances; and it washes away products of inflammation. However, there are important exceptions to this general rule. Fluids may be limited (often to 600 to 800 ml.) when there is edema, and also when there is kidney failure. If the patient's body is unable to rid itself of water efficiently, damage results from adding more to it.

When fluids are to be encouraged (often to 3,500 to 4,000 ml.), frequent, small offerings may be more palatable than large quantities which are presented less often. This is especially true for geriatric patients.

Often, the patient himself takes responsibility for his intake. It is better for the patient to help himself as much as he can, because he will feel less helpless. The nurse ascertains that the patient understands how much he should drink, how to keep track of the amount, and why the fluids are important. The nurse indicates continued interest in the patient's fluid balance even though he takes his own fluids.

The fluids may include fresh, iced water, certain fruit juices, Jello, Kool-Aid, Seven-Up, ginger ale, cola, tea, or eggnog served at intervals during the day. When it is important to limit potassium intake, certain fruit juices, tea, coffee, and chocolate beverages, all of which have a high potassium content, are limited or omitted. Juices high in potassium include grapefruit, orange, prune, tangerine, and tomato. Juices which can be included on a 1,500-mg. potassium-restricted diet include apple, cranberry, pear, peach, and pineapple (Robinson, 1970). Auxiliary personnel who may be serving fluids must be made aware of which patients have these restrictions. Overhydration (edema, wet breathing sounds) must be assessed in all patients for whom fluids are encouraged, especially those who are aged and those with potential heart or renal failure.

Because of the combination of a large intake of fluids with the symptom of frequency, the bedpan or the urinal must be kept within easy reach, especially with an older patient for whom climbing in and out of bed may be tiring and dangerous.

When fluids are restricted, the patient should understand the reason. It is unfortunate that a patient may feel psychologically denied when his condition requires that he be restricted in intake; his feelings should be respected and his expressions of hurt or anger encouraged.

Thirst is a greater problem in hot than in cool weather. Fluid intake should be spaced throughout the day, by the instructed patient. Usually one quarter of the total is given at night. Sucking on hard candy or ice may help (however, ice must be included in the total fluid intake). Mouth care can be carried out with a pleasant-tasting solution. Thirst increases as renal ability to concentrate urine decreases.

Records of intake and output should be scrupulously accurate, otherwise treatment will be based on incorrect data. Every person working with the patient should understand and agree to the method of keeping records and the amount of fluid that containers hold. If an aide believes that a glass holds 240 ml. and the nurse believes it holds 200 ml., erroneous figures will be recorded. Each source of output should be recorded separately and then totaled.

For example:

| | |
|---|---|
| Vomitus | 230 ml. |
| Cystostomy tube | 560 ml. |
| Foley catheter | 520 ml. |
| Total | 1,310 ml. |

Sodium intake is severely restricted in patients with edema. Salt substitutes containing potassium should not be used without the physician's approval. Rum, vinegar, mint, or cloves for flavoring probably will be allowed.

### Preventing Infection

Every time the patient is approached by a nurse with a catheter or an irrigating set in hand there is danger of introducing microorganisms into the urinary tract. Sterile technique must always be observed. If the catheter touches the bedclothes, for example, it must not be used. A second sterile catheter must be obtained.

### Comfort

Common causes of discomfort in the urologic patient and measures to relieve them include:

- Itching. Pruritus can occur with or without uremic frost. The physician may order an anesthetic ointment to relieve the itching. Cleanliness helps, too; perhaps this patient can have two baths instead of one a day. Although the skin is not efficient for the disposal of such waste chemicals as uric acid, it is all that the body has available when the kidneys are not functioning, and a clean skin is always more efficient and more comfortable.
- Other skin problems. Cream or lotion should be used on dry skin, not alcohol. Sheets under swollen buttocks must be taut and free from wrinkles or piercing crumbs. The patient's position must be changed frequently. Even lying on the strings of his gown can make a deep crease in the edematous back.
- Odor. Unless urine comes from a necrotic area, as in cancer, or it is infected, it is almost odorless as it leaves the body. The characteristic odor of urine is caused by ammonia, which is formed from urea by bacterial action. The more stale the urine becomes, the more malodorous. It has been said that the quality of the nursing on a urologic ward can be judged by sniffing the air. In instances of infection and necrotic tissue, odor can be combated by improved air circulation, the use of sprays, and, most important, promptly cleaning the patient as he needs it.

- Dryness of mouth. Mineral oil can be used (a touch of lemon juice with it helps). Only the smallest amount should be used on the applicator, especially in the comatose patient, since aspiration is a danger. Commercially prepared glycerine-lemon swabs are convenient. Caked blood and crusts can be removed with a mixture of hydrogen peroxide and water.
- Pain. Sitz baths, if not contraindicated, ease the discomfort of an inflamed urethra. A hot-water bottle (with the physician's order if necessary) may reduce the flank ache that sometimes accompanies disease of the kidney parenchyma or pelvis. The burning caused by cystitis is reduced by forcing fluids, thus diluting the urine.
- Long-term bed rest. A consistently quiet position leads to, among other hazards, urinary stasis, muscle deconditioning, potassium imbalance, and infection. Active or passive range-of-motion exercises should be done regularly and the gatch level of the patient's bed changed frequently. Boredom is often a problem for patients on long-term bed rest. Diversion that will interest but not strain provides relief.

  The chronicity of his illness may be very discouraging and anger provoking. Irritability may be caused by worries over hospital bills, his inability to work, over his disease—probably all. The hospital social worker may be able to help with problem solving regarding financial matters.
- Embarrassment and fear. The nurse's matter-of-fact attitude and care in not exposing the urologic patient unduly will help him to accept necessary treatments. Catheterization of male patients usually is performed by the male nurse or physician.

  A man may fear, with justification, that impotence will follow surgery. Although the patient will probably be hesitant in discussing this thought with a female nurse, the urologic nurse understands that patients do have questions regarding sexual function and can convey this information to the patient. Questions which the nurse cannot answer can be discussed with the physician or other counselor, or the information can be obtained from other appropriate sources. The nurse should encourage or assist the patient to verbalize his concerns and questions to the person who can best help him rather than doing the patient's questioning for him.

  Patients may also fear cancer and need the opportunity to talk about this.
- Appearance. The patient with generalized edema may feel self-conscious about his appearance. The edema of nephrosis gives a bloated look that, in the extreme, is startling.

### Preoperative Care

The time spent waiting for surgery can be full of anxiety, especially if the operation that is planned is mutilating or changes normal elimination patterns. The nurse should be aware of the surgeon's explanation and afford opportunities for the patient to ask questions and to talk about his adjustment to the necessary changes in his way of life, such as a different manner of voiding. For instance, other patients who have successfully lived with ureteral transplants might share their experience with the preoperative patient. However, no matter how well-informed the patient is, there will always be a question in his mind as to how he will be able to get along.

If a perineal approach is taken to any urologic surgery, the areas around the genitalia and the anus must be shaved. These are difficult areas to shave thoroughly. A good light and a sharp razor must always be used.

### Postoperative Care

**Wounds.** The three usual surgical approaches to the urinary tract are: (1) a flank incision just under the diaphragm to reach the ureter and the kidney on that side, (2) an incision in the lower abdomen above the symphysis pubis to reach the bladder, and (3) a perineal incision. Some procedures are done through the urethra. A transthoracic approach may be used for nephrectomy (excision of the kidney).

**Drains.** A tissue drain such as a Penrose drain, may be used to carry off serous fluid that accumulates when surgery results in creation of a gaping space, such as after nephrectomy. No urine will drain.

When drainage is expected from a wound, but the surgeon does not wish the dressing to be disturbed frequently, he incorporates the drain in the dressing. If the wound is infected, this drain may enter the wound superficially. Sometimes it lies near the incision line. A catheter drain is sometimes used to instill an antibiotic solution or to keep the dressing wet. Some catheters inserted into wounds are sutured in place; others should be firmly taped.

After a catheter is removed from a wound, the surgical fistula usually closes rapidly, so rapidly that if the catheter should inadvertently slip out of the wound, it may not be possible to replace it after a half-hour has elapsed; should this happen, the surgeon is notified immediately. After a catheter is removed, the site must be observed. There may be drainage from it for a short time, but it should gradually stop.

### Prevention of Complications

A flank incision is so close to the thoracic cavity that it is painful for the patient to cough and to breathe deeply. Yet he must do this to help prevent hypostatic pneumonia and other postoperative complications. Medications for pain are given as ordered and needed. When the patient gets some pain relief following medication, he can be assisted to deep-breathe and cough, while the wound site is splinted with the nurse's hands.

No drainage tube should be compressed by the patient's lying on it. Tubing must be checked each time the patient is turned.

After kidney surgery, patients may develop gastrointestinal discomfort, such as distention, due to pressure on the abdominal organs during the operation. A nasogastric tube attached to continuous suction may be used, and fluids may be given intravenously until the patient can take them by mouth.

**Hemorrhage.** The two periods when the patient is in greatest danger from hemorrhage are immediately postoperatively, and the eighth to tenth days after surgery (especially after fulguration procedures), when tissue sloughing may occur. Ambulatory patients may be returned to bed rest for these three days. Hemorrhage should be checked for vigilantly. With the patient lying on his back or his side, blood may seep under him and not appear on the top of the dressing. Because of its position, this is especially true of a flank incision. Observation for hemorrhage includes checking manually beneath the patient for dampness. The mattress should be depressed at the point of the dressing so that stains can be noted. When a draining catheter has been left in place postoperatively, it will be easier to detect bleeding if the drainage apparatus is changed every two hours. Small bottles or large test tubes can be used. These are easier to handle and it is easier to remember to change them. The time interval must be stated on the label. The bottles can be lined up with a light source, such as the window, behind them, and their colors can be compared. Normally, there is a progressive lightening from dark red to pink. If the urine remains the same color or turns brighter red, the physician should be notified. After 48 hours, the pink should give way to amber or, if the kidneys are working well and hydration is good, to yellow.

### Urinary Catheters

In addition to the urethral Foley catheter placed in the bladder after surgery to drain urine, there may also be a retention catheter in the kidney pelvis, a ureteral catheter, or one for drainage through a suprapubic wound leading to the bladder (see Figs. 48-6 to 48-8). The objective is to divert the flow of urine from above the operative site while the tissues heal. If the ureter is repaired just below its insertion into the kidney pelvis, the pelvis itself might be drained. A ureteral catheter used solely for splinting might be left in place after a plastic repair of the ureter. It is removed two to three weeks postoperatively.

A catheter that accidentally becomes dislodged from the patient should never be reinserted. It should be replaced with a sterile one, and depending on its location, it may be reinserted by the surgeon. Catheters positioned deep into the ureter or kidney pelvis through a flank incision can, at times, be replaced only by reopening the wound.

**Ureteral Catheters.** Ureteral catheters are small in diameter and are irrigated by using gravity, not plunger-pressure. A special ureteral syringe and adaptor or, a syringe and blunt needle, are used.

| Size of ureteral catheter: | 5 | 6 | 7 | 8 | 9 | 10 |
|---|---|---|---|---|---|---|
| Size of needle: | | 21 | 19 | 18 | 17 | 16 | 15 |

Ureteral catheters may become obstructed easily if there is purulent or bloody urine. For irrigation, no more than 5 ml. of sterile normal saline is instilled by gravity and it is returned by gravity. If patency of the catheter cannot be established by this type of irrigation, the surgeon must be notified.

One way to attach a ureteral catheter to drainage is to punch a small hole with a red-hot needle or pin in the rubber top of a sterile medicine dropper and thread the catheter through it. The medicine dropper is then attached to the glass or plastic connector of the drainage tubing. To prevent ureteral catheters from dislodging, an indwelling bladder catheter may be attached to them. There may be some leakage of urine around the catheters and the patient's skin care is an important nursing consideration. If there is a ureteral catheter in each ureter, they should be labeled "right" and "left" at the distal end. Newly inserted catheters draining from the kidney pelvis or the ureter should be rechecked every half-hour.

**Kidney Pelvis Catheter.** The distal end of the tube that drains the kidney pelvis always should be handled with aseptic precautions, including a sterile drainage container. The distal part of the tube near the opening should be handled with sterile forceps or the sterile gloved hand. The kidney pelvis has

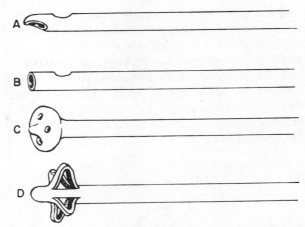

**Figure 48-6.** Some catheter tips: (A) whistle-tip, (B) hole-in-tip, (C) de Pezzer mushroom, (D) Malecot 4-wing.

a capacity of 3 to 5 ml. If a catheter draining it is blocked for a half-hour (clot stuck in the lumen, patient lying on the tube, tube kinked), urine can accumulate, causing strain on the suture line, increase in the patient's pain, and possible kidney damage.

**Urethral (Foley) Catheters.** Urethral catheters, though very useful, are said to be the major single cause of urinary tract infections and our most common nosocomial (hospital-associated infection) disease (Beaumont, 1974). The risk of infection is higher if the catheter is an indwelling one; the longer it is in place, the greater the risk of infection.

Chances of infection can be reduced by viewing each catheterization as a minor surgical procedure and using strict aseptic technique, and by preventing crossinfection by using disposable catheteriza-

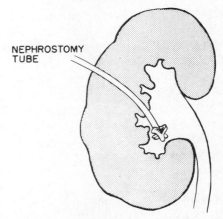

NEPHROSTOMY TUBE

**Figure 48-7.** A nephrostomy tube with a Malecot 4-wing tip draining the kidney pelvis.

tion sets and a closed drainage system (Beaumont). A closed drainage system is characterized by drainage tubing sealed to a drainage container, a bottom drain to maintain one-way flow through the system, and filtered air-vents on the container.

Catheters are measured in the French system. An adult urethra usually takes size 28 to 30 F.; but to avoid pain, size 18 to 20 F. is used for indwelling catheters.

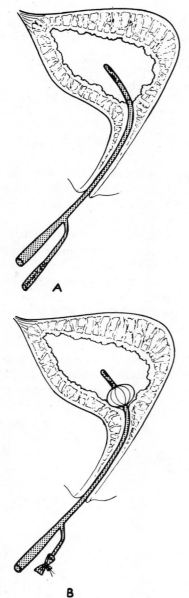

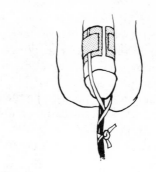

☐ = ADHESIVE TAPE

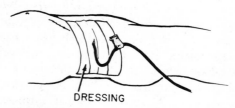

DRESSING

**Figure 48-9.** Indwelling catheters should be anchored securely to prevent pull on them.

Taping a Foley catheter to the leg of the female is done to prevent pull on the inflated balloon which would cause pressure on the bladder outlet (Fig. 48-9). In the male with a long-term indwelling catheter the penis is positioned headward to prevent erosion of the urethra from the pressure of the catheter. This position also minimizes pressure and irritation by increasing the penoscrotal angle. If the patient assumes the prone position the penis is positioned laterally toward the drainage bag.

In both male and female, the catheter exit site as well as the external genitalia must be cleansed regularly, at least once daily, to prevent secretions from accumulating and causing infection.

Infection may make the urine alkaline. The pH of the urine of patients with long-term catheters is tested frequently. A substance such as cranberry juice taken orally acidifies the urine and produces a less favorable climate for bacterial growth.

### General Principles in the Care of the Patients with an Indwelling Urethral Catheter

As soon as the urologic patient with catheters is placed in bed, each urinary catheter is connected to tubing and labeled, and the tubing is inserted in the drainage container. An intake and output record is initiated with a separate column, for each source of urine. Each drainage tube is attached to

**Figure 48-8.** Foley catheter. (A) The catheter is inserted into the bladder. (B) The inflation of the bag prevents the catheter from leaving the bladder. The inner tube that leads to the balloon is tied.

the sheet, using an adhesive tab wrapped around the tube and a pin, or masking tape alone can be used. There should be enough tubing between the anchorage and the patient so that there is no pull on the catheter when the patient turns, but not so much that the tubing will become tangled. Coiling excess tubing horizontally so that the urine does not have to flow uphill should keep it free of kinks. Tubing or a catheter should never be bent at right angles because this would clamp it off. The entire length, from insertion into the patient to the drainage bag, is checked for kinks. The drainage end of the tube must always be kept above the level of the urine. The amount of drainage is recorded at least hourly during the early postoperative period and in critically ill patients. In others it is checked at least every two hours. If urine is appearing from a catheter that should not drain, the surgeon should be notified at once. If no urine appears from a urethral Foley catheter that should drain, the following steps should be taken:

- **The length of the tubing from the patient to the drainage container is checked for kinks, pressure, and other external compression of the tube that may be obstructing the lumen.**
- **The drainage system is disconnected from the catheter and the tubing flushed through with sterile water or saline, keeping the connecting tip sterile. The flushing fluid should not be emptied into the drainage container.**
- **The catheter is "milked" from its exit to its distal end (without pulling it against the patient), feeling for gravel (sediment made of phosphates and other mineral crystals). After "milking," the flushed drainage tubing is reattached and observed for the flow of urine.**
- **The catheter is irrigated, if there is an order or policy for this.**
- **The physician may be consulted, especially if the patient is postoperative, or the catheter may be changed per standing order.**

**Drainage and Irrigation.** Usually, drainage is accomplished by gravity, though occasionally, weak suction may be used. The suction may be exerted through a bubble bottle (underwater suction) to prevent excess pressure from some mechanical difficulty. Suction may be applied to skin transplants of ureters, using a suction cup over the buds. This cup is different from the drainage cup, and the two are not interchangeable. The suction cup has an air vent that must not be occluded. When the end of the catheter is in the kidney pelvis, only gravity drainage is used.

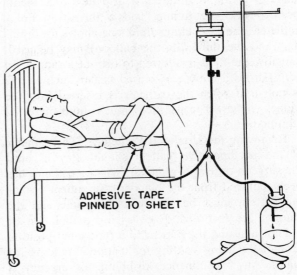

ADHESIVE TAPE PINNED TO SHEET

**Figure 48-10.** Closed irrigation of an indwelling catheter. The tube leading to the drainage bottle is compressed momentarily by hand while the few ml. of sterile fluid go from the bottle into the bladder. A clamp is not applied to this tube.

Catheters may be irrigated with sterile saline or distilled water, when there is an order or policy to do so. Irrigation is done to keep the system of tubing open and not to rinse the cavity being drained. Because every irrigation carries with it the danger of infection, sterile technique always is employed. When fluid goes in and does not return, very gentle suction may be tried *except* in recent postoperative patients and those whose catheters enter the kidney pelvis. If a return flow does not occur after initial suctioning, the tubing should be reattached to the drainage system and observed. If there is no return after an hour, the situation should be discussed with the physician. The amount of irrigation fluid not returned must be subtracted from the total output.

The amount of fluid used is ordered: a common amount for irrigating a urethral catheter is 30 ml. of sterile saline. No more than 5 ml. at a time is used to irrigate a catheter that goes into the kidney pelvis. Whenever a patient complains of pain during an irrigation, it should be momentarily halted. Irrigations should be done slowly and gently.

If irrigation is required frequently, a closed system (Fig. 48-10) may be set up to decrease the chance of infection. Intermittent irrigation can be accomplished by releasing the clamp. When constant irrigation is ordered, a drip device is incorporated into the tubing, and a three-way Foley catheter (one tube admits fluid, one allows for drainage, and the third fills the balloon) may be used. Usually, the fluid is allowed to drip at a rate of 30 to 60 drops a minute. A closed system such as this is not used when the catheter is inserted into the kidney pelvis, because too much fluid may be admitted.

**Removing the Uretheral Catheter.** The catheter of the postoperative patient should stay in until the surgeon orders its removal. When a catheter has been removed from the bladder, the patient's voiding pattern must be observed. The time and the amount are recorded. Encouraging ambulation or at least assisting the patient to a functional position promotes voiding—sitting for females, standing for males. Any incontinence, dribbling, or urgency is noted, and the bladder is palpated and percussed to check for distention. The physician may order the amount of residual urine after voiding to be determined by catheterization. Depending on the amount of residual, the catheter may have to be left in place. To avoid another catheter insertion, a Foley catheter may be used when residual urine is being checked.

Patients who go home with a catheter in place learn to irrigate it and sometimes to change it while they are still in the hospital. At home they may be helped by a community health nurse. Principles of sterile technique are taught to the patient and a family member or associate who will assist. Proper daily cleaning of drainage tubing, containers and leg bags or other devices must be learned also. Policies regarding the changing of indwelling catheters vary. They may be changed every one to three weeks, or once a month if irrigation is done regularly, or if there is odor, sediment, or obstruction. Glass or plastic connectors and tubing are changed at irrigation time. They are washed with warm soapy water and rinsed thoroughly. A weak solution of an acid, such as vinegar, will remove the coating from nondisposable catheters, tubing, or collection containers. The patient should have two drainage systems so that one can be aired and dried after cleansing.

## Rehabilitation after Surgery

The activity prescription, including return to sexual intercourse, depends on the individual pa-

tient, the surgery, and the postoperative course. Generally no heavy lifting is permitted for several weeks. The more specific the directions given the patient regarding return to full activity, the less anxious he is apt to be.

## THE PATIENT WITH URINARY BLADDER INCONTINENCE

Ordinarily, the excretion of urine is controlled by two sphincters: (1) the internal sphincter, which is close to the most dependent part of the bladder, and (2) the external sphincter, which surrounds the urethra at a lower point. As the bladder fills, nerve endings are stimulated, giving rise to the sensation of needing to void.

The anesthetized, unconscious, or senile patient may not receive these stimuli, and in these patients the urinary sphincters relax involuntarily. Also, infection of the urinary system and accidental or surgical damage to either sphincter can cause loss of control. The sphincters may not function adequately when there is local tissue damage, such as in relaxation of the pelvic floor found in some women. Interference with spinal nerves, as occurs in tumors of the spinal cord, tabes dorsalis, herniated disk, postoperative edema of the cord, and cord injuries, can interfere with conduction to the brain of the impulse to void, and result in a neurogenic bladder and incontinence. Many paraplegic patients do not know when they void because they have lost all sensation in the lower parts of their bodies. A neurogenic bladder may be spastic, preventing retention of urine, or it may be flaccid, preventing complete expulsion of urine.

Before the era of antibiotics, half of the patients paralyzed by spinal cord compression were dead within a year, mainly from urinary tract infection (Mullan). Today, the improved mortality statistics are due, in large part, to constant vigilance for signs of urinary stasis and vigorous attention to prevention of infection.

## Nursing Care

Nursing care is directed at keeping the incontinent patient catheter-free and establishing a voiding routine, when possible; when the latter is not possible, ways must be found to protect the integrity of the skin, control odor, prevent infection, and assist the patient to self-care to the extent possible, and to resocialization as he wishes.

Initially, an indwelling catheter to constant drainage may be used to prevent retention of urine and incontinence.

Later, if the bladder reflex is present, a method of bladder training may be instituted. For example, the catheter may be clamped and released every one to two hours. In this time the bladder is given a chance to hold urine and then to empty it, thus beginning to reestablish normal function. Gradually, the interval for releasing the catheter is lengthened to three to four hours, giving the bladder a chance to fill more completely. The patient can be taught to release the clamp on his own catheter at scheduled times. The retention-catheter is changed once a week.

Later the catheter is removed entirely, and the patient is instructed to void every hour. Usually he is not able to retain the urine longer initially and frequent voiding is necessary in order to prevent incontinence.

The voiding reflex can be stimulated by the patient through a number of techniques, with highly individual responses. These include tapping the bladder, stroking the thighs, and pulling the pubic hair. In the Credé technique, urine is expressed by manual pressure over the bladder.

At first many patients void in insufficient quantity, and they must then be catheterized to remove residual urine. A careful record of fluid intake and output is kept. One guideline for indwelling catheter reinsertion is that a spastic bladder should retain no more than 100 ml. and a flaccid bladder no more than 50 ml. Catheterization for residual urine may be done with a Foley catheter, which can be left in place if the residual warrants it. When the catheter is removed, the voiding interval is gradually lengthened to two, three, or four hours.

**Establishing a Schedule.** The incontinent patient and the nurse both study the urination pattern over a period of several days and together set up a schedule, so that voiding is regular and predictable. Such a program takes great patience, continued interest, encouragement of the patient, and strict attention to timing. If it is successful, it gives the patient freedom from constant odor, wetness, and the embarrassment of accidents in public. If a pattern is observed after a time chart has been kept for several days, a bedpan or commode should be available (or the patient should be helped to the bathroom if it is possible, one-half hour before the pattern shows that his bladder will empty. An association with childhood toileting experiences should not be made. This is not the same thing as toilet-training the child, and the patient's dignity should not be affronted. The process takes a great deal of patience, and accidents do happen during the retraining period. The bed should have a full-length waterproof mattress cover. When an accident occurs, linen should be changed promptly, and the patient should be assured that accidents can be expected to occur.

Fluid intake must be spaced in order for the patient to anticipate expulsion of urine. Spacing of fluids involves experimentation. If the patient limits his fluids before going to bed or going out on a social occasion, he must be sure that his intake is adequate at other times of the day. A patient with a neurogenic bladder may not void completely. Because of the danger of infection and stone formation, it is doubly important that he drink sufficient fluids—at least 3,000 ml. a day. This is the most effective means of bladder irrigation.

Until a routine is well established, a record of the time and the amount voided should be kept. Such information can help to determine if there is overflow with retention of residual urine, and it can help the patient to regulate himself. Since such frequent voiding would disturb the patient during the night, external condom drainage such as the Urosheath can be used in the male. This is placed over the penis and the distal end is connected by tubing to a drainage container. Such drainage is also useful for any bedridden incontinent male patient. During ambulation periods, the drainage tubing can be connected to a drainage bag attached by straps to the patient's leg. Condom drainage should be changed daily, and the penis cleansed, retracting the foreskin in an uncircumsized male.

Of necessity, women use a less effective method. During the night, and during the day also if bladder control is not achieved, women can wear a front-opening type of protective panty over any type of absorbent pad. (These pads should not be referred to as "diapers.") A nonabsorbent non-irritating liner worn next to the skin affords some protection, since the urine passes quickly through the liner to the absorbent pad. When the patient becomes able to retain urine longer, the voiding schedule is continued throughout the night.

Male patients usually do not achieve urinary

control as readily as do women, probably because more convenient appliances are available (Fig. 48-11). Each patient should have two urinals, one to wear and the other to wash thoroughly and hang to dry. The man's trousers cover his urinal; no one need know that he uses it. A simple urinal for the ambulatory male with a dribbling problem can be made from a disposable plastic bag that fits over the penis and can be kept in place by taping it or tying it to a gauze belt.

In one way, men are luckier, for there is less likelihood of leakage and the device is more readily concealed. However, in the long run the convenience of the device often becomes a disadvantage, because the patient becomes dependent on the equipment and is not motivated as strongly to achieve control without it.

Some incontinent patients never achieve complete freedom from catheters, others do. Success depends not only on the degree of injury but on the motivation of the patient and the amount of skillful help and encouragement he receives.

Patient and nurse should become accustomed to noting the condition of the urine. Is it cloudy? Malodorous? More concentrated than usual? Changes may indicate infection. If the patient remains incontinent and is confined to bed, his skin must be protected and the bedding arranged so that it stays dry. Condom drainage can be used for the male patient and protective panties or absorbent pads for the female. Pads placed under the patient may be disposable or washable. They should be arranged

in proper order before the patient is disturbed. A neat stack, ready for use, can be kept nearby.

Urea-splitting organisms, among them *Micrococcus ureae*, cause the urea in urine to react with water. An end-product of this reaction is ammonia, which causes both the odor of urine and the skin damage. One way to protect skin is to avoid any contact with urine. When this is not possible, an antiseptic, such as methylbenzethonium chloride (Diaparene Chloride), which kills the ammonia-forming organism in urine, may be used. The antiseptic, in ointment or powder, can be applied to the skin of the incontinent ambulatory or bed patient. Light dusting with an absorbent powder, such as corn starch, also helps to prevent ammonia dermatitis.

If powder, an antiseptic, liners, and protective pads are used, there should be no problem with odor or ammonia dermatitis. These measures should not be a substitute for scrupulous cleanliness and a change of padding as soon as it becomes wet. The buttocks and genital area of the incontinent patient should be washed with soap and water several times a day. Unlike feces, urine is not visible on the skin. To prevent skin from breaking down, the area actually must be free of urine; it is not sufficient that it appears to be clean. To avoid irritation, all soap must be removed from the skin and the skin dried thoroughly. Plastic or rubber sheets should be cleaned with soap and water at least once a day. If an ammonia dermatitis is present, the affected area is kept clean, dry, and exposed to the air. Exposure to an ordinary light bulb for 20 minutes several times a day often helps.

The continuous vigilance and the care required by the incontinent patient who is unable to care for himself may seem tiresome. Having the necessary materials right at hand and a planned routine makes quick work of the changes. The reward is a healthy, unbroken skin and a comfortable patient.

### Home Care

Sometimes the decision as to whether the patient can be cared for at home rests on managing incontinence—an embarrassing condition to the patient, and one the family may find very upsetting. Decisions about whether home care is feasible rest with the family, with the advice and support of physicians and nurses. Often what appears to professionals as a family's unwillingness to care for the

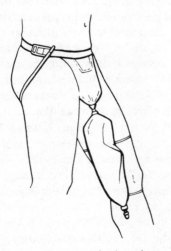

**Figure 48-11.** A leg urinal placed over the penis and held in place with a belt.

patient at home actually is fear and uncertainty about the management of such care. A family can be shown that the ambulatory patient usually can care for himself without odor or fuss, or that the bed patient can be changed quickly, easily, and inexpensively. The community health nurse who finds a convenient way to keep the patient clean and dry, can show members of the family who wish to care for the patient, but are uncertain of their skills, how home care can be carried out.

Rehabilitation of the patient with a neurogenic bladder or with urinary incontinence from other causes is often a long-term, complex nursing problem. For a more detailed treatment of the subject, specialized literature is available (see bibliography).

## URINARY OBSTRUCTIONS

An obstruction can occur anywhere in the urinary tract—from the kidney pelvis to the tip of the urethra. Obstruction may be caused by a tumor, a stone, a cyst, a kink in the ureter, stenosis or spasm of the ureters, or a diverticulum in the bladder wall that distends and blocks one or more of the three openings (two ureteral, one urethral) into the bladder. In older men, an enlarged prostate gland is a common obstructing lesion. Congenital strictures are not infrequent, though they may not be discovered until the patient is an adult.

Common congenital obstructions include strictures of the ureteropelvic (ureter and kidney pelvis) and ureterovesical (ureter and bladder) junctions, contractures at the bladder neck, and ureteroceles. The latter are cystic balloonings of the ureteral orifice that not only may block the ureter, but may be large enough to block the bladder outlet. Both kidneys then can become occluded, with serious consequences.

Acquired obstructions include surgical injuries to the ureters and urethral strictures from traumatic instrumentation. Neurogenic dysfunction of the bladder, which causes urinary stasis, is essentially an obstructive condition.

When urine cannot pass the obstruction freely, it backs up. For example, if there is closure at the orifice that leads from the ureter into the bladder, the ureter will become more and more distended as new urine passes into it from above. The back pressure moves into the kidney pelvis, which also becomes distended. Now the parenchyma of the

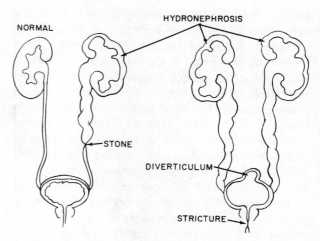

**Figure 48-12.** Hydronephrosis caused by blockage of the urinary tract. Note how dilation occurs above the point of obstruction.

kidney is squeezed between pressure from the expanding pelvis and internal pressure of the glomerulus with its continuous formation of urine. Likewise, the tiny blood vessels supplying kidney tissue are being compressed, a dangerous condition because of the possibility of permanent kidney damage. Waste products accumulate in the bloodstream. When the kidney pelvis is swollen with backflow, the condition is called *hydronephrosis* (Fig. 48-12).

The lower the level in the tract at which the obstruction occurs, the more slowly the kidney pelvis becomes distended with the backflow of urine. The more urine that can squeeze past the narrowed portion of the passageway, the less the backflow, and the slower the distention of the tract proximal to the obstruction. When the obstruction is in the urethra, the bladder distends, and finally diverticula (outpouchings) of the muscular wall form. Urine becomes trapped in these sacs, stagnates, and becomes a culture medium for bacteria. For this reason, infection accompanies obstruction. The infection may be blood-borne, such as that caused by staphylococci or tubercle bacilli, or it may enter the urethra from the outside, such as that caused by *Escherichia coli*. Control of infection is extremely difficult until the underlying obstruction is corrected.

When the obstruction is minor and pressure from backed-up urine develops slowly, there may be no discomfort. However, infection is the rule rather than the exception, and with it come pain and fever. When the kidney pelvis becomes markedly distended, a mass may be palpated through the abdomen. Advanced hydronephrosis causes renal tenderness and pain. If there is a diverticulum of the bladder, the patient may find that he can pass more urine after he empties his bladder and waits a few minutes. The final quantity of urine comes from the diverticulum sac and may be malodorous.

The aim of treatment is to establish adequate drainage of urine. The first measure may be temporary, designed to permit free flow of urine, to relieve retention, and to allow the edematous kidney to heal until it is sufficiently healthy to withstand surgery to correct the obstruction. For example, a patient with a ureteral calculus obstructing one kidney, accompanied by severe infection, may have chills, fever, and hypotension. Under these conditions, the patient may be so ill that anesthesia and surgery to remove the calculus may be very risky. Therefore, during cystoscopy, the urologist may pass a ureteral catheter above the calculus, with its tip draining the kidney pelvis. The catheter will not cure the pathology, but it will drain purulent urine from the pelvis and relieve hydronephrosis. When the patient's general condition improves, a more definitive procedure can be performed.

As soon as a way for urine to leave the body is established, the patient should be encouraged to drink fluids.

If the obstruction is so complete that a catheter cannot be passed, temporary drainage may be accomplished by inserting a tube into the kidney pelvis through a skin incision. When the acute process has subsided, surgery can remove the obstruction, repair the stricture, remove the stone, free the ureter from adhesions, or excise the tumor.

## Calculi (Stones, Lithiasis)

### Etiology

When the salts in urine precipitate instead of remaining in solution, they adhere and form stones. Stones, most of which form in the kidney, can plug the urinary tract so that obstruction with urinary stasis is frequent.

Some types of stones are derived from protein metabolism. Examples are stones composed of uric acid and cystine. Cystine stones occur secondary to an hereditary disorder, accompanied by renal excretion of this relatively insoluble amino acid. Most stones contain calcium, such as calcium oxalate. Exact conditions that cause salts to precipitate are not fully understood. Excessive excretion of calcium, as occurs in patients with hyperparathyroid disease and in some consumers of enormous quantities of milk, tends to encourage stone formation.

Infection (particularly with Proteus species) and stones tend to coexist, but in a particular patient it may not always be clear which came first. Infection can make the urine alkaline, and the result may be the precipitation of calcium. On the other hand, when the pH of urine becomes excessively acid, cystine and uric acid may precipitate. Patients with gout are likely to form uric acid stones. Osteoporosis (demineralization of bones) may be a contributing factor.

Urinary stones not infrequently occur in patients on long-term bed rest, such as those with fractures or paraplegia. When urine flow is sluggish and there is poor gravity drainage from the kidneys as the patient lies on his back, there may be disuse decalcification of bone, and stones may form. This hazard of immobility may be prevented by nursing action, such as active or passive range-of-motion exercises practiced several times a day, every day, and encouraging the patient to drink liberal quantities of fluids, if these are not contraindicated by coexisting conditions.

In most patients who have calculi, no specific reason can be found.

### Characteristics

Most calculi contain calcium, which makes them radiopaque and discernible by plain x-ray films of the abdomen, unless they are very small. The common calculus is composed of calcium oxalate, appears black to gray, is very hard, rough, and irregular. Calcium phosphate and carbonate stones are usually less rough and look like plaster. These stones, associated with infection, often contain a mixture of calcium compounds. Uric acid stones are greenish-yellow and usually smooth. The rare cystine stone is yellowish, greasy to the touch, and slightly opaque due to its sulfur content.

### Symptoms and Signs

Most small stones pass right through and cause no symptoms at all. However, some are troublesome, because they traumatize the walls of the urinary tract and irritate the lining, or because they clog the ureter or an orifice, preventing urine flow and inviting infection. The symptoms are related to number, size, and mobility of the stones.

The following symptoms may occur:

- Hematuria, gross or microscopic, as the stone traumatizes the walls of the urinary tract.
- Pyuria (pus in the urine) due to infection behind the obstruction by the calculus. The patient may experience chills, fever, and can develop serious hypotension and other signs of a gram-negative septicemia.
- Retention of urine or dysuria from blockage of the orifice between bladder and urethra. Some patients can void only in unnatural positions; others are unable to void at all.
- Flank pain or ache, related to obstruction.
- Acute renal or ureteral colic due to violent contractions and spasms as the ureter tries to pass along a stone. The severity of pain is almost inversely proportional to the size of the calculus. Smaller stones frequently travel more rapidly down the ureter, causing more forceful ureteral spasm and, therefore, greater colic.

The colicky pain is characteristic. It is agonizingly severe, coming in waves that may start in the kidney or the ureter and radiate to the inguinal ring, the inner aspect of the thigh or, in the male patient, to the testicle or the tip of the penis. In a female patient, the pain may go to the urinary meatus or the labia of the affected side. The patient may double up with pain and be unable to lie quietly in bed until it passes. The severity of the pain can cause nausea, vomiting, and shock. Often, morphine and antispasmodic drugs are given for relief. The patient must be protected from injury as he thrashes about in bed or if he finds it necessary to walk about while in pain, especially after he has been given a narcotic.

Until the kidneys and the ureters are free of stones, the colicky pain tends to recur. The violent spasm that causes the pain may move a stone along; sometimes after an attack of colic the patient may pass "gravel" or the offending stone itself. On the other hand, a spastic ureter may clamp down on a stone and hold it in place.

## Diagnosis

The diagnosis is made by the classical history, physical findings, urinary changes, the results of intravenous or retrograde pyelography, and, finally, by demonstrating the stone itself once it is out of the patient.

Most stones are radiopaque. If they are not, they may be visualized on x-ray film as lucent defects if air is injected into the renal pelvis or an opaque contrast media is used. To determine the chemical content of the urine, 24-hour urine specimens are collected. Blood is drawn to obtain uric acid levels to rule out gout, and for calcium, phosphorus, and alkaline phosphatase determinations that help to diagnose hyperparathyroidism. Gout and hyperparathyroidism are responsible in the minority of cases of kidney stones, but discovery and subsequent treatment of these diseases may prevent further stone formation.

In the hospital, urine from patients suspected of having stones should be strained through gauze to catch stones that may have been passed. A stone may be no larger than the head of a pin. At home, the patient can void into a clear glass through a small kitchen strainer lined with cheesecloth. Some stones will be sent to the laboratory for chemical analysis, because the composition of the stones will affect treatment. All stones (they may be tiny) should be saved until the physician inspects them.

## Treatment and Nursing Intervention

Most ureteral calculi, 1 cm. or less in diameter, will pass into the bladder spontaneously. Unless there is an obstruction at the bladder outlet, such as an enlarged prostate or urethral stricture, they are voided spontaneously as well. The patient newly admitted to the hospital may be observed for several days to see whether the stone will pass from his body. A large fluid intake is encouraged to reduce the concentration of crystalloids in urine and foster the passage of stones.

As soon as the acute colic subsides, the patient should be encouraged to walk as well as to drink water. An active patient is more likely to pass a stone than a quiet one. Meanwhile, concurrent disorders are treated, and drugs are given to combat infection.

If the stone does not pass spontaneously, and there is continued colic, infection above the stone, or the urologist believes there is little likelihood the stone will be passed spontaneously, surgery is generally performed. Calculi larger than 1 cm. in diameter in the renal pelvis are surgically removed.

For a stone in the renal pelvis, the surgeon may perform one of the following procedures:

- Pyelolithotomy. An incision is made into the renal pelvis, and the stone is removed.
- Nephrolithotomy. An incision is made into the parenchyma of the kidney from the outside to remove a stone in a calyx.
- Calycectomy, heminephrectomy. A proved stone-forming area is excised.

- Complete nephrotomy. The kidney is split from end to end. Each calyx is opened. This operation is most common for a staghorn calculus, a type of stone that tends to fill the kidney pelvis and to take on its shape.
- Nephrectomy. The kidney is removed if it has been permanently and severely damaged by the stone and can no longer function normally. This operation is used when unilateral kidney damage has occurred; the other kidney must have at least some healthy tissue.

Stones in the ureter may be removed surgically (ureterolithotomy). In one method a small incision is made over the stone in the ureter. A drain of the Penrose type is placed at the site of the incision, and the urine is allowed to drain from the wound until the ureter heals. The urologist may attempt to extract lower ureteral calculi with a variety of stone baskets.

Occasionally, a ureteral stone can be crushed or grasped and pulled out with a special instrument during cystoscopy. Snaring the stone is an extremely delicate procedure because the danger of rupturing the ureter is a constant threat. Usually, this cystoscopic procedure is performed under general anesthesia to avoid any sudden movement by the patient. If complications are encountered, open surgery is begun at once. If the procedure is uncomplicated and successful, the patient will have a ureteral catheter attached to straight drainage. The purpose of the catheter is to splint the ureter and to divert urine past any possible tear in the ureteral wall. It is kept in place for three to four days. At times, after a cystoscopy a ureteral catheter will be left in place for 24 hours to dilate the ureter in the hope that stones then will pass through it or be pulled into the bladder when the catheter is removed (see Care of Patient with Ureteral Catheters).

**After Ureter Surgery.** Whenever the ureters have been entered surgically—for example, to correct a stricture or to remove a stone (*lithotomy*), possible complications for which the nurse observes are infection and hemorrhage. Also, if there is no urine from the catheter on the affected side, a fistula may have formed that is diverting urine away from the urinary tract, or the catheter may have slipped, allowing urine to seep out around the sutures.

**Bladder Stones.** Bladder stones may be removed through the transurethral route, using a stone-crushing instrument called a lithotrite. The procedure (called *litholapaxy*) is suitable for small and soft stones. Larger, noncrushable stones must be removed through a suprapubic incision.

Surgery for renal calculi also includes correction of any anatomic obstructions thought to contribute to the development of stones. For example, a congenital obstruction of the ureteropelvic junction may require that the surgeon perform pyeloplasty as well as remove calculi, or stones will reform.

**Prevention.** Patients who have a tendency to form stones should ingest adequate fluids (minimum 2,500 to 3,000 ml. daily) to help to prevent a recurrence. Also, they should be instructed in methods for straining urine and should know that any stone should be brought to the physician for examination. The patient should be made aware of the importance of promptly reporting hematuria, burning, or other signs of urinary tract infection.

Patients with gout must limit their purine intake to prevent uric acid stones. Patients who have had stones of calcium may have to limit their intake of milk and milk products.

When it has been possible to determine the chemical composition of stones that have been passed or removed, dietary treatment then may be attempted to adjust the pH of the urine to keep urinary salts in solution. For example, an alkaline-ash diet may be given to prevent precipitation of uric acid and cystine crystals. An acid-ash diet may be ordered for calcium oxalate or phosphate stones. However, these diets are not fully effective, and they are not commonly used. Sometimes the desired pH can be achieved by relatively minor changes in the diet. To acidify urine, the physician may direct that the patient eliminate citrus fruits, fruit juices, other than apple and cranberry, and carbonated beverages from his diet. Tomatoes may be eaten for their vitamin C content. An acidifying agent, such as sodium acid phosphate, may be given. Vitamin C is a powerful acidifier of urine. Its indiscriminate use may result in uric acid stone formation in hyperuricemic patients.

To make the urine more alkaline, the physician may prescribe sodium bicarbonate or polycitrate solution, and 1 to 3 quarts of orange juice a day. Uric acid stones can be prevented by a low-purine diet and oral sodium carbonate to alkalinize the urine. The patient is taught how to check the acidity of urine with litmus or nitrazine paper. A further medical advance is the use of allopurinal, a xanthine oxidase inhibitor, which interferes with the endogenous production of uric acid by the body. Cystine stones can be prevented in many instances by using a vigorous fluid intake (up to 6 liters a day), stringent alkalinization of the urine, and the oral ingestion of the compound d-penicillamine.

The most effective deterrent to calcium stones, particularly calcium phosphate, is the Shorr regimen. The patient is placed on a low-calcium, low-phosphorus diet to diminish the concentration of these substances in urine. Basic aluminum hydroxide gel, 30 to 45 ml., is ingested after each meal and at bedtime to precipitate phosphorus as insoluble aluminum phosphates in the gastrointestinal tract, thus further decreasing urinary phosphate output.

**Patient Education.** Before the patient leaves the hospital he must understand and be able to carry out requirements for fluid, dietary instructions, and drug therapy. He must know the signs of infection and the resources for early treatment. It has been suggested that the patient be hydrated to the point that he voids 2,000 to 3,000 ml. per day to prevent the precipitation of stones.

Patients who have had recent kidney surgery should avoid heavy lifting.

## Urethral Strictures

Strictures are narrowings of the urethra. Because they reduce its circumference, urethral strictures act as an impediment to urinary flow and cause symptoms of obstruction. Concentric scarring, caused by traumatic instrumentation of the urethra, is the most common cause. In the past, gonorrheal infection was the leading cause of strictures in men.

As a form of obstruction, strictures are a danger to the upper urinary tract. Symptoms may include a slow stream of urine, a forked or spray stream, hesitancy, burning, frequency, nocturia, and retention of residual urine in the bladder, which may lead to distention and infection. A voiding urethrogram helps to make the diagnosis. If the patient is unable to void, a retrograde urethrogram may be done.

Urethral strictures are treated by:

- Dilation. This is done with specially designed instruments (bougies, sounds, filiforms, and followers) passed very gently into the lumen of the urethra. Although this procedure is done gently, it is still painful. Taking deep breaths may help the patient to relax. Measures previously mentioned in relation to the care of the patient after cystoscopy, such as helping him off the table and encouraging him to rest before leaving the office or clinic, are indicated.

  Since forceful stretching of the urethra may cause bleeding and further stricture formation, the urologist gently uses graduated sizes of instruments. He may start with only a 6 or 8 F. Gradually, he increases the size until a 24 or 26 F. can be tolerated. Depending on the cause of the stricture and the patient's response to therapy, the condition may subside after one or two treatments; usually periodic dilations are required indefinitely, or until the condition is corrected surgically. The nurse should help the patient to understand the importance of having these treatments regularly, as prescribed, and not waiting until the size of the urinary stream has been reduced severely or other symptoms of obstruction have developed. After a treatment, the patient may have slight hematuria and he should be told about this in advance so that he will not become frightened. If a great amount of blood appears, or if bleeding persists, he should notify the urologist immediately. Voiding will be painful for about two days after the procedure. Sitz baths help to relieve the discomfort.

- Internal urethrotomy. The urologist enters the urethra with an instrument called a urethrotome and cuts the stricture bands. A large retention catheter is then inserted and maintained in place until the urethra has healed (approximately three weeks).

- Perineal urethrostomy. For very tight, persistent strictures, a permanent opening may be constructed into the urethra through the perineum, bypassing the stricture. Following such diversion of the urinary stream, the male patient must sit to urinate. Providing privacy, emotional support, and instruction regarding hygiene after a bowel movement to prevent ascending urinary tract infection are part of the nurse's role following this surgery.

- Urethroplasty. Urine is diverted from the urethra by a cystostomy tube or perineal urethrostomy tube attached to straight drainage until the urethra has been repaired. In one method of reconstructing the urethra, the constricted area is resected, and a mucosal graft (which may be taken from the bladder) is inserted to restore the continuity of the urethra. Postoperatively, the patient will have a splinting catheter in the urethra that will remain in place until healing has taken place. This operation may be performed in two stages: urinary diversion at the first operation and plastic repair at the second.

Strictures that are most difficult to treat are those resulting from trauma. The most common cause of trauma is that inadvertently inflicted during genito-urinary surgery. Early and adequate treatment of strictures can reduce their severity and such complications as urinary tract infection and periurethral abscesses.

## Infection

A focus of infection elsewhere in the body—for example, a boil or an inflamed throat—may spread to the urinary tract, particularly the kidney, through the bloodstream or the lymphatics. An infection in the kidney can spread to tissues throughout the urinary tract. An ascending infection (one that starts in the urethra and moves upward) is commonly caused by *Escherichia coli.* In men the infection may extend to tissues of the prostate, the seminal vesicles, or the epididymis. Foreign bodies, such as stones and catheters, predispose to infection. The danger of introducing bacteria with a catheter or with an irrigating solution is so great that only the strictest aseptic equipment and technique should be used. Catheterization should be a procedure of last resort. *Klebsiella aerobacter, Proteus mirabilis,* and *Pseudomonas aeruginosa* are common organisms causing infection after instrumentation of the urinary tract or in the presence of an indwelling catheter. When an indwelling catheter is necessary for a long period, it should be changed periodically, using sterile technique. In some hospitals it is the policy to change indwelling catheters once a week. Patients who have had urinary procedures, such as dilatations, have samples of their urine tested at intervals for evidence of infection.

Treatment of all urinary tract infections includes surgical drainage of pus; identification and removal (when this is possible) of contributing factors, such as coexisting stones, obstructions, or tumors; increasing the fluid intake so that 2 to 3 liters of urine is excreted daily; and the administration of sulfonamides or antibiotics.

## Tuberculosis

Since the advent of drug therapy, tubercular infections of the urinary tract are less common than they used to be, and when found are usually secondary to lesions in the lungs. The upper pole of the kidney is usually first involved, and the disease may eventually involve the ureters, bladder, prostate, and scrotal contents. Multiple drug therapy, usually for two years, is the mode of treatment. (See Chapter 31 regarding antituberculosis drugs.)

If renal tuberculosis does not respond to drug therapy and is unilateral, nephrectomy may be done. Rest in a hospital or at home is part of the treatment. While the pulmonary lesion may no longer be active, in the early stage of treatment urine will contain the tubercle bacillus. However, only ordinary hygienic measures, such as proper hand washing, are necessary. There is no danger of transmission of tuberculosis from urine, from soiled dressings, or from bed linen.

## Acute Pyelonephritis

Pyelonephritis means infection of the renal parenchyma as well as the lining of the collecting system. In the acute form the patient is clinically quite ill. He experiences pain in the kidney, chills, fever, malaise, and nausea. The urinalysis will show pyuria. Frequency and burning on urination may be present if the bladder is also infected.

Pyelonephritis may be a complication of infection elsewhere in the body. It is often associated with pregnancy and with diabetes. The kidney becomes edematous, and the pelvic mucosa becomes inflamed and roughened. There may be multiple small abscesses.

Early treatment is important to prevent chronic infection and progressive damage to kidney tissue. The physician takes the necessary measures to relieve obstruction to urinary flow. With antibiotic treatment, fever and pain will usually subside within 72 hours. Initial choice of antibacterials will depend on the physician's judgment, since identification and antibiotic sensitivity testing of the offending organism in urine will take several days.

The patient is placed on bed rest; liberal fluid intake to keep urine dilute is urged. These patients are very sick and require attention to skin as well as mouth care, turning, and encouragement to eat. Every effort is expended to prevent both septicemia and chronic pyelonephritis. When there are no complications, the prognosis for complete cure with adequate antibacterial therapy is excellent.

## Chronic Pyelonephritis

If the treatment of acute pyelonephritis is not permanently successful (for instance, if the infection is recurrent, or if urinary stasis continues due to an obstruction), the disease may enter a chronic stage. The kidney shows irreversible degenerative changes; it becomes small and atrophic, and the pelvic mucosa becomes pale and fibrotic. Many nephrons are destroyed. If enough nephrons become inoperative, the patient will develop uremia.

Although chronic pyelonephritis may be asymptomatic, the patient can have a low-grade fever, vague gastrointestinal complaints, and anemia. There may be acute attacks; some patients will develop hypertension due to renal ischemia. Sometimes, stones form in the affected kidney.

Nothing known today can restore scarred kidney tissue. The aim of treatment is to prevent further damage. Intensive therapy with antibiotics or chemotherapeutic agents is given. Any obstruction is relieved. An effort is made to improve the patient's overall health. A nephrectomy may be done if severe hypertension develops and the other kidney can support life. The fight against chronic pyelonephritis is a long one. Prolonged medication and constant attention to general health habits may be a dull and discouraging routine for patients.

Patients with chronic pyelonephritis can develop renal failure. For care of patients with this complication, see Chapter 64.

### Cystitis

Cystitis means inflammation of the urinary bladder. Normally, the contents of the bladder are sterile. Bacteria reach it by way of infected kidneys, lymphatics, and the urethra. Because the urethra is short in women, ascending infections are more common in women than in men. Cystitis is prevented from being even more common than it is by a natural resistance of the bladder lining, which helps to prevent an inflammatory process from taking hold from the occasional invasion of the bladder by bacteria. This resistance cannot be relied on to counter the effects of introducing an unsterile catheter into the sterile environment of the bladder.

There are many causes of cystitis. It may be secondary to infection elsewhere in the urinary or reproductive tract. In men it may follow prostatitis, and it may herald an obstruction of the urethra. Straightforward cystitis in the male is rare. In women it may develop following urethral irritation after sexual intercourse. Cervicitis or pelvic inflammatory disease may involve the bladder. A cystocele may lead to cystitis because the relaxed pelvic wall prevents the bladder from emptying completely and urine stagnates. Alteration in bladder mechanics following difficult childbirth may lay the groundwork for infection. Cystitis may follow the effects of heavy radiotherapy. Poorly controlled diabetes mellitus may predispose to bladder infection, as it does to infection elsewhere.

The lining of the bladder may show only a slight increase in vascularity, or there may be edema and ulceration. In chronic cystitis the wall becomes thickened and contracted, diminishing the capacity of the bladder.

Symptoms include urgency (a pressing need to void although the bladder is not full), frequency, dysuria (painful urination), perineal and suprapubic pain, and hematuria, especially at the termination of the stream (terminal hematuria). If bacteremia is present, the patient also may have chills and fever. Chronic cystitis causes similar symptoms, but usually they are less severe.

Diagnosis is made from the patient's history, the total physical examination, and the urinalysis, including culture and the sensitivity of the offending organisms to antibiotics or chemotherapeutic agents.

Instruments are not passed into an infected bladder for fear of spreading the infection, unless it is to bypass an obstruction and to remove residual urine trapped in the bladder.

Treatment includes the correction of contributing factors. If there is partial obstruction, no cure of cystitis will be fully effective until urine can be made to drain adequately by removing the obstruction. Treatment often is prolonged, and it may require many office visits after the patient has been discharged from the hospital. For example, dilation of a contracted bladder with normal saline instillations must be repeated many times.

If the patient has a fever or other systemic symptom of infection, he may be put on bed rest. Even though he has urgency and frequency, he needs a great deal of encouragement to take large quantities of fluids. Warm sitz baths may provide some relief. Cranberry juice, which acidifies the urine and provides a less favorable climate for bacterial growth, may be offered to the patient. The nurse learns which fluids the patient prefers and provides these, if possible, so that the goal of a liberal fluid intake can be met more readily.

### Urethritis

Inflammation of the urethra caused by organisms other than gonorrhea is called *nonspecific urethritis*. Gonorrheal urethritis used to be more common than it is now. Urethritis also may be secondary to trichomonal and monilial infections in women.

The distal portion of the normal male urethra is not totally sterile. However, bacteria normally present there cause no difficulty unless these tissues are traumatized, usually following instrumentation such as catheterization or cystoscopic examination. Under such conditions, bacteria may gain a foothold to cause a nonspecific urethritis. The urethra mucosa becomes inflamed and pus forms in the tiny mucus forming glands lining the urethra. Other causes of nonspecific urethritis include irritation during vigorous intercourse.

Gonorrhea, on the other hand, is a specific form of infection that can attack the mucous membrane of a normal urethra. Usually within two or three days after contact, the patient will notice a thick purulent discharge from the meatus.

Symptoms of infection of the anterior urethra include discomfort on urination, varying from a slight tickling sensation to burning and severe discomfort. Marked urinary frequency indicates inflammation of the posterior urethra and bladder neck. Fever is not common, and its appearance in the male signifies further extension of the infection to such areas as the prostate, testes, and epididymides. Treatment includes antibiotics, a liberal fluid intake, analgesics, warm sitz baths, and improving the patient's resistance to infection by a good diet and plenty of rest.

**Prevention.** The nurse should be gentle when she is catheterizing patients, so that she does not injure the delicate wall of the urethra. Also, she should be scrupulous in maintaining sterile technique. The importance of avoiding the introduction of microorganisms with the catheter cannot be overemphasized. The patient is encouraged to drink copiously after all urethral procedures to flush out the lower urinary tract. Both nurse and patient should wash their hands well after handling the urine or urinary receptacles to avoid spreading the infection.

Cleaning by sitz or tub bath may be recommended for the ambulatory patient. The periurethral area of any patient who cannot be placed in a tub should be washed daily with soap, water, and a clean washcloth. This should be done by the nurse for patients who cannot wash themselves well. Urethritis is commonly caused by irritation from indwelling catheters, which rapidly may become infected. If a patient has an indwelling catheter, the area should be washed more frequently, especially if the patient is incontinent of feces. It is not sufficient to wash only around the anus and buttocks. Wiping must be done away from the urethra. If cotton pledgets are used, the area from the urethral meatus toward the anus is wiped downward in a single stroke and the pledget is discarded.

## Other Urinary Tract Infections

*Infected hydronephrosis* is a common urologic condition, especially in patients with a chronic obstruction. The treatment is designed to relieve both the retention of urine and the infection. *Pyonephrosis* is a suppurative destruction of the parenchyma of the kidney, which may be totally destroyed. Pyonephrosis is an end-result of infected hydronephrosis or chronic pyelonephritis. The renal pelvis becomes filled with pus and ulcerations. *Abscesses* or *carbuncles* may occur on the cortex of the kidney; usually, these are caused by staphylococci. A perinephric abscess is one that occurs in the fatty tissue around the kidney.

## TUMORS (NEOPLASIA)

### Tumors of the Kidney

The malignant hypernephroma (renal adenocarcinoma) is the most common tumor of the parenchyma of the adult kidney. Because the kidneys are deeply protected in the body, tumors can become quite large before they cause symptoms. An abdominal mass found on a routine physical examination or on roentgenograms taken for other purposes may lead to the discovery. These tumors are dangerous, because they usually metastasize early, but may present distressing symptoms only late in the course of the disease. Hematuria may occur if the tumor invades the collecting system. This is an easy symptom for the patient to ignore because it may be both intermittent and painless. Later, pain may be due to expansion of the kidney or coliclike discomfort from the passage of bloodclots.

Tumors in the pelvis of the adult kidney may be flat or papillary, benign or malignant. Papillary cancers, especially, have a tendency to seed the ureter and the bladder with malignant cells. Painless hematuria (gross or microscopic) is likely to be the first symptom. Occasionally, pieces of tumor tissue will be found in the urine.

Symptoms of a malignant tumor may include weight loss, malaise, unexplained fever, and episodes of hematuria. Sometimes, the first symptom occurs at a secondary, metastatic site. Hypertension is frequent in these patients.

Diagnosis is made by intravenous or retrograde pyelography and by renal angiography, which show deformity of the kidney, its collecting system, or its blood supply. Cystoscopy during a bleeding episode allows the urologist to observe from which ureteral orifice blood is originating and thus to determine which kidney is involved. At the same time tests are performed to demonstrate the function of the unaffected kidney—a point most pertinent to treatment. To locate the tumor precisely, nephrotomography may be done. X-ray studies of other portions of the body, particularly the bony structures, also are made in a search for metastases. Papanicolaou smears may be taken.

When cancer of the kidney is diagnosed, complete removal of the kidney (nephrectomy) and its surrounding perinephric fat may be done. If the tumor arises from the collecting system or in the ureter, a complete nephroureterectomy may be done. The kidney and the ureter as well as a cuff of bladder tissue are removed because the recurrence rate in any stump of ureter left behind is very high.

Surgery may be followed by radiotherapy while the patient is still in the hospital, or on an outpatient basis. Follow-up cystoscopic examinations are imperative to find early and newly metastasized areas in the bladder. If the unaffected kidney cannot adequately take over the function of excreting urine, or if extensive metastases are found, only palliative treatment can be given.

**Postnephrectomy Nursing.**   After a nephrectomy, a Penrose drain is left in place to catch the serous material that collects in the space left by the kidney. Since there is no kidney, no urine comes from this drain. The amount and characteristics (color, consistency, odor, and contents) of the drainage, which may be blood-tinged in the beginning, are noted and recorded.

The patient must be turned to the side when dressing observations are made. Profuse, red, thick drainage, clots, and distention of the suture line indicate hemorrhage. Slow oozing also might occur, which would not be reflected in vital signs for several hours. Drainage should stop after two days. A sterile safety pin is usually placed on the drain by the surgeon so that the drain cannot disappear into the wound. Because the surgical area is close to the pleural cavity, the patient is observed for pneumothorax. In rare instances, the pleura is accidentally nicked during the operation; air enters the pleural space from the lung and collapses the lung.

If the transthoracic surgical approach to nephrectomy is used, additional nursing care measures for the patient having open chest surgery are necessary.

Deep breathing is painful because of the proximity of the incision to the diaphragm. Narcotics are given liberally, but the patient must be assisted to deep breathe and cough to avoid atelectasis.

Positive pressure breathing treatments may be ordered. Splinting the incision with a binder, or manually, may help the patient to expand his rib cage. The patient may have a gastric tube for several days because paralytic ileus of reflex origin tends to develop. Fluids are encouraged when this tube is removed. Alertness to the possibility of hemorrhage is especially important during the immediate postoperative period and eight to twelve days postoperatively, when tissue sloughing is apt to occur.

If the hyperextended side-lying position was used for surgery, the patient may be troubled by muscular aches and pain. Pillow support and the use of prescribed muscle relaxants may give relief.

### Tumors of the Bladder

Bladder tumors may be the flat, infiltrating, or papillary type. They may be benign or malignant. The depth to which they penetrate bladder muscle bears a direct relationship to prognosis. In malignant tumors, metastases usually have not occurred so long as the muscle is not penetrated.

The most common first symptom of malignant disease of the bladder is painless hematuria (another instance of the importance of immediately investigating hematuria). Diagnosis is made by cystoscopic examination and biopsy.

Treatment varies according to the type of tumor, and the grade and stage of a malignant one. Small, superficial tumors may be cut out through the transurethral resectoscope by using an electric cutting instrument. Bleeding can be checked, or tumor tissue may be coagulated in the same manner. Fulguration may be used for small and benign tumors. Patients in whom papillomas have been removed should return for a cystoscopic examination every three months for the first year, and every six months for the next four years, so that the recurrence of a benign tumor or a new malignant growth can be discovered early.

Merits of radiotherapy for bladder malignancy are debatable at present but it may be used for palliation. Local bladder recurrences of low-grade malignant tumors have been lessened by instillations of the chemotherapeutic agent, thiotepa.

Some tumors may not be removable by the transurethral method because of their size or their location in the bladder. To remove these tumors a suprapubic incision is made and the bladder exposed and thoroughly explored. Part of the bladder may be removed (segmental resection) or all of it (cystectomy), or the bladder and adjacent tissues may be removed (radical cystectomy).

**After Bladder Surgery.** When a portion of the bladder is removed (*segmental resection*), its capacity as a reservoir is decreased. Immediately postoperatively, the patient may be able to hold no more than 50 to 60 ml. of urine. This capacity should increase to 200 to 400 ml. within a couple of months (depending on the amount of bladder removed). Fluids should be encouraged during the immediate postoperative period, and the output from both the urethral and the suprapubic catheters should be observed and recorded. The patient becomes aware of being able to hold less urine when his catheters are first removed. Prior discussion of what to expect will help to lessen surprise and anxiety. The patient will need to adjust to the smaller reservoir capacity. For example, he should learn to restrict fluids before retiring or joining a social gathering. However, it is important that his total fluid intake for the day be adequate.

Periodic spasms of the bladder may make the patient very uncomfortable for several days. Narcotics and antispasmodics are given. (See Chapter 53 for additional nursing care of the patient with a suprapubic catheter.)

After *radical cystectomy*, the patient is usually quite ill. The bladder and large amounts of surrounding tissue and pelvic lymph nodes have been removed.

In males, radical cystectomy involves removal of the prostate, seminal vesicles, and occasionally the urethra because of the possibility of recurrence. In females, the uterus and adnexa as well as the urethra are removed. The mortality rate in radical cystectomy is about 10 to 15 per cent. Sometimes a patient requires a colostomy as well as an ileal conduit, and this complicates nursing care. The emotional impact of the diagnosis of cancer and the added factor of mutilating surgery stress to the utmost the patient's ability to cope and his need for nursing support. After radical cystectomy, the male will be impotent. The vagina of the female is foreshortened, but this does not preclude sexual intercourse. However, she does have to adjust to the change in body image and function because urine will drain through an abdominal stoma (Behnke, 1973). The patient is prone to surgical shock, thrombosis, cardiac decompensation, and other circulatory disturbances. Nursing care is similar to that of the patient with major abdominal surgery. In addition, permanent urinary diversion accompanies cystectomy.

Urinary diversion may also be necessary in patients with neurogenic bladder, trauma, anomalies, or strictures.

### Surgical Procedures for Urinary Diversion

- Vesicotomy. This surgery is done for neurogenic bladder when a cystecomy is not necessary. An incision is made into the bladder, which is then moved forward, and the bladder opening is sutured to the abdominal wall. Urine is collected in a plastic pouch.
- Ureterosigmoidostomy. The ureters are attached to the sigmoid colon. The lower colon becomes the reservoir for urine. The patient voids and defecates through the rectum, which has spincter control. Complications of this procedure include infection ascending up the ureters into the kidneys from the colon, and electrolyte imbalance due to the reabsorption of various components of urine through the intestinal wall (for example, hyperchloremic acidosis). This operation is not performed if there is disease of the large bowel, such as diverticulitis, or if the anal sphincter is incompetent, since the main advantage, voluntary urinary control, is lost.
- Cutaneous ureterostomy. The ureters are brought to the skin surface. The patient wears one or two rubber collecting cups that drain the urine into a plastic pouch or leg bag, periodically emptying the bag by releasing the stopper at the bottom. This operation is a relatively safe procedure, with a low mortality rate. It is often indicated in debilitated or older patients. Stricture of the ureter at the junction with skin or fascia is one complication of the procedure. Leakage and odor problems can also occur.
- Bricker procedure (ileal bladder or ileal conduit). In this operation a small segment of ileum is resected from the intestines, with its nerve and blood supply intact. The proximal end of the segment is closed and the distal end brought out as a stoma in the lower right quadrant. The ureters are anastomosed to the pouch and drain through it. The ileal loop is no longer connected to the gastrointestinal tract. The term "ileal bladder" is a misnomer, since urine is not stored in the pouch; it only passes through it and out of the body via the stoma. The patient wears a plastic urine collecting bag over the stoma of the pouch. An infrequent complication of this procedure is electrolyte imbalance.

### Nursing Care of Patients with Urinary Diversion

Many nursing considerations in the care of a patient with urinary diversion are similar to those of a patient with a colostomy or an ileostomy. For example, in both instances there is functional loss and change in body image; the skin needs protection, and the stoma and appliances need care and cleaning. The patient needs a nurse who can encourage him by her matter-of-factness and skill as she demonstrates stoma care, teaches the patient to care for himself, and helps him to accept the stoma and adjust to a changed way of elimination. However, there are some differences. Infection is more likely to occur and a different way of voiding may be difficult for the patient to accept. In the hospital, if he is on a urologic ward, he will see others who use the same method. However, the patient may worry about how he will get along outside the hospital. His own acceptance of urinary diversion, the equipment, and its care can be increased by instructing him in self-care as soon as possible during the early postoperative period, by listening to his doubts and fears, and by having a visitor from an ostomy club talk to him. His adjustment is also enhanced by a clear preoperative explanation of what changes to expect, the nurse's familiarity with various collection appliances, expertise in skin care, teaching ability, and an introduction to other patients who have successfully undergone urinary diversion.

During the postoperative period the patient is fitted for his reusable appliance. After this is obtained, the patient is thoroughly instructed, along with another member of his family, in its application, cleaning, and care. Teaching is continued until the patient can leave the hospital confident in his ability to manage his own care alone or with the help of family members or the community health nurse.

A set of written instructions for the patient and family is helpful for home review (Winter, 1968). Anxiety in the hospital or on arrival at home may lead to memory gaps or misunderstanding.

For a more detailed description of the principles of care of a stoma, skin care, ostomy accessories and techniques, as well as the teaching and counseling roles of the nurse, see Chapter 47. Nursing considerations relative to specific types of urinary diversion follow.

**Ureterosigmoidostomy.** The advantage of attaching ureters to the bowel is that the patient is not required to adjust to caring for a continuously draining stoma on his abdominal wall. There are no appliances, and there is no need to care for the skin surrounding orifices. The lower colon acts as a reservoir of sorts (holding about 200 ml.), and the anal sphincter controls the exit of both urine and stool from the body. The amount of urine that

can be held is not so great as in the urinary bladder, and the urine liquefies the stool, but some patients learn to regulate themselves so that they can continue with daily activities.

If the ureters are to be attached to the bowel, microorganisms in the bowel will be minimized by the preoperative use of a mechanical bowel preparation with cathartics and enemas, and a drug such as sulfasuxidine or neomycin. Loss of the usual bacterial flora results in a soft, almost odorless stool. The nurse should observe the stool and chart its characteristics. Patients who have ureteral transplants to the bowel are given a low-residue diet, both before and after the surgery, to minimize the formation of fecal material that would contaminate the operative area. The patient is placed on a low-residue diet about three days before surgery, then clear fluids 24 hours before operation.

Postoperatively, a sterile rectal tube is left in place for five to ten days to keep the rectosigmoid empty and to decrease the chance of urinary leakage through the anastomosis. Ureteral catheters may be brought out through the anus and anchored to the buttocks for about ten days. During the first days after surgery, the hourly or two-hourly drainage is recorded. Later the rectal tube may be

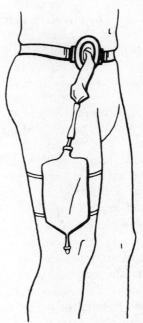

**Figure 48-13.** A rubber leg urinal collecting the urine draining from a ureter implanted into the skin. The end of the bag can be unplugged periodically during the day to empty the bag.

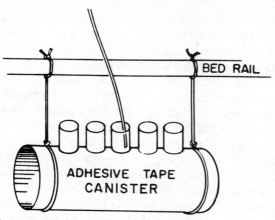

**Figure 48-14.** One way to collect hourly urine specimens. The test tubes are set in holes cut into an empty adhesive tape canister.

removed, when necessary, for defecation and reinserted. The stool at first will be liquid, but as the bowel adjusts to being a reservoir, stools become soft. A low residue diet is usually ordered until the tubes are removed.

If there are problems with the reabsorption of urinary chloride and resultant hyperchloremic acidosis, the patient is taught in the hospital and discharged with instructions to insert a rectal tube each night, anchor it to the skin, and attach it to straight drainage. The physician may prescribe oral sodium bicarbonate. To minimize the absorption of waste products the patient voids (rectally) every two to four hours. He should report symptoms of electrolyte imbalance, such as nausea, vomiting, or lethargy.

The major disadvantage of ureterosigmoidostomy is that infection of the ureters and the kidney pelvis is very frequent. The urinary tract is unprotected from organisms that normally inhabit the lower bowel. The patient should be taught to establish a regular routine of drinking 2,500 to 3,000 ml. of fluids daily, and to notify his physician on the first indication of pain, fever, or any other sign of infection. Some patients are placed on a small dose of a sulfonamide or an antibiotic and continue taking the drug for months or years in an attempt to prevent an infection of the urinary tract. Patients must be taught to tell hospital personnel on readmission that they void rectally. They do not need laxatives, and enemas would force fecal material into the ureters.

**Cutaneous Ureterostomy.** After the cutaneous implantation of ureters, the patient returns from the operating room with splinting (stenting) catheters inserted into the ureters. These catheters remain in place for at least ten days.

During surgery, the ends of the ureters are everted and attached to the skin in such a way that a circle of mucosal lining is exposed to the air. It is like rolling the end of a tube back on itself. The purpose is to prevent the ureters from closing. These stoma are called ureteral buds. For about five days postoperatively, sterile saline compresses are kept over the exposed urethral mucosa. These should be kept both sterile and wet. Saline can be added hourly with an Asepto syringe. Then the entire dressing is covered with several sterile pads to keep other parts of the patient's body from getting wet and to keep the wet dressing underneath sterile. Zinc oxide ointment and petrolatum are examples of substances used to protect the skin from maceration. The nurse notes the color of the stoma and any edema that may occlude the opening.

After the catheters are removed, a collecting device (Singer or Whitfield Cups or a pastic pouch) is placed over the buds and urine drains through tubing to a leg bag. The patient visits the bathroom at intervals during the day to release the stopper from the bottom of the bag or pouch, emptying it of urine. At night the bag may be replaced by a drainage at the side of the bed. The skin of the circumstomal area must be protected from excoriation and breakdown. As early as possible the patient assists in the care of his stoma and collecting devices with the goal of self-care by the time of discharge. He is instructed by the nurse or the enterostomal therapist (Figs. 48-13 and 48-14).

If urinary drainage stops or if the patient complains of back pain, the surgeon is notified immediately, since an indwelling ureteral catheter may be necessary. If such catheters are required on a permanent basis (for example, if buds are not formed around the orifices), the patient is taught how to sterilize, irrigate, and replace catheters.

Referral to a community nursing agency is indicated if the patient needs help to care for himself at home.

**Ileal Conduit.** Following construction of an ileal conduit (Bricker procedure), the patient may have some degree of paralytic ileus for as long as a week. Return of peristaltic activity in the isolated segment of conduit parallels that of the intestinal tract, which was reanastomosed. For this reason, some surgeons will insert a multieyed catheter into the stoma at operation, and it is not removed for five to seven days. However, the catheter lumen readily becomes obstructed by intestinal mucus and may require frequent irrigations. An alternate approach is the application of a temporary clear plastic ostomy appliance connected to straight drainage. This has an advantage in that urinary soilage of the surgical incision is less likely and the condition of the stoma can be observed through the plastic. The surgeon may insert a catheter into the conduit at times to check for residual urine (normally the conduit is nearly empty since it does not have a reservoir function) or to provide for continued drainage should there be leakage at one of the internal anastomoses. Because the patient has also had an intestinal anastomosis, he will have a gastric tube in place for several days postoperatively to prevent distention and pressure on the suture line. Symptoms of peritonitis (abdominal tenderness, fever, severe pain, distention) should be noted and reported promptly, since the intestinal anastomosis can leak fecal material, or the ileal conduit may leak urine into the peritoneal cavity. Signs of distention of the conduit with urine should be observed because this puts pressure on the suture line or back pressure on the kidneys. Pain in the lower abdomen or decreased urinary output should be promptly discussed with the physician.

The mucosa of the ileum produces mucus, which may plug the orifice and prevent urine from draining. The mucus may be removed with sterile gauze. The surgeon may dilate the stoma daily during the early postoperative period. Until the patient is able to do it for himself, the nurse frequently checks the bag to see that the urine is draining adequately, empties it before it becomes full, and changes the temporary stoma pouch as needed. Each time his position is changed, at first the nurse and then the patient, checks to make sure that the drainage system is not impeded in any way.

## OTHER URINARY TRACT CONDITIONS

### Trauma

From the back and the sides, the urinary tract is encircled by the ribs, the spinal column, and the pelvic girdle. Fracture of any of these bones should alert the nurse to watch for signs of damage to kidneys, ureters, or bladder. Any trauma to the lower portion of the body, such as a fall, an automobile accident, or a gunshot wound, may tear a portion of the urinary tract. The signs may not be immediately apparent while the more obvious wounds are being cared for. Any patient who has experienced trauma to the area should be observed for anuria; perhaps the ureters are cut through or the bladder may be ruptured. Peritonitis is possible because in the abdominal cavity urine is a foreign substance. Each urine specimen should be checked for gross or increasing hematuria. A series of specimens can be kept in test tubes for continuing comparison.

Injury to the deeply protected kidneys is usually from blunt trauma and varies from contusions to lacerations to frank ruptures. Contusions are more common, and most respond to conservative therapy with bed rest and observation. The patient is observed for signs of continued bleeding, such as hematuria, an enlarging flank mass, or signs of shock. Frank rupture or direct injury, as with a knife or bullet wound, usually requires surgical exploration, and nephrectomy is often necessary. However, the surgeon must first know the condition of the opposite kidney.

### Polycystic Disease of the Kidney

This disease is a congenital familial disorder. It is characterized by multiple, bilateral kidney cysts and may not be diagnosed until middle life. As the cysts slowly enlarge, they squeeze the functioning parenchyma between them. The kidneys may become enormous and exert pressure on nearby abdominal and pelvic organs. Nephritis, calculi, infections, and hydronephrosis may result from and complicate the condition. The patient may have hematuria, pain, pyuria, anemia, and gastrointestinal symptoms from pressure caused by the expanding kidney. The patient usually is hypertensive. The treatment is the same as that for nephritis. Emergency surgery is required, sometimes for hemorrhage. However, there is no cure for polycystic disease, and eventually uremia develops. Because the disease is bilateral, the prognosis is poor. (See Chapter 64, Care of the Patient in Renal Failure.)

## NONINFECTIOUS KIDNEY DISEASE

### Nephritis (Bright's Disease)

The term *nephritis* refers to a group of noninfectious diseases which is characterized by widespread kidney damage.

## Acute Glomerulonephritis

**Etiology.** Glomerulonephritis is a type of nephritis characterized by inflammation of the glomeruli. It has been repeatedly observed that symptoms of acute glomerulonephritis appear approximately two weeks after an upper respiratory infection, usually one that has been caused by hemolytic streptococci. Recent influenza, scarlet fever, or chickenpox also may be given in the history. The exact relationship between the respiratory infection and the nephritis is not clearly understood. The organisms are not present in the kidney when the symptoms of nephritis appear. The disease may represent an altered tissue reaction to infection, a result of host response rather than damage from infection.

Acute glomerulonephritis occurs most frequently in children and young adults.

**Symptoms.** Early symptoms may be so slight that the patient does not seek medical attention. Occasionally the onset is sudden, with generalized edema (anasarca), fever, vomiting, anuria, hypertension, and dyspnea. There may be cerebral and cardiac involvement. Most patients survive the disease without sequelae, but death from uremia may follow delirium or convulsions, or the patient may die in congestive heart failure.

More often, the patient or his family notices that his face is pale and puffy, and that he has slight ankle edema in the evening. His appetite is poor, and he is up frequently during the night to void

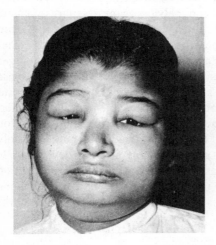

**Figure 48-15.** This patient has acute nephritis. (Vakil, R. J., and Golwalla, A.: *Clinical Diagnosis*, Bombay, Asia Pub. House)

(nocturia). He awakens with a headache (due to hypertension). His family and friends find him irritable, and he is out of breath after exertion. The patient may have only one symptom, such as a pitting, dependent edema (Fig. 48-15). Visual disturbances, often due to papilledema or hemorrhage, are common. Nosebleeds may occur. As the condition progresses, hematuria, anemia, convulsions associated with hypertension, congestive heart failure, oliguria, and perhaps anuria may appear.

The laboratory findings may include a slightly elevated blood urea nitrogen and albuminuria. There will be gross or microscopic hematuria, giving the urine a dark, smoky, or frankly bloody appearance.

**Treatment.** There is no specific treatment for acute glomerulonephritis. Therapy is guided by the symptoms and their underlying pathology. The following regimen is usual:

- **Bed rest. While the blood pressure is elevated and edema is present, bed rest may continue for several weeks. When progressive ambulation is slowly started, daily urine specimens are usually collected, and blood pressure is recorded daily. Any increase in hematuria, albuminuria, or blood pressure is an indication for a return to bed rest.**
- **Hydration. Fluids should be taken liberally. Since the glomeruli are damaged, there is a filtration problem. To get rid of waste products, the body needs ample fluids. However, in the presence of marked edema, oliguria, or anuria, fluids are limited to balance output.**
- **Diet. Sodium is restricted when edema is present. Carbohydrate intake is encouraged, especially when proteins are limited. Most physicians restrict protein intake during the acute phase, until the nitrogen balance of the body is normal. Some give a high-protein diet to replace the proteins being lost in urine. A high-protein, low-sodium supplement, such as Lanolac, may be used. Vitamins may be added to the diet to improve the patient's general resistance. Iron or liver may be needed to counteract anemia.**
- **Medication. Antibiotics may be given to prevent a superimposed infection on the already inflamed kidney. The relatively insoluble sulfonamides are contraindicated because they may lead to obstructive crystalluria and further renal damage.**

In the seriously ill patient a trial of corticosteroids may be given in efforts to alter the course of the disease. When the blood pressure climbs to high levels, antihypertensive drugs are usually given.

The patient is not considered to be cured until

his urine is free of albumin and red blood cells for six months. Return to full activity usually is not permitted until the urine is free of protein for a month.

**Prognosis.** Most patients with acute glomerulonephritis recover, usually completely. A few develop chronic glomerulonephritis. Subsequent infections with the same strain of hemolytic streptococci usually do not cause a second attack of acute glomerulonephritis. This is in sharp contrast to chronic glomerulonephritis in which upper respiratory infections must be studiously avoided to prevent exacerbations of the disease.

## Chronic Glomerulonephritis

Chronic glomerulonephritis causes permanent damage to the nephrons. Some disappear entirely. Bands of scar tissue contract the kidney and replace the functioning units. The cortex becomes distorted and shrunken.

**Symptoms.** A small number of patients with chronic glomerulonephritis are known to have had acute glomerulonephritis, but most give no such history. Symptoms are similar to those of acute glomerulonephritis, but they may be even more individualized. There may be generalized edema, headache and hypertension, visual disturbances, nocturia, dyspnea, and albuminuria. Anemia, cardiac failure, and cerebral symptoms are not uncommon. The patient who develops anasarca is said to be in the *nephrotic* stage. Generalized edema is due to the depletion of serum proteins, with loss of plasma osmotic pressure. These patients may remain markedly edematous for months or years. Quiescent periods occur between exacerbations. During this *latent stage* the patient is relatively free of symptoms and feels well, although his urine contains protein.

The course of the disease is highly variable. The patient may live for years, with only occasional acute episodes or none at all; or the disease may be rapidly fatal due to uremia.

**Complications.** Congestive heart failure, pulmonary edema, increased blood pressure that may lead to cerebral hemorrhage, and secondary infection are common and sometimes fatal complications. Blurring of vision and blindness may occur late in the disease. Anemia is usual. Increased capillary fragility causes nosebleeds, purpura, and gastrointestinal bleeding in many terminally ill patients. Bronchopneumonia is a serious danger in the nephrotic stage.

High blood pressure over a period of months or years may lead to further renal insufficiency. *Nephrosclerosis* is the term given to kidney disease caused by hypertension in its malignant phase. The resulting symptoms are those of chronic glomerulonephritis.

**Treatment.** No treatment is given during quiescent stages. Nurses are in a position to assist patients and their families to maintain a healthful regimen for the patient. Everything that can be done should be done to increase his resistance to infection, since a cold may precipitate uremia. He should rest well, eat well, and have regular health supervision.

If the patient develops an infection, prompt medical treatment is imperative. Kidney function tests may be done annually. Death from uremia is the usual outcome of chronic glomerulonephritis, but it may be delayed for years with a regimen of healthful living, hemodialysis, or, in selected patients, renal transplantation.

When the disease becomes active, often evidenced initially by hematuria and edema, the patient is put on bed rest. Dietary considerations include low sodium intake and regulation of protein intake. Sedatives, often chloral hydrate, are given for headaches, hypertension, insomnia, and irritability. Diuretics containing mercury usually are not given, because they may increase the damage to the kidneys. Intravenous hypertonic solutions may be given to reduce intracranial pressure. If the patient has congestive heart failure, treatment of that condition, with such measures as digitalis, is necessary. Anemia, if it is severe, is treated with transfusions. The symptoms often subside in about three weeks, and very gradually the patient may return to normal activity. Because restitution of renal function lags behind the patient's clinical improvement, his convalescence should be planned carefully to avoid intercurrent infection, marked exertion, and body stress that may, in turn, affect renal function.

Treatment in the nephrotic stage includes bed rest to decrease the work of the heart, diuretics, and regulation of the diet, including sodium and fluid restriction. During this phase the patient is especially prone to intercurrent infection, and he may die of bronchopneumonia. The patient needs to be protected against infection carried to him on the hands or in the throats of hospital personnel and visitors.

## Nephrosis (the Nephrotic Syndrome)

The term *nephrosis* means a degenerative, noninflammatory disease of the renal tubules. The nephrotic syndrome is characterized by edema, albuminuria, decreased plasma proteins, and blood lipid abnormalities. There may be degenerative and necrotic lesions of the distal tubules, and renal vasoconstriction. The decrease in blood flow to the kidneys may lead to anuria and uremia. If the damage has not been too severe, and the circulation has not been too greatly impaired, the tubules are capable of regeneration.

Primary nephrosis is less common in adults than in children. However, nephrotic syndrome can be caused in adults by glomerulonephritis, crushing injuries to the kidneys, thermal burns, chemical poisoning with such agents as sulfonamides and carbon tetrachloride, and infectious diseases, such as syphilis, typhoid fever, and diphtheria. It is not caused by pyelonephritis. A biopsy may be done to establish the diagnosis.

The aim of treatment is to keep the patient alive until his kidneys repair themselves. When treatment with ACTH or adrenocortical steroids is effective, diuresis occurs and loss of protein in urine decreases or ceases. If the patient is not prostrated by the disease, he is often treated at home. Bed rest may not be necessary, but he should engage in only moderate activity during the acute phase and eat a high-protein diet to replace the protein lost in urine. Because of edema, the diet probably will also be low in sodium. In the hospital, if intravenous fluids are given (to supply electrolytes), special care must be taken to regulate the rate of the intravenous drip as it is ordered and to watch for signs of pulmonary edema. A careful record must be kept of the patient's weight; he may be retaining fluid.

The disease tends to be even more serious in adults than in children. Death may occur from renal failure, hypertension, or intercurrent infection when the patient is on corticosteroid therapy. If the kidneys do not seem to be recovering, and death from uremia is impending, dialysis (see Chapter 64 on renal failure) may be performed to give the kidneys more time to heal.

## REFERENCES AND BIBLIOGRAPHY

BEAUMONT, E.: Urinary drainage systems, *Nurs. '74* 4:52, January 1974.

BEHNKE, H. (ed.): Nursing management of patients with urologic tumors in *Guidelines for Comprehensive Nursing Care in Cancer,* New York, Springer, 1973.

BERGSTROM, N.: Ice application to induce voiding, *Am. J. Nurs.* 69:283, February 1969.

BERMAN, H.: Urinary diversion in treatment of carcinoma of the bladder, *Surg. Clin. N. Am.* 45:1495, December 1965.

BOYARSKY, S.: *Neurogenic Bladder,* Baltimore, Williams and Wilkins, 1967.

CAMPBELL, M. F., and HARRISON, J. H. (eds.): *Urology,* Vols. I, II, III, Philadelphia, Saunders, 1970.

CASTLE, M., and OSTERHOUT, S.: Urinary tract catheterization and associated infection, *Nurs. Res.* 23:170, March-April 1974.

CIRKSEMA, W.: Cutaneous manifestations of renal disease, *Hosp. Med.* 9:61, September 1973.

CLELAND, V., et al.: Prevention of bacteriuria in female patients with indwelling catheters, *Nurs. Res.* 20:309, July-August 1971.

CLARK, C.: Catheter care in the home, *Am. J. Nurs.* 72:922, May 1972.

DELEHANTY, L., and STRAVINO, V.: Achieving bladder control, *Am. J. Nurs.* 70:312, February 1970.

FIRFER, R.: Prevention—the best approach to the female urethral syndrome, *Consultant* 13:74, January 1973.

FOWKER, W., and HUNN, V.: *Clinical Assessment for the Nurse Practitioner,* St. Louis, Mosby, 1973.

GARDNER, K. D., JR.: Diagnosis: Urinary tract infection, *Consultant* 14:83, January 1974.

GENTILE, R., et al.: Nurse specialist has key role in the urological care team, *Hosp. Top.* 49:73, April 1971.

GIBBS, G.: Perineal care of the incapacitated patient, *Am. J. Nurs.* 69:124, January 1969.

GIESY, J. D.: Incontinence: Causes, diagnosis and treatment, *Hosp. Care* 3:2, January 1972.

HILKEMEYER, R.: Rehabilitation needs of patients with colostomy, ileostomy, or artificial bladder, in *Rehabilitation of the Cancer Patient,* Chicago, Year Book Medical Publishers, 1972.

JOHNSON, S. B.: Understanding hyperuricemia: Nursing implications, *Nurs. Clin. N. Am.* 7:399, June 1972.

KEUHNELIAN, J. G., and SANDERS, V. E.: *Urologic Nursing,* New York, Macmillan, 1970.

KRIZINOFSKI, M.: Human sexuality and nursing practice, *Nurs. Clin. N. Am.* 8:673, December 1973.

LANGFORD, T. L.: Nursing problem: Bacteriuria and the indwelling catheter, *Am. J. Nurs.* 72:113, January 1972.

MALIN, J.: Sex after urologic surgery, *Med. Asp. Human Sex.* 7:244, October 1973.

MARSHALL, S.: Cystitis and urethritis in women related to sexual activity, *Med. Asp. Human Sex.* 8:165, May 1974.

MONROE, J., and KOMORIA, N.: Problems with nephrosis in adolescence, *Am. J. Nurs.* 67:336, February 1967.

MOREL, A.: The team approach to the care of the urological patient, *AORN* 16:68, November 1972.

————: The urologic nurse specialist, *Nurs. Clin. N. Am.* 4:475, September 1969.

MULLAN, S.: *Essentials of Neurosurgery,* New York, Springer, 1961.

MULVANEY, W. P.: Urinary calculi . . . various types of urinary calculi of different compositions, (pictorial) *Hosp. Med.* 9:50, August 1973.

OYAMA, J. H.: Kidney stones? Diet can help, *Consultant* 13:35, March 1973.

ROBINSON, C.: *Basic Nutrition and Diet Therapy,* New York, Macmillan, 1970.

SHAPBELL, N. J., and SWERGART, J.: A urinary device for patients with problem stomas, *Nurs. Clin. N. Am.* 9:383, June 1974.

STRAFFON, R.: Urinary tract infection: Problems in diagnosis and management 1973, *Med. Clin. N. Am.* 58:545, May 1974.

SR. REGINA ELIZABETH: Sensory stimulation techniques, *Am. J. Nurs.* 66:281, February 1966.

————: The scientific rationale of bowel and bladder training, *Ariz. Med.,* Janunary 1966.

SMITH, D. R.: *General Urology,* ed. 6, Los Altos, Calif., Lange, 1970.

STYKER, R.: *Rehabilitative Aspects of Acute and Chronic Nursing Care,* Philadelphia, Saunders, 1972.

SUTTON, A.: *Bedside Nursing Techniques in Medicine and Surgery,* ed. 2, Philadelphia, Saunders, 1969.

The adult female patient: Managing urinary incontinence. *Patient Care* 7:70, February 1, 1973.

TUDOR, L.: Bladder and bowel retraining, *Am. J. Nurs.* 70:2391, November 1970.

WINTER, C., and ROEHM, M.: *Sawyer's Nursing Care of Patients With Urologic Diseases,* St. Louis, Mosby, 1968.

# UNIT NINE

## Problems Resulting from Endocrine Imbalance

# The Patient with an Endocrine Disorder

## CHAPTER 49

The endocrine (ductless) glands secrete substances, known as hormones, directly into the bloodstream where they affect, to some extent, every cell of the body. The hormones are often referred to as integrators of chemical reactions within the body because of their action upon enzyme systems to promote homeostasis of the internal environment. Therefore, the endocrine glands, along with the nervous system, control and regulate the functions of the body with precision and efficiency (see Fig. 49-1).

There is a close relationship between the nervous system and the endocrine system, with two endocrine structures, the adrenal medulla and the posterior pituitary, being neural in origin and secreting their hormones in response to electrical stimulation of the autonomic nervous system. The remaining endocrine structures include: the anterior pituitary, the thyroid, the parathyroids, the adrenal cortex, the pancreas, the ovarian follicles, and the interstitial cells of the testis. The anterior pituitary secretes at least eight hormones, many of which stimulate the secretion of one of the other endocrine glands, referred to as target glands. The anterior pituitary in turn receives its stimulus from the hypothalamus, which is known to contain releasing or inhibiting factors for all hormones of the anterior pituitary. Secretions from the anterior pituitary are controlled by a negative feedback mechanism; for example, the pituitary secretes thyroid-stimulating hormone, or thyrotropic hormone (TSH), causing the thyroid gland to produce its hormone, thyroxine, which, in turn, shuts off the pituitary secretion of TSH, because of the increased concentration of thyroxine in

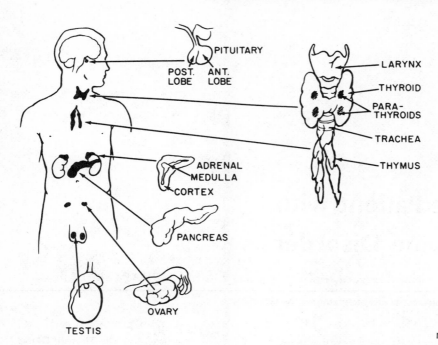

**Figure 49-1.** Location of hormone-producing glands in the body.

the circulating blood. As the blood level of thyroxine falls, the anterior pituitary again secretes thyroid-stimulating hormone.

The three primary functions of the hormones are: (1) *integrative action*, which occurs as the hormones travel in the bloodstream and reach all parts of the body, thereby permitting total response to external or internal stimuli, such as occurs with the release of epinephrine to mobilize the body defenses in threatening situations; (2) *regulation* of the internal environment of the body to maintain salt and water balance and the chemical reactions of the metabolic processes; and (3) *morphogenesis*, or control of the rate and type of growth of the organism.

The consequences of diseases of the ductless glands usually are due to overproduction or underproduction of the hormones that the glands secrete, causing a disturbance in the delicate balance that the hormones normally maintain, and often resulting in a widespread chain of pathologic events within the body.

Excess of hormone secretion may be due to overactivity of the gland itself, excessive secretion of its stimulating factor, abnormal production of hormones by tissues outside the gland, such as secreting tumors, or by inadequate deactivation and excretion of the hormone by the body. Deficiency states occur as a result of congenital absence,

idiopathic atrophy or surgical removal of the gland, or from errors of metabolism that prevent normal utilization of the hormone.

Secretion of hormones is not constant; rather, there are demonstrable rhythms to the process, with the monthly menstrual cycle in women being most familiar. The adrenocortical steroids are secreted according to a circadian rhythm, the daily pattern of activity and rest, with highest secretion early in the morning and the lowest at bedtime. When the circadian rhythm is altered, it takes the adrenal hormones about two weeks to reset to the new schedule. Rhythms and patterns of hormone secretion are being intensively studied as part of the investigation of biologic rhythms. Eventually they will provide evidence that can enhance therapy for dysfunction states, as well as advance our understanding of physiologic responses to altered circadian rhythm, as occurs, for example, in plane travel across time zones.

## THE THYROID GLAND

The thyroid gland, shaped like the letter "H," is located below the larynx and astride the trachea. The gland concentrates iodine, which is necessary for the production of the thyroid hormones thyroxine ($T_4$) and triiodothyronine ($T_3$). Ninety per cent of the hormone produced is in the form of thyroxine, which is carried in the bloodstream closely bound to plasma proteins. The thyroid hormones are necessary for cell metabolism as well as energy production and influence utilization of fats, carbohydrates, and protein. In addition, they are essential for normal growth and development, for normal functioning of the nervous system, and for maintaining water and electrolyte balance.

The thyroid gland produces a noniodinated hormone, calcitonin, discovered during the last decade. Calcitonin seems to have only one function, the reduction of plasma calcium by influencing calcium deposition in bone, thus working in opposition to the hormone secreted by the parathyroid glands.

The secretion of iodinated thyroid hormones is controlled by the hypothalamus, the anterior pituitary, and the metabolic demands of the body. The hypothalamus secretes thyrotropin-releasing factor (TRF), which stimulates the pituitary to secrete thyrotropic hormone (TSH), thus stimulating the thyroid gland to produce thyroxine. The control mechanism is the negative feedback system described above. Stress is believed to be a powerful stimulator of thyroid secretion, as is prolonged exposure to cold and increased food intake. Production of thyroxine is depressed by drugs such as sulfonamides, salicylates, phenylbutazone, and para-aminosalicylic acid, by foods with an excessively high iodine content, and by prolonged exposure to heat.

Disorders of the thyroid gland are due to deficient dietary iodine or to abnormal functioning of the hypothalamus, pituitary, or thyroid gland itself. These defects result in three possible conditions: (1) excessive output of thyroid hormone (hyperthyroidism), (2) insufficient output of thyroid hormone (hypothyroidism), or (3) an increase in the size of the thyroid gland (goiter) without obvious signs of hypo- or hyperthyroidism.

## Nursing Assessment

The patient with a thyroid disorder may have only a borderline imbalance and therefore may not exhibit all of the signs and symptoms associated with hyper- or hypofunction of the gland. Thus accurate nursing observations and recording are extremely important. In assessing this patient, the nurse should focus on the following questions:

- **Is the overall appearance of the patient one of alertness or sluggishness?**
- **Are eye movements normal?**
- **Is the voice hoarse?**
- **Does the skin appear pale and cool or flushed and damp?**
- **Does the hair appear normal or dry and thin?**
- **Is there any unusual hair growth?**
- **Does the neck appear to be swollen?**
- **Are there tremors of the hands?**
- **Does the patient exhibit sensitivity to heat or cold?**
- **Is the pulse rate rapid or slow?**
- **Is the heart rate regular or irregular?**
- **Is the patient's appetite good or poor?**
- **Has the patient experienced recent weight loss or gain?**
- **Has the patient experienced changes in menstrual cycle or changes in sex drive?**
- **Does the patient tire easily?**
- **Is the patient restless or somnolent?**
- **Is the blood pressure high or low?**
- **Have there been any changes in bowel habits?**
- **Has the patient been taking any medicines?**

The answers to these questions form part of the basis for planning the patient's care. Additional considerations include psychosocial factors, such as the kind of work the patient does, his response to the illness, his intellectual and coping abilities. The plan will differ, depending on whether thyroid function is excessive or deficient. As therapy is initiated, repeated observations must be made on a daily basis to assess the response to treatment and to make revisions in the care plan.

## Thyroid Function Tests

Tests of thyroid function most commonly employed are:

**Thyroxine ($T_4$) in Blood Serum.** This test measures free $T_4$ in blood serum and is based on the ability of nonprotein-bound hormone to pass a semipermeable membrane. Decreased values occur during pregnancy and in patients receiving estrogenic hormones.

**Triiodothyronine ($T_3$) Uptake Test.** This test assesses the interaction of thyroid hormone and plasma proteins. Tracer quantities of labeled hormone are added to a sample of the patient's serum. The amount of hormone that binds to the patient's plasma proteins is equivalent to the amount of endogenous hormone bound to plasma proteins. Uptake values are increased in hyperthyroidism and decreased in hypothyroidism.

**Protein-Bound Iodine (PBI).** Triiodothyronine and thyroxine are bound to the blood proteins that transport them. Because iodine is contained in the hormones, measurement of the PBI in a blood sample reflects the level of circulating thyroid hormone. Although the patient may be active and eat before blood is drawn for these tests, he should not have ingested any unusual amounts of iodine for several weeks. Substances containing iodine, such as some cough medicines and dyes administered for x-ray studies of the gallbladder, for intravenous pyelograms, and for bronchograms, will cause errors. Even antiseptic solutions of iodine on the skin should be avoided.

The normal concentration of PBI varies with the laboratory method used, but it is usually 4 to 8 mcg. per 100 ml. of plasma. Values below and above these figures usually indicate hypothyroidism and hyperthyroidism, respectively.

**Butanol-Extractable Iodine (BEI).** The BEI test measures the protein-bound iodine soluble in butanol. This eliminates inorganic iodides (from cough medicine, for example) and inactive iodinated proteins from measurement, since they are not soluble in butanol. Although this test can be more accurate than the PBI, it is more involved and expensive and therefore is not done routinely.

**Radioactive Iodine Uptake Test.** The fasting patient is given sodium radioiodide ($^{131}$I) either as a drink or in capsule form. Diluted in distilled water, the drug is odorless and tasteless. Then, 24 hours later, a *scintillator* (an instrument that measures radioactivity) is held over the thyroid gland to measure the amount of $^{131}$I that the thyroid has taken up. The normal thyroid will remove 15 to 50 per cent of the radioactive iodine from the bloodstream. The thyroid gland of a patient with hyperthyroidism may remove as much as 90 per cent.

**Thyroid Scanning.** The patient ingests $^{131}$I. Then a scintillator is passed back and forth across the throat, and a picture of radioactivity is recorded. The pattern of the scan indicates the concentration of iodine in the thyroid and other tissues and helps the physician to differentiate between noncancerous and malignant tissue of the thyroid when this test is used with other clinical findings.

**$^{131}$I Urine Excretion Test.** This test measures the amount of $^{131}$I excreted in 24 or 48 hours. Normally, 40 to 80 per cent is excreted, but a patient with hyperthyroidism excretes less than 40 per cent of the amount ingested. The nurse should be careful to save all urine specimens during the test period; none should be discarded. The dose is not large enough to warrant isolation precautions for radioactivity. The nurse should tell him that the amount of radiation in the tracer dose is minute and harmless.

**Radioactive $T_3$ Erythrocyte Uptake Test.** In this test the patient's blood is added to triiodothyronine that has been tagged with $^{131}$I. The amount of protein with which the hormone is bound is measured. Generally, high values are correlated with thyrotoxicosis.

**Thyroid Suppression Test.** When the results of other tests show borderline elevations, the thyroid suppression test may be used. First, a baseline measurement is made of $^{131}$I uptake by the thyroid gland. Then, fast-acting thyroid hormone is given for seven days, and the $^{131}$I uptake test is repeated. If the patient has hyperthyroidism, the hormone will not suppress the uptake of $^{131}$I by the thyroid, since in hyperthyroidism the gland is autonomous. In persons with a normal thyroid, the administered hormone decreases the amount of TSH produced by the pituitary and, therefore, decreases $^{131}$I uptake, since the pituitary-thyroid relationship is intact.

Because an abnormally high intake of iodine may harm the validity of these tests, foods high in iodine, such as large amounts of iodized table salt, are not eaten for about a week before taking any $^{131}$I tests. Also, medications containing iodine and thyroid extract are avoided.

**Blood Cholesterol.** In this diagnostic test, 5 ml. of blood are taken from the fasting patient. The normal values are 150 to 250 mg. per 100 ml. of blood. In hyperthyroidism the patient's blood cholesterol is often lower than normal, but the results of this test vary greatly. Serum cholesterol is elevated in myxedema and can be followed during treatment of this condition.

**Basal Metabolic Rate (BMR).** This test determines the rate at which an individual consumes oxygen under standard resting conditions. Because it is difficult to obtain reliable results, the BMR is infrequently used.

## Hyperthyroidism

Hyperthyroidism can be divided into two types. The first, and more common, is Graves' disease (thyrotoxicosis), and is due to a diffuse toxic goiter. The second, and much less common type, is due to toxic nodules in the thyroid (toxic nodular goiter, or Plummer's disease). It is easy to differentiate between these two conditions because the patient with diffuse toxic goiter may have exophthalmos (abnormal protrusion of the eyeball), whereas the patient with nodular toxic goiter never has exophthalmos (Fig. 49-2).

## Etiology

The etiology of Graves' disease is still speculative, but it appears to be an autoimmune disease or disorder. A substance called LATS (long-acting thyroid stimulator) has been isolated in most but not all patients with Graves' disease. This substance is presumably produced either by the pituitary or the hypothalamus; consequently an abnormal pituitary-thyroid relationship is thought to be responsible for diffuse toxic goiter and its manifestations. The toxic nodular goiter is an autonomous condition in that it originates in the thyroid gland and there is no evidence the pituitary is involved. Women are afflicted more frequently than men.

## Symptoms

Patients with well-developed hyperthyroidism are characteristically restless, highly excitable, and constantly agitated. They are emotionally labile, laughing one minute and crying the next. Often, they overreact to situations; for instance, they may take violent offense to a slight that ordinarily would be ignored. The patient may have fine tremors so that he needs help to eat. Clumsiness, due to tremors, may cause the patient to drop things. Muscular weakness and fatigability are common. The pulse may be as high as 160. Characteristically, there is an increase in systolic but not in diastolic blood pressure. The patient may experience palpitations and, if the condition is untreated, the continued excess activity may lead to cardiac decompensation.

The constant exercise and the high rate of metabolism cause the patient to lose weight, even though his appetite is usually great, and he consumes an extra number of calories. The patient with a severely overactive thyroid must satisfy his need for food and even the patient with less severe thyrotoxicosis should eat a high caloric, high carbohydrate diet.

The increased metabolic rate makes the patient intolerant of heat. This symptom can be troublesome on a ward, because ventilation that is comfortable for other patients is stifling to the patient with thyrotoxicosis; what feels comfortable to him chills the other patients. If possible, the patient

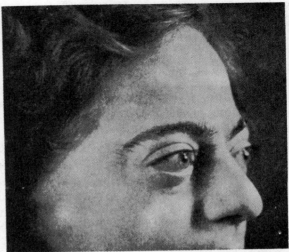

**Figure 49-2.** Exophthalmos in Graves' disease. (Cecil, R. L., and Loeb, R. F. (eds.): *A Textbook of Medicine,* ed. 5, Philadelphia, Saunders)

should have his own room in which he can adjust the temperature himself. If this is not possible, he should be placed next to the window.

Other symptoms include characteristically fine and flushed skin, menstrual abnormalities, changed bowel habits, and excessive sweating. There may be hoarseness and difficulty in swallowing due to the enlarged gland.

Many patients with hyperthyroidism exhibit exophthalmos, which gives them a permanently startled expression. This condition is not caused by an excess of thyroxine, but rather is thought to be the result of an abnormal secretion of a recently discovered pituitary hormone that increases the amount of water and fat stored behind the eyeballs. Exophthalmos sometimes occurs in the absence of the hyperthyroid syndrome and frequently this condition is unresponsive to therapy for hyperthyroidism. Usually, there is a visible swelling of the neck due to the enlarged thyroid gland.

Severe hyperthyroidism is seen less frequently today than formerly, because it is more common now for the disease to be recognized and treated earlier.

## Treatment and Nursing Care

Treatment of hyperthyroidism is directed at reducing the excessive activity of the gland and may be accomplished by administering antithyroid drugs, destroying glandular tissue by radiation, or surgically removing part of the gland.

**Antithyroid Drugs.** These agents block the production of thyroid hormone. Propylthiouracil, methimazole, or another drug of the thiourea group, may be given as medical treatment of hyperthyroidism or as preparation for surgery. The effects of the drug do not become evident until the excess thyroid hormone stored in the thyroid gland has been secreted into the bloodstream. This process may take several weeks. The usual daily dose of propylthiouracil is 100 to 600 mg. but must be individualized for each patient. The drug is excreted rapidly so that dosage needs to be given at regular intervals during the day, whether the patient is hospitalized or not. The nurse should instruct the patient to follow the physician's directions about the number of tablets to take and the intervals at which the drug should be taken. One patient who did not understand the importance of regularly spacing the medication took all the pills at once each day. The patient who is treated without surgery usually takes the antithyroid drug for at least a year, and during that time must have frequent assessment of his health status.

Toxic effects include agranulocytosis, fever, sore throat, skin rash, enlarged lymph nodes and malaise. If any of these reactions is observed, it should be reported to the physician, who may discontinue the drug. Periodic hematologic studies should be made to check the white blood-cell count and differential smear.

Another antithyroid drug, Lugol's solution, contains 5 per cent iodine and 10 per cent potassium iodide in water. Iodine causes the gland to involute and become less vascular. For this reason, to decrease bleeding during surgery, patients who are scheduled for a thyroidectomy will often have a short course of iodine treatment preoperatively. For at least two weeks before surgery, 5 to 15 minims., three times daily, of either Lugol's solution or potassium iodide are given by mouth. The drug is diluted in milk or fruit juice to prevent the iodine from burning and to make it more palatable. Drinking it through a straw will prevent the iodine from staining the teeth. The maximum effect is expected in 10 to 14 days. Toxic effects may occur if the patient receives iodine for long periods of time, but this is unusual. These effects include symptoms of the common cold, increased salivation, skin rash, fever and, occasionally, a mumpslike syndrome with swollen salivary glands.

Radioactive iodine ($^{131}I$) may be given to a patient with thyrotoxicosis to destroy the hyperplastic thyroid tissue by radiation. Because the thyroid gland is quick to pick up iodine from the bloodstream, $^{131}I$ is taken up and stored in that gland, and for this reason it is currently believed that the usual therapeutic dose does not affect seriously any other tissues of the body. No increase in the incidence of leukemia, cancer of the thyroid, or fetal abnormalities has been noted after the use of radioactive iodine in adults. However, as a precautionary measure, young patients and pregnant women usually are treated with surgery or antithyroid drugs. The dosage of $^{131}I$ is based on the estimated weight of the thyroid gland, the patient's age, his clinical symptoms, and the emanations from the gland as shown on a scintillator or Geiger counter. The drug is given once, and the patient is watched for several months. If his symptoms do not disappear, a second dose may be given, and perhaps a third. The internal irradiation allows a dose to be given without endangering the skin. There may be transient symptoms of radiation sickness (nausea, vomiting, malaise, fever), and the gland may feel tender. These reactions are rare. A more common unfortunate sequel to $^{131}I$ is hypothyroidism (discussed later in this chapter). It has been reported that as many as 43 per cent of patients treated with $^{131}I$ develop hypothyroidism when they are followed for longer than ten years. Because this complication may not occur for many years after the administration of $^{131}I$, patients must remain under medical supervision for many years.

In about six to eight weeks after the initial dose of $^{131}I$ the patient often notices that his symptoms are beginning to subside. The length of time required before the patient notices improvement is one of the disadvantages of this treatment. The patient should be instructed to avoid strenuous activity and to eat a nutritious diet.

$^{131}I$ emits gamma and beta rays. Even though gamma rays penetrate tissue (beta rays travel only a few millimeters) the dose administered in the treatment of hyperthyroidism is not large enough to constitute a radiation hazard to others. The patient may be worried about this and also about the effects on his body. The nurse can assure the patient that the medication is not a radiation danger.

**Surgery of the Thyroid.** Subtotal thyroidectomy is an effective treatment for hyperthyroidism. About seven-eighths of the glandular tissue is removed. Total thyroidectomy may be performed if malignancy is present. Because of the effectiveness of treatment with [131]I, surgery is more commonly performed when malignancy is suspected, in patients under 35 years of age and in pregnant women for whom the physicians are reluctant to use irradiation.

PREOPERATIVE CARE. The patient is given a course of antithyroid drugs, a high caloric and high vitamin diet and rest. Usually, surgery is delayed until the patient is euthyroid clinically as well as by laboratory tests. If the hyperthyroidism is not controlled before surgery, there is increased risk of postoperative thyroid crisis. The patient may be prepared for surgery in his own home or in the hospital; or he may spend several days in the hospital and then go home until he is ready for surgery. The preoperative period may be as long as several months, and the suspense is especially trying for the patient who usually feels jittery anyway because of his increased metabolic rate.

The patient should be helped by the nurse not to feel ashamed of his restlessness and irritability. The nurse can point out the temporary nature of his highly emotional state, and explain that it is related to the disease. The patient with hyperthyroidism often talks too excitedly and too much, and so the nurse should avoid garrulity. The patient's environment should be as calming as possible. The nurse may help the patient to find diversion that is both restful and enjoyable. Does he like to read? Talking quietly with the nurse may help the patient to relax and rest.

The patient's visitors should help him to rest. Suggest that visitors refrain from bringing up matters that may cause the patient any excitement or distress, and that they keep their visits short, calm, and pleasant.

To help the patient to sleep at night, the nurse should give him a back rub and straighten the bed just before the lights go out. These measures help to relieve the feeling of warmth and irritability so common among patients with hyperthyroidism.

In preparation for surgery, the patient should be encouraged to eat as much as possible. His glass should be kept full of orange juice or eggnog for snacks. A good rule to remember is that the hyperthyroid patient on bed rest needs about twice as much food as the normal person *not* on bed rest. The patient is weighed daily. His blood pressure should be recorded every day. When the nurse takes the patient's pulse, she should watch for irregularities as well as count the rate. If the patient's heart has been affected by the thyrotoxicosis, he probably will be placed on bed rest. Helping the patient to rest during this period is a great challenge. He will need help in getting comfortable, in settling down to something that interests him, and in not feeling lonely. Frequent attention to the bed is necessary because of the patient's restlessness. Preoperatively, the patient may be given oxygen to help to meet his increased need for it.

POSTOPERATIVE CARE. The patient may be placed on his back, with small, firm pillows holding his head still, so that he does not disturb the fresh wound by thrashing. He needs constant observation for mucus and frequent, prompt suctioning. When he has reacted, the head of his bed may be moderately elevated. Pillows are positioned under head, neck, and shoulders, with firm support being the objective. The patient should not move his head up and down until the wound has healed considerably. When the nurse helps the patient to move in bed, she should support his head so that it does not fall back or have any strain placed on the neck muscles (Fig. 49-3). When the patient is alone, his beverage, tissues, and whatever else he might need should be put on the overbed table in front of him, so that he does not have to reach over to the stand.

The patient usually is allowed out of bed the day after the operation. His head should be well supported while he gets into position to dangle his feet. He should hold his head still with his hands while he walks a step or two (Fig. 49-4), and it should be supported with firm pillows while he sits up in a chair. His attempt to hold his head still may cause a headache that can be relieved by rubbing the back of the neck.

Immediately after surgery the nurse watches for symptoms of respiratory obstruction. Edema or bleeding can compress the trachea, causing an inability to breathe. This catastrophe must be treated within minutes by inserting an endotracheal tube or by a tracheostomy. A sterile tracheostomy set is kept in the patient's room, ready for immediate use if needed.

Aspiration is a danger, since laryngeal and tracheal reflexes will be depressed. Suction as neces-

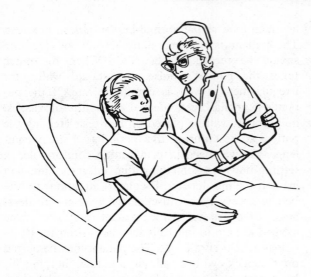

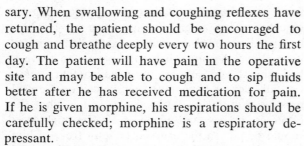

**Figure 49-3.** In helping the patient to sit up after a thyroidectomy, the nurse slides one hand under the patient's head to help to support it. The patient's back and neck are supported by the nurse's arm.

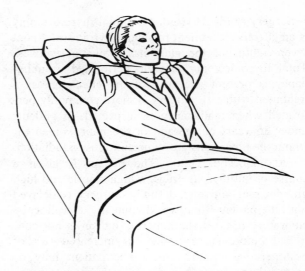

**Figure 49-4.** After a thyroidectomy the patient uses her hands to support her head while she raises herself to a sitting position. This support helps to avoid strain on the neck muscles.

sary. When swallowing and coughing reflexes have returned, the patient should be encouraged to cough and breathe deeply every two hours the first day. The patient will have pain in the operative site and may be able to cough and to sip fluids better after he has received medication for pain. If he is given morphine, his respirations should be carefully checked; morphine is a respiratory depressant.

The nurse should watch for bleeding. A small amount of blood in the wound can obstruct respirations. She should pay attention if the patient complains of a sense of fullness in the wound. Blood may not be evident on the front of the bandage, but it may ooze around to the back of the patient's neck. Periodically during the first postoperative 12 hours, the nurse should pass her hand behind the patient's neck to see whether it feels damp. When she turns the patient to his side, she should look for blood on the dressing. If the bandage encircling the neck becomes too tight, she should loosen but not remove it, and call the surgeon. She should observe for restlessness, apprehension, respiratory distress, an increased pulse or temperature, decreased blood pressure, and cyanosis. Neck swelling may be due to bleeding and accumulation of blood in the wound, distending the tissues. Physicians sometimes request that sutures be removed if blood is accumulating in the wound.

Infrequently, the recurrent laryngeal nerve is in-

jured during the operation. The patient is hoarse or may be unable to speak due to vocal cord paralysis. Respiratory obstruction may result. Hoarseness or any voice change should be reported to the physician. The patient should be encouraged not to talk much the first two postoperative days. Steam inhalations may be ordered.

Another infrequent postoperative complication is tetany (muscular hypertonia with spasm and tremor), due to a low concentration of calcium from the inadvertent removal of the parathyroid glands during thyroidectomy. The patient complains of numbness and tingling of the extremities and muscle cramps. Tetany also can cause laryngeal spasm. The method of treatment used is intravenous or oral calcium.

Thyroid crisis or storm, now a rare complication of thyroid surgery, may occur within the first 12 hours postoperatively. All symptoms of hyperthyroidism are exaggerated. The patient's temperature may be as high as 106, the pulse becomes very rapid, and cardiac arrhythmias are common. There may be persistent vomiting and extreme restlessness with delirium. The patient becomes exhausted, and not infrequently dies from cardiac failure. The treatment is intravenous sodium iodide, intravenous corticosteroids, oxygen, reserpine to slow the heart rate and cooling by applying ice, cool enemas, or a controlled thermoblanket. Morphine (or other sedation), Lugol's solution, propylthiouracil, and corticosteroids also may be ordered.

The incidence of hypothyroidism in patients subjected to surgery approximates 25 to 30 per cent in cases followed for relatively long periods. Long-term complications of thyroid surgery include hypoparathyroidism, and injury to the recurrent laryngeal nerve with vocal cord palsy (Mannix).

If the patient had a subtotal thyroidectomy, he should return to the physician periodically for re-evaluation. A patient being treated medically should be faithful in keeping his appointments with the physician, who will check on his condition and adjust drug dosage.

Since the incision for a thyroidectomy is made in a crease of the neck, the healed scar is barely visible; it is merely a thin line. If a woman patient seems concerned about it, you may suggest that she wear high-necked dresses and scarves until the scar contracts to its final tiny size. With the surgeon's approval, periodic massage of the operative scar during the first few postoperative weeks may help to obtain a good cosmetic result.

### Euthyroid Disease (Nontoxic Goiter)

In simple goiter, the thyroid gland enlarges without hypersecretion of thyroid hormones. It is caused by deficient iodine in the diet, which is necessary for the production of hormones. The gland enlarges in an attempt to produce sufficient hormone to meet metabolic demands. This condition is endemic in areas of the world where the soil and drinking water contain little, if any, iodine, such as inland and mountainous regions. In the United States, goiter is found in the Great Lakes region and in the Pacific Northwest.

Goiter can also occur from the consumption of food containing an excessively high iodine content.

Nontoxic goiter is more frequent in women than in men. It appears (sometimes only temporarily) when there is an increase in the need for thyroid hormone, and thus for the iodine to make it—at times of stress, during infection, in adolescence, and during pregnancy. In some areas of the world, a large percentage of adolescent girls have nontoxic goiters.

**Symptoms.** The thyroid gland grows noticeably larger and a sense of fullness develops in the throat. When growth is excessive, it can cause tracheal compression, but otherwise the health of the person is not impaired.

**Treatment and Prevention.** Usually thyroid extract or iodine is administered orally and after several months of treatment the size of the goiter may diminish, unless irreversible cellular changes have occurred in the thyroid tissue. Large goiters may be surgically removed.

Endemic goiter can be prevented by adding iodine to table salt. Most state boards of health request iodization of salt by manufacturers, which has greatly reduced the incidence of iodine-deficient goiters in the United States. The World Health Organization is making a similar effort in other iodine-poor areas of the world. It is known that populations in iodine-poor areas are subject to an increased incidence of other thyroid conditions.

### Thyroid Cancer

Thyroid cancer is suspected when there is an enlarged lump, which is hard to the touch, other local structures have been invaded, and when the area of the thyroid containing the lump does not concentrate [131]I as well as the surrounding normal thyroid tissue.

If the tumor is accessible, treatment is surgical and most often radical (total thyroidectomy with removal of the local lymph glands in the neck). However, considerable difference of opinion exists concerning the surgical treatment of carcinoma of the thyroid. Some surgeons advocate total thyroidectomy with radical neck dissection; others advocate the less extensive procedure of thyroid lobectomy.

After the operation thyroid replacement therapy is given in order to replace those hormones that can no longer be produced due to the absence of the thyroid gland, and to suppress pituitary TSH so that it will not stimulate the growth of residual malignant thyroid tissue.

If there is an inaccessible thyroid cancer, either local or metastatic, which can take up iodine, I[131] may be given. The malignancy will take it up and be destroyed. This effect can be enhanced by administering TSH, because it stimulates increased uptake of the radioactive iodine by the thyroid.

Approximately 80 per cent of thyroid cancer is well differentiated and has a relatively low degree of malignancy. Approximately 10 per cent of thyroid cancer falls into the group now classified as medullary thyroid cancer. This type has intermediate degree of malignancy and may be associated with other endocrine disorders such as tumors

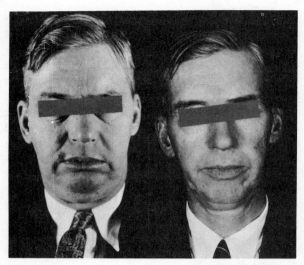

**Figure 49-5.** Myxedema. (*Left*) Before treatment. (*Right*) Appearance of patient after two years of treatment with desiccated thyroid extract. (Hurxthal, L. M., and Musulin, N.: *Clinical Endocrinology,* vol. 1, p. 430, Philadelphia, Lippincott)

of the adrenal glands or parathyroid. The final 10 per cent of thyroid cancer tends to be very malignant and is more or less incurable no matter what form of therapy is undertaken (Mannix).

### Hashimoto's Thyroiditis (Chronic Thyroiditis)

In Hashimoto's disease, atrophy of the thyroid occurs with invasion of the gland by lymphocytes, which eventually replace glandular tissue. The disease is thought to be due to an autoimmune reaction in which thyroid constituents become the antigen, resulting in destruction of the gland. Thyroid failure may result. Treatment consists of administering thyroid medications and cortisone. Thyroidectomy is frequently performed because a high incidence of malignancy is associated with Hashimoto's disease.

### Hypothyroidism

This disease is due to a deficiency of thyroid hormones, causing a lowered rate of all metabolic processes. It results in a set of symptoms called *myxedema* in the adult (Fig. 49-5). The condition may originate within the thyroid (primary hypothyroidism) or within the pituitary, manifested by a lack of TSH (secondary hypothyroidism).

### Diagnosis

In the TSH-stimulation test there is no increase in $^{131}$I uptake after TSH has been administered, when hypothyroidism is due to primary failure of the gland to function properly. If the hypothyroidism is secondary to pituitary insufficiency and a lack of TSH, then administered TSH will increase the $^{131}$I uptake. An x-ray film of the skull may be taken to examine the pituitary fossa for abnormalities, such as those that may be caused by a tumor. The results of BMR, PBI, and $^{131}$I uptake tests are low, and cholesterol is elevated.

A problem in the early recognition of hypothyroidism is that many of the symptoms are nonspecific, and may not be sufficiently dramatic to cause the patient to seek health care. This condition can go untreated for years. The nurse who notices such symptoms as puffiness of the face, chronic fatigue or intolerance to cold should refer the client to the physician.

### Etiology

Atrophy of the thyroid gland may occur after pneumonia, typhoid fever and influenza. Thyroid inflammation and surgery or irradiation for hyperthyroidism also can cause hypothroidism. Or, the deficiency may be due to an autoimmune process, in which the patient develops antibodies against his own thyroid tissue. Very often the cause is unknown. Women are affected more often than men.

### Symptoms

The symptoms of hypothyroidism are opposite in many respects to those of hyperthyroidism. Metabolic rate and both the physical and mental activity of the patient are slowed. The hypothyroid patient feels lethargic, lacks energy, dozes frequently during the day, is forgetful, and has chronic headaches. The face takes on a masklike, stolid, unemotional expression, yet the patient is often irritable. The tongue may be enlarged, the lips may be swollen, and there is nonpitting edema of the eyelids. The temperature and the pulse are decreased, and there is intolerance to cold. The patient gains weight easily. His skin is dry, and his hair characteristically is coarse and sparse, tending to fall out. A woman patient frequently has a menstrual disorder. Constipation may be severe enough to require daily enemas. The voice of the myxedema patient is low-pitched, slow and hoarse. His hearing may be impaired. There may be numbness or tingling in the arms or legs, unrelieved by change of position. Hypothyroidism may lead to enlargement of the heart due to pericardial effusion and an increased tendency toward atherosclerosis and heart strain. Anemia also may result.

## Treatment and Nursing Care

Because his metabolic processes are depressed, the patient may feel chilled in a room that is comfortable for others. In a ward his bed should not be placed next to a window, and he may need extra blankets or a robe while he is in bed. Even though his appetite is poor, he has a tendency to gain weight. The diet is usually low calorie and may be high in roughage and protein. The nurse should check daily to see whether or not he has had a bowel movement. Too many days without one may lead to an impaction. Until medication causes the patient's rough skin to soften, the nurse should apply lotion or cream, especially on the back, the elbows, and the feet.

Patients with hypothyroidism are inordinately susceptible to sedative and hypnotic drugs. If any such are ordered (a rare circumstance), the patient must be watched carefully for narcosis and diminished respirations, as he may develop respiratory failure. He should never be ignored just because he is sleeping quietly. He should be observed frequently, and his respirations counted.

Hypothyroidism is treated by replacement therapy. The patient is supplied with thyroid hormone in the form of desiccated thyroid extract or with synthetic products, such as crystalline thyroxine or triiodothyronine. Thyroid extract is very slow to act; and the dose, given by mouth, can be taken once a day. Patients may be started on 15 mg. of thyroid extract and maintained on the dose found most appropriate. The side effects of replacement therapy may include dyspnea, rapid pulse, palpitations, precordial pain, hyperactivity, insomnia, dizziness, and gastrointestinal disorders. Occasionally, a skin rash may be seen.

Before treatment has become effective, the patient's movement may be so slow that one is reminded of a slow-motion movie. If a patient with severe hypothyroidism is asked to turn over for back care, there may be a considerable interval before he responds. It is important to let these patients do things for themselves and to resist the temptation to do for them, just to get it over with. They should not be expected to move quickly, because they are incapable of doing so.

Once replacement therapy has begun, a dramatic change in the patient's symptoms may be seen in a few weeks. He feels the return of a new interest in life. His hair again becomes soft and attractive, and he can stay awake for 16 hours in one stretch. His mental and physical activities are quickened.

Because these changes in his condition may be rapid and profound, the patient may be hospitalized during the early days of treatment. The nurse has an important responsibility to observe carefully for changes in the symptoms. If the patient's heart or blood vessels have been affected by hypothyroidism, the sudden improvement in his metabolic rate may impose an additional strain on the cardiovascular system. For instance, if the coronary arteries are sclerotic, they may not be able to supply the heart with sufficient blood for its sudden increase in activity. The nurse should be alert to complaints of precordial pain, dyspnea, and changes in pulse rate, and report complaints that may indicate cardiac involvement to the physician.

These patients usually have to take thyroid extract for the remainder of their lives. A patient who is treated early and is well regulated should continue to feel well. However, periodic visits to the physician are necessary to ensure continuing the proper dosage. The nurse should emphasize to the patient the importance of keeping his appointments.

## THE PARATHYROID GLANDS

The parathyroid glands are tiny, pea-shaped bodies, usually four in number, imbedded on either side of the posterior aspect of the thyroid gland. Aberrant parathyroid tissue is often found in the mediastinum. These glands secrete parathyroid hormone (PTH), which regulates the two-way traffic of calcium between blood and bone, maintaining the physiologic levels of calcium and phosphorus in the blood. The hormone is also known to increase calcium absorption from the gastrointestinal tract, increase calcium reabsorption from the kidneys, and cause the kidneys to excrete phosphorus. As far as is presently known, the pituitary gland exerts no control over the parathyroids. Parathyroid activity appears to be controlled by blood serum levels of calcium; that is, decreased blood calcium levels stimulate PTH secretion. Calcitonin, a hormone secreted by the thyroid gland, opposes the action of parathyroid hormone and inhibits the withdrawal of calcium from bone.

Most of the calcium in the body (99 per cent)

is in the form of calcium phosphate, the hard part of bone tissue. Bone is constantly being remodeled and forms the reservoir of calcium used elsewhere in the body. Calcium preserves normal neuromuscular activity, as it affects the contractility of all muscles, including the heart, and promotes transmission of impulses at nerve junctions and between nerves and muscles. It is essential for blood coagulation, and it is necessary to meet the needs of the growing fetus during pregnancy, and of the breasts during lactation.

### Nursing Assessment

Since parathyroid dysfunction affects calcium and phosphorus metabolism, the nurse must be alert to signs associated with excess or deficient PTH secretion. In hyperparathyroidism, there will be an excessive shift in calcium stores from bone to blood with three primary results: (1) increased possibility of renal calculi formation due to the poor solubility of calcium salts, (2) demineralization of bone, and (3) slower nerve impulse transmission. Therefore, the nurse should observe the patient for symptoms of calculi formation, such as flank pain, passing "sand" during urination, or renal colic. As the bones lose calcium, the patient can be expected to evidence bone pain, difficulty with mobility, and deformity of structure. Effects on the nervous system will cause the patient to exhibit easy fatigability, weakness, and emotional changes, such as mental sluggishness, irritability, and depression. Other physiologic changes are alteration in cardiac rhythm, digestive disturbances ranging from anorexia to nausea and vomiting, stomach atony, possible development of peptic ulcers, and constipation. The patient will, of course, experience weight loss. Calcium deposits develop in small blood vessels and soft tissues, which may lead to ulceration and necrosis.

The nurse should note the results of serum calcium and phosphorus determinations, x-ray examinations, and ECG studies for deviations from normal.

In hypoparathyroidism excess amounts of calcium leave the blood, leading to increased neuromuscular excitability, manifested as a condition known as tetany. Tetany usually begins with numbness and tingling of the extremities, stiffness or cramps of the extremities, and carpopedal spasm. These symptoms may progress to laryngeal stridor

and generalized convulsions. The patient is usually emotionally labile.

The nurse assesses latent tetany by two determinations: *Chvostek's sign,* a twitch of the facial muscles when the facial nerve is tapped in front of the ear, and *Trousseau's sign,* the induction of carpopedal spasm by reducing circulation in the arm with a blood pressure cuff. The constriction is maintained for three minutes to be conclusive.

### Hyperparathyroidism

The etiology of primary hyperparathyroidism is unknown. Usually, an adenoma of one or more of the glands is discovered at surgery. Malignancy of the glands is rare. The glands are known to become hyperplastic secondary to conditions that tend to lower blood calcium levels, such as chronic renal disease or multiple myeloma, and which cause a compensatory increase in parathyroid function.

Diagnosis of parathyroid dysfunction is based on the signs and symptoms discussed above: x-ray films of the skeleton showing evidence of bone demineralization, elevated serum calcium levels, low plasma phosphate levels, increased urinary excretion of calcium, and changes in the electrocardiogram. A parathyroid hormone infusion test may be done. This procedure evaluates parathyroid function by measurement of the tubular reabsorption rate of phosphate in patients before and after the administration of parathyroid extract. For this test, the patient is instructed to drink three to four glasses of milk per day for three days before the test. The patient is permitted nothing by mouth on the morning of the test, and an infusion of 5 per cent dextrose in water is started and run over a period of twelve hours. All urine voided during this time is collected and analyzed for phosphate. A blood sample is taken after six hours of the infusion. The following day the same procedure is repeated with the addition of 200 units of parathyroid extract to the infusion. The results of phosphate excretion during the two days are compared; little responsiveness to the additional hormone is diagnostic of hyperparathyroidism.

The most reliable test for primary hyperparathyroidism is the determination by radioimmunoassay of serum parathormone levels. This technique is done only in certain institutions. However, in a situation where diagnosis is uncertain, it should be done before surgery is undertaken.

## Treatment and Nursing Care

Hypertrophied gland tissue or an adenoma is removed surgically. Postoperative care is quite similar to that given after thyroidectomy. The nurse must be especially alert to symptoms of tetany, which frequently occur in patients who have shown signs of bone disease. Infusions of calcium gluconate should be available at the bedside and may be given several times a day until calcium balance is reestablished. When oral intake is permitted, a diet high in calcium and protein is prescribed. Supplemental vitamin D may be indicated for several months after surgery. Since the patient is prone to pathologic fractures, he must be protected from injury. However, mobility will increase bone recalcification, so active and passive exercise as well as progressive ambulation are encouraged.

## Hypoparathyroidism

Hypoparathyroidism is due most often to damage to or inadvertent removal of the glands during thyroid surgery. In some instances, the glands simply cease functioning, believed by some to be the result of an autoimmune state.

Diagnosis of hypoparathyroidism is made on the basis of signs and symptoms of tetany, a fall in plasma calcium levels, and by a rise in plasma phosphates. When the disease is chronic, diagnosis is more difficult because symptoms may be vague. In patients with long-standing hypoparathyroidism, scaliness of the skin, thinning of hair on all body areas, and deformities of fingernails and toenails are evident. Cataracts are common, as are changes in the teeth.

## Treatment and Nursing Care

The treatment for hypoparathyroidism includes the administration of a vitamin D-like preparation, dihydrotachysterol (AT 10 or Hytakerol), or vitamin $D_2$ (calciferol). These drugs increase the blood level of calcium. Dosage is related to the degree of hypocalcemia, which is determined by frequent measurements of blood calcium. Urine calcium levels also may be checked.

Treatment of hypoparathyroid tetany also includes the administration of calcium salts, and, occasionally, parathyroid extract. Calcium gluconate may first be given intravenously, 10 to 50 ml. of a 10 per cent solution in 1,000 ml. of normal saline. Intravenous calcium causes vasodilation; the patient feels hot and nauseated. Calcium is never given intramuscularly, since it causes tissue sloughing. When caring for a patient receiving calcium intravenously, the nurse must be doubly careful that the needle does not slip out of the vein, spilling the solution into the tissues. If the infusion does infiltrate, it must be stopped at once.

Because the correct doses of these drugs may be difficult for the physician to estimate, the nurse should observe the patient frequently for hypercalcemia, which may occur with the administration of any of these preparations. Vomiting, usually one of the earliest symptoms, should be reported immediately to the physician. It may be followed by high fever, listlessness, and coma. Once tetany is controlled, an oral preparation of calcium will be used.

## THE ADRENAL GLANDS

The adrenal glands are paired organs of pyramidal shape, buried in the perirenal fat. Each gland is composed of an outer layer, the cortex, which is glandular in origin and produces the steroid hormones; and an inner core, the medulla, which originates from nerve tissue and manufactures catecholamines.

## THE ADRENAL CORTEX

The adrenal cortex is essential to life and produces a large number of hormones which are synthesized into steroids from the gland's store of cholesterol. The two groups of hormones produced are known as glucocorticoids and mineralocorticoids. Some sex hormones are also synthesized in the cortex of the adrenals.

The primary glucocorticoids are cortisol and corticosterone, which function to conserve glucose supplies in the body. They are essential to enable the body to respond to any type of stress, affect water and electrolyte balance, and alter the connective tissue response to injury by exerting an anti-inflammatory effect.

Aldosterone is the primary mineralocorticoid, whose action is to conserve the body's store of sodium ions. It stimulates sodium reabsorption in the distal renal tubules and excretion of potassium in the urine. Therefore, aldosterone is responsible for maintaining extracellular fluid volume as well as for maintaining blood pressure.

Both androgens and estrogens are produced by the cortex in both sexes. These hormones have the same physiologic effects as those produced by the gonads. In adrenal dysfunction diseases, the sex hormones can produce inappropriate sexual manifestations, such as decreasing male potency.

Adrenocortical secretion is controlled by the anterior pituitary, which secretes adrenocorticotropic hormone (ACTH), and by the hypothalamus, which secretes corticotropic releasing factor (CRF) by a negative feedback mechanism. During stress, the brain directly stimulates an increased output of CRF, which increases secretions of the adrenal cortex. Adrenocortical hormones are secreted in a rhythmic variation pattern each day, known as circadian rhythm or diurnal variation. The highest levels of cortisol and its derivatives occur in plasma early in the morning, with a gradual fall throughout the day. The lowest level is reached in the late evening. There is approximately a twofold difference between the highest and lowest level of secretion.

## Adrenocortical Hypofunction (Adrenocortical Insufficiency, Addison's Disease, Addisonian Crisis)

### Etiology

Addison's disease can result from destruction of adrenocortical tissue by tuberculosis or by idiopathic atrophy of the adrenal cortical tissue. It is suspected that excessive stress (overwhelming infection, surgery, or prolonged drain of the body's emergency resources) plays some role in causing insufficient steroids to be secreted. Cancer may invade the adrenal cortex. The disease can result also from the long-term use of large doses of steroids that cause adrenal atrophy by suppressing ACTH. Of course, bilateral adrenalectomy causes a deficiency of the steroids secreted by the adrenal glands. Addison's disease is comparatively rare.

### Pathology and Symptoms

Certain corticosteroids regulate absorption, distribution, and excretion of body salts and water; a decrease in these hormones leads to increased urinary excretion of sodium and retention of potassium. Dehydration, with reduction of blood plasma volume, results. The patient feels weak and easily tires. His blood pressure, BMR and temperature are low. Because he develops hypotension from sudden changes of position, such as lying down or sitting up too quickly, he may faint. He is prone to vascular collapse due to poor myocardial tonus, decreased cardiac output, and lowered blood pressure. He loses weight, is anemic, and may become cachectic. His appetite is poor, and he may suffer from a variety of gastrointestinal symptoms. He feels nervous and has periods of depression.

Patients with Addison's disease tend to have unusual pigmentation. They are perpetually tan, and this pigmentation involves creases in the palms of the hands and around the mouth. This pigmentation is extremely characteristic and many times patients who are becoming addisonian will develop pigmentation at inappropriate times, such as in the fall and winter, rather than in the spring and summer, as the normal person would. Growth of hair declines.

Because the body is deficient in hormones that facilitate the conversion of protein into glucose, episodes of hypoglycemia occur. The patient may develop hypoglycemia five to six hours after eating; the early morning, before breakfast, is an especially dangerous time. Symptoms of hypoglycemia are hunger, headache, sweating, weakness, trembling, emotional instability, visual disturbances, and, finally, disorientation, coma, and convulsions.

**Acute Adrenocortical Crisis.** Because the hormones of the cortex of the adrenal glands are prominent in effecting the body's adaptive reactions to stress, patients with Addison's disease collapse when they are faced with excess stress. Even uncomplicated surgery, such as an appendectomy, requires more physiologic adaptive ability than a patient with Addison's disease usually possesses. Unless he is given steroids, he will experience acute adrenal crisis, which is a severe flare-up of Addison's disease. His blood pressure becomes markedly depressed, perhaps so low as to be unobtainable. The patient is in *adrenal shock,* which is primarily due to lack of hormones.

Addison's crisis is an emergency; death may occur from hypotension and vasomotor collapse. Adrenocortical hormones are given intravenously in solutions of normal saline and glucose. Antibiotics may be ordered because of the patient's extremely low resistance to infection. Vital signs are taken frequently.

Vasopressor amines, such as phenylephrine (Neo-Synephrine) or metaraminol (Aramine) may be utilized when hypotension persists. The patient may have a fever and complain of headache. Morphine and insulin are contraindicated. The patient should be kept warm and as quiet as possible. He should not be permitted to do anything for himself until the emergency is over. Corticosteroids and fluids are also important aspects of therapy.

As a precaution in case of acute adrenal crisis, two 50-ml. syringes, intravenous hydrocortisone and bottles of 5 per cent dextrose in saline solution should be kept at the bedside of all patients with Addison's disease who are not well regulated. If the patient has a weak, rapid pulse, falling blood pressure, and cold, cyanotic extremities, his head should be lowered and the physician called. Salt deprivation, infection, trauma, exposure to cold, overexertion—any abnormal stress—can cause adrenal crisis. The crisis may start with anorexia, nausea, vomiting, diarrhea, abdominal pain, headache, intensification of hypotension, restlessness, or a high temperature. The nurse should watch for any of these symptoms in all of her patients with Addison's disease.

## Diagnostic Tests

The most frequently used test for Addison's disease is the adrenocortical response to ACTH. The excretion of adrenocortical hormones is measured after ACTH is administered intravenously. Normal persons have an increased excretion of 17-hydroxy-corticoids and 17-ketosteroids, whereas patients with Addison's disease show little or no increase. Also, eosinophils in the patient's blood are counted. Normally, a drop of 60 to 90 per cent in the eosinophil count occurs after ACTH is given, but there is less change in Addison's disease. The ACTH test is usually repeated over two or three consecutive days to differentiate between primary adrenal insufficiency and that secondary to pituitary ACTH deficiency. Laboratory tests in Addison's disease show a low blood sodium, a high potassium, and a low-fasting blood sugar. The size of the heart will be small in x-ray films.

## Treatment and Nursing Care

Addison's disease is treated by replacing the missing hormones. Cortisone, 12.5 mg., may be given two or three times a day. Hydrocortisone, 20 to 30 mg. a day, is sometimes prescribed.

Desoxycorticosterone acetate (DCA), 2.5 to 8 mg. by mouth, or 25 mg. every three to four weeks intramuscularly, or fludrocortisone (Florinef), 0.1 mg. daily or every other day, may be given to help to restore normal electrolyte and water balance. Toxic

symptoms of an overdose of these drugs include edema, headache, hypertension, and muscle weakness due to potassium depletion. Methyltestosterone, 5 to 10 mg. a day, may be administered orally. The patient may complain of gastric distress, which may be relieved by giving the orally administered hormones during meals. Unless orders to the contrary are given, the last dose of cortisone should be given no later than 4 P.M., since these hormones may make sleep difficult. *The nurse must be especially careful that no patient with Addison's disease receives insulin by error; he may die from hypoglycemia.* He is also extremely sensitive to opiates and barbiturates. The dose of hormones may be stabilized during the patient's stay in the hospital and continued on a maintenance basis after he is discharged.

It is imperative that the patient take the hormones as prescribed, and that he see his physician regularly. If the patient does not have active tuberculosis, and if he follows his prescribed drug regimen carefully, the outlook for his well-being is good (a prognosis that could not have been made before these hormones became available as drugs). As in diabetes, the patient's understanding of his condition can mean the difference between disability and an active life. The patient himself must be aware of his body's inability to handle stress of any sort and of the importance of seeking medical attention so that dosage can be readjusted whenever stress of any kind threatens: an infection, a car accident (even if he is not noticeably hurt), exposure to cold, an insoluble family crisis, or an excessive work load.

Part of the nurse's responsibility to the patient is to teach him and his family about the disease, how to protect his health by avoiding stressful situations when possible, and when indicated to see his physician so that his drugs can be adjusted. Despite the constant vigilance required to maintain his health, the patient with Addison's disease should not be made to feel that his condition should keep him out of the mainstream of everyday life.

The patient should carry a card stating that he is suffering from adrenocortical insufficiency. The card should include the name and telephone number of his physician. The card should contain a statement such as "... Addison's disease. In the event of illness call Dr. (name and telephone number). Give 25 mg. of cortisone every six hours by mouth. If unconscious, give 100 mg. of hydrocortisone intravenously." (Of course, the drugs and dosages are ordered by the physician.) The patient must be given a card to carry before he is discharged from the hospital.

Because of recurrent hypoglycemia, the patient may do better on five or six small meals than on three big ones. If sodium chloride pills are ordered, they may be tolerated best if they are taken with meals. Salt intake may need to be increased even more during hot weather. The patient should be instructed to add extra salt to his food if he has perspired more than usual.

When hypoglycemia occurs, it is treated by giving glucose, orally or intravenously. To prevent recurring episodes of hypoglycemia, between-meal snacks of milk and crackers are preferable to candy and other rapidly absorbed sugars. If the patient's meal is delayed by diagnostic tests, the fasting period should be kept to a minimum; he should be given breakfast as soon as it is allowed. During the fast, his activities should be limited; he should remain in bed and quiet. If he has to leave the ward, he should be taken on a stretcher or in a wheelchair.

Because of hypotension and muscle weakness, a patient with this condition is subject to falling. He should be protected with side rails unless he is well regulated and well taught. The importance of getting out of bed slowly should be emphasized. If he is dizzy on sitting up, he should lie down again. The nurse should take his blood pressure if the patient shows any symptoms, such as weakness or faintness, which would lead her to believe that his blood pressure is lower than usual. A change from the previous readings is more important than any one reading.

## Adrenocortical Hyperfunction (Cushing's Syndrome)

Excessive secretion of the adrenocortical hormones results from hyperplasia of the adrenal cortex due to adenomas or carcinomas or from overstimulation of the gland due to excessive ACTH secretion by the anterior pituitary. Bronchogenic and lung tumors of the oat cell variety are capable of secreting a hormone like ACTH, which causes adrenal hyperfunction. Cushing's syndrome also occurs as an iatrogenic disease from the use of cortisol derivatives therapeutically (Fig. 49-6).

### Signs and Symptoms

Symptoms can vary, depending on which hormones, i.e., cortisol, aldosterone, androgen, or estrogen, are secreted excessively. Most frequently, the signs and symptoms are associated with excessive cortisol production. These signs include redistribution of fat leading to pendulous abdomen, fat pads above the clavicles and buffalo hump, and a moon face. Purple striae appear on the abdomen, thighs, and upper arms. In contrast, extremities are thin from muscle wasting, the skin becomes thin, and the face is ruddy. Blood vessels are extremely fragile and the patient bruises easily. Wounds heal poorly and frequently become infected. The bones become so demineralized that the patient may have severe backache, kyphosis, and collapse of vertebral bodies. Arteriosclerosis develops rapidly, with

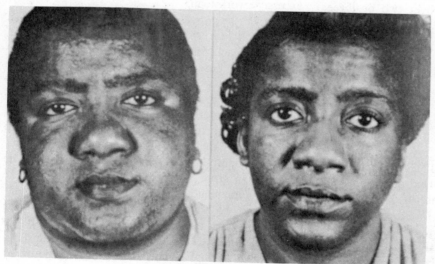

**Figure 49-6.** This patient had Cushing's disease due to benign hyperplasia of the adrenal glands. (*Left*) Before the adrenalectomy, showing the characteristic obesity, moonface, and hirsutism. These same symptoms can be seen in patients having long-term steroid therapy. (*Right*) After operation the patient has regained her normal appearance. (Novak, E. R., and Jones, G. S.: *Textbook of Gynecology*, ed. 7, p. 613, Baltimore, Williams & Wilkins)

increasing hypertension. Latent or overt diabetes mellitus is present in most patients. If sodium and water are retained, peripheral edema ensues. Symptoms of infection are masked. Therefore, the nurse must be especially alert for minor signs, a slight sore throat, or a small rise in temperature that may indicate the presence of a more severe infectious process. Vast swings in mood often occur; depression or psychosis may occur. In women, excessive secretion of cortical androgens produces masculinization with hirsutism and amenorrhea.

## Diagnosis

Urine may be examined for 17-hydroxycorticoids (17-OH) and 17-ketosteroids. The former are almost always increased, and the latter are increased or decreased, depending on the nature of the lesion. As is done in the diagnosis of hypofunction, ACTH may be given intravenously and the excretion of 17-hydroxycorticoid measured. Patients with bilateral adrenocortical hyperplasia have a marked urinary increase in 17-hydroxycorticoids. The 17-ketosteroids tend to be elevated in patients who have functioning carcinoma of the adrenal cortex. Twenty-four-hour urine samples may be collected for the measurement of urinary hydrocortisone and its major metabolites. Sometimes fractional urine samples are ordered because normally there is an increase in the excretion of hydrocortisone and its metabolites during the early morning, but this diurnal variation is not seen in Cushing's disease.

Another test is the urinary 17-hydroxycorticoid suppression test, in which a steroid, such as dexamethasone, is given to suppress ACTH from the pituitary. If, on a low dosage, urinary 17-hydroxycorticoid is not suppressed, the patient probably has hyperplasia of the adrenal cortex. If, on a high dosage of dexamethasone, there is no suppression of urinary 17-hydroxycorticoids, the patient probably has a carcinoma or an adenoma of the adrenal cortex. Hyperplasia and carcinoma may be differentiated also by giving a pituitary stimulant such as metyrapone (Metopirone). Normally and in hyperplasia, 17-hydroxycorticoid in the urine is increased when metyrapone is given, but this is not seen in carcinoma.

Occasionally, an abdominal x-ray film may show an adrenal mass, and an intravenous pyelogram may show changes in the renal shadow caused by an abnormally large adrenal gland. Skull and chest x-ray films are taken to differentiate between disease of adrenal origin and that originating in the pituitary or with a lung tumor.

## Nursing Assessment

The nurse must be aware of the signs and symptoms of cortisol excess and support the patient during diagnostic tests, which to him can seem interminable. Because of his altered body image, he is likely to manifest signs of lowered self-esteem and show frustration with his physical weakness. He needs reassurance and acceptance. The patient should be told that the unwelcome manifestations of his disease can be reversed with therapy. Because inflammatory and immune processes are suppressed, he is highly susceptible to infection, which can be overwhelming. The nurse must be alert to slight changes in body temperature, observe carefully for breaks in the skin, and listen attentively to any complaint suggestive of an infectious process, while providing a protective environment. She should monitor daily weights, observe for changes in cardiovascular status, and check urine for sugar.

Because the patient is susceptible to accidental injury, environmental hazards must be considered, with the nurse taking appropriate measures to ensure his safety. Fractures, should the patient fall, are common due to bone changes; the skin is easily traumatized and heals slowly.

A diet high in protein and low in carbohydrate should be encouraged. Sodium intake should be restricted, but extra potassium will be needed. If the patient has developed overt diabetes and is taking insulin, his diet should be planned by physician, dietitian, and nurse, with emphasis on instruction of the patient. The nurse must be alert to gastric complaints, because gastric ulcers often develop.

Rest for the patient is of prime importance but may be difficult because of the effects of increased cortisol (the patient may be tense and restless). The nurse must determine what measures best promote relaxation and when sedatives should be administered. Mood changes must be monitored and carefully recorded. Although no patient can be fully protected from upsetting experiences it is important for all who deal with him to recognize his physiologic and psychological vulnerability, and to avoid upsetting him. It is also important to teach the patient the necessity for shielding himself from stress.

## Treatment and Nursing Care

The treatment depends on whether the disease is due to a tumor or to hyperplasia, and on the views of the physician. X-ray therapy to the pituitary may be used for hyperplasia. If an adrenalectomy is to be done, adrenocortical hormone therapy may be started preoperatively in anticipation of the time when the body will be unable to produce its own hormones. However, medical opinion differs concerning the advisability of administering adrenocortical steroids preoperatively when an adrenalectomy is to be performed. Potassium chloride, 6.0 Gm. by mouth per day, may be given to counteract the effects of decreased blood potassium (hypokalemia).

After the operation the patient is treated as if he had Addison's disease—which, indeed, he now has. A postadrenalectomy syndrome of nausea, vomiting, diarrhea, muscle tenderness, and aching should be called to the physician's attention. Hypotension may be a problem, and the nurse should watch for signs of it. Also, she should observe for such complications as hemorrhage, atelectasis, and pneumothorax, since the adrenals are located close to the diaphragm and the inferior vena cava.

Because the adrenal glands and body water and electrolyte regulation are closely related, the nurse should keep careful records of fluid intake and urinary output pre- and postoperatively.

During convalescence, symptoms of diabetes show remission and the treatment necessary for residual disease must be determined. Symptoms of cardiovascular pathology usually improve. An oral cortisol preparation will be prescribed, which should be administered on a diurnal schedule. The patient must be taught to take his medication as prescribed and must know that replacement hormones will be necessary throughout his life. He should be encouraged to carry medical indentification.

CHRONIC STEROID THERAPY. Steroids are currently used in the treatment of many disease processes and in addition are used as replacement therapy in adrenocortical insufficiency. They suppress inflammatory responses of the body and excessive formation of fibrous and granulation tissue. Therefore, they tend to inhibit manifestations of disease but do not abolish its cause. Use of corticosteroids can be lifesaving in the treatment of shock and acute allergic reactions. They are used in the treatment of collagen diseases, such as systemic lupus erythematosus; in dermatologic conditions, such as pemphigus; for nephrosis; ulcerative colitis; in various types of anemia; and in ophthalmologic diseases. Topical therapy and local joint therapy are frequently used. Because of their side effects, steroid preparations are usually contraindicated for the control of chronic phases of diseases, such as rheumatoid arthritis.

Long-term therapy, utilizing supraphysiologic doses of exogenous corticosteroids, tends to produce symptoms of Cushing's disease. Minimal side effects, such as weight gain, headaches, acne, fatigue, and urinary frequency, may be tolerated if therapeutic goals are being achieved. Patients placed on steroid therapy should be informed of the side effects of these drugs and be instructed to inform their physician of signs such as dizziness, nausea and vomiting, abdominal pain, depression, nervousness, or the development of an infection.

Because therapeutic use of exogenous steroids decreases the production of endogenous steroids due to adrenocortical atrophy, these drugs must never be terminated abruptly. The patient must be told to take the drug as it is prescribed. When it is to be discontinued, dosage levels are reduced over a prolonged period of time. Gradually, endogenous production will resume. However, any patient who has been on corticosteroid therapy will not tolerate stress well for a prolonged period of time and may require cortisol if he suffers an injury or requires surgery.

Patients on long-term corticosteroid therapy appear to develop fewer side effects if the drugs are administered on alternate days and at the time of day when their endogenous secretion levels are highest, usually in the early morning.

The nurse is often responsible for teaching the patient about the complications of therapy and for observing his response to it. She must be alert to all signs of hypercorticism discussed above. She should instruct the patient to carry identification at all times, indicating that he is on corticosteroid therapy and including emergency instructions.

## Hyperaldosteronism

Aldosterone is the primary mineralocorticoid secreted by the adrenal cortex. Excessive production of the hormone, known as primary hyperaldosteronism, is rare and results in hypertension and renal loss of potassium or hypokalemia. Hypokalemia causes muscle weakness, which may progress to paralysis and polyuria. The disease can be caused by carcinoma, adenoma, or hyperplasia of the adrenal cortex. Hyperaldosteronism characteristically occurs in early middle life.

Laboratory diagnosis of hyperaldosteronism is extremely complicated and the patient needs to be thoroughly evaluated before undergoing surgery.

Treatment is unilateral or bilateral adrenalectomy. Preoperative preparation includes potassium replacement for five to seven days and a restricted sodium intake. Postoperatively, intake and output are measured and the patient observed for signs of urinary dysfunction.

## THE ADRENAL MEDULLA

The adrenal medulla's hormones, epinephrine, norepinephrine, and dopamine, are produced by the sympathetic nervous system. Although each of the hormones has a specific action, they function together to stimulate body processes in preparation for unusual activity ("fight or flight"). The body rapidly responds to the release of these hormones with heightened alertness and mobilization of energy sources. Norepinephrine (alpha-adrenergic stimulator) causes veins and arteries to constrict, resulting in increased peripheral vascular resistance, bradycardia, and an elevated blood pressure. Epinephrine (beta-adrenergic stimulator) increases coronary blood flow, increases heart rate and cardiac output, dilates the bronchi and increases respiratory rate, increases metabolic activity, and stimulates the central nervous system. The chief effect of dopamine is dilation of systemic arteries and augmentation of cardiac output, leading to an increase in renal blood flow.

### Adrenal Medulla Hyperfunction (Pheochromocytoma)

Pheochromocytoma is usually a benign tumor of the adrenal medulla, although it can occur anywhere in the sympathetic nerve chain. The tumor causes an increased secretion of epinephrine and norepinephrine and the symptoms provoked are hypertension, either sustained or paroxysmal; diaphoresis, either continuous or episodic; palpitations and tachycardia; tremors; nervousness; anorexia; weight loss; or hypermetabolism.

Pheochromocytoma may cause manifestations of other metabolic diseases, such as diabetes mellitus or thyrotoxicosis. Studies have indicated an hereditary basis for the disease. It is one form of hypertension that can be cured.

### Diagnostic Tests

X-ray examinations of chest and abdomen may reveal tumors. A specific test for the abnormal secretion of catecholamines is to determine urinary vanillylmandelic acid (VMA). In the VMA test, a 24-hour urine specimen is analyzed to determine excretion of a breakdown product of catecholamine metabolism. Three days before the test, the patient's dietary intake of coffee, tea, bananas, vanilla, and chocolate are completely restricted because ingestion of these foods alters its results. All drugs must be discontinued. The patient should rest and be protected from stress as much as possible during the test.

During the diagnostic period, the patient should be protected from attacks of severe paroxysmal hypertension. Emergency procedures should be clarified in advance by consulting with the attending physician. Usually, parenteral administration of an adrenolytic drug will be necessary to control such an attack and prevent intracranial hemorrhage or cardiac failure.

### Treatment

Surgical removal of the tumor is indicated. The operation has been dangerous, especially in the past, because wide fluctuations in blood pressure may occur during and after surgery due to the sudden liberation or abrupt cessation of epinephrine or norepinephrine. Phentolamine (Regitine) and piperoxan (Benodaine), which also neutralize epinephrine, are given in a continuous intravenous infusion preoperatively or postoperatively to counteract hypertension. Preoperatively, many physicians administer a beta-adrenergic blocker such as propanolol (Inderal) to control ventricular arrhythmias. On the other hand, if the blood pressure is too low postoperatively, norepinephrine may be administered to raise it. Surgery is less dangerous than in the past, because it is now possible to control fluctuations in blood pressure preoperatively and during surgery with phenoxybenzamine (Dibenzyline) and Regitine. In addition, the use of halogenated hydrocarbons, such as halothane, and suitable beta blockers, such as propanolol, have markedly decreased the incidence of ventricular arrhythmia, which can result in operative death. Emotional support of the patient pre- and postoperatively is especially important because high anxiety further increases the risk of surgery, and the patient may be very apprehensive about having the surgery.

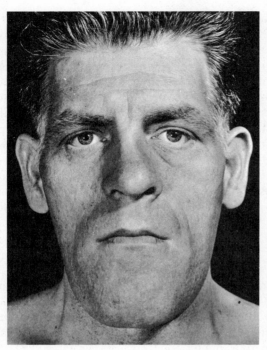

**Figure 49-7.** Typical appearance of a patient with acromegaly. (Dr. Julius Wolf and Charles Pfizer and Co., Inc., New York, N.Y.)

## THE PITUITARY GLAND (HYPOPHYSIS)

The pituitary gland is a small organ that lies in the sella turcica of the sphenoid bone behind the nose. It is attached superiorly to the hypothalamus by a delicate stalk. There are a number of distinct types of cells in the structure of the pituitary, with different types of cells being responsible for the secretion of different hormones. The gland is composed of two parts, the anterior (adenohypophysis) and posterior (neurohypophysis). There is also an intermediate lobe of the pituitary, which is quite small in man and whose importance is still somewhat obscure. The pituitary secretes many hormones and affects the function of most other glands of the endocrine system. Hyperfunction and hypofunction of the gland may be manifested in many ways, depending on which glandular cells of the organ are involved.

### The Anterior Lobe (Adenohypophysis)

The anterior lobe of the pituitary is glandular in origin. It secretes growth or somatropic hormone (STH), which acts directly on body tissues and the tropic hormones; thyroid-stimulating hormone (TSH), adrenocorticotropic hormone (ACTH), and the gonadotropic hormones; follicle-stimulating hormone (FSH), luteinizing hormone or interstitial cell-stimulating hormone (LH or ICSH), and prolactin (LTH), which act on target glands. In general, hormones of the target glands have an inhibitory effect on the pituitary by means of the negative feedback mechanism. When disorders of the pituitary occur, the feedback mechanism tends to become inoperative.

### Hypersecretion of Growth Hormone (Acromegaly)

The secretion of growth hormone is thought to be affected by serum glucose levels. This hormone facilitates the use of protein for building new tissue and to conserve glucose for use in growth rather than expending it for energy. Hypersecretion of growth hormone (somatropin) is due to hyperplasia or tumors of the anterior pituitary. When there is an excess of this hormone in children before the ends of the long bones are fully united (epiphysial union), gigantism results. Overproduction of somatropin during adulthood causes a condition called *acromegaly*, in which the bones increase in thickness because longitudinal growth is no longer possible. There are characteristic changes in appearance; the features become coarse with a large lower jaw, thick lips, bulging forehead, bulbous nose, and large hands and feet. The soft tissues hypertrophy and the skin becomes thickened. Overgrowth of bone makes the joints more susceptible to degenerative disease. The sebaceous and sweat glands increase in size and number. Headaches due to pressure on the sella turcica, when the disease is caused by a tumor, are common. The patient may become partially blind from pressure on the optic nerve. Associated endocrine imbalances frequently occur. Approximately one-third of these patients develop diabetes mellitus. Sexual function begins to fail with men becoming impotent and women developing amenorrhea. Severe problems related to body image and self-esteem are common (Fig. 49-7).

The disease is diagnosed by inspection, comparative photographs of the individual, x-rays of the skull, and laboratory determinations showing high STH plasma levels, as well as high serum levels of phosphorus and alkaline phosphates.

Acromegaly may be treated by irradiation or surgical removal of the anterior pituitary. The care of the patient after surgical treatment is similar to that of any patient undergoing craniotomy. This patient will tend to develop hypoglycemia post-operatively. Unfortunately, even though the disease may be successfully arrested, growth changes due to acromegaly are irreversible. The nurse's role involves support of the patient in coping with his appearance, and with responses of others toward him.

## Treatment of Pituitary Tumors and Nursing Care

**Diagnostic Tests.** The diagnostic procedures employed for suspected tumors of the pituitary are the same as those for any brain lesion. The patient will usually undergo skull x-rays and tomograms, lumbar puncture, and pneumoencephalogram studies. The patient often is extremely anxious regarding the outcome of the tests and may fear irreparable damage to neurologic function, if treatment is instituted. The nurse must provide careful explanations and provide the patient with the opportunity to ventilate his feelings.

Surgical treatment (hypophysectomy) will produce chronic deficiencies of the anterior pituitary hormones. Usually, the posterior pituitary is preserved. The patient will need replacement therapy with adrenosteroids and thyroid after surgery.

When irradiation therapy is employed, it may be accomplished by x-ray or by implanting radioactive yttrium 90. The implantation is a surgical procedure and, following it, the patient must be observed carefully for signs of infection, visual problems, and hormone deficiency. Implantation usually does not destroy hormone function, but x-ray therapy frequently results in hypopituitarism.

## Panhypopituitarism

Panhypopituitarism refers to a deficiency of all hormones secreted by the anterior pituitary. The most common cause of dysfunction is Sheehan's syndrome (postpartum necrosis of the pituitary). The pituitary gland enlarges during pregnancy. When women experience immediate postpartum hemorrhage and shock, the blood supply to the anterior pituitary ceases, causing ischemic necrosis. Reasons for this are not understood. Hormonal deficiencies that follow may not manifest themselves for a period of years after the incident. Usually, the patient will first show signs of gonadatropin deficiency. The genital organs involute and menses become scant. Next, signs of hypothyroidism develop and the patient appears to be aging prematurely. Finally, signs of Addison's disease develop with fatigability, weakness, and hypoglycemia. Body

hair becomes sparse and anemia develops. Fortunately, this condition is becoming increasingly rare because of improved obstetric care.

Occasionally, panhypopituitarism occurs in patients with extensive diabetic degenerative vascular disease, from sarcoid granulomas, or from tubercular or syphilitic lesions, and from surgical excision of the gland.

Panhypopituitarism is treated by replacing hormones of the thyroid, adrenals, and gonads. It is not possible at this time to restore fertility. With hormone therapy, changes in the patient are dramatic. From an almost invalid state, the individual regains strength, vigor, and vitality.

## The Posterior Lobe (Neurohypophysis)

The posterior pituitary is neural in origin. The hormones associated with the posterior lobe are synthesized in the hypothalamus, but stored and released by the pituitary. The two known hormones are vasopressin (antidiuretic hormone, or ADH) and oxytocin. Whenever body water is lost, the osmotic pressure of blood rises. This rise is detected by osmoreceptors in the hypothalamus, stimulating the release of ADH, which acts on the kidney tubules to reabsorb water; subsequently urinary output decreases.

## Diabetes Insipidus
### (Hyposecretion of Antidiuretic Hormone)

When insufficient ADH is produced, the kidney is unable to concentrate urine efficiently, causing excessive urinary output. As much as 10 to 20 liters of urine may be passed in a 24-hour period. The dilute urine has a specific gravity of 1.012 or less. The major causes of diabetes insipidus are primary or metastatic neoplasms, head trauma, local infection, and damage to the hypothalamus. In rare situations, it is an inherited defect.

The patient experiences continuous polydypsia and polyuria, which interfere with pursuit of normal activities of daily living. He may develop hypertrophy of the ureters and bladder.

Treatment consists of rectifying the underlying pathology. Vasopressin is administered to control polyuria. An aqueous solution of vasopressin (Pitressin) is administered either subcutaneously or intramuscularly. Pitressin tannate in oil is a longer-acting form of the drug, administered intramuscularly, approximately every three days. A powdered form of vasopressin may be administered by nasal insufflation; however, it tends to irritate the nasal mucosa. The objective of therapy is to reduce the patient's urinary output to 2 to 3 liters during 24 hours.

The nurse should remember that temporary diabetes insipidus may occur after head trauma or intracranial hemorrhage. Careful monitoring of intake and output and assessing cardiovascular integrity can promote prompt therapy for this complication.

## REFERENCES AND BIBLIOGRAPHY

ASIMOV, I.: *The Human Brain: Its Capacities and Functions,* Boston, Houghton Mifflin, 1963.

ASPERHEIM, M., and EISENHAUER, L. A.: *The Pharmacologic Basis of Patient Care,* ed. 2, Philadelphia, Saunders, 1973.

BLOUNT, M., and KINNEY, A. B.: Chronic steroid therapy, *Am. J. Nurs.* 74:1626, September 1974.

BRUNNER, L. S., et al.: *The Lippincott Manual of Nursing Practice,* Philadelphia, Lippincott, 1974.

COLLINS, S., et al.: Intractable pain, *Nurs. '74* 4:55, September 1974.

GLENN, R., and MANNIX, H., JR.: Diagnosis and prognosis of cushing's syndrome, *Surg. Gynec. Obstet.* 126:765, April 1968.

GREENE, R.: *Human Hormones,* New York, McGraw-Hill, 1970.

GROLLMAN, A.: *Clinical Endocrinology and Its Physiological Basis,* Philadelphia, Lippincott, 1964.

HORROBIN, D. F.: *Biochemistry, Endocrinology and Nutrition,* New York, Putnam's, 1971.

LUCE, G. G.: *Body Time: Physiological Rhythms and Social Stress,* New York, Bantam Books, 1971.

MANNIX, H., JR.: Personal Communication.

———, and LOEHR, W.: Unusual aspects of hyperparathyroidism, *Surg. Gynec. Obstet.* 126:347, February 1968.

MAZZAFERRI, E. L.: *Endocrine Case Studies,* New York, Medical Examination Publishing Co., 1971.

SAWIN, C. T.: *The Hormones: Endocrine Physiology,* Boston, Little Brown, 1969.

SPENCER, R. T.: *Patient Care in Endocrine Problems,* Philadelphia, Saunders, 1973.

SUNDERMAN, F. WM., and SUNDERMAN, F. WM., JR. (eds.): *Evaluation of Thyroid and Parathyroid Functions,* Philadelphia, Lippincott, 1963.

WILLIAMS, R. H. (ed.): *Textbook of Endocrinology,* ed. 4, Philadelphia, Saunders, 1968.

# The Patient with Diabetes Mellitus

## CHAPTER 50

Diabetes mellitus is a chronic metabolic disease of unknown etiology. While recognized as a disease of the pancreas, diabetes has a distinctive vascular component that affects large and small blood vessels; virtually every body system is affected by the metabolic derangement. Though much is unknown about diabetes, it is accepted that a relative or absolute deficiency of insulin, the hormone secreted by the beta cells of the islands of Langerhans in the pancreas, results in impaired carbohydrate, protein, and lipid metabolism.

Diabetes, which has been clinically recognized since at least 1500 B.C., affects not only humans, but domestic dogs, cats, cows, and laboratory animals as well.

The most important factor in management is a well-informed, responsible patient, able to make adjustments and accept some limitations with minimal disruption in his usual life style. The patient, who should be viewed as the crucial member of the health care team, collaborates with other team members, such as physicians, nurses, dietitians, social workers, podiatrists, and counselors in various specialties. Newer approaches to the management of the diabetic have evolved, including the exchange of "contracts" between professional health care providers and diabetic consumers of care so that each knows the expectations of the other (Etzweiler, 1973).

Because of the recognized, but heretofore often unmet, need for lifelong care and support of the diabetic patient, increasing active responsibility for the health maintenance and continuing education of the diabetic has become the role of the diabetes nursing clinical specialist. However, nurses in all settings, whether inpatient or outpatient, have diabetics among their patients and must be prepared to communicate knowledgeably with and give expert care to the known and well educated as well as the newly diagnosed patient with diabetes.

## EPIDEMIOLOGY

Diabetes is a universal disease. It is estimated that 25 per cent of the population in the United States (about 50 million people) either have, or will develop diabetes, or have a relative with diabetes.

There are approximately 4,400,000 known diabetics in the United States and about 1.6 million cases undiagnosed (*Stat. Bull.*, 54:3, December 1973). Each year more than 325,000 persons learn that they have diabetes (Public Health Service Publ. No. 1168). No age group is exempt but 80 per cent of diabetics are over the age of 40; only 5 per cent are children. Females are in the majority in every age group, and the difference increases further after the age of 45. Noncaucasian women in the United States have twice the incidence as have white women or men after the age of 45 (Skillman and Tzagournis, 1972).

The frequency of diabetes is rising, probably partly because case-finding methods are better, and people are living longer. Those women and men who previously would have died without adequate treatment now live to have children, who are more likely to develop the disease, than are children of nondiabetic parents.

Factors such as age and sex distribution of the population, national income, degree of industrialization, and the quality and extent of medical care available influence the prevalence of diabetes. There is more diabetes in urban and industrialized countries, and, generally, in more affluent societies where food is readily available and there is little emphasis on active exercise. Studies have demonstrated a decreased incidence of diabetes during periods when food was scarce, such as in Europe during World War II. Some studies show an increased incidence among Jews of certain ethnic characteristics. However, others suggest that this conclusion is based on data gathered in treatment centers utilized by a disproportionate number of Jewish people. American Indians have a higher incidence of diabetes, but this is thought to be due to inbreeding and obesity rather than ethnicity.

Eskimos, on the other hand, have a low incidence (Skillman and Tzagournis).

The highest rates of diabetes are found among obese adults with a family history of diabetes.

In 1900 diabetes was the twenty-first cause of death in the United States; in 1972 it ranked sixth, (*Stat. Bull.*, May 1973) and currently it accounts for approximately 38,000 deaths per year.

Despite the improvement in longevity due to prevention and improved management of complications such as diabetic acidosis, insulin shock, and infections the life expectancy of diabetics is reduced as compared with nondiabetics. Mortality and morbidity relate to the age at onset and the duration of the disease, being distinctly higher when the disease is acquired in childhood or early adult life; this denotes a more severe form of the disease than that which occurs in later life.

Diabetes contributes substantially to the increased mortality associated with other chronic diseases, especially those of the cardiovascular–renal system. The importance of the disease as a major public health problem is more apparent in terms of its long-term vascular complications due to involvement of large vessels in the brain, heart, kidneys, and extremities and of the small vessels, especially in the eyes and the kidneys.

## CLASSIFICATION

Primary diabetes is of two types. (1) Juvenile diabetes mellitus, also called "growth-onset diabetes" or "insulin-dependent diabetes," usually appears explosively in an individual under age 20, though it can occur in the 20's and 30's. About 10 per cent of known diabetics are of this type, which is unresponsive to oral hypoglycemic drugs and requires exogenous insulin. The course of the disease is often marked by unexplained shifts between low and high blood glucose values, leading to the descriptive term "labile." Juvenile diabetics face the probability of microvascular pathology and other degenerative complications in 20 years after onset, although good control may reduce this risk. (2) Adult-onset or "maturity-onset diabetes" appears after age 35 to 40 and usually in patients who are overweight. This type has relatively stable blood glucose levels so the patient can usually be managed with diet alone or diet and hypoglycemic drugs. About 20 to 30 per cent of adult-onset diabetics require insulin (Krosnick, 1970).

Thus, the adult diabetic whom the nurse cares for may be a juvenile diabetic who has grown to adulthood, a juvenile diabetic diagnosed in young adulthood (20's or 30's), or a maturity-onset diabetic.

"Secondary" diabetes, which is found in a small minority of patients, can usually be attributed to infection of the pancreas, chronic pancreatitis, pancreatic tumors, pancreatectomy, or other chronic diseases such as acromegaly, Cushing's disease, and hemochromatosis. Oral contraceptive drugs and steroids are diabetogenic, so women with an hereditary susceptibility to diabetes should not use them.

Primary prevention of diabetes includes counseling the diabetic to avoid marriage with a known diabetic.

## ETIOLOGY

As noted previously, in most instances the cause of diabetes is unknown. Familial aggregation studies and twin studies show that genetic factors are important in the etiology of diabetes, but there is no agreement as to the characteristics of the genetic factor. All possible modes of inheritance have been suggested, but to date no single hypothesis explains all available data (Rimoin, 1970).

It has been questioned whether a single trait is inherited—that is, a metabolic defect (insulin deficiency) to which vascular disease is due, or whether there are two traits, one for the metabolic defect and the other for premature vascular disease, which are relatively independent of each other but run along concurrently. Genetic susceptibility to diabetes is believed by many to be inherited in the manner of a Mendelian recessive characteristic. The disease does not necessarily manifest itself early in life, but (according to this theory) if both parents have diabetes, all of their children will become diabetic if they live long enough. However, only about 50 per cent of such offspring have been found to be "pre-diabetic" (Rimoin).

With this theory, the probability that a person is genetically susceptible to diabetes (if he lives long enough) is approximately 100 per cent for an individual with both parents primary diabetics and for the identical twin of a diabetic; 60 per cent when one parent and a grandparent, or an aunt or uncle, on the opposite parental side have diabetes; 50 per cent if one parent and a sibling or one parent and an aunt or uncle on the opposite parental side have the disease; 25 per cent when one

sibling has the disease, and 20 per cent when one parent is a diabetic (Steinberg, 1955). Occasionally diabetes occurs in persons with no known family history of the disease. This is usually in children and it can be anticipated that one or both parents will develop diabetes later in life.

The concept of genetic susceptibility suggests that a person who inherits the recessive genes might avoid expression of the disease during his lifetime if it would be possible to avoid or control multiple environmental or precipitating factors that influence diabetes. Such precipitating factors include aging, obesity, periods of rapid growth in children, severe mental and physical stress, other endocrine disorders, infection, pregnancy, trauma, and drugs (steroids, contraceptive pills).

The close association between the onset of juvenile diabetes and major infection has led some to question whether viruses (i.e., coxsackie-B virus, mumps virus, etc.) or other agents can destroy the islet cells, resulting in overt diabetes.

Although diabetes is classically believed to be a primary disease of the pancreas, much attention today is being given to extrapancreatic factors in the etiology of diabetes. Any one or a combination of the following factors can be involved in the relative insulin deficiency responsible for the metabolic derangement of diabetes (Mirsky, 1970):

- Impaired synthesis of insulin by the beta cells
- Synthesis of an abnormal insulin molecule with decreased hormonal activity
- An impaired pancreatic insulin-release mechanism
- Insulin-binding components of the plasma which impair the transport of insulin to tissue receptors
- Inhibitory agents in the circulation which inactivate insulin
- Increased production of agents which antagonize the physiologic effects of insulin
- Blockade of the insulin receptors of insulin dependent tissues
- Decreased cell sensitivity to the action of insulin
- Increased insulin-degradation rate

Another cause may be a decrease in the number of insulin receptors (Archer, et al., 1973).

## NATURAL HISTORY OF DIABETES

The natural history of primary diabetes suggests a progression through several stages which have physiologic and temporal characteristics.

- *Prediabetes,* a conceptual stage rather than a real entity, is the period from conception to the onset of abnormal glucose tolerance in a genetically susceptible person. The offspring of two diabetic parents, the identical twin of a diabetic, and mothers whose infants weigh over 9 pounds at birth may be characterized as "prediabetic." Evidence suggests that basement membrane thickening and abnormalities in glucose metabolism exist in the prediabetic. Fasting blood glucose and glucose tolerance tests are normal and there are no symptoms.

- These same test results and lack of symptoms are also generally characteristic of the next stage, *latent chemical diabetes*. However, here a cortisone-glucose tolerance test would be abnormal. This is also suggested by reactive hypoglycemia and by an abnormal glucose tolerance test associated with stressful situations, such as pregnancy or infection.
- In the third stage, *latent diabetes* (or *"chemical diabetes"*), fasting blood sugar is normal, but the oral glucose tolerance test is abnormal. There are usually no clinical symptoms or signs, although reactive hypoglycemia may occur.
- In the final stage—*clinical or "overt diabetes,"* abnormal amounts of sugar accumulate in the bloodstream (hyperglycemia) and subsequently are excreted in the patient's urine. The fasting blood sugar is high and the glucose tolerance test, of course, is abnormal. Overt symptoms and signs are usually present.

*Gestational diabetes* may appear during the second or third trimester of pregnancy. Frequently the woman has a positive family history and is likely to deliver a baby weighing in excess of 9 pounds. The alteration in carbohydrate metabolism usually reverts to normal about six weeks postpartum so the syndrome is considered to be a stage between prediabetes and latent chemical diabetes.

## PATHOPHYSIOLOGY AND CLINICAL MANIFESTATIONS

Diabetes is not simply a disorder of "sugar" (carbohydrate) metabolism. The major purpose of metabolism is to transfer the latent energy in food to each body cell. The process of cell metabolism also involves protein, fat, minerals, enzymes and coenzymes, insulin and other hormones, vitamins, water, complex energy transfer systems, and structural characteristics of internal tissues.

When the glucose level of the blood increases (such as after the ingestion of food), the beta cells of the pancreatic islands of Langerhans release insulin. A major action of insulin is to open passageways through the cell walls, particularly of fat and muscle, so that glucose may enter easily. Cells of the central nervous system, red blood cells, liver cells, and some others permit free entry of glucose without insulin.

Ingested carbohydrate in the form of glucose or foods readily transformed to glucose constitutes 40 to 50 per cent of the total caloric intake in most societies and is a major source of energy for cellular function. Only a small portion of ingested glucose is used immediately for energy; the remainder is stored as glycogen in the liver and muscle or as fat. Under normal conditions there is always an adequate supply of glucose for fuel. As the body needs fuel, the liver changes glycogen back to glucose (glycogenolysis) and passes it out to the bloodstream where it becomes available to muscle and other body tissues as short-term fuel for energy to protect the person in emergency conditions against a fall in blood glucose.

Insulin is an important link in this process; it promotes the formation and storage of glycogen in the liver. When ingested glucose is inadequate to meet the needs of the tissues, particularly the brain, which requires a constant supply of glucose, the liver can also provide glucose by a process called *gluconeogenesis*. This process for hepatic glucose depends on a number of factors such as amino acids, glucocorticoid hormones, and free fatty acids for energy. However, the principal coordination of the process is accomplished by insulin. In lipid and protein metabolism, insulin is essential for the conversion of carbohydrate to fat and for the formation of protein from amino acids.

A normal person has a fasting level of 60 to 100 mg. per 100 ml. of venous blood by the true blood glucose method. Within half an hour after he has eaten, some of the carbohydrate that he has ingested is digested and absorbed into the blood. The blood glucose rises to about 150 mg. per 100 ml. Two hours after eating, the blood glucose has returned to its fasting level.

In diabetes the fasting blood glucose content may be normal or elevated, but after eating it may rise to high levels (exceeding 150 mg. per 100 ml. of blood).

Whatever the reason, diabetics have less insulin available than their metabolic processes require and the ability of the liver to convert glucose to glycogen is impaired, as is the use of glucose by tissues as well as the other major functions of insulin.

Glucose accumulates in diabetes since it cannot enter muscle and fat cells normally in the absence of adequate insulin action. The condition of excess glucose in the blood is called *hyperglycemia*. With so much additional glucose in the blood, the renal tubular reabsorption mechanism for glucose is overwhelmed and some of the glucose is excreted by the kidneys. Glucose usually is found in the urine when the blood glucose level exceeds 180 mg. per 100 ml.—the renal threshold for glucose. Diabetics with renal disease may have a "high" threshold and not "spill" sugar until blood glucose reaches 250 mg. per 100 ml. The presence of glucose in the urine is called *glucosuria.*

(*Glycosuria* is a nonspecific term referring to any reducing substance in urine which could include nonglucose substances such as pentose, fructose, galactose, or lactose. *Glucosuria* denotes urinary glucose only.)

To eliminate glucose, water also must be excreted. Therefore, one of the symptoms of untreated diabetes is *polyuria* (excessive urine). The patient complains of needing to urinate frequently and of passing a large amount each time. Because so much water has been lost in the urine, the patient feels thirsty, and he drinks a great deal (*polydipsia*). Often, the amount that he drinks is not enough to compensate for the loss of water, and he becomes dehydrated.

While the needed glucose is being wasted, the body's requirement for fuel continues. The patient feels hungry, and he increases his intake of food (*polyphagia*). To meet the rising need for energy, additional amounts of fats and proteins are metabolized. He becomes hungrier and weaker, and loses weight, literally starving while overeating.

Anything that causes liver glycogen depletion and increased oxidation of fat (for instance, insulin deprivation, infection, surgery, anesthesia, and vomiting) may result in an excess of ketone bodies. Infection and surgery invite ketosis and diabetic coma because they increase the demand for insulin, which the diabetic's pancreas cannot deliver.

The metabolic situation is complicated further by overactivity of the anterior pituitary, the thyroid, and the adrenal cortex, which may stimulate the formation of glucose, reduce its utilization, and therefore elevate blood sugar levels.

Though the above symptoms and signs are considered classic for diabetes, they are relatively late manifestations and occur generally in young, more insulin-deficient patients.

Other initial symptoms are not so dramatic, yet not uncommon. Excessive fatigue or loss of strength may be the only symptom. Weight gain in the maturity-onset diabetic may be the first clue—over 75 per cent of these diabetics are overweight when diagnosed. Other symptoms include impotence in the male, blurred vision, monilial infections (especially vulvovaginitis), pruritus, postprandial drowsiness, aches or numbness in the extremities, furuncles or other skin infections, and frequent low-grade infections.

Hepatomegaly due to deposition of fat in the hepatic cells may be present if hyperglycemia is severe or prolonged. Depigmented areas or pigmented areas on the anterior surface of the legs (shin spots) should arouse suspicion.

Early in the disease in some diabetics *reactive hypoglycemia* occurs. Three to five hours after a large meal the person may experience nervousness, tremor, perspiration, and palpitations. Peak endogenous insulin level normally occurs 30 to 60 minutes after ingestion of food. Insulin release is delayed in reactive hypoglycemia to a two- to three-hour interval when blood glucose levels are high and the absorption of food nearly complete. Symptoms result from catecholamine release (epinephrine and norepinephrine) in response to a rapid drop in blood glucose or a drop to a very low level. Postprandial hypoglycemia may be treated with phenformin to prevent glucose from going up too high and triggering the marked insulin response.

## SCREENING

All nurses must be alert for the symptoms and signs of diabetes and refer suspected persons for further testing.

Attention is now being directed not only toward the discovery of persons with clinical diabetes, but also toward the use of screening measures to detect metabolic derangements before overt symptoms develop. Community health, school, or occupational health nurses often are responsible for developing and participating in programs whereby large numbers of people, such as the population of a town or the employees of an industry, are given a urine or blood test for diabetes. "Selective screening" programs are aimed at persons at high risk, such as the obese, especially over age 40; those with genetic susceptibility; and women who have given birth to infants weighing over 9 pounds.

The screening procedure of choice is a blood glucose determination made after a meal containing 75 to 100 Gm. of carbohydrate—the two-hour postprandial blood sugar. A convenient method for mass screening, which directly estimates blood glucose almost instantly, utilizes a drop of capillary blood taken from the fingertip or ear lobe rather than blood from venipuncture. The blood is applied to a test paper strip (Dextrostix) and washed off in precisely 60 seconds. The intensity of color development is compared with a chart or measured by an Ames Reflectance Meter.

A two-hour postprandial glucose value of less than 100 mg. per 100 ml. of blood is normal, using the venous blood true glucose level. Values between 110 and 140 mg. per 100 ml. are suspicious, but levels over 140 mg. per 100 ml. indicate diabetes. The diagnosis would be confirmed by a standard glucose tolerance test (see below).

Urine tests are used mainly to evaluate control of diabetes rather than for screening. Since glucose is not adequately used, it is excreted in urine. Usually glucosuria is found when the blood glucose exceeds 180 mg. per 100 ml., except in the elderly. Their renal threshold is high due to nephrosclerosis, and glucosuria may not occur until the blood glucose rises over 200 mg. per 100 ml. If fats are metabolized faster than the body can utilize ketone bodies, acetone will appear in the urine. Tests for glucose in urine can be conducted as part of routine physical examinations, but random tests are not sensitive as a screening procedure. If urine must be used for screening, a one- to two-hour postprandial specimen should be tested. However, because sugar in the urine is not always an indication of diabetes, and because not all diabetics excrete sugar in the urine, blood glucose and glucose tolerance tests are necessary to establish the diagnosis. Transitory glucosuria can be present in such conditions as stroke, myocardial infarction, acromegaly, pregnancy, and adrenal hyperfunction.

## DIAGNOSTIC TESTS

**Glucose Tolerance Test.** Normal blood sugar in the fasting person is 60 to 100 mg. per 100 ml. of venous blood by the true blood glucose method. When the nondiabetic is given glucose orally, his blood glucose level will return to normal in about two hours (when glucose is given intravenously, the level returns to normal in about an hour). If the patient is diabetic, his fasting blood glucose level may be high, and it stays even higher for more than two hours after ingesting glucose.

The usual procedure for the standard oral glucose tolerance test is as follows.

The person receives a high carbohydrate diet for three to five days before the test. The diet contains at least 150 Gm. of carbohydrate per day. This preparation for the test is important, because, without the preliminary diet, blood glucose values may be high, as in the so-called hunger or starvation diabetes.

Blood and urine samples are taken before breakfast (fasting control).

The person drinks 75 or 100 Gm. of glucose in a lemon-flavored solution or 7 ounces of Glucola, a commercial 75-Gm. carbohydrate solution. The dosage is determined by the person's weight. Some people find the drink easier to take if it is well chilled. The time when the glucose is finished is noted. If the test takes place during hospitalization, usually the nurse supervises the collection of the urine, and a laboratory technician takes the blood. Often the test is done on an outpatient basis. The individual can have nothing to eat while the test is in progress, but he may drink water.

Blood and urine specimens are taken fasting and at intervals of one hour, two hours, and three hours after the patient has had the glucose. Minimal values for a positive test are 110, 170, 120, and 110 mg. per 100 ml. at these times, using the true blood glucose method. Specimens can also be taken at the fourth and fifth hours.

There are three popular methods of evaluating the glucose tolerance test for diabetes mellitus. These are the Wilkerson point system or U.S. Public Health Service criteria, the Fajans-Conn criteria, and the University Group Diabetes Mellitus program criteria (Davidson and Henry). Before the physician establishes a diagnosis of diabetes, he must eliminate other possible causes for an abnormal test and must evaluate the patient's total metabolic status.

**Intravenous Glucose Tolerance Test.** This test is used when the patient cannot drink a large amount of glucose because of nausea or gastrointestinal problems. Twenty-five Gm. of glucose is administered intravenously over a three-minute period. Blood specimens are obtained from an indwelling needle at five- or ten-minute intervals for a period of 40 minutes.

**Oral Cortisone Glucose Tolerance Test.** A more sensitive test in the detection of latent chemical diabetes involves the administration of cortisone, eight and one-half and two hours before the oral glucose tolerance test. Dosage is dependent on body weight.

**Urine Tests.** Monitoring glucose and ketones in

**Table 50-1. Urine Tests for Glucose**

| TEST | PERCENTAGE OF GLUCOSE | | | | | |
|---|---|---|---|---|---|---|
| Tes-Tape | 0 | — | 1/10 | 1/4 | 1/2 | 2 |
| Diastix | 0 | 1/10 | 1/4 | 1/2 | 1 | 2 |
| Clinitest | 0 | 1/4 | 1/2 | 3/4 | 1 | 2 |
| INTERPRETATION | Negative | Trace | + | ++ | +++ | ++++ |

Reprinted with permission from Krosnick, A.: *The Nurse and Diabetes Control*, N.J. State Department of Health.

urine helps to determine the degree to which diabetes is controlled. Changes in drugs, diet, or activity are prescribed on the basis of the results of regular testing of urine for sugar and acetone. Until diabetes is under control and during periods of stress, such as illness, testing is done four times a day, usually before meals and before the bedtime snack. When control is established, it may not be necessary to test four times a day.

The patient is taught the selected method, and assumes the responsibility for urine testing as soon as possible after diagnosis, and continues this except when he is too ill and requires the help of others. Whatever method is used, timing must be exactly as the manufacturer's literature indicates and testing materials must be kept from absorbing moisture from the environment or perspiration from the fingers. The bathroom is not a good place to store testing materials because of its high humidity. The patient must know the differences among methods, since the results are not interchangeable (Table 50-1). He must also be taught the significance of the findings and when to bring these to the physician's or nurse's attention.

**Collection of Urine Specimen.** Since it is important to test a fresh specimen, a "second-voided" specimen is collected. The first specimen voided may contain urine that has accumulated in the bladder for seven to eight hours (as, for example, the first voided specimen in the morning). The patient is instructed to void, saving the first specimen in case he is unable to give a second specimen; a half-hour later he voids again and the second specimen is tested. This is particularly important if the dosage of insulin is to be based on the results of the test.

When a patient has an indwelling catheter it is essential *not* to take a specimen for testing from the collection bag, as this urine may have been collected over a six- to eight-hour period.

Both glucose and acetone may be present in the urine at one time of the day and absent at another.

For this reason *fractional* urines may be tested. These are consecutive specimens collected and analyzed at stated times during the day and night. The patient saves all his urine in one large bottle. At intervals a specimen is taken from the bottle. The volume is recorded, the bottle emptied and cleaned and the collection starts all over again. The usual times for collections are 7 A.M., 11 A.M., 4 P.M., and 9 P.M. Fractional urines give a picture of the pattern of the excretion of glucose in the urine, and the timing of insulin injections may be planned accordingly.

Collection of a 24-hour urine specimen gives a measure of the efficiency of utilization of the food eaten. Ideally there should be no sugar, but 4 to 10 Gm. of glucose, or less, is considered a measure of good control. An adult diabetic whose 24-hour specimen has 10 per cent or more of his total carbohydrate allowance for the day would be poorly controlled, i.e., 180 Gm. of carbohydrate—18 Gm. of glucose.

The first voided morning specimen is discarded and all specimens are saved for the next 24 hours, including the first voided specimen the next morning. The total amount is measured in milliliters and a specimen of the total amount is tested with Clinitest. The percentage of sugar is found by matching against the color chart. The total amount in milliliters is multiplied by the percentage of sugar to determine the grams of sugar lost in a 24-hour period. For example, 45 ounces $\times$ 30 ml. per ounce = 1350 ml. $\times$ .01 = 13.5 Gm. of sugar lost.

Commonly used urine testing methods for sugar include reagent tablets (Clinitest) and reagent strips (Diastix, Tes-Tape). Keto-Diastix is used for both sugar and ketones. Ketostix (reagent strip) and Acetest (tablet or powder) are used for ketones alone.

Clinitest reagent tablets have virtually replaced Benedict's solution, but the chemical reaction is the same—the reduction of blue copper sulfate to red copper oxide. Unfortunately other reducing substances (i.e., nonglucose substances, such as fructose or lactose) can give false-positive reactions for sugar when Clinitest is used. The antibiotic cephalothin (Keflin) as well as other drugs can cause a false-positive reaction with Clinitest tablets.

FIVE-DROP CLINITEST METHOD. Urine is collected in a clean receptacle. Five drops of urine is placed in a test tube, the dropper rinsed, and 10 drops of water added, followed by a Clinitest tablet. The resulting color, after boiling ceases, is graded

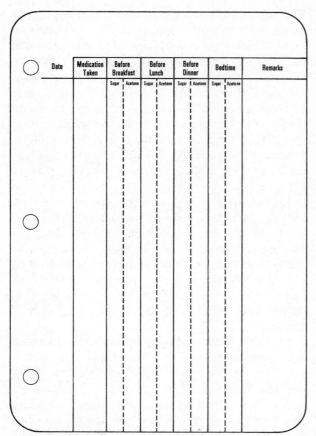

| Date | Medication Taken | Before Breakfast | | Before Lunch | | Before Dinner | | Bedtime | | Remarks |
|---|---|---|---|---|---|---|---|---|---|---|
| | | Sugar | Acetone | Sugar | Acetone | Sugar | Acetone | Sugar | Acetone | |
| | | | | | | | | | | |

**Figure 50-1.** A patient's notebook for the daily recording of urine tests.

in accordance with the Clinitest color chart after a 15-second waiting period. The tube should be observed while the reaction takes place, since a "pass-through" color phenomenon can take place making the final color an inaccurate guide. The 5-drop test is most frequently recorded with plus signs (1+ through 4+). When it is desirable to indicate glucose concentrations greater than 2 per cent (which the 4+, 5-drop Clinitest indicates) the 2-drop Clinitest (for levels up to 5 per cent) or the 1-drop Clinitest method (for levels up to 10 per cent) can be used. Special color charts with directions are available on request from the manufacturer (McFarlane et al., 1972).

Glucose-oxidase enzyme strips, such as Diastix or Tes-Tape, specifically detect glucose rather than nonspecific glycosuria. The reagent end of a Diastix strip is dipped into a container of urine or held in the urinary stream for 2 seconds and read against a series of color blocks after exactly 30 seconds.

Ketones in urine can depress the results of glucose measurement with reagent strips or sticks. An advantage of these tests is that the materials are convenient to carry. If need be, a patient can test his urine with these methods in the rest room of an airplane or while he is at a hotel.

The patient should also be taught to test urine for acetone using Acetest tablets, Ketostix, or Keto-Diastix.

Caps must be kept tight on bottles, because tablets, powder, and testing strips that have absorbed moisture from the air become useless. These testing materials can be bought in pharmacies.

The test for acetone becomes especially important when the patient has fever, vomiting, and consistent glucosuria, especially with 2 per cent or more. These are situations in which chances for the formation of ketone bodies are the greatest.

### Diabetic Records

Whether the nurse, patient, or family member assumes primary responsibility for urinary monitoring, all must understand that a daily record (Fig. 50-1) is an essential part of management and that urine testing is not just a meaningless chore. It is the chief way of assessing the level of control and the need for adjustments in insulin or diet. Daily entries should contain the record of urine examinations, insulin dosage, time of injection, and any comments about reactions, changes in exercise, or diet, or unusual stressors, such as illness or emotional upsets.

## TREATMENT

Diet therapy, education, and exercise are necessary for all diabetics; drug therapy (insulin or oral hypoglycemic agents) is necessary for some. It has been estimated that 25 per cent of diabetics can be managed by diet alone, 50 per cent by diet and oral hypoglycemics, and 25 per cent by diet and insulin.

The primary aims of therapy include the relief of symptoms; accomplishment of cognitive, affective, and psychomotor learning objectives; prevention of acute metabolic crises (ketoacidosis, hypoglycemia, hyperosmolar coma); and prevention or delay of long-term complications (atherosclerosis, microangiopathy).

Adaptation to a chronic illness such as diabetes always involves some change in the life style of the patient and, to a certain degree, the lives of others close to him. Some may be able to cope with the task adequately; others may require additional professional support to achieve adequate adjustment; while still others may lack the motivation or continuing support to make the necessary adjustment.

Generally, the better informed the patient is, the more effective will be the control of his diabetes, and, therefore, the healthier he may stay.

Treatment of diabetes must be carried out for the rest of the patient's life and it does impose restrictions and adjustments in life style. The patient (or in some instances, a family member) has the responsibility for making decisions about his day-to-day care, except during periods of illness (such as during complications of diabetes, or some other illness) when physicians and nurses temporarily carry out treatment until the patient can again assume this responsibility. Before the patient can be expected to learn factual information and technical skills, he requires assistance in accepting the fact that he has diabetes, and in dealing with his own feelings about having the disease. The nurse has an important role in helping the patient to gradually accept the condition, such as by listening to his feelings about it. She must also help to teach the patient how to carry out his treatment program. It is unrealistic to assume that these goals can be met by the newly diagnosed hospitalized diabetic, no matter how well presented the inpatient teaching program. Movement toward the goals of therapy can be initiated, but diabetic patients require long-term continuing education. Today a greater effort is made by communities to provide resources for the continuing education of diabetics using an interdisciplinary team-teaching approach (Somers, 1974).

The diabetes nursing specialist assumes a major role in the teaching and counseling of patients and in coordinating the education program.

## PSYCHOSOCIAL ASPECTS OF DIAGNOSIS

Before the various treatment modalities and the specific ways that the nurse can help the patient to apply them are discussed, several points require emphasis:

- The realization that they have diabetes is disturbing to most patients; denial, withdrawal, and depression are common responses.

    Initially, reaction to the diagnosis may be one of grief—a response to the loss of valued body integrity. Initially some patients may be relieved that their symptoms are due to a metabolic disease, rather than

to cancer, for example, but this can be followed by reactive depression when the patient feels the frustrations and resentment engendered by the discipline of the treatment program. Previously unexpressed anxieties may be intensified.

The basic personality of the patient influences the way he responds to the diagnosis. The patient should be encouraged to verbalize his perceptions of his situation and how he views the impact of the disease on his life.

- Before teaching begins it is important to assess the patient's cognitive, affective, and psychomotor strengths and limitations. What is his educational background? Is he capable of reading and understanding written learning aids, or are other methods, such as tape recordings or dial-access telephone lectures, more appropriate? Does he believe having diabetes means he will die? That he can no longer keep his job? That he will soon become blind or lose a leg? Many patients have such fears upon learning of their diagnosis. Opportunity must be provided for the patient to talk about any misconceptions.

    Do physical factors such as partial blindness or tremulous hands limit the patient's ability to give himself an insulin injection?

    Is cost likely to interfere with the patient's ability to comply with diet and drug therapy?

    What resources are available to help the patient with economic problems? Some welfare departments and other public assistance programs give an increased monetary allowance for food for diabetics.

    Are lists available of the charges made for drugs and equipment by all of the pharmacies in the area so that each patient does not have to comparison shop?

- The patient has a potentially serious illness and usually knows it. An approach which implies, "This is really nothing—all you have to do is spend a few extra moments each morning testing your urine and giving yourself insulin," serves more to relieve staff of their responsibilities to the patient, than to help the patient learn about his illness and deal with his feelings concerning it. It must never be implied that if the patient carries out his treatment faithfully, he will never experience complications. This is not true, and it can form a basis for later resentment. Treatment will help the patient feel well and avoid acute complications.

- Many patients profit from a combination of individual instruction and group teaching. The possibilities and advantages of group teaching are often not fully explored in many settings, both outpatient and inpatient. Sometimes group teaching in the hospital is not attempted because there are too few diabetic patients on one ward at a particular time but group teaching can be planned for patients from several wards.

- Coordination between physician and nurse in developing a plan for teaching the patient is essential. However, it is not appropriate for the nurse to wait for a physician's order before considering the patient's need for instruction. Ways that nurses, physicians, dietitians, social workers, vocational counselors, and others can help the patient learn about his condition require initiative and coordination on the part of the nurse. For example, as soon as the patient is admitted to the hospital, the nurse can contact the dietary department to request diet instruction at the same time that she transmits the diet prescription.

- Diabetes is especially prevalent among the elderly. Many older diabetics can learn to care for themselves if they are given sufficient time, instruction, and help in overcoming the disabilities of age (using a magnifying glass to see the markings on a syringe clearly or to read the label on a medicine bottle, for example). It is important to enlist the aid of the family or close associates, but the patient must remain the primary focus of instruction, unless it is clear that he cannot assume responsibility for his own treatment.

- The teaching staff must consider the use of words. The large number of terms that can be used to inform the patient about his diabetes can confuse and frighten him. Clear, common terms should be used. These will vary according to the educational, cultural, and experiential background of the patient, but the terms should be used consistently by all those who interact with the patient.

Before the patient leaves the hospital, it is advisable that he be able to realistically plan menus for his meals and snacks from his prescribed diet. Ideally, the patient should gradually be allowed to select and to plan his own diet, with help, during the course of his hospital stay. Accustoming himself to the size of the portions, planning when to eat, and learning to select the foods are all part of the adjustments he must make. Referral to a community nursing agency for follow-up visits by a nurse is almost always necessary. She continues teaching, checks on his progress at home, helps him with unforeseen problems that may arise, and refers him to other helpful resources in the community.

## DIET

Diet prescription is the cornerstone of treatment for all diabetics. It emphasizes a reduced and spaced intake of carbohydrate foods, lessening the strain on the patient's already inadequate insulin production. Although insulin and oral hypoglycemics may be used, no treatment will be successful without lifetime adherence to a prescribed diet.

Some diabetics, especially those who are overweight, can be controlled by reducing body weight to levels ideal for their age and body build and can then maintain control by diet alone. Diabetes is aggravated by excess weight.

Adjusting to a diet that is destined, perhaps with minor changes, to be mandatory for a lifetime, may seem to be a most dreary and discouraging prospect. Yet, if the patient's resolution vanishes in a moment of temptation as he passes a candy counter, his physiologic balance may collapse along with his resolve. If his dietary intake of carbohydrate is more than he can use or store, eventually he may develop ketosis. If he eats too little food, he ultimately will not only become malnourished but also, if he is taking insulin, be in danger of insulin shock. To prevent both occurrences, he must follow his prescribed diet, both in *quantity* and *quality*.

Diet regulation refers to a specified daily caloric intake spread over the entire active portion of the day. The regular timing of food intake and control of the proportions and quality of carbohydrate, protein, and fat in each meal or snack is important.

"Diabetic" diets do not mean special foods must be purchased. Rather each meal plan is selected from the same foods purchased and prepared for the rest of the family, provided, of course, that the family diet is nutritionally adequate.

Usually only simple sugars and sources of concentrated carbohydrates are prohibited. These include table sugar (sucrose), soft drinks, candy, honey, jams and jellies, syrups, molasses, pies, cake, cookies, pastries, and candy-coated chewing gum. Sugar-free cough syrups and cough drops are available and permitted. Alcohol may be permitted in small quantity, occasionally, but must be counted in the daily food allowance.

If a patient is following his diet and is hungry, or if he is unable to eat at all, the physician or nurse specialist must be notified immediately. A gastrointestinal upset that is minor for the nondiabetic could be a medical emergency for the diabetic, if it prevents him from eating the proper foods or causes vomiting or diarrhea.

The patient must eat no more and no less than that allowed each day, dividing the total into three meals. If snacks are included they are *counted* as part of the total daily intake.

Snacks are not arbitrary "rewards." Rather they are planned to provide additional carbohydrate and protein at a specified time each day, related to the peak of insulin action. When a long-acting insulin such as protamine zinc or ultralente is used, a bedtime snack is taken to prevent nocturnal hypoglycemia. Snacks are also permitted prior to or during a period of strenuous activity, such as football practice. Snack foods should contain protein and

### Table 50-2. Composition of Food Exchanges

| LIST | FOOD | MEASURES | GRAMS | | | |
|------|------|----------|-------|------|------|------|
| | | | CARB. | PROT. | FAT | CAL. |
| 1 | Milk Exchanges | 1/2 pt. | 12 | 8 | 10 | 170 |
| 2a | Vegetable Exchanges | as desired | — | — | — | — |
| 2b | Vegetable Exchanges | 1/2 cup | 7 | 2 | — | 36 |
| 3 | Fruit Exchanges | varies | 10 | — | — | 40 |
| 4 | Bread Exchanges | varies | 15 | 2 | — | 68 |
| 5 | Meat Exchanges | 1 oz. | — | 7 | 5 | 73 |
| 6 | Fat Exchanges | 1 tspn. | — | — | 5 | 45 |

fat as well as carbohydrate for a more sustained effect than concentrated carbohydrate would offer. An example would be two graham crackers and one-half cup of milk.

There are a number of diet "systems" in use in this country. At one extreme, the so-called "free diet," some physicians permit their patients to eat what they like, adjusting the dose of insulin according to the amount of sugar excreted in urine. On the other hand, patients at the Boston, Massachusetts, Joslin Clinic teaching center are required to weigh foods, at least as a learning exercise in the accurate measurement of food portions. The continued use of a weighed diet is recommended for juvenile and unstable diabetics.

A practical and popular approach, "Meal Planning with Exchange Lists," has been developed by The American Diabetes Association, the American Dietetic Association, and the U.S. Public Health Service (Tables 50-2 and 50-3). Food is selected in household measures from six basic exchange (substitution) lists. These are milk, vegetables (A and B), fruit, bread, meat, and fat exchanges. A number of exchanges (substitutes) are prescribed for each meal.

For example, an 1800-calorie diet might contain a dinner allotment of two meat exchanges, two bread exchanges, one vegetable exchange, one fruit exchange, and one milk exchange. The patient can exchange one item for any other in the same group and still obtain approximately the same food value. If the patient's diet allows him one meat exchange for lunch, he can look on a list and see that he can have an ounce of meat or chicken, an egg, a slice of cheese, one-quarter cup of canned fish, or a frankfurter.

The food plan for the day may be allotted in the following pattern: one-fifth for breakfast, two-fifths for his midday meal, one-fifth for supper, and one-fifth before retiring.

**The Diet Prescription.** When a diabetic meal plan is to be prescribed, a dietary history must include such factors as the age, sex, height, weight, life style, activity pattern, occupation, working hours, state of health, ethnic and cultural background, socioeconomic status, income, and insulin requirements. The patient's food preferences, likes, and dislikes must be ascertained, since compliance with diet therapy depends to a large extent on making the diet as appealing as possible for each individual.

A diabetic professional hockey player like Bobby Clarke, or a diabetic actress like Mary Tyler Moore or the baseball player Ron Santo, require different meal plans than would a writer like H. G. Wells, who also was a diabetic.

Having diabetes does not exclude intermittent strenuous activities of many different types, but does necessitate a well-balanced diet planned in accord with exercise and insulin requirements.

**Nursing Aspects.** The dietitian usually is responsible for the diet history and prepares the initial

### Table 50-3. Meal Plans and Daily Food Exchanges

| DIET | GRAMS | | | CAL. | EXCHANGES | | | | | | |
|------|-------|-------|-----|------|------|--------|-------|-------|-------|------|-----|
| | CARB. | PROT. | FAT | | MILK | VEG. A | VEG. B | FRUIT | BREAD | MEAT | FAT |
| 1 | 125 | 60 | 50 | 1200 | 1 Pt. | As desired | 1 | 3 | 4 | 5 | 1 |
| 2 | 150 | 70 | 70 | 1500 | 1 Pt. | " | 1 | 3 | 6 | 6 | 4 |
| 3 | 180 | 80 | 80 | 1800 | 1 Pt. | " | 1 | 3 | 8 | 7 | 5 |
| 4 | 220 | 90 | 100 | 2200 | 1 Pt. | " | 1 | 4 | 10 | 8 | 8 |
| 5* | 180 | 80 | 80 | 1800 | 1 Qt. | " | 1 | 3 | 6 | 5 | 3 |
| 6* | 250 | 100 | 130 | 2600 | 1 Qt. | " | 1 | 4 | 10 | 7 | 11 |
| 7* | 370 | 140 | 165 | 3500 | 1 Qt. | " | 1 | 6 | 17 | 10 | 15 |
| 8 | 250 | 115 | 130 | 2600 | 1 Pt. | " | 1 | 4 | 12 | 10 | 12 |
| 9 | 300 | 120 | 145 | 3000 | 1 Pt. | " | 1 | 4 | 15 | 10 | 15 |

*These diets contain more milk and are especially suited for children.
Meal planning with exchange lists. Reprinted with permission from, Krosnick, A.: *The Nurse and Diabetes Control*, New Jersey State Department of Health, 1970.

dietary instructions for the patient after his diet has been prescribed by the physician. However, the nurse assumes a major role in teaching fundamentals of the diet plan so she must understand the principles involved, teach certain aspects, and reinforce the teaching of other team members. In the hospital the nurse uses mealtime to review and instruct further. She must also request replacements for uneaten food items from the dietary department. Whether the patient is at home or hospitalized, the nurse must understand and help him to understand the concept of the management of diabetes on "sick days," the use of insulin at these times, variations in urine testing, and the use of liquid diet substitutes or bland, low-fiber foods when he cannot tolerate his normal diet.

**Affective Consideration.** Food, in most cultures, has certain psychologic and social meanings. For example, food may represent love, social grace, rewards, or ties to the religion, country, or family of origin. When food has a high cultural value, an attempt to take it away or ration it is a symbolic affront.

Diet regulation is especially difficult in the American culture, with its ever-increasing displays and advertising of cookies, candies, soft drinks, and ice cream. Diabetic patients with a low income may be tempted by carbohydrate-rich foods which are the least expensive items in food markets. Not only are concentrated carbohydrates routinely forbidden to diabetics but to add to the confusion, the diabetic is instructed to carry some candy or sugar on his person at all times, yet not to eat it except in a hypoglycemic emergency.

Some patients are additionally restricted, such as those on a low-sodium or low-cholesterol diet, which complicates meal planning. The services of an experienced dietitian for ongoing telephone consultation through the hospital dietary department or regional diet counseling center can be of assistance to physician, nurse, and patient when multiple dietary factors must be considered.

Many factors contribute to noncompliance with diet therapy, including an income too low for quality food expenditure, an educational level that limits the ability to comprehend food exchanges or weighed diets, misapplication of educational methods and skills by professionals, failure of professionals to consider ethnic and cultural determinants in food patterns, and the patient's inability to accept his disease. Some patients have physical disabilities limiting their ability to shop for groceries; others, especially the elderly who live alone, are lonely and lack the motivation to prepare well-balanced meals for themselves.

When it is obvious that the patient is not adhering to his diet, reasons must be evaluated and strategies developed to deal with the problem. A scolding or threatening attitude is not only not helpful, but is likely to arouse a negative emotional response and further noncompliance. Compassion, gentle persuasion, and praise for progress, however slight, encourage the patient to stay on his diet.

**Dietary Specifics.** CALORIES. Caloric intake is prescribed by using a table of ideal weights that considers age, sex, and body build as well as a multiplying factor that accounts for physical activity. This varies from 8 calories per pound per day for the patient on bed rest to 20 calories per pound per day for the person engaged in strenuous daily physical activity. The factor is 15 calories per pound per day for average physical activity. For example, 160 pounds $\times$ 15 calories equals 2400 calories per day for a man whose ideal weight is 160 pounds and whose physical activity is average.

CARBOHYDRATE. Calories from carbohydrates in the diabetic diet are reduced to 35 to 40 per cent rather than the usual 50 per cent characteristic of the average American diet, or not more than 200 to 250 Gm. per day. Foods rich in carbohydrate augment hyperglycemia. Also, carbohydrates, especially simple sugars such as table sugar (sucrose), that in soft drinks or in candy, induce hypertriglyceridemia in patients with Type IV hyperlipoproteinemia. This disorder of lipoprotein metabolism has been identified as a risk factor in premature atherosclerosis of the aorta and coronary arteries and is quite prevalent among diabetics.

Cereal, bread, rice, noodles, and spaghetti contain both carbohydrate and protein, an optimum type for the diabetic's carbohydrate source. Vegetables and fruits are advised also since they are more slowly absorbed and metabolized than simple sugars and also contain essential vitamins and minerals. Carbohydrates yield 4 calories per Gm. when metabolized and are mainly used for energy.

PROTEIN. Proteins yield 4 calories per Gm. when metabolized and are necessary to build muscles and other tissues. A minimum of 0.9 Gm. per kilogram (0.5 Gm. per pound) of high quality protein (containing the eight essential amino acids) daily is necessary for adults. Protein calories comprise about 20 per cent of the diabetic diet. Because of the increased risk of atherosclerosis, protein foods containing unsaturated rather than saturated fat may be necessary. Skimmed milk, fish, poultry, veal, and cottage cheese are recommended sources of protein.

FAT. Fats supply the most concentrated form of food energy, yielding 9 calories per Gm. If the diabetic diet is to be reduced in carbohydrate but normal in protein, it is obvious that an increase in calories from fat occurs. This essentially high fat diet cannot be used without modification for many diabetics, since atherosclerosis is the leading cause of morbidity and mortality in the diabetic. The diet must be palatable but must not raise plasma cholesterol and triglycerides. Such a diet must restrict butter, eggs, and fatty meats, such as pork. Lean beef is permitted. Vegetable oils should be substituted for saturated fats and fish and fowl used more frequently. Cholesterol intake should not exceed 300 mg. per day, and one-third of the fat calories should be polyunsaturated fats.

DIETETIC PRODUCTS. A number of sugarless products are on the market today. Most physicians believe that the diabetic patient should be educated to eat regular foods under the exchange system of diet preparation, and that there is no need to obtain special diabetic or dietetic food products, which add to the cost of food and are not necessarily advantageous nutritionally. Saccharin or other sugar substitutes may be used to sweeten tea and coffee instead of sugar, and to sweeten cooked foods after they have been cooked; otherwise, they will have a bitter taste. Various sodas are available that contain no sugar. Saccharin-sweetened puddings, cookies, and candies, and water-packed canned fruits are available. There is no added sugar in these products, but they still contain carbohydrates. There are two precautions: (1) the fats, proteins, and carbohydrates in such food still have to be counted within the framework of the patient's diet; (2) those diabetic patients who wish to buy these commercially produced foods must be instructed to *read the labels.* The sugar, fat and protein contents should be listed. "Low calorie" and "dietetic" are not synonymous with "no sugar."

DIET DURING ILLNESS. The patient needs instruction in the caloric and nutritive value of liquid and semisolid foods that can be substituted when the usual food intake pattern is interrupted due to illness. He should have such information written down for ready reference.

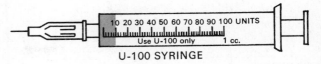

**Figure 50-2.** A U-100 insulin syringe. The nurse should always check carefully the scale on the syringe with the physician's order and the insulin bottle before drawing up the insulin.

## INSULIN

When the body does not produce enough effective insulin (endogenous insulin) the insulin must be supplied (exogenous insulin).

Before 1922 the only available therapy of severe diabetes was dietary limitation to the point of near starvation. The object of the diet was to keep the patient's blood glucose as nearly normal as possible. There was no effective treatment for diabetic coma, and death was inevitable. Most patients died five to ten years after the diagnosis was made.

In 1921 Frederick Banting and Charles Best produced the hypoglycemic factor, insulin, from dog pancreas. In the following year humans were first treated with it. Now, treatment with insulin can achieve good metabolic control of diabetes, prevent ketosis, and prolong the patient's life.

Commercial insulin is made from the pancreas of hogs and cows, and some from fish pancreas; a small amount of human insulin is available for research. Insulin, a complex protein, has been synthesized but not perfectly since it does not act like insulin when used in the human body. Insulin must be injected since it is inactivated by the digestive juices. It is measured in units—1 unit being the amount necessary to lower blood glucose in a fasting rabbit, weighing 2 kg., from a normal level to 45 mg. per 100 ml. In the past, insulin was prepared in solutions of various strengths, such as U-40 or U-80. At present, U-100 insulin is being marketed and after 1975 U-40 and U-80 insulin will be discontinued.

Units are clearly marked on the bottle and on the insulin syringe. U-40, U-80, and U-100 insulins, respectively, contain 40 units, 80 units, and 100 units per milliliter (Fig. 50-2). The bottles and syringe markings are color coded: red for U-40, green for U-80, and orange for U-100.

The patient needs to understand that the number of units he takes of U-100 insulin, using a U-100 syringe, is the same number of units he took from a U-40 bottle using a U-40 syringe or a U-80 bottle

**Table 50-4. Forms of Insulin**

| TYPE | EFFECT STARTS WITHIN | PEAK EFFECTS | EFFECT LASTS FOR |
|---|---|---|---|
| *Short-Acting* | | | |
| Regular | | | |
| Crystalline | 1/2–1 hr. | 2–4 hrs. | 6–8 hrs. |
| Semilente | 1/2–1 hr. | 2–4 hrs. | 6–8 hrs. |
| *Intermediate-Acting* | | | |
| Globin | 1–2 hrs. | 8–10 hrs. | 12–16 hrs. |
| NPH | 1–2 hrs. | 8–10 hrs. | 12–16 hrs. |
| Lente | 1–2 hrs. | 8–10 hrs. | 12–16 hrs. |
| *Long-Acting* | | | |
| Protamine Zinc | 4–8 hrs. | 14–20 hrs. | 36–72 hrs. |
| Ultralente | 5–8 hrs. | 14–20 hrs. | 36–72 hrs. |

using a U-80 syringe. The difference is one of volume only. U-100 is more concentrated than U-80, which, in turn, is more concentrated than U-40. Thus a smaller volume of U-100 insulin is needed for injection; this also represents an economic savings.

A patient requiring more than 100 units of U-100 insulin can use a standard 2-ml. syringe for measuring and injecting the dose.

The physician usually specifies both the dose and unit type of insulin to be used; for example, NPH Insulin 20 U of U-100.

When the insulin syringe is held, the first thing to do is to match the correct scale to the bottle and the patient's ordered dose. Twenty units of U-40 insulin measured on the U-80 scale would give the patient only half his correct dose. One advantage of change to a single concentration of insulin (U-100) and a syringe marked on a U-100 scale is the reduction in dosage errors related to the use of multiscale syringes.

**Forms of Insulin.** Insulin preparations are classified as rapid, intermediate, and long-acting according to the time of their peak hypoglycemic effect and duration of action after subcutaneous injection (Table 50-4).

In general, rapid-acting insulins (regular, crystalline, semilente) are used to supplement other forms of insulin, or in situations where rapid control of diabetes is essential, as in ketoacidosis, during and after surgery, and where the response to insulin is unpredictable.

Because the short-acting forms do not last throughout an entire day, a means of prolonging the action is necessary, so such substances as zinc, globin, and protamine are added. NPH (neutral protamine Hagedorn) is an intermediate-acting insulin; PZI (protamine zinc insulin) and ultralente are long acting. Some patients can get along with only one long-acting injection a day, and still not become hyperglycemic at night. However, because of the danger with long-acting insulins of nocturnal hypoglycemia and in order to give smoother control of blood sugar, insulin preparations whose effects are intermediate in time, such as NPH and lente, are used more frequently than the long-acting forms. Recent studies indicate that the use of two doses of intermediate-acting insulin (morning and late afternoon or early evening) gives better control in some patients (Guthrie and Guthrie, 1973). The long-acting forms (PZI and ultralente) usually are not given alone; supplementary regular insulin may be necessary to achieve control during parts of the day. "Hangover effects" from previous injections can also occur.

Both NPH and PZI contain protamine, a protein which delays absorption and also fixes the pH at 7.2. The lente family of insulins is not combined with protein but is mixed with an acetate buffer, which determines absorption. The lente family of insulins can be intermixed and can be combined with crystalline insulin. Other combinations of insulins may alter pH, change the absorption pattern, and cause irregularities, so compatibility must be known before mixing. Since the lente family is not combined with protein, these insulins are less likely to cause an allergic response, as compared with NPH or PZI.

PZI contains a large excess of protamine. If regular insulin is added, the excess protamine combines with regular insulin to form more PZI—hence the rapid action may be negligible. If these are to be given together, the physician must compensate for this reaction when ordering the dose of each insulin, such as using a ratio of 2 units of regular insulin to 1 unit of PZI. NPH insulin can be mixed with regular (crystalline) insulin because the protamine is completely bound.

Before withdrawing it into the syringe, PZI and NPH must be mixed by rotating the container between the palms and gently turning it end over end. They are not shaken since this would create a froth that would make it difficult to withdraw the insulin into the syringe. If the insulin is not mixed well, the dosage received by the patient will vary from injection to injection. Rapid-acting insulins are administered 15 to 30 minutes before a meal, so the insulin reaches the cell receptors at about the same time as does the glucose; long-acting insulins usually are given 30 minutes to one hour before the patient eats. It is the nurse's responsibility to safeguard the hospitalized patient by insuring that the interval between insulin injections and meals is correct. This is one medication that should always be given on time. If the patient is fasting for a blood sugar test or a glucose tolerance test, or does not eat for any other reason, his insulin is not given until 15 to 30 minutes before his meal is certain to be served. Exact timing is most important. If the patient's usual meal pattern would be very upset due to his fasting for a minor surgical procedure, for example, he may be managed on regular insulin for that day.

**Indications.** Insulin must be supplied for all patients in diabetic acidosis; for those with juvenile diabetes; as initial therapy for diabetics of any age who have ketonuria and other intense symptoms; in stable diabetics undergoing severe stress, such as major surgery, infection, or pregnancy; and when diet and oral hypoglycemics fail to bring about control in the maturity-onset diabetic.

**Intravenous Insulin.** Insulin is almost always given subcutaneously. Regular insulin is generally used intravenously only as the first dose in a severely ill diabetic in acidosis. It has a low pH (acid). Its reaction when added to an intravenous solution is unpredictable. It must be mixed well or it may crystallize out and some may be adsorbed on the tubing.

**Patient Education.** Almost all diabetics who need insulin can and should be taught to inject it themselves. A member of the patient's family or a close associate should also be taught, in case the patient becomes unable to help himself. It is also recommended that diabetics who receive hypoglycemic drugs be taught how to inject insulin so that they are prepared when the need arises, as in the event of infection. Because injection is a daily procedure, it is important that the insulin-dependent diabetic patient be independent and have control over his own regimen. Teaching can start as soon as his symptoms have been relieved, a treatment regimen has been established by his physician, and his cognitive, affective, and psychomotor strengths and limitations have been assessed. The teaching pace must be regulated by the patient's understanding and acceptance of his condition and his associated physical limitations.

It is not easy to learn to insert a needle into the flesh of another person. For many people it is even harder, initially, to give an injection to themselves. For the first injection into his own skin, the nurse may wish to guide the patient's hands. Although injections are commonplace in the nurse's work, this familiarity is not so for most others. Yet, with support, 9-year-olds and 90-year-olds have overcome their distaste for the procedure, and in some cases, children have taught their parents.

Some patients find the Busher Automatic Injector helpful. This device automatically inserts the needle at a proper depth and angle. It can be used or adapted for use with any B-D (Becton, Dickinson and Company) self-contained disposable insulin syringe or insulin syringe/needle unit. It is widely available and reasonably priced.

Blind or nearly blind patients can be taught to inject themselves but need to have the syringe filled for them. For convenience, a five-day supply can be prepared by the community health nurse or sighted associate of the patient and kept in the refrigerator.

Most patients must be taught all phases of the injection process, including how to inject air into the bottle (or both bottles if more than one insulin is used in one syringe) before any insulin is withdrawn; to eliminate bubbles; and to ascertain that a blood vessel has not been entered.

If he is not going to use disposable equipment, he must be taught how to boil the syringe and the needle for ten minutes, to examine the needle for burrs and dullness before sterilizing it, and how to sharpen it when it is necessary.

It is recommended that insulin be given at a 90-degree angle, with the needle held perpendicular to the skin, instead of the more common 45-degree to 60-degree subcutaneous angle. For obese patients a three-quarter-inch 25-gauge needle may be needed. In thin patients, injecting insulin into a skin fold pinched between the fingers helps to prevent an intramuscular injection. The objective is to place the insulin deep in the subcutaneous tissue, not into the skin, and not intravenously.

**Site of Injection.** The rate at which insulin is absorbed is influenced by the site of injection and the amount of subcutaneous tissue. Absorption is more rapid from the upper extremities than from the lower. The degree of muscle work also influences absorption. For example, a runner who injects into the thigh preceding a race will have a different rate of absorption than he will have on a day when he is not racing.

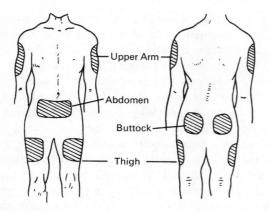

**Figure 50-3.** Recommended sites for insulin injection. A diagram can be made to help the patient remember the rotation pattern.

The patient must be taught to vary the site of injection on a regular schedule to avoid *lipodystrophies* (Fig. 50-3). The importance of this precaution cannot be overemphasized. A given area, 3 to 4 cm. in diameter, should receive insulin no more than once in three or four weeks.

*Atrophy* of subcutaneous fat in the arm, thigh, or abdomen occurs particularly in girls and young women.

*Hypertrophy* or bulging of subcutaneous tissue occurs mostly in boys and young men. Hypertrophic sites have the appearance of developed muscle but are actually avascular fibrous scar tissue, partially or totally anesthetic. Because of this lack of sensation, these sites may be unwisely selected, particularly by unsupervised children, to avoid pain. Absorption of insulin is very poor.

Lipodystrophic tissue can return to normal, though very slowly, if injections at the site are stopped. Because the cause of lipodystrophy is not clear, the patient may prefer to give his injections into lesser exposed subcutaneous tissue, such as the abdominal wall. Lipodystrophy is said to be less marked in patients using U-100 insulin.

**Insulin Dosage.** There is no certain way for the physician to select the ideal dose of insulin for a newly diagnosed diabetic. One way to arrive at a dose is to subtract 100 from the fasting blood sugar and divide this result by 5. Another way is to simply start with 10 to 20 units of an intermediate insulin and supplement this with regular insulin according to fractional urine tests and to 24-hour quantitative urine glucose and blood glucose determinations.

The morning dose is gradually increased based on the amount of regular insulin needed. A week to ten days is often necessary before the ideal dose is reached (but it is not necessary for a patient to be hospitalized all this time).

**Monitoring Glycemia and Adjusting Insulin Dosage.** Studying the pattern of response to insulin, diet, and exercise is necessary to assure that a satisfactory pattern of glycemia is achieved, rather than peak highs or lows.

The patient's record of sugar and acetone tests of the "second voided" specimen four times a day is one method of assessment. Urine testing, combined with the convenient method of measuring capillary blood glucose with the use of Dextrostix and Reflectance Meter (which can be done even in the home), or measurement of venous blood glucose at expected periods of hyperglycemia and hypoglycemia gives more accurate information as well as an indication of renal threshold. Occasionally the physician may request a 24-hour urine specimen for glucose measurement. The patient can do this at home simply. A continuous monitor for 24-hour monitoring of blood glucose is presently in research use (Guthrie and Guthrie).

It should be recognized that completely predictable response to insulin, diet, and exercise is rarely achieved and that there are often day-to-day fluctuations in the same compliant patient.

The so-called "coverage method" of giving regular insulin in a dose based on the amount of sugar in fractional urine specimens is only taking care of an event that has already occurred, whereas study of the pattern of response may indicate the need for a change in the type as well as the dose of insulin. For example, some possible alternate prescriptions for a patient on NPH insulin, who is hyperglycemic in the early morning and hypoglycemic at night include changing to PZI with a dose of regular insulin before breakfast; changing to lente insulin with a small amount of ultralente for night effect; or the dose of NPH or lente insulin could be split, giving three-quarters in the morning and one-quarter at night.

A patient receiving an intermediate-acting insulin, who is hyperglycemic before breakfast, might have his dose of insulin increased, ultralente insulin added, or changed to a two-dose (A.M. and P.M.) schedule of NPH or lente insulin.

A midafternoon low glucose could mean that the

early morning dose of intermediate insulin is too high or the luncheon food intake is too low. If the glucose is high at midafternoon, the morning dose of intermediate insulin may need to be increased.

A patient with an extremely high prelunch glucose with normal fasting and late afternoon levels might require a morning dose of regular insulin along with his intermediate-acting insulin or a combination of lente and semilente.

Cooperative, alert patients can be taught to modify their insulin dosage, according to written guidelines developed by the physician supplemented by telephone consultations between visits with the physician or nurse specialist. The amount of sugar in second-voided specimens over two or more days and symptoms of hypoglycemia are indicators of the need for insulin dosage adjustment. Different guidelines are necessary for patients taking insulin in two daily doses rather than one. The patient must not only know the duration and peak of action of the insulin he is taking but must understand the significance of his urine test results to be able to modify his dosage properly.

**Insulin on Sick Days.** During illness, even when the patient is unable to eat, the liver continues to manufacture glucose (gluconeogenesis), which requires insulin for its metabolism. It is a common *error* to presume that since no food is eaten, insulin should not be taken. It is urgent that the patient or responsible associate understand that the *usual daily dose of insulin must never be omitted.* During any illness, the patient must test his urine four times a day, since additional insulin may be required. Any illness in a diabetic should be viewed as a possible prelude to diabetic coma. A vial of regular insulin should always be kept on hand. The patient, as well as a responsible close associate, must be instructed in and provided with written guidelines for sick days.

Patients on oral hypoglycemics can also develop diabetic acidosis, though this is uncommon, and may require insulin treatment during illness. For this reason instruction about insulin should be part of the curriculum for all diabetics.

**Storage of Insulin.** The diabetic should make it a practice to study the product literature that comes with his insulin. Storage directions are included. Generally, it is recommended that the reserve supply of insulin be refrigerated to maintain its potency until the expiration date. At room temperature (68 to 75 degrees F) a bottle of insulin in current use will maintain its potency if used within a few weeks. Extremes of temperature (below 34 or over 75 degrees F) must be avoided as loss of potency can occur. Physical changes in insulin may make it difficult to withdraw the proper dose of insulin. Insulin which has changed in appearance or is difficult to draw into a syringe should not be used.

Insulin travel kits are available. The traveler to another country should take sufficient insulin with him if he is not certain that the correct type can be purchased at his place of destination. Not all types are available in every country. A vacuum bottle can be used to protect insulin, if extremes of temperature are anticipated.

**Continuing Education.** Not only do newly diagnosed diabetics require instruction and supervision, but the manner in which the patient is caring for himself should be evaluated periodically.

The necessity for periodic evaluation of self-care cannot be stressed too strongly. In one study of 162 diabetic patients from three clinics and 22 private practices, it was found that 58 per cent of 115 patients taking insulin made dosage errors (Watkins, et al., 1967a). The same study showed that, of the 47 patients taking oral drugs, 23 per cent made potentially serious errors. Errors and misunderstanding concerning sterilization of equipment, urine testing, and adherence to prescribed diet were also prevalent (Watkins et al. 1967b). Too often a brief program of instruction is given to the newly diagnosed diabetic without necessary followup. Often the patient is uncertain about aspects of his self-care and soon begins to make mistakes. Such errors can be triggered, for instance, by a neighbor who explains that it is better and cheaper to buy disposable syringes, and then boil them, so that they can be reused. (The markings quickly become indistinct, and the patient may then measure his insulin incorrectly.)

When the patient's ability to carry out his own care is evaluated, it is more effective to ask him to explain what he does and demonstrate how he does it, than for the nurse merely to repeat to him the instructions he may have heard many times but may misunderstand or apply incorrectly.

**Insulin Resistance.** After pancreatectomy in nondiabetic patients, the insulin requirement is only 20 to 50 units daily, whereas patients with diabetes sometimes require 80 or 100 units or more daily. Often this need cannot be related to diet, activity, or infection. When patients require more than 200 units daily for at least two days in the absence of any known cause, the term *insulin resistance* is used. It has been hypothesized that insulin resistance may be due to the binding of insulin by antibodies in circulating blood, tissue unresponsiveness due to antibodies against insulin present in tissues, or insufficient available insulin receptors at the cellular level.

Treatment may include a shift to pure pork, pure beef, or fish insulin. Steroids may also be given.

**Insulin Allergy.** Redness and itching at the injection site or generalized urticaria (hives) are indications of allergy to insulin. Although this usually clears without treatment or with antihistamine drugs, it requires prompt treatment if respiratory embarrassment or anaphylactic shock appears. Insulin allergy usually occurs in those who resume injections after they discontinued exogenous insulin for a period of time. The treatment may involve the use of antihistamines, such as diphenhydramine (Benadryl), switching to plain pork, or plain beef, or fish insulin, or desensitizing the patient by using dilutions of insulin.

**Fluid Shifts.** When insulin therapy is instituted initially, or given to a patient who had been grossly out of control for some time, rehydration and restoration of electrolyte balance can cause edema of the feet and legs, or more dramatically, blurred vision due to swelling of the optic lens. The edema abates after several days of therapy; a change of eyeglass lenses should not be made for several months until a stable state is achieved.

The patient recovering from acidosis should be asked whether his vision is clear or blurred.

## EXERCISE

Regular exercise is an essential part of therapy. Physical exertion enhances peripheral utilization of glucose as a source of energy in muscle cells and other tissues. Where practical, exercise should be prescribed as diet and drugs are prescribed, taking into account the individual's age, sex, occupation, life style, interests, environmental limitations, and other health conditions. Walking for exercise is available to almost all, but sudden spurts of physical exertion should be avoided.

Those who engage in very active intermittent muscular work, such as football players, can be taught to vary their diet pattern to provide for periods of exertion or reduce their insulin dosage on heavy exercise days, or both. For example, before playing, the diabetic may take slow-acting carbohydrate, such as milk with crackers or bread and supplementary feedings every one to two hours while actively engaged in exercise. Concentrated forms of carbohydrate ("sweets") may also be permitted during strenuous exercise.

## WEIGHT REDUCTION

Except in the case of complicating illness, the obese maturity-onset diabetic patient may be able to achieve control by reducing his weight to that recommended and by adhering to his prescribed diet and exercise program. If diabetes is still uncon-

Table 50-5. Oral Hypoglycemic Drugs

| GENERIC NAME | TRADE NAME | SIZE (MG.) | USUAL DAILY DOSE | APPROXIMATE DURATION OF ACTION (HRS.) |
|---|---|---|---|---|
| *Sulfonylureas* | | | | |
| Tolbutamide | Orinase | 500 | 0.5–3.0 Gm. | 6½ |
| Tolazamide | Tolinase | 100, 250 | 0.1–1.0 Gm. | 6–18 |
| Chlorpropamide | Diabinese | 100, 250 | 0.1–0.5 Gm. | 24–60 |
| Acetohexamide | Dymelor | 250, 500 | 0.25–1.5 Gm. | 12–24 |
| *Phenethylbiguanide* | | | | |
| Phenformin (tablets) | DBI Meltrol-25 | 25 | 25–200 mg. | 4–6 |
| Phenformin (timed-disintegration capsules) | DBI-TD Meltrol-50 Meltrol-100 | 50, 100 | 50–300 mg. | 8–14 |

trolled, then he may respond to an oral hypoglycemic agent.

## ORAL HYPOGLYCEMIC DRUGS

Oral drugs may be prescribed when weight reduction, diet, and exercise fail to produce control in the diabetic over age 40 who has had the disease less than five years. Oral hypoglycemics are of no value in juvenile diabetes or in the symptomatic adult with acetonuria; in these cases insulin is essential.

There are two groups of oral hypoglycemic agents; the sulfonylureas and the phenethylbiguanides. Phenformin is the only drug of the latter group in current use in the United States (Table 50-5). The sulfonylureas are thought to act by stimulating the beta cells of the pancreas to secrete or release more insulin; and the biguanides act at the cellular level, promoting the utilization of glucose by muscle and other peripheral tissue. The latter may also act on the intestine by decreasing its rate of glucose transport and thus absorption. The exact action of the oral hypoglycemics is not fully understood, however.

The sulfonylureas include tolbutamide (Orinase), chlorpropamide (Diabinese), tolazamide (Tolinase), and acetohexamide (Dymelor). These agents cannot lower blood sugar in a patient who has no pancreas, or in a patient whose pancreas cannot be stimulated to release more insulin. They are not used in patients with gastrointestinal disturbances that interfere with absorption, or in those with previous toxic reactions to any sulfa drug; they may not work well if certain other drugs such as the thiazide diuretics and birth control pills are being used. Since tolbutamide, chlorpropamide, acetohexamide, and tolazamide are metabolized by the liver, they should not be used in patients with hepatic disease since unmetabolized drug can accumulate in the blood and result in hypoglycemic coma. Kidney disease is also a contraindication to the sulfonylureas, especially chlorpropamide whose metabolic breakdown products are still pharmacologically active; this is less of a problem with tolbutamide. Oral hypoglycemics are contraindicated during pregnancy because of possible teratogenic effects that have as yet not been clarified.

Severe hypoglycemia can occur when sulfonylureas are taken by patients who are chronic alcoholics. In addition, chlorpropamide exerts a disulfiram effect with alcohol ingestion, causing acute illness (sweating, weakness, apathy, nausea, and vomiting).

Longer-acting sulfonylureas should be avoided in the elderly because in this group hypoglycemia often presents with central nervous system symptoms initially. When there is liver disease or arteriolar nephrosclerosis (common in the elderly), hypoglycemia may be misdiagnosed as a cerebral vascular accident, wasting valuable treatment time. Blood glucose should be determined immediately in elderly patients in coma.

Mild side effects associated with the sulfonylureas include dermatitis and gastrointestinal upset; severe side effects include hepatotoxicity and bone marrow depression. These potential effects should be monitored by blood counts and liver function studies.

There are two types of phenformin: tablets and timed-disintegration capsules. Because an anorexogenic effect of phenformin often diminishes food intake and promotes weight loss, it may be the drug of choice for the obese maturity-onset diabetic. Since these patients often have normal or excessive amounts of insulin, as determined by immunoassay, there is no point in stimulating insulin further by using the sulfonylureas.

Phenformin enhances the formation of lactic acid in diabetics, so it is important that patients receiving phenformin routinely test their urine for ketone bodies as well as glucose. Plasma bicarbonate levels may be required in these patients if symptoms suggestive of acidosis appear. The side effects of phenformin include a "metallic" taste in the mouth and gastrointestinal disturbances, i.e., nausea, vomiting, and diarrhea. The patient must report these symptoms if they occur, since dehydration, electrolyte imbalance, and acidosis can result.

With some patients a maximal dosage of oral drugs fails to reduce blood sugar ("primary failure"). Others may initially obtain a good response but later fail to respond ("secondary failure"). In secondary failure, a different sulfonylurea may be tried or a combination of a sulfonylurea with phenformin. This latter combination is especially useful when a high but necessary dose of phenformin alone causes intolerable diarrhea. Adding a sulfonylurea may bring control with a lower dose of phenformin. Phenformin can also be tried with the insulin-dependent diabetic to enable him to achieve control with less insulin. In primary failure, insulin must be administered.

A danger of oral hypoglycemic drugs is that the patient may underestimate the danger in the progression of his disease; he may fail to remain under medical supervision, or he may neglect his diet, his foot care, or his urinalysis. He may erroneously reason that his disease can be ignored, because taking a pill is so much simpler than the injections taken by others with the same diagnosis. In talking with the patient the nurse should help him to recognize the need for care, but to lessen anxiety that can interfere with his ability to care for himself.

Oral hypoglycemics are more expensive than insulin. The patient may have to be referred to a social service agency for information regarding sources of financial assistance.

The nurse should be aware of the possibility of drug potentiation or drug incompatibility when other medications are taken by the patient. For example, the hypoglycemic effect of tolbutamide is increased by phenylbutazone, long-acting sulfa drugs, bishydroxycoumarin, probenecid, salicylates in large doses, propranolol, and the monamine oxidase inhibitors.

**The University Group Diabetes Program Study (UGDP).** During the 1960's a prospective study of 8½ years involving patients in 12 geographically separated medical centers was aimed at determining if the vascular complications of diabetes could be delayed or prevented by diet, oral drugs, or insulin. A higher statistical incidence of cardiovascular deaths in subjects treated with diet and tolbutamide and diet and phenformin has created a controversy over the use of such agents, although no cause and effect relationship was established. Diabetologists who continue to prescribe these drugs cite inappropriate case selection, inadequate therapeutic regimens due to a fixed dose of drug, and inappropriate biostatistical techniques as supportive of their rejection of the UGDP study conclusion that the use of oral hypoglycemics is accompanied by an increased risk of cardiovascular deaths.

**Parameters of Control.** There is some agreement that "good control" of diabetes would be characterized by little or no glycosuria; a two-hour postprandial glucose at or near normal (less than 150 mg. per 100 ml.); infrequent and minimal hypoglycemia; absence of ketonuria and ketonemia; normal serum lipids; and normal growth and development.

## SHORT-TERM COMPLICATIONS

### Insulin Reaction (hypoglycemic reaction; insulin shock)

When there is too much insulin in the bloodstream in relation to the amount of available glucose—in other words, when blood glucose goes below about 50 mg. per 100 ml. of blood—hypoglycemia results. The cause can be too much insulin, too little food, or more than the usual amount of physical activity. Reaction occurs around the time of predicted peak effect of the specific insulin the patient is receiving. Hypoglycemia can also occur in those receiving oral hypoglycemic drugs, especially the elderly (see also section on Oral Hypoglycemics).

The initial signs and symptoms are due to the liberation of epinephrine as the body's homeostatic mechanism attempts to elevate the low blood sugar level by releasing liver glycogen as glucose.

**Symptoms and Signs.** The pattern of insulin reaction varies from patient to patient, depending on the degree of hypoglycemia, the patient's individual reaction, and the type of insulin taken. For example, with the long-acting insulins, the symptoms may be headache, nausea, drowsiness, and a feeling of malaise. Many patients who are having an insulin reaction initially experience weakness, nervousness, hunger, tremors, and excessive perspiration. Some patients have personality changes characteristic for them. One may become combative and negativistic; another, weepy. Confusion, aphasia, numbness of the lips and hands, delirium, a staggering gait, or vertigo may occur. If the hypoglycemia is not relieved, symptoms may progress to difficulty with coordination, and the patient may have double vision. If he still is untreated, he may have convulsions and become unconscious; if he is neglected further, he may suffer permanent brain damage, and, in very rare cases, he may die. Symptoms are variable, but they tend to be repeated in the same person whenever he has relatively too much insulin and too little food. The sequence may be extremely rapid, with the patient convulsing or dropping into unconsciousness before any other symptoms are noticed.

It is important to teach nursing aides, the family, and anyone else who may be with the patient that personality change may represent a hypoglycemic reaction and should be treated as such.

Patients who develop personality reactions are

often not able to treat themselves with sugar, so someone else must do it. While the patient who feels faint and weak often is viewed as sick, the one who becomes obstinate or aggressive may not be treated as promptly. Asking such a patient, "Would you like to have some sugar?" usually evokes the response, "No!" Instead, he should be given the sugar, assisted to take it, and his response should be observed. If he does not respond after a second dose is given ten minutes after the first, the physician should be notified.

A hypoglycemic reaction can occur when the diabetic is in a deep sleep. Signs may include nightmares, sleepwalking, restless tossing about, or calling out. If awakened, the patient may be hostile and combative or may exhibit other behavior atypical for him.

**Treatment.** Suspected insulin reaction demands immediate treatment with a fast-acting sugar. Examples are:

4 ounces of orange juice or regular ginger ale
2 lumps of sugar
6 to 7 Lifesavers or 4 Charms
2 teaspoons of a concentrated syrup such as Karo, cola, or honey
4 ounces of a commercially prepared solution such as Glucola or Dexcola

Ten minutes should be allowed for these to act, and if there is no improvement the same dose should be repeated.

Because of the danger of aspiration, liquids must not be given to the unconscious hypoglycemic person. The treatment alternatives include Instant Glucose, glucagon, intravenous 50 per cent glucose solution, or a rectal retention enema containing 3 to 4 ounces of concentrated syrup such as Karo, cola, or honey. Instant Glucose (Reactose) is a thick sweet substance that can be absorbed when placed inside the cheek.

*Glucagon* is a product of the alpha cells of the pancreas, which, when injected, acts on the liver to change glycogen to glucose, provided the liver has adequate glycogen reserves. If the patient has been out of control, with a consistently high blood sugar, the liver's store of glucose may be depleted and treatment with glucagon will not be effective.

Commercially prepared glucagon is available by prescription. The adult dose is 1 to 2 mg. subcutaneously or intramuscularly, in the form of a solution made by dissolving the lyophilized powder in the solvent that comes with it. Since glucagon is pre-

pared from animal extract, sensitization reaction is possible, though rare.

Ordinarily the patient responds in 5 to 20 minutes if glycogen stores are not depleted. Glucagon can be repeated once or twice at 20-minute intervals. When the patient wakes, he should be given orange juice or another quick-acting carbohydrate.

If the patient does not respond he requires the immediate attention of a physician so that glucose, 50 per cent, can be administered intravenously.

When the hospitalized patient requires glucagon, blood should be drawn for glucose determination whenever possible, while the nurse is preparing the medication.

Any institutional unit that has diabetics among its patient population must have fast-acting carbohydrate and glucagon quickly available. In the home a family member or other associate of the patient should know how to administer glucagon in the event a physician or nurse is not immediately available.

A night-time insulin reaction can go unrecognized, but the body's homeostatic response may cause the morning urine test for sugar to be unexplainably high. Obviously, giving more insulin would worsen the situation. A decrease in intermediate- or long-acting insulin or an increase in the bedtime snack is indicated.

Insulin reaction is as much a medical emergency as is diabetic coma. The nurse stays with the patient, observing him and participating in therapeutic measures. After such an episode the regulation of the patient's metabolism is very difficult for about 24 hours, and he should be under close observation for further symptoms of imbalance. If the reaction is severe, cerebral edema can result, with signs persisting for several days. Brain damage is a possibility.

PREVENTION OF INSULIN REACTION. The patient must understand and practice uniformity from day to day with regard to insulin, diet (including meals and snacks), and exercise. He should be positive about the type and dose of insulin he requires and know when the peak hypoglycemic effect should occur. Unusual exercise must be offset by a decrease in insulin or by additional food. Selected patients can be taught to decrease their dose according to rules.

Every diabetic should carry on his person at all times a source of concentrated carbohydrate and a means of identifying himself as a diabetic, such as

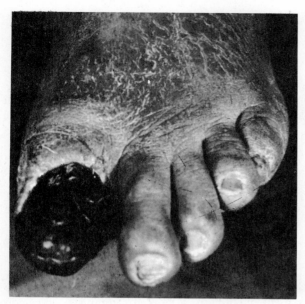

**Figure 50-4.** Gangrene of the toe. (Dr. W. L. Lowrie, Detroit)

an American Diabetes Association card or Medic Alert emblem. It is recommended that the insulin-dependent diabetic not operate a motor vehicle for more than one hour without taking carbohydrate, and the diabetic on intermediate insulin should have a midafternoon snack to avoid an accident if driving home from work. Diabetics who drive should not delay or skip meals and should pull off the road and get help at the least symptom of a reaction.

A full insulin reaction can be a terrifying experience for a patient. Each incident can be used as a learning experience if the nurse reviews the entire episode with the patient, who is often well motivated to prevent such drastic imbalance in the future.

## Infections

Patients with diabetes are highly susceptible to infections, infections heal slowly, and the diabetes itself becomes more difficult to control while the infection persists. The most frequent foci of infection are the urinary tract (pyelonephritis) and the skin (furuncles and carbuncles). Vulvovaginitis, balanitis, prostatic abscess, upper respiratory infection, and infections of the feet are also more frequent. The latter includes infected corns and fungus infection of the nails and toes. Ulcer forma-

tion with cellulitis and gangrene (Fig. 50-4) may result in loss of part of the foot or leg. Tuberculosis is said to be more frequent in diabetics than in nondiabetics.

Prevention of infection must be emphasized in the education program and in care given by the health care team. So that the condition can be diagnosed accurately and treatment started promptly, symptoms of infection should be reported to the physician without delay. An increase in body temperature should be thoroughly investigated. The patient must take his insulin as usual and test his urine for sugar and acetone at least four times a day. If infection is severe, an increase in insulin dose or a shift from oral hypoglycemics to insulin may be necessary.

## The Diabetic Undergoing Surgery

Major surgery and general anesthesia produce certain stresses that interfere with usual diabetic control; other factors are the underlying disorder requiring surgery, changes in nutritional requirements, and the route of food intake postoperatively. Until these stresses are relieved, therapy is planned to prevent marked hyperglycemia or ketosis and hypoglycemia. Generally, the last dose of an intermediate- or long-acting insulin is given the day before surgery. Until oral intake is permitted, small doses of regular insulin are given every four to six hours, together with intravenous glucose infusion. The dose of insulin is determined by testing urine for glucose and acetone or by estimating capillary glucose with Dextrostix. Generally the same total amount of insulin is necessary as the patient's usual daily dose.

Maturity-onset diabetics, controlled by diet alone or by diet and hypoglycemic drugs, may require small doses of regular insulin until oral feedings can be resumed. The amount is prescribed according to the results of urine tests or blood glucose analyses.

## Diabetes and Pregnancy

Female diabetics in the child-bearing years are often concerned about their chances for motherhood and diabetic problems related to pregnancy. Often diabetics are not candidates for adoptive motherhood because of their health problems.

Diabetes mellitus may be clinically evident before pregnancy or it may be discovered during pregnancy and persist after delivery. In gestational diabetes, the patient reverts to a latent chemical diabetes, or even to normal carbohydrate tolerance, after delivery.

With modern expert management, fertility, maternal mortality, and spontaneous abortion are not appreciably different in diabetics and nondiabetics (Carrington, 1970). However, medical and obstetric examinations may be required every two weeks during pregnancy, and every week in the terminal stage. Diabetes in pregnancy is managed by diet and insulin in virtually all cases, although gestational diabetes may require only diet. Additional dietary modifications include restriction of sodium and total calories, adequate protein, and supplementary vitamins and minerals. Insulin need increases during the second and third trimesters, presumably due to the production of insulin antagonists by the placenta.

Because of the potential for sudden development of ketoacidosis, common conditions associated with pregnancy, such as nausea and vomiting or urinary tract infection, must be treated early and aggressively. Poor diabetes control, associated with obstetric complications such as fluid retention, hydramnios, and toxemia, increases the risk of fetal death. The ideal time for delivery is about the thirty-seventh or thirty-eighth week, preferably by induced vaginal delivery rather than cesarean section. Measures of fetoplacental function, such as determination of 24-hour urinary estriol excretion rates, are used to assess fetal welfare and to schedule delivery. After delivery, the insulin requirement is reduced, sometimes by as much as 50 per cent.

The newborn infant of a diabetic mother tends to be of high birth weight (about 9 pounds), with a puffy, cushingoid appearance. The reasons for this are presently not clear. A pediatrician is usually present at delivery and the newborn usually requires intensive nursing care and observation for several days.

When the mother goes home from the hospital, her insulin requirement may still be unstable, and the demands of the newborn may militate against establishing a meal and sleep schedule. Referral to a community nursing agency, household help, and instructions to the father and others in the care of both mother and infant is required. Breast feeding is not contraindicated, but diet and insulin must be adjusted.

## DIABETIC ACIDOSIS (KETOSIS) and COMA

Diabetic acidosis is the end-result of uncontrolled diabetes. It is potentially fatal. Too little effective insulin, too much food over a period of days, infection, injury, emotional stress, pregnancy, or illness may precipitate diabetic acidosis.

This dreaded complication now occurs less often than formerly, because of more effective regulation of the disease and greater emphasis on teaching patients and families. In some instances coma develops in spite of the patient's having carefully followed his physician's recommendations. Such patients may be in the group of severe diabetics whose disease is hard to control. On occasion a patient is admitted to the hospital in diabetic coma who had not known previously that he was a diabetic. Diabetic coma also occurs with greater frequency among persons who have inadequate medical care. One of the most common causes of diabetic coma is infection.

Poor regulation of carbohydrate metabolism, with the dangers of diabetic coma, may also be brought about by ignorance or carelessness or by extreme emotional stress. Or, a patient who has been well regulated may become depressed and not care any longer; he may fail to keep his diet or refuse to test his urine and to take his insulin. A gastrointestinal upset with vomiting may force him to eat less. He may then reason that he needs less insulin, and cut down on his daily dose. This is a dangerous fallacy, and it may lead to ketosis, because illness often increases the need for insulin. Nurses should teach diabetic patients that any slight illness, such as a head cold, is an indication for more frequent testing of the urine, and for particularly careful adherence to the regimen of diet and insulin, or oral hypoglycemic agent. If ketonuria is present, or if the slight illness persists or grows worse, the patient should contact the physician or nurse specialist.

### Pathophysiology

A deficiency of insulin action results in a decrease in the utilization of glucose by the cells, decreased energy production, and decreased protein synthesis. It also promotes gluconeogenesis and glycogenolysis, hence a high level of hyperglycemia. A common range for blood glucose in acidosis is 400 to 800 mg. per 1000 ml. The high blood sugar acts as an osmotic diuretic, causing intracellular and extracellular water loss (dehydration) and a depletion of blood volume (hypovolemia). Large amounts of chloride, sodium, potassium, and other constituents are lost with diuresis. With volume depletion, blood flow to the kidneys and their ability to excrete glucose and ketones are reduced. Ketones accumulate when the body tries to provide a substitute fuel for glucose and utilizes fats.

Normally, when fat is metabolized, ketone bodies are formed in the liver and transported to muscle and other tissue, where they serve as a source of energy. (Ketone bodies are chemical intermediate products in the metabolism of fat.)

The more fat that is metabolized, the more ketone bodies are formed. With increased fatty acid breakdown and interference with the utilization of acetyl Co A, there is an increase in ketone bodies —beta-hydroxybutyric acid, acetoacetic acid, and acetone.

When these substances are produced faster than they can be oxidized in tissues, they accumulate in tissues and body fluids. Ketone bodies are strong organic acids and so the acidity of the blood (hydrogen ion concentration) is increased. Ketone bodies are buffered by the bicarbonate buffer system but this compensatory mechanism ultimately fails if the condition is untreated.

### Signs and Symptoms of Ketosis

The early symptoms of ketosis may be vague, but they become more definite—and serious—as more and more ketone bodies accumulate in the bloodstream unchecked. Initially, the patient may be weak, and have excessive thirst. Anorexia, nausea, and vomiting are common. When the patient must stop his oral intake of water and salt because of nausea, vomiting, or abdominal pain, a critical point is reached. The continued use of body water in excretion of glucose and ketones results in dehydration, a rapid rise in hydrogen ion concentration, and extracellular volume depletion. Chloride and sodium are lost in the vomiting that accompanies acidosis, and calcium and potassium are also wasted. If treatment is not given and compensatory mechanisms fail, the outcome is circulatory collapse, renal shutdown, unconsciousness, and death. This complex is known as *diabetic coma* (though severe ketosis can be present without the patient's being comatose).

Clinically, diabetic acidosis is reflected in extreme weakness and decreased reflexes and in mental ob-

tundation progressing from drowsiness to stupor to coma. Dehydration and loss of electrolytes is evidenced by tachycardia, hypotension, dryness of mucous membranes, flushed dry hot skin, and decreased intraocular tension. Acetone, being volatile, can be detected by the fruity odor of the breath. As the lung attempts to get rid of carbonic acid by blowing off $CO_2$ the rate and depth of respirations increase. This noisy hyperventilation pattern characteristic of diabetic acidosis is called Kussmaul's breathing.

### Diagnostic Assessment

The patient's history and clinical state make the diagnosis rather obvious. However, when diabetes is known or suspected, blood and urine samples are taken and glucose and ketone bodies, electrolytes, pH, BUN, and hematocrit are determined to confirm the presence and the degree of diabetic acidosis. If the patient is comatose, he is catheterized and a retention urinary catheter is left in place. Catheterization is avoided whenever possible because of the high risk of infection.

The $CO_2$ combining power of plasma is an indirect measure of the acidity or alkalinity of blood. Since $19/20$ of the total carbon dioxide in the plasma is in the form of bicarbonate, the $CO_2$ combining power is principally a measure of plasma bicarbonate. The normal $CO_2$ combining power is 58 ml. per 100 ml. of plasma or 58 volumes per cent. Metabolic alkalosis is manifested by an increase to 70 volumes per cent or higher, while in severe metabolic acidosis the $CO_2$ combining power may be as low as 10 volumes per cent.

The pH of the blood depends on the ratio of alkaline and acidic substances, and not on the absolute amounts. Studying arterial blood gases and pH provides for more accurate assessment of the patient in ketoacidosis than does the study of $CO_2$ combining power. In metabolic acidosis, there is a lowered pH, a low $P_{CO_2}$ and lowered serum bicarbonate. The low $P_{CO_2}$ results from hyperventilation (Kussmaul's breathing). The lung attempts to compensate for the increased carbonic acid level of the blood by "blowing off" $CO_2$ and water. The kidney attempts to compensate by retaining serum bicarbonate and excreting excess hydrogen ions. When compensatory mechanisms fail, pH falls below the normal 7.4. If the patient's metabolism has produced ketone bodies, there will be less base in the bloodstream, because base unites with the acid ketone bodies (see Chap. 60).

The severity of ketosis is determined by the degree of ketonemia (ketones in the blood). Bedside determination of acetone (with Acetest or Ketostix) in serial dilutions of plasma with water (1:1 through 1:16), is being used for the initial diagnosis and for evaluating the response to treatment.

When weighing the diagnostic data, the physician must rule out nonketotic hyperosmolar coma, lactic acidosis, uremic coma, cerebral vascular accident, and head trauma (Skillman and Tzagournis, 1972).

## Treatment

Usually the patient in suspected diabetic coma is admitted to an intensive care unit because he is critically ill.

Immediate treatment includes provision of insulin, fluid and electrolytes, glucose, and alkali to correct metabolism of carbohydrate, protein, and fat and to restore volume and pH to normal. Since great variability exists among patients, an individual assessment and treatment plan must be devised.

Supportive treatment includes gastric aspiration if there is distention, abdominal pain, or vomiting. The gastric contents of a dilated stomach may be vomited and aspirated by the partially comatose patient. An enema may be necessary. Treatment for circulatory collapse may require whole blood or plasma and vasopressor drugs. Infections, often the precipitating factor in acidosis, must be identified and treated with antibiotics.

**Insulin.** Insulin lessens the production of ketones by making carbohydrate available for oxidation by the tissues and restoring the liver's supply of glycogen. Regular insulin is given for a rapid effect. The initial dose of regular insulin may be given intravenously. The amount is determined by the plasma acetone level, which indicates the degree of severity. One hundred to three hundred units can be given by the physician. Subsequent doses are determined by hourly plasma acetone; or the Dextrostix and Ames Reflectance Meter can be used at the bedside to monitor the patient's blood glucose response to insulin therapy. Insulin is reduced when the degree of ketonemia is minimal (trace in undiluted plasma), since hypoglycemia can occur.

**Fluids and Electrolytes.** The patient who is hypovolemic may require plasma, whole blood, or rapid infusion of intravenous isotonic fluids. Depending on the severity of acidosis and volume depletion up to 4 liters of fluid may be necessary during the first six to eight hours of treatment. Physiologic saline may be used initially. An alkali solution such as ⅙ molar sodium lactate may be ordered if the $CO_2$ combining power is very low, or sodium bicarbonate solution may be added to the primary intravenous solution.

Hypokalemia may be manifested by shallow respirations, skeletal muscle weakness, and cardiac arrhythmias; electrocardiographic monitoring and measurement of serum potassium guide the physician's prescription of potassium, which may be ordered after the first four to eight hours of therapy. If the patient can drink, orange juice and beef broth are good sources of potassium. Potassium chloride 40 mEq., may be added to a 1000 ml. intravenous solution of 5 per cent glucose in water and infused slowly with electrocardiographic and serum potassium monitoring.

With intensive treatment and supportive care, the patient usually shows dramatic improvement in six to eight hours, but with overzealous, rapid treatment sorbitol—the alcohol of glucose—can accumulate in the central nervous system, resulting in cerebral edema.

As the patient recovers and is able to take fluids by mouth, he is started on salty broth, orange juice, milk, or oatmeal. Specimens of blood and urine continue to be tested for glucose and ketones at frequent intervals; treatment with insulin and carbohydrate feedings (to prevent insulin shock), fluids, and electrolytes continues until the diabetes is regulated.

## Nursing Assessment and Intervention

Observation must be acute; action, swift and organized.

The nurse observes for a patent airway and suctions mucus away when necessary, keeps the patient flat in bed, and notes changes in his condition that indicate deepening coma or response to therapy. The nurse keeps an intake and output record as a guide to therapy and an estimate of kidney function. She works closely with the physician and laboratory personnel in keeping an accurate flow sheet of significant events, including vital signs, blood and urine levels of glucose and ketones, amount and time of insulin administration, and level of consciousness. She may examine the abdomen, to detect gastric dilatation and paralytic ileus, and the urinary bladder for distention. The lungs are auscultated for signs of aspiration or volume overload. Signs of potassium depletion must be noted. The patient's safety must be provided for and complications of bedrest prevented.

The patient recovering from acidosis may have blurred vision. Fluid shifts and changes in equilibrium between the lens and vitreous cause a change in lens contour. This is a temporary condition. Eyeglasses should not be changed for several months until the condition is stabilized.

After recovery, long-term management with diet and insulin resumes, with emphasis on patient education including a review of events leading up to the crisis so that the patient and family learn from the experience.

## LONG-TERM COMPLICATIONS

Today, deaths from acute complications of diabetes are relatively rare. Mortality and morbidity associated with diabetes result chiefly from chronic vascular disease, primarily premature atherosclerosis, and microangiopathy.

**Atherosclerosis.** Atherosclerosis and medial arteriosclerosis occur earlier in life in the diabetic, and the distribution of the lesions as well as the magnitude of involvement is greater. Circulating concentrations of plasma lipids (cholesterol, triglycerides, and phospholipids), which are associated with a higher incidence of atherosclerosis, are generally higher in the diabetic. Adult-onset diabetes is often associated with several risk factors for myocardial infarction, including obesity, high blood cholesterol and uric acid levels, and hypertension. As in nondiabetics, coronary atherosclerosis is the leading cause of death.

Atherosclerosis is also manifested clinically by cerebral vascular disease and peripheral vascular disease (arteriosclerosis obliterans). Disease can involve numerous arteries—the carotid, subclavian, aortic, iliac, femoral, and distal ones as well. Amputation of an extremity because of gangrene in the past has been approximately twenty times more frequent in diabetics than in the normal population, but this has decreased with preventive measures, vascular surgery, and so on.

Nursing care involves those measures used to attain and maintain diabetic control as well as prevention, assessment, and participation in treatment of the vascular complication. (See chapters on coronary artery disease, myocardial infarction, cerebro-vascular disease, peripheral vascular disease, and amputation for care of these patients.)

**Microangiopathy.** Diabetics are uniquely susceptible to a microvascular abnormality involving the arterioles, venules, and capillaries and characterized by deposition of collagenlike material within the basement membrane of certain tissues. This small vessel disease is thought to be the morphologic basis for the major long-term complications of diabetes—retinopathy, neuropathy, and glomerulosclerosis. Vessels of the lower extremities, heart, brain, pancreas, vasa vasorum, skin, and periodontal structures can also be involved.

The pathogenesis of microangiopathy is unknown. Some diabetologists believe that microangiopathy is genetically determined, unrelated to the control of blood sugar levels and an inevitable consequence of diabetes. Others believe microangiopathy results from poor control of diabetes.

**Retinopathy.** The associated retinopathy of diabetes is now the most common cause of blindness in the United States. Unfortunately strict control of diabetes does not always prevent this devastating complication. Among those who have had diabetes for 20 years it is estimated that 75 per cent will have significant diabetic retinopathy, and the percentage increases with the duration of the disease (Zweng, 1972).

ASSESSMENT. Ophthalmoscopic examination reveals characteristic changes. In the early, asymptomatic stage, there is venous dilatation and tortuosity, bullet-shaped or round red capillary microaneurysms, and small and discrete yellowish waxy exudates or punctate hemorrhages. Loss of vision occurs when the vascular lesions extend beyond the retina and enter the vitreous region or preretinal space. *Retinitis proliferans,* the most advanced stage, is characterized by large and more numerous hemorrhages into the retina and vitreous, the formation of thick intravitreous scars, new blood vessel formation, secondary glaucoma, retinal detachment, and ultimate blindness.

Because it was thought that a pituitary factor, possibly growth hormone, is responsible for the progress of the lesion, an endocrinologic approach to treatment has included pituitary suppression therapy as well as surgical destruction of the anterior lobe of the pituitary. Recently, photocoagulation of multiple points of the retina itself with the laser beam has replaced the more complicated pituitary destruction with encouraging results regarding preservation of visual acuity. Photocoagulation is the transfer of light energy into heat energy. Two pigments (melanin in the retina and hemoglobin in the retinal vasculature) absorb light and convert it to heat, creating a burn scar that destroys those parts of the retina that are the sites of diabetic lesions.

While the nurse specialist or physician should do a funduscopic examination during each visit, in the diabetic this examination must be done through a dilated pupil by an ophthalmologist at least every two years after diabetes is diagnosed, more often if retinopathy is present. Blurred vision, cataracts, and a form of glaucoma are also associated with diabetes. Neuropathic involvement of the eyes can cause double vision.

A blind or a near-blind diabetic has the same need for independence as the sighted diabetic. Perhaps his need is even greater. He should be assisted to rely on himself. Some can use the sense of touch to test for sugar in urine. A quarter teaspoon of baker's yeast is placed in a plastic tube (such as the Ames Urin-Tek Tube), which is then filled with urine. Then a rubber fingercot is placed over the tube (it will hang limply from the top of the tube), and the tube is vigorously shaken. If sugar is present, carbon dioxide released by yeast fermentation of the sugar will cause the fingercot to inflate. At room temperature, glucose concentrations as low as 0.25 per cent can be detected in 20 to 30 minutes (Diabetes in the News, November-December 1973).

The blind or partially sighted diabetic can have a five-day supply of insulin prepared in separate syringes by a community health nurse or sighted helper. The injections can be kept in the refrigerator. The patient needs to know how to protect himself from injuries that may cause a break in the skin and infection. The family can help by keeping obstructions out of the way and seeing that furniture is in its accustomed place. Some diabetics with poor vision use guide dogs with great success. (See also Chapter 26, The Patient with a Visual Problem.)

**Nephropathy.** The renal lesions of diabetes were described by Kimmelstiel and Wilson 15 years after the discovery of insulin. This is about the length of time it takes for symptoms of nephropathy to appear in the insulin-treated diabetic.

The glomerulus, the renal tubule, and the arterial vessels may be involved. Diffuse glomerulosclerosis, capillary basement membrane thickening, and arteriosclerosis of the major renal arteries and their branches are examples of the renal lesions.

During the early stage of diabetic nephropathy (10 to 15 years after the onset of diabetes), there are virtually no clinical symptoms. Urinalysis might reveal mild hematuria, albuminuria, and waxy or granular casts. The middle stage (2 to 10 years after the first) is also called the phase of the nephrotic syndrome. There may be hematuria, albuminuria, and a low level of serum albumin, causing decreased plasma osmotic pressure and its clinical manifestations of edema, particularly of the face, around the eyes, and in the lower extremities. Elevated blood cholesterol and triglycerides, and hypertension also are found.

Progressive renal insufficiency usually is limited to those who have been diabetic for a long period of time. Eventually the patient with nephropathy reaches the late stage and develops the uremic syndrome. This stage is managed symptomatically, such as by restriction of dietary protein and sodium, antihypertensive drugs, and hemodialysis. Some patients, particularly in the 40- to 50-year age group, are candidates for kidney transplant, but for many juvenile diabetics, renal failure is the eventual cause of death. (See also Chapter 64, The Patient in Renal Failure.)

NEUROPATHY. The diabetic, especially with advancing age, is subject to a variety of neurologic disorders. Sensory, motor, and autonomic nerves may be involved. The cause of this manifestation of diabetes is not clear, but defects in glucose and lipid metabolism in nerve tissue as well as microangiopathy affecting the vasa vasorum of peripheral nerves have been suggested. Generally, the course of diabetic neuropathy is slow and progressive, but rapid deterioration or rapid improvement of a specific syndrome can occur. Symptomatic treatment is often helpful as is maintaining good diabetic control. Diabetic neuropathy mimics other nervous system diseases, and these must be ruled out.

Though any nerve tissue may be affected, the most common clinical manifestation is peripheral neuropathy of the lower extremities characterized by pain, paresthesia (the patient may feel as though he is "walking on sponges"), and hypasthesia. The patient may complain of a burning sensation, itching, numbness, tingling, and pain (which is often aggravated at night but relieved by walking). The skin may become so sensitive that the weight of bedclothes may be intolerable. There may be a loss of sensation so that he does not feel intense heat, and he can be burned without realizing it. Ability to drive a motor vehicle may be impaired since he may not feel the pressure of his foot on the brake or gasoline pedal.

The examiner would find loss of tendon reflexes, diminished or absent sensation of touch, vibration, pain, position, and thermal recognition. Measurement of motor nerve conduction velocity may be done.

Circulatory impairment may also be manifested by "shin spots," which are pigmented or depigmented areas on the anterior surface of the legs, and by the absence of hair on the toes.

*Neuropathic ulcers* can occur and, in the absence of pain or temperature sensations, are often first noted by the discharge on a sock or stocking. Occurring at weight-bearing joints, particularly under the metatarsal heads and on the joints of the toes and feet, these ulcers must be distinguished from the ulcers of occlusive vascular disease. Usually the neuropathic ulcer has a granulating base reflecting adequate circulation, the foot is warm, and arterial pulses are palpable.

Treatment includes curtailing or temporarily eliminating weight bearing, antibiotics, and trimming the callus that precedes ulcerous breakdown.

ASSESSMENT. The feet should be observed by the patient during his bath and by the nurse or physician at each office or clinic visit. The presence or absence of hair on the toes should be noted. The examiner should check between the toes for fissures and ulceration, and should check the toenails for thickness, discoloration, and infection. Substances such as commercial corn and callus removers or corn plasters or disinfectants should not be used. A softening agent, such as lanolin or petroleum jelly, can be used. Lamb's wool can be used between the toes to absorb moisture. Calluses, corns, or warts should be removed only by the surgeon or podiatrist.

At each visit the dorsalis pedis and posterior tibialis pulses should be felt.

Buerger-Allen exercises or walking may be prescribed to maintain or improve muscle tone. (See Chapter 38 for further considerations of nursing care of the patient with peripheral vascular disease.)

Surgical removal of the metatarsal head eliminates a source of pressure. This may also be accomplished by the use of a plastic innersole molded to the individual foot.

The diabetic should be advised to purchase supporting shoes of proper length and width.

**Other Neuropathies.** There may be postural hypotension, facial paralysis, atony of the urinary bladder with the threat of ascending infection to the kidney, gastric atony with retention of food, and neuroarthropathy (Charcot's joint). Explosive, repetitive, unexpected "diabetic diarrhea" may cause the patient to restrict his social activities because of the realistic fear of an accident in public.

A particularly distressing occurrence is neurogenic impotence. Studies have shown that approximately 50 per cent of diabetic men are impotent —a three- to fivefold greater frequency than in nondiabetics. Psychogenic causes account for 90 per cent of the impotence in the latter group (Ellenberg, 1973). Though the libido remains intact, nerves from the parasympathetic plexus, which control dilatation of the penile arteries necessary for engorgement of the corpora cavernosa and corpus spongiosum that produce erection, are involved in the neuropathic process; prognosis is very poor. One method of treatment is a surgical procedure involving the implantation of a silicone prosthesis which gives the penis sufficient rigidity to permit intercourse (Lash, 1972). One study reported that 35.2 per cent of diabetic females have complete absence of orgasmic response (Mourad and Chiu, 1974).

## PROGNOSIS

Although diabetics do not have as long a life expectancy as nondiabetics, there has been a significant increase in their life expectancy as a result of modern therapy, and, in part, probably as a result of emphasis among the population as a whole on such health hazards as obesity and smoking. Patients whose disease is treated within the first year of its discovery outlive those whose treatment is delayed. The patient who understands his disease and accepts it is better able to keep his diabetes in control than one who lacks knowledge or attitudinal change. The patient whose morale is high is better able to keep his diabetes in control than is the depressed patient.

## PSYCHOSOCIAL ASPECTS

Prejudice against hiring diabetics is common. Many employers fear that insulin reaction or coma will occur on the job, or that time will be lost due to illness. Therefore, diabetics often have difficulty obtaining employment commensurate with their abilities and their financial needs. The prejudice seems unjustified. While there is some restriction, such as a job that exposes a diabetic, prone to hypoglycemia, to injury from open machinery, well-regulated diabetics can enter a variety of occupations, such as teaching, nursing, medicine, and carpentry. However, employers or school personnel should know that a person is diabetic, just in case he should need care while at work. The prejudice against employing diabetics causes the patient to conceal the fact at times.

Diabetics need not be conspicuous socially. They can travel widely, and, with practice, can eat in restaurants or the homes of others without difficulty by knowing the ingredients of foods, the kinds of food offered, method of preparation, and the appropriate amounts of food.

At times the diabetic may feel helpless or become depressed. Fear of premature aging, chronic fatigue, dread of blindness or amputation, awareness of shortened life expectancy, and the need to cope daily with restrictions and at times with complications are reality factors that can make adaptation difficult for even the most well-motivated individual.

Individual or group psychotherapy or family therapy is recommended when the patient's capacity to cope and that of those close to him are overtaxed. Emotional stress influences the quality of diabetic control and strains significant interpersonal relationships. Not much study has been done of marital adjustment and diabetes, though it is known that adaptation to a chronic illness of one member involves other members of a family as well. Diabetics do have a lower marriage rate.

Diabetes clubs or groups that meet on a regular basis to share new ideas and approaches to common problems and to plan group social activities permit participants to share strengths and peer support in their long-term struggle to stay in control.

Conditions such as diabetes may or may not become disabilities. The patient can influence this outcome to a considerable extent, but he cannot wholly control it. The patient who carefully regulates his diet and his insulin is making the experience of an insulin reaction less likely; however, despite careful adherence to his treatment, he may later develop complications, such as impaired circulation to his feet and legs. The patient's ability to cope with any long-term condition is fostered by an attitude of respect for the condition. It cannot safely be ignored, it will not go away, and it has power to harm, particularly if the patient does not follow the treatment.

Helping the patient to acknowledge the condition and to adapt his way of life accordingly, is a challenge for the nurse. Assisting the patient to recognize the choices open to him (for instance, the choice between learning to follow a diet, and becoming ill from unregulated diabetes) and helping him to learn from his own experiences are measures that can help him to deal effectively with his condition. Too often threats and dire warnings are used in an attempt to frighten the patient into compliance with therapy. While the threat of complications is real, threats can be used in a nonthreatening way.

Sometimes the nurse adopts a "policemanlike" role, searching the patient's bedside stand periodically for forbidden food. Such measures are largely ineffective. Decisions about self-care and the will to abide by them must be fostered within the patient, since in most instances he carries the responsibility for his own care.

Unfortunately, in the past almost all instruction was concentrated at the time the patient first discovered that he had diabetes, and was largely confined to rather didactic teaching of facts. Today emphasis is on lifelong continuing education. As the patient experiences fluctuations in his state of well-being, and as he begins to link cause and effect, he can be helped to establish for himself the boundaries within which he must function. He learns what he can tolerate and what he cannot, and becomes increasingly able to predict consequences of his actions upon his health. It is important to continue nursing care, including teaching, over a long period so that the patient is helped to learn experientially, on the basis of his body's reactions to diabetes and its therapy, how to regulate his daily activities to follow his treatment.

## PATIENT EDUCATION

An initial and ongoing educational plan should be designed for the individual diabetic, which considers his cognitive, affective, and psychomotor strengths and limitations. The educator must select appropriate teaching methods. Particular tasks for consideration in each domain of learning are delineated below.

### Cognitive.

- Definition of diabetes and how it is controlled.
- The basics of dietary control, including the importance of achieving ideal weight; the selection of meal and snack foods and beverages (including alcohol) at home, in a restaurant, at work, or when traveling, which are consonant with the substitution (exchange) allowances in a meal plan.
- Adjustment of food intake in relation to an increase or decrease in activity.
- Menu planning and the assessment of convenience foods according to the label.
- The principles of urine testing, the significance of results, and the plan of action based on results.
- The action of insulin, the type and dose, and when and how to make adjustments in the dose of insulin, such as on sick days or heavy exercise days.

- The action, type, dosage, and side effects of prescribed hypoglycemic agents.
- Understanding the causes, signs, symptoms, prevention, and treatment of acute complications, i.e., hypoglycemia (insulin reaction) and hyperglycemia (acidosis).
- Understanding the causes, prevention, and treatment of long-term complications.
- Understanding the role of regular exercise in the management of diabetes and the exercise prescription.
- Understanding the reasons for lifelong periodic health surveillance.
- Becoming aware of resources in the community that can offer assistance, such as diabetes clubs or group teaching and counseling sessions.

### Affective.

- Achieve acceptance of diabetes.
- Demonstrate the level of acceptance by willingness to identify oneself as a diabetic; attend diabetes education classes; ask questions to clarify areas of lack of understanding; be willing to adjust food selection on social occasions and in restaurants.

**If unconscious or acting strangely I may be having a reaction to insulin or to an oral medicine taken for diabetes.**

# I HAVE DIABETES

If I can swallow give me sugar, candy, fruit juice or a sweetened drink. If this does not bring recovery or I can not swallow call a physician or send me to a hospital quickly for administration of glucose or glucagon.

Distributed by
**AMERICAN DIABETES ASSOCIATION, INC.** • 18 East 48th St. • New York, N.Y. 10017

| NAME | | PHONE | |
|------|------|------|------|
| ADDRESS | | | |
| (Street) | | (City) | (State) |
| PHYSICIAN | | PHONE | |
| ADDRESS | | | |
| (Street) | | (City) | (State) |

| INSULIN | DOSAGE | TIME | ORAL MEDICATION | DOSAGE | TIME |
|---------|--------|------|-----------------|--------|------|
| Regular | | | Orinase | | |
| PZI | | | Diabinese | | |
| Globin | | | Dymelor | | |
| NPH | | | Tolinase | | |
| Lente | | | DBI | | |
| Semilente | | | DBI-TD | | |
| Ultralente | | | | | |

DATE _____    © 1966

**Figure 50-5.** Identification card for diabetics. (American Diabetes Association, New York, N.Y.)

- Verbalize anxiety or concerns about complications to members of the health care team.
- Verbalize perception of the impact of the diesase on his life style and his response to the diagnosis.
- Seek help when economic burdens interfere with compliance with treatment.
- Maintain a record of diabetes control parameters.

Clues to the level of acceptance can be assessed by the physician or nurse by history of control or lack of control, verbal and nonverbal expressions regarding the diagnosis, and the patient's perception of the impact of the disease on his life. Since the disease is lifelong, remotivation to follow the treatment plan may be required.

The diabetes educator should recognize that some diabetics may consciously or unconsciously reject the disease and manifest this by an unwillingness to assume the responsibility for self-management or even to accept what is regarded as essential. A diabetic may deny that anything can be done to change the course of the disease. His feelings should be accepted as having a cause and an environment should be created which remains open to the patient's discussion of his feelings. Some patients require a long period of time before they accept their disorder, while others may never reach this stage.

The adult diabetic with immature personality development can attempt to control others by using his illness as a weapon. Or, anger and frustration can be expressed covertly through mismanagement of the disease.

### Psychomotor.

- Test urine for sugar and acetone after instruction in the appropriate method.
- Keep a written record of urine test results, insulin dosage, and comments.
- Prepare equipment for injection of insulin and inject it correctly, rotating to recommended sites; follow-up care of insulin and syringes.
- Store and take oral hypoglycemics regularly.
- Inspect and bathe feet daily, drying well, especially between the toes.
- Trimming toenails as instructed.
- Wearing well-fitting shoes and socks or stockings.
- Carry out other aspects of general care, such as genital hygiene and care of the teeth and gums.
- Carry identification as a diabetic at all times (Fig. 50-5).
- Carry out the exercise prescription.
- Contact appropriate professionals by telephone for emergencies or questions.

- Make and keep appointments for regular health maintenance visits and visits to specialists, such as the ophthalmologist or podiatrist when indicated.

## NURSING ASSESSMENT

In addition to the general points of a nursing history, supplementary aspects for a diabetic being admitted to any health care service should include the following data:

- History of the disease in the individual.
- Management of the disease, including the usual daily pattern of insulin or oral hypoglycemic drug and what was taken on the day of admission; the prescribed diet, meal plans, food allergies, food preferences and dislikes, and food intake on the day of admission; the usual daily pattern of physical activity, including type of job and work attendance record.
- Complications, past or present, and any functional disabilities.
- Methods of monitoring control.
- Usual medical or nursing supervision.
- Usual pattern of hypoglycemic reaction and the usual management.
- General hygienic routine.
- Personality characteristics.
- Developmental needs and tasks.
- The degree of self-management of the disease and the degree of assistance from significant others; who the significant others are.
- Cognitive, affective, and psychomotor strengths and limitations.
- Cultural and socioeconomic factors.
- Patient's perception of his learning needs.
- Any coexisting illnesses or conditions.

The nurse participates in physical assessment according to her level of preparation. An initial and interim health maintenance assessment should include the following:

- Height and weight.
- Vital signs (temperature, pulse, respiration, and blood pressure).
- Percussion, palpation, and auscultation of the heart, lungs, and abdomen.
- Emphasis on target organ screening, including examination of the lower extremities including pulse taking and oscillometric readings; inspection of nails and feet for absence of hair, infection, corns, calluses, warts, color, temperature, sensation, shin spots, and varicose veins.
- Ophthalmoscopic examination for venous dilatation, aneurysms, exudates, background retinopathy, hemorrhage, and new blood vessels.
- Neurologic examination and assessment of functional disabilities.

- Screening for kidney disorders by eliciting symptoms and ordering urinalysis and kidney function tests when indicated.

The patient's record is reviewed and any difficulties with or questions about the management program or compliance with it are discussed. The continuing education plan is implemented.

**The Diabetes Nursing Clinical Specialist.** A nurse with specialized preparation in the care of diabetic patients has many important roles and functions. Working in collaboration with the physician, nutritionist, and others, she may be the primary care provider in a diverse number of settings, such as the hospital outpatient department, neighborhood health center, or community nursing association. Her functions include history taking, physical assessment, patient and family education (individually or in groups), supervision of the diabetes management program, evaluation and treatment of acute and chronic complications, and patient and family counseling. She becomes involved in patient care wherever the patient is, including the intensive care unit, the general hospital ward, the clinic, the office, or the patient's home. She also acts as patient advocate and liaison in his relationships with schools or employing agencies and as a consultant to occupational health or school nurses. She is also available as a "hot line" consultant to her patient population.

## REFERENCES AND BIBLIOGRAPHY

ARCHER, et al.: Insulin receptors in human circulating lymphocytes, *J. Clin. Endocrinol.* 36:215, February 1973.

ARNOLD, H. M.: Elderly diabetic amputees, *Am. J. Nurs.* 69:2646, December 1969.

BENOLIEL, J. Q.: The developing diabetic identity: A study of family influence, In *Communicating Nursing Research: Methodological Issues,* Boulder, Col. WICHE, 1970, pp. 14-32.

BURKE, E. L.: Training program in diabetes care, *Nurs. Outlook* 19:548, August 1971.

————: Insulin injection: The site and the technique, *Am. J. Nurs.* 72:2194, December 1972.

CARRINGTON, E.: Diabetes in pregnancy, Chap. 32, In Ellenberg, M., and Rifkin, H. (eds.): *Diabetes Mellitus: Theory and Practice,* New York, McGraw-Hill, 1970.

Consider a patient with intracranial hemorrhage, diabetes, hypertension, fever and dehydration. What judgments do you need to assess his fluid and electrolyte changes? *Nurs. '72,* 2:6, March 1972.

DAVIDSON, J.: Diabetes Mellitus in adults, in Conn, H. (ed.): *Current Therapy 1974,* Philadelphia, Saunders, 1974.

DAVIDSOHN, I., and HENRY, J.: *Todd-Sanford Clinical Diagnosis by Laboratory Methods,* ed. 15, Philadelphia, Saunders, 1974.

*Diabetic Complications: New Concepts and Controversies,* Geigy Symposia Series, March 1972.

The diabetic foot: Ischemic or neuropathic? *Patient Care* 5:38, January 30, 1971.

Diabetic out of control. *Nurs. '73,* 3:10, May 1973.

Diabetics speak out: What patients say they aren't taught about self-care. *Nurs. Update* 4:11, May 1973.

ELLENBERG, M.: Impotence in diabetics: a neurologic rather than an endocrinologic problem, *Med. Asp. Human Sexuality,* 7:12, April 1973.

————: Diagnosis and management of neuropathies, Kalamazoo, The Upjohn Company, October 1973.

ELLENBERG, M., and RIFKIN, H. (eds.): *Diabetes Mellitus: Theory and Practice,* New York, McGraw-Hill, 1971.

ETZWEILER, D. (ed.): *Education and Management of the Patient with Diabetes Mellitus,* Elkhart, Ind., Ames Company, 1973.

Giving diabetics control of their own lives, *Nurs. '73,* 3:44, September 1973.

GRIM, R. A.: Mr. Edward's triumph, *Am. J. Nurs.* 72:480, March 1972.

GRANCIO, S.: Nursing care of the adult diabetic patient, *Nurs. Clin. N. Am.* 8:605, December 1973.

GOLDSTEIN, H.: *Diagnosis and Management of Diabetic Nephropathy,* Kalamazoo, The Upjohn Company, 1974.

GUTHRIE, D., and GUTHRIE, R.: Coping with diabetic ketoacidosis, *Nurs. '73,* 3:14, November 1973.

————: Juvenile Diabetes Mellitus, *Nurs. Clin. N. Am.* 8:587, December 1973.

HUANG, S.: Nursing assessment in planning care for a diabetic patient, *Nurs. Clin. N. Am.* 6:135, March 1971.

Insulin reactions in a brittle diabetic, *Nurs. '72,* 2:6, May 1971.

JORDAN, J. D., et al.: The primary health care professional was a nurse. *Am. J. Nurs.* 71:922, May 1971.

KOZAK, G. P., et al.: Skin disorders in diabetes (pictorial); Part 1: *Hosp. Med.* 8:64, July 1972. Part 2: *Hosp. Med.* 8:8, August 1972.

KROSNICK, A.: *The Nurse and Diabetes Control,* New Jersey State Dept. of Health, Rev., 1970.

————: The diabetic driver, *Public Health News,* New Jersey State Department of Health 52:70, May 1971.

LAUGHARNE, E., et al.: Gestational diabetes—when teaching is important, *Canad. Nurse* 69:34, March 1973.

LASH, H.: Surgical management of diabetic impotence in *Diabetic Complications: New Concepts and Controversies,* Geigy Symposia Series CVIII, March 1972.

Managing vascular disease in the diabetic, *Patient Care* 4:87, December 15, 1970.

MARBLE, A., et al. (eds.): *Joslin's Diabetes Mellitus,* ed. 11, Lea and Febiger, 1971.

McFARLANE, J., et al.: Two-drop and one-drop test for glycosuria, *Am. J. Nurs.* 72:939, May 1972.

MIRSKY, I. A.: Certainties and uncertainties in diabetes mellitus, Ch. 48, in Ellenberg, M., and Rifkin, H. (eds.): *Diabetes Mellitus: Theory and Practice,* New York, McGraw-Hill, 1970.

MOSS, J. M.: How emotions affect your diabetic patients, *Med. Insight* 3:22, January 1971.

MOURAD, M., and CHUI, W.: Marital-sexual adjustment of amputees, *Med. Asp. Human Sexuality,* VIII: 47 February 1974.

NICKERSON, D.: Teaching the hospitalized diabetic, *Am. J. Nurs.* 72:935, May 1972.

Recent developments in diabetes. *Metropolitan Life Stat. Bull.* 54:4, May 1973.

REDMAN, B.: The Process of Patient Teaching in Nursing, ed. 2, New York, Mosby, 1972.

Regional variations in mortality from diabetes. *Metropolitan Life Stat. Bull.* 54:3, December 1973.

RIMOIN, D.: The genetics of diabetes mellitus, Chap. 22, In Ellenberg, M., and Rifkin, H. (eds.): *Diabetes Mellitus: Theory and Practice,* New York, McGraw-Hill, 1970.

ROSEN, D.: Argon laser photocoagulation for retinal vascular disease, *Canad. Nurse* 69:36, May 1973.

SCHUMAN, D.: Coping with the complex, dangerous, elusive problem of those insulin-induced hypoglycemic reactions, *Nurs. '74,* 74:56, April 1974.

Simple exercises for patients with diabetic foot lesions, *Patient Care,* 5:49, January 30, 1971.

SKILLMAN, T., and TZAGOURNIS, M.: *Diabetes Mellitus,* Columbus, Ohio State University, 1972.

SOMERS, A.: Educating the consumer: it can mean better health, lower costs, *AMA News,* May 27, 1974.

STEINBERG, A.: Heredity and diabetes, *Eugenics Quart.* 2:26, 1955.

STONE, S.: Hypophysectomy for diabetic retinopathy, *Am. J. Nurs.* 73:632, April 1973.

STUART, S.: Day-to-day living with diabetes, *Am. J. Nurs.* 71:1548, August 1971.

TANI, G., and HANKIN, J.: A self-learning unit for patients with diabetes, *J. Am. Diet Assoc.* 58:331, April 1971.

TRAYSER, L. M.: A teaching program for diabetics, *Am. J. Nurs.* 73:92, January 1973.

U 100 insulin, *Nurs. Clin. N. Am.* 8:369, June 1973.

WATKINS, J., et al.: Observation of medication errors made by diabetic patients in the home, *Diabetes* 16:882, December 1967a.

————: A study of diabetic patients at home, *Am. J. Pub. Health* 57:452, March 1967b.

WATKINS, J. D.: Diabetes consultation and education service. Nursing assessment of the patient's management of diabetes mellitus, *ANA Clin. Sess.* 23:9, 1970.

WILLIAMS, S. M.: Diabetic urine testing by hospital nursing personnel, *Nurs. Res.* 20:444, Sept.-Oct. 1971.

ZWENG, H. C.: Preventing blindness in diabetics, In *Diabetic Complications: New Concepts and Controversies,* Geigy Symposia Series CVIII, March 1972.

# UNIT
# TEN

## Disturbances of Sexual Structures or Reproductive Function

# The Female
# Reproductive Pattern

## CHAPTER 51

## THE ROLE OF THE NURSE

### Emotional Support

Care of gynecologic patients presents many challenges for the nurse. *Because* most nurses are women, it is sometimes easy for them to recognize and to empathize with some of the concerns of women who experience disorders of reproductive function. On the other hand, because she too is vulnerable to these disorders, the nurse may avoid listening to these concerns lest her own anxiety about such disturbances be aroused. An important aspect of gynecologic nursing involves the ability to listen to the patient with concern as she expresses anxiety.

Several themes recur repeatedly among the concerns gynecologic patients express.

- **Fear of damage to or loss of reproductive capacity and reproductive organs.**

- **Anxiety that the capacity to respond sexually may be impaired or lost, thus affecting not only the patient, but her relationship with her partner.**

- **Concerns about pregnancy: for example, loss of the fetus if abortion threatens; worry over another child if the patient discovers she is pregnant when she did not wish to be.**

Attitudes about sexual organs are highly emotional. Women's attitudes toward gynecologic procedures are both realistic reactions to the physiologic discomforts or after effects and irrational attitudes connected with the area's symbolic meanings. Unconscious or denied fears become more conscious and sometimes are more easily

913

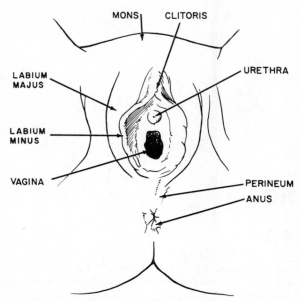

**Figure 51-1.** Diagram of female external genitalia.

verbalized after operative procedures. While reactions vary greatly, most women believe that gynecologic surgery may affect their sexual desires and behavior. They may continue to believe this emotionally even after health care personnel reassure them that a particular procedure will have no physiologic effect. Women fear impairment of sexual functioning and drive. They also fear that it may result in rejection and isolation from human contact and relatedness. Gynecologic procedures also may threaten the sexual identity of the involved partner. Psychiatrists are well acquainted with neurotic manifestations in husbands after gynecologic operations performed upon their wives. Many women depend on their husbands to reinforce their self-concept of femininity. Thus, gynecologic surgery can have significant emotional effects upon each member of the couple and upon their relationship.

While care of gynecologic patients sometimes seems very routine to the nurse, experiencing a gynecologic disorder is an acutely stressful experience for most patients. Many promptly become physically independent in caring for themselves. In fact, this may be a barrier to the patient's receiving *any* effective nursing, if the nurse views her role primarily in terms of physical care. For example, the woman who undergoes dilatation of the cervix and curettage of the uterus (D and C) is often subject to nursing neglect because her hospitalization is brief and she requires relatively little

physical care. However, many patients have this minor surgical procedure to help determine whether more radical surgery is indicated. Others have a D and C because they have just aborted a fetus, and the procedure is necessary to remove products of conception that, if left in the uterus, would cause continued vaginal bleeding. Such patients require sensitive, empathic nursing care and, because their hospitalization is brief, they need nurses who can quickly tune in to them as women undergoing stress.

Fear of cancer is prominent. Many patients know, when they enter the hospital for various diagnostic procedures, that cancer may be found. Some patients discuss this fear, others do not; it is important to create an atmosphere that allows the patient to bring up this topic if she wishes. Fear of cancer is not confined to any particular age group. Younger women experience it, although concern about the possibility of cancer usually increases with age, as does the likelihood of developing cancer among women during and after menopause. It is helpful to remember that allowing the patient to express her fears does not mean the nurse must be able to answer all questions or completely remove the fears. The nurse should provide emotional support for the patient. If the patient *does* ask a question that the nurse cannot answer, the nurse should refer it to the appropriate person. If the patient is afraid of the possibility of cancer, the nurse cannot remove this fear, but by listening supportively she may be able to lessen it, and also to help the patient think through just what it is she fears. Is it the possibility of surgery, the possibility of death, or both? It may be unrealistic or unnecessary for the nurse to think of herself as helping the patient singlehandedly with such problems. Rather, she can be one of the persons in whom the patient may confide, and by so doing the patient may gain confidence so that she is more ready to discuss some of her anxieties with others with whom she has professional and personal relationships.

### Patient Education

To the nurse, with her understanding of human anatomy and physiology, it may seem startling that in this era of scientific enlightenment many women have little understanding of their own body processes (Figs. 51-1 and 51-2). Nevertheless, many women, even among the younger age groups, have gleaned most of their information about female re-

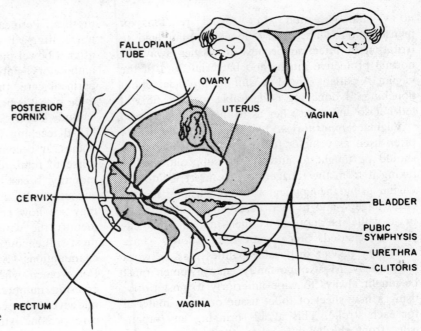

**Figure 51-2.** Anatomy of female reproductive organs.

productive functions from mothers, sisters, and peers who are ill-informed and steeped in superstition. This is especially true of those who are educationally and economically disadvantaged. Many such patients enter and leave a gynecologic unit without significant instruction—a situation urgently requiring nursing intervention. How many patients believe bathing or shampooing is harmful during menstruation? How many take douches daily, using strong and potentially harmful solutions? How many believe that masturbation is harmful? Various physiologic and mental problems are sometimes erroneously attributed to masturbation. Worry and guilt about it can be far more harmful than any physical effects, which authorities say are nonexistent. How many patients know that it is vitally important for every woman to have a yearly gynecologic examination with a vaginal smear? Does the couple know that frigidity (inability to become sexually aroused) is most frequently of psychic origin, and that it often can be helped? With the nurse's help, admission to a gynecologic service can provide women an opportunity to learn desirable health practices, as well as the opportunity for treatment. Such teaching can also occur in schools and camps, in adult community groups, and so on. Group teaching is a very useful supplement to individual teaching because women are often helped by realizing that others have similar questions and concerns, and they thus become bolder in seeking information.

Some women may be reluctant to ask questions of a man, even a physician, whereas they may feel more comfortable in approaching a female nurse. The nurse must be approachable, gentle, and tentative, especially if resistance is felt. A woman who is uninformed may fear or be unable to ask questions important to her.

**Hygiene Sprays and Douching.** The nurse must be prepared with the correct information. It must be made easy for the patient to talk in privacy. She can be encouraged to express her ideas and to voice her questions. For example, advertisements stress the importance of feminine "cleanliness." Feminine hygiene sprays are not only unnecessary, but in many women cause severe allergic reactions. Such products are now required to have a printed warning that they should not be used except externally. The nurse can reassure a woman who is using such a product that the body cleanses itself naturally. There will be no odor if baths are taken at regular intervals.

Douches are usually unnecessary. Some women may still believe douches are helpful as contraceptives. In such cases it should be pointed out that sperm may have entered the uterus before a douche can be given, and that douches enter only the vagina.

The normal, healthy vagina ordinarily requires

no vaginal irrigation after sexual relations or menstruation. Unnecessary douching may lead to irritation or infection because it washes away the normal protective mucus and bacterial flora of the vagina. A patient should consult her physician about douching. If douching is desirable for her, he will tell her so and advise her as to the solution to use.

**Vaginal Suppositories.** Vaginal suppositories are often used as vehicles for medication. The patient should be taught to unwrap the suppository after taking it from the refrigerator, to insert it into the vagina using the applicator or by pushing it with clean fingers, and to then lie down for 20 minutes or so while the suppository melts and the medication is released. Since some suppositories stain, a sanitary pad or disposable panties may be worn temporarily. Most importantly, many women must be taught always to wipe anteriorly to posteriorly, using a new sheet of toilet tissue or other material for each stroke. This avoids bringing any organisms from the anal area to the vagina or the

urethra. Perineal care should be given by the nurse after a bedpan has been used and especially after a bowel movement in bed rest patients. If the ambulatory patient is taught to give her own perineal care, the nurse should check periodically to be sure it is being done correctly.

**Body Care.** As more and more books are published teaching women how to care for their own bodies, it becomes increasingly important for the nurse to reinforce useful health practices, such as monthly breast self-examination. The nurse can encourage the use of a mirror so that the woman may see how her body is formed and be able to identify the various anatomical structures. Nurses must still encourage women to have yearly physical examinations given by a professional practitioner. For women who are embarrassed, there are increasing numbers of female physicians or nurse midwives who can serve as their primary health care person. Although many self-help clinics are being formed and women are being encouraged to

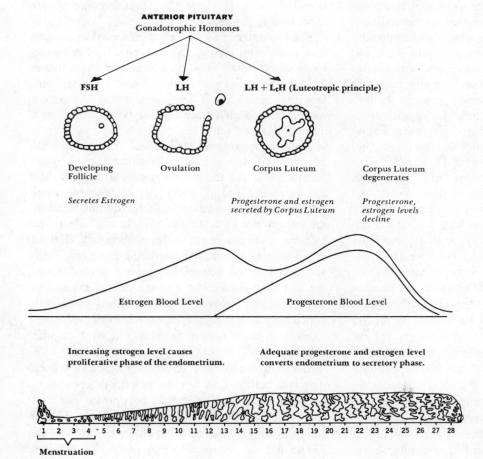

**Figure 51-3.** Simplified version of the normal menstrual cycle. (The Upjohn Company, Kalamazoo, Mich.)

become more self-aware, it is important that ties to the health care system not be broken. Nurses may demonstrate their support by serving as volunteers in such settings. Nurses encourage women to examine a speculum and how it works, explain various procedures, and give expert input on avoiding such commercial products as "do-it-yourself" pregnancy tests, which so far have been very unreliable. Many of them have been legally removed from the market.

## THE MENSTRUAL CYCLE

Many women are glaringly uninformed about the exact nature of the female reproductive system and the menstrual cycle (Fig. 51-3). Many companies that sell sanitary napkins and tampons also have free literature available for distribution to women.

### Physiology

Under the influence of the follicle-stimulating hormone (FSH) of the anterior pituitary, the ovarian follicle matures along with the ovum inside it. With the release of a second pituitary hormone, the luteinizing hormone (LH), the mature follicle ruptures and discharges the ovum, which is drawn into the end of the fallopian tube. This process is called *ovulation*, and occurs about every 28 days during the period between menarche and the menopause.

After the ovum is shed, the ruptured follicle is transformed into a small body filled with yellow steroid-producing tissue, the *corpus luteum*.

If the ovum meets a spermatozoon in the fallopian tube and is fertilized, it moves down to the uterus and implants itself in the *endometrium*, the highly vascular glandular tissue lining the inside of the uterus, which is prepared to receive it. If fertilization does not occur, the ovum is expelled from the body by way of the uterus and the vagina.

Whether the ovum is fertilized or not, the endometrium prepares itself for a possible pregnancy. The development of the uterine endometrium is governed by the hormone estradiol produced by the maturing ovarian follicle which is under the influence of FSH. Estrogen production is, in turn, probably regulated by LH. After the follicle has ruptured, the resultant corpus luteum produces another hormone, progesterone. This stimulates a change in the endometrium, making it richer and thicker in preparation for a possible fertilized ovum. The production of FSH is now inhibited.

If the ovum is not fertilized, the prepared endometrium degenerates and menstrual flow begins about two weeks after ovulation. After menstruation the endometrium again begins to grow, becoming thicker and more vascular. Because of these cyclical, hormone-dependent changes, the microscopic picture of the uterus is almost constantly changing. Thus it is important that each gynecologic specimen sent to the laboratory (such as vaginal smears or curetting obtained by scraping the uterus) be marked with the date of the beginning of the patient's last menstrual period.

When conception occurs, the corpus luteum persists during early pregnancy. When conception does not occur, it degenerates and shrinks; the endometrium, which has become swollen with blood to nourish the fertilized ovum, sheds its outer layers with some bleeding. Menstrual flow usually lasts four to five days, with a loss of 30 to 180 ml. of blood.

### Menarche

The start of menstruation (menarche) usually occurs between the ages of 10 and 14. If menses—even if they are irregular at first—have not begun by the time a girl is 15 or 16, the parents should be advised to take her to a gynecologist who will look for endocrine imbalance, an imperforate hymen, or congenital anomalies. The hymen normally contains an opening adequate to allow the menstrual flow to occur, but occasionally this opening is not present, and the menstrual flow is held back.

Menarche is preceded by physiologic changes that may be puzzling to the girl and fraught with emotional significance. The breasts develop, body fat is redistributed, and pubic and axillary hairs grow. Nurses are sometimes consulted for advice, and they can help girls to understand what is happening to them and how to care for themselves. Misconceptions can be corrected, and physiologically accurate explanations given.

A frequent problem is that not all adolescents develop secondary sex characteristics at the same time. Some girls in seventh-grade may be menstruating regularly; others may not have begun to experience the obvious body changes that occur at puberty, and one group may be as embarrassed and as concerned as the other. The nurse can help these girls to know that they will have caught up with one another long before they graduate from high school. A girl may wonder, but not ask, about the normal vaginal secretion that occurs between menses. If she knows that most women have this discharge, she may be saved some worry.

Young girls need accurate information concerning personal hygiene, and the school nurse is in a position to teach them how to care for themselves during menses. (The need for such teaching is of course not limited to girls, but is often required by older women who may receive instruction from the community health or hospital nurse.) Discussion of the use of external pads and of tampons is often helpful to adolescent girls who are establishing patterns of self-care during menstruation.

The amount of discomfort experienced during menses is often significantly related to attitudes toward menstruation and femininity. Obviously this does not rule out the possibility of disease or abnormality. Any woman, regardless of her age, who experiences severe painful menstruation (dysmenorrhea) should be advised to have a gynecologic examination. The four or five days of discharge should be accompanied by little or no discomfort other than a sense of fullness in the pelvis and mild lassitude. Breasts may become enlarged and tender, particularly during the few days before menstruation, and there may be mild cramps or backache. There is no reason to curtail activities during menstruation. Many women swim during this period, and athletes not only enter athletic contests, but win them. A daily shower or a bath should be taken. Bathing in warm water is not only safe but desirable, to lessen odor. There is no reason not to shampoo the hair.

It is at this time that the girl may also start thinking of herself as a woman, not as a child.

## Dysmenorrhea

Dysmenorrhea is often not a serious medical problem but does affect many women. It is frequently caused by ovulation and the secondary effects of progesterone on uterine muscles and blood vessels. Individual reactions are influenced by a heightened awareness of discomfort or by having been conditioned to believe that menstruation will be uncomfortable. Often dysmenorrhea is idiopathic. Mild symptoms are intensified by fatigue, cold, and tension. For some women, discomfort is intensified by an emotional need for more satisfying human contacts, and dysmenorrhea is one way in which this need is communicated. Others fear menstruation, or are convinced that they really are sick during this time.

Menstruation, by its regular occurrence, calls attention to a woman's femininity, and in some instances dysmenorrhea is related to difficulty in accepting feminine identity and role. One way of helping some women who have dysmenorrhea is to help them think through and accept the physiologic phenomenon as a part of their physical selves.

Women nurses, particularly those in school, college, community health, and industry, are especially likely to be consulted about dysmenorrhea. They should urge the patient to visit the gynecologist to uncover any possible pathology.

Dysmenorrhea may be secondary to other pathology, such as endometriosis, displacement of the uterus, or narrowing of the cervical canal. For some conditions, exercises may be suggested by the gynecologist. For example, if dysmenorrhea is related to retroversion of the uterus (the uterus tilts backward), the knee-chest position may be prescribed. Surgery may sometimes be necessary (e.g., in severe endometriosis). However, every effort is made to preserve child-bearing function. The main consideration in therapy for dysmenorrhea is helping the woman to feel well throughout her menstrual cycle so that she can continue her accustomed activities without interruption.

If no pathology is present, the estrogen test is performed. Stilbestrol or conjugated estrogenic hormones (Premarin) is given for a month. This causes an anovulatory period, during which the bleeding will be painless, if the dysmenorrhea is due to the effect of progesterone on the uterus. If menstruation is still painful, the causes must be assumed to be psychosomatic. This does *not* mean the pain is imaginary, but rather that it can be relieved through comfort measures, such as mild analgesics or antispasmodics, e.g., lututrin (Lutrexin). Whatever measures the individual has found to be helpful may be continued, such as knee-chest position, exercising, hot-water bottle to the lower abdomen, or even just resting for an hour or two. If the medications did allow painless bleeding, birth control pills are sometimes prescribed to inhibit ovulation, thus relieving the dysmenorrhea.

For women in whom emotional difficulties seem to play a prominent part in causing painful menses, psychotherapy may be helpful.

## Premenstrual Tension

This is a more severe discomfort than normal, caused by sodium and fluid retention during the premenstrual phase of the normal cycle. The woman feels physically, mentally, and emotionally tense. In severe cases complaints may include headaches, inability to sleep, fatigue, breast swelling and painfulness, abdominal and pelvic pain, and discomfort in other areas. Severe cases are usually due to psychic factors but are often also aggravated by an estrogen-progesterone imbalance. Treatment consists of limiting salt intake and possibly the use of diuretics. Progesterone may be given during the latter part of the cycle. Cytran is frequently used since it contains progestin, a mild diuretic and a mild tranquilizer.

A girl may approach the nurse with a simple question, but she may wish really to know something that is more complex, especially if she has heard discussions in class or from her friends that conflict with what she has learned at home. She may be poorly informed as to why she menstruates, or how babies are born.

## Problems Requiring Intervention

Amenorrhea is the absence of menstrual flow. It is expected before menarche, at pregnancy, after menopause, and after an hysterectomy or other procedures due to severe pathology. Other causes include chromosomal problems, endocrine imbalance, nutritional problems such as severe malnutrition or marked obesity, chronic diseases, and psychosomatic influences. Oligomenorrhea refers to infrequent menses. There are variations in the extent to which emotional reactions affect menses. Some women miss a period when they become moderately anxious, while for others only severe emotional disturbances affects the menses. Some women do not menstruate for several months after they have moved to a different climate. The woman who misses periods should see a gynecologist who will initiate studies to determine the cause.

Menorrhagia, excessive bleeding at the time of normal menstruation, may be caused by endocrine imbalance, fibroid tumors, and a variety of other pelvic abnormalities. Unchecked it can lead to anemia. Because the amount of blood loss is difficult to describe, a rough estimate can be made by asking the patient how many pads or tampons she uses a day. Menorrhagia is a symptom that should cause the patient to consult a gynecologist.

Metrorrhagia, bleeding at a time other than a menstrual period, may consist of a slight pink or brownish spotting, or it may be frank bleeding. It can be caused by various abnormalities. Spotting can occur in early pregnancy, and sometimes it is a warning symptom that abortion is imminent. Metrorrhagia should always be brought to the attention of a physician because it may be an early indication of cancer. Postcoital bleeding may be an early symptom of cancer of the cervix. It is not the amount of blood that is important; it is the fact that it occurred when no bleeding was expected. The seriousness of the underlying condition is not implied by the slightness of this symptom. Nurses should explain the necessity for a visit to the physician, stressing the importance of an examination but making every effort not to frighten the patient. Most women are aware of the possibility of cancer when they experience gynecologic symptoms, and fear of this diagnosis can militate against their seeing the physician. The nurse who shows concern for the patient is more likely to persuade the patient to visit the physician than is a nurse who uses "scare techniques." Metrorrhagia may be difficult for the menopausal woman to identify, if her periods have become irregular. Is the spotting a scanty menstrual flow or an abnormal symptom? When she is in doubt, she should consult a gynecologist, because intermenstrual bleeding is not a normal characteristic of the climacteric (see below).

## FIRST INTERCOURSE

Sooner or later every girl faces the question of whether to retain her virginity or to engage in sexual intercourse. While a discussion of the pros and cons of premarital intercourse is beyond the scope of this text, it should be pointed out that young people often seek counsel on this matter from persons in authority whom they trust. Often these young people seem to want to be told, "do not engage in this behavior." When such questions arise, the nurse must listen closely to assess what approach is likely to be helpful. For example, information and opportunities to discuss values related to sexual conduct may be needed. If they have decided to engage in sexual intercourse, the nurse should ask whether they are planning to avoid pregnancy. She should also point out that, just as soon-to-be-married couples have premarital physical examinations and blood tests to guard against venereal infections, so should young people who plan

**Table 51-1. Methods of Contraception Currently Used**

| | PILL | IUD | DIAPHRAGM | FOAM AND CONDOM | RHYTHM |
|---|---|---|---|---|---|
| *Description* | Synthetic hormones, estrogen and/or progesterone | Small plastic device introduced into uterine cavity through the cervical os | Circular, flexible rubber dome with flexible rim filled with contraceptive jelly or cream, which when inserted rests above and behind the pubic bone in front and extends over the anterior vaginal wall and the cervix to the upper end of the vagina. The jelly lies between the cervix and the diaphragm. | *Condom:* thin rubber sheath  *Foam:* white, aerated cream | Calculation of fertile days during menstrual cycle and abstinence from intercourse during this time (estimated as 6-7 days before ovulation) |
| *Action* | Prevents ovulation | Thought to irritate uterine lining and prevent implantation of fertilized egg | Blocks entrance to uterus, jelly chemically destroys sperm. | *Condom:* collects sperm, preventing entry into vagina  *Foam:* chemically destroys sperm; physically blocks cervical os | Pregnancy cannot occur without intercourse. |
| *How Used* | One pill daily for 21- to 28-day cycle | Inserted by physician or other person. Woman checks for presence of IUD string at cervical os weekly. Many physicians prefer to replace IUD every year or two and request annual checkups. | Diaphragm filled with jelly inserted into vagina before intercourse. If properly fitted cannot be felt by either partner. | *Condom:* rolled on over penis  *Foam:* inserted into vagina, to cover cervical opening | Estimate ovulation based on length of menstrual cycle and basal body temperature (BBT). BBT should be taken and recorded each morning before arising; it is slightly lower than normal at time of ovulation, and rises 0.3-0.5 degrees 24 hours after ovulation. |
| *Effectiveness* | 99.9% if taken correctly | 97% | 88-95% if properly fitted and correctly placed before each act of intercourse | Condom and foam: 97%  Condom: 85%  Foam: 80% | 76% if the principles are understood |
| *Contraindications* | Thrombophlebitis, cardiac or renal dysfunction, diabetes, liver disease, carcinoma, abnormal vaginal bleeding | Pelvic infection, uterine abnormality, uterine tumor, pregnancy | Certain uterine positions, poor vaginal tone, frequent urinary tract infection | Allergy to condom or foam | Inability to calculate fertile period, irregular menstrual periods, unwillingness to avoid intercourse for the necessary 1-2 weeks per month |
| *How Obtained* | Physician or family planning clinic | Physician or family planning clinic | Correct size must be fitted by physician or member of family planning clinic. Must be refitted after childbirth or after a 10-lb. gain or loss in weight. | Purchase without prescription in any drug store | Basal thermometer can be purchased in any drug store without a prescription |
| *Disadvantages* | Breast enlargement, nausea, weight gain, decreased menses, slight increased tendency to intravascular clots | Menorrhagia, dysmenorrhea, metrorrhagia, expulsion, uterine perforation, infection | Allergic response possible; may become dislodged during intercourse | Allergic response to condom or foam | Possible mental or physical strain for some couples caused by abstinence |

on living together. During this examination birth control can be discussed.

## RAPE

For many years rape has been a taboo subject in our society. Myths are that the woman involved either wanted to be raped or provoked the incident. Even today most cases are not reported since the victim may feel guilty about having been raped.

Until recently, health care usually focused only upon emergency medical treatment and a gynecologic examination in case the victim decided to press charges. However, since the incidence of rape has been increasing at an alarming rate and women have begun to assert themselves, health care professionals are beginning to respond more positively to the needs of the victims. Basic physical needs are still met through a physical examination to repair any tear or other trauma and confirm the presence of sperm. The nurse should stay with the woman throughout the examination to comfort and reassure her. She should also talk with the woman about possible pregnancy prevention measures. Medication is also given to prevent venereal disease. The woman must understand that she will need a follow-up blood test within six weeks to detect possible syphilis.

In addition to physical needs, the victim will require a great deal of emotional support. Rape is a crisis situation, in which the act of violence is often accompanied by threats of physical harm or murder. Since the woman's safety and life were seriously threatened, she may need very strongly to feel that she is now safe. The nurse can help the victim to identify what she is feeling at this time. Most women are still frightened, anxious and, in a sense, denying what has happened. Therapeutically the nurse might ask a few questions and then listen as the woman verbalizes her feelings. After her concern about pregnancy is relieved, she may begin to wonder about whom she should tell of her experience. Rape victims often have a deep need to talk to someone. At present many cities are developing rape crisis centers staffed by women who have been victims of rape. Often these paraprofessionals are willing to come to the victim, answer her questions, offer counseling, and encourage her to come back for follow-up services.

## BIRTH CONTROL

Today women have the opportunity to control their fertility. Not only can they decide whether they will ever bear children, but also how many children they will have and how frequently they will have them.

Such major decisions can only be made by women themselves after considering factors that may be important to them: personal life goals, self-image, age, feelings of the male partner, finances, medical status, social, cultural and religious background, and so on.

The nurse must respect each woman's individual attitudes and must not impose her own personal beliefs. However, she can provide factual information about available contraceptive methods, the effectiveness, advantages, and disadvantages of each, and instructions for correct use. In many settings, nurses who have extra training, for example, nurse-midwives and pediatric and family nurse practitioners, are able to add to this counseling role the ability to provide such direct care as a breast and pelvic examination, and instructions for diaphragm fitting, and IUD insertion. (For methods of contraception currently used, see Table 51-1.)

### Sterilization

Sterilization is the only method of preventing pregnancy which is 100 per cent effective and irreversible. A bilateral tubal ligation is the most common technique for achieving sterility in females.

**Tubal Ligation.** A small section of each fallopian tube is removed and the remaining ends tied off. Ovulation continues to occur, but the egg disintegrates in the blocked tube and can never unite with a sperm. There are three approaches for tubal ligation:

1. Abdominal. This operation is performed through a low abdominal incision with the patient under general anesthesia. Because it is major surgery, hospitalization is required for four to five days.
2. Laparoscopy. A slender instrument with lights and lenses is inserted into the abdominal cavity through a tiny incision near the umbilicus. A second instrument is passed through another incision located above the symphysis pubis. Using these tools and general anesthesia, the physician can perform a tubal ligation. Two Band-aids are the only dressing required. Usually, the patient stays in the hospital for three days, but in some areas the procedure is performed on an outpatient basis.

**3.** Vaginal. Tubal ligation is less commonly accomplished through an incision in the upper posterior vaginal wall. Only one to two days in the hospital is recommended after this surgery.

In all 50 states today, voluntary sterilization is legal. The nurse functions as a resource person. Not only might she be asked to explain the technique, but she also has the responsibility for clarifying the implications of sterilization. Informed consent is of *particular* importance, and the nurse must be sure the woman understands, before she consents. Women seeking this procedure must realize that its effect is lifelong. They also need to be reassured that tubal ligation will not change their hormonal balance, menstrual cycle, physical appearance, or sexuality. Individuals seeking information can be referred to a private physician or to the Association for Voluntary Sterilization, Inc., 14 West 40th St., New York, New York 10018 (212-524-2344).

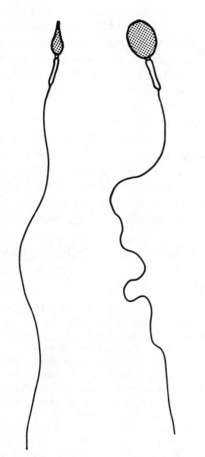

**Figure 51-4.** Two normal spermatozoa. The long tails give the sperm motility.

## INFERTILITY

A primary concern of gynecologic care is helping the woman to achieve a satisfying sexual life and, if she wishes, to prepare for motherhood. This care requires the nurse to discuss with the woman her sexual concerns and feelings about her own femininity and motherhood. Nurses are increasingly teaming up with physicians to provide male/female discussion leaders to help couples discuss and deal with sexual concerns. But even without formal counseling sessions the nurse must be prepared to answer questions about sexual concerns. Since it is difficult to become expert in this area, and most nursing schools do not offer such courses, the nurse is referred to the books written by Masters and Johnson and other publications on this subject, for more detail. She is encouraged to continue her education in addition to that required by the basic nursing program, such as by courses and workshops on human sexuality and marriage and the family.

Infertility is a problem in approximately 15 per cent of married couples. Both husband and wife will be examined, since it is their reproductive capacity as a biologic unit that determines their relative fertility.

### Etiology

Infertility may be caused by cervical problems, tubal problems, a lack of or a deficiency of sperm, hormonal problems, or the presence of antibodies to sperm. Obvious factors are the age of the woman and that of the man, how often they engage in intercourse and its timing, and the length of time they have been attempting conception. For optimal fertility, intercourse should be engaged in every other day. Attempts to become pregnant should be continued for 18 months before medical evaluation for infertility is sought.

### Physiology

Sperm are manufactured in the testes. They pass in tubules through the epididymis into the vas deferens, and they are discharged into the urethra and out of the body by rhythmic contraction of the muscles of the vas deferens and the penis during the sexual climax. Accumulated fluid from the male reproductive organs that carry the spermatozoa is called *semen*. This fluid is alkaline; spermatozoa are rapidly immobilized in an acid environment. Human males produce spermatozoa

922

continuously (Fig. 51-4), even though they leave the body only periodically.

High in the fundus of the uterus are two openings for the fallopian tubes along which ova travel from the ovaries to the uterus, and which sperm enter from the uterus. The tubes are about 4 inches long. After the ovum is shed from the ovary, movement of the cilia at the fimbriated end of the fallopian tube and muscular contractions of the tube itself draw the ovum along toward the uterus. If the ovum is not fertilized, it degenerates and is shed.

The volume of normal ejaculate is 2.5 to 3.5 ml., which contains an average of 100 million spermatozoa. For conception to occur, it is necessary for a spermatozoon to make its way, by movement of its tail-like portion, up the entire length of the uterus and into the fallopian tube. Fertilization occurs when a sperm pierces the outer coat (zona pelluciuda) of the ovum. Although actual fertilization is by one spermatozoon, it is probably necessary for more than one sperm to be present to dissolve the zona pellucida sufficiently to allow one spermatozoon to enter the ovum.

Usually, the ovary ejects only one ovum during each ovulation, although it is probable that many spermatozoa find their way into the fallopian tubes. Ovulation apparently occurs midway between menstrual periods, but in individuals the time of ovulation probably varies from month to month. Women are fertile (capable of becoming pregnant) soon after ovulation. A married couple who wish to have a baby may be advised by their physician to have intercourse every other day, from the tenth through the sixteenth day after the first day of the woman's menstrual period. Every other day, instead of every day, is suggested to allow for sperm buildup. Couples who wish to conceive may not know about ovulation, and they may limit sexual intercourse to the times just before and just after menses when conception is least likely to take place, thus inadvertently practicing rhythm control of conception (see Table 51-1).

Although men are sometimes reluctant to accept the fact, in about one-half of all couples who experience reproductive difficulty, the problem lies with the male. Causes of sterility in men can be general debility, hypopituitarism, hypothyroidism, obesity, infection, absence of a genital organ, undescended testicles (even when they are corrected), orchitis after mumps, irradiation of the testes, and mental stress. Conception can occur when the sperm count is as low as 2,250,000 spermatozoa per milliliter of semen, but the chance of a sperm contacting an ovum is less than when the count is higher. In normal semen, 15 per cent or less of the sperms are nonmotile, and 20 per cent or less are formed abnormally. When these percentages rise above 15 and 20, respectively, the chance of conception decreases.

Women, as well as men, may be infertile from systemic causes. In addition, women may have problems interfering with normal ovulation, such as a variety of endocrine disorders. Occluded tubes are a significant cause; gonorrheal, streptococcal, or other infections can cause tubal strictures that prevent the ova from traveling up the tubes. Endometriosis is a common cause of infertility in women. In both men and women psychologic factors sometimes play an important part in causing infertility.

### Diagnosis

When a couple is unable to conceive after several years of married life, both should be examined by a physician. He probably will give them a complete physical examination, including basic laboratory tests to rule out a possible systemic cause. The husband may be examined first, because his examination is made more readily.

**Semen Examination.** After four to six days abstinence (preferably), the man collects his semen, usually in a clean dry glass jar, and immediately takes it to the physician. The sperm cells are counted and note taken of their motility and the presence of abnormal forms, such as those with two heads or two tails. Some deficiency observed in one examination of the semen does not indicate the husband is sterile. Physical illness, prolonged emotional stress or fatigue, and too frequent intercourse can lower the number of spermatozoa temporarily. A man is considered infertile only if spermatozoa are absent in repeated examinations. When the sperm count is low, it means only that there is less chance of conception, not that conception is impossible.

**Endometrial Biopsy.** In women, it must first be determined whether ovulation occurs and whether the endometrium prepares for implantation.

A basal body temperature chart maintained for several months, will show either a curve demonstrating ovulation or irregular curves indicating irregular or lack of ovulation.

Endometrial biopsy confirms ovulation and whether the endometrium is suitable for implantation. This is done shortly before or on the first day of the menstrual period. It may be done in the physician's office. A small curette is passed through the cervix and a few specimens of endometrium are taken from various areas. Microscopic examination of the tissue shows whether or not the endometrium has been prepared for implantation of the fertilized ovum. If it has, ovulation is assumed to have occurred. A series of biopsies may be taken to show a pattern of endometrial change. This test provides information about hormonal balance, as reflected in the state of the endometrium, and is also employed to help diagnose the cause of severe dysmenorrhea and amenorrhea. During and after the procedure, the patient may have some cramping sensations due to cervical dilatation. The discomfort can be relieved by aspirin, which may be ordered by the physician, and by applying warmth to the lower abdomen.

**Vaginal Smears.** Vaginal cytologic smears are taken to examine the cervical mucus and determine its glucose content. A commercial Tes-Tape test is available so the patient may test herself for "normality."

Current research seems to demonstrate that electrovaginal potentials can be measured and the time of ovulation definitely established. However, this technique is not yet ready for office use.

If ovulation appears to be occurring normally, tests are done to determine whether the fallopian tubes are normal and patent.

**Rubin's Test.** A Rubin's test is usually done immediately after menstruation. It may also be repeated, since tubal spasm may interfere and cause the tubes to appear obstructed.

For this test a sterile cannula is introduced into the uterus and gas (carbon dioxide) then forced through the uterus, the fallopian tubes, and into the peritoneal cavity to determine whether the tubes are patent or closed. The physician, or his assistant, listens with his stethoscope for the swish that tells him that the gas has escaped into the peritoneal cavity. He also records the pressure necessary to force the gas through the tubes. If the manometer reaches 200 mm. of mercury, occluded tubes are suspected. The pressure usually is not increased beyond that because of the danger of rupturing a tube. If the gas does pass through the tube, the patient experiences referred pain to her shoulder or scapula on that side, a sign of air or gas under the diaphragm. Atropine 1/100 gr. may be given to decrease tubal spasm.

After the test, if the patient assumes the knee-chest or Trendelenburg position, the gas will rise into her pelvis, and she will be more comfortable sooner than if she stands up.

A helpful consequence of this diagnostic procedure is that in some instances of tubal occlusion, the obstruction may be cleared and the patient become fertile.

**Hysterosalpingography (uterosalpingography).** This test is an x-ray study of the uterus and the fallopian tubes made by introducing a radiopaque dye. The patient may take a laxative the night before the test and an enema in the morning, so that bowel distention does not distort the picture and she may be catheterized before the dye is injected.

Culdoscopy allows the physician to see the pelvic organs directly. It is more accurate and more informative than tubal insufflation or hysterosalpingography and therefore is beginning to be used most often. The patient assumes the knee-chest position, a local anesthesia is injected, and a culdoscope is inserted into the posterior fornix of the vagina.

**Sims'-Huhner Test (Postcoital Test).** In this test vaginal and cervical secretions are aspirated six to twelve hours after intercourse.

Finally the cervical mucus is examined to see if it allows penetration, survival, and motility of the husband's sperm. The cervical mucus sample may demonstrate poor sperm quality, poor seminal fluid due to partners' chronic inflammation, or poor quality cervical mucus due to chronic endocervicitis or hormonal imbalance. The test is usually done two or three times before it is considered to be conclusive.

In some couples a specific immunologic factor may be responsible for the infertility. Immune antibodies are not only in the blood but also in body secretions. The wife may have an antibody that attacks the husband's antigen, thereby killing all of his sperm. In these cases the husband's semen may be inserted directly into the uterus when ovulation is believed to have just occurred or to be just about to occur.

## Treatment

Physical techniques used to enhance fertility include ovulating agents (such as clomiphene and human menopausal gonadotropin), management of hormonal deficiencies of the corpus luteum, surgery for tubal reconstruction and uterine defects, therapy for immunologic incompatibility, and the use of artificial insemination.

If the physician believes that a systemic disorder is causing the infertility, he will treat the underlying disorder. Tubal strictures may be treated by surgery, although the operation is rarely successful. A low-grade infection may be treated with antibiotics.

In some infertile couples no physiologic defect can be found. There is a psychic factor in fertility that is poorly understood. Sometimes a pregnancy occurs only after the couple has given up hope of conceiving and has adopted a child.

Nurses can help couples wishing to conceive by making sure that they know how and when the ovum is fertilized, so that intercourse is not avoided at the midpoint between menses. Does the woman douche immediately after intercourse? Normally at this time douching is not necessary or advisable; it might wash the semen away. The woman whose physician has advised her to douche for whatever reason or who feels that she must douche, should wait until the next morning to do it.

Approximately 50 per cent of infertile couples can be cured of their sterility. However, for the remaining 50 per cent the nurse may want to discuss with the couple their feelings regarding artificial insemination or adoption. There is growing acceptance of varied life styles, and less pressure toward social conformity. Some married couples are enjoying childlessness. In some areas groups are formed that discuss feelings about this issue. Popular bestsellers help couples determine how much they themselves desire a child and how much they feel they *should* have children. Some couples freely admit relief when total sterility has been definitely proven, since they can now relax and quit trying. They are then able to readjust their marital goals and focus their attention elsewhere.

## MENOPAUSE AND LATER LIFE

The term menopause means the cessation of the menstrual cycle. The term climacteric is the long period during which ovarian activity gradually ceases. The terms are often used interchangeably, and this period of time is also called the "change of life." Menopause normally occurs between the ages of about 45 to 55.

## Physiology

Ovulation gradually ceases and with it, the menstrual cycle and reproductive function ends. The change usually is not sudden; rather, the menses become scanty (or sometimes unusually copious) and irregular for a time before they stop permanently. The uterus, the vagina, and the vulva decrease in size. As ovarian function diminishes, so does the production of estrogen and progesterone. The resulting endocrine imbalance leads to the cardinal symptoms of menopause: hot flashes, flushed skin, and intense sweating. These symptoms occur even more when heat production is increased, such as when the woman is exercising, eating, upset and tense, or when heat loss is impaired, such as in warm weather or when the woman is wearing lots of clothing.

As estrogen supply decreases, the skin arteries dilate and body heat is reduced. The resulting hot flashes may be so mild and so transitory that they almost escape notice, or they may last as long as 2 minutes and occur every 10 to 30 minutes around the clock. In some instances the hot flashes are disturbing enough to interfere with sleep. Night sweats frequently occur during menopause. Their cause should be medically evaluated, however, to rule out the possibility of disease, such as tuberculosis.

It should be added that menopause often occurs at a time when there are many other changes in a woman's life. Her children may be grown and leaving home, her husband may be at the peak of his involvement in his employment, and home responsibilities may be decreased. Many women find other necessary and interesting jobs, often outside the home. They need no longer worry about pregnancy. For some women there is a sense of well-being and their general health improves. However, for other women, cessation of menses may represent loss of femininity and hence a threat to their self-esteem. These women may be much more aware of symptoms, such as nervousness, irritability, headaches, fatigue, and so on.

Since normal and abnormal changes may readily

be confused, it is especially important for women to have regular gynecologic examinations during this period.

## Emotional Reactions

Depression is a common reaction to menopause and has both physiologic and emotional causes. Many women find that the depression lifts when they are treated with supplementary estrogens. It seems likely, therefore, that depression is, to some extent, related to ovarian insufficiency. Depression is also a reaction to loss: cessation of reproductive capacity constitutes a serious loss for most women. This aspect of the woman's experience is often rationalized by discussions of how many children she has, or, if she has none, by how busy she is at work, thus obscuring an irretrievable loss in capacity, which can contribute significantly to depression. Other aspects of loss are also evident during this period of life: the woman's appearance changes as wrinkles, gray hair, and differences in the figure appear. These changes are especially disturbing in a culture such as ours, which is obsessed with the importance of a youthful, attractive appearance.

The meaning of the loss experienced at menopause and the woman's reaction to it vary with the individual's level of personal development as well as with the circumstances of her life. Inability to bear more children may be viewed quite differently by a woman who has several children than by a woman who has none. The woman who is absorbed in a career that holds her interest and offers her satisfaction may deal with her children's growing independence more effectively than one whose life has been immersed in the role of mother. Generally, the reaction to menopause is one of stress and loss, and how well the woman handles it depends on her ability to cope: to recognize, acknowledge, and assimilate the losses, and to find new avenues of expression for her creative abilities and new sources of satisfaction and meaning for her life. The woman who has gradually sought experiences and satisfactions in addition to caring for her home and family is in a better position to continue this development during the climacteric than the woman whose interests and satisfactions have been focused almost exclusively on her home and children.

Nurses have many opportunities to help women experiencing the climacteric. Superstitions abound concerning this period of life, and one important service the nurse can render is to help women obtain correct factual information. Does the patient believe that women "go crazy during the change"? Does she think that women's bones become suddenly soft? These and many other superstitions are voiced by women when they are given an opportunity to discuss their ideas about menopause. As is often the case, superstitions contain some element of fact. Thus, the added stress of menopause may be the "final straw" that results in psychosis after a lifetime of impaired personal development and difficulty in coping with life's demands. Osteoporosis *is* more common among women after menopause, but this does not mean that women's bones suddenly "go soft." Group discussions are useful in teaching women in clinics, inpatient services of hospitals, and in various community groups about menopause. It is essential for nurses to take the initiative in guiding and teaching women about this period of life.

Helping women to talk about their feelings concerning menopause is another contribution nurses can make when working with individual patients and groups of patients. A superficial "cheer-up" campaign, concentrating on hair styles and community activities, is unfortunately a common approach and can leave the woman feeling more isolated and lonely than before. (Practical suggestions for improving appearance and finding new interests are useful, however.) Among some of the anxieties commonly expressed are:

Loss of role ("My children don't need me any more.")
Concern for marital relationship ("Maybe my husband won't want me.")
Loss of attractiveness and femininity
Fear of physical or mental disability ("Getting cancer" or "Having a nervous breakdown")

Verbalizing such fears does not remove them, but it can help the woman move ahead with measures to begin dealing with her fears and can help her realize that others have similar concerns. Instead of just worrying that she may have cancer, she can go to the clinic twice yearly for a Pap smear and breast examination. Instead of withdrawing from her husband and wondering what his attitudes are about change of life, she can perhaps begin to talk with him about it, voicing some of her concerns and listening to his. The views of others who are significant to her, such as her husband and children, have important effects upon the woman who is going through the menopause. If others whose esteem she values believe that a woman's life is over at 50, she will have the additional burden of experiencing these attitudes toward her. The nurse can help the patient to consider what her own attitudes are toward menopause and aging. Often the woman is hampered by not sufficiently delineating her own views on this matter of vital concern.

Assisting women to deal with daily discomfort and to develop habits which help counteract depression and bring more satisfaction is important. Group or individual discussion can help the patient who is irritable or who cries easily to review situations that elicit this behavior and to try to find other means of responding that foster improved relationships with family and friends. Also, the patient may find that she is more even-tempered after she consults her physician and begins taking estrogens.

A regular program of exercise (enjoyable exercise, not just more housework if the woman is already bored by it) can counteract the tendency to weight gain and muscle flabbiness, as well as provide zestful pleasure.

Branching out in her tastes, activities, and style of dress can help the woman look and feel more attractive, confident, and energetic. When she communicates this attitude of optimism to others, she receives a more positive response from them, and this helps her break out of a circular pattern of depression and poor relationships with others to a more positive regard for herself and for others.

Community activities begin to absorb the time and attention of many middle-aged and older women, and can render valuable service to others as well as provide the women with an outlet for their talent and energy. Work that is truly satisfying requires commitment—of energy, time, and interest. This is true whether it is volunteer community service or paid employment. Sometimes it is difficult for women in this age group to begin to develop themselves in preparation for their work so they can derive satisfaction from it. Programs to help older women up-date their skills are important, so that they can develop the skills needed to become meaningfully involved with work. Glib advice to spend an afternoon a week as a volunteer in a service organization (valuable and satisfying as that may be) is not usually the whole solution to the problem of the woman who needs to discover or rediscover a new expression of herself.

Alertness for symptoms of depression among menopausal women is essential for nurses who work with these patients in hospitals or in the community.

Depression can be so immobilizing that the patient is unable to carry on any of her usual activities, and it can lead to suicide. The nurse should be especially observant for such communication from the patient as:

- feelings of worthlessness and uselessness
- feelings of emptiness and hopelessness
- lack of interest in others and in usual activities

The nurse should talk promptly with the patient's physician if she observes such indications of serious depression, so that the patient can be referred promptly for psychiatric treatment. It is difficult to relate to depressed persons; the tendency is to withdraw. Realizing this, the nurse should make a particular effort to make contact with the depressed patient and to show concern for her. She should continue this concern while the process of referral is occurring until the patient is receiving treatment for depression.

**Other Aspects of Later Life.** The time of menopause coincides with other aspects of aging. Gray hair, wrinkles, or perhaps the onset of a degenerative disease, such as arthritis or a cardiovascular disorder, may call attention to passing time. The endocrine changes that occur during menopause cause a shift in the distribution of the body fat. The woman gains weight easily, with the greatest increase in hips, abdomen, and buttocks. Her breasts become less firm, and if they are large, they have a tendency to become pendulous. The vaginal mucous membrane becomes thinner and more readily irritated.

Some women attribute all symptoms to the menopause, when a symptom may be due to a coexisting disorder. Menopause is only one aspect of the aging process, albeit one that sharply directs a woman's feelings to herself.

**Treatment.** There has been considerable discussion and some disagreement still exists among physicians concerning the use of supplementary estrogens for menopausal and postmenopausal women. Some physicians consider the postmenopausal state virtually a deficiency condition and believe that supplementary estrogens should be prescribed much in the way that insulin is prescribed for diabetics. Physicians who subscribe to this view believe that the woman's overall health will be improved by estrogen administration and that the incidence and severity of some diseases of later life, such as osteoporosis, can be lessened by long-term estrogen therapy.

A more widely held view at present is that decisions concerning estrogen therapy must be individualized.

The vaginal cytogram or Maturation Index is the most simple procedure to determine the extent, if any, of an estrogen deficiency. A specimen of cells is taken from the vaginal wall and a slide prepared. Microscopic examination shows the percentage of mature cells present, which depends on estrogen. This test may be used as a guide to estrogen therapy. Some of the questions the physician considers are whether, by administering estrogens, there is a possibility of stimulating growth of cancer cells in the uterus or breast. A patient with a history of uterine or breast cancer is not treated with supplementary estrogen, and patients who do receive estrogen supplements are examined regularly for any sign of cancer of the uterus or breast. Some patients experience little discomfort at this period and do not require estrogen therapy. The primary consideration in therapy of menopause, according to physicians who advocate highly individualized treatment, is helping the woman to feel well, physically and emotionally, and to carry out her various roles as wife, mother, and worker effectively. Estrogens, sedatives, tranquilizers or mood-elevating drugs, such as the amphetamines, may be prescribed at various times to alleviate symptoms. The effects of long-term estrogen therapy remain to be evaluated. Many years are required to follow women so treated to determine, for example, the relative incidence of myocardial infarction, osteoporosis, and cancer of reproductive organs contrasted with those who do not receive this treatment.

When the patient is receiving exogenous steroids, uterine bleeding may or may not occur. Because bleeding also is an early symptom of cancer, it is especially important that the patient knows if and when bleeding is expected on her particular regimen. When androgen therapy is used, watch for masculinizing side effects, such as a deepening of the voice and an increase in facial hair. Usually, the dosage given is too small to produce these symptoms.

The climacteric can be precipitated by the surgical removal of the ovaries and by the radiologic destruction of ovarian function. Because of the suddenness of artificially induced menopause, replacement therapy sometimes is given to supply the hormones of which the patient's body has been so abruptly deprived.

Menopause does not mean the end of a woman's "motherliness" or sexual life. Many women find even more joy in being foster grandparents or biologic grandparents than they did with their own children. With all her achieved wisdom and practical experience, the woman can often be extremely helpful to other younger, more inexperienced women, both her own daughters and other women in the neighborhood. In a similar fashion, now that they have more time and energy for intimate relationships, older women may find that sexual behavior has even more enjoyment and pleasure than formerly. An asset at this stage of life is that the older woman can focus more on her own needs and on the needs of others who are important in her life.

## REFERENCES AND BIBLIOGRAPHY

See end of Chapter 52.

# The Woman with a Disorder of the Reproductive System

Treatment of the gynecologic patient is undertaken with two objectives: (1) to preserve or restore the woman's health, and (2) to preserve her childbearing capacity if she so desires. The first objective is operative throughout the patient's lifespan and the second, until she has passed through menopause or decides that she prefers not to be fertile.

Regardless of when pathology occurs, early diagnosis and medical attention are essential. The nurse familiar with normal function can often help women to understand the importance of regular gynecologic examination and of when to seek medical help.

Disorders of a woman's reproductive organs cause a powerful emotional impact. The emotions aroused depend on what these structures mean to a particular woman, with her unique background, life situation, and personality.

Thus, it is important that the nurse recognize that deep feelings are involved. A permissive atmosphere should be provided for the patient, so that she can come to grips herself with her own emotions. This kind of atmosphere is achieved by recognizing the patient's feelings. The nurse must be sensitive to expressions of emotion (clear or subtle) and be calm and efficient, so that the patient can feel the security of being with a professional person who knows what she is doing. If a patient raises a great fuss over some minor procedure, the nurse should listen carefully. This may be her way of communicating more significant fears.

The patient should be told what to expect. Many will be grateful for an explanation of the terms they hear but cannot interpret.

929

## ASSESSMENT OF THE GYNECOLOGIC PATIENT

The following are examples of areas requiring assessment:

- The patient's illness and what results are likely from the illness and its treatment.
- The patient's understanding of her condition and its treatment.
- The patient's emotional response to the diagnosis, to therapy, and to the experience of having a gynecologic disorder.
- The patient's general physical condition (nutritional status, weight, presence of other illnesses, age, and so on) in relation to reproductive capacity; in relation to the specific disorder (e.g., vaginal discharge, presence of a palpable uterine tumor); and in relation to treatment (e.g., response to drugs, surgery, radiation, and so on).

- The patient's family relationships, both supportive and dependent. What effect will her condition have upon such relationships (e.g., future child bearing)? If family ties are weak or if there is no family, are there close friends to whom she can turn for help?
- Available resources for convalescent care, if needed (e.g., convalescent home, family, or visiting nurse or homemaker).
- The long-range prognosis. Is recovery likely? If not, what is the patient's level of awareness of and response to the prognosis?
- The effect of the patient's philosophical and religious convictions (e.g., in relation to termination of pregnancy).
- The patient's views of herself as a woman and the effect of the disorder and its treatment upon these views. Does she equate womanliness with weakness or with strength and competence?

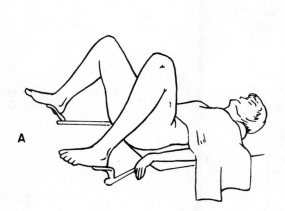

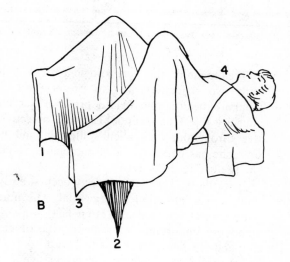

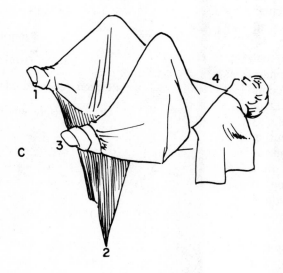

**Figure 52-1.** Draping a patient in the lithotomy position.

(A) The patient is placed in this position while she is under a sheet (which was removed for this drawing). Note that the patient's hips are right at the edge of the table.

(B) The sheet is turned on the diagonal. One corner (4) is placed under the chin, the opposite corner (2) hangs down between the legs, and the other corners (1 and 3) go over each foot.

(C) Wrap corners (1) and (3) around the feet. When the physician is ready for the examination, corner (2) is folded up, and only the patient's vulva is exposed.

● **The effects of the patient's role(s) and life style upon her plans for convalescent care and rehabilitation.**

## DIAGNOSTIC PROCEDURES

### The Gynecologic Examination

Most women dread a gynecologic examination. They are embarrassed and fearful about being examined. They not only fear exposure, but also what the examiner may find. The patient usually feels less embarrassed when the nurse moves and acts in a matter-of-fact fashion. It may help if the nurse asks the patient what specifically is frightening or embarrassing her. The nurse can then find ways to possibly lessen the fear and embarrassment. For example, if the patient states that she fears the pain of the examination, the nurse can explain the procedure and have her practice the deep-breathing and muscle-relaxing measures that will lessen the discomfort. If the patient says she fears venereal disease, it would be helpful for the nurse to explain that, whatever the difficulty, the patient will have the opportunity to speak with the examiner about the diagnosis and the treatment that is needed.

**Preparing the Patient.** A nurse *always* remains in the room the *entire* time that a patient is being examined by a physician. In some situations, the nurse who has the necessary skills carries out pelvic examinations. She should check that all needed equipment is available before the examination begins. The patient will be asked about any problems she may be having so that she can express her feelings in her own way, stressing what is important to her. Specific questions will focus on her menstrual history, her pregnancies, any problems concerning sexual relationships, any abnormal pelvic pain, and any bleeding or discharge she may have noted. The patient should be encouraged to give a full history. Many patients do not mention certain aspects because they feel too embarrassed to discuss them fully. The nurse should explain what will be done during the examination.

The patient is instructed to remove her underclothes from the waist down and to loosen anything tight around the waist. A sheet can be wrapped around her until she is positioned on the examining table. The patient must void, since a full bladder may interfere with the examination. A distended bladder, for example, may lead to confusion as to the presence or absence of an ovarian cyst or tumor.

**Positioning the Patient.** The most common posi-

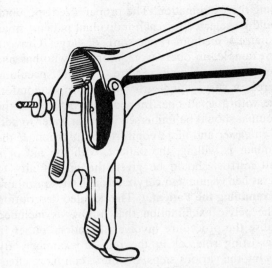

**Figure 52-2.** A bivalve speculum. With the mouth of the speculum closed and well lubricated, the speculum is passed into the vagina. Then it is opened to give the physician a clear view of the cervix. Specula come in various sizes.

tion for the gynecologic examination is the lithotomy position (Fig. 52-1). It is uncomfortable for anyone to maintain. With a sheet around her, the patient sits at the edge of the examining table and lies back. The nurse helps the patient to lift both legs at the same time, and places the patient's feet in the stirrups. If the stirrups are metal, the patient should wear shoes for a better grip and more even distribution of pressure on the soles of her feet. Then the nurse helps the patient slide to the edge of the table. By draping her securely, the nurse reassures her that her modesty will be protected. Sims' and genupectoral (knee-chest) positions are used occasionally for this examination.

**Equipment.** Although the vagina is not a sterile cavity, equipment is sterilized each time it is used to prevent any introduction of pathogens. Both for preventing infection and for aesthetic considerations, the patient must have a fresh sheet to lie on and the examiner must wash his hands after examining a patient and before handling equipment in preparation for the next patient. A bright spotlight should be set up behind the examiner's stool. On occasion, a flashlight held by an assistant must be used.

A bivalve speculum is needed to visualize the vaginal walls and the cervix (Fig. 52-2). The patient should be familiarized with the instrument beforehand so that she will not be frightened and tense during the examination. The proper sized speculum should be selected for each individual patient: small (pediatric), medium (Pederson), or large (Graves). For example, an obese woman or one who has had several children may require a large speculum, whereas a very young girl would be more comfortable with a small one. Immediately before use the speculum should be immersed in warm water to permit an easier and more comfortable insertion. If the examiner is willing, the patient, with the aid of a small mirror, should be given the opportunity to look at her vagina and cervix through the speculum.

**Examining the Patient.** The detailed description of the pelvic examination that follows is included because the procedure involves the nurse, either in an assisting role, or in the role of examiner. By knowing the various steps, the nurse can more effectively prepare the patient for the examination and support her while it is being performed. However, the order in which the examiner performs various aspects of the pelvic examination varies. It is considered preferable to begin the examination by observation, first of the external genitalia and adjacent structures, and then of the vaginal walls and the cervix of the uterus through the bivalve speculum. When observing the external genitalia the examiner searches for discharge, irritation, inflammation, edema, and malformation of the external structures; he observes the state of the hymen and the perineum. The examiner places one or two fingers of his gloved hand into the vagina. By palpation, the structures beyond the orifice are examined, including the vaginal walls and Bartholin glands, the base of the bladder, the pelvic floor, and the cervix. Without removing his gloved fingers from the vagina, the fingers of the other hand are placed on the patient's lower abdomen for the bimanual examination, and the position, the size, and the contour of the uterus, the ovaries, and other pelvic structures palpated between the two hands. Any abnormal mass in the pelvic area may thus be felt. At the end of the examination, the examiner may place a gloved and lubricated index finger into the patient's vagina and the second finger into the rectum, as high as the level of the posterior surface of the uterus can be felt. The presence of hemorrhoids, fistulas, and fissures can also be noted. Examination of the breasts is ordinarily carried out before or after the pelvic examination (see Chap. 54).

Although the gynecologic examination is uncomfortable, the patient should not feel pain unless disease is present. The more relaxed the lower abdominal muscles are, the better the examiner can palpate internal organs. The patient should be asked to make her lower abdomen soft. Breathing deeply through the mouth also may help to relax the abdominal muscles. A staff member should concentrate on the patient—helping her to relax, preventing her from wriggling to the head of the table, talking to her, or holding her hand if that seems to give comfort.

**Care after the Examination.** The perineum should be cleaned of lubricating jelly. The patient should be helped to slide her hips back from the edge of the table, removing both feet from the stirrups at the same time to prevent strain, and helped off the table. After she has been in the lithotomy position, she may wish to rest for a few moments on a stool or chair before she gets dressed. She should be given a tissue or gauze to wipe off the remaining lubricating jelly, and allowed a moment of privacy. Although the nurse may wipe the perineum after the examination, the patient usually prefers to finish the job. She should be given a fresh sanitary pad, if she needs one, and wrappings in which to dispose of the old one. She should be shown where to dispose of it, and where she may wash her hands. If the physician used gentian violet, the patient will need a pad to prevent the dye from staining her underclothing. Considerations such as these smooth the way and convey acceptance and caring.

Used equipment must be rinsed in cold water, to prevent secretions from sticking, scrubbed with soap and water, and resterilized. The hands must be washed after cleaning the perineum or touching used equipment. The nurse must keep her hands away from her face especially, to protect the eyes from such infectious organisms as the gonococcus.

If the patient has a discharge, she should have been instructed not to douche before the examination. The examiner may want to see the discharge and to take a specimen for more detailed study.

## Cytologic Test for Cancer (Papanicolaou Test)

Since about 25 per cent of all malignant disease in women arises in the genital tract and since such cancer is particularly likely to be treated with success, the Pap test should be done at regular intervals to detect early cancer. All women over age 20 should be tested since 10 to 15 per cent of cervical cancer occurs in women age 20 to 29.

For the Pap test, cells that have exfoliated are picked up, spread on a slide, stained, and examined for malignancy (Fig. 52-3). Secretions from various body parts are also studied microscopically to determine the presence of malignant cells. The Pap test is used mainly to detect early cancer of the cervix, which is the most common form of malignancy of the reproductive tract in women. The lining of the fallopian tubes, the uterus, and the cervix constantly shed cells into the pool of vaginal secretions. If a smear of secretions from the vagina is examined under a microscope, abnormal cells can be detected before symptoms develop, thereby improving prognosis by early therapy. This test gives more reliable results for cells from the cervix, however, than for cells shed from higher up in the reproductive tract.

Papanicolaou smears may be taken in the following manner. The patient should have been instructed not to douche for two or three days before the test, because irrigation may remove the exfoliated cells. The speculum used to expose the cervix is lubricated only with tap water, because lubricant may interfere with the accuracy of the test. A small amount of secretion is obtained from the posterior fornix with a Pap stick, spread on a glass slide, and immediately immersed in a solution of one part 95 per cent alcohol and one part ether. A solution called Spraycyte may be used instead. It is dispensed in a pressurized bottle and sprayed directly on the slide. To take an endocervical smear, one end of a Pap stick is used to scrape the cervix.

Some experts prescribe the test every six months; others, yearly. A positive test (one in which abnormal cells are found) requires further study, such as a biopsy of tissue from the cervix. A negative test merely means that no abnormal cells were found in these specimens. A questionable classification means that cells are found that cannot be readily classified as normal or abnormal. A specimen that is considered questionable requires further investigation.

Cultures for bacteria and viruses are taken when there is a question of possible infection. A fresh smear or a culture swab rubbed on the area may be used.

**Followup.** Cervical biopsy is the usual followup when a cytologic test is positive or questionable. When the physician suspects cancer, he may take a tiny piece of the cervix for laboratory examination. This procedure may be conducted in the physician's office or in the clinic. Preferably, it should be scheduled approximately one week after the pa-

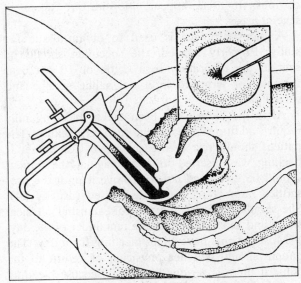

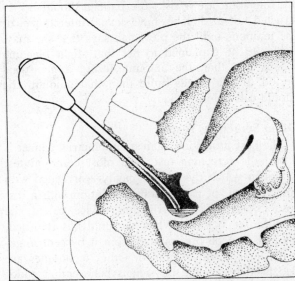

**Figure 52-3.** The Papanicolaou test. A vaginal smear can be taken with a pap stick applicator. (*see inset*) A cervical smear can be taken with a pap stick. The smears are spread on a glass slide and "fixed."

tient's monthly menstrual flow has ceased, when the cervix is least vascular. The patient may have some discomfort, but the procedure is not painful since the cervix does not have pain receptors.

A Schiller's test involves painting the cervix with iodine solution, dated as having been made within the past month and stored in a dark brown bottle. Abnormal tissue will not stain brown. (A similar test using toluidine blue dye may be done on the vulva.) Abnormal areas are thus made more obvious. If none appear, biopsies are taken at several areas.

A biopsy forceps is used to obtain tissue for study. Properly labeled, the specimen should be sent to the laboratory in a bottle of 10 per cent formalin or wrapped in a wet saline sponge and waxed paper.

After the biopsy has been taken, bleeding may require additional treatment, such as packing. The patient should rest before she leaves for home. If packing was inserted into the vagina, the patient should be instructed not to remove it until the prescribed number of hours has passed (usually 24). She should be instructed to avoid unusual physical strain and heavy lifting for the remainder of the day.

Most patients have slight bleeding for a day. The patient should call her physician or return to the clinic if there is serious bleeding. Because bleeding and infection are a risk, the patient should be instructed not to douche, have sexual intercourse, or use tampons until the physician says that she may. It should be explained to her that slight bleeding means less than the amount during a menstrual period. If she bleeds more than that amount, she should call the physician.

### Other Screening Tests

The best protection against endometrial cancer is a periodic screening test. The most common test is that in which the uterine cavity is irrigated with about 30 ml. of normal saline solution with a disposable suction-type irrigation device called the Gravlee Jet Washer. When the fluid has returned, the cells can be precipitated from it by centrifugation, stained, and examined. Other techniques are also available. Some physicians believe that endometrial carcinoma is best diagnosed by dilating the cervix and curetting the uterus (D and C). Endometrial smears are another diagnostic measure used to determine the presence of carcinoma. In some areas endometrial biopsy is the preferred screening test.

An endometrial biopsy is done by the physician inserting a speculum, wiping any mucus from the cervix, painting on Schiller's solution, and grasping the cervix with a tenaculum. A uterine sound (a metal tube) is inserted to determine the direction and length of the cervical canal and the uterus. The nurse should tell the patient that she may feel slight discomfort similar to a menstrual cramp. A curved curette or suction instrument is inserted into the uterus and a bit of tissue is scraped or aspirated. This test is done immediately before the menses if for a fertility study. After this test the patient may have a cramped feeling that usually can be relieved by heat over the uterine area or by a mild analgesic.

Culdoscopy is examination of the pelvic organs by inserting a trocar and then a culdoscope into the posterior fornix of the vagina while the patient is in the knee-chest position (Fig. 52-4). Local anesthesia is used. The only after care necessary is to instruct the patient not to douche or to have intercourse for approximately two weeks.

## DILATATION OF THE CERVIX AND CURETTAGE OF THE UTERUS (D AND C)

*Dilatation* refers to stretching the mouth of the cervix; *curettage* means scraping the lining of a cavity (in this instance the endometrium). This common gynecologic operation is often performed to find the cause of abnormal bleeding and, also, to examine the patient for malignancy and fibroid tumors. (The scrapings are sent to the laboratory for investigation.)

Although endometrial biopsy is equally helpful, a D and C may be done as part of an investigation into the cause of sterility. In this instance it is performed before menstruation. When the scrapings, which are sent to the laboratory along with the date of the last menstrual period, are examined microscopically, the physician can determine whether ovulation occurred during that menstrual cycle, the adequacy of the endometrial lining, and the state of hormonal balance. Cervical dilatation is performed initially to permit uterine curettage, though it is also done to relieve stricture or stenosis of the cervical orifice, to permit tubal insufflation and, in selected instances, to relieve dysmenorrhea. The procedure is done in the operating room, under general anesthetic, with the patient in the lithotomy position. Curettage is usually avoided when vagina, cervix, or fallopian tubes are infected because the infection could spread.

### Preoperative and Postoperative Care

Preparation for a D and C includes care similar to that of any patient about to receive general anesthesia: food and fluids withheld for 12 hours prior to surgery; rest; skin cleansing; and safety precautions. Opinions concerning whether the patient's vulva and perineum should be shaved prior to

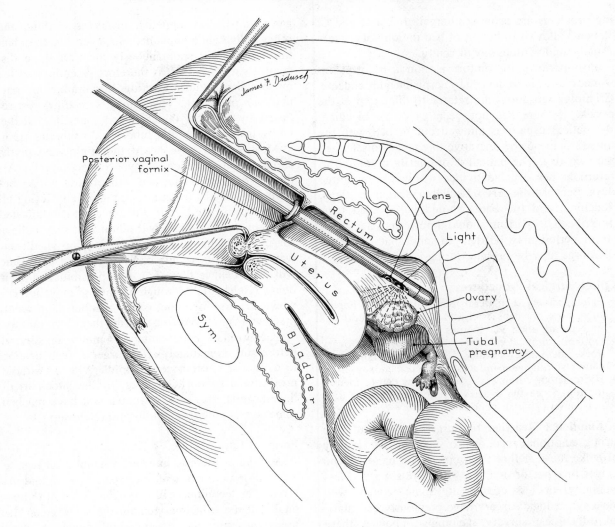

**Figure 52-4.** Culdoscopy. Sagittal section showing culdoscope viewing pelvic viscera. (Te Linde, R. W.: *Operative Gynecology*, ed. 4, Philadelphia, Lippincott, 1970)

D and C vary among different gynecologists. Usually there is no prep or enema. Because of their proximity to the operative area, the bladder and lower bowel must be emptied on the morning of surgery. If the patient has lost a significant amount of blood, for example, during an incomplete abortion, a transfusion may be started.

Although some consider the procedure a simple one, no operation that requires anesthesia and surgical intervention is without danger. The patient faces the physical and emotional trauma associated with surgery and also may be anxious about the outcome of diagnostic findings.

When the patient returns from the operating room or the recovery room, she may be wearing a sterile perineal pad, but she probably will not be wearing a belt to hold it in place. She should be given a belt or a T-binder to keep the pad in place so that she can be comfortable and the sheets will not be soiled. She will have a serosanguineous discharge for several days. Packing occasionally may be placed within the vagina and the cervical canal. When it is used, it is removed the next morning. Postoperatively, the nurse should investigate the perineal site and note the drainage on the perineal pad. Immediately after surgery the pad should be observed every 15 or 20 minutes for the first two or three hours.

Voiding should be checked. The time and amount of the first voiding should be charted. However, voiding problems are usually minimal after a D and C. Patients allowed to be out of bed the day of surgery usually void without any difficulty.

Postoperative discomfort is minor in most instances and is relieved by aspirin and codeine. Cramping sensations are related to dilatation of the cervix. If there has not been excessive bleeding, the patient usually is allowed out of bed with the nurse's help on the operative day and is discharged the next day. The patient is ordinarily permitted to return to her usual activities within two or three days. Because the cervix is dilated, sexual relations, douching, and tub baths should be avoided temporarily. The patient should know that her menstrual period may be delayed, and that a vaginal discharge may be present during convalescence.

## Other Surgical Procedures

- Salpingectomy. Unilateral, removal of one fallopian tube, does not cause sterility, although bilateral salpingectomy does. The menses continue.
- Oophorectomy. Unilateral, removal of one ovary does not cause sterility. Bilateral oophorectomy causes sterility and induces artificial menopause.
- Hysterectomy. Removal of the uterus causes menses to stop. Since the ovaries are not removed, it does not cause artificial menopause.

**Emotional Reaction to Surgery.** Women have strong emotional reactions to such surgery. It may provoke the fear that the woman's husband will no longer love her or that she will be less worthy, less womanly, or less competent. Some women who have gynecologic surgery have previously had marital difficulties; surgery seemingly enhances these difficulties. Feelings of defeminization seem particularly common among women who define themselves primarily as wives and mothers.

Although professionals may view the situation as a physiologic need, the woman often will focus more on the fertility aspects than on the disease process necessitating the surgery (Nehring, 1972). It must be emphasized that the *ability* to have children is sometimes much more crucial than the actual *desire* to have them.

About the third or fourth day after surgery, women often cry, feel withdrawn, and are depressed. While the nurse might expect this, due to the grieving process, the woman involved is often not only surprised, but quite confused by the intensity of her feelings.

Gynecologic patients are uncomfortable. They do not sleep well, have quite a lot of discomfort, gas cramps, poor appetite, problems voiding, and other individual complaints. However, less than half the women will spontaneously mention these discomforts (Nehring). It is therefore essential that the nurse make a point of asking. Gas cramps are particularly prevalent. These may sometimes be relieved by charcoal tablets taken four times a day or by inserting a rectal tube for 20 minutes p.r.n.

Most women have heard the frightening myths about the after effects of gynecologic surgery. Although the better-educated will profess not to believe these myths (such as gaining weight, losing all sexual desire, etc.), it is difficult not to be affected by them. Most women will admit that they believe surgery will change their lives in some significant way. Some will become badly frightened and some will even believe there is a real possibility of their dying (Nehring). Although a patient may not cry when a nurse or other staff member is present, many will cry at some time during their hospital stay.

The woman needs intense emotional support before and immediately after surgery. Verbalization to a listener is often very helpful. With or without professional support, however, by the later part of their hospital stay, many women will have reached some sort of tentative equilibrium (Nehring).

## Perineal Care

As long as there is sufficient vaginal discharge to warrant a perineal pad, perineal care should be given. The technique will vary from hospital to hospital, but the principles remain the same: keep the area clean and the patient comfortable. A clean rather than a sterile technique is considered adequate in many instances (before proceeding with perineal care or teaching the patient to do it, the nurse finds out which technique is required). Because the perineal area is not sterile, and because simplifying techniques often encourage their employment, many hospitals use a clean method employing a disposable washcloth, especially for ambulatory patients. This procedure is easily taught to patients, who then can do their own perineal care. Some hospitals use cotton balls or paper pledgets: a fresh one for each stroke. The teaching should begin as soon as the patient becomes ambulatory.

In some hospitals perineal care is given as a warm sitz or tub bath. Most hospitals use disposable plastic basins for the sitz bath which the patient may later take home with her, thus making it easier for her to continue the treatment at home.

The tub bath, relaxing in itself, is often preferred by the patients. Of course, the tub is scrupulously cleaned between patients. To many patients, perineal irrigation is particularly comfortable. Sterile or clean water, 100 to 105 degrees F, is poured over the vulva from a pitcher no higher than 6 inches over the patient. The perineum can be dried with sterile cotton balls or a clean washcloth, depending on the technique used. In many hospitals, warm water is placed in a plastic bottle. Ambulatory patients are taught to give themselves an external irrigation of the genital area by squeezing the bottle, after each voiding and each change of perineal pad.

The nurse should give perineal care during at least the first 48 hours postoperative. Giving perineal care affords the nurse an excellent opportunity to observe the surgical area. Perineal care always should be done after a bowel movement and after voiding. When there are sutures in the perineal area the nurse should examine the area several times a day. When packing is in the vagina, the nurse should give the perineal care, being especially careful not to dislodge the packing. Draping, ensuring privacy, and sure movements minimize embarrassment to the patient.

If a patient can administer perineal care herself, she should have all the necessary equipment at her bedside, including paper bags in which to dispose of the waste, and should be instructed to wipe herself with downward strokes toward the rectum, with clean tissue for each stroke.

Perineal care is not only a protection against infection, but also a source of comfort to the patient.

Since the vagina is not sterile, vaginal irrigations or douches are usually done with a clean technique. In comparison, catheterization of the bladder is always a sterile procedure.

- When catheterizing female patients, the nurse must remember that the urethral opening is below the clitoris and just above the vagina. She should have a good light, and look for these landmarks before attempting to insert the tip of the catheter. If the vagina is entered accidentally, it will be necessary to take a new catheter before proceeding, since the vagina is not sterile. Because the clitoris is a very sensitive organ, poking it with the catheter may cause the patient discomfort. The nurse spreads the labia first, placing her fingers carefully so that their position need not be changed during the procedure.
- Because the urethral opening is so close to the vagina, postoperative care of surgical perineal wounds is often complicated by voiding problems. Dressings should be changed whenever they become wet. After

gynecologic surgery patients may have a catheter in place, and catheterization may be ordered preoperatively to empty the bladder fully and to avoid accidental trauma to the bladder during surgery.

## ABORTION

Abortion is the termination of a pregnancy before the fetus is viable. The term *abortion* is used to designate interruption of pregnancy before the fetus weighs more than 500 Gm. (about 20 weeks of gestation). Between this time and a full-term delivery, expulsion of the fetus is referred to as a *premature birth*.

### Types of Abortion

**Spontaneous Abortion.** About 10 per cent of all pregnancies result in spontaneous abortion ("miscarriage" is the layman's term), usually before the twelfth week. (The nurse might keep in mind when talking to patients that for some people the word "miscarriage" may be more acceptable.) Abnormalities of the fertilized ovum or the placenta, inconsistent with life, are believed to be the most frequent cause. Maternal disease, such as a severe acute infection, endocrine imbalance, or a chronic wasting disease, may be a cause. Physical trauma rarely causes abortion; emotional trauma may cause it. In searching for a reason for losing the baby, it is easy to remember a recent shock or bump, and easy to forget similar incidents that had no such effect.

Abnormal uterine bleeding in any woman during her childbearing years may indicate an abortion in the early weeks of gestation—so early in her pregnancy that she is unaware that she was pregnant. Pain and bleeding are common symptoms. The pain may be so mild that it is disregarded or as severe as labor pains. Bleeding may range from spotting to hemorrhage. Generally, spontaneous abortion occurs six weeks or so after the fetus has died.

**Threatened Abortion.** Bleeding or spotting may indicate that abortion is threatened. Other signs may be cramps or backache. Only about half the women who have these symptoms lose their babies; in the others the pregnancy may proceed entirely normally.

**Incomplete Abortion.** Some of the products of the pregnancy are expelled, and some (usually a portion of the placenta) are retained. Incomplete separation of the placenta from the uterine wall causes hemorrhage. In *complete abortion* all of the products of conception are expelled.

**Missed Abortion.** The fetus dies, but is not expelled. It may be retained two months or longer.

**Habitual Abortions.** Such abortions occur repeatedly without apparent cause. Improved nutrition, bed rest, and hormonal therapy have helped some women who habitually abort to carry a fetus to term. Emotional support can be an important factor in helping the patient carry the baby to term. If abortion does occur, support from the physician and nurse can assist the patient to deal with the loss of her baby. The fear of being unable to carry a baby to term is very common among women who have once suffered a spontaneous abortion.

### Treatment and Nursing Care

A pregnant woman should report the first signs of vaginal discharge, bleeding, or cramps to her physician. He probably will recommend bed rest, put her on a light diet, and warn her against any straining, such as when she moves her bowels. She should save all formed vaginal discharges for the physician to examine. The physician may order a sedative or a tranquilizer to help her rest quietly. If the bleeding stops, he may allow her out of bed in several days, but only for quiet activity. If abdominal pain becomes severe or uterine bleeding increases, abortion may be imminent, and the physician probably will hospitalize the patient. An incomplete abortion is treated by curettage. The patient may enter the hospital, bleeding profusely. Blood typing and cross-matching are done, and a transfusion started. In missed abortion the uterus usually is allowed to empty itself. Occasionally it is necessary to remove the dead fetus. In incomplete abortion drugs, such as oxytocin and ergonovine, are frequently used to make the uterus contract and to control bleeding.

If the abortion is threatening, there is the possibility that a quiet stay in bed will save the baby. If the abortion is imminent or incomplete, bed rest will prevent increased bleeding with activity. The patient should be observed carefully and repeatedly for hemorrhage. The nurse must check the patient's vital signs and observe the perineal pad for amount and character of discharge. Is there bright red blood? Dark blood? Clots? Pieces of tissue? The nurse should save all large clots and tissue for the physician to examine. The patient should not use the toilet; instead, she should use the bedpan to avoid passing the fetus or placenta unnoticed. If the patient begins to have cramps, the nurse should inform the physician immediately.

A patient with a threatened abortion may remain on bed rest for a long period of time. A few women spend the major part of the nine months in bed, although they may not be in the hospital for the entire time. Many of these women carry the infant to term, but the husband or a relative has to take care of the household. For a woman who wants a baby, the suspense of a threatened abortion is very difficult, but she is usually motivated to follow the prescribed treatment, including bed rest, if necessary. She may be resentful that other women are able to carry a baby without having to stay in bed. She may feel guilty because she has to be waited on and cannot contribute to the work of the household. Because she has little exercise in bed, her diet should be light but nutritionally sound.

Nursing care after an abortion is similar to that given after a D and C or that given any time after the cervix has been dilated. Perineal care is given as long as there is a discharge; because the cervix is dilated, the patient should not have douches or sexual intercourse.

A woman who has aborted may grieve over the lost baby. Her emotional reaction will be governed by many factors; for example, it will make a great difference whether the patient is 20 years old or nearing the end of her childbearing period. She may feel that in some way she has contributed to the abortion, perhaps by thinking of the baby as an additional financial burden or by strenuous exercise or injudicious eating. If she gives any hint of such feelings, the nurse should let her talk them out and inform her that medical science has not found any proof of the idea that exercise, eating, or thoughts can cause abortion. If she seems bitter over losing the baby, the nurse can encourage her to recognize this emotion. She will still be angry, but being listened to will give her some relief. If there is likelihood that the patient can again become pregnant, the physician explains this to her. Although knowledge that she is likely to conceive again does not take away the loss of the fetus, some believe it can help the patient deal with her grief and begin to look forward to becoming pregnant again.

**Criminal Abortion.** This is the illegal termination of pregnancy. The incidence has decreased because of the availability of legal abortion. Women who seek this procedure usually either attempt it themselves by taking large amounts of drugs and thus run the risk of poisoning themselves (this approach almost always fails to empty the uterus), or put themselves in unskilled hands for a crude curettage. There are three outstanding dangers to the latter procedure: rupture of the uterus, infection, and hemorrhage. If the nurse believes a woman is considering a criminal abortion, she should counsel her that legal abortion is available, and help her to consider all the alternatives open to her.

Women who consider abortion may need help thinking through whether or not to continue a pregnancy. The nurse can be helpful both as a listener and as a source of information and referral.

Women interested in therapeutic abortion can be referred to their local office of Planned Parenthood or they can contact a nationwide referral service called Abortion Information Data (AID) Bank, P.O. Box 26462, San Francisco, California. (415-398-6222).

For women who would like to keep their pregnancy but are in need of assistance, other agencies exist. Birthright, the Salvation Army, and the Florence Crittendon League all offer counseling, housing, and obstetric care or referral.

The nurses' association of the American College of Obstetricians and Gynecologists suggests these guidelines for nurses working with patients who have abortion or sterilization. (1) The nurse has the responsibility to discuss with her employer her personal views concerning abortion and sterilization, and the right to expect employers to discuss the agency's policies and practices regarding sterilization and abortion. (2) Nurses have the right to refuse to assist in the performance of abortions or sterilizations, because of their own ethical or religious beliefs, except in emergency situations. (3) It is especially important for the nurse to confront her own feelings honestly concerning abortion and sterilization, so that she does not unwittingly convey punitiveness to patients whose views differ from her own. The patient needs to feel accepted and cared for. Often these women will be very hesitant to express their feelings because of their fear of rejection. Their need for an understanding listener who can help them explore their own views is often particularly important.

## Therapeutic Abortion and Abortion on Demand

With a woman's consent, therapeutic abortion is purposely induced by a physician. Until recently, the procedure could only be done if the life of the mother was threatened by medical complications, if her mental health was threatened, or if the fetus was thought to be radically deformed.

Because of a 1973 Supreme Court decision which made abortion on demand legal in the United States, women now have the opportunity to decide for themselves whether or not to carry a pregnancy to term. Some women feel strongly that they have the right to control over their own bodies and the course of their lives. This view enhances the possibility that every child born will be a wanted child.

State laws vary on the requirements for women to be eligible for abortion. Likewise, religious sects, social groups, and individuals have diverse opinions on the acceptability of abortion on demand. Therefore, the nurse needs to be familiar with the guidelines and attitudes prevalent in her community, as well as her employing agency, and with her own feelings. It is important to recognize that some people believe that the fetus is a developing, individual human person, however immature, with the right to life and protection by society; this view is held as a moral imperative by some persons despite changing legal views.

Following abortion the nurse also has the responsibility for educating or referring patients who want information on the methods available for the prevention of future unwanted pregnancies.

### Techniques of Abortion

**Morning After Pill.** Within the three days following an unprotected intercourse in midmenstrual cycle, a woman may obtain a prescription for 50 mg. of diethylstilbestrol (estrogen) to be taken for five days. This medication affects the uterine lining and makes implantation of the fertilized egg impossible. It may also cause severe nausea.

**Menstrual Extraction.** Prior to the fifth week after conception, a small, flexible tube (called a Karman cannula) can be inserted into an undilated cervix. Attached to the tubing is a syringe that sucks out the fertilized egg and endometrium. In this way, the "missed period" is induced.

**Suction Curettage.** The cervix is dilated to allow insertion of a small tube which is attached to a suction machine. In less than five minutes, the products of conception are pulled from the uterus, causing minimal cramping and bleeding. The procedure is most commonly done under paracervical block in an outpatient clinic for women who are less than twelve weeks pregnant.

**Intraamniotic Injections.** In the hospital, under local anesthesia, saline or prostaglandin solution is injected into the amniotic cavity. Labor usually occurs within 24 hours and the patient, who is 16 to 24 weeks pregnant, delivers the fetus in bed.

**Hysterotomy.** This is a major surgical procedure in which the fetus is delivered through an abdominal incision. It is employed only when a saline abortion has failed or when a patient must be delivered immediately, as in severe sepsis. Future childbirths may have to be by cesarean section.

## Complications of Abortions

Any abortion, whether therapeutic or spontaneous, can be complicated by hemorrhage, infection, and partial retention of the fetal-placental unit. The nurse should be alert to any of the following signs: heavy blood loss, blood clots, foul-smelling discharge, increased temperature and pulse, severe cramping, nausea, and vomiting.

## ECTOPIC PREGNANCY

This term refers to the implantation of the fertilized ovum outside the uterus. The fallopian tubes are the most common ectopic site, but implantation may occur elsewhere, such as in the abdominal cavity. Tubal pregnancies occur about once in every 200 or 300 pregnancies. Any condition, such as salpingitis or congenital anomaly of the tube, that narrows the lumen of the tube or causes blind pockets in it predisposes to implantation of the fertilized ovum in the tube instead of in the uterus. The fetus starts to develop just as it would in the uterus. In most cases the patient has all classic signs of pregnancy. In addition, she may complain of spotting and pain in the lower abdomen.

Because there is so little room for expansion in the tube, the enlarging fetus and the placenta will rupture it. The diagnosis of a tubal pregnancy is rare until rupture occurs. The patient has a sudden, sharp pain, and often is admitted to the hospital in severe shock from hemorrhage. Profuse bleeding occurs both vaginally and into the abdominal cavity. The patient is taken immediately to the operating room, and a salpingectomy is usually performed, although attempts can be made to save the fallopian tube. Because of the rapidity with which the patient can become exsanguinated, the staff, both

surgeons and nurses, have to move quickly. Preparing the patient for the operating room has to be accomplished with speed. Treatment for shock and hemorrhage is instigated immediately. Blood transfusions are given as soon as blood typing and cross-matching are done.

After the operation, careful and frequent observation of vital signs is imperative until they are well stabilized. The nature and the quantity of the vaginal discharge should be noted and perineal care given as long as there is any vaginal discharge. Preoperative bleeding into the abdominal cavity may cause peritonitis postoperatively; therefore abdominal pain, nausea, and vomiting should be reported to the physician. Rupture of a tubal pregnancy is a sudden and shocking event not only for the patient but also for the family. The patient probably will need some time postoperatively to assimilate the experience and to accept the fact that she has lost the baby.

A woman who has had one tubal pregnancy has an increased possibility of having another. However, a normal pregnancy is possible as long as she has one functioning ovary and one patent tube left, and this fact should be pointed out to women who desire to have children.

## PERINEAL PRURITUS

The vulva or perineal area is highly sensitive; vulvitis or vulvar inflammation may arise from many causes.

For obvious reasons there is no worse place to itch than the perineum. This itching may be due to an irritating vaginal discharge and is very common among diabetics due to their increased susceptibility to monilial infections. It may also develop secondary to urinary incontinence, an inflammatory skin disease, or local skin infection, such as moniliasis, scabies, and pediculosis pubis. Allergic reactions to fabric, dye, or "feminine hygiene" products can produce or contribute to the pruritus, which is a symptom, not a specific disease. It is seen in many genital conditions, both in the presence and in the absence of a vaginal discharge.

The treatment is directed at the underlying cause. Ninety per cent of vulvar itches are due to specific infections of trichomonas, monilia, or lice. Obese patients are especially prone to suffer pruritus, because as they walk, skin surfaces rub against each other. In such cases a light dusting with cornstarch may help to decrease the friction. Itching may be severe. If the patient does scratch, the itching will often become even worse. Often applying pressure to the area for about 10 seconds may relieve the intense itching momentarily. Underclothing should be light, nonrestrictive, and made of cotton washed only in mild soaps. It may help to avoid perineal pads, synthetic fabrics, and any harsh soap or perfumes, including vaginal sprays. Loose girdles or pants with long legs keep the skin surfaces separated and are particularly helpful in hot weather. If itching continues after the above measures are tried, the physician may prescribe a hydrocortisone ointment or lotion.

## INFECTIONS

### Vaginitis

The normal acidity of the vaginal secretion at maturity (pH 3.5 to 4.5) is a natural defense against infection. Nevertheless, a variety of pathogenic organisms can invade and infect the vagina—most commonly the protozoon *Trichomonas vaginalis,* the fungus *Candida albicans,* and certain bacterial species.

An abnormal vaginal discharge is a prominent symptom of vaginal infection. It may be copious, malodorous, and is often irritating, causing itching and redness of the perineum and the anus. If the mouth of the urethra is affected, the patient may have urinary symptoms, such as burning on urination and the feeling that she has to void frequently. Also, there may be some discomfort in the lower abdominal region. In contrast with an abnormal discharge, a normal vaginal discharge has little odor and is colorless.

Normal vaginal discharge changes in character and amount during the menstrual cycle, usually becoming more noticeable at ovulation and before menses. It varies from clear to cloudy.

*Trichomonas vaginitis* can cause a thin yellow-brownish, highly irritating leukorrhea, and candida infection can cause a leukorrhea that has the consistency of cottage cheese and itches intensely.

The patient often is treated as an outpatient. Diagnosis of trichomonas vaginitis is made upon microscopic examination of the vaginal secretions. The patient should not douche before the examination, since washing away the secretions will prevent the physician from noting their characteristics and from taking an adequate smear. After determining

the cause of the infection, the physician may swab the infected area with a cleansing solution, using cotton balls on a Kelly clamp. A vaginal jelly or suppository may then be inserted, or tampons may be prescribed to absorb the discharge.

Döderlein's bacillus, by favoring the production of lactic acid, serves to maintain an acid medium as a natural defense mechanism. Trichomonas prefers an alkaline climate. Vinegar douches may be ordered for cleansing and esthetic reasons. The douche is always taken before any medication is instilled, not afterwards. Oral beta lactose may be ordered. Metronidazole (Flagyl), a specific drug for the treatment of trichomonas vaginitis, is taken orally. A treatment course may be ordered for ten days. Diiodohydroxyquin (Floraquin) vaginal tablets may also be prescribed. If a vaginal cream is prescribed, its use is continued throughout the menstrual period, because this is the time when the secretions become more alkaline.

Monilial vaginitis, caused by the fungus *Candida albicans,* is a common infection during pregnancy and after broad spectrum antibiotic treatment (the antibiotics destroy the normal vaginal flora). It also is frequent in diabetics whose urine contains sugar (the monilial fungus is supported by carbohydrates) and is occasionally seen after long-term corticosteroid therapy. A marked increase in the incidence of monilial vaginitis has accompanied the use of oral contraceptives (effect is similar to pregnancy).

Nystatin (Mycostatin), an antibiotic fungicide, may be given orally and in suppositories, one at bedtime for fifteen nights. When the perineum is badly irritated, an antibiotic-antimycotic-corticosteroid (Mycolog) cream may be applied locally. If the patient has diabetes, eliminating glycosuria by controlling the diabetes is an aspect of the treatment. A gentian violet (Gentia-Jel) or gentisic acid (Gentersal) cream may be applied vaginally for two to four weeks. Sodium perborate douches (one teaspoon to a quart of water) may be prescribed.

The physician may wish to examine the sexual partner to determine if he is infected with the same organism. Often the man and woman may continue to reinfect each other. If infection is present or seems to be recurring, the male sexual partner is instructed to use condoms for a few weeks and may also be given oral medication.

In menopausal vaginitis (senile vaginitis) the atrophied vaginal membrane is traumatized by cracking and infection. There is pruritus and some vaginal discharge. Estrogenic preparations may be given to improve the condition of the vaginal mucosa.

If the vaginal smear shows bacteria and pus but no particular causative organism, the resulting infection may be called "nonspecific" vaginitis, although many physicians believe such infections are caused by *Hemophilus vaginalis*. Treatment consists of vinegar douches (one cup vinegar to two quarts of water), nitrofurazone (Furacin) vaginal suppositories and hexetidine (Sterisil) vaginal gel applied every night. Other medications may also be prescribed.

**Teaching a Patient the Aspects of Treatment and Self-Care.** Before the patient leaves for home, be sure that she understands every detail of what she needs to do. In most instances the treatment will be performed by the patient at home. Can she obtain the vaginal suppository if one is ordered? Does she know that she should wash her hands before inserting a vaginal suppository? Does she know that she should be in the dorsal recumbent position, use her longest finger, and aim up and back toward the posterior fornix? Some suppositories and creams come with long applicators that the patient may not know how to insert. She needs to learn how to hold the applicator, to lie down on a bed with her hips elevated on a pillow, how to insert the applicator, and to stay in this position for 10 to 15 minutes when cream or suppository is used so that it will melt and the dissolving medication will cover the vaginal vault. A good way to use a vaginal suppository is to insert it while lying in bed upon retiring. It probably will not dislodge and will melt during the night. The next morning a perineal pad may be worn or a tampon inserted if the pad is irritating to the already infected perineum. When douches form a part of the treatment they are used before the suppository is inserted.

Can the patient fit the prescribed home treatment into her schedule? Does she have any feelings regarding the treatment that will prevent her from carrying it out faithfully? Even in a busy clinic or in a physician's office, the nurse should take the time to sit down with the new patient and go over, step by step, the procedures that she needs to carry out. This should be done in a private nook or a corner, so that she will not feel embarrassed by being overheard by passers-by or patients who are waiting. The nurse may discover at this time that the patient has overused douching in the past. Perhaps she had made it a part of her daily hygiene.

Some authorities feel that such frequent douching removes the normal vaginal flora, alters the pH, and destroys Döderlein's bacillus, thereby establishing an environment receptive to pathogenic invasion.

Vaginitis can be stubborn and discouraging. Vigorous early treatment may overcome its tendency to become chronic. At best, the patient can expect at least six weeks of treatment before she is cured. At worst, vaginitis persists for years, recurring at the very moment when it appears to be cured. Patients with long-term vaginitis are understandably discouraged. They are tired of the malodorous discharge, of wearing perineal pads every day of the month, of going to the physician for treatment.

Attention to an overall health regimen may help to combat the infection. If the patient is not getting enough sleep, perhaps her schedule can be rearranged so that she can. An adequate diet and exercise may help. Personal hygiene may need attention: the importance of perineal cleaning each time she goes to the bathroom, wiping from front to back, and the need for hand washing before and after each perineal pad is changed. Frequent bathing and frequent change of the sanitary napkin or tampon, with perineal care each time, will reduce the odor and irritation.

The treatment may be uncomfortable. For example, a bivalve speculum is often used to provide a greater viewing surface of the vaginal vault and to apply medication. When in place, the speculum is rotated to observe whether all vaginal surfaces are covered with medication. Turning the speculum over the already irritated vaginal mucosa is painful. The patient will need the nurse's support while undergoing this and similar procedures. Later, she will need to know that a perineal pad or tampon is necessary to absorb the draining medication. She may note some bloody discharge (a little less each time she changes the pad) for the next several hours. Inform her that the discharge will be colored by the medication, and will be blood stained due to traumatization of the inflamed vaginal cavity by the procedure. An awareness of what to expect will save the patient some anxious hours. Many patients worry silently, fearful to call the physician to ask whether a discharge is expected.

The nurse should be available if the patient needs someone to talk to about her vaginitis, or if she needs to talk with someone who is not involved in her family life about how to set up a more healthful regimen for herself. A discharge is in itself upsetting, and to many it suggests uncleanliness. An infection of the genital area is often linked with venereal disease, even if it is not venereal. The patient may ask whether or not it is infectious and a hazard to her family; and if it is not a venereal disease, what is it? The patient may ask whether she should use the same toilet seat as the rest of the family. Most infections are not transmitted this way. Of course if some discharge drops on the seat, she would wash it off with soap, water, and some antiseptic cleansing agent.

## Cervicitis

Cervicitis (inflammation of the cervix) may be caused by a number of infectious organisms. Almost all women have a minimal degree of cervicitis after childbirth but this causes no problems. If present, it is usually caused by a mixed flora from the vaginal area. Eventually it may cause a discharge or discomfort when the patient is engaged in intercourse (dyspareunia) or upon menstruation.

Unless acute cervicitis is treated promptly, it has a tendency to become chronic and difficult to cure. Examination of the cervix six weeks after giving birth, in addition to regular gynecologic examination for all women, is important in discovering the condition before it becomes chronic. Inflammation, erosion, and a viscid discharge from the cervical orifice can be seen by the doctor through the vaginal speculum, sometimes before the patient experiences symptoms. That the constant irritation of chronic cervicitis from any cause can lead to cancer is under investigation.

**Treatment and Nursing Care.** Acute cervicitis may be treated with douches and antibiotics locally and systemically. Chronic cervicitis may be treated with electrocautery. The procedure is usually done in the physician's office or in the clinic five to eight days after the end of the menstrual period. The patient is put in lithotomy position, a vaginal speculum inserted, and the cervix painted with an antiseptic. The nurse should be sure that the physician has a good light. He may first take a biopsy for microscopic examination for cancer cells. The eroded tissue is touched with a thin electrical rod, burning strips around the mouth of the cervix, destroying any cysts present. Usually no anesthesia is used, since there is no pain. If the cautery blade is inserted into the cervical canal, there may be a momentary cramping sensation. When performed with anesthesia, a more complete cauterization can be accomplished. Because of its thoroughness, often one treatment is all that is necessary. Without anesthesia a less extensive treatment is performed, making it necessary to repeat the treatment several times, at intervals of approximately six weeks. Sometimes silver nitrate sticks are used instead of the electrocautery.

For a day or two after electrocautery the patient should rest more than usual. No straining or heavy lifting should be undertaken. If slight bleeding occurs, the physician may advise bed rest. Frank bleeding should bring the patient back to the physician. Cervical or vaginal packing, or electric coagulation of the bleeding vessel, may be necessary. The nurse must be sure that the patient knows to expect a gray-green slough (discharge) for about three weeks after cautery. The discharge is watery at first and as the burned tissues become necrotic, the discharge becomes malodorous. Slight bleeding may occur about the eleventh day. The physician will wish to reexamine the cervix two to four weeks later. Dilatation is done if there is cervical stenosis. Sexual relations should not be resumed until adequate healing has occurred. Healing takes six to eight weeks.

Severe chronic cervicitis may be treated by *conization* (removing the diseased portion of the cervical mucosa). The procedure is done with an electric instrument that simultaneously cuts tissue and coagulates the bleeding area. The patient usually is hospitalized, but not always, and anesthesia may or may not be given. The tip of the instrument is placed at the external os and rotated. It penetrates the cervical tissue to the degree required, removing the diseased area. The part that has been enucleated is free of blood because the bleeding vessels have been coagulated. After-care is similar to that following simple cautery. The discharge usually starts about the fourth day, and it is blood-tinged. If a gauze wick is placed in the cervical canal, it usually is removed the next day. Again, the nurse should check for bleeding that may occur when the packing is removed. If the patient is going home, she should be instructed to return to the hospital or the physician if bleeding starts. As with cautery, approximately six to eight weeks are required for healing. The follow-up visits (usually about every two weeks) to the physician are most important, so that he may observe the patency of the cervix. Successful treatment eliminates distressing leukorrhea, may aid fertility, and eliminates constant irritation.

## Puerperal Infection

Puerperal infection is the term given to an infection that follows childbirth. Often due to *E. coli,* the infection often centers in the endometrium, but it may spread anywhere in the pelvic and peritoneal cavities. It can cause generalized sepsis after the organisms enter the bloodstream. Puerperal infection is a grave danger of criminal abortion during which unsterile instruments are used. Retention of bits of placenta after a normal delivery provides a good culture medium for pathogenic organisms. Also, rupture of the membranes several days before delivery, and delivery of a baby under unsterile conditions may lead to puerperal infection. Careful technique to prevent infection is extremely important once the patient's membranes have ruptured. For example, after rupture of the membranes the patient is especially vulnerable to infection that can be transmitted by unsterile instruments or by personnel who have not thoroughly scrubbed their hands.

Puerperal infection is relatively rare today; but in the Vienna Lying-In Hospital in the 1840's, when physicians habitually went from the autopsy room to the obstetric ward without realizing the need for washing their hands, one ward reported 1,989 deaths from the disease in a six-year period. Dr. Ignaz Philip Semmelweiss noticed that the ward handled by midwives, who did not do autopsies, had only 691 deaths from puerperal fever in the same period of time. When he instructed his staff to wash their hands before attending patients, he cut the mortality from childbed fever on his ward to 0! He tried to teach that the simple act of washing the hands could save thousands of lives a year, but in spite of the solid evidence of his statistics, he was laughed at and ignored. He died from septicemia—the very infection that he had campaigned against—brokenhearted, and before the world recognized that he was right.

The patient with a puerperal infection is febrile and, if the endometrium is involved, she will have tenderness in the area and a vaginal discharge. Antibiotics are given to combat the infection. If placental fragments are retained, a D and C is performed. Change of position is encouraged to facilitate pelvic drainage and to help prevent thrombophlebitis in the legs. The patient is usually given a supportive high vitamin diet. Thorough hand washing by the personnel caring for the patient is necessary before and after any procedure in which the genital area is touched. Frequent perineal care and changes of the vaginal pad provide some comfort to the patient and help to prevent the infection from spreading.

## Pelvic Inflammatory Disease (PID)

This is a term that describes an infectious process within the pelvic cavity. The most probable cause is gonococcus although some 10 per cent are due to other organisms.

There may be inflammation of the ovaries (oophoritis) or of the fallopian tubes (salpingitis); pus in the fallopian tubes (pyosalpinx); and inflammation of the pelvic vascular system or of any of the pelvic supporting structures.

Infection may enter these structures through the peritoneum, the pelvic organs, the lymphatics, and the bloodstream.

Symptoms of PID may include a malodorous discharge that is infectious and should be handled with care by both patient and nurse to prevent the disease from spreading. There may be backache, severe or aching abdominal and pelvic pain, a bearing-down feeling, fever, nausea and vomiting, menorrhagia, and dysmenorrhea. Pain may be felt during sexual intercourse or a pelvic examination. Severe infection may cause urinary symptoms or constipation.

The patient with acute pelvic inflammatory disease usually is hospitalized and kept in bed. Often the bed is adjusted to a semisitting position to facilitate pelvic drainage and to help prevent extension of the infection upward. Antibiotics usually are administered, and warm lower abdominal applications may be ordered. Heat improves circulation to the area. Warm sitz baths may be given. The tub should be well scrubbed afterward to prevent the spread of infectious organisms. Douching is usually avoided because there is danger that the infection will be spread by it.

If there is leukorrhea, the perineal pad should be changed frequently. It should be wrapped in paper before discarding it, or the patient should be given bags in which to deposit it. The patient, and any auxiliary personnel who care for her, must wash their hands well after changing the perineal pad. When there is copious discharge, perineal care should be given each time that the pad is changed and after the patient uses the bedpan. When the causative organism is particularly infectious, as in gonorrhea, the patient is placed on isolation precautions, and whoever gives the patient perineal care should wear gloves. Amount, color, odor, and appearance of the discharge should be recorded daily on the nurse's notes. Tampons should not be used, because they may obstruct the flow of discharge. If the infectious process of PID is not treated early, it may localize and form an abscess.

One way of preventing PID is early medical attention for such symptoms of infection in the genital or urinary tracts as a feeling of pressure in the pelvic area, burning on urination, and leukorrhea. Early treatment may prevent the infection from moving up the genital tract. When early treatment of acute pelvic inflammatory disease is delayed or inadequate, the infection may become chronic. The symptoms may come and go. A chronic infection anywhere in the body robs the patient of vigorous health. Often, salpingitis results in sterility, which lasts after the infection is cured. Frequently, the purulent exudate causes the formation of adhesions that block the fallopian tubes.

Antibiotics are given. If the symptoms are not reduced markedly, a total hysterectomy with bilateral salpingo-oophorectomy may be done. In some instances, an ectopic pregnancy may result when a tubal stricture prevents a fertilized ovum from proceeding down the fallopian tube to be implanted in the uterus.

After discharge from the hospital the patient should refrain from sexual intercourse as long as leukorrhea or any other abnormality exists, since intercourse tends to extend the infection and may also result in reinfection from the untreated sexual partner.

## ENDOMETRIOSIS

This is a condition in which tissue that histologically and functionally resembles that of the endometrium is found outside of the uterus—most frequently on the ovaries, commonly elsewhere in the pelvic cavity, and occasionally in the abdominal cavity. Endometrial tissue has been reported even in the thigh and the forearm. The ectopic tissue responds to estrogen, and perhaps also to progesterone, stimulation. It "menstruates," shrivels after menopause, and may regress during pregnancy. Endometriosis is serious, since the tissue bleeds into

spaces that have no outlets. The free blood causes pain and adhesions. During menstruation, dysmenorrhea may be severe and bleeding copious. The fallopian tubes may be occluded, causing sterility. If the endometrial tissue is enclosed in an ovarian cyst (chocolate cyst), there is no outlet for the monthly bleeding.

Other symptoms may occur ranging from menorrhagia, metrorrhagia, dyspareunia, or even pain upon defecation. However, many women will have no symptoms at all. The condition may be discovered accidentally or during an infertility examination. Occasionally the ovarian cyst may rupture, causing the old blood to spill out, generalized peritonitis, and hence an acute abdominal emergency. Culdoscopy is done to confirm diagnosis, and to see if the disease is not so far advanced that conservative treatment would be just a waste of time.

Conservative treatment consists of progesterone (Progestin) to keep the patient in a nonbleeding phase of her menstrual cycle for a prolonged time, such as nine months. Sometimes this therapy controls the ectopic tissue, so that the patient is symptom-free for several years. Small doses of testosterone (5 mg. a day) may relieve the symptoms without making the patient infertile. Synthetic oral progestins prevent ovulation while the patient is taking the hormone, but pregnancy can occur when the drug is discontinued. Large doses are required to prevent breakthrough bleeding. Often physicians prescribe continuous norgestrel (Ovral) or medroxyprogesterone (DepoProvera). Since this is, in effect, a pseudopregnancy, patients taking these birth control pills may experience nausea, vomiting, and diarrhea. Taking the tablets with food may reduce the nausea. Breasts may become tender, and there may be dizziness, weight gain, and stomach cramps. Patients should be taught good leg care (such as not using round garters, not sitting for long periods with legs crossed, and using supportive stockings if there are varicosities), because the estrogen content of the birth control pills may cause thromboembolic phenomena. If the patient notices vaginal bleeding during hormonal therapy, she should notify the physician. The dosage may need to be increased.

Because many women with the diagnosis of endometriosis become infertile, usually they are advised by the physician to complete their families as quickly as possible.

This condition is relieved by menopause: natural,

surgical, or radiologic. However, because it is a disease of women in their child-bearing years, an artificially induced menopause raises many problems. Surgical treatment often is designed to remove the cysts and as much of the ectopic tissue as possible, and to free the adhesions caused by bleeding without destroying the child-bearing function. Endometriosis that is widespread throughout the pelvic organs may necessitate extensive surgery, such as panhysterectomy (removal of the uterus, both fallopian tubes and ovaries). Sterility of course results.

## TUMORS

### Ovarian Cysts and Tumors

Cysts commonly occur on the ovaries. Follicular cysts, caused by retention of fluid, often are symptomless and may disappear. Occasionally, they are needled and aspirated, or they are removed surgically; usually, however, they require no treatment. Luteal cysts form when the corpus luteum fails to regress after the ovum is discharged. These cysts may disturb menstruation. Either type may cause a sensation of heaviness and a dull ache or hemorrhage which is seldom severe; either type may rupture, or twist (when a pedicle is present), and cause lower abdominal pain. If the symptoms necessitate surgery, in most instances the corpus luteum can be removed and the rest of the ovary saved. Dermoid cysts (benign cystic teratomas) may contain such substances as bone, nerves, skin, and hair. It is presumed that dermoid cysts originate from embryonic cells in the ovary at birth.

Oophorectomy may be required if the cyst is twisted, necrotic, or torn. In the operating room, the cysts are opened and examined. The surgeon may send a specimen to the pathologist, who searches for malignancy.

Ovarian tumors may have a masculinizing effect, causing menstruation to cease, hirsutism, atrophy of the breasts, and sterility. Treatment is surgical removal of the tumor; in some instances an oophorectomy, uni- or bilateral, may be required. Sexual changes are gradually reversed after the tumor is excised, to the vast relief of the patient.

A cancerous growth of an ovary may become huge—larger than a full-term fetus—and cause ascites. There may be urinary frequency and urgency, due to pressure on the bladder, and a sense of heaviness in the pelvic region. Sharp pain

results if there is torsion of the pedicle of the tumor. In the late stages, the patient experiences weight loss, severe pain, and gastrointestinal symptoms. Treatment of choice is panhysterectomy followed by a full course of deep x-ray therapy or chemotherapy. In some instances, polyethylene tubes are left in the abdomen postoperatively and chemotherapeutic agents injected through them. If the cancer is detected before it has spread, and the patient wishes to have children, a unilateral oophorectomy may be performed.

Cancer of the ovaries is an extremely dangerous disease because it frequently is unnoticed until it has spread. The best protection is regular gynecologic examination. Because the ovary does not have a direct connection with the fallopian tube, the Pap smear is of less value than in detecting malignancy lower in the reproductive tract.

### Benign Tumors of the Uterus

*Myomas* (fibroids) in the uterine wall are the most common tumor of the female pelvis. The development of these tumors is believed to be stimulated by estrogen. They may be small or large, single or multiple. Growth is usually slow except during pregnancy. Fibroid tumors can occur in various locations in the uterus: subserous, intramural, and submucous. The latter are frequently associated with excessive menstrual bleeding.

Sometimes this benign tumor causes no symptoms, and the woman is unaware of its existence. When there are symptoms, menorrhagia is the most common. Also, the patient may have a feeling of pressure in the pelvic region, dysmenorrhea, anemia (from loss of blood), and malaise. Although multiple myomas are not necessarily incompatible with pregnancy, a disturbance of the childbearing function may be caused mechanically, for example, by fibroids that grow over the openings of the fallopian tubes. Abortion is somewhat more common in women with fibroids than in those without. A large myoma near the cervical canal may complicate the delivery of the baby through the vaginal canal and necessitate cesarean section.

A very large tumor may press on surrounding structures; pressure on the urethra can prevent the free flow of urine, causing retention. The bowel can be squeezed, causing constipation. Pain occurs if the tumor becomes infected or twisted on its pedicle, or if it rests on pelvic nerves. When a tumor is attached to the uterus by a pedicle, torsion of the stem can reduce circulation, so that the tumor becomes necrotic.

The treatment of benign uterine tumors is governed by a number of factors. An asymptomatic tumor in a woman who wishes to have children is usually watched closely by her gynecologist, but it is not treated. The patient is re-examined every three to six months, and a Pap smear taken at least once a year.

Because such tumors usually grow quite slowly, it is often possible for the physician to merely observe and be sure it remains asymptomatic until the natural menopause. It is not uncommon for the tumor to diminish in size after the menopause. If symptoms do occur, a myomectomy or hysterectomy will be done, essentially according to whether the woman wants more children.

When the patient has had abnormal bleeding, she may be admitted to the hospital, and a D and C performed to determine the cause of the bleeding, which may be a coexisting condition, unrelated to the fibroid. Sometimes, a curettage is performed to control the bleeding. Although it does not remove the tumor, it preserves the uterus, and it may make immediate, more extensive surgery unnecessary. Surgical removal of the tumor (myomectomy), which also preserves the uterus, may be performed. These operations are done only when the physician feels sure that the tumor is benign. Further surgery may be required—if possible, after the patient's family is complete. An hysterectomy may be performed when the symptoms are severe and incapacitating. Myomectomy or hysterectomy may be done through either a vaginal or an abdominal approach.

### Cancer

**Cervical Cancer.** The most common malignancy of the female reproductive tract is cancer of the cervix. Only cancer of the breast exceeds it in frequency. There is a relationship between cervical cancer and the Type II herpes virus. This cancer is more prevalent in women who have had a greater number of sex partners. Routine inspection of the cervix, with Pap smears and biopsy of suspicious tissue, is imperative for early diagnosis. When cancer is suspected or diagnosed, the physician may do a Schiller's test in which the cervix is painted with an iodine preparation. Biopsies are taken of all unstained tissues, since cancerous tissues are among those that remain unstained.

Cure is possible if the disease is discovered before it has spread. When the cellular change is still confined to the mucosal layer of the cervix, it is called *carcinoma in situ*. Invasion of surrounding tissue may not occur for five or more years after the preinvasion period. In this early stage there are no symptoms. Even when the cancer has begun to invade the cervix, there still may be no symptoms. Bleeding is the most prominent symptom.

At first, there is spotting, especially after slight trauma, such as douching or intercourse. Later, if the condition is still untreated, the discharge continues, growing bloody and malodorous as the cancerous tissue becomes necrotic. There may be pain, symptoms of pressure on bladder or bowel, and generalized wasting of advanced cancer. Malignancy of the cervix often spreads more quickly than does malignancy of the fundus, making it imperative that the disease be detected early.

If the patient wants children, and the disease is still *in situ*, it may be treated by a cone-shaped amputation of the cervix, leaving the fundus in place for childbearing. Postoperatively the patient is monitored with frequent Pap smears. Usually, however, an hysterectomy is performed if the cancer has not spread. If the cancer is invasive, it is treated by radical surgery, such as hysterectomy with pelvic node dissection and radium inserts, x-ray or radioactive cobalt therapy, or drug perfusion. The average age of women with carcinoma in situ is about 38; of those with invasive cancer, almost 50. When cancer is untreated, the average time between the onset of symptoms and death is less than 21 months. The rate of cure when there is regional involvement is 44 per cent; the potential rate of cure for carcinoma in situ is 98 to 100 per cent. Theoretically, all cancer of the cervix begins in situ. It may take 10 to 15 years to become invasive. Therefore, regular Pap smears are very important for women in their 20's. The means are theoretically available for completely eliminating cancer of the cervix as a cause of death.

**Cancer of the Fundus.** Cancer of the fundus is second only to cancer of the cervix as a site of malignancy of the female genital organs. The relative incidence of cancer of the fundus to cancer of the cervix appears to be growing. Only a small percentage of untreated fibroid tumors become malignant; most carcinoma arises in the endometrium and not in fibroid tumors (myomas). Myomas may coexist with cancer in the same uterus. Carcinoma of the fundus occurs most frequently, and yet not exclusively, in menopausal and postmenopausal women. Bleeding is the earliest and most common symptom. Before the menopause it may appear as menorrhagia. All vaginal bleeding after the menopause must be investigated, as must any unusual bleeding in women before menopause.

When cancer is suspected after a gynecologic examination and a Pap smear, the patient may be admitted to the hospital for a diagnostic curettage. If malignancy is revealed, the treatment is directed at removing the tumor. An hysterectomy may be done; radium, in a rigid applicator or interstitial needles, may be inserted into the uterine cavity, and/or deep x-ray therapy may be given to the pelvis. If the tumor is large, it may be irradiated before surgery to reduce its size. Radiation may follow surgery if metastases are suspected.

This type of cancer occurs most frequently in women past their 50's, who because of other complicating diseases (obesity, hypertension, diabetes) may be poor surgical risks. For example, a patient with a serious cardiac disease may be such a poor surgical risk that she is treated solely by irradiation, although improvements in anesthesia and surgical technique make operation on the poor-risk patient more feasible than it was formerly.

Because of the absence of pain, all too frequently cancer of the uterus is brought to the attention of a physician too late for cure. The patient may not have a family physician, or perhaps she dislikes going to the clinic. She may have noticed a slight watery discharge that has gone away. She would not think of going to a physician about it—unless she knows that it could be serious. It can be.

Death from cancer of the uterus is believed to be largely preventable if frequent examinations of uterine secretions by Pap smears are made, and if patients have regular, thorough pelvic examinations. The greatest reliability of Pap smears is in relation to cancer of the cervix.

People often have difficulty giving sufficient attention to their physical selves because of the heavy demands of other responsibilities on their time, money and energy. The drawn-out suspense of repeated reports of atypical cells is a source of worry, and a woman may find the necessary follow-up both emotionally and physically taxing. A nurse's understanding of the many and varied reasons (such as fear, inertia, lack of money, ignorance, pressure of time, other emotional upsets) why women do not have regular Pap smears is a prerequisite to any educational program encouraging them to do so.

**Cancer of the Vulva.** This is a relatively rare malignancy usually occurring in women past their 60's. Intense pruritus is the most frequent early symptom. Later, there may be pain, tenderness, a slight bloody discharge, enlarged nodules (as the adjacent lymph nodes become involved), ulceration, edema and a visible mass; finally, there is severe pain. As the cancer ulcerates, there may be a bloody, perhaps purulent, discharge from the vulva.

Diagnosis is confirmed by biopsy. Vulvectomy with removal of the inguinal lymph nodes (radical vulvectomy) is the treatment of choice. After five years 60 to 75 per cent of the patients are alive and considered to be cured. The patient usually is very uncomfortable after vulvectomy, and she probably will need frequent administration of analgesics for at least two weeks. Because the urethra is involved in the operation, the patient will return from surgery with a Foley catheter inserted into her bladder. A record should be kept of urinary output. Placing the patient in a semirecumbent position may relieve some of the pressure on the sutures, which will probably be taut. However, she should not remain in one position, even if a comfortable one is found. When she is on her side, the upper leg should be bent and supported with pillows to prevent pull on the operative area. She should do leg exercises frequently—at least once an hour—during the early postoperative period. She should be assisted with passive movements until she can move her legs herself. Straining at stool should be avoided. The patient will be given enemas preoperatively and a low-residue diet postoperatively. After she does have a bowel movement, the nurse should avoid contaminating the wound when cleaning the anal region.

The initial pressure dressing is held in place with a T-binder. After this dressing is removed, the patient is given frequent perineal care (sterile technique, usually). Sterile saline, peroxide, or an antiseptic solution may be ordered for cleaning the surgical area. If drains are inserted, they should not be disturbed; drainage from them should be noted and recorded. Heat-lamp treatments are used to dry the area after perineal care and also to improve circulation, thus promoting healing. After the sutures have been removed, warm sitz baths may be given. Also, these may help the patient to urinate after the Foley catheter has been removed. She should be assured privacy during perineal care, heat-lamp treatments, and sitz baths.

The groin wounds may be exposed to the air. The appearance of the area may be shocking to the patient. The nurse should not allow her facial expression to change when she sees the wounds, since the patient will be watching her reaction. Wounds will heal slowly in the older patient because of the extensive surgery. The slow healing, the pain, and the mutilation of surgery often are especially distressing to the patient. It is a long hospitalization, a time filled with pain and worry—a long interruption in the patient's life. At discharge, it still is not over; the patient is often weak and worn, and an extensive period of convalescence is required.

When cancer of the vulva is inoperable, wet dressings and perineal irrigations with a deodorizing solution may help to control the odor and infection that so often occurs in the ulcerating neoplasm.

## General Nursing Care of Patients With Gynecologic Tumors

Because gynecologic tumors can be a threat both to life and reproductive power, the patient should receive as much emotional support as possible from the nurse. It is helpful to the patient if the same nurse cares for her consistently, so that rapport is established and the patient will feel free to discuss her thoughts. The desire for children, the fear of returning to the physician for observation of a fibroid, the fear of cancer, the dread of mutilation, and of the loss of femininity are emotions that lie deep. Sterility, resulting from some gynecologic surgery and usually from gynecologic irradiation, often requires severe adjustments by the patient. Postoperative tearfulness, which is fairly predictable, may be based on hormonal changes as well as a feeling of depression. If it seems helpful, discuss the patient's reactions with the family, so that they, too, can support her while she makes her difficult adjustment. Lend an empathic ear to the husband, since his wife's condition has a special meaning to him as well. Perhaps you can help him to help her.

Preoperative preparation may include vaginal suppositories and catheterization to minimize the chance of damaging the bladder (or, perhaps the order will read to make sure that the patient voids). She is usually given an enema. The peri-neal preparation of the skin usually is done with the patient first in the lithotomy position and then in Sims's position to shave the anal region.

An hysterectomy or the removal of a large tumor causes sudden shifts in body spaces, and distention is a frequent and uncomfortable complication. A heating pad and a rectal tube may be ordered, and the patient usually is kept on a light diet until peristalsis is reestablished. An enema may be ordered about the third postoperative day.

A patient with a vaginal hysterectomy will wear perineal pads. In some hospitals, sterile pads are used. These pads should be changed frequently, and the patient should have a T-binder or sanitary belt to hold them in place. There will be some serosanguinous drainage, particularly if a radical operation was done. The patient should have frequent perineal care, including after each use of the bedpan. The ambulatory patient who gives herself perineal care still needs the nurse to observe the operative area at least once every eight hours. The nurse should watch for hemorrhage. With both a vaginal and an abdominal hysterectomy, there should be no more bleeding than is seen in a normal menstrual period. Check the perineal pad every 10 to 15 minutes during the first few postoperative hours, and then every hour for the rest of the day. There will be a moderate to a slight amount of drainage for the first one or two days, and some spotting for about two weeks. Frank bleeding is not expected. Bleeding may, of course, be internal; thus, observation of vital signs is essential.

Patients who have had perineal surgery may have discomfort from perineal stitches. Heat in the form of a lamp, sitz baths, or warm perineal irrigations may be ordered.

Inability to void is a frequent postoperative complaint because the urinary tract is in the operative area. There may be edema, inflammation, and loss of muscle tone of bladder and urethra. A Foley catheter usually is inserted preoperatively, and removed on about the fourth postoperative day. After it is removed, the patient is often catheterized immediately after each spontaneous voiding to note the amount of residual urine, until there is no more residual than 50 to 80 ml. The nurse should note and record the first few times the patient voids spontaneously. Is the amount adequate? Is it bloody? (Occasionally, surgical injury to the ureter or the bladder occurs during gynecologic surgery.)

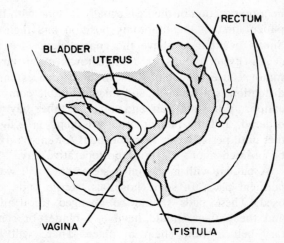

**Figure 52-5.** A fistula between bladder and vagina (vesicovaginal fistula).

Decreased urinary output and a low backache may indicate that a ureter has been ligated. Also, a large tumor of the uterus can exert such pressure on the urinary system that there is a backflow of urine, resulting in hydronephrosis. A poorly functioning kidney often does not withstand the shock of surgery well.

Thrombophlebitis is a common complication of hysterectomy. The surgery itself, or the position of the patient during surgery (the lithotomy position is used for vaginal hysterectomy) may interfere with circulation. Frequent turning and active exercises of the legs are in order. To avoid the pooling of blood in the pelvis and pressure on leg veins, the nurse should help the patient to exercise. Elastic stockings are often used postoperatively to help prevent venous stasis. The knee gatch should not be raised. The patient should lie flat for short periods during the day. She probably will be out of bed, with help, the day after surgery.

Occasionally, a patient will have the entire contents of her pelvis removed (*pelvic exenteration*). This operation includes a panhysterectomy, a cystectomy, removal of the rectum, and an abdominal-perineal resection. A colostomy is done and the ureters are transplanted into the skin or into the ileum. Both the physical and the emotional trauma resulting from this extensive surgery can well be imagined, considering the radical alterations in physiology and the extensive adjustments in activities of everyday living. If the patient is not already past the menopause, she will have surgical menopause. Because of the severity of the operation,

water and electrolyte regulation will be upset. After vaginectomy the patient will be unable to have sexual intercourse, unless there is sufficient remaining vagina to permit it. Weakness and fatigue will be all-consuming for some time after surgery. In addition, the patient has to adjust physically and emotionally to both a colostomy and a ureterostomy.

On returning home after any kind of gynecologic surgery, the patient should know that heavy lifting, straining, or active sport should not be undertaken for several months. Swimming is usually permitted, but horseback riding is not. Any constrictive clothing, such as a panty girdle, which binds in the area of the groin, should not be worn.

The surgeon will advise when the patient may resume driving a car and climbing stairs. An aspect of discharge planning involves assisting the patient to obtain answers to specific questions concerning activities she may undertake when she goes home.

## VAGINAL FISTULAS

A fistula complicating cancer of the pelvis is not uncommon (Fig. 52-5). The opening may be between a ureter and the vagina (*ureterovaginal* fistula); between the bladder and the vagina (*vesicovaginal* fistula); or between the rectum and the vagina (*rectovaginal* fistula). Fistulas may be congenital or a result of obstetric or surgical injury, but the most frequent cause in adults is a breakdown of tissue due to cancer or irradiation.

A large fistula causes the patient endless distress. An opening between the urinary tract and the vagina means that there is continuous leakage of urine from the vagina. The vaginal wall and the external genitalia become excoriated, and often they become infected. The patient may not void at all through the urethra, since there may be no accumulation of urine in the bladder. As soon as this fistula develops, the patient is given urinary antiseptics and acidifying agents to prevent infections. Since tampons or sanitary napkins usually are not adequate for controlling wetness, the Tassette menstrual cup of appropriate size can be inserted into the vagina as a collecting vehicle. This keeps patient dry, comfortable, and ambulatory. The urine collects in the cup and drains down an attached tubing. The nurse must teach the patient to remove and clean the cup daily before reinserting it.

Rectovaginal fistulas cause fecal incontinence

and discharge of flatus through the vagina. The feces added to the leukorrhea already present, or initiated by the passage of stool over the vaginal mucosa, are so distressingly odorous that the patient quietly withdraws from social contacts. Frequently, the tissues are in such poor condition that surgical repair is not possible.

## Treatment and Nursing Care

Surgery is performed under only as close to optimum conditions as possible: when inflammation and edema have disappeared. This may mean months of waiting. Unfortunately, surgery for a rectovaginal fistula is frequently unsuccessful.

When operation is done for a rectovaginal fistula, both preoperatively and postoperatively the patient is placed on sulfasuxidine or sulfaguanidine to clean the bowel of colon bacilli. She is given a light, low-residue diet preoperatively, to keep the stool soft, and an enema and a cleansing vaginal irrigation the morning of surgery. Postoperatively, the patient may be kept on clear fluids for several days to inhibit bowel activity, and then she may be graduated first to a light, low-residue diet and then to a general diet. Paregoric may be given to constipate the patient during the early postoperative period. The genitalia must be kept clean. Warm perineal irrigations and perineal heat-lamp treatments may be ordered to promote healing and to lessen discomfort. Because patients with vaginal fistulas often are debilitated, they need attention to overall health measures, such as an adequate diet, fluids, and rest.

After repair of a vesicovaginal fistula, a Foley catheter will be inserted. Its drainage should be carefully noted. If the tube becomes blocked and the bladder is allowed to fill, the pressure may break down the surgical repair and cause the fistula to reappear. If irrigations are ordered, they should be done very gently so that no pressure is applied to the suture line. Vaginal serosanguinous drainage is expected. The absence of urine in the vagina indicates the fistula is healing. If douches are ordered, pressure should be kept to a minimum.

When the fistula cannot be repaired, as in advanced cancer, frequent sitz baths and deodorizing douches help to control infection and odor and to make the patient feel cleaner. A perineal pad or rubber pants will be needed. Before she joins a social gathering, a woman with a rectovaginal fistula may give herself a low, gentle cleansing enema. If the enema is to be effective, the tube must be inserted above the point of the fistula, and directed away from the opening.

The patient with a fistula usually is discouraged and uncomfortable. It is difficult for her to feel clean. She is always wet with urine, which perhaps is mixed with feces. Not only does she feel the opposite of fastidious, but her skin becomes raw and irritated. There is a constant odor about her. Sexual relations are hindered. How can she comfortably sit at the breakfast table with her family? How can she ride in a car with others or invite a friend in for a chat and be relaxed? The patient may feel too embarrassed to be with people and withdraws.

Although the problems remain serious as long as the patient has the fistula, certain measures may help to make her more comfortable. She may wear an absorbent material, such as a perineal pad. Frequent changes of the pad and sitz baths help to reduce odors and lessen skin irritation. Wearing a liner next to her skin helps to keep the urine off the skin. Some patients are soothed by a light dusting of cornstarch. Waterproof underpants are sometimes worn to protect clothing and furniture.

## RELAXED PELVIC MUSCLES

When the muscles and fascia that support a structure relax, that structure sags. After unrepaired postpartum tears, childbirth, multiple births, or sometimes from a slight congenital weakness, the floor of the pelvis relaxes, and the uterus, rectum, or bladder may herniate downward. Bulging of the bladder into the vagina is called a *cystocele*, the most common type of poor pelvic support. Herniation of the rectum into the vagina is called a *rectocele*. Downward displacement of the uterus is called *prolapse*. A cystocele and a rectocele usually accompany uterine prolapse. The presence of the uterus low in the vaginal vault is spoken of as a *first-degree prolapse*; a *second-degree prolapse* is the extension of the cervix beyond the vaginal os; and when the entire uterus hangs outside the body, a *third-degree* or *complete prolapse* (procidentia uteri) is present. The improved obstetric care now available to many women before, during, and after delivery has greatly reduced the incidence of postpartum pelvic relaxation due to childbirth.

Kegal exercises are taught routinely to women both before and after childbirth, and to any woman experiencing relaxation of pelvic muscles. These have been found to be effective in reducing the incidence of pelvic support muscle relaxation. These exercises also achieve control in mild cases. Essentially, Kegal exercises consist of tightening all pelvic floor muscles about ten times or so each time the woman voids. She may also be taught to stop the flow of urine momentarily.

Symptoms may include backache, pelvic pain, fatigue, and a feeling that "something is dropping out," especially when lifting a heavy object, coughing, or with prolonged standing. A cystocele may cause difficulty in emptying the bladder, resulting in stagnation of urine and possible cystitis. There may be stress incontinence: a little urine seeps out every time that the woman coughs, bears down, or strains. A rectocele can cause difficulty in evacuation; constipation can result. In some instances, the patient may need to put her finger into her vagina and apply pressure to the posterior vaginal wall to reduce the herniation before she is able to evacuate the stool collected in the pocket.

In severe prolapse the tissue that protrudes below the vaginal orifice is subject to irritation from clothing or rubbing against the thighs in walking. This is especially seen in second- and third-degree prolapse. Ulceration and infection frequently follow. These symptoms are annoying and they may be incapacitating. They may forbid standing for a long time, walking with ease, or lifting and other activities that are difficult to avoid. Stress incontinence requires the continuous use of perineal pads. The activities of a housewife, for example, are markedly curtailed when she cannot stand for any length of time, cannot lift, and climbing stairs is a torture. Nevertheless, some women are reluctant to seek medical help because of excessive modesty, expense, or fear of surgery.

### Treatment and Nursing Care

The surgical repair of a cystocele is called *anterior colporrhaphy*. Repair of a rectocele is called *posterior colporrhaphy*. Repair of the tears (usually old obstetric tears) of the perineal floor is called *perineorrhaphy*. The operations are done vaginally. A vaginal hysterectomy may be done to remove a completely prolapsed uterus.

Patients may be admitted to the hospital several days before surgery.

The patient may be kept on bed-rest for one or two days before surgery to decrease any edema of the area. The bed should not be placed in a high sitting position, which would increase congestion to the pelvic region. Before posterior colporrhaphy, an enema is given to empty the bowel.

Postoperatively, perineal dressings are not commonly used; rather, perineal care is given several times a day and always after the patient has urinated or defecated. A heat lamp is sometimes ordered to dry the area and to promote healing. Every effort is made to prevent pelvic pressure and stress on the suture line. An ice pack may be ordered to relieve edema and pain, and this should be placed so that the weight of the pack lies on the bed and not on the patient. Sitz baths may be given. About the third or fourth postoperative day, the patient may be given a suppository or a cathartic. She is instructed not to strain when having a bowel movement. When the patient does her own perineal care, the nurse should inspect the area daily. She observes for redness, edema, and whether or not the Foley catheter is in position.

After an anterior colporrhaphy, a Foley catheter usually is inserted to keep the bladder empty, since overdistention could weaken the repair. The Foley catheter often is attached to straight drainage, while the patient is in bed. When she is ambulatory, the nurse should find out whether the catheter is to be clamped or whether straight drainage is to be continued. Clamping may be ordered to allow the bladder to fill to increase its muscle tone. However, it should be released every four hours to prevent overdistention. If the patient does this herself, the nurse should check it.

After the catheter is removed (two to seven days postoperatively), the nurse should observe for adequate voiding. The patient should urinate every four hours, but she may have frequency without adequately emptying the bladder. Catheterization for residual urine may be ordered. Urinary output should be measured for the first day or two. If the patient is consistently voiding only 50 ml. at a time, the physician should be informed. If the patient is ambulatory, a basin is placed under the toilet seat, to collect the urine so that it can be measured. This arrangement is also useful in helping the patient to assume a natural position, if voiding into a bedpan in bed is difficult. Fluids should be encouraged, especially if the patient has cystitis or a Foley catheter. The patient who has frequency may voluntarily restrict fluids, and she should be told to force them instead.

Urinary problems after an anterior colporrhaphy can be especially distressing. For example, two patients who had had cystoceles repaired had their Foley catheters removed on the same day. One patient voided adequately and went home several days later. The other patient could not void, became frightened, said that she felt that she would never urinate again, and had to have the Foley catheter reinserted. The physician promised her that she could go home as soon as she could void. Eventually she did both, but her discharge from the hospital had been delayed for almost a week. In addition, the stress incontinence may require that the ligaments about the neck of the bladder be shortened through a suprapubic incision.

Because these conditions are most frequently found in older women, sometimes there are complicating diseases that make surgery too great a risk to be undertaken. Under such circumstances the displacement may be reduced by inserting a pessary, which repositions the uterus (Fig. 52-6). The pessary should be kept as clean as possible to avoid infection. A sterile lubricant should be applied to it before it is inserted. Once the pessary is in place, the patient should feel nothing. Discomfort may indicate that it is placed incorrectly or is causing irritation. The appearance of leukorrhea may indicate an infection, in which case the patient should see the physician immediately. The pessary usually is kept in place for six weeks at a time. The patient should return to the physician one week after it is inserted and then about every two months. If the pelvic floor is very relaxed, and there is danger the pessary may fall out, a string may be attached to it and pinned to the clothing. Hard rubber or plastic pessaries have less tendency to become soggy than soft rubber ones. Assuming the knee-chest position for a few minutes once or twice a day helps to keep the genital organs and the pessary in good position. Modern surgical techniques, and concern over the possible harmful effects of chronic irritation from the pessary, have limited their usefulness.

Pelvic relaxation develops over the years. It is not uncommon for a woman to tolerate the increasing discomfort until a more "convenient" time for surgery. She may wait until complications are well developed. All nurses, and particularly those in public health and industry, are in a position to urge early medical attention before complications become severe and the condition is incapacitating.

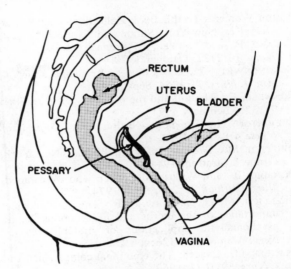

**Figure 52-6.** Ring pessary in place.

## UTERINE DISPLACEMENT

In some women the position of the uterus is abnormal. Displacement usually is congenital; sometimes backward displacement is due to childbearing. *Anteflexion* is the term given to a uterus that is bent forward at an acute angle. In *retroversion* the uterus tilts backward. In *retroflexion* the fundus is bent backward on the cervix (the opposite of anteflexion).

Displacement may be asymptomatic or it may cause backache, sterility, or other problems. The condition usually requires no treatment, since it is usually asymptomatic. Occasionally use of a pessary or surgical uterine suspension may be required.

## SUMMARY

The woman with a gynecologic problem may or may not be physically seriously ill. She always has many feelings and stresses due to the strong feelings women have about their sexual organs. The gynecologic nurse must not only give excellent physical care, but she must allow the woman to focus most of her energy on dealing with the emotions aroused by her illness.

## REFERENCES AND BIBLIOGRAPHY

AVERY, W., et al.: Vulvectomy, *Am. J. Nurs.* 74:453, March 1974.
BENSON, R. C.: *Handbook of Obstetrics and Gynecology,* Los Altos, Lange Medical Publications, 1971.

Boston Women's Health Book Collective: *Our Bodies, Ourselves,* New York, Simon and Schuster, 1973.

CELANO, P., and SAWYER, J.: Vaginal fistulas, *Am. J. Nurs.* 70:2131, October 1970.

CHRONENWETT, L., and CHOYCE, J.: Saline abortion, *Am. J. Nurs.* 71:1754, September 1971.

CONNELL, E.: The pill and the problems, *Am. J. Nurs.* 71:325, February 1971.

CREIGHTON, H.: The new abortion ruling, *Supervisor Nurse* 4:8, July 1973.

DEUTSCH, M.: *The Psychology of Women,* New York, Grune & Stratton, 1944.

DONADIO, B., and WHITE, M.: Seven who were raped, *Nurs. Outlook* 22:245, April 1974.

DRELLICH, M. G., and IRVING, B.: The psychological importance of the uterus and its functions: Some psychoanalytic implications of hysterectomy, *J. Nerv. Mental Dis.* 126:4, 1958.

FRANCES, G.: Cancer: The emotional component, *Am. J. Nurs.* 69:1677, 1969.

GREEN, T. H.: *Gynecology,* Boston, Little, Brown, 1971.

GONZALES, BETTY: Voluntary sterilization, *Am. J. Nurs.* 70:12 (Dec. 1970) 2581-2583.

GUTTMACHER, A. F.: Family planning: The needs and the methods, *Am. J. Nurs.* 69:1229, June 1969.

HELLMAN, L., and PRITCHARD, J.: *Williams Obstetrics,* New York, Appleton-Century-Crofts, 1971.

ISENMAN, A., et al.: *Seminar in Family Planning,* Chicago, The American College of Obstetricians and Gynecologists, 1972.

JANIS, I.: *Psychological Stress,* New York, Wiley, 1958.

KELLER, C., and COPELAND, P.: Counseling the abortion patient is more than talk, *Am. J. Nurs.* 72:102, January 1972.

KISTNER, R.: The infertile woman, *Am. J. Nurs.* 73:1937, November 1973.

LEROUS, R., et al.: Abortion, *Am. J. Nurs.* 70:1919, September 1970.

LORD, E.: My crisis with cancer, *Am. J. Nurs.* 74:647, April 1974.

MANISOFF, M.: Intrauterine devices, *Am. J. Nurs.* 73:1188, June 1973.

MASTERS, W. H., and JOHNSON, V. E.: *Human Sexual Inadequacy,* Boston, Little, Brown, 1970.

————: *Human Sexual Response,* Boston, Little, Brown, 1966.

MATHIS, J. L.: The emotional impact of surgical sterilization on the female, *J. Okla. State Med. Assoc.* 62:141, 1969.

MCBRIDE, A. B.: *The Growth and Development of Mothers,* New York, Harper and Row, 1973.

OB/Gyn nurse group takes stand on abortion, *Am. J. Nurs.* 72:1311, July 1972.

SIEGLER, A.: Tubal sterilization, *Am. J. Nurs.* 72:1624, September 1972.

SORKA, C.: Gynecologic cytology, *Am. J. Nurs.* 73:2092, December 1973.

STEPHENS, G.: Mind-body continuum in human sexuality, *Am. J. Nurs.* 70:1468, 1970.

WEISS, S. M.: Psychosomatic aspects of symptom patterns among major surgery patients, *J. Psychosom. Res.* 13:109, 1969.

WILLIAMS, C., and WILLIAMS, R.: Rape: A plea for help in the hospital emergency room, *Nurs. Forum* 12:388, 1973.

# The Male Patient with a Disorder of the Genitourinary System

## CHAPTER 53

Anatomy and Physiology

Nursing Assessment

Prostatic Obstruction

Disorders of the Testes and
Their Adjacent Structures

Infertility

Embarrassment, fears of impotence, and feelings of loss of manly self-esteem frequently make a disorder of a reproductive organ hard for the patient to bear. It is important for the nurse to realize that although the patient may more readily discuss his concerns with a knowledgable man, for example the physician, the nurse should show a willingness to listen to the patient. (Sometimes the firm belief that the patient does not wish to discuss these concerns with the nurse has more to do with her discomfort over the topic rather than with the patient's reluctance to discuss it.) The nurse who plans to work in urology may need to obtain special preparation to become skilled in the sexual aspects of the counseling role of the nurse (see Bibliography).

If the patient appears worried about his illness or an impending operation, the prepared nurse can let him know that his fears are neither strange nor unexpected, and that he may discuss any matters that he wishes. If the patient seems unduly shy or hesitant, the nurse might mention her observations to the physician so he may open the subject with the patient. In addition she herself should spend time and show concern for the patient. The patient himself decides how he wishes to proceed.

## ANATOMY AND PHYSIOLOGY

The male lower urinary tract and reproductive system are so closely associated that disorders in this area frequently affect both systems. This is in contrast to the female where, although close together, these sys-

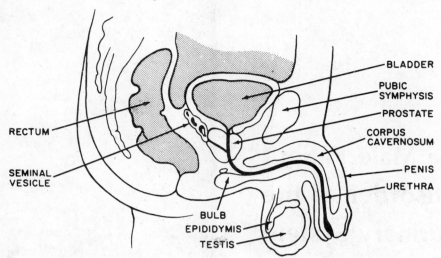

RECTUM

SEMINAL
VESICLE

BULB
EPIDIDYMIS
TESTIS

BLADDER
PUBIC
SYMPHYSIS
PROSTATE
CORPUS
CAVERNOSUM
PENIS
URETHRA

**Figure 53-1.** Male genito-urinary tract.

tems are somewhat more separate. The male genital system consists of the testes which produce sperm, and the epididymidis and vas deferens, which deliver the sperm to the prostate and seminal vesicles. The bladder urine and seminal fluid are both discharged, although separately, to the outside through the urethra, which traverses the penis. (Fig. 53-1).

## NURSING ASSESSMENT

The nursing history should include questions relative to planning nursing care. The patient should be told how sharing such information is necessary for his care. The urinary pattern and habits are elicited, including frequency, "dribbling" (retention with overflow), dysuria, polyuria, oliguria, urgency, hesitation, nocturia, hematuria, pyuria urethral discharge, incontinence, aids to elimination, or urinary diversion. Further significant aspects of the patient's medical history may include sexual problems, stone formation, testicular pain or swelling, and venereal disease.

Signs of bladder distention include swelling of the abdomen; a tense highly sensitive area can be determined on palpation. A "kettle-drum" sound is elicited when the swollen area is percussed.

The urine should be observed for amount, color, degree of opacity, odor, sedimentation, mucus, clots or shreds of material, or other unusual constituents.

A complete individual nursing assessment is essential. Since most of these patients are in the older age group and are prone to other conditions, such as pulmonary, metabolic, or cardiovascular disorders, a complete medical evaluation is usually planned by the physician.

## PROSTATIC OBSTRUCTION

### Benign Prostatic Hypertrophy

The prostate gland is an accessory sex organ that produces most of the seminal fluid. This fluid contains zinc, invert sugars, and other substances necessary for the nutrition of sperm.

The prostate is located just below the urinary bladder. The urinary stream travels through the center of the gland in the prostatic urethra. With advancing age and seemingly under the influence of male sex hormones, the periurethral glandular tissue undergoes hyperplasia, with gradual enlargement of the gland. This outward expansion is not of any clinical importance. However, inward encroachment of this tissue, which diminishes the diameter of the prostatic urethra, certainly is.

Benign prostatic hypertrophy is so common among elderly men that they half-anxiously and half-jokingly regard the onset of symptoms as a sign of old age. Not all men who acquire benign prostatic hypertrophy require surgery. An enlarged prostate may be discovered during a physical examination and the patient may then be referred to a urologist.

Symptoms of "prostate trouble" are all secondary to an increasing impediment to urinary flow and appear gradually. At first the patient may notice that it takes more effort to void and there is decreasing force and narrowing of the urinary stream. As the residual urine remaining in his bladder accumulates, the bladder fills more quickly, and the patient finds that he has the urge to void more and more frequently. Urgency, to the point of incontinence, is common. At night he awakens for trips to the bathroom. There may be difficulty in starting the stream, and hematuria when it does start. Residual urine is a good culture medium for bacteria, and if infection results, symptoms of cystitis also will be present. The combination of hesitancy, narrowed stream, straining to void, frequency, urgency, and nocturia is known as prostatism. Any obstruction in the lower urinary tract can cause these symptoms, but the most common is prostatic enlargement.

### Diagnostic Assessment

Diagnostic tests include a rectal examination, catheterization for residual urine, cystoscopic examination, and pyelography. A digital examination through the rectum is an important part of the urologist's diagnostic workup. The prostate gland and seminal vesicles can be palpated in this way.

Before the examination the patient empties his bladder. He is placed in the knee-chest position or the examination can be performed with the patient bending over the table. The patient can be told that if he relaxes his perineal muscles and takes slow deep breaths, the examination will be less uncomfortable and over more quickly. The woman nurse rarely stays during the examination—her presence would embarrass many patients. A rubber glove or a fingercot and lubricating jelly is used for the examination. If the patient has prostatic hypertrophy, the examiner will feel the gland to be enlarged and elastic. Cystoscopy will reveal the extent of the infringement on the urethra and the effects on the bladder. Pyelography will give information about the possible damage to the upper urinary tract due to the backup of urine. Blood chemistry tests are done to reveal kidney malfunction. Measurement of significant quantities of residual urine (usually at least 60 ml.) adds to the data confirming the diagnosis.

The nurse assists the patient by explaining diagnostic procedures and their preparation to him, by providing for privacy during examinations, rest afterwards if indicated, and by participating in the diagnostic assessment when prepared to do so.

### Treatment, Nursing Assessment, and Intervention

Decompensated benign prostatic hypertrophy is treated by surgically removing the obstruction. This involves removing part of the prostate gland. Unless the patient has marked symptoms or is totally unable to void, a urethral catheter is not inserted preoperatively. The history will tell whether the patient has had an acute episode of retaining his urine, or whether he has been building up larger and larger residual amounts over a long period of time. If the patient has gone into sudden acute retention, a urethral catheter is inserted and connected to straight drainage. If, on the other hand, the history suggests a gradual worsening of chronic retention, a rapid complete emptying of the bladder may have dire consequences. These include profound hematuria due to rupture of numerous stretched mucosal blood vessels and postobstructive diuresis. In a chronically obstructed patient, the sudden, complete relief of obstruction by means of a catheter may be followed by marked diuresis with loss of large amounts of sodium in the urine. If unnoticed and unreplaced, the salt and water loss may be serious enough to cause the patient to go into shock.

Consequently, if the retention is chronic, the bladder is decompressed slowly (over a period of hours) to avoid the bleeding that sometimes accompanies rapid withdrawal of urine from a bladder that has been chronically distended. Decompression drainage causes the bladder to empty gradually and also helps to maintain bladder tone, because the urine, with free flow maintained through the catheter, must be pushed uphill. As shown in Fig. 53-2, the top end of the Y-tube is left open to the air as a safety vent, should intravesical pressure (pressure in the bladder) become too high. The apex of the Y-tube is placed 6 to 8 inches above the level of the pubis. The Y is gradually lowered 1 inch an hour until it is at bladder level. Eventually it is replaced by straight drainage. The two most important precautions are to ascertain that the entire tubular passageway from the patient to the bottle is patent, and that the level of the Y-tube is as ordered.

**Preoperative Period.** During the preoperative period, the patient is put on a healthful regimen, with emphasis on copious fluids (unless medically contraindicated), a good diet, and rest periods. Other illnesses are treated, such as regulation of diabetes and digitalization for heart failure. Although

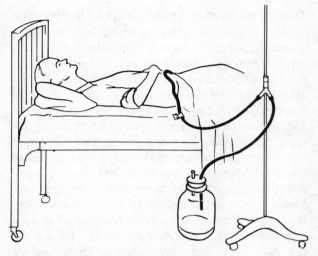

**Figure 53-2.** Decompression drainage. In this instance the Y-tube is placed at the level of the patient's body. There are two airways in the system: the top of the Y-tube and the glass tube in the collection bottle. The tubing is pinned to the bed.

an indwelling catheter will induce and continue urinary infection simply by its presence, most physicians believe that the advantages of adequate urinary drainage for the symptomatic patient usually outweigh the disadvantages of any infection induced.

If catheter drainage is not provided, the patient is taught to measure his urine, and keep a record of the time and amount that he voids. Each day's intake and output is recorded on his chart. An abnormal pattern that will be fairly consistent from day to day for this patient may be evident.

If during the preoperative evaluation period significant damage to the upper urinary tract is found, the urologist may perform a suprapubic cystostomy (a small suprapubic incision into the bladder through which a catheter is inserted). This type of urinary drainage bypasses the prostate until renal function recovers adequately and a definitive operation on the prostate can be performed safely. A suprapubic catheter for long-term drainage prevents epididymitis and other serious infections associated with prolonged use of a urethral catheter. The patient may be sent home with this drainage for several months. He and a family member need instruction in the care of the catheter and skin before he is discharged from the hospital.

### Types of Surgery

As benign prostatic hypertrophy develops, the hyperplasia of the periurethral glands forms an adenoma, which comprises the bulk of the prostate. The adenoma thins and compresses the surrounding true capsule of the gland. Between the adenoma and capsule there is a plane of cleavage that can be developed easily by the surgeon. The aim of all surgical procedures for benign prostatic hypertrophy is to remove the adenoma, leaving the true capsule behind. Subsequently, the patient urinates through this fossa. Healing, by re-epithelialization, occurs over a two- to three-month period. At open operations (retropubic, perineal, or suprapubic prostatectomy), the surgeon develops the cleavage plane between the adenoma and capsule either by finger or sharp dissection. The adenoma is removed along with the mucosa of the prostatic urethra. The transurethral method accomplishes the same objective, except that the adenoma is removed, piece by piece, through an instrument inserted through the urethra.

The surgeon's preference, his experience with various techniques, the general condition, and in-

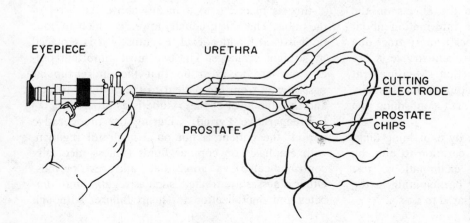

**Figure 53-3.** A transurethral prostatectomy in progress. The prostatic chips will be washed away in the periodic irrigations during the surgery.

formed consent of the patient play a part in the type of operation performed. An open operation is generally performed for large adenomas (50 Gm. or larger). If the patient is very obese, the transurethral or perineal approach rather than an abdominal one may be selected. A patient may become discouraged if he observes another patient who entered at the same time with the same complaints going home one week after a transurethral resection. Such a patient can be helped to understand that the transurethral approach would not have been the best procedure for him, and that results, even with the same operation, differ from patient to patient.

## Transurethral Prostatectomy
## (Transurethral Resection: TUR)

Using a modification of the straight panendoscopes described in Chapter 48, the surgeon removes slivers of prostatic adenoma until he has resected down to the inner aspect of the prostatic capsule throughout the gland. The instrument utilizes one of various models of "working units" which incorporate a wire electrode directed through the tissue under visual control. By utilizing currents produced by an electrosurgical generator, the surgeon can cut tissue or fulgurate bleeding points by selecting his currents with a double pedal foot switch. During the procedure irrigating solution constantly enters the bladder through the instrument to wash away blood and debris. Since electrical current is involved, the solution must be nonelectrolyte in order not to disperse the electricity. (Otherwise, the current would not be directed to the area of electrode contact.) The fluid is also isotonic with body fluid to avoid hemolytic reactions in the blood, should too much of this liquid be resorbed into the circulation from the operative site. The solutions are prewarmed to body temperature to avoid hypothermic reactions. As the bladder becomes full, the surgeon removes the inner working unit and empties the bladder of solution and tissue chips. This process is repeated many times during the operation until the resection is completed (Fig. 53-3).

Another transurethral method is the "cold punch" technique. The instrument contains a tubular knife, which is manipulated to cut off pieces of tissue directed into the opening of the sheath. Hemostatis is accomplished by electrical fulguration. *Cryosurgery* of the prostate is presently an experimental procedure. Liquid nitrogen is circulated through an especially designed urethral probe. The adenoma is

thus frozen and a urethral catheter is inserted. Subsequently, the enlargement sloughs and the patient is able to void.

After TUR, the patient returns to the ward with a urethral catheter. The catheter is removed as soon as the urine is clear of blood for 24 hours. This usually takes three to five days. Then, the patient should measure and record his urinary output for several days. Most patients are discharged in one week postoperatively. Patients are instructed to contact the surgeon promptly if hematuria reappears. This may happen ten days or longer after surgery, and it represents sloughing of the fulgurated blood vessels. A catheter will be reinserted until the urine no longer shows traces of blood.

Transurethral prostatectomy is the easiest of the four operations, for the patient, since there is no external wound. It is performed most frequently on patients with complicating conditions, such as heart disease and advanced age, and those with a small amount of prostatic hypertrophy.

## Suprapubic (Transvesical) Prostatectomy

The surgeon makes a lower abdominal incision, identifies the bladder, and opens it near its dome (the superior portion). He inserts his finger into the prostatic urethra through the bladder neck, and cracks the urethral mucosa anteriorly until he reaches the plane of cleavage. The adenoma is enucleated by sharp or blunt dissection. A urethral Foley catheter is inserted and its balloon expanded either in the prostatic fossa, as in Figure 53-4, or inside the bladder. Most surgeons prefer the latter positioning for two reasons: (1) the muscle in the prostatic capsule contracts, similar to a postpartum uterus, and thus stops much venous oozing; (2) the prostatic arterial blood supply enters at the bladder neck. Therefore, traction on a catheter with its balloon blown up inside the bladder can sometimes be used to tamponade arterial bleeding. The bladder opening is sutured. At the dome, a second catheter, such as a Malecot, is inserted and brought out through the abdominal wall. Advantages of this operation are that it is rapid, allows the surgeon to explore the bladder and to correct any abnormalities (stones, diverticula) found there. A technical disadvantage is that the surgeon controls bleeding by indirect methods, such as catheter traction, rather than direct suturing or fulguration.

The urethral catheter may be removed on the second to fourth day, but the suprapubic cystostomy

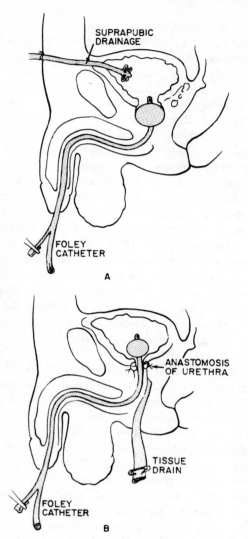

**Figure 53-4.** Drainage after prostatectomy. (A) The Foley catheter provides pressure in the prostatic fossa. In this instance there is a suprapubic drain. (B) After a perineal prostatectomy the Foley catheter supports the operative site, supplies tamponade and a passageway for urine. A tissue drain is inserted through the site of the incision.

tube is used for seven to ten days. Early removal of the urethral catheter diminishes the incidence of urethritis and fever, and the patient is much more comfortable. After the urethral catheter is removed, the patient voids normally in larger and larger amounts.

After removal of the suprapubic tube, the wound frequently leaks urine for a few days; it should be kept very clean and dry because it easily becomes infected. The wound heals slowly. Depending on the overall health of the patient, it may not close for a month. When the wound is infected, healing is even slower.

The convalescent period is longer than that for a transurethral prostatectomy because the bladder has been entered.

### Retropubic Prostatectomy

Through a lower abdominal incision the surgeon exposes the anterior prostatic capsule in the space behind the pubis. The capsule is divided transversely and the adenoma dissected out. A urethral Foley catheter is inserted. The bladder is not entered to perform the operation, but the surgeon may insert a cystostomy tube for additional drainage. The capsule is reapproximated, followed by closure of the abdominal incision. As with suprapubic prostatectomy, the urethral catheter may be removed on the second to fourth day, but the cystostomy tube may be left in the bladder for seven to ten days. Convalescence is often shorter than for the suprapubic procedure. Bladder spasm also tends to be less, since the bladder is not operated on, and less pressure for hemostasis at the sphincter is required. Retropubic prostatectomy is especially applicable to enlarged prostate glands that do not extend into the bladder. Another advantage is that the surgeon can look directly into the prostatic capsule to control bleeding by suture ligature. Although there may be greater blood loss at operation, the ultimate control of bleeding is more secure.

### Perineal Prostatectomy

The patient is placed in the extreme lithotomy position so that the perineum is parallel to the floor. A semicircular incision is made from one ischial tuberosity to the other between the scrotum and anus. The surgeon dissects the anterior rectal wall off the underlying posterior capsule of the prostate. Once adequate exposure has been obtained, the capsule is incised and the adenoma enucleated. A urethral catheter is inserted, the capsular defect repaired, and the incision is closed. An advantage of this approach is that the surgeon can take a biopsy of any suspicious appearing areas, and if the pathologist's report reveals malignancy, radical surgery can be performed at once. The patient with a simple perineal prostatectomy will return to his bed with a urethral catheter and a drain inserted into the perineal tissues and not into the urinary tract. Recovery from the procedure is usually rapid. The perineal incision is less painful than the abdominal approaches.

Although most patients retain potency following operations for benign prostatic hypertrophy, there is a significant percentage in whom it is impaired after perineal surgery. This must be explained to the patient by the surgeon in order for him to obtain informed consent. Consequently, the perineal approach is reserved either for the elderly or for patients in whom there is a strong suspicion of cancer and a radical prostatectomy may be planned. There is also some danger of injury to the rectum resulting in incontinence and possible fistula formation. Following simple perineal prostatectomy, patients generally do not require catheter drainage for longer than one week.

Preoperatively, many surgeons will order a bowel prep to decrease postoperative fecal wound contamination.

**Vasectomy.** Many surgeons perform vasectomy as a routine part of prostatectomy. The term *vasectomy* does not mean complete removal of the vas, a tube 10 inches in length, but rather its interruption near its origin from the epididymis in the scrotum. The usual technique is to isolate the vas in the scrotum, excise a segment approximately half an inch in length, and ligate the ends.

The purpose of the vasectomy, under these circumstances, is to ward off retrograde infection down the vas from the postoperative prostatic bed, with a resultant epididymo-orchitis. This complication of an acutely tender, swollen scrotum accompanied by chills and fever, particularly in elderly patients, is one to be avoided and may be severely disabling.

Vasectomy for contraceptive purposes in younger men is becoming increasingly popular and acceptable. This is probably the safest and simplest method of contraception available today. The procedure is usually performed under local anesthesia on an ambulatory basis. Postoperative discomfort is minimal. The patient is advised to avoid strenuous physical activity for 24 hours after which normal living can be resumed. This includes all forms of bathing. Sexual intercourse can be resumed, but the patient is advised to continue the same type of contraception as before until the surgeon can check the seventh or eighth ejaculate to be sure all previously manufactured sperm distal to the point of vasal interruption have left the patient's body.

Preoperatively the procedure is discussed with the patient, and preferably his wife, if she can be present. He is advised that vasectomy will not affect his potency and his ejaculation volume will remain essentially the same, since most of his seminal fluid is produced by the prostate and seminal vesicles. He is advised that he should consider this a final procedure, although it is reversible. The results of reconstruction are not very good since there will be some eventual diminution in spermatogenesis and technical factors cause difficulty in reanastomosis of such small structures.

A question has been raised by some observers regarding possible long-term deleterious effects of vasectomy. Others note, however, that this is an operation that has been performed by urologists as a part of prostatectomy since the turn of the century. Admittedly it has been done on older patients, many of whom have survived for quite a number of years after their operations. Furthermore, many men in the older age group are active sperm-formers, as witnessed by the study of testicles removed for hormonal treatment of cancer of the prostate. Although the age groups are not strictly comparable, those who perform vasectomy proceed on the belief that the final analysis will not show any long-term undesirable consequences of vasectomy for contraceptive purposes.

## Nursing Assessment and Intervention After Prostatectomy

No matter which surgical approach is used, there are general principles of care applicable to postprostatectomy patients.

When the patient returns to the ward, his catheter or catheters are attached to the appropriate type of drainage. Hourly output of each is recorded separately as well as all intake. Intravenous fluids are given for 24 to 48 hours after surgery.

The patient may also return to his bed with a Penrose drain inserted into the tissues of the operative site. This drain does not enter the urinary tract. The drain removes blood and urine that have leaked into the area. The Penrose drain is removed when all drainage has ceased.

A program of pulmonary hygiene, movement in bed, and early ambulation are essential to prevent deconditioning and cardipulmonary complications.

The following are matters of considerable import for the nursing assessment.

**Bleeding.** Clear urinary drainage following any type of prostatectomy is rare. Hematuria is generally present. However, frank bleeding is a serious emergency and a potential complication for several days after surgery. The color of the urine and the presence of any clots must be noted. Bright red blood indicates an arterial bleeding source, while a deep black red suggests venous oozing. Clots can obstruct the catheter, causing spasm, pain, and further bleeding. Therefore, the catheter must remain patent at all times. The bladder must be palpated and percussed for fullness and tenderness. If these are present, the bladder could be distended with clots and the surgeon should be promptly notified.

To control arterial bleeding, the surgeon may apply traction on the urethral catheter. One method used is that of taping the catheter to the thigh. The traction may be maintained for six hours, but after this there is danger of damage to the bladder sphincter causing temporary incontinence. The surgeon may order the tension to be decreased gradually or may reapply more gentle traction overnight.

The patient who has a Foley catheter bag inflated for purposes of hemostasis has a sensation of having a full bladder, even though it is empty. If he tries to void around the catheter, the bladder muscles contract causing a painful spasm. The nurse can explain to the patient that the bladder is kept empty by the catheter and that trying to void causes irritation to the bladder mucosa. Encouraging fluid intake (if permitted) helps to decrease bladder mucosal irritation because there is a constant passage of fluid over the irritation. Explaining to the patient why he feels this need to urinate may help him not to worry about it. Careful observation is made of vital signs. Since many older men are hypertensive, postoperative blood pressure must be assessed in terms of the patient's usual pressure taken preoperatively. Any drop in blood pressure may be significant. Hypotension, pallor, and other signs of shock warrant emergency measures.

**Drainage and Irrigation.** Usually there is straight drainage without irrigation. Overzealous irrigation may induce further bleeding and cause frequent and uncomfortable bladder spasms. The surgeon leaves orders regarding when to irrigate as well as how much and what kind of solution to use. Irrigation is generally kept to a minimum and used only when necessary. If gentle irrigation or "milking" the catheter does not establish drainage, the surgeon is consulted.

In selected patients, continuous irrigation, regulated by a drip mechanism, is ordered. The continuous gentle flow of fluid helps to prevent clots from forming in the bladder and plugging the catheters. The drip is regulated to maintain drainage at a light pink. The danger of bleeding is increased if the irrigating fluid is continued when the outflow is obstructed by clots. When this through-and-through irrigation is ordered, the urethral catheter is usually used for inflow and the cystostomy tube for outflow. Decompression drainage is usually not effective for arterial bleeding, but it may be ordered for venous oozing because the small amount of urine in the bladder can act as a tamponade.

Normal saline is preferred for irrigation, especially if large volumes are necessary, to prevent blood from being diluted by absorption of the irrigating solution.

When the urethral catheter is removed, the time and amount of each voiding should be recorded for several days. The patient may be instructed to do this. Urgency and dribbling may occur for several days after the removal, but this is generally temporary. Occasionally, if urinary function does not progress satisfactorily, the catheter may have to be reinserted.

**Bladder Spasms.** It is important that the nurse distinguish between catheter obstruction and bladder spasm. Usually with catheter and, consequently, bladder obstruction there is gradual and increasing discomfort with absence of urinary output. The bladder becomes distended and is tender on palpation. Relief of the obstruction is urgent. If there is an order for catheter irrigation by the nurse, she should do this gently. If patency is not achieved, or there is no order for irrigation, the surgeon should be consulted.

When bladder spasm without catheter obstruction is present, the patient will have a urinary output, but pain may be constantly present or intermittent. Some bladder spasms are extremely painful, but fortunately each spasm lasts only a few seconds. Narcotics do not seem to lessen the spasms, but they will help to decrease pain from the operative area. An antispasmodic drug such as propantheline (Pro-Banthine) may be ordered. Bladder spasms generally lessen in severity after 48 hours.

**Dressings and Wounds.** The nurse changes cystostomy and perineal dressings as frequently as necessary to keep the patient clean and dry. Care must be taken not to disturb any tissue drains. Montgomery straps simplify frequent dressing changes. Strict aseptic technique is essential to prevent wound infection.

After a cystostomy tube is removed, the suprapubic wound frequently leaks urine for a few days. A saturated wet dressing, smelling of urine, and wet bed clothes can be very uncomfortable and embarrassing to the patient. If his dressings are not changed promptly when necessary, he may attempt to keep dry by restricting his fluid intake. The nurse encourages liberal fluid intake (when the patient's medical status permits) by demonstrating to the patient that he will have his dressings changed promptly and by attempting to provide the type of liquids most appealing to him.

The amount of urine that comes from the wound is observed and recorded as is the condition of the skin surrounding it. To prevent irritation, the skin should be washed frequently. A medicated powder or ointment may be prescribed if irritation develops. The wound heals slowly, depending to a great extent on the general health of the patient. If it becomes infected, healing is even slower.

Although a perineal wound may not be as painful as an abdominal incision, the patient may experience some discomfort when sitting, for the first week or two. A male T-binder is used to support the dressing. In some instances, beginning on the second or third postoperative day, special wound care consisting of cleansing the incision with surgical soap and water followed by exposure to a heat lamp is performed three times daily. The procedure is completed by applying an antiseptic and a dry sterile dressing. Sitz baths may be ordered after removal of the drains. By ten days after operation, perineal wounds are well on their way to healing in most instances. Early postoperative patients should have help in cleansing after a bowel movement to avoid contaminating the wound. Much of the nursing care after a perineal prostatectomy involves principles similar to those following any perineal or rectal procedure: for example, promoting cleanliness and healing through sitz baths after the drain has been removed.

**Rectal Precautions.** Generally, the use of rectal tubes, rectal thermometers, and enemas is not resumed until at least a week after prostatectomy to avoid perforation or hemorrhage. This precaution is observed especially for patients who have had perineal surgery.

**Bowel Hygiene.** After prostate surgery the patient should be cautioned to avoid straining to have a bowel movement because this can cause prostatic hemorrhage. Stool softeners, daily, or a mild cathartic may be ordered after the third day. Copious fluids and dietary roughage, as permitted, help to prevent constipation.

**Emotional Needs.** Since most patients that have prostatic surgery are in the older age group, surgery can be a severe strain and one more contributory factor to preexisting depression. Personality change as a result of the increased emotional and metabolic stress should be anticipated after surgery. As the patient gropes for a return of emotional balance, the nurse, rather than avoiding him, makes an effort to make him feel wanted and valued. An aspect of her relationship with the patient is established by nonverbal communication: her frequent appearance at his side when he feels most desperate, the good physical care she gives, the expression on her face, and the way she moves, all convey to the patient that she wants to care for him, no matter what his mood. Continued emotional support of the depressed patient is not always easy for the nurse. If the patient does not respond immediately, she may feel helpless and not know what to do next. It is then all too easy to avoid the patient.

## The Convalescent Period

Depending on the type of surgical approach as well as the general health and response of the patient, the length of the convalescent period varies. After discharge from the hospital, the patient should continue to follow established fluid and bowel routines and the surgeon's orders for physical activity. Generally, no lifting or straining is permitted for several weeks.

Patients may be instructed to do exercises to restore bladder control, such as starting and stopping the urinary stream. The nurse can suggest that fluids be limited during the evening if nocturia is present. This is generally only a temporary problem.

Many patients that have had a prostatectomy will be single, retired, living alone, and confronting the myriad problems of the elderly in our society. A referral to the social worker or community nursing agency and other community resources may be indicated.

## Cancer of the Prostate

Prostatic carcinoma is most common in men over the age of 50. As life expectancy increases, more and more men live to the age group of highest incidence of this disease. Its incidence is close to that of cancer of the lung and gastrointestinal tract in men. But recent survival information shows improvement—66 per cent for localized cancer and 53 per cent for cancer with regional involvement are the five year survival figures.

**Symptoms.** At first there are no symptoms, and none may occur for years. The disease usually starts as a nodule in the posterior lobe of the gland, which is furthest away from the urethra. If the tumor grows large enough, it will obstruct urinary flow and cause the attendant symptoms of frequency, nocturia, and dysuria. Thus, a patient with cancer of the prostate who has urinary symptoms usually has a more advanced stage of the disease. Many patients who have prostatic cancer also have benign prostatic hypertrophy, and the symptoms of urinary obstruction may be due to the latter condition. Spread of the cancer is by way of the bloodstream and lymphatics to the pelvic lymph glands and skeleton, particularly the lumbar vertebrae, pelvis, and hips. The first symptoms may be back pain or sciatica due to metastases to the nerve sheaths.

## Prevention

Because early cancer of the prostate is asymptomatic, and because cure is possible only when the disease is discovered early, regular annual or biannual rectal examinations of all men over 50 are as important as are regular gynecologic and breast examinations for women. Men (especially those over 50) who complain of a backache or pain that travels down a leg must have prompt medical attention, including a digital rectal examination.

**Diagnosis.** Rectal examination reveals a solitary hard nodule or the majority of the gland may be replaced by a diffuse, hard irregularity indicative of extensive tumor. Cancer of the prostate, unlike that of certain other areas, does not tend to become necrotic and to form weeping ulcers; there may be no symptoms at all until the malignant cells have spread and set up tumors in other sites in the body (especially lungs, liver, and bones).

Cystoscopy may show the effects of prostatic enlargement on the urinary tract due to compression of the bladder neck, but it does not reveal the cause of the prostatic enlargement. During the rectal examination the urologist may massage the prostate, thus expressing some fluid from it that is sent to the laboratory for a microscopic search for cancer cells (Papanicolaou technique). Blood may be drawn for phosphatases (enzymes that split inorganic phosphates). Increased acid phosphatase in the blood indicates in 75 to 80 per cent of cases that prostatic carcinoma has metastasized. An elevated alkaline phosphatase means that new bone formation is taking place in the body, and therefore it may mean metastases to bone. The tests are used as a guide to the progress of disease rather than as ways of establishing the diagnosis. When the acid phosphatase is elevated, radical prostatic surgery usually is not contemplated, since the tumor has most likely metastasized. X-ray films of the bones may demonstrate characteristic osteoblastic metastases. Since the patient may have metastases with pain for several months before radiographic changes, a radioactive strontium scanning of the skeleton may aid in early diagnosis.

Definitive diagnosis is made by biopsy of prostatic tissue. With clinically obvious cancer, a perineal needle biopsy may be deemed sufficient, but for the solitary nodules—should the biopsy be negative—the surgeon may be concerned about sampling errors. If the nodule is positive and the patient potentially curable, there is some danger of spilling cancer cells into the needle tract. Fifty per cent of suspicious nodules of the prostate eventually turn out to be benign. If the patient has clinically extensive prostatic cancer with obstructive urinary symptoms, diagnosis may be confirmed from a transurethral resection specimen.

**Treatment and Nursing Care.** The outlook for most patients with prostate cancer is relatively good in that many men who are obviously incurable may experience prolonged palliation on conservative therapy. The prognosis seems to be quite dependent on the degree of histologic differentiation of the cancer; some do progress rapidly. Prostate cancer was historically the first cancer in humans demonstrated to be hormonally dependent. Many such tumors will progress under the influence of androgens and regress with estrogens. Following the decrease in androgens by castration (bilateral orchiectomy) and treatment with estrogens, 50 per cent of men with "incurable prostate cancer" will be reasonably comfortable and well five years later. Manipulation of the patient's hormones may give surprising, if temporary, relief of symptoms. Where there had been severe pain, there may be none; where there was bladder neck obstruction, urine may flow freely.

The prescription of any of the synthetic estrogens commonly used is guided by demonstrating a full estrogen effect in the patient, such as slight gynecomastia (enlargement of the breasts) or breast tenderness. If there has been no clinical response on reaching this end-point, a further increase in estrogen dosage usually is of no value. Because of fluid retention problems associated with estrogen therapy, the patient with congestive heart failure must be very carefully observed. A low salt intake is recommended.

As androgens are decreased, and estrogens are given, the patient's voice may become higher, and his hair and fat distribution may change. Also, gastrointestinal disturbances may occur. Because the dosage is regulated according to the response of the patient, it is important that the nurse's observations be especially accurate and the patient's record up-to-date. The patient can be taught to keep a record of his subjective responses and bring it with him on a follow-up visit.

If, even after drug therapy, the tumor obstructs the bladder neck, a transurethral prostatectomy may be necessary to establish urinary drainage. Occasionally, permanent suprapubic drainage will have to be established.

Once the suppressive effects of estrogen treatment wear off (a period which may be quite a few years), the disease progresses more rapidly. For some patients, a second remission, although not as pronounced, may be obtained by hypophysectomy (removal of the pituitary).

**Radical Perineal Prostatectomy.** In the presence of a solitary nodule in a younger patient (usually under 70 years), an open perineal biopsy with frozen section may be done. The surgical approach is as for simple perineal prostatectomy. If the nodule is benign and the patient has symptoms of prostatic obstruction, a simple prostatectomy can be performed at that time. If the nodule is seemingly localized cancer, a radical perineal prostatectomy can be performed. In contrast to prostatectomy for benign disease, the so-called radical operation involves en bloc removal of the entire prostate with its capsule and the seminal vesicles. The bladder neck is sutured to the membranous urethra over a Foley catheter, which is left indwelling for 10 to 14 days. Disadvantages of the operation include virtually guaranteed impotence (versus a chance to be cured of cancer) and some serious difficulty with urinary control in 5 to 10 per cent of patients.

**Preoperative Aspects.** The patient who is to have radical surgery for cancer of the prostate has many problems to deal with. The diagnosis of cancer and the factor of probable impotence combine to stress the patient's psychic resources to the utmost. He needs to discuss both of these problems, and others as well, but may require a great deal of assistance. The urologic nurse understands that these are concerns of the patient and helps him to verbalize them and to get his questions answered. It is helpful for the wife to be present for discussions regarding change in sexual functioning as a result of surgery. The patient, at this time of life, is often retired, or on the verge of retiring and looking forward to enjoying relaxation and reasonable financial security. He may have a strong need to ventilate feelings of anger. He may also feel guilty about putting what he perceives to be a burden on other family members. If the patient is to have radical surgery through a perineal approach, bowel preparation usually includes enemas, a liquid diet the day before the operation, and a drug such as Neothalidine (Sulfathalidine [phthalylsulfathiazide] and neomycin). After surgery the patient is kept on a low-residue diet until healing occurs, so that he does not strain at stool. He may be given camphorated tincture of opium to constipate him for several days immediately postoperatively.

The patient returns to his unit with a Foley catheter placed so that the balloon supports the urethral anastomosis to the bladder neck. Care must be taken that the tube is not displaced from this position. Because the Foley catheter is not used for tamponade, as it is after transurethral prostatectomy, there usually are fewer bladder spasms. Also, there is less bleeding than after a transurethral prostatectomy, but the nurse remains watchful for hemorrhage. She notes and records the color of the urine. The Foley catheter is removed in 10 to 14 days. The patient will have a tissue drain. Initially, there may be seepage of urine through the wound, but this should stop in about two days.

Perineal irrigations may be ordered to help keep the wound clean and to decrease pain and inflammation. After the sterile dressing is removed, the nurse irrigates very gently with the solution that is ordered, often a mild antiseptic such as hydrogen peroxide. This treatment gives the nurse an excellent opportunity to observe the wound's progress in healing and to look for signs of disturbance in the healing process. Additional wound care and nursing measures are similar to those carried out for the patient after rectal or perineal surgery.

The perineal dressing is very close to the rectum.

It must not be permitted to remain soiled with fecal matter. Since a fistula easily develops in the fragile tissue of the operative site, nothing is inserted into the rectum—no rectal thermometers, no rectal tubes, no enemas—unless specifically ordered by the surgeon. Fluids should be encouraged to 3,000 ml., a day, unless there are medical contraindications.

Often, patients are assisted out of bed the second postoperative day. They should sit on a firm, even surface. They should never sit on a rubber ring or an air mattress, either of which could cause compression of or congestion in a portion of the operative site.

If urinary or fecal incontinence results, some patients may be helped to regain control by doing perineal or bladder exercises to improve muscle tone and by regulating their diet. Perineal exercises may be done by contracting and relaxing the gluteal muscles. The patient is taught to observe the effects of various foods and instructed in an adequate diet. He should avoid only particular foods that cause diarrhea, and not any important food groups. Dietitian, surgeon, and nurses work with the patient to help him to establish a dietary regimen that results in good nutrition and regular, formed bowel movements.

The thought of urinary incontinence for the rest of his life may be very depressing to the patient. He can be taught how to keep himself dry and odorfree, so that he will not be reluctant to mix with other people. Teaching the patient to care for himself should start early during the postoperative period. One objective is to make self-care as simple and routine as possible, so that the patient will be relatively free to concentrate on matters other than his condition.

In the late stage of the disease, there may be severe pain, which may be treated by chordotomy. Radiotherapy may give some relief from painful metastases. (See Chapter 10 for care of the patient in pain and Chapter 18 for care of the patient having radiotherapy.)

## DISORDERS OF THE TESTES AND THEIR ADJACENT STRUCTURES

### Cryptorchidism (Hidden Testicle)

Failure of the testicle to lie in the scrotum is known as cryptorchidism (or undescended testicle). At least one testis must be in its normal position in the scrotum for the patient to have reproductive function. The undescended testis may lie in the inguinal canal, abdominal cavity, or rarely in the perineum or femoral canal. If undescended testes are not placed in the scrotum by age five or six, the likelihood of their being good sperm producers diminishes markedly. Undescended testes have a significantly higher incidence of malignant degeneration, whether or not they are placed in the scrotum, but the overall incidence of tumors of undescended testes is low. In some individuals, undescended testicles find their way into the scrotum without treatment during childhood or at puberty.

The treatment may consist of a short (one week) trial of hormone (gonadotrophin) therapy. If there is no response within three weeks, surgery may be performed (orchiopexy). After orchiopexy the patient may have three wounds: inner thigh, scrotal, and inguinal. The surgeon makes an inguinal incision and locates the testis. It is held in the scrotum on tension to a taped rubber band attached to a suture through the lower pole of the testis and to the skin of the upper thigh. The suture is usually removed in five to seven days. Often there is an associated congenital hernia, which is repaired at the time of orchiopexy. The patient can move his leg, but, undue pressure should not be placed on this traction. The nurse should inspect the traction, which will be outside the dressings, several times a day to make sure that it is functioning well.

Adolescent boys who have this operation may be particularly embarrassed to have a female nurse present during dressing changes or to have her inspect the dressings. If there is a male on the nursing team, the patient may feel more comfortable in his care. Some young people in their embarrassment will joke excessively. A matter-of-fact but friendly and accepting manner on the nurse's part may help them to reestablish poise.

### Epididymoorchitis

Infection and inflammations of the testis and epididymis usually occur simultaneously. Presently, the most common cause is infection ascending via the vas deferens and its surrounding lymphatics from a prostatitis. A less common cause of acute epididymitis is untreated gonorrhea.

The symptoms are chills, fever, scrotal pain, and tenderness. The scrotal skin may be erythematous and tense. A markedly swollen testis and epididymis can be palpated. Elevation of the scrotum relieves the pain considerably by lessening the weight of the testes. The scrotum may be elevated with a 4-tail bandage or on adhesive taped across the upper thighs (Bellevue Bridge) (Fig. 53-5).

Strict bed rest usually is ordered during the early stage. An ice bag may be ordered to help to relieve the pain. It is placed under the tender scrotum, not on top of it or leaning against it. The cold bag should not be kept constantly next to the skin, because it may damage tissue. On an hour off a half-hour is one routine that may be followed. Heat is not applied to the scrotal area because spermatozoa are damaged by heat even a few degrees above body temperature. (Normal temperature of the scrotum is lower than that of the rest of the body.) As with any infection, copious fluid intake is encouraged. Antibiotics may be ordered. Oxyphenbutazone may be prescribed to speed up resolution of swelling.

Tuberculosis may be a factor in chronic forms of epididymitis. Antitubercular drugs are used for primary therapy. Rarely is excision or drainage necessary.

Orchitis without epididymal involvement is most often caused by mumps occurring after puberty. This viral orchitis may result in testicular atrophy and sterility. For this reason men who have not had mumps as children and who are exposed to it are advised to receive immediate medical attention. The administration of gamma globulin may have the effect of lessening the severity of mumps if it develops. Commonly, there will be a sudden onset of chills, fever, and testicular swelling one or two weeks after the parotid swelling. Urethritis may also be present. Besides local treatment, corticosteroids may be prescribed.

Bilateral epididymitis frequently leads to permanent azoospermia (absence of sperm), especially when the infection recurs frequently or becomes chronic. Vasectomy (removal of the vas deferens) prevents recurrent attacks but causes sterility if it is performed bilaterally.

## Torsion (Twisting of the Spermatic Cord)

This condition occurs in prepubescent boys and men whose spermatic cords are (congenitally) unusually unsupported in the vaginal sac and are freely movable. The precipitating cause of the twist may be a sudden contraction of the cremaster muscle. Torsion may follow severe exercise, but it also may

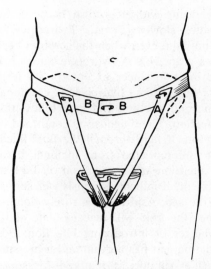

**Figure 53-5.** Four-tail bandage that supports and elevates the testes. The B tails are pinned firmly over the iliac crests. The A tails are brought from the back and snugly hold a small towel in place.

occur during sleep or following such a simple maneuver as crossing the legs. There is a sudden, sharp testicular pain and local swelling. The pain may be so severe that nausea, vomiting, chills, and fever occur. Characteristically, the testis is extremely tender and the examiner may find the usually posterior epididymis located anteriorly. In contrast to inflammatory conditions, elevation of the scrotum will increase the pain by increasing the degree of twist.

Treatment consists of prompt recognition of the disorder and immediate surgery to prevent atrophy of the spermatic cord and to preserve fertility. At that time, the torsion is reduced, excess tunica vaginalis (the membrane surrounding the testis) excised, and the testis is anchored with sutures in the scrotum. Since the condition can be bilateral in at least 10 per cent of patients, a similar prophylactic procedure may be performed on the opposite side.

## Hydrocele

The testis is surrounded by a membrane called *tunica vaginalis*. Normally, there is a small amount of fluid in the space between the testis and this membrane. A large accumulation of fluid in that space is known as *hydrocele*. This common cause of scrotal enlargement may be due to an infection, commonly epididymitis or orchitis, or trauma; the majority occur without known cause. When fluid accumulates slowly (chronic hydrocele), there is usually no pain, even when the scrotum becomes as large as a grapefruit. A hydrocele causes few symptoms in most instances except for its weight and unsightly bulk. Acute hydrocele is accompanied by both pain and swelling and may follow trauma or local infection. The diagnosis is confirmed by transillumination of light through the fluid-filled sac. It must be differentiated from inguinal hernia with scrotal extension and a neoplasm of the testicle.

Treatment, if indicated, consists of surgical excision of the sac. Aspiration is rarely done, particularly since the fluid will reaccumulate and there is a real danger of introducing infection. Postoperatively, the patient has a drain and a pressure dressing. A snug support is required for some weeks afterward.

If aspiration is done, the nurse should observe for bleeding, which may be internal into the scrotum, causing it to enlarge.

## Varicocele

This condition usually occurs on the left side of the scrotum and consists of dilation and tortuous clumping of tributaries of the spermatic vein. Swelling and a dragging pain are the major symptoms. Very rarely does a varicocele per se cause enough symptoms to warrant surgery. In certain instances of infertility, correction of a varicocele has resulted in significant improvement in the semen specimens, for unknown reasons. The surgery involves an inguinal exploration of the spermatic cord with ligature and division of the major spermatic vein tributaries in this region.

## Cancer of the Testis

Malignancy can occur anywhere in the male reproductive system but is not common in the testes. However, testicular tumors tend to metastasize early, and the first symptoms may be related to the secondary site of growth. The symptoms may be abdominal pain, general weakness, and aching in the testes.

Occurring chiefly in young men, the overall cure rate is 60 to 70 per cent (Behnke, 1973). Gradual or sudden swelling of the scrotum always should receive medical attention.

The diagnosis is most often made when the examiner discovers a hard, nontender scrotal swelling. If cancer of the testis is suspected, an orchiectomy is performed for a resectable tumor through an inguinal incision. Biopsy risks spilling tumor cells, and these tumors are highly malignant.

In the embryo the testes originate in association with the kidneys. Thus, the lymph nodes that drain the testes are not in the groin but along the aorta and vena cava. Metastasis from a testicular tumor is to the retroperitoneal regional node system, which must be the target area for surgery or radiation.

Depending on pathology, further treatment may be radiotherapy to the lymph glands (para-aortic nodes) and surgical removal of these glands followed by radiotherapy, or chemotherapy with actinomycin-D. When radical lymph node dissection through a thoracoabdominal incision is done bilaterally, the procedure involves extensive surgery and the patient is very uncomfortable postoperatively. Because the tissue supporting the kidneys may have been removed, the patient may be kept in a Trendelenburg position for a week or two to help to maintain the kidneys in good position. In this position it is difficult to eat, to read, to urinate, and to defecate and a great deal of nursing assistance is required.

A major side effect of retroperitoneal lymph node dissection is that seminal emission, and thus fertility (though not potency), is lost. This, in addition to the impact of the diagnosis of cancer in a young person, necessitates a high level of interpersonal skill on the part of the nurse, if she is to be supportive of the patient.

## INFERTILITY

See Chapter 51 for a discussion of male and female infertility.

## REFERENCES AND BIBLIOGRAPHY

American Cancer Society: '74 Cancer Facts and Figures, New York, 1974.

BEHNKE, H., et al.: Nursing management of patients with urologic tumors, in Guidelines for Comprehensive Nursing Care in Cancer, New York, Springer, 1973.

BORS, E., and COMARR, A. G.: Neurological Urology, Baltimore, University Park Press, 1971.

CAMPBELL, M. (ed.): Urology, ed. 3, Philadelphia, Saunders, 1970.

CONNORS, M.: Ostomy care: A personal approach, *Am. J. Nurs.* 74:1422, August 1974.

FLINT, L., and HSIAO, J. H.: Radical prostatectomy for carcinoma: A review and perspective, *Surg. Clin. N. Am.* 47:695, June 1967.

FOREMAN, J. R.: Vasectomy clinic, *Am. J. Nurs.* 73: 819, May 1973.

GRABSTALD, H., and GOODWIN, W.: Devices and surgical procedures in the treatment of organic impotence, *Med. Asp. Human Sexuality* 7:113, December 1973.

JACOBSEN, L.: Illness and human sexuality, *Nurs. Outlook* 22:50, January 1974.

KROOK, J.: How to deal with patients who act out sexually, *Nurs. '73* 3:38, December 1973.

KASSELMAN, M. J.: Nursing care of the patient with benign prostatic hypertrophy, *Am. J. Nurs.* 66: 1026, May 1966.

KEUHNELIAN, J., and SANDERS, V.: *Urologic Nursing,* New York, Macmillan, 1970.

KRIZINOFSKI, M.: Human sexuality and nursing practice, *Nurs. Clin. N. Am.* 8:673, December 1973.

MALIN, J.: Sex after urologic surgery, *Med. Asp. Human Sex.* 7:244, October 1973.

MOREL, A.: The urologic nurse specialist, *Nurs. Clin. N. Am.* 4:475, 1969.

STRYKER, R.: *Rehabilitative Aspects of Acute and Chronic Nursing Care,* Philadelphia, Saunders, 1972.

WILCOX, R.: Counseling patients about sex problems, *Nurs. '73* 3:44, November 1973.

WILLIAMS, G.: An approach to transsexual surgery, *Nurs. Times* 69:787, June 21, 1973.

WINTER, C., and ROEHM, M.: *Sawyer's Nursing Care of Patients with Urologic Diseases,* St. Louis, Mosby, 1968.

# The Woman
# with Breast Disease

## CHAPTER 54

Breast disease, manifest by infections and benign or malignant tumors, is one of the most frequent and emotionally upsetting health problems confronting women. Education concerning breast abnormalities must be available to health professionals and the public alike. Information is at times fragmentary and promotes controversy, such as in the treatment of cancer of the breast. Many believe that valid data regarding diagnosis and treatment should not be discarded and replaced by unproven regimens that appeal more to femininity than potential longevity of those affected.

## PHYSIOLOGY OF THE BREAST

The breast is a complicated glandular organ that produces milk after pregnancy. Considerable space in the breast is devoted to a network of ducts that carry milk to the nipple; the lymphatic and blood supplies are rich.

The breast manufactures milk from elements in the blood. Amino acids and glucose in blood are transformed to the proteins and lactose in milk by a chemical process not yet fully understood. To make 30 ml. of milk, it has been estimated that the breast must process 12,000 ml. of blood.

Although the most dramatic changes occur in the breast during its preparation for its primary function—lactation—the mammary glands are a part of the female reproductive system, and thus they respond to the hormonal cycle associated with menstruation. Estrogen, secreted by the ovaries, brings about the growth and development of the duct systems and suppresses lactation. Progesterone, secreted by the corpus luteum of the

Physiology of the Breast

Epidemiology of Breast Disease

Signs and Symptoms

Diagnosis

Cystic Disease

Breast Surgery

Patient Education

Complications of Breast Surgery

Treatment of Metastatic Cancer

Breast Abscess

**970**

ovary, stimulates lactation, as does prolactin, an anterior pituitary hormone.

Recent studies have shown that prolactin, chorioembryonic antigenlike materials, and many enzymes are components of breast tissue and fluids. They vary in neoplastic tissues, but the significance of their presence is not understood.

## EPIDEMIOLOGY OF BREAST DISEASE

Information as to the cause of benign and malignant breast disease is fragmentary. However, studies indicate that endocrine metabolism, marital status and parity, hereditary background, preexistence of specific benign neoplasms and dysplasias, ionizing radiation, and racial background are all etiologic factors in the development of carcinoma of the breast. The degree of their importance as to who does or does not develop carcinoma of the breast should not be considered specific. All too often a woman will develop cancer of the breast and have no family history of such cancer or any of the other so-called high-risk factors.

The American Cancer Society estimated that 90,000 American women would be found to have breast carcinoma during 1974. This is a substantial increase in the incidence of ten years ago (63,000).

One of every 15 women with breast masses has cancer. Breast cancer is diagnosed most frequently between the ages of 48 and 60, but cancer is found in the 20- and 80-year brackets also (Table 54-1).

**Table 54-1. Breast Cancer Survival Among White Females by Age, Diagnosed 1950-1964***

| AGE AT DIAGNOSIS | 3 YEARS | 5 YEARS | 10 YEARS |
|---|---|---|---|
| *All Stages of Disease* | 72% | 61% | 48% |
| Under 45 | 75 | 64 | 52 |
| 45-54 | 73 | 63 | 51 |
| 55-64 | 71 | 59 | 45 |
| 65-74 | 72 | 59 | 43 |
| 75-84 | 69 | 59 | 52 |
| *Localized Disease* | 90% | 83% | 73% |
| Under 45 | 90 | 83 | 75 |
| 45-54 | 91 | 85 | 75 |
| 55-64 | 91 | 84 | 72 |
| 65-74 | 90 | 81 | 64 |
| 75-84 | 88 | 82 | 79 |

*Metropolitan Life Insurance Company, *Statistical Bulletin*, New York, March, 1969.

Benign breast tumors are most frequent in younger women. Fibroadenomas occur during the years of active menstruation. Solitary gross cysts usually occur five years or less prior to or after menopause. Infections are probably most common during or immediately after pregnancy, but can occur at any time.

## SIGNS AND SYMPTOMS

**Pain.** At times breast pain may be normal. It is not uncommon for the breasts to become enlarged, lumpy, and tender during the period immediately before menstruation. These physical changes probably are associated with hormonal changes during the reproductive cycle and may be due to an increase in extracellular fluid tension, but the mechanism is not fully understood. Women with cystic disease also frequently experience fullness, tenderness to the touch, and some pain in the breast immediately before menstruation.

**Lumps.** This is one of the prime symptoms of breast disorder. The chief importance of self-examination lies in the discovery of lumps. A lump may be a cyst, a benign tumor, or a malignancy. Many lumps disappear at the time of menses and only those present postmenstrually are significant. Characteristically, malignant lumps are painless during their early stages. The differential diagnosis can be made by a physician, but only if the lump is brought to his attention. Rarely is a lump in the axilla the first sign noticed in malignancy. In those women who do not regularly have breast examinations, most lumps are discovered by accident. For example, a woman receives a sharp blow to her breast. That night the area is still tender, she puts a hand up to it, and discovers a lump. The lump was not caused by the blow, but its discovery was.

**Nipple Discharge.** A discharge that spots the brassiere or drips out without being elicited requires medical attention immediately. Cheesy and milky discharges are usually of no significance. Bloody, brown, or clear-fluid discharges should be checked immediately.

**Change in Appearance.** A breast with an adhering lump near the surface may *dimple* the skin outside or it may cause the nipple to *retract*.

A deep-adhering cancer may fix the breast tissue to the underlying pectoral muscle. There may be a change in *firmness*, *redness*, *chapping of the areolar area*, *erosion*, or *edema*.

## DIAGNOSIS

Available data reveal that a combination of self-examination by the patient, physical examination by a physician or specially prepared nurse, and mammographic examinations of the breasts will demonstrate the presence of most breast lesions that should be biopsied. Self-examination, taught by a health professional, is available to all. Nearly 90 per cent of lumps eventually biopsied are detected in this manner. The physician informs the patient when a lesion should be biopsied. The patient who has not reached menopause should examine herself once a month and during the week following menstruation because the breast is in its most normal state during this time. Prior to menstruation, many nodules exist that later disappear. A thickening or lump during the postmenstrual phase of the cycle should be taken seriously. Frequently, these masses are cysts that can be aspirated and fluid withdrawn. However, a physician should be consulted regarding what should be done.

Mammography is a procedure that can detect lesions too small to be found by the patient or her physician. It is not 100 per cent accurate in determining whether a cancer exists but will frequently discover cancers that are microscopic in size. Several types of equipment are used. The xerograph and conventional mammograph are both effective radiographic units. Even though one of these reports is interpreted as negative for cancer, a biopsy of a lump or thickening is indicated unless the mass is proven to be a cyst.

### Examination

**Self-Examination.** To discover carcinoma of the breast early enough so that its excision will be life-saving, all women should examine their breasts regularly. The best protection against cancer is effective early action. Most lumps are not cancer, but a patient cannot make the differential diagnosis. If every woman in the United States visited her physician every three months for an examination of her breasts, the death rate from this disease would drop. But such frequency of medical visits is not practical.

The following technique is suggested for self-examination of the breasts:

- Sit or stand in front of the mirror, with your arms relaxed at your sides, and examine your breasts carefully for any changes in size and shape. Look for any puckering or dimpling of the skin, and for any discharge or change in the nipples.
- Raise both arms over your head, and look for exactly the same things. See if there has been any change since you last examined your breasts.
- Lie down on your bed, put a pillow or a bath towel under your left shoulder, and your left hand under your head. (From here on, you should feel for a lump or a thickening.) With the fingers of your right hand held together flat, press gently to feel the inner, upper quarter of your left breast, starting at your breast bone and going outward toward the nipple line. Also feel the area around the nipple.
- With the same gentle pressure feel the lower inner part of your breast. Incidentally, in this area you will feel a ridge of firm tissue or flesh. Do not be alarmed. This is perfectly normal.
- Now bring your left arm down to your side, and still using the flat part of your fingers, feel under your armpit.
- Use the same gentle pressure to feel the upper, outer quarter of your breast from the nipple line to where your arm is resting.
- And, finally, feel the lower outer section of your breast, going from the outer part to the nipple.
- Repeat the entire procedure as that described above on the right breast.
- Examine your breasts every month right after your period. Be sure to continue these checkups after your menopause.
- Additional information may be obtained by examining one's breasts while in a shower. Wet fingers are more sensitive and palpation may detect thickenings not discovered when the fingers and breast are dry. If you find a lump or a thickening, leave it alone until you see your physician. Most breast lumps or changes are not cancer, but only your physician can tell.

In spite of the excellent educational program of the American Cancer Society, there has not been a significant drop in the death rate due to cancer of the breast. Many women are not aware of what they themselves can do to discover early disease. Some women have not been exposed to the idea of self-examination. Others have, but fail to attend to it. Small early cancers can only be found by regular examinations.

**Cognitive and Affective Factors.** In the education of women for protecting themselves from death due to cancer of the breast, imparting knowledge is not enough. The educator also must understand why there is resistance to action, and how people may be helped to overcome their apparent indifference. Apathy, fear, and the magical belief that cancer will happen to the other person and not to oneself lead women to resist regular examinations of the breasts in the search for lumps. Fear may lead to "forgetting" or refusing to do the monthly examination; or, on the other hand, it may induce such concentration on the breasts as to lead to daily examinations. One woman said, "I'd hate to examine my breasts. I couldn't do it! Both my mother and my father died from cancer. Last night I dreamed about it and woke up in a cold sweat from the nightmare. I have a terrible phobia about it. I'm so frightened that I hate to wash under my arms, I'm so afraid that I'm going to feel something there. Of course, I do wash, but never without thinking about cancer." Instead of examining herself, this woman visits her physician regularly every six months. A wise nurse would encourage this woman to continue her regular visits, without pushing her on the point of self-examination. The nurse should be flexible, accepting the compromise, lest her patient's fear take the form of resistance to any type of examination.

The knowledge that two-thirds of all breast operations are for benign lesions is not necessarily reassuring. The patient knows that she may be in the other third. Those who have seen a close relative die of cancer of the breast may find self-examination especially difficult.

Some women fear the cure as much as the disease. Breast amputation is mutilating; irrevocably it alters a woman's body. Particularly significant is the fact that it affects a part of her body intimately associated with sexual fulfillment and childbearing. Concern with appearance after surgery may be mitigated only partly by the use of prosthetic devices. The change in her body is one that the woman herself must learn to accept and cope with, regardless of what measures she may use to conceal the disfigurement from others.

These are deep and significant feelings, not to be ignored. Nurses should help women to come to grips with these feelings by listening to them. Without prying, the woman can be helped to identify exactly what it is that troubles her and be assisted to talk to the nurse or physician without feeling ashamed. She should be provided with the factual information that she needs. The patient needs a great deal of support from the physician, nurse, office secretary, friends, and family.

Fear of cancer is not limited to those outside the medical and nursing professions. The United States culture is one that places high value on the female breast as a primary source of identification with the feminine role. Since most nurses are women, some may find the care of patients with breast cancer threatening and anxiety producing because of their vulnerability to this disease. Unwittingly, they may avoid the patient except for highly structured activities, such as teaching postmastectomy exercises. If the nurse is to support patients she must have the opportunity to become aware of her own feelings and reactions.

Some women seem to survive surgery for breast cancer without damage to their self-concepts. One woman who had had a bilateral mastectomy said, "My breasts weren't me. The me is still there." This woman did not suffer postoperative depression and says that when she is dressed she does not feel that her appearance is markedly altered.

**Diagnostic Assessment.** All women should have their breasts examined by a physician or nurse specialist at least once a year. Those over 30, those with cysts, and those who have a relative who has had cancer should be examined every six months. Women should go immediately to a physician when a lump in the breast is discovered.

To investigate a lump in the breast the doctor completely palpates the breasts and nodes. Palpation of adjacent (such as axillary) lymph nodes helps the physician to determine evidence of cancer that has spread; the spread to lymph nodes sometimes is diagnosed by biopsy. The physician inspects the breasts from every angle, with the patient sitting, standing, and bending. *Mammography*, or soft tissue roentgenography of the breast without the injection of a contrast medium may be ordered. On these films it is possible for the radiologist and the surgeon to distinguish, with considerable accuracy, a benign from a malignant lump, and to discover lesions that are still too small to palpate.

When a malignancy is suspected, the surgeon usually takes a biopsy to confirm the diagnosis. *Aspiration biopsy* can be done in the physician's office under local anesthesia. For this procedure a large-bore needle, attached to a syringe, is inserted into the tumor. By applying suction, the physician draws a core of tissue into the bore of the needle. The material is smeared on a glass slide, fixed and stained, and sent to the pathologist.

Recurrent cysts may be aspirated periodically to facilitate examination of the breasts in the search for a new lump that may be cancerous. Malignancy in the breast seems to be somewhat more common in patients with cystic disease than in women with normal breasts (Davis, 1964). The most important point in the nursing care of these patients is to encourage them to have regular examinations. The search for new lumps is complicated by the already existing ones caused by the cysts, but the woman who becomes familiar with her own breasts by periodic examination often can identify new growths.

*Incisional biopsy* is performed in the operating room and the tissue removed is submitted for histologic study. While the patient is still anesthetized, the pathologist examines a frozen section. His report guides the surgeon in his treatment of the patient.

*Thermography*, an additional diagnostic method under investigation, is based on the principle that neoplastic tissues produce more heat than do surrounding tissues due to their high metabolism. The heat is transmitted to overlying skin, the infrared radiation detected, and a heat "image" produced by scanning devices. Temperature difference between normal and malignant tissue is in the range of 2 degrees F.

Roentgenograms may be taken to determine whether or not there are metastases to bone.

## CYSTIC DISEASE

Chronic cystic mastitis is not inflammatory (as the word *mastitis* would imply). In this disorder normal breast tissue proliferates and forms many masses throughout the breasts. The masses become fibrotic and block the ducts, causing cysts to form.

Cystic disease of the breast may cause no symptoms other than lumps, or the breast may be tender, especially premenstrually. There may be shooting pains one or two days before menstruation. A well-fitted brassiere may be advised by the physician. During periods when the breasts are tender, the patient may feel more comfortable if she wears a brassiere during the night as well as the day. Multiple cystic disease sometimes is treated by simple mastectomy. The areola may be saved, and reconstruction surgery may be done with fat and fascia or a plastic insert to preserve the appearance of the breast (augmentation mammoplasty).

A single breast cyst may develop, frequently with the bluish color that prompted the name *blue-*

*domed*. Cysts usually are movable in the surrounding breast tissue. They have far less tendency to adhere and to cause retraction than does cancer.

## BREAST SURGERY

### The Breast Cancer Controversy

A benign tumor usually is excised. When there is malignancy, the surgeon usually removes the pectoralis major, the pectoralis minor, and the entire breast along with the adjacent lymph nodes in an attempt to remove all of the cancer cells from the patient's body: this procedure is a *radical mastectomy*. In recent years, some surgeons have advocated less radical procedures on a selective basis. Unfortunately, patients are difficult to classify since there are many factors involved in the origin and metastasis of breast cancer—age, the size of the tumor, node involvement, immune status, hormone balance, heredity, viruses, for example. A *simple mastectomy* is removal of a breast without lymph node dissection. Some surgeons might advocate *lumpectomy* (removal of the tumor) with radiation. In *partial mastectomy* the cancer is removed with at least 1 inch of the healthy tissue surrounding it. In *subcutaneous mastectomy* the breast tissue is removed but the skin and nipple preserved. In women with palpable nodes, simple mastectomy may be combined with radiotherapy to the axilla and internal mammary lymph nodes. A *modified radical mastectomy* involves removal of all of the breast tissue and lymph nodes in the axilla but without removing the pectoralis muscles.

Other procedures for malignancy include extended radical mastectomy with chest wall resection, and super-radical mastectomy in which the sternum is split and the lymph nodes dissected from the mediastinum. Since the latter two procedures involve opening the thoracic cavity, additional postoperative care is required.

Because long-term data are not available regarding the merits of alternative procedures vs. radical mastectomy, particularly with regard to longevity, many surgeons believe radical mastectomy is the best treatment for all patients with cancer of the breast. Other surgeons are involved in studies in which women meeting certain study criteria are randomly assigned to a management protocol and their progress followed.

The woman should ask her surgeon to discuss all

of the methods available for the treatment of breast cancer and the advantages and disadvantages of each so they can decide on a mutually acceptable approach. Of course, many women would rather put their trust in the decision of an experienced surgeon.

A few years ago most surgeons recommended radical mastectomies whenever the biopsy revealed that carcinoma was present and the preoperative workup showed that the cancer was clinically limited to the breast and adjacent axillary lymph nodes. Some modifications have resulted from controlled studies of patients with specific situations. It has been established that a majority of breast carcinomas are multicentric in origin, regardless of whether they are noninvasive or invasive. Therefore, the least that is recommended is a total mastectomy and removal of the adjacent axillary nodes. Data reported by proponents of partial mastectomy show that their local recurrence rate is higher than among those patients who have had the entire breast removed. In addition, the ten-year survival for patients subjected to partial mastectomy is nearly half that of women subjected to conventional therapy (34 vs. 60 per cent). It is noted that many of those with partial mastectomy were subsequently subjected to additional surgery. The inability to accurately determine clinically the presence or absence of metastatic axillary lymph nodes (an error of 33 per cent) makes it imperative that adjacent axillary nodes be removed (Robbins).

Specifically, most breast surgeons remove the breast and axillary nodes if the patient has noninvasive breast carcinoma. When the lesion is invasive, less than 1 cm. in diameter, and is located in the outer one-half of the breast, the same procedure is used (a modified radical mastectomy). If the dominant tumor mass is located in the inner half or in the center of the breast, the internal mammary lymph nodes may be involved. Therefore, they are removed surgically or subjected to postoperative radiation therapy. Other patients with invasive, potentially curable carcinoma of the breast are subjected to a radical mastectomy, provided there are no medical complications considered contraindications for such surgery (Robbins).

Prophylactic postoperative radiation therapy is utilized in specific situations, depending on the extent of disease found at the time of surgery.

## Preoperative Care: Nursing Assessment and Intervention

In surgery for a lump in the breast, the patient is prepared for the more extensive operation because until the surgeon receives the pathology report he does not know whether the lesion is benign or malignant.

The spread of cancer is capricious and inconstant. It may begin early or late. At first it is microscopic and not detectable grossly. Since cancer spreads through the lymphatics and blood vessels, a very small lump in the breast may have sent some cancer cells along the lymphatics to the axillary nodes.

Before surgery the patient should be told, by the surgeon, if a radical mastectomy may be necessary. The operative permission includes consent for radical surgery, if it is indicated. In this case, skin preparation includes the axilla. Blood typing and crossmatching are done.

During this time the patient often is tense and in suspense. She does not know whether she will awaken from the anesthesia with only a benign lump removed, or an entire breast removed and a diagnosis of cancer. She must be helped in every way possible to face the impending operation.

It may be easier for the patient to talk to a woman about her fears than to a man. It is essential that the nurse know what the surgeon has told her. She may not know that cancer is the disease in question (although that would be rare today), and the word should not be used first by the nurse. The nurse listens to the patient's perception of her situation. Some prefer not to mention the word "cancer," even though they are aware that it is a possible diagnosis. She can be assured that her breast will not be removed, unless the surgeon believes that this operation will be necessary for her health. If she has doubts about this subject, either preoperatively or postoperatively, she should be encouraged to express them but the nurse should continue to convey the idea that the operation may be necessary. When the patient seems unable to accept the surgery, this should be discussed with the surgeon before the operation is performed to lessen serious postoperative sequelae, such as severe depression, or the patient's inability to recognize and to acknowledge that a breast has been removed.

When there is no doubt that a radical mastectomy must be done, a short visit from a recovered patient may help the patient to accept the surgery more readily.

## The Operation

The patient is prepared for a radical mastectomy and is kept under general anesthesia while the biopsy specimen is being examined. The pathologist requires about 15 minutes to make his diagnosis from the tiny piece of tissue. If the diagnosis is benign tumor, the surgeon will simply excise the lump and close the wound.

Excision of a benign breast tumor is minor surgery. If it were not for the possibility of performing a radical mastectomy, many benign tumors could be removed under local rather than general anesthesia. The surgery is over quickly, and the incision is small; the patient usually goes home after two or three days in the hospital.

**Radical Mastectomy.** If at operation the pathologist's report shows that the lesion is malignant, the surgical drapes are changed, the operating team rescrubs and proceeds with a radical mastectomy.

Drainage by Penrose drains or a Hemovac system is instigated beneath the skin flaps to prevent the collection of fluid in the wound. A skin graft (often from the anterior thigh) may be required to close the resulting wound. When there is a graft, a drain is left in the axilla to drain fluid that may form under the graft and prevent its "take." If a graft has been done, pressure dressings are applied on both the donor and the recipient sites.

If the cancer is so far advanced that there are metastases to other portions of the body, removing the breast will not cure the disease and a mastectomy may not be done. A simple mastectomy may be performed to remove a grossly enlarged, draining breast to make the patient more comfortable.

The combined operations—radical or modified radical mastectomy and bilateral oophorectomy for node metastases are performed in premenopausal women by a significant number of surgeons. Because the ovaries are removed to eliminate the source of estrogen from the body, no replacement estrogens are given to relieve the distressing symptoms of surgical menopause. The sudden lack of estrogen frequently causes more severe menopausal symptoms in these patients than those associated with natural menopause.

The two operations, singly or in combination, are threatening to a woman's image of herself, especially for women of childbearing age. The one operation prevents a woman from having children, the other mutilates her appearance.

Because some surgeons believe the risk is high for the development of another primary cancer in the remaining breast, the surgeon may recommend that the remaining breast be removed.

## Postoperative Nursing Assessment and Intervention

Patients who have had a radical mastectomy frequently discover their diagnosis for themselves when they are beginning to recover from anesthesia. Unlike many other types of surgery, this operation makes the diagnosis evident to the patient. The surgeon and the family have no time to talk over how, if, and when to break the news to the patient. The patient, whose emotional and physical resources have been lowered by anesthesia, surgery, drugs, and suspense, needs a nurse to be there to help her at the time she discovers the breast has been amputated. The patient should not be left to grope alone. When the recovery room nurse sees that the patient is beginning to respond from anesthesia, even though hazy, she should remain with her, talking to her quietly and gently, as the patient feels the dressing and comes to the grim realization that her breast is gone, with all the loss portends for the future.

**Arm Position.** Because in radical surgery the incision is extensive, disturbing the integrity of a large area of skin and muscle, excessive motion of the upper arm on the affected side is prevented immediately after surgery, especially abduction. That arm may be bandaged to the body, with the elbow bent at a right angle, especially if grafting has been done. Motion might pull the graft free of its attachments. Whether the arm is bandaged or not, its abduction on the affected side is not permitted. The arm must be kept especially still when grafting has been done. One or two pillows are placed under the arm to help to support it and to elevate it above the level of the remaining breast at least for the first day. The elbow should be slightly higher than the shoulder. This aids in preventing the lymphedema that commonly develops postoperatively from interference with the circulatory and lymphatic systems. If the arm is bound to the body, the hands must be observed for signs of impaired circulation (swelling, cyanosis, coldness, tingling). If such signs occur, the surgeon should be notified.

**The Incision.** Drains may be inserted at the time of surgery to remove the serous fluid that collects under the skin, thereby delaying healing and predisposing to infection. A drainage tube may be attached to low-pressure suction, such as the Hemovac, which enables the patient to be easily up and about and eliminates the need for constantly reinforcing dressings. Drainage tubes are irrigated daily by the physician to free clots. Drainage is measured every eight hours or as ordered.

Wound drainage may be copious; its color, amount, odor, and consistency, whether from a tube or tissue drain should be observed and recorded. The dressing should be checked for bleeding also, and any evidence of this reported to the surgeon. Since fluid seeping from the wound may not be visible on the front of the bandage, but may flow underneath the patient, this area must be felt and inspected. The dressing is checked at least every 15 minutes immediately after surgery. On the second and the third postoperative days it should be checked, though not disturbed, at least three times a day. The dressing, which is bulky so as to hold the skin flaps down, usually is left in place until the fifth to ninth day after the operation, depending on whether a graft was used and the surgeon's preference. At that time the dressing is changed.

The patient needs to be prepared for the initial dressing change. Talking about it prio. to the experience can make the situation easier for the patient to handle. The nurse can initiate discussion when the patient is given an approximate time for the first dressing change by asking the patient what she expects to see. (In addition to the incisions, stab wounds for drains are also present.) The overall appearance can greatly upset the patient who may react with hysteria, anger, crying, depression, or withdrawal. Helping the patient involves anticipation of and sensitivity to her reaction, such as allowing for the expression of anger or letting her cry.

Every effort should be made to encourage the patient to look at the incision before going home, but she should not be pushed into this at the time of the first dressing change. Timing the encouragement requires assessment of the patient's state of readiness. Helping her focus on something specific and positive, such as signs of wound healing or less swelling, may ease the way towards acceptance.

A primary nurse assigned to the patient is especially helpful in providing an opportunity for the growth of a trusting, accepting relationship.

When the patient's refusal continues, a lead such as "You seem not to be able to look at the incision," can be helpful in initiating discussion. Chiding the patient that she'd best be prepared before she goes home is not helpful. Sometimes, having the husband, daughter, or other person who will help the patient at home, come to the hospital for the dressing change is beneficial. The nurse can offer support and answer questions.

The patient needs to know that in time, redness, swelling, and irregularity disappear, the scar becomes less prominent, and the tissues more normal in color. The healing period for the wound is four to eight weeks for most patients. Pressure dressings may be continued after the initial dressing change and dressings are changed daily until healing occurs.

**Helping the Patient Toward Self-Sufficiency.** Since dressings tend to constrict the chest, the patient needs to be helped to cough deeply. Pain is considerable and narcotics are given liberally, as ordered by the physician. Because movement of the chest is painful and opiates depress respirations, the patient may require assistance to take full breaths after medication for pain has had its effect.

Ambulation is encouraged as soon as possible after surgery and the patient who had radical surgery, with or without drainage, is helped to walk as soon as those who have had a simple mastectomy. Therefore it is not unusual to help the patient out of bed for the first time on the operative night or the next day. If the patient needs assistance as she walks, she is supported on the *unaffected* side. She will have a tendency to splint the operative site and to balance herself by hunching that shoulder, but she must be encouraged to keep the shoulder level and the muscles relaxed. For approximately two weeks (the length of time varies with the surgeon's preference) the arm on the affected side is usually supported in a sling whenever the patient is out of bed.

Once the patient has been out of bed, she may feel that she can ambulate safely by herself. She should be assured that the nurse is available to help her while she is still unsteady on her feet.

Postoperatively, the patient should be helped with those activities that she cannot do for herself, for example, cutting her meat. To avoid placing her in the dependent and embarrassing position of having to ask for this service, the need for it should be anticipated. However, as soon as it is possible, the patient should be helped towards independence by encouraging her to do everything for herself that she can. This must be done in such a way that she will not misinterpret the staff's intentions to mean that they do not want to be bothered with her.

## PATIENT EDUCATION

### Affective Factors

Teaching exercises, wound and arm care is important but it should not be the focus of the nurse-patient relationship. The feelings and reaction of the patient afford the framework in which the nurse teaches. A perfect teaching plan can be a failure if the patient is not ready to learn or is so anxious that her perception is distorted. Because patients vary in their reactions to grief, some may be too depressed to be able to meet the nurse's expectations for participation in self-care activities. The normal healing processes of grieving cannot be accelerated and some patients need more time, artful listening, gentle suggestion, and sometimes passive exercises by the nurse before they are able to accept changes in themselves and be ready to learn. As the patient's mourning and depression lessen, she will be able to be more aware of how the exercises and self-care activities are helping her and become a more active participant in the learning process.

Nurse-led group sessions can help patients to recognize and deal with their feelings, to share their experiences, and to gain support from the nurse as well as from each other. Talking with and doing exercises with other women who have the same difficulties can help a patient to realize that she is not odd or clumsy, but that she is one among others who share a common problem and have common goals.

### Cognitive and Psychomotor Factors

Teaching can be on a one-to-one basis or group teaching can be carried out in any hospital where there is more than one postmastectomy patient. The nurse teacher explains and demonstrates exercises with daily progression, discusses and demonstrates wound and arm care and the prevention of infection and lymphedema, and talks about and

demonstrates the types of breast forms available. The physical therapist and social worker may also participate. A rehabilitated mastectomy patient from the local chapter of the American Cancer Society's *Reach to Recovery* program can answer many questions about adjustment to usual life style. This visitor also brings a booklet, *Reach to Recovery* (American Cancer Society, 1972) and information about purchasing brassieres, prostheses, bathing suits, and so on.

*Exercises* of the affected arm will be ordered by the physician and in some institutions begin about the third or fourth postoperative day. With grafting, no exercise is used without definite written orders from the surgeon. In patients who do not have grafts, exercises are frequently preceded from the first postoperative day by such activities of daily living as brushing the teeth, washing the face, and combing the hair with the affected hand. Squeezing a rubber ball stimulates circulation and helps restore function. Exercises prevent shortening of muscles, contractures of joints, and loss of muscle tone.

Active exercises are always more effective than passive ones. As soon as the surgeon has given his permission, the patient starts on a regular program that can enable her to perform all the activities in which she used her arm preoperatively. The first exercises may be opening and closing the hand, flexing and extending the fingers, and bending the wrist forward and backward. In some hospitals no order is needed to commence these exercises, and they are started on the first postoperative day. There is a psychological as well as a physiologic point to starting active exercises soon after surgery. This is something that the patient herself can do to aid in her recovery. When the drains are removed, and the first dressing is changed, the surgeon may consider that the wound has healed sufficiently so that the patient can abduct her arm. Raising the elbow away from the body may be started. If fluid collects in the wound, exercises are delayed.

Whenever the exercises start, it is important for the return of full function that they be practiced regularly. The removal of the pectoral muscle causes some temporary loss of strength, but no loss of arm function. Though the arm on the affected side will present the most difficulty, exercises should be bilateral to avoid pain and postural change resulting from inconsistent development and consequent structural change.

All exercises in the hospital, and later at home, should be done in comfortable clothes and shoes, in loose sleeves and from a starting point of good posture (standing position) (Fig. 54-1). As in all exercises for rehabilitation, they should be stopped before the point of fatigue.

Some of the exercises that the physician may wish the patient to do include:

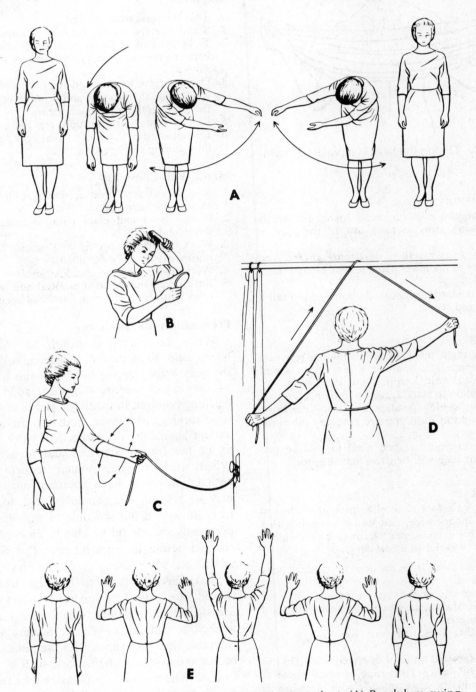

**Figure 54-1.** Exercises for the postmastectomy patient. (A) Pendulum-swinging exercise. (B) Hair-brushing exercise. (C) Rope-turning exercise. (D) Rope-sliding exercise. (E) Wall-climbing exercise.

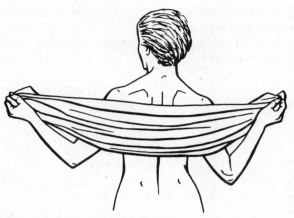

**Figure 54-2.** Drying the back is a practical alternative to rope sliding.

## Pendulum Swing

1. Start in standard position. Bend forward from the waist, allowing arms to hang toward the floor by gravity.
2. Swing both arms together, describing an arc from one shoulder to the other. Do not bend elbows. Keep arms parallel.
3. Return to standard position and allow arms to fall to sides. Rest and repeat.

## Hair Brushing

1. Sit beside a night table. In the beginning rest your arm (on the operated side) on a few books. Comb and brush your hair, keeping your head erect.
2. One side will do to start. Little by little, release your arm from its resting position and work the brush around your head until you are covering the entire scalp.
3. Rest whenever you feel you need to, but be persistent. (Your hair will benefit from this, too!)

## Rope Turning

Equipment: A six-foot clothesline rope or six feet of bandage, three inches wide, tied to a doorknob with a double knot. This exercise may seem to be difficult at first, but it will be easier in a few days.

1. Stand four feet away from the door in standard position. Face door.
2. Take the loose end of the rope in the hand on your operated side. Make a knot to put between your third and fourth fingers.
3. Place the other hand on your hip to help your balance.
4. Extend arm forward on your operated side. (Do not bend elbow or wrist.) Turn rope in small circle at first and gradually work into as wide a swing as possible.
5. Rest and repeat given number of times. (Try the same exercise with your other arm occasionally.)

## Pulley Motion (Rope Sliding)

Equipment: A six-foot rope or six feet of bandage, three inches wide; a shower rod or similar rod above your head. Place knots in rope at ends and at two intervals.

1. Toss the rope over the rod.
2. Stand directly behind the rope in standard position.
3. Hold the end of the rope in each hand with knots between your third and fourth fingers, and raise arms sideways.
4. Using seesaw motion and with arms stretched sideways, slide the rope up and down over the rod until the knots in the rope touch the rod.
5. Return to standard position, rest and repeat.
6. Do not bend at the waist. Keep your feet flat on the floor during this exercise.

## Hand Wall Climbing

1. Start in standard position, facing wall, with toes as close to wall as possible.
2. Bend elbows and place palms against the wall at shoulder level.
3. Work both hands up the wall parallel to each other until arms are fully extended.
4. Work hands down to shoulder level.
5. Return to standard position. Rest and repeat. (It will relax you a bit if you rest your head against the wall.)

## Preparation for Discharge

While the patient is still in the hospital, she needs help to plan for continuing exercise after she goes home. Drying her back with a towel (Fig. 54-2) provides exercise as good as rope sliding; the reaching required in making a bed is as adequate as rope turning. Moreover, both are productive. The patient should be encouraged to work slowly into all of her former activities and to avoid fatigue. When she first goes home, frequent relaxation periods, in which she is stretched out on her bed, may be helpful. She should be told not to expect to begin with a full schedule of activities, but that eventually she should be able to do everything that she did before the mastectomy. The surgeon will advise her when she may play tennis or golf.

**Skin Care.** After the bandage has been removed, the patient is taught to care for the skin area herself. She should wash it gently with a soft washcloth and soap. Wound healing takes considerable time and varies with the patient's state of health and complicating factors, such as wound infection. Whereas some patients heal in two months, others may require six to eight months for complete healing. It is not unusual for patients to have some discomfort in the operative site for several months.

One described the discomfort thus: "It pinches and pulls and feels as if it is bandaged with sandpaper." Cold cream, pure lanolin, or any emollient may be applied to the scar. Talcum powder may relieve itching.

**Affective Factors.** The emotional significance of a mastectomy varies from patient to patient. To some it is only a surgical experience and life continues as before. To others it means the first signal of the death process. Many women are occupied with thoughts of death, but find no one with whom to discuss their feelings freely. One study shows that the impact of the significance of surgery is more likely to be felt fully once the patient has returned home (Quint, 1963). Yet family and friends understandably tend to avoid conversations about death, and the patient is expected to carry on as before. Not only are family and friends emotionally involved with the patient, but a conversation about another's impending death is a reminder that one, too, will die.

The postmastectomy patient often feels isolated, with no one to help her face the annoying problem of the healing incision and the larger problems of social acceptance and worry about death. The community health nurse, the independent nurse practitioner, the clinic nurse, or the office nurse must assume continuing responsibility for assessment and appropriate intervention with regard to the patient's emotional state as well as her physical needs.

How effectively the patient maintains her contacts with family and friends when she returns home is determined by her prior relationship with them and by her attitude, and theirs, to the surgery. Most wives worry about their husband's reaction.

They, too, have to deal with their feelings regarding the diagnosis of cancer, their fears about death, and their feelings about their wife's disfigurement. Some men, particularly those who react negatively to the idea of a less than perfect body, are in need of help themselves if they are to be supportive of the patient. The nurse can detect clues of a strained marital relationship and provide counseling, if she is prepared for this role, or suggest sources of help.

The nurse can encourage the patient to maintain her ties with friends and family during hospitalization by showing courtesy to the patient's visitors and by assisting the patient, if she needs help to write letters or to make telephone calls. Perhaps the greatest help that the nurse can render the patient and which will help her to maintain her ties with others after she leaves the hospital is to show that she accepts the patient and wants to help her come to grips with the impact of surgery. The skillful nurse allows her patient to express what she wishes concerning the meaning of the operation to her, without suggesting what it should mean, might mean, or has seemed to mean to other patients.

If the patient learns to care for her skin while she is still in the hospital and has support and interest, she may have less tendency to shun the scar once she gets home. If she is repelled by the sight of it, she should be allowed to express this. Its progress of healing can be pointed out and she can be told that the scar will become less noticeable in time (Fig. 54-3). For example, the married patient who can begin to accept her scar before she leaves the hospital can help her husband to feel less shy or embarrassed about it, and then in turn he can help her to feel more comfortable about it.

**A Prosthesis.** The patient is seldom ready to

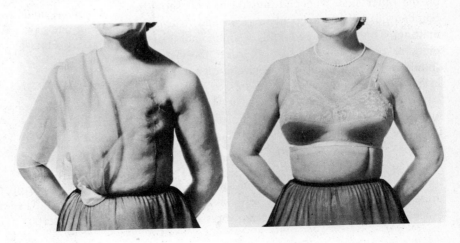

**Figure 54-3.** (*Left*) Radical mastectomy scar. The slight irregularity is typical. (*Right*) Same patient fitted with a prosthesis. (Identical Form, Inc., New York, N.Y.)

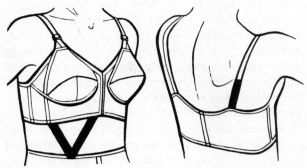

**Figure 54-4.** Elastic inserts that prevent the breast prosthesis from riding up.

wear a commercial prosthesis for about three months because the wound is not healed. In the hospital the patient can wear a nylon-lace "sleep bra" stretch type unit. Light air-filled plastic forms may also be used for cosmetic appearance and comfort, especially for those with bilateral mastectomy. (Perhaps the more acceptable word to the patient will be "falsie.") Until a prosthesis is obtained, and when the surgeon approves, a makeshift one can be fashioned to wear over the dressing, using the patient's brassiere. For example, the nurse can suggest that the patient tack a sanitary pad or cotton padding into the cup that fits over the affected side (providing her, of course, with the padding and the sewing implements). One end is sewed to the middle section of the brassiere and the other end to the back, so that the padding extends under the arm and fills in the space left by the lost muscle and glandular tissue. Some absorbent cotton is then fluffed and stuffed into the area between the brassiere and the padding until the contour of that side is similar to that of the breast on the other side. The pad and the cotton should be changed daily to keep them clean and to avoid matting. This improvised "falsie" must not exert pressure on the shoulder. If it does, the patient should be given a small strip of elastic tape to insert in her shoulder strap. When she dresses in her own clothes, and before she is allowed to wear a commercial prosthesis, a V-shaped elastic insert from her brassiere to her girdle will prevent that side of the brassiere from riding up (Fig. 54-4). This is a very important point, because if the patient feels that the cotton is about to pop out from the neck of her dress, she will be unnecessarily self-conscious, have a tendency to keep pulling at her brassiere, and

refrain from using her arm on that side freely and naturally.

In the beginning, at least before she is fitted with a commercial prosthesis, some women may feel more comfortable wearing dresses with high necks, loose sleeves, and perhaps a jacket, a scarf, or a stole.

When the surgeon tells the patient that she may wear a commercial prosthesis, she has her choice of several different types. Some are made of foam rubber; others are inflated with air or filled with fluid. Sponge rubber is light and easily washable. Excessive heat and, of course, careless handling should be avoided. If a rubber prosthesis is worn under a bathing suit, it can be squeezed dry unobtrusively with the forearm while the woman dries her face with a towel. Any prosthesis in a bathing suit should be tacked in. Prostheses that are filled with water assume natural contours, in keeping with those of the other breast, as the woman changes position. These prostheses feel more like a normal breast and even assume body warmth.

It is especially important for nurses to know where to refer their postmastectomy patients, since it is frequently the nurse to whom the patient will turn for help.

Some surgical supply houses and corsetiers who sell breast prostheses have an experienced female prosthetist who can give the patient a correct fit and instruct her in the care of the prosthesis. Such stores may be found in the yellow pages of the local telephone directory. Many large department stores carry prostheses. Some companies have excellent pamphlets prepared for postmastectomy patients. The Reach to Recovery program supplies an extensive list of prosthesis types, manufacturers, availability, and cost as well as suggestions for making one's own form. (See also Supportive Care for the Postmastectomy Patient.)

## COMPLICATIONS OF BREAST SURGERY

**Pain.** Some postmastectomy patients develop sympathetic pain in the other breast. The patient should be told to call this symptom to the attention of her surgeon. It usually does not represent organic disease. At times the remaining breast becomes larger postoperatively.

**Infection.** The amputation site may become infected or serous fluid may collect beneath it. During dressing changes, and after the dressing is no longer necessary, the wound should be inspected at least daily. Pockets of swelling, redness, discharge, odor, and breaks in the suture line should be reported to the surgeon.

**Lymphedema.** Slight and transitory swelling of the arm is relieved, usually as soon as the arm regains function. However, in some postmastectomy patients lymphedema is disabling. It may develop shortly after the operation or years later. The cause is unknown, but it is believed that an infection that obstructs lymphatic flow can cause this distressing complication. Radiation may aggravate it. Because infection may play a role in its etiology, and because the complication may occur years later, women who have had a mastectomy should be taught how to avoid infection and to treat as serious even slight infections of that arm and that hand. The healthy unbroken skin is the best protection against a minor infection that may lead to the major complication of edema of the arm. The following points should be emphasized in the patient education program*:

- **Cuticles should be pushed back rather than cut to avoid the risk of infection. The patient should exercise care not to break the skin when she cuts her nails, and hangnails should be cut, if at all, by a physician. Most women are understandably reluctant to go to a physician to have a hangnail cut, but they must be warned not to pull or bite it, to keep it very clean, and to report to the physician the slightest sign of soreness or infection.**
- **Canvas gloves should be worn for protection when gardening and rubber gloves should be worn when using steel wool or abrasive cleansers.**
- **Burns should be guarded against by wearing an asbestos padded glove(s) when reaching into a hot oven and, in those who smoke, by holding the cigarette in the unaffected hand. Tanning the skin gradually rather than risking a sunburn is a must.**
- **Pressure and swelling should be avoided by keeping dress sleeves, watch band, and jewelry loose on the operative arm.**
- **To avoid nicks, scrapes, or punctures of the skin an electric razor rather than a blade razor should be used for shaving, and a thimble should be worn when sewing.**
- **Heavy purses and packages should be carried on the unaffected side.**
- **The unaffected arm should be used for blood pressure measurement as well as for injections or vaccinations.**

*Adapted from *Breast Carcinoma Monograph,* Memorial Hospital for Cancer and Allied Diseases, 1973, p. 70.

- **Though lotions or creams can be used to keep the skin soft, beauty creams containing hormones must have the physician's approval.**
- **A break in the skin, no matter how small, should be washed immediately with soap and water and covered with a Band-Aid. Any symptoms of infection of the hand or cellulitis of the arm (heat, pain, swelling, reddening, or red streaks on the arm) should be brought to the physician's attention immediately.**

Edema of the arm is treated by antibiotics to abolish the underlying infection; however, this treatment is effective only if it is applied before fibrosis has blocked lymphatic outflow. Often the patient is hospitalized, and her arm is kept elevated on a pillow. An air pressure machine (Fig. 54-5) may

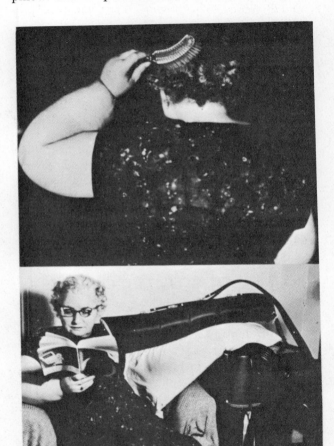

**Figure 54-5.** (*Top*) Lymphedema of the arms. (*Bottom*) The Circulator (Circulator Therapeutics, Inc.) is used to treat lymphedema. This patient spends four hours a day using the sleeve. In eight months her upper arm was reduced in circumference from 18½ inches to 15 inches. The patient positions her arm so that gravity aids the mechanical pressure. She makes sure that the tubing is not kinked.

be used. It automatically fills the segments of the sleeve with air, exerting progressive cumulative pressure on the arm. The most distal portion of the sleeve fills first, then the next portion, and so on, forcing fluid past incompetent lymphatic valves toward the heart. After all the segments are filled, the air is released, and the cycle starts over again. The machine is set approximately 5 mm. below the diastolic blood pressure. This treatment must be used several times a day to be effective. Significant arm edema can be controlled in some cases with an elastic sleeve or Ace bandage. Patients who are obese will need help in losing weight, as obesity complicates the reduction of edema. Low sodium diets and diuretics are sometimes prescribed.

**Metastasis.** The spread or recurrence of breast cancer is an ever-present possibility. Cancer cells can spread to any structure in the body. Metastases often cause pain in the new site. Sometimes, the discomfort can be lessened by radiation to the affected area. When bone becomes involved, there is danger of pathologic fracture (fracture after slight or no trauma). The patient is taught to take precautions against falling and to avoid bumps. Without frightening her, or discouraging her from normal activities and hobbies, she must be encouraged to examine the remaining breast regularly and to report any changes, as well as keep regular appointments with her physician.

## TREATMENT OF METASTATIC CANCER

It is estimated that slightly over two-thirds of the individuals affected with mammary cancer will sometime during their lifetime have disseminated mammary cancer. Lymph nodes are most commonly involved in metastasis, with bone and pulmonary involvement following in order. Many organs and systems can be affected before death. Variables regarding the clinical course of the patient include: the presence of metastatic carcinoma in the axillary lymph nodes at the time of surgery, the size of the primary tumor, the characteristic of tumor margins, histologic type and, also, in the event of spread, the length of the "free" interval between mastectomy and recurrence (Perez, 1967).

Treatment varies with the specific type of metastasis and is aimed at providing the greatest period of palliation for the patient. Physicians differ in their treatment preferences. All forms of treatment

carry the possibility of unpleasant side effects and complications.

**Hormonal Therapy.** Normal function of the mammary gland depends on the action of several stimulating hormones, including progesterone, prolactin, somatrophin, the growth hormone mammogen, and especially estrogen. Changing the hormonal environment of the body should inhibit growth of the primary tumor, or metastatic tissue derived from the primary tumor, elsewhere in the body. The hormonal environment of the body can be changed by *ablation* (removal) of an endocrine organ or by the *addition* of exogenous sex hormones.

Endocrine ablative procedures include prophylactic or therapeutic destruction of the ovaries or testes (castration) by surgery or radiotherapy. Since the adrenal gland is capable of producing estrogen, bilateral adrenalectomy sometimes is performed in women who have estrogen-dependent metastatic cancer, and whose vaginal smears continue to demonstrate a high level of estrogen activity. This operation may cause the cancer to regress and the patient to feel less distress. Lifetime replacement of cortisone, adjusting the dosage in times of stress, is necessary after adrenalectomy.

Removal of the pituitary gland (hypophysectomy) may be done in the treatment of estrogen-dependent tumors to suppress both the adrenal glands and the ovaries. Other endocrine glands will be suppressed as well, and the patient may require adrenal and thyroid replacement therapy. After both adrenalectomy and hypophysectomy the nurse should observe the patient for polyuria and other water and electrolyte balance disturbances. Additional stress may bring about symptoms of adrenal or pituitary insufficiency. (See Chapter 49 for nursing care in these conditions of endocrine imbalance.)

Additive hormonal therapy to change the internal environment includes the use of androgens, estrogens, progesterone, and cortisone.

Large doses of estrogen and testosterone are used sometimes to help alleviate the pain, the weight loss, and the malaise of metastatic cancer in postmenopausal women. Estrogen is contraindicated in premenopausal women, for whom large doses of testosterone propionate may be ordered for its antagonistic effect. Hormonal treatment does not cure cancer that has spread, but it may increase the lifespan by months or even years, and it makes some patients more comfortable during much of this time. Why the hormones have this effect is unexplained.

Estrogen therapy can cause nausea and vomiting, pigmentation of the remaining nipple and areola, and uterine bleeding. Stress incontinence is frequent. Sodium may be retained, leading to excessive storage of intercellular fluid and edema. To help to relieve this situation, diuretics and a low-sodium diet may be ordered. Large doses of estrogen sometimes cause mobilization of calcium into the bloodstream. When this happens, the kidney may be damaged during the process of excreting excess calcium.

Intramuscular and oral androgen (testosterone) therapy are used, especially when there are metastases to bone. Patients may have increased bone pain after the first few injections, but as therapy continues, pain frequently is lessened, there is some recalcification of bone, and the patient gains appetite and weight. Androgen therapy may cause fluid retention and distressing symptoms of virilization, such as a deeper voice and hirsutism; increased libido may result also.

The results of therapy aimed at decreasing the amount of estrogen in the patient's body may be observed by vaginal smears and studies of the urinary excretion of estrogen and calcium.

**Radiotherapy** may be given preoperatively or postoperatively. If the surgeon finds that the axillary nodes contain cancer cells, a series of x-ray treatments may be ordered prophylactically, even though the nodes have been removed. The rationale is the likely presence of microscopic deposits of malignant cells in the lymph node bearing areas of the breast. Postmastectomy exercises should continue during the x-ray treatments. There is some question whether such radiotherapy increases survival time (Mercado, 1967). For palliative purposes, radiotherapy may be directed to treatment of primary tumors; regional or distant metastases, especially to bone; or local recurrence to the chest wall.

**Chemotherapy.** Metastases to soft tissue and bone are most responsive to chemotherapeutic agents. The purine antagonist 5-fluorouracil (5-FU) and the alkylating agent thio-TEPA (N, N′, N″—triethylenethiophosphoramide) are the most useful chemotherapeutic agents for the treatment of mammary carcinoma. These drugs may cause bone marrow depression, granulocytopenia, anemia, nausea and vomiting, hypotension, dermatitis and malaise, diarrhea, and stomatitis.

Any of the above measures may prolong the patient's life and make her more comfortable. Many will eventually succumb to the disease, but some will die from other causes. Though breast cancer is a milestone in life, it is not necessarily a tombstone. Some patients are symptomfree for long periods and lead relatively comfortable and fruitful lives. Unfortunately, others, like the young woman with galloping metastases, may die quickly. Still others might have to endure long periods of suffering before they succumb. The victims of breast cancer offer to nursing unlimited challenge.

## BREAST ABSCESS

Abscesses occur most frequently as a postpartum complication (Fig. 54-6). Fissures and cracks in the nipple provide an entry for organisms, especially staphylococci, which thrive in milk. The patient

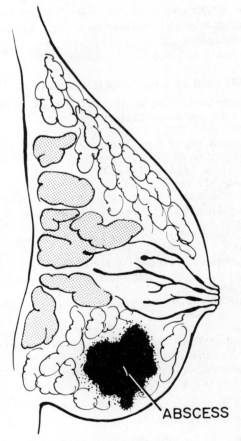

**Figure 54-6.** A breast abscess.

usually is hospitalized, placed on isolation precautions, and treated with antibiotics. A localized lesion may be incised, drained, and packed. Because the soiled dressings are highly infectious, the nurse should keep a separate dressing tray at the patient's bedside.

Montgomery straps can be used so that the frequent removal of adhesive tape will not irritate the skin. If warm soaks are ordered, vaseline is applied to the surrounding skin to avoid maceration. Massaging the neck and shoulder muscles on the affected side may help to decrease the pain by relaxing those muscles. The arm and the shoulder should be supported with pillows. The patient is instructed not to shave axillary hair on that side until healing is complete. She also needs to be taught how to prevent spread of infection to other body parts and to other persons.

A postpartum patient admitted to the hospital with a breast abscess is often worried about the new baby she had to leave in someone else's care at home, and about the added expense of a second and an unexpected hospitalization. The social service department may be able to arrange for temporary assistance.

## REFERENCES AND BIBLIOGRAPHY

American Cancer Society, 1972, *Reach to Recovery*. 1973, *A Breast Check*.

ANDERSON, D. E.: Familial factors in breast cancer and their implications, *Hosp. Pract.* 7:107, June 1972.

BAILEY, A. G., et al.: Paget's disease of the nipple, *Hosp. Med.* 8:7, May 1972.

BARD, M., and SUTHERLAND, H.: Psychological impact of cancer and its treatment. IV. Adaptation to radical mastectomy, *Cancer* 8:656, July-August 1955.

*Breast Carcinoma Monograph,* New York, Memorial Hospital for Cancer and Allied Diseases, 1973.

DAVIS, H. H., et al.: Cystic disease of the breast: Relationship to cancer, *Cancer* 17:957, 1964.

DIETZ, J. H., JR.: Rehabilitation of the cancer patient, *Med. Clin. N. Am.* 53:607, May 1969.

EGAN, R.: Mammography, *Am. J. Nurs.* 66:108, January 1966.

FOSS, G., et al.: Postmastectomy exercises, how to make them painless, more effective, *Nurs. '74* 4:23, June 1974.

GRIBBONS, C. A., et al.: Treatment for advanced breast carcinoma, *Am. J. Nurs.* 72:678, April 1972.

HARRIS, H., and SPRATT, J. S., JR.: Bilateral adrenalectomy in metastatic mammary cancer, *Cancer* 23:145, January 1969.

HARTLEY, I., and BRANDT, E.: Control and prevention of lymphedema following radical mastectomy, *Nurs. Res.* 16:333, Fall, 1967.

HARRELL, H. C.: To lose a breast, *Am. J. Nurs.* 72:676, April 1972.

LEIS, H. P., JR.: Surgical procedures for breast cancer, (Pictorial) *RN* 37:OR-ED 1, January 1974.

Mastectomy's challenge: Nursing grand rounds, *Nurs. '72* 2:7, June 1972.

*The Mastectomy Controversy.* Kemmerer, W.: For radical mastectomy. Cruz, A.: For modified mastectomy. *Nurs. '72* 2:12, June 1972.

MAYO, P., and WILKEY, N.: Prevention of cancer of the breast and cervix, *Nurs. Clin. N. Am.* 3:229, June 1968.

McCORKLE, M.: Coping with physical symptoms in metastatic breast cancer, *Am. J. Nurs.* 73:1034, June 1973.

MERCADO, R.: Radiotherapy, in Spratt, J., and Donegan, W.: *Cancer of the Breast,* Philadelphia, Saunders, 1967.

Metropolitan Life Insurance Co.: *Statistical Bulletin,* Vol. 50, March 1969.

OWEN, M.: Special care for the patient who has a breast biopsy or mastectomy, *Nurs. Clin. N. Am.* 7:373, June 1972.

PEREZ, M. D.: Pathology of mammary carcinoma, in Spratt, J., and Donegan, W.: *Cancer of the Breast,* Philadelphia, Saunders, 1967.

The post-mastectomy patient: Emotional and physical rehabilitation. *Patient Care* 4:102, December 15, 1970.

QUINT, J. C.: The impact of mastectomy, *Am. J. Nurs.* 63:88, November 1963.

ROBBINS, G.: Personal Communication.

ROBERTS, M. M., et al.: Simple versus radical mastectomy, *Nurs. Digest,* 2:85, January 1974, abstracted from *The Lancet,* May 19, 1973.

RODMAN, M.: Anticancer chemotherapy, Part 2, Against solid malignant tumors, *RN* 35:61, March 1972.

Supportive care for the postmastectomy patient. Ch. 8:6 in *Breast Carcinoma Monograph,* New York, Memorial Hospital for Cancer and Allied Diseases, 1973.

The treatment of women with advanced breast carcinoma: additive and ablative methods. Ch. 9:72, in *Breast Carcinoma Monograph,* New York, Memorial Hospital for Cancer and Allied Diseases, 1973.

WAKELY, C.: Tumours occurring in the male breast, (pictorial) *Nurs. Mirror,* 137:26, August 17, 1973.

# The Patient with Venereal Disease

## CHAPTER 55

Venereal diseases spread primarily through sexual relationships. Classically, there have been five venereal diseases: gonorrhea, syphilis, granuloma inguinale, lymphogranuloma venereum, and chancroid. However, today there is growing awareness that practitioners dealing with venereal diseases see many other diseases that are transmitted through sexual relationships; in fact in many places the term sexually transmitted disease has replaced the term venereal disease (Table 55-1). Although most texts on venereal disease concentrate on syphilis and gonorrhea, as is the case with this chapter, the nurse must realize that patients may have a variety of health problems due to sexual relationships. Patients with any sexually transmitted disease need medical and nursing care, and such care should not be limited to the classic venereal diseases, as is unfortunately still the case in some treatment facilities.

### Table 55-1. Sexually Transmitted Diseases

| TYPE OF ORGANISM | DISEASE |
| --- | --- |
| Viruses | Herpes genitalis |
| | Condylomata acuminata (venereal warts) |
| Chlamydia | Lymphogranuloma venereum |
| | Nonspecific urethritis* |
| Bacteria | Syphilis |
| | Gonorrhea |
| | Chancroid |
| | Granuloma inguinale |
| Fungi | Candidiasis |
| Protozoa | Trichomoniasis |
| Large parasites | Pediculosis pubis (crabs) |

*The chlamydial etiology of nonspecific urethritis is not considered to be proven.

## GONORRHEA

Gonorrhea is the most common of the sexually transmitted diseases, and has been known since antiquity. It is a bacterial disease that mainly affects the genital tract, but can spread to more distant sites. Gonorrhea is a common cause of sterility in both men and women. Its control is made difficult due to reluctance of patients and physicians to report it.

### Etiology

Gonorrhea is caused by infections with the bacterium *Neisseria gonorrheae*, commonly called the gonococcus. This organism is a gram-negative diplococcus. On smears of pus from patients with gonorrhea, pairs of gonococci are generally seen within leukocytes, but the organisms can also be found extracellularly.

The gonococcus has fastidious growth and survival requirements. A carbon dioxide atmosphere is necessary to initiate growth on culture and this creates problems in obtaining adequate cultures away from the laboratory. In addition, the gonococcus needs moisture for survival, and is destroyed easily by drying. Therefore, it is very difficult for gonorrhea to be spread on inanimate objects, and almost all gonorrhea, with the exception of some disease in children, is spread by sexual contact.

### Clinical Features

To appreciate the consequences of gonococcal infection, it must be realized that a large percentage of people infected with the gonococcus are asymptomatic or have symptoms of such a mild nature that they do not seek medical care. About three-quarters of the women with gonococcal infections are asymptomatic, and it is now thought that many males with gonococcal infection may also be asymptomatic or have very mild symptoms. Such asymptomatic individuals can unknowingly spread the infection.

The classically described picture of gonorrhea is that of the male patient with acute gonococcal urethritis. The incubation period is generally three to five days, although it can be between one day and two weeks. The earliest symptoms are an uncomfortable sensation in the urethra, followed by frequency of urination. This is followed, often in a matter of hours, by a purulent, yellow urethral discharge. The inflammation generally starts in the anterior urethra, but if untreated, can spread back to the posterior urethra, prostate, seminal vesicles, and epididymis.

In the female the initial infection usually involves the cervix, Skene's glands, Bartholin's glands, and the urethra. Although most infections in the female are asymptomatic, when local symptoms do occur, they are related to these structures. Spread of the disease in the female leads to pelvic inflammatory disease, which may occur soon after acute infection or may be delayed for several months. When it occurs, the fallopian tubes are frequently affected. The purulent inflammation of the fallopian tubes may become trapped, forming a pyosalpinx; may escape into the abdominal cavity resulting in peritonitis; or may result in scar tissue blocking the tubes. These tubal strictures may prevent the ovum from passing through the tubes, resulting in ectopic pregnancy or sterility.

Symptoms of primary gonococcal infection are not infrequently seen in extragenital locations. Rectal gonorrhea in the male is usually the result of homosexual contact, while in women proctitis may be due to direct spread from vaginal discharges as well as from genitorectal exposures. Acute gonococcal pharyngitis is now commonly seen and is usually the result of fellatio with a male who has a urethral infection.

In addition, gonococci can be spread through the bloodstream and cause symptoms distant from the genital tract. These distant complications occur in approximately one in 100 cases, but because of the high incidence of gonorrhea, they are not rare events in facilities giving medical care to these patients. Before effective antibiotic therapy became available complications were more prevalent in men than in women, but today they are more common in women, probably because men are more likely to develop symptomatic gonorrhea and are more likely to receive treatment for early symptoms.

The most common distant complications of gonorrhea are arthritis and a cutaneous eruption, which can occur together. Rarer complications are meningitis and endocarditis.

The gonococcus may also affect the eyes, particularly those of the newborn infant who becomes infected when passing through the birth canal of an infected mother. The infant develops severe gonococcal conjunctivitis, called *ophthalmia neonatorum*. Silver nitrate solution or antibiotic ointment is usually instilled into the eyes of newborn infants to prevent ophthalmia neonatorum. Home deliveries, where this method may not be used, present increased risk of this complication.

## Laboratory Diagnosis

In men with acute purulent gonococcal urethritis, a stained smear of the urethral exudate usually provides the diagnosis. Gram-negative diplococci are seen on the smear. These smears are inadequate in the female, and required bacteriologic cultures are usually taken from the cervix. Today cultures are also taken from the rectum and pharynx as well, when clinically or epidemiologically indicated, and to diagnose asymptomatic or mildly symptomatic gonorrhea in males.

While several media are used for bacteriologic culture of gonococci, that used most often is Thayer-Martin medium, which must be incubated in a carbon dioxide atmosphere (usually obtained by using a candle jar). Various other media are available for transporting and culturing gonococci, but most systems are not completely satisfactory in all respects.

No reliable blood test for gonorrhea is available, although research efforts are being made to develop such a test.

## Treatment

Primary treatment for uncomplicated gonorrhea, recommended by most authorities, is aqueous procaine penicillin, 4.8 million units, plus 1.0 Gm. of probenecid. This regimen gives a very high blood level of penicillin, and, thus far, has proved to be very effective, even against penicillin-resistant gonococci. It is also effective in preventing incubating syphilis. However, the large dose required, the possibility of penicillin allergy (particularly life-threatening anaphylaxis), and the occasional psychotic reaction observed to the large dose of injected procaine, are disadvantageous. The injection of penicillin must be given in facilities and under circumstances where emergency treatment can be given should serious complications develop.

Alternative oral therapy is 3.5 Gm. of ampicillin combined with 1.0 Gm. of probenecid administered simultaneously. For patients allergic to penicillin, 2.0 Gm. of spectinomycin in the male and 4.0 Gm. in the female can be given. Alternative oral therapy is tetracycline, 1.5 Gm. initially and 0.5 Gm. four times a day for four days (total 9.5 Gm.), with equivalent doses of tetracycline

analogues. The disadvantage of this last therapy is that it cannot be given at one time and patient cooperation is needed for the complete course. Because social stigma causes many persons to seek treatment from friends or through a sexual partner, many receive inappropriate drugs or dosage.

## SYPHILIS

Syphilis (lues) is one of the most serious of the sexually transmitted diseases, because, if untreated, it may produce seriously damaging and life-threatening complications many years after the original infection.

### Etiology

The causative organism of syphilis is a delicate spirochete, *Treponema pallidum,* found in lesions and in the bloodstream. Moisture and the warmth of the body are necessary for its survival. The organism is transmitted by direct contact with infectious lesions, and usually involves some form of sexual relationship. Syphilis is almost never spread by inanimate objects. The lesions of primary and secondary syphilis are highly infectious, while those of late syphilis, which may contain some spirochetes, are not considered to be so. During the latter half of pregnancy, syphilis can also be transported across the placenta from mother to fetus.

### Clinical Features

The incubation period of syphilis ranges from 10 to 90 days, with an average of 21 days. The lesion of *primary syphilis* is called a chancre, a relatively painless, highly infectious ulcer swarming with spirochetes (see Plate 3). The chancre usually develops at the site where the spirochetes enter the body and is found most often on the genitalia, for example, on the penis, the wall of the vagina, or in the area of the rectum or mouth. Occasionally a chancre will be found elsewhere on the body.

The patient with primary syphilis is generally well, but often has enlarged lymph glands in the area draining the chancre. In the female, a small chancre may not be noticed and the patient will infect others, but even if untreated, the chancre will eventually disappear, generally in two to five weeks, and the patient remains highly infectious to others.

The *secondary* stage of syphilis occurs between

six weeks to six months after onset. There can be many manifestations of secondary syphilis, the most common of which is a rash that can take a variety of forms and is often diffuse (see Plate 4). On mucous membranes, as in the genital region or in the mouth, highly infectious luetic plaques (condylomas) develop. Sometimes the patient loses hair in patches, giving the head a moth-eaten appearance. There is often generalized enlargement of lymph glands, and there may be a variety of other rarer symptoms, such as fever, headache, and malaise, but the patient may feel completely well. Symptoms of secondary syphilis generally disappear in a few weeks, although they may reappear only to disappear again after a short time. It should be emphasized that the primary and secondary stages are the infectious stages of syphilis, and it is at this time that the patient is in danger of transmitting the disease to others.

During the *latent period* of the disease, the patient has no signs nor symptoms, and the presence of syphilis can only be determined by a positive blood test. About two-thirds of the patients with latent syphilis will never be troubled by the disease again, but the remaining one-third, if untreated, will eventually develop additional symptoms anywhere from one year to twenty or thirty years later.

Symptomatic syphilis at this stage is known as *late syphilis* or the *tertiary stage* of syphilis. Whereas lesions of early syphilis usually are merely annoying to the patient (although they are infectious to others), the late complications are feared. Late syphilis is generally not infectious, but it does lead to serious disability and even death.

The most serious life-threatening complication of late syphilis is cardiovascular syphilis, which most often strikes the aorta. Patches of necrosis occur in the wall of the vessel causing the wall to thin and an aneurysm to develop. The aneurysm may grow as the aortic wall thins, eventually bursting so that the patient bleeds to death. In the heart, the spirochetes may invade the aortic ring or aortic valves, causing narrowing of the coronary vessels and coronary insufficiency, or valvular damage and aortic insufficiency.

In terms of disability, late neurologic complications of syphilis are varied and severe. For example, syphilitic lesions of the nervous system occasionally cause meningitis, which responds to antiluetic therapy. Another manifestation of central nervous system involvement is general paresis, a chronic

syphilitic meningoencephalitis. In these cases the patient exhibits slight changes in personality, which may begin ten or twenty years after the original infection; memory and judgment become impaired. The mental state varies from euphoria to depression to paranoia. Often these patients require hospitalization in a psychiatric institution. If the disease progresses, optic atrophy with blindness may occur and the patient becomes totally helpless, both physically and mentally, and eventually dies.

Another neural complication of syphilis is tabes dorsalis, in which the posterior spinal nerve roots, the posterior columns of the spinal cord, and posterior root ganglia become infected and degenerate. This syndrome may appear five to twenty years after the original infection, and the first symptoms are frequently pain and loss of position sense. Very often the pain is severe, knifelike, and burning. Tabetic crises, acute attacks of severe abdominal pain with vomiting, may occur. The patient with tabes dorsalis has eye involvement, i.e., the eyes accommodate to near and far vision, but the pupils do not react to light (Argyll Robertson sign). Optic atrophy with blindness may occur. A further complication of tabes dorsalis is the Charcot joint, in which the joint atrophies, due to syphilitic involvement of its innervation, becomes excessively motile, and will not support weight. The knee and the spine are most frequently involved.

Gummas, well-defined local lesions, develop in tertiary syphilis. The gummas contain far fewer spirochetes than the chancre of early syphilis; they may develop in any tissue, but they appear most frequently in skin, bones, liver, larynx, and testes. Whenever these lesions occur, they may give rise to symptoms of dysfunction of the affected organ.

Congenital syphilis, which occurs when the fetus is infected during pregnancy, may occur at any stage of the disease in the mother. *Treponema pallidum* can cross the placenta during the last half of pregnancy. Therefore a pregnant woman with untreated syphilis risks spreading the disease to her baby. The disease can also result in a miscarriage, the birth of a full-term stillborn infant, or a baby with congenital syphilis.

There are both early and late lesions of congenital syphilis. The early lesions generally appear during the first few weeks after birth although they may appear up to the age of two. They include skin lesions that are frequently vesicular, as well as cutaneous lesions that resemble those of acquired syphilis. The mucous membranes of the nose and pharynx are frequently involved with a heavy mucoid discharge referred to as the "sniffles." Both skin and mucous membrane lesions are teeming with spirochetes and are therefore infectious. Bone involvement as well as anemia, enlargement of the liver and spleen, and abnormal spinal fluid findings, can also occur.

Many years later there can be lesions of late congenital syphilis. These occur because of continued activity of the disease process or they may be due to scarring. Late congenital syphilis is not infectious. The lesions include an interstitial keratitis in which the cornea of the eye becomes opaque. There are also lesions of the teeth resulting in so-called Hutchinson's teeth and mulberry molars, or there can be bone involvement, one of the most prominent being sabre chins, and lesions of the skin. The patient with congenital syphilis can also have neurosyphilis, cardiovascular lesions, and gummas.

Congenital syphilis is treated as would be the appropriate stage of acquired syphilis, except that reduced doses of antibiotics are used in infants. The most important thing about congenital syphilis is its prevention. A mother with syphilis who is treated during the first half of pregnancy will not infect her infant, as she will be cured before the spirochetes can cross the placenta. Since penicillin also crosses the placenta, treatment of a mother after the fetus has been infected will also cure the fetal infection, although previous damage to the fetus may not be repaired.

### Laboratory Diagnosis

There is no practical way to grow *Treponema pallidum* in a bacteriology laboratory. Laboratory diagnosis of syphilis is made by visualizing the spirochetes on a smear or by serologic tests.

Since early lesions of syphilis usually swarm with spirochetes, those in fluid from the primary chancre or from a moist lesion of secondary syphilis can be seen under a microscope. A darkfield condenser must be used on the microscope and the moving spirochetes viewed against a dark background. This examination is particularly important in primary syphilis, because serologic tests frequently are not positive during the early stages of the disease and the darkfield examination may be the only way to diagnose syphilis.

The serologic tests for syphilis can be divided into two types, nontreponemal and treponemal tests. The nontreponemal tests are generally easier to perform and less expensive than the treponemal and are therefore better suited to large-scale screening. The antigen used in these tests has no biologic relationship to the treponeme, but is similar antigenically. There are numerous nontreponemal tests, each named after the individual or laboratory that first devised it. The original test was the Wassermann but the test used most often today is the VDRL (Venereal Disease Research Laboratory) test. These nontreponemal tests are very sensitive in picking up syphilis and are also useful in following the results of therapy in early syphilis. Unfortunately, they are not always specific for syphilis. Many other conditions can give a positive serologic test, in which case the result is referred to as a biologic false-positive (BFP) test. A persistently positive BFP can signify serious disease, such as a collagen disease like lupus erythematosus. Therefore, every initially positive nontreponemal test should be followed by a treponemal test.

The early prototype treponemal test was the treponema pallidum immobilization test (TPI). This is a difficult test that only a few laboratories are able to do. Several other tests have subsequently been developed, the most recent ones being the fluorescent antibody tests. The most commonly used test today is the FTA-ABS test, which is much more specific for syphilis than are the nontreponemal tests, although false-positive reactions also occur with the treponemal tests. A combination of a positive nontreponemal test and a positive treponemal test is presumptive evidence that the patient has had a syphilitic infection. A positive test may remain positive throughout life and so does not necessarily indicate current infection.

Serologic tests should be performed on all patients with lesions even remotely suspicious of syphilis. Contacts of syphilitic patients should receive serologic tests as well as all patients thought to be at some risk of acquiring syphilis. For example, all patients with gonorrhea should be tested for syphilis.

### Treatment

Penicillin is the drug of choice in the treatment of syphilis. Unlike the situation with gonorrhea, very high levels of penicillin are not necessary, but it is important that penicillin be in the bloodstream for many days to give adequate treatment. There is no evidence that *Treponema pallidum* has become penicillin resistant.

The generally recommended treatment is a single injection of 2.4 million units of long-lasting penicillin, such as benzathine penicillin G. Adequate treatment can also be accomplished by giving aqueous procaine penicillin (600,000 units for ten days). For patients who cannot take penicillin because of an allergy, erythromycin or tetracycline can be used, although tetracycline should not be used in a pregnant woman. Periodic followup is indicated, and serologic tests should be repeated every three months for one to two years.

During the late stages of syphilis, penicillin is still the treatment of choice, but larger dosages of drugs are given. Organs already damaged by syphilis cannot be repaired and therefore treatment with penicillin can only halt the process but will not restore the damaged organs.

Specific measures for other care are also indicated in patients with late syphilis, such as cardiac care for the patient with cardiovascular syphilis or specific neurologic supportive care for the patient with neurosyphilis.

## GRANULOMA INGUINALE

Granuloma inguinale is a slowly progressive disease of the skin and mucous membranes, with some involvement of the lymph nodes. Ulcerative, nodular, and scarring forms occur, with gradual extension over the genital and inguinal areas. Severe mutilating effects are seen in untreated patients, who have an increased likelihood of developing carcinoma in the involved areas. The causative organism is *Calymmatobacterium granulomatis*. Aggregates of the organism, noted in biopsy, form what are called *Donovan bodies*. Tetracycline, ampicillin, and streptomycin have been used effectively in treatment.

## LYMPHOGRANULOMA VENEREUM

Lymphogranuloma venereum (LGV) is caused by the organism chlamydia, which was once thought to be a virus, but because they have a more intricate structure and metabolism than do true viruses, they are now classified separately. Chlamydia are also responsible for such diseases as trachoma and psittacosis.

The symptoms of LGV are variable, ranging from very mild to severe illness. A typical course of illness starts with mild ulceration, usually on the genitalia but sometimes in the mouth or anus. This usually disappears, but is soon followed by enlarged lymph nodes draining the primary area, usually the inguinal nodes in the male. In the female various nodes in the genital and rectal areas are involved. Abscesses form, which become necrotic, and many suppurate through the skin. These lesions are called buboes. The patient feels weak and has fever, chills, and anorexia. If untreated, late persistent edema (elephantiasis) of the genitals, and rectal strictures may result.

Laboratory diagnosis is made by a skin test known as the *Frei test,* and by a serologic test (a complement fixation test). Neither test is highly sensitive and false-positive results for LGV have occurred in patients infected with other chlamydia. Tetracyclines or sulfonamides are used in treatment. Fluctuant lymph nodes may be aspirated, but never incised. Surgery may have to be undertaken to correct polypoid masses, elephantiasis, and rectal strictures.

## CHANCROID

Chancroid is a very common disease about the world, although it is not seen too often in the United States. It is an acute disease characterized by large multiple ulcerations of the genitals. Regional lymph nodes are also involved with abscess formation. The causative organism is *Hemophilus ducreyi*. This bacterium is difficult to isolate and diagnosis is frequently made on the basis of the clinical findings and the exclusion of other venereal diseases, such as syphilis. Chancroid is not infrequently found in association with another venereal disease. Sulfonamides and tetracyclines are effective therapy for chancroid.

## CANDIDIASIS

Candidiasis is usually caused by the yeast *Candida albicans*. Susceptibility to infection is influenced by a variety of host factors, including oral contraceptives, pregnancy, and the use of broad spectrum antibiotics.

Women often complain of itching, in the vulvar and anal area, associated with a white vaginal discharge. A dermatitis frequently develops on the skin around the external genitalia, thighs, and perineum. The vaginal wall may also be inflamed, and the patient may have pain on urination and on sexual intercourse. The male often has urethritis and the skin of the penis, scrotum, or thighs is involved.

Diagnosis is made by observing the small budding spores and mycelia in scrapings from lesions. Topical treatment, which consists of nystatin or amphotericin B creams or nystatin vaginal inserts for vaginitis, is generally used (see Chap. 52).

## TRICHOMONIASIS

Trichomoniasis is an infection with a flagellated protozoan, *Trichomonas vaginalis*. While trichomoniasis of the vagina has been recognized for a long time, it is now well established as a sexually transmitted disease. Trichomoniasis occurs frequently in association with gonorrhea.

Women may be asymptomatic, but usually complain of an irritating vaginal discharge. There may be pain on sexual intercourse and on urination. The vulva may be infected with excoriation of the thighs. The vaginal discharge has a yellow color, musty odor, and frothy consistency. There may be red spots on the mucosa of the cervix and the vaginal wall is often involved. Most males with trichomoniasis are asymptomatic, although some may have urethritis and other symptoms related to the genitourinary tract.

*Trichomonas vaginalis* is usually identified on a fresh moist slide preparation from the discharge. It is best observed with a darkfield microscope, the motile protozoan being seen in the preparation. There are also culture techniques for the organism. Oral metronidazole is used for treatment of trichomoniasis. If reinfection is to be avoided, it is important that the sex partner also be treated (see Chap. 52).

## HERPES GENITALIS

Herpes genitalis is caused by *Herpesvirus hominis* (herpes simplex). This virus has two antigenic types: Type I, which causes herpes labialis (the common cold sore), and Type II, which causes herpes genitalis. Herpes genitalis is a serious sexually transmitted disease because (1) it produces a painful, inflammatory dermatosis, (2) it can cause extremely severe illness and death in infants born to a mother with genital herpes, and (3) it may lead to the development of cervical carcinoma.

Genital herpes infections can be grouped into primary and recurrent infections. A primary infection may be asymptomatic and only become apparent when recurrent infection later develops. When symptomatic, the primary infection is accompanied by systemic symptoms of fever, headache and malaise. The lesions are vesicular, often progressing to deep ulcers with surrounding inflammation. The draining lymph nodes are involved and may be extremely tender. Recurrent herpes also has vesicular lesions, but the extent of the lesions, the pain and discomfort associated with them and draining lymph nodes is less than with primary infection. Constitutional symptoms are also less severe with recurrent herpes.

Laboratory diagnosis can be made by obtaining a smear from the lesion, and, after appropriate staining, visualizing multinucleated, giant cells under the microscope. The herpes virus can also be grown in a laboratory equipped for the diagnosis of viral infections. Treatment for herpes is not completely satisfactory because it is nonspecific. Local compresses of 0.25 per cent silver nitrate, 1:6000 potassium permanganate, 1:4000 benzalkonium chloride, or boric acid solution are often used.

Of particular concern is herpes genitalis infection in the pregnant woman. If the infant becomes infected, it can suffer an overwhelming, often-fatal virus infection, that most often occurs through the birth canal. The situation is particularly dangerous when there is prolonged rupture of membranes. Cesarean section should be performed on women with active genital herpes infection at the time of labor.

In recent years there has been a good deal written about the relationship between genital herpes and cervical carcinoma. Although the mass of evidence suggests the two diseases are related, it is not conclusive.

## VENEREAL WARTS (CONDYLOMATA ACUMINATA)

Condylomata acuminata, or venereal warts, are caused by a virus that is thought to be similar to the virus causing common skin warts. The warts tend to appear one to three months after the infecting sexual intercourse. In men, the most commonly affected areas are about the penis; in women, the area about the vaginal opening is commonly affected, although deeper vaginal and cervical lesions can be found. Venereal warts can also be found about the anus and in the mouth, following anal or oral intercourse.

In moist areas, the warts are usually pink, or red and soft with an indented cauliflowerlike appearance. Warts can be single or multiple. On dry skin, they are more often small, hard, and yellow-gray, resembling ordinary skin warts on other parts of the body. The diagnosis is generally made by the appearance of the lesions. If warts are small, they can be removed easily by applying podophyllin. Larger warts may have to be removed surgically.

## NONSPECIFIC URETHRITIS
## (NONGONOCOCCAL URETHRITIS, NSU)

A large number of infections of the lower urogenital tract present a syndrome for which no specific etiology has been found. They are grouped together as nonspecific urethritis or nongonococcal urethritis. In many European countries, patients with nonspecific urethritis constitute the largest number of those with a sexually transmitted disease.

There have been many attempts to find the cause of nonspecific urethritis. In recent years most attention has focused on chlamydia and mycoplasma organisms, particularly the former. It is possible that nonspecific urethritis syndrome may involve more than one etiology.

In the male the usual symptoms are low-grade urethritis, with scanty or moderate mucopurulent discharge and some discomfort on urination. The clinician can usually distinguish this syndrome from gonococcal urethritis, but occasionally nonspecific urethritis will manifest itself as a more severe urethritis, resembling that caused by the gonococcus. Conversely, the illness may be so mild as to be discovered only on careful examination of a sex contact. The chief complication of nonspecific urethritis in the man is prostatitis.

In the woman the disease is often asymptomatic, or of a very mild nature that may be disregarded. Acute or recurrent cystitis, such as "honeymoon cystitis," may be related to this syndrome.

The diagnosis of nonspecific urethritis is one of exclusion, by demonstrating a urethritis with no specific cause being found. The best treatment available is the use of tetracyclines for at least a week, although this is not always satisfactory. A great deal still remains to be learned about this disease, which is becoming one of the most important sexually transmitted diseases.

## EPIDEMIOLOGY OF VENEREAL DISEASE
## IN THE UNITED STATES

Syphilis, gonorrhea, chancroid, granuloma inguinale, and lymphogranuloma venereum are reportable diseases in most health jurisdictions in the United States. The last three diseases are relatively rare in the United States. The other sexually trans-

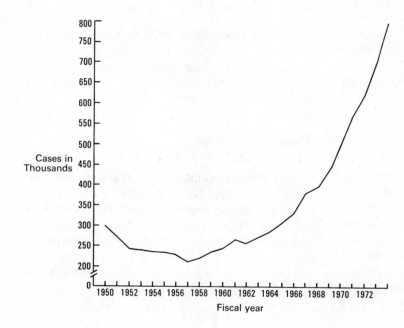

Source: Public Health Service

**Figure 55-1.** Reported cases of gonorrhea in the United States, fiscal years 1950-1973. (Courtesy, American Social Health Association)

mitted diseases are not reportable and there is very little data on their occurrence. However, most clinicians dealing with sexually transmitted diseases believe that there has been a real increase in the incidence of all of these diseases. In many venereal disease clinics, patients with syphilis and gonorrhea represent only a minority of the patients seen with sexually transmitted diseases.

Although gonorrhea is a reportable disease, reporting practices of physicians are poor. It is estimated that only one of every ten cases of gonorrhea is reported. Venereal disease clinics maintained by public health departments are much more likely to report cases than are physicians in private practice. Data therefore are biased toward cases occurring in cities, where most clinics are located, as contrasted with suburban and rural areas. Syphilis is more likely to be reported than gonorrhea, although statistics are still far from complete. Adequate reporting is available only for early syphilis, and since infectious syphilis is the most important in establishing public health trends, only the more reliable data on primary and secondary syphilis will be discussed here. There are no reliable data on the prevalence of cardiovascular and neurosyphilis in the population, but it is generally believed that these conditions are far less prevalent at this time than in the past.

Gonorrhea is the most frequently reported disease in the United States. As can be seen in the graph in Fig. 55-1, the incidence of gonorrhea has increased markedly during the past decade. Some of this increase is due to fuller reporting of gonorrhea and to special programs to find new cases, but there has undoubtedly been a real increase in gonorrhea. It has become popular to talk about the current epidemic of gonorrhea. One hopeful sign is that in the past year the rapid rise in the incidence of gonorrhea appears to have reached a plateau.

As shown in Fig. 55-2, from a sharp drop in incidence in the 1950s, the incidence of primary and secondary syphilis rose in the early 1960s and then leveled off, with slight ups and downs. This has been disappointing to public health authorities and to all concerned with health, because it was hoped that large scale programs initiated in the 1960s would bring a marked decrease in the incidence of syphilis.

Venereal diseases occur in all areas of society and in all types of communities (Fig. 55-3). However, in allocating our health care resources, it is

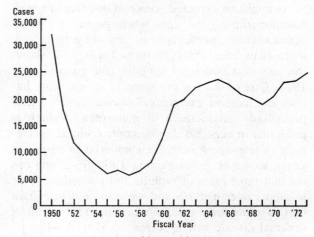

Source: Public Health Service

**Figure 55-2.** Reported cases of primary and secondary syphilis in the United States, fiscal years 1950-1973. (Courtesy, American Social Health Association)

important to be aware that there are areas of higher venereal disease incidence. Despite reporting biases, cities have a higher incidence of most venereal diseases than more outlying areas, and therefore cities need more resources to control these diseases than do other areas.

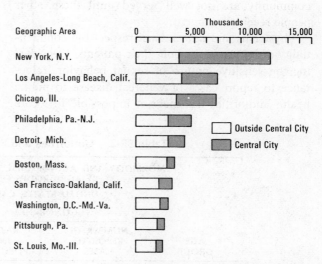

A standard metropolitan statistical area (SMSA) is a county or group of contiguous counties that are socially and economically integrated with at least one central city of 50,000 inhabitants or more, or with "twin cities" having a combined population of at least 50,000.
Source: Reports from the Bureau of the Census, the National Center for Health Statistics, and the Virginia State Department of Health

**Figure 55-3.** Population in leading standard metropolitan statistical areas, April 1, 1970, including reported corrections to April 1, 1972. (Courtesy, Metropolitan Life Insurance Company)

As might be expected, venereal diseases are most common during the ages when people are more active sexually, particularly in terms of activity with more than one sexual partner. Table 55-2 shows the age distribution of syphilis and gonorrhea in 1972. One of the big problems in recent years has been the increase in venereal disease in teen-agers, particularly an increase in gonorrhea. Numerous programs in venereal disease control aimed specifically at teen-agers have been undertaken in recent years. However, by examining Table 55-2, one can see that most cases of syphilis and gonorrhea occur in adults over age 20, and we must not lose sight of this older age group in our desire to control venereal disease among teen-agers (Fig. 55-4).

## Public Health and Preventive Aspects of Venereal Diseases

The responsibility of physicians, nurses, and other health care personnel does not end when a particular patient receives proper treatment. A patient with a sexually transmitted disease was infected by another person who may also have infected others. Thus, other people must be examined and appropriately treated. The patients and the community are not well served until these other people receive treatment.

Physicians and nurses must respect the confidentiality of information about their patients. Considering the sensitive nature of sexual behavior, reluctance to report cases of venereal disease to public health authorities has made it impossible to locate for treatment the sexual contacts of patients. Aside from the fact that it is a violation of the law not to report certain venereal diseases, this attitude generally does not serve the patient nor the public well. If a patient's contacts are not treated, especially if it is a spouse or a regular sexual partner, that contact can reinfect the patient. In addition, a person in close relationship to the patient may have, or be incubating, a venereal disease, and should be treated early before complications develop. Privacy during the physical examination and during the interview are essential. Reluctance to seek treatment may stem, for example, from a marital partner's dismay at having to reveal infidelity. Sexually transmitted disease may affect children who acquire the disease from an adult in the home. Under such circumstances, there may be particular reluctance to report the child's symptoms. The school nurse or community health nurse may be the first to notice the symptoms. Disease transmitted by homosexual contact presents particularly distressing problems because, despite the greater openness of recent years, society's attitudes often continue to be harshly rejecting and punitive. Patients who have contracted a venereal disease often show emotional responses of guilt, fear of exposure, and its possible consequences upon their personal and coworker relationships, anger, and shame.

A mother, upon discovering she has gonorrhea, may become overanxious about the possibility of transmitting the disease to her children. A marital partner may respond with rage, not only at having

**Table 55-2. Gonorrhea and Primary and Secondary Syphilis**

| AGE GROUP | MORBIDITY AND AGE—SPECIFIC RATES PER 100,000 POPULATION BY AGE GROUPS OF REPORTED CASES UNITED STATES, CALENDAR YEAR 1972 | | | |
|---|---|---|---|---|
| | GONORRHEA | | PRIMARY AND SECONDARY SYPHILIS | |
| | NUMBER OF REPORTED CASES | RATE PER 100,000 POPULATION | NUMBER OF REPORTED CASES | RATE PER 100,000 POPULATION |
| 0-9 | 2,191 | 6.1 | 20 | .1 |
| 10-14 | 7,777 | 37.4 | 212 | 1.0 |
| 15-19 | 204,635 | 1,035.4 | 4,035 | 20.4 |
| 20-24 | 311,051 | 1,813.5 | 7,216 | 42.1 |
| 25-29 | 135,220 | 921.6 | 4,811 | 32.8 |
| 30-39 | 79,789 | 347.2 | 5,232 | 22.8 |
| 40-49 | 19,897 | 84.6 | 1,986 | 8.4 |
| 50+ | 6,655 | 12.9 | 917 | 1.8 |
| Total | 767,215 | 371.6 | 24,429 | 11.8 |

Source: Public Health Service

the disease, but at the realization that the partner originally acquired it from a third party. Persuading patients to accept treatment and to assist in tracing contacts must be done with sensitive recognition of the patient's emotional response and of the repercussions of the situation upon his life. For one person, a case of gonorrhea may be considered a joke; another may feel overwhelmed with shame.

The nurse can have an important role in case finding and in assisting patients and their sexual contacts to receive treatment. The school nurse and community health nurse are in situations that require their sensitive concern and astute observation for possible symptoms of venereal disease. As the nurse assumes broader responsibility as primary care-giver, her role in detecting significant signs and symptoms and in referring the patient are extremely important.

It is essential to stress to the patient that persons with whom he has had sexual contact require prompt examination, since they can become ill, infect others, and reinfect the patient. Many patients require instruction concerning the possible consequences of untreated disease, so that they do not mistakenly assume that, because a chancre disappears, or a vaginal discharge abates, there is no need for therapy.

A special situation exists in regard to syphilis. Over the years, a large-scale program has been developed for the control of syphilis by the U. S. Public Health Service, cooperatively with state and some local health departments. The program involves the use of trained investigators to interview patients about sexual contacts, and then to find the contacts and bring them to treatment.

The investigators also attempt to find people who, while not direct sexual contacts of the patient, are at a relatively high risk of having syphilis. This is called "cluster testing." The interviewer attempts to ask the patient about other people who might be at risk of having syphilis, such as those with lesions of secondary syphilis or whom the patient knows have had sexual contact with others who might be harboring syphilis.

These investigators are trained in motivational techniques and in the ability to find contacts and clusters, often with relatively scanty information. They are usually far better qualified to perform this job than a physician or a nurse. Therefore, in most health jurisdictions where there is a well-developed syphilis control program, a physician or a

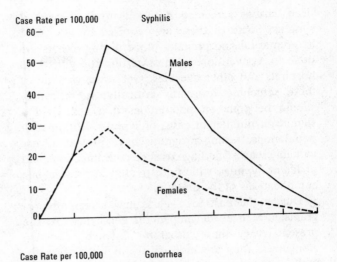

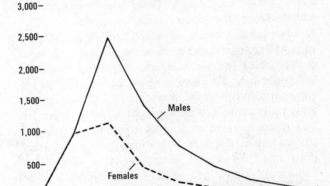

Source: *Morbidity and Mortality* 21, 53, Ann. Supp. Summary 1972, Center for Disease Control, Atlanta, Ga., June 1973

**Figure 55-4.** Incidence of venereal disease by age and sex in the United States, 1972. (Courtesy, Metropolitan Life Insurance Company)

nurse should promptly inform the public health authorities so that the trained investigators may do this work.

The issue of confidentiality must be dealt with. It is important for health personnel to explain to the patient existing policies and procedures concerning efforts to bring infected persons to treatment, and the reason this is necessary. Explanation at the time the patient first receives treatment is essential if he is to maintain a sense of trust in personnel.

In addition to direct case-finding programs involving sexual contacts of patients with venereal diseases, there are a number of screening programs that attempt to find patients with certain sexually transmitted diseases. For many years, there have been various screening programs to find cases of syphilis. Some of these are required by law, such as premarital and prenatal blood testing, others are done by convention, such as testing the patient in hospitals and other agencies. One must view all of these screening programs critically, in that they should be done on populations that will yield a significant number of cases of syphilis. Within such populations, testing programs have proved a very valuable way of finding cases of both infectious and of latent syphilis, which are treated to prevent late complications of the disease.

During the past few years, new screening programs have been developed for gonorrhea. At the present time, these programs involve screening women, as they are more likely to have asymptomatic gonorrhea. Patients who are having pelvic examinations for other purposes, such as in a family planning clinic, in a prenatal clinic, as part of a gynecologic examination, or as part of a general physical examination, are also being screened for gonorrhea. The screening procedure requires a smear for culturing the gonococcus and the culture must be examined in an appropriate laboratory.

The nurse who functions as a primary care agent (for example, the nurse who does pelvic examinations upon women to detect signs of disease or abnormality) must be aware of the need for, and be skilled in, carrying out tests for venereal disease: for example, in taking a culture for the presence of gonorrhea and referring the patient as necessary.

In the matter of prevention of venereal disease, unfortunately there is currently no vaccine available for these diseases. The primary preventive measure is to render a patient noninfectious. In this way, no matter what the sexual activities of the patient, he or she cannot infect another person. Thus, when a patient with syphilis or gonorrhea receives appropriate penicillin therapy, that patient is soon noninfectious, and thereby a preventive action has been performed for all persons with whom the patient has sexual contact. For this reason, any patient with infectious syphilis or gonorrhea should receive treatment as soon as possible, because an infectious person may have sexual intercourse in the very near future and will infect others unless treatment is accomplished promptly.

Another method of prevention is to treat patients who are possibly incubating a venereal disease. For example, a patient who has had known sexual contact with a person with proved infectious syphilis may be incubating the disease and still not show clinical or laboratory evidence of syphilis at the time the patient is first seen. Such a person should receive preventive therapy against syphilis, which is the same as that given for early syphilis. A similar situation exists with the patient who has had contact with a known case of gonorrhea and is still in the incubation period of the disease but has not developed symptoms. This patient should receive appropriate prophylactic therapy for gonorrhea. It is as important to prevent these diseases as it is to treat patients who have already developed signs and symptoms of gonorrhea.

Additionally, there is a variety of advice that can be given to patients for the prevention of venereal disease. Sexual abstinence is a preventive measure, although it usually is not a very practical means of prevention. Statistically speaking, people who have sexual relationships with one partner are much less likely to develop venereal diseases than are people who have had sexual relationships with several partners.

There are some mechanical means of prevention, such as the use of a condom. The condom is thought to be somewhat effective in lowering the incidence of some venereal diseases, when it is used properly. This means that the condom must be used through the entire period of sexual intercourse, and be removed properly. People often recommend the condom for persons who will have frequent sexual relationships with different partners. However, it should be stressed that the condom must be used properly, that it cannot be relied on as being an absolutely safe measure of preventing venereal disease, but only that it might help to lessen the chance of contracting some of the sexually transmitted diseases.

## VENEREAL DISEASE EDUCATION

Venereal disease education is a field in which the nurse plays a very active and widening role. Venereal disease education is very actively being presented to school-age populations, particularly teen-agers, and there is a definite need for the school nurse, as well as for the community health nurse, to participate actively on the venereal disease control team.

A nurse working with any patient who has a sexually transmitted disease has an essential educational role. It is important that the patient understand about his or her disease, about the complications of the disease, and the manner in which the disease was contracted. The patient should be encouraged to return for appropriate follow-up examinations, be informed of any possible preventive measures, and be aware of the need to bring sexual contacts to treatment.

The main purpose of venereal disease education is to acquaint people with the signs and symptoms of venereal disease, to acquaint them with the knowledge of how venereal diseases are acquired, to talk about possible preventive measures where applicable, and, most important, to encourage people to seek treatment if they suspect they might have a venereal disease. This involves encouraging people to see their private physician or to seek help in a clinic that treats sexually transmitted diseases. The nurse should know the location of these clinics so that she can direct patients to them. It is helpful to know the staff (or some member of the staff) and to refer the patient, who may be very embarrassed, to a specific staff member for the initial professional contact.

A nonjudgmental accepting attitude in all contacts with teen-agers can foster their seeking help with such problems as venereal disease. Often, those of this age group do not see parents as resources for information concerning sex. Sometimes information (and misinformation) is acquired from the peer group, and the adolescent experiences considerable pressure to conform to the norms of his peers. For this reason it is especially useful to deal with students through group discussions of venereal disease and sexuality, so that students can support one another and learn together. In almost every state in the United States it is now possible for minors to receive treatment for venereal disease without parental consent or knowledge. It is important for young people to know this, so that they are not deterred from seeking treatment by fear of punishment from their parents. Such fear, when it precludes treatment, places the young person's health and reproductive capacity in jeopardy, and poses a threat to others with whom he may have sexual contact.

Because of the prevalence of venereal disease among teen-agers, it is necessary to appeal to a younger age group in all preventive and case-finding measures. The use of mass media has been very effective.

An additional measure needed is available screening facilities in areas where young people are most likely to be found. It is desirable to combine screening programs in one location to appeal to a wide range of age groups and avoid stigmatization. For example, birth control information, screening for sickle cell anemia, tuberculosis, suspected pregnancy, and venereal disease could be available in one location. An important point to remember is that young people need assistance long before the premarital physical examination. Facilities for VD screening and treatment are not enough, however. Personnel should be available for patient conferences and for tracing contacts. Both individual and group conferences may be necessary. In the group setting as many as ten to twenty young people may be involved in discussions about VD facts, the influence of beliefs and attitudes about VD and sexual activity. The nurse sees people in their homes, at school, at work, in clinics, or in inpatient settings. Establishing and maintaining contact with people in these various settings provides a valuable source of accurate information and a resource person for young people. Frequently the nurse is called upon to talk with teen-agers, particularly those involved in organizations such as the Girl Scouts or Boy Scouts. In providing information about health matters she can also at this time discuss areas of sex education and clarify any misconceptions the young people may have.

An additional point is that young people who are sexually active should have the benefit of an intensive testing program. It is generally felt more profitable to interview young men for their contacts, since they are more likely to seek treatment. When girls are found to be infected on examination, they should also be interviewed for their contacts. All sexually active persons should be encouraged to seek testing when they change sex partners or when they doubt the fidelity of a sex partner.

## NURSING MEASURES FOR THE HOSPITALIZED PATIENT

Routine isolation precautions are unnecessary for patients with gonorrhea or syphilis. Instead, precautions are taken as necessary in light of the patient's condition and the possibility of transmitting the organism. The unnecessary use of such precautions as gowns and masks can lead the patient to feel rejected. Because of the stigma associated with venereal disease, it is especially important to convey acceptance to the patient and to avoid measures likely to cause him to feel isolated. There is no reason, for instance, to place the patient in a private rather than in a semiprivate room (unless the patient has chosen admission to a private room). Sometimes, previously undiscovered gonorrhea will be noted in a patient admitted to the hospital for another illness. While this patient has a discharge, contact with the discharge while it is still wet is avoided. For example, the nurse should wear gloves if she gives an enema, the patient should wash his hands after going to the bathroom, and the female patient should wash her hands after changing the perineal pad she wears while she has a discharge. Because the gonococcus has special predilection for the eye (gonorrhea used to cause a large percentage of the world's blindness, infecting newborn babies when they passed through the vagina), both the nurse and the patient should be especially careful to wash their hands before touching the face, after coming in contact with the discharge. In some hospitals the linen is considered contaminated for the first one or two days after treatment for gonorrhea is started. However, this organism dies so quickly on drying that the danger of spread of the disease by any means except direct contact with the still-wet discharge on a mucous membrane or an open cut is practically nonexistent.

Patients with primary syphilis who enter the hospital for another condition may not, while they are hospitalized, be identified as having syphilis. If serology is done, the patient may be discharged from the hospital before the results are returned, because it takes some time for the report to be returned from the laboratory. These patients with positive serology should be followed up by the appropriate public health agency so that they receive treatment for syphilis. If a patient known to have untreated primary syphilis is admitted to the hospital, precautionary measures are applied to avoid direct contact with the lesion during the brief period that the spirochetes are still alive in it after treatment has been instituted. For example, the nurse should wear gloves if she gives care that requires touching the chancre.

In one hospital it was noticed that the aides and orderlies would not enter the room of a patient with gonorrhea, although they entered the rooms of patients with other types of infections. The social stigma is such that unrealistic fears of contracting venereal disease overcome the logic of scientific precautions. The organisms are not airborne, as is the pneumococcus. They do not live outside of their warm, moist environment, as do tubercle bacilli.

Venereal disease is not limited to any socioeconomic group, although the patient in a high socioeconomic class will probably be treated by his own physician, rather than in the clinic. The patient who comes from a high socioeconomic class and who secures private treatment is probably less likely to have his disease reported to health authorities than is a lower-class patient who seeks care at a clinic. In some groups the acquisition of gonorrhea is considered halfway between a joke and a sign of virility. This attitude may not be acceptable to the nurse with a middle-class background, yet this patient also will need her teaching and understanding. This patient will also require help in realizing that gonorrhea is a serious disease that can cause severe illness and disability.

## REFERENCES AND BIBLIOGRAPHY

BENELL, F.: Drug abuse and venereal disease misconceptions of a selected group of college students, *J. School Health* 43:584, November 1973.

BRAVERMAN, S.: Homosexuality, *Am. J. Nurs.* 73:652.

BROWN, M. A.: Adolescents and VD, *Nurs. Outlook* 21:99, February 1973.

CLEERE, R. I., et al.: Physicians' attitudes toward venereal disease reporting, *JAMA* 202:941, 1967.

COHEN, R.: Suggested directions for effective future planning in regard to venereal disease control, *J. N.Y. State School Nurse Teachers Assoc.* 3:20, Winter 1973.

CONLEY, JOHN A., and THOMAS, W. O'ROURKE. "On improving instruction in sex education," *Journal of School Health,* 43(9):591-593.

*Criteria and Techniques for the Diagnosis of Gonorrhea,* Center for Disease Control, Department of Health, Education and Welfare, Venereal Disease Branch, Atlanta, Georgia, June 1973.

Editorial: Treatment of gonorrhea, *J. Infec. Dis.* 127:578, May 1973.

FLEMING, W., et al.: National survey of venereal disease treated by physicians in 1968, *JAMA* 211:1827, March 16, 1970.

HINMAN, A. R.: Venereal disease, *J. N.Y. State School Nurse Teachers Assoc.* 3:17, Winter 1972.

HOLMES, K. G.: Gonococcal infection: Clinical, epidemiological and laboratory perspectives, G. H. Stollerman (ed.), *Advances in Internal Medicine,* Vol. 19, Yearbook Medical Publishers, Inc., 1974.

JEROME, E., et al.: Gonorrhea at a teenage medical service, *Minn. Med.* 57:245, March 1974.

*Morbidity and Mortality,* Vol. 23, No. 7, week ending February 16, 1974, Center for Disease Control, U.S. Department of Health, Education and Welfare.

*Morbidity and Mortality,* Vol. 23, No. 24, week ending June 14, 1974, Center for Disease Control, U.S. Department of Health, Education and Welfare.

Metropolitan Life Insurance Company, *Statistical Bulletin* 54:5, November 1973.

ROBINSON, R. C. V.: Congenital syphilis, *Arch. Dermatol.* 99:599, 1969.

RUDOLPH, A. H.: Control of gonorrhea, guideline for antibiotic treatment. *JAMA* 220:1587, 1972.

TERMINI, B. A., and MUSIC, S. I.: The natural history of syphilis: A review, *South. Med. J.* 65:241, 1972.

*Today's V.D. Control Problem 1974:* American Social Health Association, New York, 1974.

TOP, F. H., SR., and WEHRLE, P. F. (eds.): *Communicable and Infectious Diseases,* ed. 7, St. Louis, Mosby, 1972.

U.S. Department of Health, Education and Welfare, Public Health Service: *Syphilis: a Synopsis,* Washington, D.C., U.S. Government Printing Office, 1968.

WARREN, C. L., and ST. PIERRE, R.: Sources and accuracy of college students' sex knowledge, *J. School Health* 43:588, November 1973.

WEBSTER, B. (ed.): Symposium on Venereal Disease, *The Medical Clinics of North America,* Vol. 56, No. 5, Philadelphia, Saunders, September 1972.

# UNIT ELEVEN

## Common Problems Involving Disfigurement

# The Patient with a Dermatologic Condition

## ASSESSMENT OF THE SKIN

Systematic examination of the skin is an essential aspect of physical assessment, whether or not the patient is suffering from a dermatologic condition. Observation of the skin yields important data relevant to the patient's physical status and sometimes to his emotional status as well. Thus, cool sweaty skin of the hands is a frequent indicator of anxiety. Skin color may be pale, which may indicate anemia, or yellow, as in jaundice. Areas of hyperpigmentation, occurring in the inner surfaces of elbows and knees or the creases of the neck, often indicate chronic eczema. Temperature of the skin, to touch, may be increased in infection involving the skin, and in burns. Cool moist skin (e.g., in a postoperative patient) may indicate shock. Skin normally loses some elasticity (ability to return quickly to normal position and contour when stretched) with aging. Elasticity of the skin is decreased by such factors as dehydration, and rapid weight loss. Firm, glistening, shiny skin, for example, of the ankles, accompanied by swelling of the underlying tissues, is often indicative of edema. Hair is indicative of general health and of the care given it. Damage to hair often results from injudicious use of dyes or bleaching agents. Patchy loss of hair may indicate such conditions as secondary syphilis. The nails may undergo changes with systemic disease, or in relation to dermatologic conditions—for example, clubbing of the nails may be seen in patients with chronic obstructive pulmonary disease; fungus infections sometimes involve the nail bed. It is essential when examining the patient's skin to be aware of implications for dermatologic conditions and for possible indicators of systemic disease.

Disciplined examination is important. Thus, many practitioners begin by examining the skin of the face, neck, scalp, and external ears, moving methodically downward in the examination to include inspection of the lower extremities. The patient is draped so that only the skin area being examined is exposed. A good light, a comfortably warm environment, and privacy for the patient are essential.

In addition, the following guidelines offer examples of important facets of nursing assessment for any patient with a dermatologic condition.

SOME GUIDELINES FOR ASSESSMENT OF THE PATIENT WITH A DERMATOLOGIC CONDITION

1. **Affective.** Patient's response to the lesions, to changes in appearance, to stress from the condition, such as itching. Response of family and close associates, to the patient; (accepting, repelled, fearful of contagion).
2. **Cognitive.** Patient's understanding of the condition and its treatment; ability to use his understanding to help himself. Previous learning which patient can apply (such as from previous episodes of the condition).
3. **Physical.** Appearance of the lesion (color, exudate), distribution of the condition on the body; indications of secondary infection. Symptoms experienced by patient: itching, feeling of dryness, tautness.
4. **Socioeconomic.** Effect upon patient's work, home, and social life.
5. **General health status.** Nutrition, rest, sleep, presence of other illnesses.
6. **Capability of carrying out prescribed care.** (Most patients are treated on an outpatient basis; this ability is essential from the start.)
7. **Long-range considerations.** Is the condition acute and of short duration? Likely to recur? Is it made worse by environmental factors, such as the material from which clothing is made; emotional factors, such as anger and conflict?

## THE CARE OF NORMAL SKIN

Since the skin is in constant contact with the environment, it is unusually subject to injury and irritation. Nurses are in a strategic position to help others to maintain a normal, healthy skin. In bathing a hospitalized patient or in teaching patients in outpatient departments, industry, or their homes about sound practices in skin care, the nurse can help others to avoid abusing the skin and subjecting it to disease or injury. The nurse is often consulted about everyday problems concerning personal hygiene and grooming, as well as about the commonplace discomforts or diseases that affect the skin. She is frequently asked such questions as "What's good for dry skin?" or "Can estrogenic hormone creams keep wrinkles away?" or "How often should I shampoo my hair?" or "What's good for acne?"

The nurse who gives primary health care can bring patients to treatment for dermatologic conditions. For example, basal cell carcinoma of the skin is common in older age groups. When treated early it usually has an excellent prognosis, and there is little or no ensuing disfigurement from surgical removal. Particularly in nursing homes and retirement communities, it is essential for the nurse to be alert for such lesions when she carries out physical assessment. The nurse can also apply her knowledge to the care of her own skin and to the avoidance of practices that present particular occupational hazards.

Probably no other organ in the body is as subject to self medication as the skin, and because of its accessibility such self-treatment is commonplace. Although most people recognize the importance of healthy skin as an asset to personal appearance, those who unhesitatingly seek medical advice for other symptoms try a variety of nostrums on skin lesions, often making the condition worse. The idea that skin disease is never serious and therefore can be trifled with is far from the truth.

**Cleanliness.** Our culture values cleanliness, beauty, and the avoidance of body odors. Skin diseases of all sorts are often attributed to poor personal hygiene, and a vigorous program of scrubbing and cleansing is sometimes undertaken to "clear the condition up." Popular advertising reinforces this idea by emphasizing the wonderful properties of various soaps and cleansers.

Countless bacteria, most of them nonpathogenic, normally exist on the skin. Although thorough scrubbing with soap and water or a detergent will temporarily reduce the number of bacteria, the number rapidly returns to previous levels. Because most skin disorders of adults in this country are not related to germs and dirt, vigorous cleansing is not a cure-all. In fact, many conditions, such as those related to excessive dryness or to allergy, are made worse by preparations that increase skin dryness by removing natural oils, or that further irritate a sensitive skin with a variety of perfumes and colorings. People with oily skins need to bathe more frequently than those with dry skins. Older people, especially women, tend to have dry skins. Often, they cannot tolerate the drying effect of a hot tub bath daily. Instead, they may sponge-bathe the hands and the face, the axillae, the genital region, and the feet daily, and take a tub bath or a shower two or three times a week. Using lukewarm water and bathing quickly are also less drying, because they avoid prolonged contact with hot, soapy water. Adding a little oil to the bath water also lessens the drying effect.

Sweat glands are present over the entire body, but they are especially abundant in axillae, forehead, palms, and soles. In adults perspiration in the axillary region has an odor that is considered unpleasant. Deodorants are commonly used by both men and women to banish it. When bathing a patient, the nurse should apply the patient's deodorant if he is unable to do so or, if he wishes to purchase some, help him to obtain information about whether and where it is sold in the hospital.

**Preventing Dryness.** The sebaceous glands, which surround the hair follicles, secrete sebum, an oily substance that protects the hair and skin from becoming excessively dry. However, some persons produce less sebum than desirable for keeping the skin soft. This is particularly common during later life.

Heredity is important in determining the type of skin that a person will have. It is often noted that very dry or oily skins are most common among persons who have a family history of these conditions.

Creams help to keep the skin soft and smooth by reducing the loss of moisture from the skin, particularly during cold weather, when moisture is lost more quickly. But regardless of additions of estrogenic hormones, creams cannot "restore youthful beauty." Their value lies primarily in the cream, rather than in the hormones. Most people, as they grow older, find that creams and lotions applied to face, hands, elbows, and feet help to keep the skin smooth and soft. Wearing rubber gloves when using soaps and detergents for laundry and dishwashing also helps to prevent dryness. Such simple measures can greatly reduce chapping and cracking, which make the skin not only unattractive and uncomfortable, but also vulnerable to infection and rashes.

**Dandruff.** People with oily scalps need to shampoo their hair more frequently than do those with dry scalps. Pronounced oiliness and the shedding of greasy scales (commonly described as dandruff)

require advice and treatment by a dermatologist. This condition is quite common, and many people either neglect it entirely or indulge in self-medication. If neglected, dandruff can be a factor in the thinning and the loss of hair. Regular brushing and shampooing and the avoidance of such constricting apparel as tight hat bands and tight wigs are important in preserving a healthy scalp.

**Sunlight.** Tanning by exposure to sunlight helps to protect the skin from the damaging effects of excessive ultraviolet light. But effects of exposure to sunlight vary, depending on the condition of the patient's skin and on the length of the exposure. For example, acne is usually improved by exposure to sunlight, but prolonged exposure, particularly of fair-skinned persons whose skins do not tan effectively, can cause a painful sunburn. Adolescents and young adults tolerate exposure to sunlight better than older persons do, because the skin becomes thinner, drier, and less protective with increasing age. Prolonged exposure to sun eventually causes the skin to become coarse and leathery, and increases the risk of skin cancer. People who must work outdoors can avoid unnecessary exposure by wearing wide-brimmed hats and by covering the skin (wearing a T-shirt as well as trunks or slacks). Sun-screening lotions are also advised for those who enjoy or are obliged to have considerable exposure to sunlight. This is especially important for fair-skinned persons and for those known to have had skin cancer.

The condition of the skin reflects a person's general health. Good health habits help to keep the skin, as well as the rest of the body, in good condition. Plenty of sleep, relief of worry and tension, regular exercise, and an optimum diet are important.

## Nursing Considerations

What particular dermatologic problems are often encountered by the hospitalized patient, and how can the nurse help to prevent them?

- **The nurse should remember that the alkalinity of ordinary soaps sometimes causes irritation, especially in older, bedridden patients. The physician may suggest a soap substitute of neutral pH, such as Dermolate or Lowila.**
- **When giving a bed bath, the nurse should rinse the soap off with clear water. The soap should never be left in the bath water, because it makes the water soapy and also wastes soap. A soap dish should be used. If one is not available, a folded paper towel**

will do. The water in the basin should be changed frequently, so that the process of rinsing is not actually a reapplication of soap.

- The nurse should use the method that provides the best possible rinsing compatible with the degree of activity permitted the patient. A patient who can have a tub or a shower with assistance should have this rather than a bed bath.
- Instead of giving "routine baths," especially for long-term patients, the nurse should plan ahead and allow time for shampoos and care of the nails. To give a complete bath daily, but to allow no time to give a shampoo for two months reflects lack of planning. Shampooing the hair of a helpless patient is often made easier by placing him on a stretcher and taking him to the sink, where, with the end of the stretcher protected by a rubber sheet, his hair can be washed conveniently under running water. The patient's brush and comb should be washed periodically. This detail often is overlooked.
- The nurse should keep the patient's elbows covered by seeing that the sleeves of his gown or pajama top stay down over them. Creams and lotions applied to the elbows and the knees help relieve dryness. A footboard keeps the patient from sliding down in bed and avoids friction. Elbows and knees often are chafed due to the friction of the bed sheets as the patient moves himself up in bed. Digging the elbows into the bedding when the patient is moving up in bed irritates them.
- If she notices skin lesions, the nurse should avoid washing them with soap and water. She should not try to clean off any scales or exudate, since the appearance of the lesions is important in making a diagnosis.
- The nurse should assess the appearance of lesions carefully. When taking the health history, she should be alert for medications the patient is taking, or has recently taken, since dermatologic problems sometimes occur in response to medication. If the patient is hospitalized, it is important to review medications he is receiving.

The nurse can apply these measures to safeguard the health of her own skin, and, she can also take the following special precautions against specific occupational hazards:

- She should avoid unnecessary contact with medications; many of them can cause allergic skin reactions. Careful handling of syringes, needles, and medicines can greatly reduce physical contact. If a medicine spills on her hands, the nurse should wash it off promptly.
- Thorough hand washing is important in preventing the spread of infection. Because she must wash her hands so often, the nurse should use hand cream or lotion liberally, and always dry her hands well after washing. These precautions will help to prevent chapping and cracking of the skin.

- If a patient has a skin disease, the nurse should determine whether or not it is contagious. If it is, she should follow the necessary medical aseptic technique. (This rule applies, of course, to any contagious condition.)

## INJURY AND DISEASE OF THE SKIN

By the time that he has reached adulthood, almost everyone has had some contact with one or more of the common skin disorders. For example, hormone imbalance during adolescence is believed to be responsible for acne.

The following are some common causes of skin diseases with examples of the resulting conditions.

- Allergy—urticaria (hives)
- Congenital lesions—nevus (mole)
- Emotional disturbances—neurodermatitis (a form of eczema)
- Hormonal imbalance—acne
- Infection—furuncle (boil)
- Malignant growth—malignant melanoma
- Trauma—accidents: burns, lacerations; radical surgery, such as that for cancer of the head and neck

Disorders of the skin may also be classified according to the degree of the involvement of the entire body. For example, a burn may be small and produce only local symptoms; or it may cover a large area of the body and produce systemic as well as local symptoms, because of the marked physiologic disturbance accompanying it. Some skin diseases produce only local manifestations (e.g., acne). On the other hand, many systemic diseases, for example, measles and syphilis, produce dermatologic symptoms. Certain diseases included in this chapter are systemic diseases with symptoms manifested by the skin as well as by other organs of the body (e.g., systemic lupus erythematosus and scleroderma). Both of these diseases affect collagen, a connective tissue widely distributed in the body.

## THE PROBLEM OF DISFIGUREMENT

Our society places a high premium on youthful beauty, and advertising continues to stress an ideal which, though patently unrealistic, is nonetheless highly persuasive. What effect has this on the person whose skin is disfigured from disease or trauma? Skin diseases have long been associated with immorality, uncleanliness, and contagion. Despite the fact that these associations are usually unjustified, an inflamed and pimply skin does not convey the look of fresh cleanliness that a clear skin does. Some skin lesions exude serum that has an unpleasant odor, further adding to the impression of uncleanliness. Few skin diseases are contagious; nevertheless, many persons are afraid to touch the person with skin disease, or even to be near him. People whose faces have been scarred by burns or cuts may be severely disfigured.

It is not difficult to understand why people who suffer severe facial disfigurement often undergo personality changes. They become painfully aware of the stares, the avoidance, and even the revulsion of other people, and they tend to withdraw from social and business contacts. Many occupations are closed to those who are disfigured, particularly jobs that emphasize personal attractiveness (e.g., those of a receptionist, an airline stewardess, or salesman).

Today disfigurement is more common than it was in the past. Cancer of the head and neck is treated more often by radical surgery, as new advances in surgical techniques are developed. Although the malignant cells may be removed successfully, the problem of disfigurement remains. People with severe injuries of the face and the neck have a better chance of survival, because of such treatments as antibiotics and parenteral fluids. Plastic surgery has helped many of these patients—by such methods as reconstructing an ear so skillfully that it scarcely can be distinguished from the normal ear. Nevertheless, some patients are so severely mutilated that they remain disfigured despite all that plastic surgeons can do for them. Rehabilitation must emphasize function, but appearance is important, too.

Learning to accept those who are disfigured is a challenge. Often, the nurse is the one who is with the patient when he becomes aware of the change in his appearance. While it is easy to preach acceptance, it is not always easy to practice it, because, like others, nurses are not immune to prejudice. The points listed below may seem too commonplace to deserve mention; but because the care of disfigured patients is often difficult, the list will help to spell out some of the things which can be done to help the patient to feel accepted.

- **When dressings or treatments are required, the nurse should not hesitate to touch the part as she ministers to the patient. She should use only the logical and the necessary protective techniques. For example, gloves should be worn only if the skin disease is contagious, and their purpose should be explained to the patient. Even if the patient is physically able to carry out his own treatments, the nurse should arrange to do some part of the care of the lesions herself as a way of demonstrating acceptance of the patient and his condition. Understanding the disease will help her to feel sure of herself, so that she can use a firm rather than a gingerly touch.**
- **The nurse should neither stare at the patient's disfigurement nor avoid the sight of it. She should try to look at the total patient, including his rash or his scar, in the same way that she would look at any other patient.**

First experiences with severely disfigured persons can be trying. At first the nurse may feel shock, or pity, or revulsion. Recognizing how she feels will help her to control the expression of her feelings to the patient. Gradually, in working repeatedly with the same patient, or with others who have a similar disability, she will find that the changed appearance can be accepted more easily as a temporary, or even a permanent, part of her patient. Although his appearance may differ from that of others, his needs for acceptance, companionship, affection, and a chance to do useful work are the same as those of other people.

Having begun to recognize and to cope with her own feelings, the nurse can understand more readily the reactions of the patient's family, friends, and coworkers to his condition. Part of her task lies in helping them. She can:

- **Demonstrate by her behavior that she accepts the patient, with his changed appearance. Her assurance as she approaches and ministers to him can convey this.**
- **Give the family members an opportunity to talk with her away from the patient, as well as in his presence. They may fear that others will stigmatize the patient, and this dread can be a powerful threat.**
- **Show the family members how they can help to care for the patient—for example, in applying dressings or ointments. Allow them to ask questions concerning communicability of the disease so that they can be spared unnecessary fears but be instructed in whatever precautions are necessary.**

## Treatment of Skin Disease

Both local and systemic treatment may be used in skin disease. Lotions, powders, and ointments may be applied to soothe and to soften the skin (*emollients*), to relieve itching (*antipruritics*), to protect the lesions, to provide a vehicle for other medications, and to stimulate the healing of chronic lesions. In addition, local preparations may be keratolytic (dissolving thickened or horny skin), antiseptic, or antiparasitic. The following list contains an example of each of these types of preparation:

- Emollient—lanolin
- Antipruritic—calamine lotion
- Protection—zinc oxide ointment
- Vehicle for other medication—bacitracin ointment
- Stimulation of the healing of lesions—coal tar ointment
- Keratolytic—salicylic acid plaster (contained in many corn plasters)
- Antiseptic—potassium permanganate solution
- Antiparasitic—undecylenic acid (Desenex powder)

Local preparations for the skin often are combinations of several ingredients carefully chosen for their specific effect. Patients who have similar skin disorders may respond very differently to a particular preparation.

The action of preparations that stimulate healing is not fully understood, but they seem to act as counterirritants, helping chronic lesions to heal and helping thickening of the skin to disappear. Stimulating ointments should be rubbed in, whereas ointments applied for their soothing effect should be gently dabbed on, or spread on a piece of gauze and laid on the skin. The application of excessive amounts of ointment should be avoided, because it is wasteful and it soils the patient's clothing. Lotions that settle with standing must be shaken before each use.

Systemic treatment is usually part of the patient's management. Most skin disorders grow worse when the patient is tired or under emotional stress; therefore, rest and sleep are an important part of treatment. Rest may mean different things in different situations. For one patient it may mean rest in a hospital bed, away from a tense home situation. For another it may mean a vacation from his job.

Diet may also be an important part of treatment. For instance, most patients with acne find that the condition grows worse after eating chocolate. A patient may develop hives (*urticaria*) from eating fish, and therefore he may have to eliminate it from his diet.

Since some skin diseases are manifestations of systemic disorders, the variety of drugs given is as broad as the study of pharmacology itself. The following are some commonly used preparations:

- Corticosteroids help to relieve many severe skin diseases. They do not cure the disease, but they often relieve the symptoms, sometimes with dramatic speed. As is true of their use in other diseases, these drugs can have serious toxic effects. Therefore, they are used primarily to relieve acute attacks. Continued use in long-term conditions brings greater risk, and it is justified only when the disease itself is very serious and cannot be relieved by other treatments. It is sometimes very difficult to help the patient to understand the necessity for reducing or discontinuing doses of corticosteroids when the physician recommends this. The patient is usually so grateful for the relief obtained that he is understandably reluctant to discontinue use of the drug. It is important to help him understand the necessity of following the physician's recommendation.
- Antihistamines frequently are prescribed when allergy is a factor in causing the disease, and for the relief of itching.
- Sedatives and tranquilizers are used to help the patient to relax and rest.
- Antibiotics are used to treat infection.

Sunlight is important in the treatment of some dermatologic problems. For example, its effects—bacteriostasis, drying, and mild peeling of the skin—are helpful in acne. Exposure to ultraviolet light can produce a similar effect in much less time, and ultraviolet treatments are often given by dermatologists. Usually, only the part being treated is exposed to the light. Any type of heavy cloth or opaque paper can be used to protect the other parts of the body from exposure.

## NURSING CARE OF PATIENTS WITH SKIN DISEASE

When assessing the patient's condition it is essential that the nurse examine the skin over the patient's entire body. Although the condition may be especially severe in the area indicated by the patient, evidence of it, or of other dermatologic conditions, may be noted elsewhere. A good light and careful draping of the patient are essential. Only those areas being examined at the time should be exposed, because patients with skin diseases usually are particularly sensitive to being examined. The examination may not be limited to the skin. Any aspect of physical examination may be required. The necessity for diagnostic tests must be carefully explained to the patient, who may see no connection between the tests and the lesions on his skin.

## Itching

Although itching (*pruritus*) is a common and very distressing symptom of many skin diseases, the mechanism of itching is still somewhat obscure. The itch impulse probably has a lower frequency and intensity than the pain impulse, thus differentiating the feeling of pain from the sensation of itching. Certain factors tend to make itching worse: excessive warmth (as from too many blankets); rough, prickly fabrics; emotional stress; and idleness. Itching usually is worse at night, probably because the patient's attention is not occupied, and he is therefore more aware of the sensation.

Severe itching is agony. Scratching leads to trauma and excoriation, and often it leads to infection. Helping the patient with severe pruritus to obtain some degree of comfort and to avoid scratching is a challenge to all who care for him. Reminders not to scratch are little help; usually, all that is accomplished is that the patient grows tired of being scolded, and the nurse is irked, because he does not stop scratching. Instead of scolding the patient, the nurse should try to:

- **Divert his attention from the itching. A game of cards with another patient or painting a picture can work wonders. Here is a word of caution: the materials that the patient uses should not irritate his condition. A patient who is allergic to wool obviously should not knit a woolen sweater.**
- **Provide enough clothing and bedding for comfortable warmth, but avoid overheating. Carefully check the temperature of the room to avoid chilling or excessive warmth.**
- **Encourage the patient to keep his nails short and very clean. This will minimize trauma and infection from scratching.**
- **If the patient scratches while he is asleep, have him wear white cotton gloves at night.**
- **Help the patient to cope with emotional problems.**
- **When the sensation of itching is acute, and the patient cannot resist the impulse to touch his skin, have him press his finger or hand against it, without scratching. Sometimes, this pressure will lessen the itching. Some patients find that clenching their fists tightly and counting to ten helps them to avoid the impulse to scratch.**
- **Help the patient to sleep. A back rub, a snack or a chance for some quiet reading may help him to relax and go to sleep.**
- **Note carefully any bedtime treatment or medicines ordered to relieve the itching or to promote sleep.**

A variety of treatments may be prescribed to alleviate itching. The treatment of the disease itself, thus eliminating the cause of the symptom, is, of course, the most effective. However, in waiting for curative treatment to take effect, or in treating conditions in which complete cure is unlikely, much relief of itching can be achieved by symptomatic treatment. Wet dressings or starch baths often help. The relief of emotional tension helps to reduce itching; sedatives and tranquilizers often are ordered for this purpose. Soothing lotions, such as calamine, often give temporary relief. When allergy is a factor, antihistamines may provide considerable relief.

## Dressings

If dressings are needed, they should be applied so that they fit snugly and yet do not bind. Dressings applied to open, denuded areas should be sterile. Cotton should not be placed next to the skin, because of its tendency to stick to moist surfaces. Gauze or cotton cloth may be used. Tubular cotton gauze, which is thinner but similar to the stockinette used under casts, is easy to apply, and it stays smoother than roller gauze. If this material is not available, a long, white cotton stocking or a sock will serve. The foot should be cut out of the stocking, making a tubular dressing that can be applied over an arm or leg. Adhesive tape should not be applied directly to the skin, because it can cause trauma and irritation.

**Wet Dressings.** When applying a wet dressing, the nurse should determine first whether the procedure is to be clean or sterile. The nature of the lesion (acute or chronic; open, weeping, or dry) helps to determine whether sterile technique must be used. In either case, scrupulous cleanliness is important. The following are some points that should be remembered in contrasting the clean and the sterile technique for a wet dressing:

| CLEAN | STERILE |
|---|---|
| 1. Clean bowl, washed, dried and reused by the same patient; sterilized before it is used by another patient. | 1. Sterile bowl, used only once and then resterilized. |
| 2. Gauze, or cotton cloths. Gauze may be remoistened and reused by the same patient. Discard when it is soiled. | 2. Gauze or cotton cloths that have been autoclaved. Use during one treatment only. |

CLEAN

3. Dressing may be handled by patient or nurse after washing hands thoroughly.

STERILE

3. Two sterile forceps, to use when placing compresses in solution, wringing them out, and applying them. Depending on the size and the location of the area to be covered, and the amount of handling of the dressing that is necessary, sterile gloves may be needed, so that dressings can be handled directly with the gloves.

Wet dressings have a cooling and a soothing effect, produced by the evaporation of the moisture from the dressing. To avoid chilling, the nurse should make certain that the rest of the patient's body is kept warm.

Wet dressings may be applied by either the open or the closed method:

CLOSED

Moist compresses are applied and then covered with waterproof material, such as plastic sheeting or waxed paper.

OPEN

Moist compresses are applied and left open to air. Do not cover the part with bedclothes. The foundation of the bed is protected by laying a rubber or a plastic sheet, covered by a cotton draw sheet or treatment towel, under the part.

For dermatologic patients, the open method is usually preferable, because it permits greater evaporation, thus increasing the soothing and the cooling effects of the treatment. The closed method, by preventing evaporation, lessens this effect, and if it is used for prolonged periods, it causes maceration of the skin. Whether the open or closed method is used is an essential aspect of data regarding the treatment.

Moist dressings may be prescribed for varying periods of time. During the acute phases of the disease they may be ordered continuously. As the condition improves, they may be used two or three times daily for 20 or 30 minutes. In any case, the dressing must be kept wet during the entire time that it is in place. The dressing needs to be moistened more frequently when the open method is used than when the closed method is used.

Several points must be considered in keeping the dressing wet:

- **A dressing that is completely dry should never be moistened by pouring solution over the dry, outer layers of the gauze. The solution may not even penetrate to the gauze next to the patient's skin, and the solution can carry dirt inward from the surface of the dressings. The dressings should be removed completely, and the treatment resumed by immersing fresh dressings in a bowl of solution and applying them.**
- **An open dressing that is changed frequently enough to prevent soiling and is not allowed to dry out usually may be remoistened at intervals using an Asepto syringe.**
- **If the dressing is not only dry, but also stuck to the skin, the outer layers of gauze should be removed first, the inner layer moistened with solution, using an Asepto syringe. The nurse should never pull roughly at a dressing that is stuck, because this action will cause pain and trauma.**
- **A closed dressing that is protected by outer wrappings may usually be remoistened by squirting solution on it with an Asepto syringe, provided that the dressing has not dried out.**

Often, the patient can assist in keeping the dressing moist, provided that the sterile technique is not necessary; the area is one that he can reach; his physical condition permits; he is shown how to do it; and the necessary supplies are provided for him. Permitting the patient to care for his own dressing without considering each of these factors is a frequent reason for neglect of the treatment. The nurse is always responsible for seeing that the treatment is carried out, whether or not she performs every aspect of it herself.

**Starch Baths.** Starch baths (colloid baths) are useful in relieving itching. Usually, they are used at bedtime to help the patient to sleep. The patient may be able to carry out the treatment with only a little help, as long as he is physically able. He should be carefully instructed, and there must be an effective call system in the bathroom, so that he may signal for help if he needs it.

The nurse fills the bathtub with lukewarm water, adds one pound of cornstarch or laundry starch, and stirs the water so that the starch is mixed through it. The patient immerses his whole body by stretching out full length in the tub. A washcloth or a compress may be used to apply the solution to the face and any other parts not covered by the solution. The cloth or compress should be applied gently, without rubbing the skin. Soap is not used with the starch bath.

Although the primary purpose of the bath is soothing, it also helps to cleanse the skin. Unless this fact is explained to the patient, he may reach for the soap, and its use could irritate his skin. The bath often is taken for 20 to 30 minutes at a time. The bathroom should be comfortably warm, and more hot water should be added occasionally to prevent the patient from becoming chilled. When the treatment is over, the skin should be patted dry. Rubbing should be avoided, since this causes irritation.

Whatever local medication is prescribed should be taken to the bathroom and applied immediately after the patient's skin has been dried. Irritation and increased itching may result if application is delayed after the bath. The patient should not clean up the bathroom. Instead he should go right to bed so that the soothing effect of the treatment will not be lost. Often, patients with a skin disease are susceptible to chilling, particularly after a bath. Therefore, it is necessary that the patient wears his bathrobe and his slippers to and from the bathroom.

A feeling of relaxation and the relief of the itching should result from the bath. The nurse can help to assure these results by:

- **Providing for privacy and lack of hurry. Other patients should not be allowed to knock at the door. They should be told that the bathtub is being used for a treatment and will be free in half an hour. A sign on the outside of the door may help to avoid interruption.**
- **Offering assistance as needed. Usually attendance is not necessary if the nurse shows the patient how to signal, and assures him that it is all right to do so.**

## Patient and Family Education

Most dermatologic patients are treated as outpatients and are hospitalized only for acute exacerbations of the condition. Therefore, the patients and their families need to learn how to carry out the prescribed treatment at home. Specific treatments, such as application of medications and dressings, must be explained and demonstrated. Successful treatment frequently depends on the willingness and the ability of the patient to carry out his treatment. Thus the instruction should be as simple and concise as possible, and the patient should be allowed time to ask questions, and given written directions to take home with him. The nurse in private practice may assist patients to carry out therapy, working with a dermatologist. The nurse who has her own practice carries a particularly important respon-

sibility in early detection of skin problems. For instance, careful examination of geriatric patients can result in prompt detection of lesions which may be malignant, and the patients can then be promptly referred to a dermatologist.

## COMMON DERMATOLOGIC CONDITIONS

### Acne

Acne is one of the most widespread skin conditions. The cause is not fully understood, but acne characteristically occurs during adolescence, and it is believed to be related to the hormone changes during that period of life when the secondary sex characteristics are developing. Other factors can aggravate the condition, although they alone do not cause it. Fatigue, emotional stress, and eating too many rich foods, such as chocolate and ice cream, are examples. Girls often notice that the condition grows worse at the time of the menstrual period.

The skin of the affected areas (usually face, chest, and back) is excessively oily. The lesions consist of comedones (blackheads), papules (pimples), and pustules (pimples filled with pus). In severe cases, cysts sometimes occur, appearing as large, reddish swellings. The severity of the condition ranges all the way from an occasional pimple, which during adolescence is so common that it is considered to be almost normal at this age, to a face that is covered with bright-red pimples and peppered with blackheads. Severe acne, if neglected, can lead to the formation of deep, pitted scars that leave the skin permanently pock-marked. Oiliness of the scalp and the shedding of greasy scales (seborrhea) often accompany acne. Infection and the formation of pustules are fostered by picking and squeezing the lesions.

Seeking care for acne seems foolish to many people. "She'll outgrow it" is a commonly expressed attitude. In one sense, acne usually is a self-limited condition that disappears in the late teens or early 20's. But what of the girl who develops acne at age 10, and whose face is covered with pimples until she is 20? Ten years is a long time—particularly to a young person who longs to be pretty and popular. Acne can also be difficult for boys, who are just beginning to show concern about personal appearance. The possibility of scarring from severe acne is too often overlooked. These scars are *not* outgrown, and they can spoil a complexion for life. But the emotional scars may be just as important.

For some young people these matters mean just temporary distress, but for others who feel less secure, who already have difficulty in making friends, severe or unusually prolonged acne can interfere seriously with their developing into poised, confident adults. Acne that is in any way pronounced or unsightly should be treated—the more prompt the treatment, the less likelihood of scars, physical or emotional.

**Treatment.** Despite the fact that there is as yet no swift and certain cure, a great deal can be done to relieve the symptoms and, in time, to help them to disappear. Instruction in personal hygiene from a person whom the patient considers to be an authority on health matters is heeded more often than the advice, however kindly, of parents and neighbors. Because the adolescent normally is striving for independence from his parents, he may consider their suggestions irritating and restrictive, whereas he may follow eagerly the same advice from a physician or a nurse.

The dermatologist can remove the blackheads and drain the pustules with special instruments. This process should never be attempted by the patient or by family and friends, because infection and scarring can be caused by unskilled manipulation. "Hands off" is an ironclad but difficult rule that the patient must learn to follow. The patient is instructed to keep his fingernails short and clean, since this helps to prevent infection of the skin lesions. He should wash his hands thoroughly before applying medication or carrying out any other treatment of the lesions. His self-conscious preoccupation with the condition often tempts him to pick and squeeze the lesions, and to peer into the mirror at them. Patients should be discouraged from constantly inspecting any skin lesion, since such preoccupation with the condition may actually aggravate it and at least may make it seem to be more severe and conspicuous.

Thorough washing of the affected areas with mild soap is important in the treatment, since it helps to reduce oiliness and temporarily cuts down the number of bacteria, thus helping to prevent infection. Mild soaps that do not irritate are preferable to hard or highly perfumed varieties. Medicated preparations should be used only as prescribed. Some physicians recommend washing the skin with an antibacterial soap to keep the number of staphylococci on the skin to a minimum. Sometimes, an abrasive soap, rubbed in gently, helps in peeling the skin. The diet should exclude any foods that the patient has found make the condition worse. Chocolate and nuts are common offenders, as are other fatty foods, such as salad dressing, fried foods, and bacon.

Healthful living can help to relieve acne. The skin of a young person whose lunches have consisted mainly of jelly sandwiches, soft drinks, and candy bars, and who habitually stays up late, often improves after such everyday treatment as plenty of fresh air and exercise, improved diet, and more sleep.

Exposure to sunlight is beneficial, because it lessens oiliness, reduces the number of infection-causing bacteria, and causes peeling of affected skin. The combination of increased exercise, relaxation and sunlight often makes acne improve during the summer. But the exposure to the sun should do no more than produce slight pinkness and peeling; a painful sunburn is not beneficial. Short treatments with ultraviolet light provide similar benefits, and they have the added advantage of year-around application and controlled dosage which helps to prevent burning.

White lotion (lotio alba) is useful in drying the skin and decreasing the severity of the lesions. It is applied each night and washed off in the morning. Local treatment of the scalp to decrease oiliness and scaling is also important (see treatment of seborrheic dermatitis below).

Other treatments sometimes used for acne include antibiotics and vitamin A. Contraceptives are sometimes given to prevent ovulation and the formation of progesterone, since progesterone aggravates acne. The scarring that has already occurred from acne lesions can be made less conspicuous by *dermabrasion*. Lotions containing corticosteroids have been effective in treatment of severe acne. Corticosteroids are sometimes administered orally for this purpose. In general, face creams are to be avoided, since they increase oiliness.

## Seborrheic Dermatitis

The common term for mild seborrheic dermatitis is *dandruff*. The symptoms are familiar: oily scalp, formation of greasy scales, itching, and irritation. Severe cases have inflammation with redness, swelling and, sometimes, exudation and pyogenic infection. Seborrheic dermatitis frequently accompanies acne, but unlike acne it is not limited typically to adolescence. Often, it persists throughout adulthood. It affects the scalp primarily, but it may spread to the eyebrows, the skin around the ears, the sides of the nose, and the forehead near the hairline, causing the skin in these areas, as well as the scalp, to be red, oily, and scaly.

Normally, new cells are constantly being formed and pushed to the outside of the skin, where they die and are gradually and imperceptibly shed (*keratinization*). In the presence of certain diseases, such as seborrheic dermatitis, keratinization is speeded up, and scaling becomes visible.

Like acne, mild seborrheic dermatitis is often either neglected or treated with a variety of cosmetic preparations. The condition is uncomfortable and unattractive. The itching leads to picking and scratching, which result in showers of scales on clothing. The excessive oiliness of the scalp results in greasy hair, which, together with visible scales, spoils the appearance. Severe or prolonged seborrheic dermatitis is frequently accompanied by premature loss of hair.

Why so many people suffer from oily scalps and dandruff is not understood clearly. Sometimes, the condition appears, together with acne, during adolescence. Prompt and persistent treatment often results in great improvement, to the degree that only good scalp hygiene is required to avoid a return of the condition. However, many people are not so fortunate and continue to require regular treatment to control the symptoms. These individuals have chronically overactive sebaceous glands; the condition may be related to heredity, emotional tension, a diet too high in fat, or endocrine imbalance.

**Treatment.** Treatment includes regular cleansing, application of local medication between shampoos, and a regimen of healthful living. When the oiliness is severe, daily shampoos may be needed. Although the scales are removed by washing, they promptly accumulate again until the condition is controlled. The dermatologist should be consulted about the selection of a shampoo. An antiseborrheic shampoo such as Selsun, or Fostex cream, is often recommended. When the condition is unresponsive, mildly antiseptic lotions or medicated ointments may be prescribed for use between shampoos. The lotions should be applied directly to the scalp rather than to the hair. Application to the hair does no good and is messy. The patient should be taught to part his hair temporarily, and then to apply the medication directly on the scalp until the entire

scalp has been reached. If the solution is thin, a medicine dropper, gauze or cotton pledgets can be used for this purpose. The nurse should explain the importance of this systematic application of medication to the patient. Just enough lotion to cover the affected area should be used; otherwise, the medicine will run down the patient's neck, and into his eyes and his ears. Regular exercise, sufficient rest, and relief of emotional tension are important aspects of therapy.

Although the condition improves with treatment, the symptoms often return when treatment is interrupted. Faithful adherence to the treatment regimen plus good hygienic care of the scalp usually can keep the condition under control. Hygienic care of the scalp and the hair includes:

- Cleanliness. Persons with dry hair require shampoos less often than patients with oily scalps, who may have to wash their hair almost daily. Brushes and combs should not be shared and should be washed regularly.
- Brushing and massage of the scalp. Both help to improve circulation to the scalp and are important in maintaining the scalp and the hair in healthy condition. Massage should be done by holding the fingers tightly against the head and then moving the scalp, rather than by rubbing the fingers over the scalp. Regular brushing with a soft-bristle brush also helps to keep the hair clean and glossy. Too stiff a brush or too much force can break hairs.
- Avoidance of constriction that could impair circulation, such as that caused by tight hat bands, tight hair nets, or wigs.
- Avoidance of substances that can cause irritation or possibly allergic reactions. Some hair dyes are in this category, as are dry shampoos containing powdered orris root. People with a history of allergy must be especially careful in their choice of cosmetics.

## Allergic Reactions of the Skin

The skin is one of the organs most frequently affected by allergy. The allergic response of the skin is characterized by dilation of the blood vessels, causing redness and swelling, and sometimes by vesiculation (blister formation) and oozing. Itching is a prominent symptom.

Allergic reactions of the skin are commonly caused by substances with which the skin has contact, such as cosmetics, fabrics, or chemicals. The resulting disorder is called *contact dermatitis*. The condition also may be caused by drugs (dermatitis medicamentosa) and foods. Penicillin frequently causes urticaria.

Irritants are differentiated from contact allergens

in that an irritant, if it is used in sufficient quantity, causes skin inflammation in almost everyone, whereas an allergen provokes a reaction only in people who are hypersensitive to that particular substance.

Patch tests, in which small amounts of various substances are placed in direct contact with the skin, may help to identify the causes of the reaction. A variety of substances may be used, such as a sample of the patient's lipstick or nail polish. A careful history is very important in any allergic condition. For example, it may be discovered that the patient has taken some new drug or has tried a new cosmetic.

### Urticaria (Hives); Angioneurotic Edema

The most familiar example of urticaria is a mosquito bite. The skin reacts to the insect's bite with a *wheal* (a roundish, white elevation) that is surrounded by an area of redness and itches furiously. Imagine being covered with mosquito bites, and you will have some idea of the misery of a severe case of urticaria. The wheals are a result of localized edema, due to increased capillary permeability. Urticaria is often an allergic response, although among adults emotional stress often causes the condition. Edema in some areas of the body, although acutely uncomfortable, is not a threat to life. However, if it involves certain critical areas, such as the larynx, life may be threatened.

In *angioneurotic edema* the part shows an all-over swelling rather than the patchy swellings of hives. The lips may be swollen to three times their normal size, or the tissues around the eyes may be so edematous that the patient cannot open them. Patients with allergic reactions must be observed for symptoms of respiratory obstruction, because edema of the larynx may interfere with respiration.

The treatment of urticaria and of angioneurotic edema includes avoidance of the allergen and the use of antihistamines and epinephrine and, in severe cases, corticosteroids. Cold compresses applied to the affected areas help provide relief. When angioneurotic edema and urticaria are associated with emotional tension, counseling, tranquilizers, and sedatives are useful.

### Eczema

The term *eczema* refers to a group of skin diseases that tend to be chronic and are related to heredity, allergy, emotional stress, and, possibly, endocrine disorder. The lesions consist of tiny vesicles (blisters) on reddened, itchy skin. The vesicles sometimes burst, causing the area to weep and later to form crusts from the dried fluid. The skin of the affected areas is red, dry and scaly. Leathery thickening (lichenification) and darkening of the skin result from continued irritation and scratching. A form of eczema called *infantile eczema* occurs in children under the age of two. The following discussion will be confined to the chronic type of eczema frequently seen in adults. It is called *atopic eczema*, or *neurodermatitis*.

This type of eczema is related closely to allergy and to emotional strain. Usually, the patient has a family history of allergy. Typically, other members of the family have suffered from eczema, hay fever, or asthma. The patient himself may have asthma or hay fever as well as eczema. Often, the skin disorder appears in early childhood, and it may be aggravated by exposure to specific allergens, such as certain foods. As the patient grows older, the importance of emotional stress in causing attacks seems to increase; exacerbations seem to be related more often to stress and strain than to allergy. Eczema that appears at the time of the menopause is believed to be related to endocrine changes.

Eczema typically occurs in the folds of the elbows and the knees and on the neck and the face. During acute attacks it may spread widely to other parts of the body. The symptoms tend to vary in severity. The patient may have a severe flare-up that necessitates absence from work or school. Several months later he may have no symptoms of the disease, and he may remain symptom-free for months or even years. However, the condition tends to recur. Frequently, an exacerbation of eczema can be traced to an emotional upset. At other times the immediate cause of the attack is obscure. People with chronic eczema frequently have patches of thickened, dark skin in the bends of their elbows and knees or on their necks. These patches persist long after the acute attack subsides. During an acute attack these areas become red, scaly, oozing, and crusted, and later they revert to their darkened leathery appearance. A form of eczema occurs in the perineal region, causing itching and inflammation. Sometimes, the condition is referred to as *pruritus ani* (itching of the anus) or *pruritus vulvae* (itching of the vulva).

**Treatment.** Caring for the patient with eczema demands the utmost skill and understanding. Medical treatment includes local creams and ointments that are soothing and antipruritic, such as hydrocortisone cream. If the skin is very inflamed, wet dressings or starch baths may be ordered. Antihistamines often help to relieve the symptoms. Sedatives and tranquilizers may be necessary to calm a tense, restless patient. Corticosteroids are sometimes administered orally when symptoms are very severe. Rest and sleep are essential in the treatment, and yet they are difficult to provide because of the severe itching and the discomfort. Sedation can help to break the cycle of insomnia, tension, itching, and scratching.

More is required than physical treatment for the successful management of eczema. The re-education of the patient, and sometimes of his family, is often the foundation on which other treatments must build. When emotional factors play a major role in causing the condition, ignoring them makes lasting improvement doubtful. Most patients respond to a program of treatment that includes patience, medication, and counseling. Psychotherapy may be effective.

The nurse can play an important role in helping the patient to learn to manage his condition. The following are some suggestions:

- **Avoid talking down to the patient.**
- **Try to understand some of the social and the emotional pressures that may affect the patient besides his physical discomforts.**
- **Help the patient to feel less tense. Give him a chance to talk; help him to find diversion and to obtain adequate sleep.**
- **If emotional tension seems to play a large part in causing the condition, avoid giving the patient the impression that you think he could snap out of it, or that he has purposely brought it on himself. Help him to learn to cope more effectively.**
- **Remember that eczema is not contagious. Do not be afraid to go near the patient.**
- **If allergy plays a major role in causing the attacks, learn specifically what allergens the patient must avoid, keep them away from him when he is in the hospital, and teach him to recognize and avoid them when he goes home.**

The control of eczema is a lifelong challenge. The primary responsibility must rest with the patient. Learning to know oneself is, after all, a life task of every person, and not just of those who have illnesses related to stress. Nevertheless, the task seems particularly urgent for these people, because recovery from illness so often depends on it.

The following are some everyday problems of self-care with which the patient may need help or instruction:

- Prescribed ointments should be applied sparingly; otherwise, they will be wasted and cause clothing to become unnecessarily soiled.
- If the trunk or genital region is involved some soiling of underwear is inevitable while the condition is acute. Wearing white cotton undergarments is helpful. (Cotton is more absorbent than nylon or an elasticized fabric.) If the weeping of the lesions is severe, a perineal pad may be necessary until the condition improves.
- Toilet tissue, especially if it is rough or highly colored, may be irritating to an already inflamed skin. After a bowel movement, soft cotton pledgets and plain water may be used for cleaning.
- Soap should not be used, because it irritates the lesions Nonirritating detergents may be prescribed.
- For aesthetic reasons, cleaning and drying should be carried out with some soft disposable material like cotton. All that is necessary is the observance of good practices of personal hygiene, such as not sharing towels and careful hand washing, since the condition is not contagious.

## Other Common Dermatologic Conditions

**Psoriasis.** Although both men and women are affected by psoriasis, usually during young adulthood and middle life, men are affected more often than women. The cause is unknown. It may be related to metabolic disorder, heredity, or emotional conflict.

The disease is characterized by patches of erythema (redness), covered with silvery scales, usually on the extensor surfaces of the elbows and the knees, the lower back, and the scalp. Itching is usually absent or slight, but occasionally it is severe. The lesions are obvious and unsightly; the scales tend to shed (see Plate 5).

The following measures are used to treat psoriasis:

- Local medication. A variety of ointments, such as those containing ammoniated mercury, salicylic acid, and coal tar are used.
- Diet. Avoidance of alcohol is recommended.
- Actinotherapy. Exposure to sunlight or to ultraviolet light helps.
- Systemic medication. Vitamin A, sedatives, tranquilizers, antihistamines, and corticosteroids are sometimes administered. Folic acid antagonists, such as methotrexate, are sometimes given.

The prognosis is guarded. Some patients respond very well to treatment. However, the condition tends to recur. Some patients obtain little relief from therapy and are easy prey for a variety of widely advertised remedies promising quick relief.

**Rosacea.** More common in women than in men, rosacea typically occurs during middle life. Emotional stress, anxiety, tension, endocrine disturbance, hypochlorhydria, and coexisting seborrheic dermatitis may all play a part in causing rosacea.

The symptoms include flushing of the face, particularly of the cheeks and the nose. Papules and pustules form on the flushed skin.

Treatment includes:

- Local medication. Sometimes, white lotion (lotio alba) is prescribed.
- Diet. Coffee, tea, chocolate, nuts, and alcoholic beverages are restricted, as are highly seasoned foods.
- Exposure to sunlight or ultraviolet light may be helpful.

The administration of hydrochloric acid is often helpful. Estrogenic hormones and corticosteroids are sometimes employed. Antibiotic therapy may be given on a long-term basis.

Patients who are willing and able to accept counseling and to take the prescribed medication often obtain relief of the symptoms.

**Self-inflicted Lesions (Dermatitis Factitia).** Self-inflicted lesions can occur at any period of life. They are a manifestation of emotional disturbance, which causes the patient to injure himself.

Often the lesions are bizarre, and they do not resemble any typical dermatologic condition (for instance, a lesion may be produced in the arm or the face by an acid burn). Sometimes, the lesions closely resemble those of other skin disease and may be hard to differentiate from them.

Symptomatic treatment is given to heal the lesion; the application of an occlusive dressing may be necessary to prevent the patient from touching it. Psychiatric treatment for the underlying disorder often is necessary.

**Dermatitis Venenata.** This condition is caused by contact with a substance that produces inflammation of skin; the oleoresins (plant oils and juices) of poison ivy, poison oak, and poison sumac are common offenders in this country.

Dermatitis venenata can occur at any age, but it is more common in children (who are likely to touch the plants during play outdoors, and who often do not recognize the plant or know of its power to cause dermatitis). Individuals differ greatly in their sensitivity. Some people react violently to contact with minute amounts of the oleoresin, whereas others may experience no symptoms even after considerable exposure.

Dermatitis venenata can be prevented by:

- Learning to recognize the plants and to avoid them.
- Wearing clothing that protects the skin from contact when a person is obliged to walk through areas where the plants exist (slacks, closed shoes, and socks rather than open sandals, no hose, and shorts or a skirt).
- Prompt and thorough cleaning of the exposed skin with soap, followed by application of alcohol, helps to remove the oleoresin from the skin after exposure. The cleaning should be done preferably within the first few minutes after contact, as the oleoresin later becomes fixed in the skin, and can no longer be removed.
- Desensitization by repeated administration of minute quantities of an extract of the oleoresin; this method of prevention is reserved for persons who are extremely sensitive to a particular plant.

Symptoms include redness, itching, formation of blisters, and edema. Usually, symptoms are limited to the point of contact—for example, legs or hands. In unusually severe cases, the eruption may involve large areas of the body, and the edema may be severe. Symptoms usually subside in about seven days, although in severe cases they may last longer.

Wet compresses of potassium permanganate solution or Burow's solution may be ordered to soothe and to lessen itching. Lotions, such as calamine, may also be ordered. Injections of the plant extract are not given during an acute attack, because they may cause exacerbation of the symptoms.

**Impetigo Contagiosa.** More common in children than adults, impetigo is caused by a streptococcal or a staphylococcal infection of the skin. The symptoms include erythema and vesicles that rupture and are covered with a sticky yellow crust (see Plate 6). Face and hands are common sites.

Impetigo is highly contagious, and contact by other persons with the lesions or the exudate should be avoided. The patient should never share his towel or bed linen. Meticulous hand washing after applying any medication is important. The patient should avoid touching the lesions unnecessarily. Because the condition can be spread from one part of his body to another, as well as to other people, he should wash his hands immediately after any touching of the lesions.

The crusts should be removed with soap and water, or with mineral oil, before any local medications are applied. It is important to remember that applicators or gauze used for this purpose must be wrapped carefully and immediately discarded. Various preparations may be ordered, such as neomycin-bacitracin ointment, ammoniated mercury ointment, or gentian violet. The systemic administration of antibiotics is frequent.

Usually, the condition is cured in a week. However, it can be especially severe in the newborn, and it can even cause death.

**Verrucae (Warts).** Warts are caused by a virus, which may enter the body as a result of an injury to the skin. Susceptibility to warts varies greatly, and they can occur at any age.

A wart appears on the skin as a small lump that has a roughened surface, and that may become yellowish or brownish (see Plate 7). Sometimes a single wart appears; at other times there may be a whole crop. The wart or warts may persist for months or years. Sometimes, they disappear spontaneously. Warts are usually painless, except for plantar warts. This particular type usually occurs on the soles of the feet, and because of pressure from the weight of the body, they grow inward, causing considerable pain.

Warts are removed by electrodesiccation (destruction of the lesion by short, high-frequency electric sparks). Warts sometimes may be made to disappear by suggestion, although how or why this treatment works is not understood. Acids, such as dichloracetic or nitric acid, are sometimes used to treat warts. The acid is applied deep into the root of the wart, after the thick, horny outer tissue has been carefully pared away. Rarely, x-ray therapy may be given.

Warts are benign lesions; however, they can spread, and treatment is almost always advised.

*Mosaic warts* are lesions which appear most commonly on the sole of the foot. They can also occur on the hand. The lesion consists of multiple small warts, growing in a cluster. The warts burrow deeply into the foot, causing pressure and pain. The patient notes a swelling, over which grows thick skin resembling a callus. When the physician removes this layer of skin the mosaic of multiple warts is visible underneath. Treatment of the con-

dition is slow and the outcome somewhat uncertain. Unless all warts are removed the condition recurs. Some patients are treated by applications of 40 per cent salicylic acid plaster and friction with a pumice stone. The plaster is left on for 48 hours. When it is removed, the dead skin, including the warts, is pumiced "down to the quick." The warts gradually come to the surface and more of them are removed by the pumice stone with each treatment. This process may take several months. Patience and perseverance are necessary. The patient, if properly instructed, can carry out the treatment himself. Other measures, more drastic, which are sometimes used to remove the warts are x-ray therapy and surgery.

**Herpes Simplex (Cold Sore).** Herpes simplex is caused by a virus. It is believed that many people harbor the virus, and that a variety of factors, including colds, fever, emotional upsets, and menses may precipitate the appearance of herpes simplex.

A group of blisters occurs on reddened, inflamed skin, usually near the month, or on the genitals. Usually, pain and burning accompany the lesion. Herpes simplex often is called a cold sore or a fever blister. The lesions subside in about a week. Some people are especially susceptible to herpes simplex, and they have frequent recurrence of the lesions.

Usually, the symptoms are mild, and the condition subsides without treatment. No specific treatment is available that can shorten the duration of the lesion. Sometimes smallpox vaccine is administered in an effort to control recurrent eruptions of herpes simplex.

**Herpes Zoster (Shingles).** Herpes zoster is caused by a virus. The virus is the same one that causes chickenpox. The cutaneous lesions usually follow the course of a sensory nerve (see Plate 8).

Before skin lesions appear, the patient usually experiences fever and malaise. Erythema and vesicles then appear, usually on the trunk or the face, along the course of a sensory nerve. Neurologic pains occur, and they may be severe, particularly in elderly persons. The condition subsides in about three weeks; however, the neuralgia may persist for months or even longer.

No specific treatment is available. Analgesics are ordered for the relief of the pain. Local applications like calamine lotion are used to soothe the lesions.

In older people systemic corticosteroids may be given. Clothing should be loose and nonirritating.

**Corns and Calluses.** The skin protects itself against friction by growing protective layers of epithelial tissue. Corns and calluses are familiar examples of local thickening of the skin in response to friction or pressure. Corns are hard, raised areas, which often are painful. Calluses are flat, thickened patches. Corns and calluses frequently form on the feet, due to constant pressure from shoes. Calluses also may form on the hands.

The relief of pressure or friction is the only treatment that is permanently effective. Various remedies usually contain a keratolytic agent, like salicylic acid, which helps to remove thickened, hard skin. However, if the pressure is not relieved, the corns and the calluses return. Rubbing cream into calluses may help to soften them.

**Furuncle, Carbuncle, Furunculosis.** Streptococci, staphylococci, and other pathogenic organisms sometimes exist harmlessly on the surface of the skin, but when the normal protective functions of the skin are impaired these pathogens may cause infection. For example, dryness and chapping of the skin may result in cracking, which allows microorganisms to enter and to cause infection. These lesions usually are caused by staphylococcal infection. Often, an injury, such as that caused by squeezing a pimple, is the immediate cause, since it allows infection to enter through a break in the skin. Furunculosis is frequently due to lowered resistance, poor general health, and poor diet. Sometimes virulent strains of hospital-type staphylococci are the cause.

The descriptive symptoms of these conditions are:

- Furuncle: A whitish, raised, painful lesion, surrounded by erythema. The area feels hard to the touch. After a few days the lesion exudes pus, and later a core. It heals, leaving a tiny scar. Neglect or mismanagement can cause a larger, obvious scar.
- Carbuncle: A large swollen lesion, often on the back of the neck, surrounded by erythema. It is acutely painful; it has several openings through which pus drains.
- Furunculosis: In addition to multiple boils, the patient may have fever, anorexia, weakness, and malaise.

Hot soaks are used to localize the infection. Often, for a single boil, this is the only treatment necessary. Antibiotics, such as penicillin or erythromycin, may be ordered to control the infection. Often, large doses are prescribed when fever is present, or if the lesion is a carbuncle. Incision and drainage may be necessary. When boils recur frequently, staphylococcus toxoid and autogenous vaccine (vaccine derived from the organism infecting the patient) may be given. Measures to improve general health are important in treating furunculosis. Often the condition occurs in people who are chronically fatigued, who are diabetic, or who eat a diet high in carbohydrate and fat but lacking other essential nutrients, like protein and vitamins. Rest, improved diet, and relief of emotional stress are important in increasing the patient's resistance.

The patient never should pick or squeeze a boil, as this practice favors spread of the infection to surrounding tissues or even to the bloodstream, causing septicemia. The exudate should be allowed to escape through the opening without the patient's squeezing the lesion or picking the top off. Drainage from a boil is infectious; strict medical aseptic technique is essential to prevent the spread of the infection to other parts of the patient's body or to other persons.

A single boil usually heals readily. Furunculosis may persist for many weeks or even months before the condition is controlled. Carbuncles, unless they are promptly and skillfully treated, can cause severe scarring and severe systemic as well as local symptoms.

**Acute Paronychia.** Paronychia is caused by an infection that enters the tissues around the nail through a break in the skin. Streptococci and staphylococci are the usual causative organisms. A painful, red, swollen area appears next to the nail. If it is neglected, it can spread completely around and even under the nail. Hot soaks are used to localize the infection. Antibiotics may be given to control the infection. Incision and drainage may be necessary. Usually, recovery occurs promptly, provided that the patient has adequate treatment.

**Sebaceous Cysts.** Sebaceous cysts are caused by obstruction of the duct of a sebaceous gland. The gland continues to secrete sebum despite the obstruction, thus causing accumulation of an oily secretion in the blocked duct. A swelling appears which at first is small, but which can grow to be large and unsightly. Treatment of the condition is surgical excision of the cyst, or cysts. If the lesion is small it may be removed outside the hospital; larger cysts must be dealt with in a hospital operating room.

**Hair Loss.** Hairs are constantly falling out and being replaced by new ones. An excessive loss of hair leads to thinning and to baldness. The reason for male baldness is not understood clearly, but it is believed to be related to endocrine function and to hereditary factors. Commercial claims notwithstanding, no scalp treatment now known can reliably prevent or cure baldness.

*Alopecia areata* is a condition of unknown cause characterized by patchy loss of hair. Emotional strain and endocrine factors may, it is believed, be implicated. Usually, the scalp is affected, although sometimes the eyebrows and the beard are involved. There is no specific treatment. If any factors, such as emotional upsets, are noted, the patient may receive treatment to relieve the underlying condition. Usually, the condition disappears spontaneously after six to eight months. Often, the new hairs growing over bald patches are white, but they later regain normal color. Occasionally, the hair loss continues until total baldness results, a condition called *alopecia totalis.*

**Ichthyosis.** Persons with ichthyosis have a congenital deficiency of oil and sweat secretions of the skin. The condition varies in severity. In the mild form the skin is very dry, scaly and rough, and somewhat thickened. The condition is worse in winter, when the dryness is especially pronounced, and leads to itching and discomfort. In more severe forms of ichthyosis the body is covered with irregularly shaped scales (hence the name *ichthyosis,* which means fish skin).

There is no cure. The dryness can be lessened by minimizing use of soap and hot water, particularly during winter months, since these increase the dryness and discomfort. Bath oils are helpful. Creams and lotions should be used liberally. Overexposure to sunlight also accentuates the dryness of the skin, and should be avoided.

**Intertrigo.** Intertrigo is characterized by reddening and irritation of opposing skin surfaces, such as those under the breasts, in the axillae, or in the groin. The main factor in treatment is to separate the skin surfaces, thus removing the friction, and to provide for drying by exposure to the air. The parts should be gently cleaned, and measures should be taken to keep the skin surfaces from rubbing together. For the patient with pendulous breasts, a properly fitting brassiere can keep the skin surfaces under the breasts apart. Pants or panty girdles with

long legs can serve the same purpose if the affected area is the upper, inner aspect of the thighs. Intertrigo is a particular problem among obese persons and is especially likely to occur during hot weather.

**Miliaria Rubra (Prickly Heat).** This condition is characterized by eruption of tiny red papules and blisters, which itch and burn. It is common in hot weather and is related to the profuse perspiration which many persons experience in hot climates. Cooling baths, using mild soap, and gentle drying of the skin are helpful. Absorbent underclothing, such as cotton, should be worn and changed frequently. For some patients, dusting powder applied after the cooling bath helps to minimize the irritation. Cornstarch, which is inexpensive, may be used. When applying the powder teach the patient to dust lightly, because a heavy layer of powder caught between two moving skin surfaces tends to roll into tiny balls that exert pinpoints of pressure on the skin and irritate it further. Use of air conditioners is likewise effective both as treatment and prevention.

**Lichen Planus.** Lichen planus is a condition of unknown cause in which there is eruption of itchy flat papules. The condition can affect wide areas of the body. It does not, however, occur on the face, palms or soles. Treatment includes use of lotions and ointments to relieve itching, and corticosteroids to provide relief. Though uncomfortable, the disease is not serious. The lesions disappear, in time, even without treatment.

**Dermatophytosis (Athlete's Foot).** Dermatophytosis is a fungus infection most common in young adults. Usually, dermatophytosis first affects the toes, and particularly the skin between them. The affected skin becomes red, scaly, cracked and sore. Sometimes, the condition also affects the sides of the toes and the soles of the feet. Sometimes it spreads to hands, axillae, and groin. The nails may become involved also and are characteristically yellow, friable and opaque.

The treatment includes benzoic and salicylic acid ointment (Whitfield's ointment) and undecylenic acid (Desenex powder and ointment). Many other remedies are available. (Before local medication is applied, scales and dead skin should be gently removed.) An antibiotic, grisofulvin, is useful in treatment. Grisofulvin is given orally in doses of 125 mg., four times daily. The drug may be required for many weeks in order to eradicate the infection.

Side effects include urticaria, headache, nausea, and diarrhea. In severe cases corticosteroids may be administered for a limited time (such as one week) to lessen the inflammation.

The disease may be transmitted from person to person through towels, locker room, and bathroom floors. Towels and slippers should not be shared, and those using locker rooms or "community" bathrooms in dormitories should avoid going barefoot. Early diagnosis and treatment are important in preventing spread. Keeping the feet (particularly the area between the toes) dry increases resistance to the infection. People whose feet perspire freely often find that powdering between the toes helps to keep the area dry. Washing and drying the feet, putting on clean, dry socks and a different pair of shoes after coming home from work is another aspect of personal hygiene that helps to keep the skin of the feet healthy.

Because the fungus can survive in shoes, slippers, and socks and these can constitute a source of reinfection, socks should be boiled after each use; slippers and shoes may have to be discarded. The fewer articles that the patient touches with his feet, the less is the problem of disinfection, and the fewer are the chances of reinfection. For example, it is preferable for the patient to wear clean socks at all times, even at night, rather than to place his bare feet in contact with slippers and bedding. Shared bath mats can be a source of infection for others. If the patient uses a separate towel as his bath mat, it can be more easily boiled and laundered than a heavy bath mat or a rug—and is therefore less likely to spread infection. The patient should clean the tub or the shower floor with a disinfectant, such as creosol (Lysol), after each use.

Treatment for dermatophytosis is tedious, but meticulous adherence to it usually controls the condition in time. However, patients who are careless of their personal hygiene often reinfect themselves and spread the condition to others.

**Infestation and Bites.** An infestation with pediculi (lice) results in *pediculosis*. The following terms are used to describe pediculosis:

- Pediculosis capitis—infestation of the hair or the scalp.
- Pediculosis corporis—infestation of the body surfaces with a louse larger than the one that affects the scalp and the hair. This parasite and its eggs may be found also in the patient's clothing—particularly within cuffs and seams.

- Pediculosis pubis—infestation of the pubic area with a very tiny louse shaped like a crab—hence the lay term, *crabs*. Although this condition occurs primarily in the pubic area, it may occur also in the hairy areas of the axilla.

The symptoms of pediculosis include itching, scratching, and irritation of the skin. Scratching denudes the skin, making it susceptible to infection. Eggs are deposited on the hair near the scalp, and they may be confused with dandruff. These eggs, often called *nits,* cannot be brushed out as dandruff can; they are attached firmly to the hair. The lice are tiny, grayish-brown creatures that may be seen when they move on the scalp.

Benzyl benzoate and benzine hexachloride are contained in a variety of ointments, powders, and lotions that are effective in killing pediculi. Kwell lotion and shampoo are commonly used preparations. Although pediculi can be promptly killed by these modern remedies, repeated infestations are likely if the individual continues to have close contact with others who harbor the parasities, and if personal hygiene is poor. Pediculosis capitis can be spread by shared toilet articles, like combs, and by close personal contact, such as that occurring in crowded places. Pediculosis pubis can be transmitted by toilet seats and by sexual intercourse.

*Scabies* is caused by infestation with the itch mite (*Sarcoptes scabiei*). Symptoms include intense itching, which usually is worse at night, accompanied by excoriation and burrows (the lesion caused when the female itch mite invades the skin, burrowing underneath, leaving a dark line). The lesions occur most often between the fingers and on the forearms, the axilla, the waistline, women's nipples, men's genitals, the umbilicus, and the lower back.

Kwell or benzyl benzoate in lotions and ointments are highly effective in treating scabies. Thorough bathing, clean clothing, and the avoidance of contact with others who have scabies are essential in preventing recurrence. Before any treatment is started, the patient should have a thorough bath. After medication has been applied, he should have a complete change of clothing.

The itch mite can be transmitted readily from one person to another by close personal contact and by sharing towels and clothing.

*Bedbug bites* are caused by tiny, dark-brown insects that infest mattresses and wooden bed frames. In heavily infested dwellings, bedbugs may live in crevices of the woodwork or in upholstered furniture. Although they are more common in crowded, unsanitary homes, bedbugs may be brought into any home on clothing or even on newspapers. The symptoms of bedbug bites include the appearance of wheals (hives) with central points or dots. These lesions may appear on any part of the body, but they are most commonly found on the wrists, the ankles and the buttocks. Usually, the bites require little local treatment. Sometimes, calamine lotion or witch hazel is applied to soothe the lesions. The services of an exterminator are frequently required to get rid of the bugs.

SOCIAL AND EMOTIONAL IMPLICATIONS. The diagnosis of pediculosis, scabies, or bedbug bites often causes embarrassment and is difficult for many people to accept. This is true whether the patient comes from a clean home in a suburban neighborhood, or whether he lives in a slum. To the poor person who lives in a crowded, dirty environment, the condition may be viewed as further evidence of economic and social disadvantages. Whether or not this is true, he will be sensitive to the attitudes of those who care for him. Indications of disgust and distaste will serve to make the patient less willing to seek treatment the next time that he needs health care. If the nurse sees the condition as a willful neglect of personal hygiene, or as a result of laziness and irresponsibility, her attitude of condemnation will show through—despite her attempts to hide it.

However, if the nurse recognizes the interdependence of social, economic, and health factors, she will be better able to understand the degree to which people can be the victims of poverty and lack of opportunity. The nurse who can accept the patient—even the one with pediculosis—has taken the biggest and most important step in helping that patient to recover from the condition and to learn to prevent its recurrence. Such instruction must be handled with great tact.

The person who has excellent personal hygiene and high living standards may also acquire parasites. Bedbugs and lice ask no questions about their host's social position! One fashionable young woman (tan and barelegged) went to the movies in the summertime and returned home with bedbug bites all over the backs of her legs. (Apparently they were acquired from infested upholstery at the theater.) She was painfully embarrassed when she learned the diagnosis. No bedbugs could have survived the strenuous cleaning and spraying to which she immediately subjected her apartment and her clothing. Such patients need to be told that these things can happen to anyone—and that the diagnosis itself implies absolutely nothing about the patient—except that he has acquired a parasite.

## SYSTEMIC CONDITIONS WITH DERMATOLOGIC SYMPTOMS

### Three Conditions with Similar Nursing Problems

**Pemphigus.** Fortunately, pemphigus is neither common nor infectious. Of unknown cause, it can affect men and women of any age, although it is more likely to occur during middle life.

Bullae (large blisters) appear on the skin and the mucous membranes. The bullae rupture, leaving a raw, crusted, weeping lesion with an offensive odor. There may be severe itching.

Local treatment is designed to clean, soothe, and relieve the itching. Baths or wet dressings, in which such mildly antiseptic solutions as potassium permanganate 1:25,000 are used, may be ordered. Neocalamine lotion is sometimes used to relieve itching. A high protein diet is given, because body protein is lost through the weeping areas of the skin. Pressure dressings are applied sometimes to the exuding areas. Antibiotics may be given, since raw skin surfaces predispose to infection. Corticosteroids, although they do not cure the disease, suppress the symptoms. However, the drugs must be continued for a considerable period to control the symptoms. Toxic effects from long-continued use of corticosteroids are common, but the risk seems justified by the nature of the disease and its prognosis.

Most patients eventually have exacerbation of the disease, although corticosteroids temporarily may cause a remission. Patients who develop pemphigus now live much longer and more comfortably because of the relief afforded by corticosteroids.

**Systemic Lupus Erythematosus.** This disease affects the collagen (an important constituent of connective tissue, widely distributed throughout the body). Because of the wide distribution of the affected tissues, the symptoms affect many different parts of the body. It is believed that systemic lupus erythematosus is an autoimmune disorder (i.e., that it is caused by a disorder of the patient's immunologic mechanism in which the antigen-antibody reaction occurs between substances of the patient's own body). Some hereditary predisposition to the condition may exist.

Recent investigations have indicated that the disease is not so uncommon as was believed formerly. The discovery of an abnormal cell (LE cell) in the blood has facilitated diagnosis. Young women are affected most often.

The disease is protracted; its course is characterized by exacerbations and remissions. The symptoms reflect dysfunction of many organs, including skin, kidneys, joints, lungs, and heart. Not all patients experience all symptoms. One patient may have considerable kidney involvement and yet may not show any skin lesions. The symptoms include erythema, characteristically in a butterfly pattern over the cheeks and the bridge of the nose; painful joints; edema, fever, and anemia.

There is at present no specific treatment for the condition. Adrenocortical steroids are helpful in relieving the symptoms. The patient may require treatment over a prolonged period, and side effects from steroid therapy are not uncommon. ACTH and cortisone do not cure the condition; when they are withdrawn, symptoms usually reappear. Symptomatic treatment is important (e.g., salicylates are given to relieve joint pains and to reduce fever). Antimalarial drugs like atabrine and chloroquine are sometimes very helpful.

The prognosis is guarded. Although corticosteroids have not cured the condition, they have helped to make the patients with this disease more comfortable.

**Scleroderma (progressive systemic sclerosis).** Scleroderma is a progressive, systemic disease of unknown cause, characterized by sclerosis (hardening) of collagenous tissue. Relatively uncommon, the condition is most likely to occur during middle life. Some evidence suggests an autoimmune cause of this illness.

Usually, many organs are involved, including skin, muscles, bowel, heart, and lungs. The skin becomes smooth, hard, and tight. Movement becomes difficult, due to the inelasticity of skin and muscles. The face may become expressionless. The movement and the function of the heart and the lungs may be impaired, causing dyspnea, cyanosis, and edema. The disease is slowly progressive, leading often to severe disability and death. The course

of the disease is characterized by periods of exacerbation, and remission. Although the skin manifestations are the most easily visible, the most serious changes are those that occur internally and interfere with the functioning of vital organs.

There is no specific treatment. Symptomatic treatment includes ointments, massage, heat, physical therapy, and hydrotherapy in an effort to relieve stiffness and inelasticity. Cortisone may provide temporary relief.

**Nursing Care.** The nursing care of patients with pemphigus, systemic lupus erythematosus, and scleroderma is a challenge to any nurse's skill and understanding. These conditions present similar nursing problems in that:

- The disease is prolonged.
- The prognosis is grave.
- Specific, curative treatment is not available.
- The symptoms often can be relieved for considerable periods by corticosteroids. Because these drugs are administered for long periods, be alert for side effects.

The nursing management of these patients involves helping them to maintain as much independence as possible for as long as possible. They also need help in adjusting to restrictions in activity when their condition makes limitations necessary. Because these illnesses tend to be long-term, many patients remain at home during part of the course of the disease. Family members need help in understanding how to care for the patient. Homemaker services, home-care programs, and community nursing services may make it possible for the patient to remain at home during much of the illness.

Particularly, patients with pemphigus need to be shown that others are willing to care for them— and are willing to minister to their very great physical needs, as well as their emotional needs. Because the lesions of pemphigus cause oozing, secondary infection, and unpleasant odor, these patients may feel that others are unwilling to go near or even touch them.

Being "there" is one of the most demanding and rewarding aspects of nursing. It is one of the privileges of nurses to stay with, to help, and to support patients and their families during prolonged illness. This aspect of nursing is taxing, both physically and emotionally. The nurse must try to recognize her own feelings in demanding situations. This self-awareness will help her to control her reactions and to identify and to concentrate on the patient's needs when she is with him.

Meticulous care can greatly minimize the patient's discomfort. For instance, the patient with pemphigus may require frequent gentle cleansing of his mouth if the lesions occur there. Local treatments ordered by the physician, such as compresses or baths, help to soothe, to clean, to lessen odor, and to minimize secondary infection. Because these patients are especially vulnerable to infection, techniques to prevent infection must be followed scrupulously.

## Other Conditions

**Erysipelas.** Elderly persons are especially susceptible to this condition, which is caused by the hemolytic streptococcus. The symptoms include chills, fever, headache, and a raised reddened area of the skin, which spreads quickly and is sometimes accompanied by blistering. The face frequently is affected.

Erysipelas is treated by antibiotics, such as penicillin, after which most patients recover quickly. If these drugs are not given, the outlook is serious.

**Erythema Nodosum.** This condition is characterized by development of red, tender nodules in cutaneous and subcutaneous tissues. The areas over shins, thighs, and forearms are commonly involved. The patient may have fever and malaise. The cause of the condition is not fully understood, but it is believed to be an allergic reaction to drugs or to viral or bacterial infections.

Treatment involves identifying and, if possible, removing the cause. In addition, the condition is treated symptomatically by salicylates, bed rest, and, occasionally in severe cases, by corticosteroids. The condition usually disappears in several weeks to a month. Occasionally, a patient is troubled by recurrent episodes of erythema nodosum.

**Polyarteritis (periarteritis nodosa).** This condition is characterized by nodules that appear along the course of arteries. Arteries of medium and small caliber are usually involved. Symptoms often include widespread areas of the body in which the arteries are affected. There may be muscle and joint pain, nausea, vomiting, diarrhea, and abdominal pain. Fever and weight loss are common. Treatment is symptomatic and includes analgesics, rest, and corticosteroids; the latter often produce marked

relief of symptoms. The prognosis is guarded. When the arteries of the heart, lungs or kidneys are extensively involved, the condition is usually fatal.

**Erythema multiforme.** This condition is a systemic illness that manifests itself in a variety of symptoms, prominent among which is an eruption of red macules, vesicles, papules, and bullae. Skin areas over the wrists, hands, ankles, feet, knees, elbows, and face are commonly affected. Mucous membranes may also be involved. Fever, malaise, pains in muscles and joints, and symptoms of gastrointestinal disturbance may accompany the skin lesions. Symptoms of disturbed functioning of urinary, respiratory, and nervous systems sometimes occur.

The cause of the condition is not fully understood. Some physicians consider it secondary to other conditions, such as drug reactions and infections. Others believe that it is a separate disease, the cause of which may be an infectious agent, unidentified as yet. The condition is quite common, particularly in its mild form.

Treatment includes eradication of any underlying illness, application of soothing lotions, such as calamine, to the lesions and administration of antihistamines. Severe forms of the illness may require administration of corticosteroids. The wide variety of symptoms which may occur are treated symptomatically.

## PREMALIGNANT AND MALIGNANT SKIN LESIONS

The public has become so aware of the problem of cancer that any growth appearing on the skin may cause a great deal of alarm, and it may precipitate extreme reactions. One patient may insist that a benign lesion be removed instantly, because he is sure that it is cancer. Another may be so fearful of the possibility of cancer that he refuses to see a physician.

Skin lesions usually are readily observable, thus facilitating prompt diagnosis and treatment. Nurses have a responsibility to teach people to seek medical advice for any lesion that persists. If it is malignant, prompt treatment often can prevent spread and cure the condition.

Several factors predispose to malignant changes in the skin:

- Prolonged, repeated exposure to ultraviolet rays. Sailors, farmers, overzealous sun bathers, and others who are exposed to a great deal of sunlight are particularly vulnerable.
- Exposure to radiation.
- Ulcerations of long duration and scar tissue. Both are prone to malignant changes.

**Precancerous Lesions.** Some lesions are considered precancerous. *Leukoplakia* is characterized by shiny white patches that usually occur on the mucous membrane of the mouth or the female genitalia. If leukoplakia occurs in the mouth, smoking is definitely contraindicated, because it makes the condition worse. Rough, jagged teeth should be replaced, so that they do not irritate the lesion. Surgical excision of the lesions often is recommended because of the danger of cancer. The lesions also may be removed by electrodesiccation.

*Birthmarks* (*nevi*) are of various kinds, including vascular nevi (*angiomas*), brown moles, and black moles. The lesion may not be visible at birth; however, the beginnings of the lesion are present at birth and may appear later. Black, smooth moles are the most likely to become cancerous. However, any mole that becomes irritated, bleeds, or begins to grow larger should have prompt medical attention. Surgical removal usually is recommended. Light brown moles that are not located where irritation from clothing is a problem usually do not have to be removed unless it is desirable for cosmetic reasons. Tattooing of flat angiomas is used sometimes to make them less conspicuous.

*Senile keratoses* are brownish, scaly spots appearing on the skin of older persons. They are most likely to occur on exposed portions of the skin, such as the face, the ears or the hands. Patients who develop senile keratoses should be advised to seek medical attention. Because the lesions are common and seem to be insignificant, they often are disregarded. But they may become malignant, and their removal usually is recommended.

**Malignant Lesions.** Malignant growths of the skin usually are primary lesions. The spread to other parts of the body may be prevented by prompt removal of the malignant tissue. *Epithelioma* is a common type of skin cancer. It arises from the surface layers of the skin. If promptly treated by surgical excision, electrodesiccation, or x-ray therapy, these lesions usually are controlled promptly. On the other hand, *malignant melanoma* is a highly malignant, rapidly spreading lesion. Usually, it is coal-black. Wide surgical excision may be attempted to save the patient's life; however, because of the rapid spread, the prognosis is poor. *Squamous-cell carcinoma* is another dangerous type of lesion, because it tends to metastasize to internal organs. This type of cancer often occurs on the tongue or the lower lip. (Chronic irritation from pipe smoking is a common causative factor in lesions involving the lower lip.) Depending on the size and the location of the lesion, the treatment may involve electrodesiccation, surgical excision, or x-ray therapy.

## REFERENCES AND BIBLIOGRAPHY

ABEL, T. M.: Facial Disfigurement, *in* GARRETT, J. F. (ed.): *Psychological Aspects of Physical Disability,* Washington, D.C., U.S. Government Printing Office, (n.d.).

ALLEN, L. G.: Facts and fancies about cosmetics and aging skin, *Nurs. Clin. N. Am.* 2, 2, Philadelphia, Saunders, 1967.

BAER, R., et al.: Changing patterns of sensitivity to common contact allergens, *Arch. Derm.* 89:3, 1964.

BOWDEN, L.: Current trends in treating malignant melanoma, *AORN* 17:84, March 1973.

BUTTERWORTH, T., and STREAN, L.: *Manual of Dermatologic Syndromes,* New York, McGraw-Hill, 1964.

CAHN, M. M.: The skin from infancy to old age, *Am. J. Nurs.* 6:993, July 1960.

CUNLIFFE, W. J.: Itching—mechanism, causes and treatment, *Nurs. Times* 68:356, March 1962.

DAVE, V. K.: Contact dermatitis, *Nurs. Times* 67:504, April 1971.

DUBOIS, E. (ed.): *Lupus Erythematosus,* New York, McGraw-Hill, 1966.

GOLDMAN, L.: Prevention and treatment of eczema, *Am. J. Nurs.* 64:114, March 1964.

GRIESEMER, R. D.: The emotional impact of fatal skin disorders, *Med. Insight* 4:28, January 1972.

JOHNSON, S. (ed.): *The Skin and Internal Disease,* New York, McGraw-Hill, 1967.

LEIDER, M., and ROSENBLUM, M.: *A Dictionary of Dermatological Words, Terms, and Phrases,* New York, McGraw-Hill, 1968.

LEIDER, M.: Some principles of dermatologic nursing, *RN* 35:48, May 1972.

LEWIS, G. M., and WHEELER, C. E.: *Practical Dermatology,* ed. 3, Philadelphia, Saunders, 1967.

MACKENNA, R. (ed.): *Modern Trends in Dermatology,* Washington, D.C., Butterworth, 1966.

MAIBACH, H. I., and STOUGHTON, R. B.: Topical corticosteroids, *Med. Clin. N. Am.* 57:1253, September 1973.

MARTEN, R. H.: Skin, tough but vulnerable, *Nurs. Mirror* 129:34, November 1969.

MOHS, F. E., et al.: Chemosurgery and skin cancer, *AORN* 13:89, February 1971.

MONTAGU, A.: *Touching: The Human Significance of the Skin,* New York: Columbia University Press, 1971.

MUSAPH, H.: *Itching and Scratching,* Philadelphia, Davis, 1964.

NICHOLS, E. G.: Jeanette: No hope for cure, *Nurs. Forum,* 111:97, 1972.

RICE, A. K.: Common skin infections in school children, *Am. J. Nurs.* 73:1905, November 1973.

RODMAN, M. J.: Drugs for allergic disorders, *RN* 34: 53, July 1971.

SARKANY, I.: Detergents and hand eczema, *Nurs. Times* 67:1211, September 1971.

SAUER, G. C.: *Manual of Skin Disease,* ed. 2, Philadelphia, Lippincott, 1966.

THOMSON, W.: Occupation and the skin, *Nurs. Times* 68:873, July 1972.

THORNE, N.: The problem of the black skin, *Nurs. Times* 65:999, August 1969.

UTTLEY, M.: Sweat glands and perspiration, *Nurs. Mirror* 133:35, November 1971.

WEXLER, L.: Gamma benzene hexachloride in treatment of pediculoses and scabies, *Am. J. Nurs.* 69: 565, March 1969.

WINKELMANN, R. K., et al.: Chronic aeral dermatitis, *JAMA* 225:378, July 1973.

# The Patient Undergoing Plastic Surgery

The terms *plastic surgery* and *reconstructive surgery* often are used interchangeably to refer to the repair of defects that may be congenital or acquired through injury or radical surgery. (See Chapter 56, which deals with dermatologic problems, for further discussion of disfigurement.) The repair may have been performed for cosmetic purposes or to improve function. For example, a crooked nose may be straightened, or contracted scar tissue in the axilla may be freed to restore normal motion to the arm. A deformed hand may be totally reconstructed by repair of tendon, bone, nerve, or skin. An eyelid that has been damaged by trauma or by surgery for cancer may be repaired by means of a pedicle graft or advancement flaps. The four main kinds of conditions treated by plastic surgery are:

1. Congenital deformities, such as harelip and protruding ears, spina bifida, hypospadius.
2. Deformities resulting from trauma, such as burns and automobile accidents, especially injuries to the hands and face (see Plate 11).
3. Conditions for which the patient seeks cosmetic surgery, such as face lifting and body contouring.
4. Disfigurement resulting from malignant disease, such as cancer of the head and neck and breast (see Plate 10).

## NURSING ASSESSMENT

The following areas are particularly revelant to nursing assessment in plastic surgery. This is not meant to be inclusive, but represents some major areas for concern.

**1028**

| AREA | ASSESSMENT |
|------|-----------|
| Psychosocial/mental/ emotional | Perception and understanding of illness and disfigurement |
| | Perception of need for plastic surgery; cosmetic and/or functional |
| | Expectations regarding singular outcome of surgery |
| | Previous reactions to illness |
| | Major areas of concern regarding illness/surgery |
| | Affect: emotional response to disfigurement and to attempts to correct it |
| | Self-esteem |
| | Response of significant others to the patient's surgery |
| Neuro/sensory/motor | Movement and feeling in target area |
| | Response to stimuli |
| | Range of motion |
| Circulatory | BP; pulse; presence of edema |
| Skin | Color; intactness; scars |
| | Operative site: dry, drainage, odors, dressing |
| General health status | Nutrition, rest and sleep, elimination; ability to carry out aspects of personal hygiene |
| Needs for postoperative instruction (especially important, since these patients are often discharged after brief hospitalization) | Care of operative area when at home |
| | Resumption of function of the part (e.g., hand) |
| Possible effects of changed appearance upon his work, home, and social life | Ability to cope with responses of colleagues, friends, neighbors, if there is considerable change in appearance |

## PLASTIC SURGERY: APPEARANCE AND FUNCTIONAL IMPROVEMENT

Plastic surgery holds the promise of a more normal appearance and improved function for many patients. This highly specialized treatment combines art and medicine. Both appearance and function are important considerations; however, their relative importance varies with the part of the body involved. For instance, function is a prime consideration in reconstructive surgery on the hand, and appearance is of particular significance in surgery involving the face. Surgical treatment that produces the greatest functional improvement may not be the same as that which leads to the most satisfactory cosmetic result.

Plastic surgery is not new, but advances in surgical techniques and the control of infection produce results that never before were possible. The large number of combat injuries during World Wars I and II stimulated interest in and study of plastic surgery. The need for plastic and reconstructive surgery is not limited to war injuries, but it forms an important part of the treatment of civilians who are burned or cut or suffering from traumatic amputation of some part of the body. Patients who undergo radical surgery for the treatment of cancer often require plastic surgery to repair the defect left by the extensive excision of malignant tissue.

The following are examples of plastic surgery to improve function:

**Hand Reconstruction.** Because all tissues in the hand are vital for essential function, reconstructive surgery requires orthopedic surgery, neurosurgery, peripheral vascular surgery, and plastic surgery. The basic goals sought for hand function include push, pull, pinch, and hook.

Because of recent advances in microvascular repair, re-implantation of amputated digits, and even arm re-implantation are technically feasible. Return of function is a more realistic goal because of techniques which permit reconstruction of nerve injuries.

**Midfacial Retrusion.** This more recently developed surgery allows for the advancement of the middle third of the face to produce a more functional dental occlusion as well as a more normal profile. This type of surgery requires the teamwork of dental surgeons, orthodontists, and psychologists.

**Cosmetic Surgery.** In cosmetic surgery the aim is not to produce beauty as such, but beauty in the sense that the changed appearance is appropriate for the particular patient and blends unnoticeably into his features, producing as natural an appearance as possible.

When we think of cosmetic surgery, we usually think only of the face and the neck. Although these areas are involved frequently in plastic surgery, it is by no means limited to them. The degree of disfigurement can range from slight to marked; however, it may not be a reliable indicator of the patient's reaction to his condition. A very tiny flaw may seem like a huge blemish to a person who is very sensitive about his appearance. Cosmetic surgery may bring great relief to patients who are very conscious of, for example, a hooked nose; correcting the nose may bring the person a new feeling of poise and assurance.

However, people who tend to blame all their failures and disappointments on what may seem to others a barely noticeable blemish have unrealistic expectations of what plastic surgery can accomplish. Although it can remold a nose and remove some wrinkles, it cannot suddenly change the patient's whole personality or make him young again. Sometimes, plastic surgery is contraindicated if the patient's dissatisfaction with his appearance seems to be an expression of a deeper emotional problem. Such a patient is likely to be disappointed with the results of plastic surgery, since the operation cannot reasonably fulfill all his expectations. Hence, careful screening of candidates for plastic surgery is essential. Psychologists, psychiatrists, social workers, and nurses sometimes participate in the screening process. Those patients whose difficulties seem to be more an indication of emotional problems than of physical disfigurement may be referred for psychotherapy.

The pressures on people to conform to demanding standards of personal appearance are mounting with urbanization (and the resultant increase in the number of persons with whom they have contact), and with the growing emphasis on personal attractiveness in holding jobs, winning friends, and establishing an enduring marriage. Many people who consult plastic surgeons do so in an attempt to compete more successfully in job or other situations in which an attractive appearance is especially important. Improved appearance can also increase one's poise and confidence.

Although in the past use of plastic surgery, particularly to lessen the appearance of aging, was considered primarily a woman's concern, there are now many men who seek plastic surgery in order to compete more successfully in a business and social world which places a premium on youthful appearance.

The following are a few examples of plastic surgery performed for cosmetic purposes:

"FACE LIFTING" AND BLEPHAROPLASTY. Most of the incision for face lifting is made in the hairline. Wrinkles are removed by the tightening of fascia and skin and the removing of excess skin. Most of the fine scar, resulting from surgery, is concealed by the hair. Modern face-lifting techniques produce results that are longer lasting than was the case with formerly used techniques. Although more time is necessary to evaluate how long the results of these newer procedures last, it is believed that one face-lifting procedure will suffice for many years.

Frequently blepharoplasty (eyelid reconstruction) is carried out as part of the surgical procedure, in an effort to remove the aged appearance which frequently sets in at about the age of 50 when fibers of the dermis lose their elasticity, and some of the subcutaneous fat that produces a youthful look becomes absorbed. In eyelid reconstruction, incisions are made which are hidden in normal crease-lines. The excessive eyelid skin and orbital fat (if necessary) are removed. The result is a more balanced, symmetrical, and, hence, more attractive appearance of the face.

RHINOPLASTY. Since the nose is the most exposed part of the face, it is frequently injured, often without the individual's remembering the accident. Reconstruction of the tissues has developed to a fine art. Usually within two to three weeks after the surgery the patient's improvement in appearance, breathing, and senses of smell and taste are apparent. With these improvements come greater poise, assurance, and improved morale.

DEFORMITIES OF THE EXTERNAL EAR. Congenital anomalies of the external ear include macrotia (excessive size), microtia (small size), and protruding ear, as well as complete absence of the external ear. The cosmetic deformity may be severe, particularly in young boys and men who wear short hair styles. The more successful plastic surgery has been that done to reduce the excessive size of the ear and replace the ear in its proper position. Less successful have been attempts to construct a normally appearing ear.

ARTIFICIAL PARTS. Artificial parts may be used to camouflage defects. For instance, part of a nose or an ear may be made of plastic to match the patient's features so exactly that it is hard to tell which is the prosthetic part, and which is the natural. Plastic materials are also used as framework or supporting structures over which the patient's tissues grow. For instance, a plastic material, such as silicone rubber, may be used beneath the skin to correct an underdeveloped chin. Plastic materials used in this way must be chemically inert and nonirritating and should retain their shape and consistency when inside the patient's body. Whether such implants may prove to be carcinogenic is a question that must await long-term study of patients who have received such implants. Studies to date indicate that the plastics in current use are noncarcinogenic.

Tissues, such as skin, bone, cartilage, and heart are being intensively studied in the field of organ transplantation. Improved methods are being developed by combining serological techniques with cell mediated techniques. It has been proven that the development of specific cellular immunity (antigen-antibody reaction) is directly proportional to clinical graft rejection. Techniques are being developed to predict which patients will reject particular grafts.

BODY CONTOURING. There has been an increase in demand for body contouring including mammoplasty, abdominal lipectomy, buttock reduction, thigh reduction, and arm and forearm reduction. In all of these procedures care must be taken in screening patients to determine their individual needs and expectations.

There are instances, in which the plastic surgery is done in conjunction with necessary surgical procedures. For example, there are situations in which the augmentation surgery is collateral to surgical removal of the breast for some reason. An example of body contouring follows:

*Mammoplasty* may be performed to change the size and the shape of the breasts (Fig. 57-1). Very large breasts may make a woman self-conscious,

contribute to poor posture, and interfere with breathing. Excess tissue is removed surgically under general anesthesia. Afterward, the patient must wear a firm supporting brassiere for several months until healing is complete, and the tissues are firm. Surgery is sometimes undertaken to enlarge small breasts (augmentation mammoplasty). Tissues from the patient's own body, such as a buttock, or plastic materials, such as silicone gel within a silastic bag, are used as an implant between the chest wall and the breast. Placing the material between the chest wall and the breast, rather than inside the breast, has two advantages: (1) the function of the breast is unimpaired: the woman can lactate normally; and (2) the possibility of carcinogenesis from introduction of foreign materials into breast tissue is obviated.

DERMABRASION. This is a technique for removing surface layers of scarred skin. It is useful in lessening such scars as the pitting from severe acne. The outermost layers of the skin are removed by sandpaper, a rotating wire brush, or a diamond wheel. A local anesthetic, such as ethyl chloride-freon mixture may be used during the procedure. Afterward, the skin feels raw and sore, and some crusting from serous exudate occurs. Patients frequently say that the discomfort is much like that from a burn. The patient is instructed not to wash

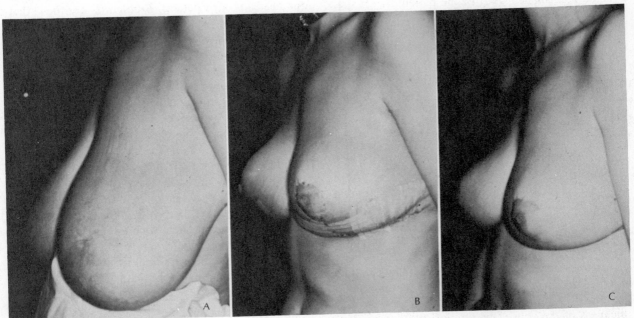

**Figure 57-1.** (A) Hypertrophy of breasts with ptosis partially due to pregnancy. (B) Patient two weeks following mammoplasty: removal of excess breast tissue, formation of a "skin brassiere." (C) Patient two months postoperatively. (Courtesy, Dr. Robby Meijer, Livingston, N.J.)

the area for five or six days, until sufficient healing has occurred. He should avoid picking or touching it, since this contact might cause infection, or produce marking of the tissues.

TATTOOING. This technique is used to change the color of the skin. Pigments are blended to just the right shade for the patient's skin and then are implanted into it. The treatment is useful in covering up dark-red birthmarks (port wine stains), and in matching the color of grafted skin to its surrounding skin more exactly. However, the pigments may shift position beneath the skin so that they are no longer effective in covering up the blemish. Also, the pigments sometimes look different in environments of various temperatures. For example, a tattoo that is not noticeable at room temperature may become noticeable, due to color change, when the patient goes out into the cold.

Tattooing and dermabrasion usually are carried out in the physician's office or in a clinic.

## SKIN GRAFTS

Skin grafts (see Plate 9) may consist of *autografts* (skin transplanted from one part of the patient's body to another) or of *homografts* (skin transplanted from one person to another). Only autografts or skin transplanted from one identical twin to another can become a permanent part of the patient's own skin. However, homografts are useful in temporarily closing large defects, thus preventing further loss of tissue fluid. Although the homografts slough away after one or more weeks and must be replaced by autografts, they tide the patient over the critical period of his illness and help him to recover enough to permit the use of autografts.

Considerable study is in progress in an effort to develop measures that will prevent the body's rejection of homografts, which is related to the body's immunologic mechanisms for protecting itself against foreign substances. It has been found that administration of antihistamines, which lessen the intensity of the body's immunologic reaction to foreign substances, enables the body to retain a homograft longer than would otherwise be possible.

**Thickness.** Skin grafts vary in thickness. The Ollier-Thiersch graft consists of large pieces of skin varying in width from one-half to nearly the full thickness of the skin. This type of graft, also called a *thick split skin graft,* is widely used. Large slices of skin may be removed by a *dermatome,* a me-

chanical cutting device that can be adjusted so that precisely the desired thickness of skin will be evenly removed.

*Pinch grafts* consist of small cones of skin that are lifted, cut off and transplanted to the graft area. They look like little islands, or dots of skin, set on the recipient site. The pieces of skin grow together, so that when healing has occurred, the entire area is completely covered. Pinch grafts do not give as smooth an appearance as other grafts; the skin appears rough and pebbly. Therefore, such grafts are used on areas of skin that will be covered by clothing.

*Full-thickness grafts* (Wolfe-Krause grafts) are composed of a full depth of skin. They give the best cosmetic appearance, and therefore they are used for face, neck and hands when feasible. The supply of skin from the patient's own body that is suitable for use as full-thickness grafts is limited. Sufficient skin for this purpose may be procured when the defect is small, but it may be difficult to obtain enough suitable full-thickness skin to repair a large defect. The surgeon must consider also matching the skin for color and texture. For example, color and texture of skin from the abdomen are quite different from those of the skin of the face.

**Types.** Several different types of skin grafts are in use. The physician selects the kind best suited to the needs of each patient. *Free grafts* are those that are completely severed from the donor site and transferred to the recipient site. In *pedicle* or *tube grafts* two or three sites may be involved. A piece of skin is freed at one end, and the free end is allowed to grow onto the recipient site, while the other end is still attached at the original site. The flap of skin receives its blood supply from the original site until the blood supply is sufficiently well established for it to be transferred to the recipient site.

Pedicle grafts are used when thick pieces of skin that could not survive an interruption of blood supply are transplanted. Pedicle grafts can carry tissues other than skin with them, such as bone and fat.

For grafts to "take," there must be a sufficient blood supply to the part and an absence of infection. The graft must stick close to the tissues on which it is to grow; excess blood or serous fluid can cause the graft to become separated from the tissues and to fail to grow. Sometimes warm, moist saline compresses are placed on pedicle grafts. The skin being transplanted by a pedicle has blood supplied from the donor site. The warmth transmitted to the recipient bed through the graft is believed to favor the development of blood circulation in the graft. Such drugs as tolazoline (Priscoline) and alcohol are sometimes administered because they, too, cause vasodilation, thus increasing the blood supply in the recipient bed.

Usually, it takes about three or four weeks for sufficient blood supply to be established to permit severing the skin completely from the donor site. Meanwhile, depending on the location of the parts involved, the patient may have to be in a very awkward position. Sometimes, a cast is used to fix the parts in the proper position and to prevent movement until the flap can be freed from its original site. For instance, a cast may hold the arm to the chin, so that a skin flap can grow from the arm to repair a defect of the chin. Nutrition is also important to the success of the graft. The patient must be helped to take plenty of protein and vitamins and sufficient fluids, so that his body tissues will be as healthy as possible.

**Dressings.** Skin grafts may be covered by a variety of dressings, or, occasionally, by no dressings at all. (Some surgeons believe that the grafts heal more quickly and with less chance of infection if they are left exposed to the air.) Fine-mesh petrolatum gauze is a popular type of dressing. Moderate pressure may be applied to help to hold the grafts in contact with the recipient site by placing sponge rubber or cotton pads over the petrolatum gauze and holding them firmly in place with a bandage.

## NURSING CARE OF PATIENTS WHO HAVE PLASTIC SURGERY

Classifying surgery as *minor* or *major* has many pitfalls. Much of plastic surgery is referred to as minor, because the areas involved usually are superficial and readily accessible. Nevertheless, the success or the failure of the surgery has grave consequences *for the patient*.

Whether the patient has skin grafting or reconstructive surgery of some feature, such as his nose, it is important for him to understand what to expect from the surgery. The surgeon will discuss the operation with the patient in advance, but there may be many times during his recovery when the patient will turn to the nurse for repeated explanation and reassurance. Sometimes, moving pictures portray the removal of a dressing after plastic surgery as though it were the unveiling of a beautiful statue. Everyone stands by, breathless, and the hush is broken by someone saying, "Oh, doctor, she's beautiful." If this is what the patient and his family expect, they are certain to be disappointed. Plastic surgery, like every other kind of surgery, causes some trauma in the process of helping the patient. For instance, immediately after plastic repair of the nose (rhinoplasty), the patient's nose may be swollen and bruised. His first thought may be that he looks worse than ever. He should be helped to understand that he cannot evaluate the results of the surgery until the healing has taken place. The swelling will disappear and so will the black-and-blue spots.

The nurse must be especially careful not to respond to the patient's apprehension concerning the outcome of surgery with promises of favorable results. Because most patients feel considerable tension about the outcome of plastic surgery, they may question the nurse repeatedly about matters which can be answered only by the surgeon. The patient should be allowed to express his concerns, and it should be explained to him that he will have the opportunity to discuss the matter further with his physician. Because some patients are hesitant to voice some of their worries to the physician, it is important for the nurse to mention to the physician the questions which the patient has raised, so that he can talk further with the patient about them.

The nurse has an important part to play in insuring the success of a plastic-surgery procedure. She must guard carefully against conditions that would interfere with the success of a graft. For instance, care must be taken to avoid excessive pressure that might impair circulation. (A bandage that is too tight can interfere with circulation.) The part must be protected from injury. The patient should not lie on or bump the area. The most meticulous aseptic technique is necessary to prevent infection. If a warm, moist dressing is ordered, the nurse should make sure that the solution is sterile, that it is poured into a sterile basin, and that it is wrung out and applied with sterile forceps. It should be about 105 degrees F. A dressing that is too hot could damage the tissues rather than help them to grow. A dressing should never be changed unless the physician specifically requests it; removing the dressing may take the graft with it. The nurse should report to the physician any evidence of bleeding or of pus on the dressing.

Patients with skin grafts have two sites to be cared for before and after the surgery—the donor site and the recipient site. Usually, the skin of the donor site is shaved before the patient goes to the operating room. The surgeon will specify which area (often the upper thigh) is to be prepared. The recipient site is the wound or the defect to which the grafts will be applied. The surgeon will specify the particular care needed for this area, too. Postoperatively, the nurse must observe both the donor area and the recipient area. For instance, a sheet or a slice of skin may have been removed from the anterior thigh by a dermatome, leaving a raw, weeping surface. Often, petrolatum gauze is placed over the wound and covered by a dry dressing. The nurse must observe this area for any sign of infection or bleeding, and she must protect it from injury until it has healed.

Permanent grafts must be obtained from the patient's own skin; yet, when large areas of a patient's skin have been destroyed by trauma, such as a severe burn, the amount of healthy skin available for grafting is limited. The failure of the graft to grow can mean that another operation is necessary, or that the procedure cannot be repeated because of the scarcity of healthy skin. Most patients who undergo plastic surgery already have suffered a great deal (e.g., the patient whose life was endangered by severe, mutilating burns, or the one whose face has been deformed from an auto accident). Because of what they have already been through, the disappointment of an unsuccessful skin graft may be almost too much to bear. Many of these patients feel that their whole future is staked on the success of the surgery—a difficult but important point for the nurse to understand.

When the patient should first be permitted to see the results of the surgery is a perennial and much debated question. If he does not see the area during the immediate postoperative period, he will be spared the shock of seeing the part before its appearance has improved. For this reason, the dressings may be left on somewhat longer than is absolutely necessary.

Attempts to remove mirrors seem quite unrealistic, since many patients are ambulatory shortly after the surgery and can readily find a mirror in the bathroom or obtain one from another patient or a visitor. However, if the disfigurement is one that is not likely to show rapid improvement (for example, when the plastic surgery must be postponed for a considerable period, or when the defect is so marked that even after plastic surgery the deformity is obvious), the patient must be helped gradually to accept his changed appearance. Becoming aware of the change by seeing it himself is a difficult but essential part of this process. Banishing mirrors is not a kindness to this patient, who must later face a world with many mirrors—the ones on walls and those on the faces of others.

The patient's reaction to the change in his appearance may sometimes seem baffling—particularly when the surgery results in a considerably improved appearance. Instead of immediately showing pleasure and gratitude, the patient may cry. (Even when a change in his body is a cosmetic improvement, some loss of the patient's "old self" is inevitable, and grief can occur over the loss, even of a deformity.) Ordinarily, grieving is short-lived when the surgery results in improved appearance. It is important during this period that the patient be helped to realize that his reactions are acceptable and not unusual. The nurse should give her patient opportunity to talk about his feelings concerning his changed appearance. Another possible reaction after plastic surgery is hostility, which the child may show by tantrums and fighting with neighborhood children, but which in an adult is more likely to be expressed as crankiness, impatience, and general dissatisfaction. Reasons for such behavior are individual, and each patient must discover these and deal with them himself. An accepting, concerned listener can help him to do so. Possibly he has stored up anger as a result of many years of humiliation over a deformity, and once it is removed, so too is the muzzle he has placed on the expression of his anger.

Sensitivity is required in helping the patient to resume his contacts with others after surgery. This is especially problematic if the patient's appearance has been altered for the worse. For example, a patient who has been badly burned may have his disfigurement only partially alleviated by plastic surgery, and this improvement may be the result of numerous operations over a period of many months. The patient may dread being seen by family and friends but be badly in need of the encouragement and support their visits can bring. Often the nurse can help in such situations, by gently preparing visitors before they enter the room for the first time. Such preparation may involve a brief explanation, such as, "You will notice that his face is covered with dressings. He must lie quite still now until more healing has occurred. I've put a chair beside his bed, where he can see you easily without raising his head." The nurse should also be available when visitors leave the patient's room, so that they may express their concerns. She should advise them to consult the surgeon about questions they may have concerning the procedure and what may be expected in relation to the patient's appearance.

Tactfully encouraging the patient's contact with other patients on the unit can also help lessen his isolation. Careful assessment of the patient's readiness, and that of other patients, is important. For example, a patient who is painfully self-conscious about his appearance may tolerate and then begin to enjoy the visits of a quiet person who comes to offer some brief service, such as sharing a newspaper, but be overwhelmed by being wheeled to a solarium where a group of patients is gathered.

The period of recovery may be brief (as is usually the case after such procedures as rhinoplasty), or prolonged, as occurs when the patient requires multiple operations to deal with severe disfigurement following trauma. Skilled nursing care can help assure success of the surgical procedure, and can assist the patient to deal with resultant changes in his appearance and bodily functions.

## REFERENCES AND BIBLIOGRAPHY

ABEL, T. M.: Facial disfigurement, in GARRETT, J. F. (ed.): *Psychological Aspects of Physical Disability*, Washington, D.C., U.S. Government Printing Office, (n.d.).

ALSOP, J. A.: Augmentation mammoplasty, *Nurs. Times* 66:1617, December 1970.

BARSKY, A.: *Principles and Practice of Plastic Surgery*, ed. 2, New York, McGraw-Hill, 1964.

CONLEY, J.: New face, same owner, *RN* 35:1, January 1972.

CONWAY, H., and NAYER, D.: Skin grafts, *Am. J. Nurs.* 64:94, November 1964.

DAVID, D. J.: Skin grafting, *Nurs. Times* 68:1473, November 23, 1972.

EDWARDS, B. F.: Endoprostheses in plastic surgery, *Am. J. Nurs.* 64:123, May 1964.

GIBSON, A.: A severely burned patient, *Nurs. Times* 69:791, June 21, 1973.

GIBSON, T. (ed.): *Modern Trends in Plastic Surgery*, Washington, D.C., Butterworth, 1966.

GILL, S. A.: Nursing the plastic surgery patient, *AORN* 18:505, September 1973.

HAMM, W. G.: Nursing care in surgery of the head and neck, *NCNA* 2:475, September 1967.

HURWITZ, A.: About faces, *Am. J. Nurs.* 71:2168, November 1971.

MANCUSI-UNGARO, A. P.: The surgical management of macrotia with protrusion, transactions of the Fourth International Congress of Plastic and Reconstructive Surgery, Rome, 1967, p. 1102.

————: Rhytidectomy, a new concept, presented March 1974, American Society Aesthetic Plastic Surgery, New Orleans, La. (unpublished).

MACGREGOR, F. C., et al.: *Facial Deformities and Plastic Surgery*, Springfield, Ill., Thomas, 1953.

MCGREGOR, I., and REID, W. H.: *Plastic Surgery for Nurses*, Baltimore, Williams and Wilkins, 1966.

PEET, E., and PATTERSON, T.: *The Essentials of Plastic Surgery*, Philadelphia, Davis, 1963.

SHERMAN, J., and FIELDS, S. K.: *Guide to Patient Evaluation. History Taking, Physical Examination and the Problem-Oriented Method*, Flushing, N.Y.: Med. Exam. Publ. Comp. Inc., 1974.

TROWBRIDGE, J. E.: Caring for patients with facial or intra-oral reconstruction, *Am. J. Nurs.* 73:1930, November 1973.

WOOD-SMITH, D., and POROWSKI, P. (eds.): *Nursing Care of the Plastic Surgery Patient*, St. Louis, Mosby, 1967.

ZAYDON, T. J., and BROWN, J. B.: *Early Treatment of Facial Injuries*, Philadelphia, Lea and Febiger, 1964.

# UNIT TWELVE

## Acute Life-Threatening Physiologic Crisis

# Intensive Care Nursing

The concept of intensive care involves a concentration of highly specialized medical and nursing staff and allied health personnel specially prepared to assess, treat, and evaluate the progress of critically ill patients with the assistance of various kinds of technology. The lifesaving benefits of such units have been clearly demonstrated.

In an intensive care unit (ICU) the patients may have the same diagnosis, such as acute myocardial infarction. Or, in a mixed unit there can be patients in acute renal or respiratory failure, patients after cardiac surgery or severe trauma, patients with third-degree burns, septicemia, postsurgical complications, or metabolic crises such as diabetic ketoacidosis, among other diagnoses.

Because of the need for close and constant observation and the potential for deterioration of the patient's condition, the ratio of nurses to patients is high. But a high nurse-patient ratio is not the essence of intensive care nursing. Rather its essence is the personal support of the patient and his family or associates through the illness experience so that integration of the experience and consequent learning take place (Fig. 58-1). Because of the patient's requirements, physicians and nurses work closely together, thus creating many opportunities for professional colleague relationships.

Intensive care nursing is a blend of expertise in the technical-judgmental skills and the interpersonal skills exercised in behalf of the patient and family caught in a life-death crisis, many for the first time. For example, should cardiac arrest occur, each nurse team member knows exactly what to do and how to do it, whether it be to perform defibrillation, or external cardiac mas-

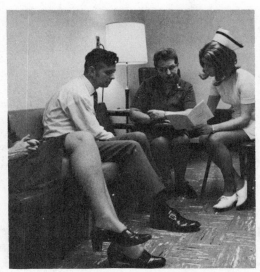

**Figure 58-1.** Nurse meeting with patients' relatives. Visitors' room at the Paul Felix Warburg Cardiac Care Unit at the New York Hospital—Cornell Medical Center.

sage, or to prepare intravenous drugs. The complete resuscitation team, however, could have as a member one nurse assigned in advance to speak with the other patients and with the frantic visitor in the waiting room who may have heard the "code" call and seen some team members rush by. It is unrealistic to expect that a nurse working with the patient can leave him to assume this aspect of the nursing role.

The cardiac arrest survivor needs to discuss the experience in order that fantasy and delusion formation be minimized. Posthospital insomnia or terrifying dreams represent attempts to master the terror he has been through. Discussion of the event should be initiated even in the face of an avoiding tendency on the part of the patient (Heller, 1974). Discussion should take place as close to the time of arrest as is reasonable, preferably within the first 24 hours. The patient should be assured that his body was alive during the time of heart (or respiratory) arrest.

In intensive care nursing, it is essential that the nurse know the significance of laboratory reports such as arterial blood gases and implement a predetermined course of action or notify the physician promptly, rather than wait for him to come in. The nurse may change the settings on a patient's respirator quite competently in response to lab reports, but fail to tell the patient what changes to antici-

pate. For a person dependent on a respirator who comes to personalize his own machine, a change in the sound or rhythm of the machine can signify a change in himself. If his anxiety mounts, his breathing can be affected and a vicious cycle ensues.

The importance of performing technical tasks in a knowledgeable, precise, and manually dexterous manner with necessary adjustments to the individual patient cannot be overestimated. The nurse who traumatizes a patient because of an unskilled attempt at nasal or oropharyngeal suctioning can cause the patient to resist or refuse to be suctioned again, despite his need.

In a fast-paced, highly technical environment it is possible to overlook some of the more traditional but essential components of nursing care. A patient suffering from automobile-accident trauma has enough to deal with without a raging urinary tract infection acquired from an unsterile catheterization procedure. And the coping capacity of the patient with acute myocardial infarction is taxed sufficiently without acquiring a decubitus ulcer or joint contracture as well. With pain so frequent, the nurse who functions in an automatic manner can simply dispense narcotics repeatedly for pain when a more accurate assessment of the patient's need would indicate a necessity to discuss the pain with him and reduce it by other means. (See Chapter 10, The Patient in Pain.)

## THE ENVIRONMENT

The sights, sounds, and smells which surround his small living space in the intensive care unit are foreign and threatening to the patient. It is hard to distinguish night from day when lights are on all the time and activity is constant. Restrained from moving by intravenous lines, monitoring electrodes, and various kinds of other devices, and separated from family and friends, the acutely ill patient faces a fearsome burden. Nursing assists the patient to cope with all of these strange and threatening conditions so that his major efforts can be directed toward the work of healing. Noise can be reduced, curtains can be drawn in such a way that the patient can be seen by the staff but shielded from offensive sights. The room can be aired and deodorized. Excreta and other odor-producing substances can be removed promptly. Lights can be dimmed except where the nurse is actually working. To some extent the typical ICU stressful environment can be compensated for by the humanizing elements of the nurse-patient relationship (Fig. 58-2). In addition, familiar bedside objects such as clocks, radios, photographs, or even art work can reduce both sensory monotony and the patient's sense of isolation.

## THE FAMILY

At times the family may require more assistance than the patient because the patient may be unconscious or lacking temporarily the awareness of the nature of his illness. Since the critically ill patient is often unable to be interviewed extensively on admission, the family or visitor is sought out as the resource for the nursing history and the initiation of the written nursing care plan. To be truly committed to the patient, the intensive care nurse must be committed to the family as well.

The experience of an intensive care unit head nurse whose father was admitted to a reputable ICU illustrates a valuable learning experience gained from being "on the other side of the fence." Having spent much time waiting in the visitor's room outside the ICU, she was amazed at the wide variety of emotional responses among the other visitors. The process of grieving in its various stages was evident. Some relatives of newly admitted patients were stunned and shocked, unable to grasp the full import of what was happening and, because of their composed outward appearance, seemed "well adjusted." Others, comprehending the possibility of final separation with their loved one through death, wept openly. Some showed marked physiologic symptoms of overwhelming stress, such as wailing, pacing, hand wringing, or hyperventilation. Others castigated themselves, such as the young father whose wife was admitted after a suicide attempt with barbiturates. Some relatives were ambivalent, regretting the illness and suffering of the sick person, but at the same time being annoyed with him for subjecting them to a crisis which might have been prevented if advice had been followed. Still others, having been through crisis after crisis before, had experienced anticipatory grief and seemed somewhat resigned to the possible fatal outcome. Though distressed, some were relieved that the burdens of care and decision making were in more competent hands.

The visitor-nurse recounted her utter frustration at reading a "cold" list of visitor's rules and at

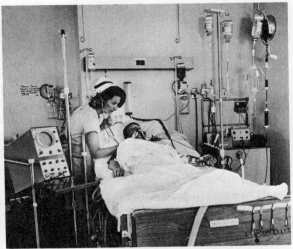

**Figure 58-2.** Nursing the patient in a modern intensive care unit. (Winter, P., and Lowenstein, E.: Acute respiratory failure, *Sci. Am.* 221:23, November, 1969; courtesy of Edward Lowenstein, M.D., Massachusetts General Hospital)

having to inquire into an intercom box on the wall about her father's condition, and being repeatedly answered in stock phrases by a ward clerk. Significantly, no nurse ventured beyond the domain of the ICU to speak personally to a visitor. The visitor-nurse watched, somewhat guiltily, the husband separated from his wife for the first time in 30 years, who tried repeatedly to "flag down" a nurse to talk with about his wife. Unfortunately, the highly technically competent nurses had not learned to deal with their own feelings about the hopelessness of the situation and were unable to provide any measure of support for the man. Small wonder that he cried to the nurse-visitor that uneducated clerks in a junk store would show more awareness of and sensitivity to a plea for help.

This nurse watched in horror the hysteria of a woman who had tried for three hours to see her husband in cardiogenic shock and had been repeatedly told that the staff was busy "working on him." When someone did approach her, it was an intern to ask for an autopsy and tell her she could view her deceased husband's body.

Though visitors provided each other with a modicum of support, and clergy assisted some, the nurse-visitor could not sufficiently separate herself from her role as a nurse-observer to deny the physical and psychological pathology being promoted in visitors who, when finally allowed in, approach the bedsides with tachycardias, palpitations, distorted perception, and a host of other symptoms of anxiety which adequate preparation and communication might have reduced. Undoubtedly some of their anxieties were communicated to already anxious patients. Nor could this nurse ignore the physical and emotional strain involved for older visitors who felt compelled to wait around the hospital for hours and then to stand for their five-minute visit every hour when a longer visit twice a day, sitting, would have been better for both them and the patient. She was distressed when a harassed husband was ushered out after his one five-minute interval because he could visit his wife only when he was on his way home from work to take care of their children.

As her father's condition improved, this nurse had time for reflection. She found it difficult to understand, though she had behaved previously in a similar manner herself, why her nurse colleagues, who were used to making judgments which affected the lives of very sick people, would not take the responsibility to make exceptions for more flexible visiting routines when necessary. For example, they could have advised the elderly lady to come twice a day for 15 minutes and to rest at home between visits. She wondered what fostered the behavior that led nurses to make their only communication with visitors the communication of "rules" or the announcement that "time is up." She wondered why, if the concept of teamwork operates, physicians communicate their expectations to nurses, but nurses do little to communicate their expectations of physicians to physicians. For example, it is reasonable to expect that the physician communicate directly with the patient, if possible, and the family any changes in the patient's condition; and that he keep the nurses informed of what he has told the patient and family regarding the current status and prognosis of the patient. She questioned why the nursing staff felt free to request classes which updated their technical skills, but did not request classes on the why's and how's of providing emotional support.

It is hoped that each nurse will not have to go through the experience of being an ICU visitor; but unless the nurse views family care as part of nursing care, she will resent the questions of visitors and view their visits as interference with her work instead of as their basic right. One creative aspect of the professional nurse's role could be that of intermediary between visitors and professional staff. The nurse's good judgment will also be rendered in behalf of the patient if she terminates a visit that is harmful. For example, when unanticipated illness occurs, family members or business associates can attempt to coerce a very sick patient to sign a will or other legal document against his better judgment. In such a situation, the visit should be curtailed and the matter should be called to the attention of the patient's physician and the hospital's legal authority.

## THE NURSE

For the staff the intensive care unit also poses problems. There may be small working space, with the nurses' station in hearing or viewing range of some patients, thus decreasing the nurses' privacy. There is a constant state of heightened tension with peak crisis periods which increase anxiety in team members who may tend to take their feelings out on each other. The work is fast-paced, often with little opportunity afforded for relief breaks. Mortality is high, and feelings of helplessness in the professional staff, at times, can be overwhelming. Heller notes that the danger for the nurse is callousness, the result of a protective noninvolvement with patients.

Just as one needs specialized education to deal with newer technical aspects of care, so do the members of the intensive care staff need continuing assistance to deal with their own and patients' psychological problems and emotional responses. This help, which has been highly successful when provided by some institutions, can take the form of staff conferences with a psychiatric nurse specialist or other prepared leader who can help nurses deal with their own feelings (and those of other staff members) so that they can be more helpful to patients and families.

The argument that there is no time for emotional support in an ICU because there is always a crisis impending is unsound, and it is also factually untrue. Lack of emotional support can play a large part in the occurrence of crises. The nurse who does not understand the emotional factors involved in a clinical situation where mortality is high and crises are frequent and always threatening may be doing an admirable job technically, but is not viewing intensive care nursing in its full perspective. If she does not recognize or understand her own feelings and receive help to deal with them, she may protect herself by preoccupation with the technical aspects of care and unwittingly ignore the person to whom the care is given. Continuing education programs for intensive care nurses must include programs for the development of the nurse in the counseling and teaching roles as well as in the technical-judgmental skills.

Interdisciplinary conferences can help staff to deal with issues of assumption of authority, complex patient care problems, staff morale, and ethical issues. The latter includes the patient's right to give informed consent and considerations regarding withdrawal of life support for particular patients.

There is considerable challenge and satisfaction in intensive care nursing. Many lives are saved by a caring, competent team. Newer treatment modalities offer new opportunities for learning, sharing, and collaboration between physicians and nurses in the interest of quality patient care.

Many people make demands on the nurse who cares for the critically ill, and she must know what needs to be done first, and what can be delegated to others. The situation calls for a nurse who moves quickly without adding confusion, who can function as a member of a team, and who can translate compassion for the patient into effective action and soothing words. To be prepared for all of the demands made in this situation, the nurse must be familiar with biomedical technology and must undergo many supervised patient care experiences.

If the patient dies, or if any acute condition exists that in itself is not always fatal but in a certain instance proves to be fatal, the staff faces problems that are different from those encountered in the care of a patient with an acknowledged terminal illness, such as metastasized cancer. Many physicians and nurses never forget the memories of certain patients for whom they cared and who, they believe, should not have died. Sometimes these thoughts are irrational, and whether or not they may be justified can never be ascertained. Occasionally, a nurse will try to relieve her own hurt by blaming her colleagues. To prevent such situations requires a continuing team commitment to quality care for every patient as well as recognition of the fact that life and death are not wholly in the control of physicians and nurses.

A high level of anxiety in nurses and physicians (as in everyone else) in addition to other emotions, such as anger and frustration, interfere with optimal functioning. An interdisciplinary review of problematic episodes helps team members to learn from such situations so that they are not repeated.

In her own interests as well as those of the patient, the nurse may have to provide the impetus for such review.

## THE PATIENT

The patient admitted in an emergency to an intensive care unit has special problems different from the patient admitted electively, such as the postoperative open-heart surgery patient. (See Chapter 63.)

An illness requiring admission to an ICU is most often acutely disruptive of work or home life. The nature of the patient's admission by ambulance with siren screeching, the rush of personnel, and the emergency therapies, serve to reinforce the message which his pain, or dyspnea, or bleeding, or vomiting has already conveyed to him—that he is gravely ill and may even die.

Providing emotional support for the ICU patient is as much a part of sound physiologic care as is the overtly technical procedure. The patient's psychological response to an acute physical problem stresses his cardiovascular, respiratory, and endocrine systems. Increase or decrease in heart rate, cardiac arrhythmias, hyperventilation with subsequent shift in pH, and the outpouring of catecholamines from the adrenal gland are examples of physiologic responses to stress. The experience of pain, difficulty in breathing, sudden trauma, or whatever else prompted the patient's admission to the hospital may have provoked certain defense mechanisms which protect the patient from overwhelming anxiety. It is part of nursing to know what these mechanisms are, to be able to observe the mechanism in action as it manifests itself, and to be one of the professionals who discuss the situation and decide upon intervention when the "defense" is not serving the patient. For example, the patient with severe chest pain uses denial when he unconsciously puts off seeking prompt medical assistance and resorts to old home remedies. When his symptoms become so urgent that they can no longer be ignored, he seeks or accepts help. Very often, a family member, nurse, or physician must say a decisive, "You have to go to the hospital," because to go along with the patient's "defense" could directly lead to his death.

What the patient does not need is to be scolded for his delay. The nurse continually presents the facts of the current situation as the patient can tolerate them, and when, through supportive nursing care, the patient becomes more comfortable and less threatened, he can begin to cope with reality. Because high anxiety levels result in the distortion or preclusion of sensory intake, the nurse understands that explanations to the patient and his family may need to be repeated many times before understanding is reached.

Physical presence and physical ministration by the nurse, though reassuring if the performance is competent and confident, are not sufficient for true communication with the patient. If at all possible, he must be engaged in conversation regarding what is happening to and around him if he is to understand that he, and not the machines, exerts the priority. Lack of privacy, strange noises, and offensive odors are often part of his experience when he needs all of his energy to cope with his own illness. Witnessing other patients having convulsions or cardiac arrest gives him more and more difficult things to cope with when extraneous stressors need to be kept to a minimum. Since the entire situation is such a contrast from the patient's normal experiences, any cultural preferences or rituals which may approximate and preserve some aspect of the patient's life style should be incorporated into the nursing care plan. For example, a religious medal can be tied to the bed, or the family can bring in ethnic foods when instructed about the dietary prescription.

Though the patient may be quite ill and temporarily very dependent, he should not be treated as a nonentity but as a living human being who can participate to some degree in the direction of his life. Thus he should be expected to participate in his personal care and grooming to the extent permitted by the nature of the illness.

The seemingly unconscious patient may still hear, and attempts at explanation of what is to happen to him should not be denied him. It is quite distressing for a sick patient to be examined by the physician and nurse who then withdraw out of earshot to talk about their findings rather than communicate with him.

Inevitably, some patients will die. They and their families need as much support and dignity as the situation permits. The other patients need an honest answer to their question, "Where is Mr. Jones?" Such an answer is, "Despite all we could do for him, Mr. Jones died this morning." To attempt to give a false answer such as "The patient was transferred" destroys the patients' confidence when the truth is inevitably found out.

Sudden death means that the patient's family has had no time to prepare for it; the news may be overwhelming. Family members should be afforded privacy, and the chaplain called if that is desired. The physician should see them and explain what happened. Usually, there are all sorts of matters that make the situation even harder for the family. They may have no money on hand and no idea about how to arrange for an undertaker. In their shock and sorrow they may feel aggressive toward the hospital staff. The nurse should understand their reaction, even though it may be difficult for her to listen to them, and explain that everything possible was done for the patient. The bedside environment should be straightened, and the deceased person prepared for immediate viewing by the family if that is their desire.

The surviving patient's stay in the ICU is generally a short one, and he is transferred as soon as possible to a general hospital area. Study has shown that the patient who is not prepared for this transfer through early anticipation of the time of transfer, discussion of the meaning of the move, weaning from equipment such as a cardiac monitor on which he may have developed a degree of dependence, and acceptance by a knowledgeable new nursing staff, may experience sufficient stress to cause a major setback (Klein, 1968). In addition to patient preparation, the staff on the general nursing unit needs a full nursing history, a transfer summary of his ICU course, and a well-developed, written nursing care plan so that nursing care can continue without disruption.

## REFERENCES AND BIBLIOGRAPHY

BILODEAU, C.: The nurse and her reactions to critical-care nursing, *Heart Lung* 2:358, May-June 1973.

CASSEM, N.: Confronting the decision to let death come, *Crit. Care Med.* 2:113, May-June 1974.

HELLER, S.: Psychological needs of the cardiac patient, Chap. 3 in McIntyre, M. (ed.): *Heart Disease: New Dimensions of Nursing Care,* Garden Grove, California, Trainex Press, 1974.

KIELY, W. F.: Critical-care psychiatric syndromes, *Heart Lung* 2:54, January-February 1973.

———: Psychiatric aspects of critical care, *Crit. Care Med.* 2:139, May-June 1974.

KLEIN, R., et al.: Transfer from a coronary unit: Some adverse responses, *Arch. Intern. Med.* 122:104, 1968.

KORNFELD, D., et al.: Psychological hazards of the intensive care unit: Nursing care aspects, *Nurs. Clin. N. Am.* 3:41, March 1968.

OBIER, K., and HAYWOOD, L. J.: Enhancing therapeutic communication with acutely ill patients, *Heart Lung* 2:49, January-February 1973.

SCZEKALLA, R. M.: Stress reactions of CCU patients to resuscitation procedures on other patients, *Nurs. Res.* 22:65, January-February 1973.

STORLIE, F.: Double entendre in a CCU, *Am. J. Nurs.* 74:666, April 1974.

STRAUSS, A.: The intensive care unit: Its characteristics and social relationships, *Nurs. Clin. N. Am.* 3:7, March 1968.

VERSTEEG, D.: If I could hold your hand, *Am. J. Nurs.* 68:2554, December 1968.

WEINBERG, S.: Toward humane care for the critically ill, *Heart Lung* 2:43, January-February 1973.

# The Patient in Shock

## CHAPTER 59

Normally, the pathways of the vascular network are adjusted from moment to moment to direct the body's limited supply of blood. They are manipulated constantly to serve tissues with the amount of blood suited to their various states of rest or exertion. Why blood vessels occasionally fail to maintain the balanced constriction that maintains normal pressure is not completely understood. It is known that master adjustment centers in the brain can be impaired by drugs, by hypoxia, by anesthesia, and by trauma, among many examples, and that poor vascular tone can result. Despite much investigation, agreement on the exact pathophysiologic disturbances involved in shock or on modes of treatment has not been reached. It is agreed that shock is a complicated series of interwoven events—vascular, hormonal, neural, metabolic, and hemodynamic.

Shock is a clinical syndrome indicating inadequate circulation that results from a variety of causes. Inadequate circulation leads to tissue hypoxia. Regardless of the cause, prolonged shock is incompatible with life. The faster the shock state can be reversed, the greater the chance of uncomplicated recovery for the patient. There are few instances in the care of patients where careful attention to nursing assessment and intervention is as important to recovery as in the management of the patient in impending or actual shock.

## ETIOLOGY AND PATHOPHYSIOLOGY

In health, the intact circulatory system delivers essential elements, including oxygen, to all tissues of the

Etiology and Pathophysiology

Prevention

Clinical Assessment

Treatment and Nursing
Care Implications

Prognosis and Complications

body and removes the waste products. In shock, there is interference with this basic physiologic process of effective perfusion of blood to the tissues, leading to hypoxia. As poor perfusion and hypoxia persist, normal metabolism cannot take place. The body then resorts to anaerobic (nonoxygen consuming) methods of metabolism, and metabolic acidosis develops.

A decrease in cardiac output is a problem common to all types of shock. Fall in blood pressure stimulates baroreceptors in the heart and great vessels, and the response is one of adrenergic or sympathetic defenses. Norepinephrine from adrenergic terminals and epinephrine from the adrenal medulla attempt to preserve cardiac output by increasing the rate and contractile force of the heart. Arteriolar constriction raises blood pressure. Venous constriction decreases the venous reservoirs in an attempt to augment venous return to the right ventricle. The spleen, for example, can contribute 500 to 700 ml. of blood to the general circulation.

Among the many additional homeostatic mechanisms are the secretion of pituitary antidiuretic hormone (ADH) and aldosterone from the adrenal cortex, which act to conserve salt and water.

The adrenergic response is valuable as an early defense mechanism, but continued or exaggerated response causes prolonged decreased organ blood flow and contributes to the development of "irreversible shock." For instance, when the amount of hemorrhage is small, vasoconstriction can compensate for this. If the volume loss continues, body compensatory mechanisms lose their effectiveness, resulting in harm to vital organs, such as heart, brain, and kidney, and in a poor prognosis.

## Hemodynamics

Circulatory integrity can be viewed as a resultant of three basic components:

1. The pump (heart)
2. The blood volume
3. The vascular bed, consisting of
   a. Resistance vessels—arteries and arterioles containing about 20 per cent of normal bood volume
   b. Exchange vessels—the capillary network containing about 5 per cent of normal blood volume
   c. Capacitance vessels—veins and venules containing about 75 per cent of total blood volume

In the shock state, insufficient tissue blood flow (perfusion) results from a depressed cardiac output due either to

1. Factors that interfere with the ability of the heart to pump blood. This can be called "cardiogenic shock," or "pump failure." It can result from
   a. Factors that interfere with cardiac filling, such as pericardial tamponade, severe mitral stenosis, tachyarrhythmias
   b. Factors that interfere with cardiac emptying, such as myocardial infarction, myocarditis, heart block, severe aortic stenosis

or

2. Factors that cause inadequate venous return
   a. Decreased blood volume
      (1) From external loss—hemorrhage, dehydration, burns, vomiting, diarrhea
      (2) From internal loss—hemothorax, retroperitoneal hemorrhage, peritonitis, intestinal obstruction, fractures, angioneurotic edema
   b. Increased vascular bed vasodilation and pooling
      (1) Gram-negative bacteremia
      (2) Anaphylaxis
      (3) Central nervous system depressants such as anesthesia, barbiturates
      (4) Spinal cord transection

or

3. Impediments to blood flow, such as massive pulmonary embolism or vena cava obstruction

In any given patient there may be certain elements of each of these with the hemodynamic state representing a resultant of several related factors.

## Etiologic Classification

In addition to this hemodynamically oriented approach, shock can be classified according to etiology:

**Hypovolemic shock,** in which there is a reduction in the volume of circulating blood. This type of shock may be caused by hemorrhage, in which blood is spilled from the usually closed system of arteries and veins. Other causes include severe burns, in which a large amount of fluid seeps from the circulatory system into the injured area; and the loss of large amounts of fluid in vomitus and diarrhea. In hypovolemic shock the volume of blood filling the vascular channels is low. Hemorrhage into a cavity, such as thoracic or abdominal, may be hidden from sight, but it is just as deadly as the hemorrhage one can see from an external wound.

**Cardiogenic shock,** in which the circulatory failure involves faulty pumping of the heart. A common cause of cardiogenic shock is acute myocardial infarction. Despite advances in therapy, the mortality rate from this complication remains about 85 per cent. Destruction of 40 per cent or more of the left ventricle is almost always associated with cardiogenic shock.

**Vasogenic shock,** in which there is diffuse vasodilation, resulting in an increase in the size of the vascular bed. The dilated vessels afford so much room for blood that it does not easily move along. While remaining in the vessels, this blood is just as unavailable to the circulatory effort as if it had been lost through hemorrhage. When blood becomes trapped in small vessels and in the viscera, it is lost temporarily to the mainstream of circulating fluid. The skeletal muscles and the viscera may become engorged with blood, while the volume of circulating blood is reduced dangerously. This type of shock is *normovolemic.* That is, the amount of fluid in the tubes of the circulatory system is not reduced, but it is not circulating in such a way that permits effective perfusion of the tissues. Anaphylaxis is an example of vasogenic shock. (See Chapter 9 for a discussion of anaphylactic shock.)

**Neurogenic shock,** which results from an insult to the nervous system. Intracranial damage and certain drugs can cause neurogenic shock. Vasodilation is a prominent feature.

**Psychic shock,** in which pain or severe fright or other strong emotion interferes with normal vascular control. Excitation of the parasympathetic nerves to the heart (vagus) slows the heart and thereby reduces arterial pressure and cardiac output. A frightened patient makes a poor surgical risk.

**Septic shock,** which may be seen in any overwhelming bacterial infection, usually occurs in the patient who is succumbing to his infection. Septic shock is more common in patients whose bacteremia is caused by gram-negative organisms. Endotoxins released by the organisms probably are a major cause of bacteremic shock, but other, as yet undefined, factors may also be involved.

This etiologic approach to the diagnosis of shock may not be as critical as a hemodynamic or physiologically oriented approach. For example, it may be presumed that the cause of shock in an elderly patient with an indwelling urinary catheter and pyuria is due to gram-negative sepsis. Antibiotic and vasopressor therapy might not be sufficient to reverse this, however. What may not be so obvious is the role that cardiac decompensation is playing in the production of hypotension.

## PREVENTION

Careful preoperative preparation, both physical and psychological, is important in preventing shock. Estimation of the patient's blood volume and its replacement, if needed, by transfusions preoperatively are important. Only surgery that in itself is necessary to save the patient's life is undertaken while a patient is in shock. For example, in arterial hemorrhage, stopping the bleeding is the first step in treatment to prevent continued blood volume loss. Surgery may be a mandatory step to reach the bleeding vessel.

Nurses should become expert at estimating fluid loss, both in and out of the operating room. How many ml. are in a puddle of vomitus on the floor? How many ml. are soaked into the bed linen after a severe nosebleed? How much fluid can a saturated four-inch square sponge hold? One way to train the eye is to take a known amount of fluid and pour it on the floor, in a sheet, or on a sponge and see what it looks like. Another way to estimate fluid loss is by weight. For example, in the operating room a dry sponge can be weighed. Then a blood-soaked one is weighed and the difference noted.

A healthy adult can lose up to about 500 ml. of blood without need for replacement. The ill, the elderly, or the poorly nourished need replacement therapy for less blood loss. Central venous pressure monitoring is one way of assessing fluid balance in the elderly patient undergoing surgery in order to better evaluate volume replacement needs.

It is difficult to estimate the capacity of a patient to adjust to circulatory impairment. Most blood donors do not faint. Why does a particular donor faint after contributing a pint of blood? How much of the effect was due to fear? How much to reduced blood volume? How much to an inadequate ability to react to signals that usually produce adjustment? Some people can adjust to rapid loss of a quart of blood without evidence that their bodies had to resort to a massive response to accomplish adjustment.

The ability of an individual to avoid shock cannot be predicted. The patient who has undergone a known cause of shock is safer when cared for as if shock might develop. All accident victims and patients with acute myocardial infarction, for example, should be treated as if shock were imminent. All postoperative patients belong in this category. Even if the surgical procedure involves practically no blood loss, the stress of undergoing surgery, anesthesia, and the necessary trauma of the surgical incision are influences that can contribute to shock. However, hypovolemia is more significant as a cause of shock than such factors as anesthetic agents and psychic stress.

The patient should be moved gently. A horizontal position is usually ordered because blood can move back to the heart more easily without having to overcome gravity factors. Light covers and a warm room protect body warmth, but heat is not applied to the body because of its undesirable vasodilating effect. There is careful use of sedatives and analgesic drugs because they tend to depress brain centers, respiration, and muscle tone, and operate in opposition to effects that promote the control of blood pressure. A quiet, calm atmosphere and staff who instill confidence and give the patient a sense of security are basic to the patient's protection.

Frequent observations of the patient and his vital signs to maintain an appraisal of the circulatory state are ordered until the occurrence of shock is no longer considered probable. The nurse must watch for signs that the body is being forced to call on major defensive mechanisms to maintain blood pressure. Although deep shock can develop in minutes, more often there is a warning period. In hypovolemic shock the rate of volume loss is most directly related to the speed with which the symptoms of shock appear. For example, the patient whose aorta ruptures progresses almost instantaneously to profound circulatory collapse, whereas the patient sustaining a venous hemorrhage will go into shock in a more orderly, step-by-step fashion through the sequence of symptoms indicating impending circulatory collapse.

## CLINICAL ASSESSMENT

Nursing management of a patient in severe shock requires a high level of knowledge and expertise. However, nurses who care for patients who are at risk of developing shock should have basic knowledge such as the types and mechanisms of shock, the characteristic signs and symptoms, basic parameters of patient monitoring, and methods of prevention, treatment, and nursing intervention.

## Pulse

Cardiac output, a function of heart rate and stroke volume, is depressed in shock because of a drop in stroke volume. A compensatory tachycardia occurs in an attempt to raise the output. This is frequently the first change in vital signs to appear.

*Pulse pressure* is the difference between the systolic and diastolic blood pressures. In shock, a fall in systolic blood pressure with a rise in diastolic pressure results in a narrowed pulse pressure. The small spurts of blood passing in the artery feel more like a quiver than the thump of a full pulse. It is often described as a "rapid, thready pulse."

Tachycardia associated with easy compression of the radial pulse is an early sign of shock. It precedes the thready nature of the pulse in established shock. In the later stages of shock, the pulse is imperceptible.

In some cases such as in shock following myocardial infarction, reflex vagal stimulation can override the sympathetic response and the patient may present a bradycardia rather than a tachycardia. The quality of the pulse (which an electrocardiographic monitor cannot determine) is an important parameter in the evaluation of the patient.

## Blood Pressure

Blood pressure is a valuable but not an infallible index of shock. Organ blood flow, not blood pressure, is the critical determinant.

Systolic blood pressure falls, due to reduced cardiac output. For some adult patients, the situation is:

|  | SYSTOLIC BLOOD PRESSURE |
|---|---|
| Average, normal | 110 to 130 mm. Hg |
| Impending shock | 90 to 100 mm. Hg |
| Shock | Below 80 mm. Hg |

For someone with a normal systolic blood pressure of 180 mm. Hg, a pressure of 120 mm. Hg could represent severe shock, whereas the lower figure might be a normal pressure for someone else. The usual pressure of the patient should be known. Regardless of the numerical figure, the consistent progressive fall of blood pressure with a rapid, thready pulse is a serious sign. In the early stages of shock the blood pressure may not yet have fallen. It may fall later if the tachycardia isn't fully compensatory. A rapid pulse, apprehension, or air hunger may be the only indication of impending shock.

If the patient is in the supine position, the initial signs of a developing hypovolemia may be masked. The nurse who has a clinical suspicion of impending problems can perform a simple "tilt" test. The patient is placed in a sitting position and his vital signs are taken. Increased pulse rate and decreased blood pressure when the patient is sitting (compared to supine) may be the earliest clue to impending shock and should not be ignored.

The physician should be made aware of any fall in systolic blood pressure below 100 mm. Hg or any fall of 20 mm. Hg below the patient's usual blood pressure when this is an unexpected occurrence.

The systolic blood pressure level may be ascertained by palpation, using a sphygmomanometer with the fingertips on the radial pulse. After the cuff has been inflated sufficiently to obliterate the pulse, the column of mercury is reduced sufficiently for blood to begin flowing through the radial artery. The systolic blood pressure is recorded as the point at which the radial artery is palpable. Also, the femoral arterial pulse should be palpated. This may be of good quality.

When intensive vasoconstriction is present, cuff blood pressure measurement may be difficult or even impossible to obtain or may give falsely low readings. This is particularly true of those patients with peripheral vessel arteriosclerosis compounded by the effects of vasopressor drugs. *Intra-arterial blood pressure* monitoring is becoming more commonplace because it is more accurate than the usual indirect auscultatory method. It allows for beat-to-beat analysis, permits recording of mean pressures, and eliminates interrupting the patient's rest. As an invasive procedure, however, it carries the risk of infection and thrombi and may cause some discomfort.

## Central Venous Pressure

Central venous pressure (CVP) is the pressure of the blood in the right atrium or venae cavae. It serves to distinguish relationships among the hemodynamic variables in shock—the venous return, the quality of the pump, and vascular tone. Thus it is a valuable though not infallible guide in the management of the patient in shock. Normal central venous pressure is 0 to 4 cm. of water in the right atrium and 6 to 12 cm. of water in the venae cavae with a reference point at the midaxillary line.

An isolated CVP reading is of little value unless

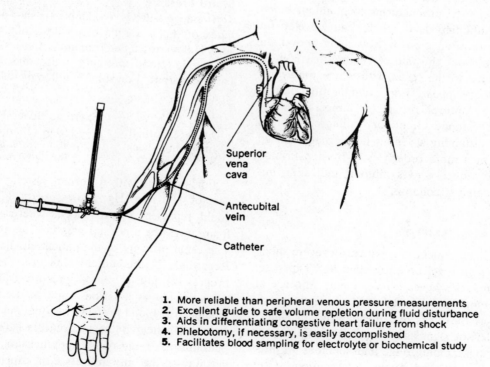

Superior vena cava

Antecubital vein

Catheter

1. More reliable than peripheral venous pressure measurements
2. Excellent guide to safe volume repletion during fluid disturbance
3. Aids in differentiating congestive heart failure from shock
4. Phlebotomy, if necessary, is easily accomplished
5. Facilitates blood sampling for electrolyte or biochemical study

**Figure 59-1.** Advantages of central venous pressure catheterization. (Elek, S.: Use of pressor agents in shock following myocardial infarction, *Hosp. Med.* 4:4, May, 1968)

it is unusually high or low. Central venous pressure is best used by obtaining a baseline value and then taking frequent readings. The response of the patient to drug therapy or to volume expansion or contraction can then be evaluated. In a "fluid challenge," 100- to 200-ml. boluses of a parenteral solution are administered intravenously over a short period of time by the physician, and the CVP is monitored to determine if the patient will benefit from volume expansion. Since left ventricular overloading may not be reflected in CVP measurement, the patient must be carefully observed for signs of congestive failure such as rales, tachypnea, restlessness, and $S_3$ gallop. Pulmonary capillary wedge pressure (PCWP; see below) provides more accurate assessment of left ventricular activity than CVP. Fluid challenge may be indicated if CVP is lower than 8 or PCWP lower than 12.

A high CVP indicates heart failure or cardiac tamponade. Vasoconstriction or increased circulatory volume produces a high CVP if congestive heart failure is also present.

Low CVP indicates hypovolemia due to fluid or blood loss. Examples are:

1. Fluid loss
   a. External—vomiting, diarrhea, burns
   b. Internal—rapid ascites formation, angioneurotic edema, or loss into a gangrenous loop of bowel
2. Blood loss
   a. External—frank hemorrhage
   b. Internal—retroperitoneal hemorrhage or bleeding into the thigh following a fractured femur

CVP is significant only when interpreted in relation to the patient's overall condition (Fig. 59-1). For example, a normal CVP reading in a patient with known decreased blood volume would indicate that the decreased volume has been compensated for by a decrease in the vascular bed secondary to sympathetic activity.

For the very critically ill patient, CVP readings should be taken every five minutes or every 100 ml. of fluid. To be accurate, the zero level on the manometer must always be at the same height in relation to the patient's right atrium. As the patient's position varies from the initial reading, so should the manometer baseline.

### Pulmonary Artery and Wedge Pressures

Central venous pressure reflects right ventricular filling pressure which may or may not coincide with left ventricular filling pressure. The latter is the

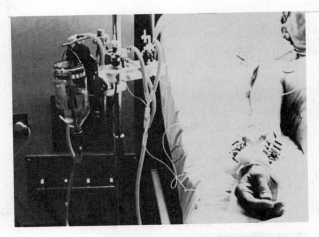

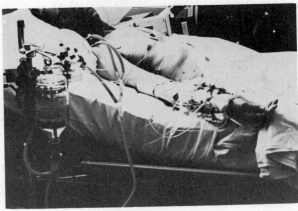

**Figure 59-2.** A Swan-Ganz catheter with the manifolds, connections, pressure transducers, and flushing system, illustrated in a patient with an acute myocardial infarction. The pressure transducers are mounted on a bedstand to reduce weight on the patient's arm and to provide a stable reference point while the patient is recumbent. (Rackley, C. E.: *Invasive Techniques for Hemodynamic Measurements,* American Heart Association, 1973; by permission of the author and The American Heart Association)

more important since it mirrors left ventricular performance and more precisely indicates left ventricular failure which may lead to pulmonary edema, an especially important consideration in shock following myocardial infarction, which is primarily a disease of the left ventricle.

A measure of left ventricular performance is the pulmonary artery pressure or the pulmonary capillary wedge pressure. In this measurement a flow-guided balloon catheter (Swan-Ganz) is passed into the pulmonary artery and wedged into a small distal arteriole (Fig. 59-2). Inflating the balloon with air seals off the forward flow of venous blood from the right ventricle, and establishes hemo-dynamic communication with the left side of the heart. Since the pulmonary wedge pressure reading is a reflection of left atrial pressure (thus a mea-sure of left ventricular end-diastolic pressure) the data obtained is more accurate than CVP. Normal pulmonary capillary wedge pressure is 6 to 8 mm. Hg. Elevation may indicate change in compliance of the left ventricular wall due to acute myocardial infarction or left ventricular failure; low PCWP may indicate hypovolemia.

Pulmonary artery pressure is optimally measured by the transducer-oscilloscope method, which per-mits a continual display of the pressure readings on the oscilloscope screen. Nursing measures in addi-tion to recording pressure readings include reporting sudden or gradual changes in pressures, preventing the formation of microemboli through the use of a flush solution of heparinized saline, and caring for the catheter insertion cutdown site (Gernert and Schwartz, 1973).

### Peripheral Vascular Resistance

Peripheral blood vessels constrict to direct blood from the skin to more vital organs. Ischemia ren-ders the skin pale and cold. It is clammy due to activation of the sweat glands. There may be cyano-sis especially of the fingernail beds, lips, and ear-lobes. Cyanosis means severe tissue hypoxia. Its absence, however, does not mean the absence of hypoxia. Recognition of cyanosis may be obscured by deep skin pigmentation, anemia, and poor light-ing conditions.

One way to monitor peripheral blood flow as well as the onset of shock through temperature reduction is through the use of the thermistor. This is an electronic device applied to the underside of the great toe of each foot which measures temperature (Delano, et al., 1971).

### Effects on Vital Organs

**Kidney.** Vasoconstriction in shock contributes to a marked reduction in renal blood flow. Many physicians believe that the rate of urine formation is the most important indicator of the status of the shock patient. The patient in shock or impending shock needs an indwelling urethral catheter and hourly measurement of urine output. The physician should be notified of urinary output below 30 ml. per hour so that therapy may be initiated promptly to promote adequate renal perfusion.

With rapid reversal of the shock, urine output usually returns promptly. Continued oliguria after reversal of shock indicates renal damage secondary to ischemia and may indicate the onset of complete renal failure and anuria.

**Brain.** The highly specialized nerve cells of the brain are more vulnerable to damage from the lack of oxygen than are the cells of other organs. Altera-tion in cerebral function is often the first sign of impaired oxygen delivery to the tissues. Mild anx-iety, increasing restlessness, agitation, or other change in behavior can be clues in advance of the more obvious signs of shock. As the condition de-teriorates, the patient becomes listless, stuporous, and finally unconscious.

**Heart.** Being both central pump and peripheral tissue, the heart is in a vulnerable position.

Minimal essential myocardial perfusion pressure to maintain coronary artery blood flow is considered to correspond to a systolic pressure of about 80 mm. Hg. Below this the myocardium becomes in-creasingly hypoxic.

Since blood flow to the coronary circulation oc-curs mainly during diastole, the diastolic blood pressure at the root of the aorta is one important determinant of coronary blood flow, regardless of systolic blood pressure.

Though other body tissues can be maintained temporarily by anaerobic metabolism, the mechani-cal contractions of the heart muscle cannot be main-tained by anaerobic means. The force of myocardial contraction decreases and the potential for danger-ous cardiac arrhythmias, including ventricular fibril-lation, increases.

The very structures responsible for directing and carrying out defensive reactions, particularly the heart and the nervous system, are impaired by ischemia. As these organs are weakened, the blood pressure falls further. The effectiveness of vital organs is reduced further, and the overwhelmed defense forces become contributors to the state of shock, which can proceed to circulatory collapse and death.

**Lung.** A specific form of pulmonary pathology following trauma and shock from any cause has been designated as "shock-lung" (Kamada and Smith, 1972). Pathologically the lung appears en-gorged, atelectatic, and hemorrhagic. The lung changes are manifested by clinical symptoms and signs of progressive respiratory failure, falling $Po_2$ levels, increasing tachypnea, dyspnea, cough, cyanosis, respiratory acidosis, and physical signs of pulmonary congestion or pneumonia. The exact cause is uncertain, but causative factors may be microemboli, loss of pulmonary surfactant, oxygen toxicity, and volume overload. Should "shock-lung" develop, it may preclude any chance for recovery from shock.

The repair of tissue trauma as soon as possible and good ventilatory therapy as part of the prompt overall management of the shocked patient are essential.

## Fluid and Electrolyte Balance

All patients who are at high risk for shock should have a keep-open intravenous infusion; intake and output from all routes should be measured and recorded. An indwelling catheter is inserted, and urinary output is measured at least hourly. Specific gravity determinations may be ordered every four hours, as well as additional laboratory examinations. Intravenous fluids may be ordered to be titrated to maintain the patient's urinary output at 30 ml. per hour. Intravenous fluids are continued until the patient's condition stabilizes; then a keep-open rate may be used as a precautionary measure.

## Respiration

In shock, the tissues are receiving less oxygen. In response, the patient tries to gain more oxygen by breathing faster (tachypnea). Rapid respirations are helpful in moving blood along in the large veins toward the heart. The respirations are shallow and there may be grunting. In earlier stages the patient is hungry for air, but in profound shock the respiratory rate decreases to two or three a minute.

To treat hypoxia, humidified oxygen is given. Pure oxygen can be given only for short periods without adverse effects on the lungs. Oxygen at concentrations of 40 to 60 per cent is usually prescribed.

When a patient is kept in the same position, sections of the lungs are not fully ventilated. Continued perfusion of these poorly ventilated areas leads to the return of unoxygenated blood to the left atrium. This is called venoarterial shunting.

Normal individuals avoid this by sighing automatically every 5 to 15 minutes. Collapsed alveoli are opened by these brief, deep inspirations. The nurse assists the patient in shock to have optimum lung ventilation by changing his position and by encouraging sighing and deep breaths.

## pH and Blood Gases

The measurement of hydrogen ion concentration (pH), oxygen tension ($Po_2$) and carbon dioxide tension ($Pco_2$) in arterial blood is becoming more commonplace in the monitoring of the shock patient. Specimens are usually obtained from an indwelling arterial catheter. Newer laboratory techniques allow more frequent reporting of results. These studies are used for assessing the adequacy of tissue oxygenation and, more importantly, indicate the degree of hypoxia, which will provoke myocardial ischemia and irritability and compromise left ventricular function.

The arterial oxygen tension ($Po_2$) reflects the amount of oxygen that has diffused into the arterial blood from the walls of the alveoli and capillaries. The normal value is 95 to 100 mm. Hg.

Arterial $Po_2$ levels are always depressed in shock states and are not normally elevated even by the administration of 100 per cent oxygen, thus indicating some degree of venoarterial shunting, probably caused by interstitial and alveolar edema.

The arterial carbon dioxide tension ($Pco_2$) is normally 35 to 45 mm. Hg.

In shock, with subsequent anaerobic metabolism and the accumulation of lactic and other acids, pH falls below the arterial norm of 7.39 to 7.45. Bicarbonate and other buffer stores are decreased. Since the body does not tolerate relatively minor shifts in pH, an alkalinizing solution such as sodium bicarbonate may be necessary (see Chap. 60).

## Temperature

Heat-regulating mechanisms are depressed in shock and heat loss is increased by added diaphoresis. With the possible exception of bacteremic shock, subnormal temperature is characteristic. Since there is a definite temperature range for cellular function and enzyme activity, the patient should be kept comfortably warm through control of environmental temperature and light blankets. Direct heat to the skin should not be used since it causes vasodilation, further increasing heat loss and reducing the flow to critical organs. Heat also raises the metabolic rate, which raises the tissue requirement for oxygen.

## Restlessness and Pain

Restlessness in shock is caused more often by hypoxia than by pain and may be relieved by oxygen administration. Pain can cause or enhance shock, and it lessens the patient's adaptive response.

Narcotics cause further respiratory and circulatory depression. Opiates administered subcutaneously or intramuscularly to patients already in shock often are not absorbed effectively from the tissues because of the diminished circulation. If several injections of narcotics are given during shock, a double or triple dose may be absorbed when the patient's circulation improves, causing serious toxic effects. This result can happen with any drug given by an intramuscular or subcutaneous route. When symptoms of shock are present, the nurse should call the physician and in the meantime withhold all previously ordered drugs. Narcotics should be given very judiciously to a postoperative patient whose blood pressure is falling, or to a patient who shows other symptoms that may indicate the approach of shock. In such situations these drugs are best given intravenously in a diluted bolus dose slowly, titrated to the patient's response.

## TREATMENT AND NURSING CARE IMPLICATIONS

The complete picture of well-developed shock is far easier to recognize than its insidious early signs, but the alert nurse who has recognized the early warnings can bring help to the situation while the body's defenses are still in control. If a patient shows early warning signs of shock, the physician should be notified. While waiting for him, the nurse monitors the vital signs and administers oxygen. An intravenous line should be opened for drug therapy. Obvious causes, such as external hemorrhage, should be controlled. A nurse should remain with the patient to observe him and to reassure him.

The treatment of shock depends on the clinical assessment of the patient and the complex hemodynamic variables involved. Treatment of hypoxia, pain, and cardiac arrhythmias proceeds concurrently with treatment of the shock state.

Treatment also depends on the school of thought to which an individual physician subscribes. One who considers further alpha adrenergic response to be beneficial may use vasopressors. Another may consider further alpha adrenergic stimulation to be harmful and order a pure beta adrenergic stimulator. Or at times both may be used together or alternately depending on the clinical condition of the patient.

There are some guidelines, however. If central venous pressure is low, volume replacement should be the first therapeutic step and the more potent circulatory drugs are deferred until CVP has been raised to 12 to 15 cm. of $H_2O$. Vasopressor drugs are more effective once the circulation has been primed (filled). Drugs which cause vasodilation can overexpand an already underfilled vascular bed and further compromise perfusion.

### Replacement Therapy

Hypovolemic shock is best treated with the type of fluid that is being lost. In hemorrhage, this is whole blood; in burn shock, plasma; in extreme vomiting and diarrhea, solutions containing electrolytes. When blood is given, the physician usually orders that the transfusion run rapidly while the blood pressure is low, and that the rate of administration be slowed to the usual 40 drops a minute when the blood pressure rises. At times, in order to keep pace with blood loss, several simultaneous transfusions are given. Blood may be forced by pressure into a vein to achieve more rapid introduction into the circulation than could be accomplished by free flow of the blood. When whole blood is desired but not available, the intravenous infusion may be started with plasma, concentrated albumin, low molecular weight dextran, or saline, until blood can be obtained.

When the CVP or PCWP is initially elevated or rapidly rises to high levels with volume increments of fluid, intravenous fluids are deferred. Efforts to improve the pumping effectiveness of the heart (positive inotropic action) are then made. Drugs such as digitalis, levarterenol (Levophed), or isoproterenol (Isuprel), as well as mechanical circulatory assist devices, can be employed to this end.

**Pulmonary Edema.** The nurse remains alert for symptoms of overdose of fluids into the vascular system. Sudden elevation or a significant steady rise in CVP or PCWP indicates the inability of the heart to accept a further fluid load. If more fluid arrives at the right than the left side of the heart can hold and move forward, blood accumulates in the lungs. Its rising pressure in the pulmonary vessels squeezes some fluid from the vessels into alveoli. This fluid (pulmonary edema) can drown the patient. During hypovolemic shock, when an inadequate volume of blood is reaching the heart, the infusions of blood or other replacement therapy are providing the heart with something to pump. As the blood pressure improves, and as the fluid of the infusions, plus the body's own blood supply, reach the heart effectively, an overload may develop. The nurse will notice that the patient feels as if he cannot breathe well, and his respiration will be rapid. Rales can be heard with the stethoscope or lung sounds may be grossly audible. Frothy pink sputum may be coughed up. All these signs point to the complication of pulmonary edema, and without immediate help this can be as serious as the shock state. The head of the bed should be elevated, oxygen administered, the infusion stopped, and the physician notified.

## Position

In the shock position, the legs and the feet are raised, keeping the knees straight. The trunk is kept horizontal and the head elevated on a pillow. Usually the position is accomplished by elevating the foot of the bed on shock blocks, or by turning a crank that raises the foot of the bed (not the knee gatch, but the whole bottom of the bed). The slope should be gentle, because too great a tilt will throw the patient's abdominal viscera up against his diaphragm and impede breathing. The simple maneuver of elevating the patient's legs might return as much as 500 ml. of blood to the general circulation. Therefore, in impending shock, if the patient's legs have been up, as in a lithotomy position, they are not put down without conferring with the physician.

Patients in shock from conditions resulting in increased intracranial pressure (after brain surgery, for example) are positioned flat in bed, or even in a low sitting position, because lowering the head could result in further increase in intracranial pressure.

Patients in cardiogenic shock may benefit from a low Fowler's position. Respiratory excursion and pulmonary expansion are enhanced when the diaphragm is lower. Also, the slight degree of gravity aids pulmonary venous emptying into the left atrium which tends to relieve pulmonary congestion.

## Drugs

It is postulated that the effects of the sympathetic nervous system are mediated by receptors located throughout the body called adrenergic receptors. Adrenergic receptors are classified as alpha and beta on the basis of their characteristic responses.

When stimulated, alpha receptors cause constriction of the smooth muscle of blood vessels supplying skeletal muscle, the splanchnic vascular bed, skin, and mucosa.

Beta adrenergic stimulation results in excitation of the S-A node resulting in increased heart rate, increased cardiac conduction (positive chronotropic effect) and increased myocardial contractility (positive inotropic effect). Also, the smooth muscles of the arteries, veins, and bronchi are relaxed, resulting in dilation.

Alpha and beta adrenergic blockers prevent the effects of alpha and beta stimulators, respectively.

Alpha and beta adrenergic stimulating drugs as well as alpha adrenergic blocking agents can be used in the treatment of shock.

| ACTION | DRUG |
|---|---|
| Alpha stimulator causing vasoconstriction | methoxamine (Vasoxyl) phenylephrine (Neo-Synephrine) |
| Beta stimulator causing vasodilatation and positive inotropic effects | isoproterenol (Isuprel) |
| Alpha and beta stimulator causing vasoconstriction and positive inotropic and chronotropic effects | levarterenol (Levophed) metaraminol (Aramine) mephentermine (Wyamine) epinephrine (adrenalin) dopamine (Intropin) |
| Alpha adrenergic blocker causing vasodilatation | phenoxybenzamine (Dibenzyline) phentolamine (Regitine) chlorpromazine (Thorazine) |

## Alpha and Beta Adrenergic Stimulators

**Levarterenol (Levophed).** Using the 0.2 per cent commercially prepared levarterenol bitartrate solution, 4 ml. may be added to 1,000 ml. of glucose in distilled water, or a greater concentration may be ordered. The solution is titrated intravenously using a microdrip administration set, and the blood pressure is checked every five minutes to prevent wide swings. The rate of administration depends on the patient's blood pressure, the desired blood pressure ordered by the physician, and the concentration of the solution.

For example, the physician may request that the patient's blood pressure be kept as close to 100/70 as possible. If the systolic pressure falls below 100, the nurse speeds up the flow of levarterenol; if it rises above this figure, she slows the flow down. A patient receiving this drug requires constant monitoring by the nurse. If his blood pressure suddenly shoots up, he is in danger of a cerebral hemorrhage.

If a solution containing levarterenol infiltrates the tissues, the infusion should be discontinued immediately. The drug causes such profound vasoconstriction that the tissues it contacts directly become severely ischemic. The tissues can become necrotic and slough away, leaving a serious wound to be treated. For the moment, treatment of shock takes precedence over all other problems. However, if the patient's condition allows attention to the injury produced by the infiltration, the physician may inject a vasodilating drug, phentolamine (Regitine), into the area, or he may ask the nurse to keep the wound covered with ice-water dressings or an icebag. Another venipuncture site must be selected.

**Metaraminol (Aramine).** Metaraminol may be given intravenously in a dose of 50 to 200 mg. in 1,000 ml. of 5 per cent dextrose in water at a rate of 1 to 2 micrograms per minute, or intramuscularly in a 2- to 10-mg. dose. The dosage is regulated to the patient's response, especially his blood pressure.

Administration of metaraminol has to be regulated very carefully, as the effects can accumulate. The maximum effect may not be in evidence until ten minutes after the drug is given. Overdose can lead to hypertension and cerebral hemorrhage. Metaraminol is given intramuscularly only when shock is mild, and there is sufficient circulation to absorb it; if it is given in profound shock, not only will the drug fail to produce the intended effect, but it will remain in the tissues to be picked up by the bloodstream when the patient's circulatory state improves, at which time an overdose might be received.

Metaraminol produces its pressor effects by releasing stored epinephrine from nerve endings rather than by acting directly on arteriolar receptor sites as does levarterenol. Patients previously treated with reserpine or guanethedine may have reduced or depleted catecholamine (epinephrine and norepinephrine) stores and be refractory to metaraminol.

**Epinephrine (adrenalin)** may be given in anaphylactic shock. It increases the output of the heart and the force of the cardiac contraction; it constricts the blood vessels of the skin and increases blood pressure. It may be given intravenously in the dose of 0.5 ml. of a 1:1,000 solution diluted with 10 ml. of saline or dextrose solution. Tremors, dyspnea, chills, increased apprehension, nausea, vomiting, cyanosis, perspiration, and headache may follow the administration of epinephrine. Epinephrine is a dangerous drug in hypovolemic shock or any other physiologic state in which the cardiac muscle is ischemic, because the drug may cause death by ventricular fibrillation. One of the actions of epinephrine is to increase cardiac irritability, and this action is enhanced whenever myocardial oxygenation is compromised. Its use in shock usually is limited to anaphylactic shock.

**Dopamine (Intropin).** This drug has a beta-adrenergic effect on the myocardium, and produces direct nonadrenergic dilation of the renal and mesenteric vascular beds. Also, its alpha-adrenergic stimulating effect causes skeletal muscle vasoconstriction. Blood pressure rises as a result of enhanced cardiac output. It is administered intravenously, 200 mg. (5 ml.) in one liter of 5 per cent dextrose in $H_2O$ at an initial rate of 0.04 to 0.10 mg. per minute.

Beta Adrenergic Stimulator

**Isoproterenol (Isuprel).** The pure beta stimulator drug isoproterenol (Isuprel) is another useful therapeutic agent in shock. Its vasodilating effect promotes increased skin, renal, coronary, and cerebral blood flow. Because it increases heart rate and speed of conduction and is a myocardial irritant, patients receiving isoproterenol require careful monitoring for increased heart rate above that ordered by the physician, and for signs of ventricular irritability manifested by dangerous forms of ventricular premature beats. Since vasodilation can lead to further hypotension, isoproterenol is used in conjunction with volume replacement and CVP or PCWP monitoring. The drug is titrated intravenously in a concentration of 1 to 4 mg. per liter using a microdrip administration set.

Because of its potency, a low volume fluid reservoir is added to the infusion setup to avoid accidental overdosage. The patient receiving isoproterenol should not be left alone. The drug is ordered to be discontinued if tachycardia at a specified rate, ventricular irritability, or further hypotension develops. The response of the patient receiving isoproterenol is not evaluated strictly in terms of blood pressure but rather in regard to evidence of improved perfusion. Increase in urinary output and "pinking" of the skin are positive signs.

## Alpha Adrenergic Blocking Agents

These drugs are not vasodilators, but act as such by reversing norepinephrine-induced vasoconstriction. They may increase organ blood flow. Phenoxybenzamine (Dibenzyline), phentolamine (Regitine), and chlorpromazine (Thorazine) are useful as alpha blocking agents. Because they produce marked venodilation and increase the volume of the venous reservoir, central venous pressure has to be monitored carefully when they are used. Adequate quantities of a plasma expander should be available at the bedside.

## Steroids

Even though there is no deficiency of steroids in the body during shock, corticosteroid therapy seems to help to maintain blood pressure. Particularly in septic shock, which has not responded to the usual supportive measures, intravenous hydrocortisone may be given. Dosage may be as high as 2.0 Gm. a day.

Some practical points about drug therapy in shock are:

1. **Blood pressure should be raised no more than 20 to 30 mm. Hg below the preshock normal level. If this is not known, systolic blood pressure should be kept between 90 to 100 mm. Hg. Excessive elevation of blood pressure produces marked vasoconstriction, reduces cardiac output, and increases cardiac work and irritability.**
2. **Prolonged use of vasopressors is not recommended and the dosage should be reduced or the patient weaned from them as soon as possible. They should be used as emergency drugs only. Their continued use leads to enhanced capillary transudation of fluid and eventually to depletion of intravascular volume. If efforts are not made to restore this "lost" volume, prolonged hypotension with difficulties in weaning from vasopressors frequently occurs.**

3. **In terms of their effect as alpha or beta stimulators, some adrenergic drugs are dose dependent, that is, there is some evidence to suggest that the beta adrenergic (vasodilating) action of metaraminol and levarterenol is more prominent at lower dosages, the alpha adrenergic (vasoconstricting) effects more pronounced at higher doses.**

Pharmacologic agents used for the shock patient are potentially hazardous. Regardless of the physician's choice of drug or combination of drugs, the nurse must realize their benefits as well as their hazards, meticulously administer them, and intelligently observe the patient's response.

## Activity

The patient in shock needs to have his metabolic activity kept to a minimum without introducing further hazards of immobility. Physical and emotional activity increase cellular needs for oxygen and nutrients and increase the formation of metabolites. Positioning, lifting, and turning are done gently by the nurse. Care should be planned so that the patient has some periods of uninterrupted rest. He needs to be protected from unnecessary and controllable stimulation. Visitors are limited. Understandably, they are distressed and need to be approached humanely and counseled regarding the rationale for rest.

## Mechanical Assistance Devices

Conventional medical therapy has not appreciably reduced the high mortality rate in cardiogenic shock (85 per cent). The short-term use of mechanical assistance devices is aimed at reducing myocardial oxygen demands and improving coronary artery blood flow while supporting the systemic circulation. This would allow time for recovery of ischemic cardiac muscle and, hopefully, improved ventricular function after mechanical assistance is withdrawn. The use of this approach is not widespread and has been primarily on a research basis. One invasive method utilizes the concept of counterpulsation. A balloon attached to a catheter is inserted into the descending thoracic aorta. Rapid inflation of the balloon during diastole augments coronary blood flow by raising ascending aortic diastolic pressure. On deflation during systole there is reduction of resistance to left ventricular ejection, enhanced ventricular outflow, and reduced myocardial oxygen demand. Another invasive approach has been through the use of modified total cardiopulmonary bypass techniques.

Noninvasive external counterpulsation devices are currently being tested and include the lower extremity body boot or wet suit, and a system of arm and leg cuffs for sequenced pulsation of the extremities (Amsterdam, et al., 1973).

## Cardiac Surgery

Ventricular angiography and coronary arteriography are sometimes performed on patients in cardiogenic shock to determine if an emergency surgical procedure would be likely to be effective. Mitral valve replacement, repair of a ruptured interventricular septum, infarctectomy, or saphenous vein bypass are examples of such procedures. (See Chapter 63 for care of the cardiac surgical patient.)

## PROGNOSIS AND COMPLICATIONS

When shock has progressed too far before treatment is started, or when, despite prompt treatment, the patient fails to respond, or when the underlying condition, such as a huge infarction of the myocardium, cannot be effectively treated, death follows.

Fortunately, when shock is treated adequately and promptly, the patient usually recovers. As vital signs return to normal, careful withdrawal of therapeutic measures can be made gradually.

An important indication of the patient's welfare is the urine output. Kidney function during shock is expected to fall or even to cease. A grave complication is the failure of the kidneys to resume work after blood pressure improves. The nurse records both the amount of urine and the time of voiding. She should inform the physician if no urine is excreted and blood pressure has been satisfactory for two hours, or if less than 30 ml. per hour is being put out.

Other complications may occur that are not always observable until the patient has recovered from shock. There may be kidney damage, or a clot that formed in the slow-moving blood. Even in uncomplicated recovery the patient requires a period of convalescence to end the effects of the changes the body commanded when it called out its defensive reactions to fight shock.

Caring for the patient in shock presents a formidable nursing challenge. The physician depends on the nursing assessment and evaluation to guide his choice of therapy. The patient, acutely threatened with death, depends on the nurse for almost total support of his life processes. Surrounded as he is with many intrusive devices—catheters for urine output, venous pressure and arterial pressure, intravenous fluids, oxygen equipment, electrocardiographic monitor—the patient is reassured by the nurse's technical competence as well as her humane concern for him. It is possible in the midst of high-powered action and equipment to overlook the person to and for whom the action is directed. Families, too, need attention and support during this critical time.

## REFERENCES AND BIBLIOGRAPHY

AMSTERDAM, E., et al.: Evaluation and management of cardiogenic shock. Part I. Approach to the patient, *Heart Lung* 1:402, May-June 1972. Part II. Drug therapy, *Heart Lung* 1:663, September-October 1972. Part III. The roles of cardiac surgery and mechanical assist, *Heart Lung* 2:122, January-February 1973.

AYRES, S., et al.: *Care of the Critically Ill*, ed. 2, New York, Appleton-Century-Crofts, 1974.

BELAND, I.: *Clinical Nursing: Pathophysiological and Psychosocial Approaches*, ed. 2, New York, Macmillan, 1970.

BETSON, C.: Blood gases, *Am. J. Nurs.* 68:1010, May 1968.

BETSON, C., and UDE, L.: Central venous pressure, *Am. J. Nurs.* 69:1466, July 1969.

CHANDLER, J. G.: The physiology and treatment of shock, *RN* 34:42, June 1971.

DELANO, A., et al.: Monitoring the acutely ill cardiac patient, *Cardiovasc. Nurs.* 7:61, January-February 1971.

FRAZEE, S., and NAIL, L.: New challenge in cardiac nursing: The intra-aortic balloon, *Heart Lung* 2:526, July-August 1973.

GERNERT, C., and SCHWARTZ, S.: Pulmonary artery catheterization, *Am. J. Nurs.* 73:1182, July 1973.

GUYTON, A.: *Textbook of Medical Physiology*, ed. 4, Philadelphia, Saunders, 1971.

KAMADA, R., and SMITH, J.: The phenomenon of respiratory failure in shock: The genesis of "shock-lung," *Am. Heart J.* 83:1, January 1972.

KUHN, L.: Clinical management of cardiogenic shock, *Bull. N. Y. Acad. Med.* 50:366, March 1974.

LISTER, J.: Nursing intervention in anaphylactic shock, *Am. J. Nurs.* 72:720, April 1972.

MARCHIONDO, K.: CVP: The whys and hows of central venous pressure monitoring, *Nurs. '74* 4:21, January 1974.

NIELSEN, M.: Intra-arterial monitoring of blood pressure, *Am. J. Nurs.* 74:48, January 1974.

PREGAS, L. S., et al.: Use of the Swan-Ganz catheter in the diagnosis of ventricular septal defect after myocardial infarction, *Heart Lung* 2:539, July-August 1973.

RACKLEY, C., and RUSSELL, R.: *Invasive Techniques for Hemodynamic Measurements,* New York, The American Heart Association, 1973.

ROYCE, J. A.: Shock: Emergency nursing implications, *Nurs. Clin. N. Am.* 8:377, September 1973.

SEDLOCK, S.: Assessment of the patient with heart disease, Chap. 4 in McIntyre, M. (ed.): *Heart Disease: New Dimensions of Nursing Care,* Garden Grove, Colo., Trainex Press, 1974.

SLADEN, A.: Pathogenesis of the shock lung, *RN OR/ICU* 34:OR-1+, December 1971.

SPENCE, M. I., et al.: Shock following acute myocardial infarction, *Heart Lung* 2:582, July-August 1973.

————: Cardiogenic shock, *Heart Lung* 2:738, September-October 1973.

Suited for shock, *Emerg. Med.* 5:120, November 1973.

SUMMERS, E., et al.: Combined pharmacologic, pump support and surgical attempts to salvage patients in cardiogenic shock, *J. Cardiovasc. Surg.* 13:313, 1972.

SUN, R. L.: Trendelenburg's position in hypovolemic shock, *Am. J. Nurs.* 71:1758, September 1971.

SWAN, H. J., et al.: Catheterization of the heart in man with use of a flow directed balloon-tipped catheter, *New Eng. J. Med.* 283:450, August 27, 1970.

What CVP can and cannot tell you about patients in shock, *Patient Care* 5:102, March 15, 1971.

# The Patient with Ventilatory Insufficiency and Failure: Acidosis and Alkalosis

By their very nature, conditions that result in respiratory distress are anxiety producing for the nurse and the patient. Only when normal breathing is compromised does the realization that disruption of breathing leads quickly to death enter awareness. Disturbances of respiratory function can have great psychic impact, and matters of psychic importance can disturb respiratory function. Measurements of breathing are frequently useful indicators in studies of emotion and personality.

The acute disruption of breathing and increasing anxiety go hand in hand. An instant reaction to one's incapacity to breathe is panic, and one of the major symptoms of an acute anxiety attack is the feeling that one cannot breathe. Regardless of the cause, survival is threatened and the human organism reacts swiftly and strongly to respiratory threats with emergency neural adaptive mechanisms. As breathing is facilitated, anxiety is reduced, and as anxiety lessens, breathing improves.

The patient with continued respiratory distress has the double task of dealing with the underlying disease process and the anxiety generated by it. The symptom of dyspnea is related to the amount of work involved in breathing and the amount of pressure generated by the respiratory muscles. The dyspneic patient spends much of his energy on the work of breathing. The additional energy directed to control and eradicate his anxiety as well can leave him exhausted and handicapped in coping with the basic exigencies of life, such as eating.

The major objectives of nursing care for the patient in respiratory distress are to facilitate ventilation ($O_2$

intake and $CO_2$ removal) and to reduce the work of breathing. Competent observation, judgment, technical ministration, and emotional support of the patient are the ingredients of nursing care of the patient in respiratory distress. By facilitating ventilation through providing good respiratory care, including interpersonal skills, anxiety can be reduced to the point where it is possible for the patient to respond to the teaching and counseling aspects of nursing care that he may require.

The nurse's anxiety is reduced when she is knowledgeable and confident in her clinical judgment, skilled in the sophisticated technical aspects of care, and secure in her relationships with other members of the respiratory care team.

However, regardless of how competent the nurse is, it is still disquieting to observe and care for a person in severe respiratory distress. Few conditions convey so poignantly man's vulnerability and helplessness, and have such power to arouse empathic concern and anxiety in others. The nurse's supportive presence is a powerful factor in relieving apprehension. One important consideration in care of patients in respiratory distress involves the nurse's assessing her own anxiety when confronted with such patients and seeking ways to control it, so that she does not communicate her anxiety to the patient.

Facial expressions are as powerful as words. The patient should never read hopelessness or helplessness from the nurse's face. She should remember, too, that actions speak louder than words. How a task is accomplished is often as important as what is accomplished.

Because life processes depend on the continuing availability of oxygen to the mitochondria of each body cell, all intensive care patients, regardless of whether they are admitted with burns, poisoning, after trauma or surgery, with myocardial infarction, or any other life-threatening condition, can be considered to be respiratory patients as well. Some will have respiratory disease as their major problem; all require nursing action which prevents respiratory complications. The encouragement of periodic sighing and coughing, deep breathing maneuvers, correct positioning with a regular routine of turning, and chest physiotherapy (see Chap. 30) within the limitations of the individual patient become part of the care plan for each patient in the intensive care unit.

## LUNG FUNCTION

The main function of the respiratory system is to exchange oxygen and carbon dioxide between ambient (atmospheric) air and the blood. Usually it has sufficient reserves to maintain normal partial pressures or tension of these gases in the blood during times of stress. If, however, there is too much damage in part of the lung, or if the patient's reserves are inadequate, respiratory insufficiency develops. Disturbances in ventilation, perfusion, distribution, diffusion of gases, or the production of surfactant, a lipoprotein substance secreted by the alveolar cells and necessary to decrease the surface tension of the fluids lining the alveoli and respiratory passages, can be involved.

*Ventilation,* the movement of air in and out of the lungs in volumes sufficient to maintain normal *arterial* oxygen and carbon dioxide tensions (partial pressures—$P_{O_2}$ and $P_{CO_2}$) can be reduced by brain damage, narcotic or sedative drugs and general anesthesia, paralysis of the respiratory muscles, injury to the chest, or painful breathing such as that following gall bladder surgery, or obstruction of the airways such as in pulmonary emphysema. Because gas exchange is below normal, these conditions result in alveolar hypoventilation.

*Perfusion* of the lungs is the filling of the pulmonary capillaries with venous blood returning from the systemic circulation via the right ventricle. These capillaries are in intimate contact with the alveoli. Normal perfusion of the lung results in a fairly constant ratio of ventilated alveoli to the pulmonary capillaries. In many disease states, marked discrepancies in ventilation-perfusion ratios occur. One part of the lung can be poorly ventilated, but normally perfused with blood. Another part of the lung can have adequate ventilation, but be poorly perfused with blood. In either case, part of the unoxygenated blood going to the lungs from the right side of the heart returns to the left side of the heart still unoxygenated. Instead of pure arterial blood entering the systemic circulation, venous blood is mixed with it. This is called a venoarterial shunt. In normal individuals this blood would comprise 2 to 3 per cent of the cardiac output, but in the critically ill patient, progressive atelectasis can result in a venoarterial shunt comprising 30 to 50 per cent of cardiac output with resulting severe hypoxemia.

*Diffusion* is the process whereby oxygen and carbon dioxide are exchanged across the alveolar-capillary membrane. Diseases that cause loss of lung surface area, such as pulmonary emphysema or loss of part of the lung as in lobectomy, result in diminished gas transfer. Also in conditions such as sarcoidosis, the alveolar membrane can become thickened or fibrosed, thus impeding oxygen passage. Anemias also result in lessened diffusion. The chief function of red blood cells is to transport hemoglobin, which, in turn, carries oxygen from the lungs to the tissues. When red blood cells are deficient, there is, in turn, diminished diffusion and, therefore, decreased oxygen transport to the tissues.

In patients with shock or other causes of diminished pulmonary blood flow, the production of *surfactant* is decreased. Surfactant prevents alveoli from collapsing as they get smaller and from rupturing as they expand. Sighing or other mechanisms which increase alveolar inflation stimulate alveolar cells to produce surfactant.

*Distribution* is the delivery of ambient (atmospheric) air to the separate gas exchange units in the lung. It is accomplished by the successive bifurcation of the tracheobronchial system. Airway obstructions in any part of the system would interfere with normal distribution.

## RESULTS OF LUNG DYSFUNCTION

Abnormalities in ventilation, perfusion, diffusion, or distribution lead to the following conditions:

*Hypoxia,* or the diminished availability of oxygen to the cells of the body

*Hypoxemia,* or reduced oxygen in the body fluids (refers particularly to oxygen in arterial blood)

*Hypercapnia,* or excess carbon dioxide in the body fluids

*Hypocapnia,* or lessened carbon dioxide in body fluids

Some hypothetical patient situations illustrate these abnormal states.

The patient who is *hypoxemic but normocapnic* (without hypocapnia) would have a low arterial oxygen tension. He is not receiving sufficient oxygen into the pulmonary capillaries. A frequent cause of this is atelectasis and venoarterial shunting (some blood that passes through the lungs does not participate in gas exchange). The patient would be expected to be restless, anxious, and to have tachypnea (rapid respirations) and tachycardia. As the condition progresses, the patient would show other signs, such as duskiness, sweating, and cardiac arrhythmias, and he might be combative or confused. One of the first signs of tissue hypoxia is confusion, disorientation, or other behavioral changes. The brain tissue is most sensitive to a lack of oxygen.

The usual color of a hypoxic patient (if hypoxia is of pulmonary origin) is ashen white or clammy gray, *not* blue. If cyanosis is present, it indicates a very advanced pathophysiologic abnormality. Therapy aimed at improving gas exchange by such measures as vigorous suctioning, supplemental oxygen, chest physiotherapy, humidification, or bronchoscopy to remove mucus plugs is instituted.

Frequent position changes are essential. The patient's position in bed is an important determinant of the ventilation and perfusion pattern in the lungs. Mucus has a tendency to be retained in the dependent portions of the lungs and therefore interferes with normal gas exchange.

The patient who is *hypoxemic and hypercapnic* has a low arterial oxygen tension and elevated carbon dioxide tension. This is a result of alveolar hypoventilation. As carbon dioxide accumulates in the blood, the patient develops headache and becomes successively drowsy and then comatose. The hypoxia is the last remaining stimulus to respiration since the respiratory center becomes narcotized or "anesthetized" from excessive carbon dioxide. The patient is in a state of respiratory acidosis. To give the patient oxygen only would take away his last stimulus to respiration and, though his color might improve temporarily, he could die from respiratory arrest. Treatment consists of assisted or controlled ventilation with intubation and a mechanical respirator. Evacuating carbon dioxide allows adequate oxygenation to take place. Because mechanical ventilators are very powerful, the reduction of carbon dioxide should take place slowly over several hours rather than several minutes. If there is a precipitous rise in pH by ventilatory removal of $CO_2$, there can be dangerous fluctuations in myocardial potassium with serious cardiac arrhythmias. What had been the state of respiratory acidosis could swiftly become metabolic alkalosis.

The patient who is both *hypoxemic and hypocapnic* would be one, for example, in serious shock where all body processes are depressed. Attempts to control the patient's ventilation and maintain adequate alveolar gas exchange are accomplished by a volume-cycled ventilator.

## ACIDOSIS AND ALKALOSIS
### (Acidemia and Alkalemia)

The kidney, as well as the lung, together with the body fluids and electrolytes and several buffer systems, acts and reacts to keep the arterial pH (hydrogen ion concentration) within the normal limits of 7.39 to 7.45. Since normal pH is essential for correct enzyme action and cellular metabolism, the body's ability to make adjustments is of critical importance. Life cannot be maintained for more than a few moments when pH falls to 7.0 or rises to 7.8.

Alveolar ventilation determines the amount of carbon dioxide in the body. An increase in carbon dioxide, present in body fluids primarily as carbonic acid, decreases the pH below the normal of 7.4 (acidemic). A decrease in carbon dioxide increases the pH above 7.4 (alkalemic). The hydrogen ion concentration, or pH, on the other hand, affects the rate of alveolar ventilation by a direct action of hydrogen ions on the respiratory center in the medulla oblongata.

The kidney contributes to the normal pH by maintaining serum bicarbonate between 24 to 26 mEq. per liter and excreting excess hydrogen ions.

The lung and kidneys combine to maintain the carbonic acid to bicarbonate ratio at 1:20, fixing the pH at about 7.4:

$$\frac{H_2CO_3}{HCO_3^-} \text{ or } \frac{\text{lungs}}{\text{kidney}}$$

In the critically ill patient, various homeostatic mechanisms operate to compensate for altered physiology. Buffer ratios shift, the lung can "blow off" carbonic acid as carbon dioxide, or the kidney can excrete more bicarbonate in an attempt to maintain normal pH. Compensatory mechanisms, however, can become overstressed and fail, and dangerous clinical conditions develop which in the intensive care patient are generally superimposed on an already serious underlying condition. The patient's condition is said to be compensated as long as the ratio of carbonic acid to bicarbonate remains 1:20. (To determine the ratio [the same units must be compared] multiply $P_{CO_2}$ by .03.) In uncompensated acidosis, the ratio is greater than 1:20 and the pH

is a lower number. In uncompensated alkalosis, the ratio is smaller than 1:20 and the pH is a higher number. By convention, disturbances in pH which involve the lung and carbonic acid levels which result from dissolved carbon dioxide are termed respiratory; the other disturbances are termed metabolic. At times, metabolic and respiratory derangements coexist.

Formerly, assessment of acid-base balance by laboratory method was indirect. For example, the $CO_2$ combining power was used as a general measure of the acidity or alkalinity of the blood. An increase in $CO_2$ combining power (normal range is 50 to 70 volumes per 100 ml. of serum) usually indicates alkalosis, while a decrease is usually indicative of acidosis. Since the pH of the blood, however, depends on the ratio of basic and acidic substances and not the absolute amounts, changes in $CO_2$ combining power do not always represent changes in pH of the blood. Today, blood gas studies done on a sample of arterial blood determine the acid-base balance dependably and rapidly. The blood may be withdrawn by single arterial puncture or repeated samples may be drawn from an indwelling arterial catheter. A heparinized syringe is used and, after careful filling to avoid bubbles, it is capped with a syringe cap or a round toothpick. If delay in analysis is anticipated, the syringe is immediately immersed in ice. This decreases the metabolic activity of the blood cells and prevents oxygen consumption in the syringe.

Some laboratory values of importance in the care of the respiratory patient or other patients requiring assessment of acid-base balance are:

| ARTERIAL BLOOD | |
| --- | --- |
| pH | 7.39 to 7.45 |
| $P_{O_2}$ | 100 mm. Hg breathing room air |
| | 300 to 600 mm. Hg breathing 100 per cent oxygen |
| $P_{CO_2}$ | 35 to 45 mm. Hg |
| $O_2$ saturation | 96 to 100 per cent (per cent oxygen attached to hemoglobin compared to how much could be attached) |
| $HCO_3^-$ (Bicarbonate) | 20.0 to 29.0 mEq./L. |

Laboratory diagnostic tests are useful only when they are related to the overall clinical picture of the patient. Also, because of the numerous ways in which individuals can vary in their response to illness, laboratory tests serve as guides, but are not black and white indicators of the overall clinical condition of the patient.

The physician makes the medical diagnosis from laboratory and clinical data and orders the treatment. The nurse collects data necessary for making the diagnosis and activates a predetermined communication system with the physician when significant laboratory reports are returned or clinical observations are made. Laboratory reports of blood gases, for example, require prompt decision making; they cannot be relegated to a spindle for the physician to look at the following morning. In some hospitals respiratory nursing clinical specialists assume an expanded role in the care of patients with respiratory insufficiency and failure. For example, they assess the laboratory and clinical data and make adjustments in therapy in collaboration with the physician and inhalation therapist. Close observation of the patient, including his general behavior, state of consciousness, skin turgor, urinary output, rate and depth of respiration, muscle function, intestinal function, and abdominal distention, is an essential nursing activity. Concern for the safety and comfort of the patient and his ongoing needs for explanation and emotional support provides a continuing nursing challenge. With this in mind, the following brief narrative will summarize some of the key points in disturbances of acid-base balance.

## Metabolic Alkalosis

In this condition there is bicarbonate excess due to increased renal reabsorption, or excess loss of acids due to vomiting or gastric suction. Excess intake of alkaline salts such as sodium bicarbonate can also precipitate this state. It is associated with severe depletion of body potassium stores even though serum potassium can be normal.

**Compensation.** The body attempts to raise the level of carbonic acid in the blood through retention of $CO_2$ by alveolar hypoventilation. Shallow breathing is a characteristic symptom. The kidney excretes sodium bicarbonate in the urine, making it alkaline, and depresses the mechanism for the excretion of hydrogen ions.

**Signs and Symptoms.** The patient may show symptoms of central nervous system hyperexcitability. Peripheral nerve symptoms such as tingling or numbness, muscular twitching, facial twitching, or the total bodily involvement of tetany can occur.

**Treatment.** Depleted potassium and other electrolytes are replaced and fluid balance is restored. Irrigation of gastric tubes should be done carefully with small quantities of solution to avoid loss of chloride ion, or only normal saline should be used for irrigation. Diuretics can also cause chloride depletion.

Blood Gas Example

| | | |
|---|---|---|
| pH | 7.60 | pH is above normal which |
| $P_{CO_2}$ | 40 | indicates alkalosis. The bi- |
| $HCO_3^-$ | 40 | carbonate ($HCO_3^-$) is mark- |
| $P_{O_2}$ | 96 | edly elevated, which indi- |

cates metabolic disturbance. $P_{O_2}$ and $P_{CO_2}$ are normal. The report indicates metabolic alkalosis.

## Metabolic Acidosis

This state can be caused by loss of upper intestinal secretions with a high bicarbonate content or severe diarrhea.

Uncontrolled diabetics can develop this along with fluid and electrolyte depletion when, because of failure to metabolize adequate quantities of glucose, the production of sulfuric and phosphoric acids and incompletely oxidized fatty acids is increased.

Following cardiac arrest, or in conditions such as shock or major arrhythmias where there is a severe reduction of cardiac output with tissue hypoxia, anaerobic metabolism takes place with the accumulation of lactic acid.

**Compensation.** The hyperventilation following heavy exercise is an attempt to repay the oxygen debt accrued when anaerobic pathways are used. The Kussmaul's breathing of the diabetic in ketoacidosis is an attempt to lower blood carbonic acid by "blowing off" $CO_2$. Urinary output is increased and the urine is acidic in reaction. Sodium and potassium are also lost.

**Signs and Symptoms.** Such a patient would have dry skin with flushing and poor skin turgor. The eyeballs can even lose fluid and become soft. Restlessness and abdominal pain may be present.

Signs of central nervous system depression characterized by disorientation and coma may be present. There would be increased rate and depth of respiration due to pulmonary hyperventilation.

**Treatment** is directed at the underlying conditions and would include infusion of an alkalinizing solution to restore the hydrogen ion concentration to normal. These include sodium bicarbonate, sodium lactate, or THAM buffer.

BLOOD GAS EXAMPLE

| | | |
|---|---|---|
| pH | 7.24 | pH is below normal, which |
| $PCO_2$ | 37 | indicates acidosis. The bi- |
| $HCO_3^-$ | 16 | carbonate is lowered, which |
| $PO_2$ | 95 | indicates a metabolic disturbance. $PCO_2$ is in the lower range of normal. $PO_2$ is normal. |

## Respiratory Alkalosis

This occurs when there is decrease in carbonic acid or hydrogen ion concentration in the blood in proportion to the bicarbonate. In hyperventilation, when the rate and depth of respiration is increased, too much $CO_2$ is blown off. Also, because the hydrogen ion concentration is lowered, the level of ionized calcium is lowered and the patient can develop tetany.

**Compensation.** The kidney attempts to compensate by increasing the excretion of bicarbonate.

**Signs and Symptoms.** The patient may be lightheaded or complain of dizziness. Peripheral nerve symptoms or the more severe signs of tetany can be present.

**Treatment** is directed toward the underlying condition. Rarely do pathologic disorders cause this condition. The low oxygen content of air after an ascent to a high altitude may cause a person to breathe faster and deeper, which causes excess loss of carbon dioxide. Psychoneurotic persons can overbreathe to the extent of alkalosis. The level of carbon dioxide in the alveoli and thus in the blood can be raised by holding the breath for a few minutes or rebreathing air in a paper bag.

BLOOD GAS EXAMPLE

| | | |
|---|---|---|
| pH | 7.60 | pH is above normal limits, |
| $PCO_2$ | 20 | indicating a state of alkalosis. Since the $PCO_2$ is far below normal limits, the causative factor is said to be in the lungs. The $PO_2$ and bicarbonate are within normal limits. |
| $HCO_3^-$ | 20 | |
| $PO_2$ | 95 | |

## Respiratory Acidosis

A slight decrease in alveolar ventilation which reduces arterial oxygen tension can cause carbon dioxide tension to soar. $PCO_2$ rises considerably in chronic obstructive lung disease, obesity, chest-wall trauma, and neurologic or drug-induced depression of the respiratory center. Increase in the metabolic rate due to anxiety, fever, or muscular work increases the amount of carbon dioxide which the lung must handle. In persons with normal lungs, hyperventilation decreases the arterial carbon dioxide tension. However, in patients with emphysema, for example, voluntary hyperventilation causes increased carbon dioxide output from the work of the respiratory muscles, and the diseased lung cannot handle the additional load. Carbon dioxide accumulates in the blood as carbonic acid and the arterial pH falls.

**Compensation.** Quick changes in the serum bicarbonate–carbon dioxide tension ratio buffers the sudden increase in carbonic acid to keep the pH compatible with life. The kidney then helps by increasing the reabsorption of bicarbonate. The $PCO_2$ may remain elevated but pH is restored to almost normal.

Patients with long-term respiratory insufficiency and chronically elevated arterial carbon dioxide tension have blood pH close to normal since their elevated blood bicarbonate maintains the 1:20 ratio.

**Signs and Symptoms.** The patient with impending respiratory acidosis or $CO_2$ narcosis is an ashen white or clammy gray color. Cyanosis, if present, indicates a severe physiologic derangement. Finger twitching may be present at rest but disappears on movement. Drowsiness, mental dullness, and confusion increase if treatment is not initiated promptly.

**Treatment.** The patient with alveolar hypoventilation in respiratory acidosis is drowsy. (The patient with atelectasis and hypoxemia due to venoarterial shunting is usually restless and anxious. The arterial carbon dioxide tension does not rise appreciably in these patients.) Increasing drowsiness leading to coma results from the anesthetic effect of retained carbon dioxide. *Mechanical ventilation* is the only means of reversing the hypercapnic state.

Though the patient's dusky appearance and vague or confused manner are symptoms of hypoxia and would seem to indicate the need for oxygen in high concentration, the administration of oxygen without provision for relieving the hypercapnia could prove fatal. Mechanical ventilation permits oxygen to relieve the severe hypoxemia and blows off $CO_2$.

Initially the increasing level of carbon dioxide in the blood is a stimulus to respiration. When the medulla becomes overloaded with $CO_2$, however, respiratory depression occurs. Then the only remaining mechanism to drive the respiratory center is the hypoxic stimulus.

If this is removed by conventional oxygen therapy, the patient's color may improve but progressive coma and death ensue.

Mechanical ventilation, however, must be carefully administered. Today many patients with chronic respiratory acidosis take diuretics for coexisting heart failure. Since some are potassium-depleting drugs, the patient with a compensated respiratory acidosis (chronic high carbon dioxide tension) who becomes hypokalemic due to potassium-depleting diuretics may have an alkaline pH due to metabolic alkalosis. This is induced by the kidney's increased reabsorption of bicarbonate in response to low serum potassium. When a powerful mechanical ventilator is used, it can decrease carbon dioxide tension from 60 to 40 mm. Hg in ten minutes, but since serum bicarbonate remains elevated, the unbalanced ratio results in a profound metabolic alkalosis driving serum potassium into body cells. Severe cardiac arrhythmias develop as serum potassium falls. This is prevented when the $P_{CO_2}$ is lowered slowly at a rate of about 10 mm. Hg per hr. The body does not tolerate rapid changes in homeostatic responses.

Another mode of therapy is the use of the carbonic anhydrase inhibitor, acetazolamide (Diamox), which reduces the plasma bicarbonate and therefore the $CO_2$ content of the blood through increased excretion of bicarbonates in the urine.

BLOOD GAS EXAMPLE

*Compensated* Respiratory Acidosis

| | | |
|---|---|---|
| pH | 7.37 | The pH is below normal, which indicates acidosis. The $P_{CO_2}$ is markedly elevated but the pH does not reflect this major elevation. In an attempt to compensate for the elevated $P_{CO_2}$ the bicarbonate ($HCO_3^-$) is also elevated, thus keeping the ratio of carbonic to bicarbonate at 1:20. |
| $P_{CO_2}$ | 62 | |
| $HCO_3^-$ | 35 | |
| $P_{O_2}$ | 96 | |

*Uncompensated* Respiratory Acidosis

| | | |
|---|---|---|
| pH | 7.31 | The pH is below normal, which indicates acidosis. The $P_{CO_2}$ is elevated, which indicates respiratory origin of the acidosis due to severe hypoventilation. The normal bicarbonate shows no compensation for the high $P_{CO_2}$. The $P_{O_2}$ is low, indicating hypoxemia. Since there is alveolar hypoventilation with elevated $P_{CO_2}$, oxygen to correct the hypoxemia should not be administered without mechanical ventilatory assistance. |
| $P_{CO_2}$ | 66 | |
| $HCO_3^-$ | 28 | |
| $P_{O_2}$ | 50 | |

## ACUTE RESPIRATORY FAILURE

Acute respiratory failure, or acute ventilatory failure, is a life-threatening complication in which alveolar ventilation becomes inadequate to maintain the body's vital need for oxygen supply and carbon dioxide removal. Though the signs are not specific, the patient initially may be restless, agitated, confused, and diaphoretic, and may have tachycardia. Cardiac arrhythmias and signs such as "flapping tremor" (asterixis) may develop. Though laboratory confirmation of acute respiratory failure will show different correlations with each patient's clinical condition, one general guideline is that acute respiratory failure will reveal a $P_{O_2}$ of less than 50 mm. Hg, a $P_{CO_2}$ of more than 50 mm. Hg, and a pH of less than 7.30 (Nett and Petty, 1967).

The most frequent circumstance of acute respiratory failure is when a patient with moderate to severe chronic obstructive lung disease (see Chap. 30) develops an acute bronchopulmonary infection, is oversedated, undergoes general anesthesia, has chest trauma, or incurs some other type of insult to his already embarrassed pulmonary reserve. Injudicious use of bed rest may precipitate pulmonary complications that may progress to respiratory failure.

Other patients with neurological disorders, acute poisoning, or surgical intervention (especially abdominal operations) are susceptible to respiratory failure.

At first the patient may be alert, but he is apprehensive, dyspneic, wheezing, but rarely cyanotic. There may be use of the accessory muscles of respiration. In the advanced state of respiratory failure the patient may appear to be quite comfortable or asleep. Though the patient initially often looks as if he would benefit from sedation because of his apprehension, therapy is directed toward relieving the patient's symptoms by improving ventilation. Sedation, alone, can further depress respiratory effort. In the presence of continued hypoventilation, cardiac arrhythmias, hypotension, and congestive heart failure can develop. The ensuing clinical state of the patient depends partly on his pre-existing state, particularly his renal and cardiopulmonary status. Not only is the level of blood gases a factor, but also the rapidity with which increased hypoxemia and hypercapnia develop. If $CO_2$ retention develops slowly, there is time for the kidneys to excrete chlorides and reabsorb bicarbonate and sodium ions, thus maintaining the pH within normal limits. If the renal mechanisms fail to compensate for rapidly accumulating $CO_2$, the pH falls below the normal 7.39 and respiratory acidosis develops.

## Patient Care

A program of care is planned for the patient which encompasses the following aspects of management:

- **Clearing the airways**
- **Combating bronchospasm**
- **Giving oxygen for hypoxemia while assisting or controlling ventilation**
- **Humidification**
- **Combating infection**
- **Monitoring clinical and laboratory values**
- **Treating cardiac and circulatory status**
- **Maintaining fluid and electrolyte balance**

Essential to nursing management of the patient is understanding the aims of therapy, explaining these to the patient as they are about to involve him, skilled observation and judgment, technical expertise with various forms of equipment utilized by the respiratory care team to enhance the objectives of care, and establishing effective communication with the patient so that he knows what is expected of him and knows what he can expect of others. The patient's fear is lessened when he is assisted to remain in control of his situation for as long as possible. When he can no longer do so, he must have the confidence that he can temporarily relinquish the control to others who are concerned and competent to do the job for him.

### Airway Maintenance

Cough is the major mechanism for clearing the tracheobronchial tree of abundant, tenacious mucus. Effective coughing requires that the patient be assisted to a position (usually sitting with knees flexed and feet supported) which facilitates exhalation and compression of the thorax. Before coughing, secretions must first be mobilized to the region of the carina through a series of slow expiratory efforts while bending forward. When the patient is ready to cough he takes a deep abdominal breath through the nose, then bends forward and controls a soft, staged, staccato cough with his mouth and glottis open (Lagerson, 1973). In the event that the patient's cough is ineffective but he is conscious and cooperative, coughing may be stimulated as a last report by tracheal irritation with a catheter. The use of the intermittent positive pressure respirator serves to inflate the lungs and enhance the ejecting mechanism of the cough by driving air past mucus secretions. Simply giving the patient an IPPB treatment is not enough. After the treatment, the patient must be assisted to cough or the treatment will be ineffective. Thus, he requires nursing attention even if another member of the respiratory care team, such as the inhalation therapist, actually turns on the machine. Encouraging fluid intake within the maximum limits of the patient's treatment regimen aids in preventing the drying of secretions. Turning and positioning the patient every hour and performing chest physiotherapy aid in directing mucus to the main airway from whence it can be expelled.

### Liquefying Secretions

Secretions often must be thinned to be expectorated. To be most effective, sterile solutions or medications must be delivered to the mucous-covered surface. However, nebulization therapy is the least traumatic and most effective method of providing water. Water particles must be small enough to be deposited on the distal bronchioles rather than be evaporated into the air. To accomplish this, the vapor pressure of sterile distilled water can be reduced with a substance such as propylene glycol. Also, humidified air can be heated and a mist produced which creates an excess of water particles to deposit in the bronchi, such as with the Puritan heated nebulizer. Nebulizers can be powered by hand, by compressed gas, by an intermittent positive pressure breathing machine, or by a power-driven compressor. Heated nebulizers can be used continuously with semiclosed or closed inhalation systems and hold up to 500 ml. of fluid. Smaller nebulizers with a 25-ml. capacity can be used intermittently. Ultrasonic nebulizers produce very fine particles through the use of high frequency sound waves. As much as 1 liter of water can be delivered to and absorbed by the lungs in 24 hours by this method. Caution must be taken to prevent the patient from becoming overhydrated.

Nebulization is also used to deliver medication directly to the distal airway membranes. Bronchodilators such as isoproterenol (Isuprel) or epinephrine (Vaponefrin), mucolytic agents such as sodium ethasulfate (Tergemist), or acetylcysteine (Mucomyst) may be ordered. A wetting agent such as tyloxapol (Alevaire) or corticosteroids such as dexamethasone (Decadron) may also be ordered.

Since the primary purpose of nebulization is to thin secretions for easy expectoration, the patient may need help by assisted coughing, postural drainage, or suctioning. Every precaution must be taken that the nebulizer is sterile. Bronchopneumonia can directly result from breathing aerosols produced by a contaminated nebulizer. Intravenous theophylline ethylene diamine (aminophylline, 500 mg. in 500 ml. of 5 per cent dextrose in water over a one-hour period by intravenous drip) may be ordered as a parenteral bronchodilator.

### Intratracheal Suctioning

When the patient cannot cough effectively despite therapy, nasal-tracheal suction may be utilized. Passage of the suction catheter is facilitated if the patient is sitting upright and leaning slightly forward with his jaw extended. An assistant can grasp the patient's tongue. A 16-inch, size 18 to 24 F. catheter, lubricated with a water-soluble substance, is inserted gently, without suction, into the nostril. As the patient coughs or pants repeatedly, the glottis opens and permits the catheter to be passed between the vocal cords and into the trachea. The catheter is attached to a suction apparatus with a "Y" connection. As the opening of the "Y" is occluded, gentle suction (40 cm. of water) is applied. The catheter is rotated between the left thumb and forefinger to sweep the walls. Suction is applied for no longer than 15 seconds at a time. The catheter can be guided into either main bronchus by turning the patient's head to the side opposite that to be catheterized. Sterile normal saline, 5 to 10 ml., can be inserted into the trachea through the catheter once it is in place. The catheter can be left in place between periods of suctioning, but oxygen is given during these intervals. As the catheter is withdrawn, suction is applied to clear the oropharynx of secretions. Suctioning can result in reflex vagal stimulation. The effects can be noted on the cardiac monitor or in the patient's pulse. Bradycardia or any degree of heart block relative to suctioning should be promptly reported. Suctioning may have to be less frequent or less vigorous, or the physician may order a drug such as atropine sulfate to override the vagal effect.

### Endotracheal Intubation

Suctioning can be accomplished also through an endotracheal tube which the physician inserts through the nose or mouth (Fig. 60-1). It can remain in place for several days, and when its cuff is inflated to provide a tight connection, it can be attached to a respirator for controlled ventilation. The patient, however, cannot speak and may have difficulty swallowing. Sedation may be ordered for him as long as respiration is controlled. Suctioning is not as effective as when tracheostomy is done, but the time delay, surgical trauma, and complications of tracheostomy are avoided. Once the patient is intubated with an endotracheal tube, the following points are important considerations:

**Placement of the Tube.** If the tube is not anchored securely to the exterior, it can slip into the right main stem bronchus. Then the left lung would not be ventilated and is actually completely obstructed from the flow of air. When the patient is intubated, both sides of the thorax should rise evenly during inspiration. Because this is not always a reliable sign, both sides of the lung should be auscultated with a stethoscope to hear the flow of air. The physician or nurse can do this.

The tube can also be misplaced and pass into the esophagus. If the patient is still breathing spontaneously, breath sounds will still be heard in both lung fields. The physician can check correct placement of the tube by attaching it to an "Ambu" bag or other type of anesthesia bag and, while squeezing the bag, simultaneously auscultate the thorax.

**Obstruction of the Tube.** Absence of breath

sounds in either or both lungs can indicate obstruction of the tube. The tube can become obstructed by: (1) secretions; suctioning and liquefying secretions is required; (2) kinking of the tube; (3) biting down on the tube by the patient; this can be prevented by the use of a bite block or an oropharyngeal airway; (4) the cuff, which, when inflated, provides a tight seal between the tube and the trachea; it can slip down and occlude the orifice; and (5) the distal end of the tube, which may press on the wall of the trachea. All of the above situations demand emergency action because of the immediate danger of asphyxiation.

### Removal of the Tube

- Accidental removal by the patient must be guarded against as this can result in laryngeal edema or spasm and predispose to respiratory arrest.
- The physician makes the decision to remove the tube when the patient's vital capacity, measured with a ventilometer, is adequate (see succeeding section). Blood gas values are also used as a guideline for tube removal.
- The endotracheal tube should be removed only by a person who can replace it if necessary. The necessary emergency equipment should remain at the bedside.
- Before the cuff is deflated, the pharynx is aspirated so that secretions do not gravitate downward. The tube is usually removed with the patient in semi-Fowler's position. Laryngospasm can occur. If so, air is given by positive pressure with an "Ambu" bag; the physician may reintubate the patient, and may order muscle relaxants.

### Postextubation Care

- High or semi-Fowler's position promotes chest expansion and optimal alveolar ventilation.
- The patient's posterior pharynx may be dry and he may be hoarse. Humidification aids in preventing further complications. Candy "Life Savers" or sour balls may be comforting.
- The patient should be observed carefully for signs of laryngeal edema or increased respiratory distress.

## Tracheostomy

An opening into the trachea with insertion of a cuffed tracheostomy tube provides a good portal for suctioning, and the tube also can serve as a good connection for a respirator. There is less interference with swallowing than with the endotracheal tube. Talking, if permitted, can be accomplished with occlusion of the tube and release of the cuff; trauma to the larynx is lessened, and easier trials of extubation by plugging the tube can

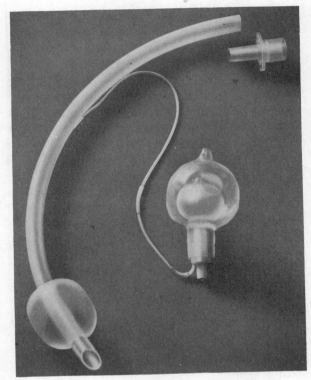

**Figure 60-1.** Disposable Lanz controlled pressure cuff endotracheal tube. (Marketed by Extracorporeal Medical Specialties, Inc.)

be achieved. Complications of tracheostomy include infection, bleeding, tracheal trauma, and pneumothorax. Humidification is necessary to prevent drying and incrustation of the mucous membrane in the trachea and the main stem bronchus. Crusts can break off, obstruct the lower airway, and cause asphyxiation.

Ideally, a new disposable suction catheter and disposable sterile glove should be used each time the patient is suctioned, and these are then discarded. The frequency of suctioning depends on the amount of secretions present.

The period of suctioning should be as brief as possible, not exceeding 15 seconds. Severely hypoxic patients should receive a few breaths of 100 per cent oxygen prior to insertion of the suction catheter (Selecky, 1974).

Because of the danger of necrosis of the tracheal wall, the cuff of the tracheostomy tube should be deflated on a regular basis. The amount of air injected into the cuff should be just enough to pre-

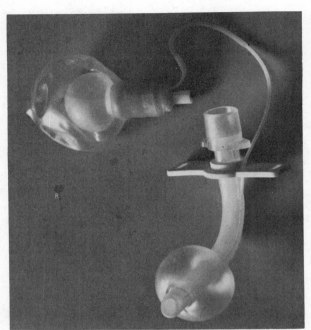

**Figure 60-2.** Disposable Lanz tracheostomy tube with controlled low-pressure, integral cuff and external pressure-control balloon with pressure-regulating valve to minimize tracheal pressure. (Marketed by Extracorporeal Medical Specialties, Inc.)

vent an air leak around the tube or through the mouth.

To avoid tissue ischemia and tracheal necrosis, high volume-low pressure cuffs are used today (Fig. 60-2).

### Oxygen

Supplemental oxygen is often necessary for adequate tissue perfusion, especially of the heart and brain.

Supplemental oxygen is a drug. It must be administered in a specific amount to treat a specific condition. This can be determined only by arterial blood gas analysis.

Compensatory responses to hypoxia, such as increased cardiac output, with hypertension and tachycardia, peripheral sympathetic overactivity, tachypnea (rapid breathing) and hyperventilation, can reach a maximum of usefulness and then the patient's condition deteriorates. Therapy should be afforded the patient before this point.

The exact oxygen tension (or partial pressure of oxygen in the arterial blood) at which observable signs of lack of oxygen develop varies among patients. When $Po_2$ decreases below the normal of 95 to 100 mm. to about 80, the patient may become tachypneic with a rate of about 25, breathe with his mouth open, and be short of breath on walking. With further decrease, restlessness, hypotension, diaphoresis, and combativeness are likely to be present. Serious cardiac arrhythmias and cardiac arrest can develop quickly.

Generally, optimum arterial oxygen tension is maintained between 80 and 120 mm. Hg. An oxygen tension of 70 is of concern and an oxygen level below 60 in the acutely ill patient is dangerous. For example, a $Po_2$ of 60 mm. Hg may be detrimental for a patient who has just had gallbladder surgery (and who does not have pulmonary disease). However, many patients with chronic pulmonary disease ambulate quite well with a $Po_2$ of 60.

Recently it has been noted that oxygen toxicity can be as great a problem as hypoxia. Levels of oxygen tension over 120 mm. Hg are unnecessary and may lead to oxygen toxicity. High levels of oxygen depress respiration and also damage the surface membrane of the lung and lead to progressive atelectasis.

The physician orders the technique of oxygen administration, though the effect of therapy is continuously monitored by the nurse. For the hypoxemic but normocapnic patient (low $Po_2$ but normal $Pco_2$), oxygen can be administered by nasal cannula. The oxygen flows through two prongs of the tubing into each nostril. At an oxygen flow rate of eight liters per minute, the nasal cannula can deliver 32 per cent oxygen at the oropharynx in the normal individual. The nasal mucosa can become quite dry at a flow rate over ten liters.

The nasal catheter gives a similar concentration of oxygen, but is more reliable because it is inserted into the oropharynx and taped in place. The catheter must be changed to the other nostril at least every 12 hours.

The "Venti-Mask" (Venturi mask) is designed to deliver oxygen of predictable concentration. This is of great importance in the patient with chronic airway obstruction. It must be observed that the vent holes in the plastic face mask are not occluded in order to prevent accumulation of carbon dioxide and change in oxygen concentration.

The Puritan nebulizer delivers heated or cold aerosol therapy with varying concentrations of oxygen. At a flow rate of ten liters of oxygen, three settings provide for 40, 70, or 100 per cent oxygen.

After the dilution with room air, the patient receives a concentration of 36, 48, or 65 per cent oxygen.

An oxygen mask with a rebreathing reservoir, if secured tightly to the face, can deliver oxygen concentrations over 70 per cent. The liter flow of oxygen must be high enough to keep the bag inflated on inhalation.

If airway clearance and conventional oxygen therapy are not sufficient to maintain adequate oxygenation above 50 to 60 mm. Hg and removal of carbon dioxide, a respirator (ventilator) attached to a cuffed endotracheal or tracheostomy tube may be ordered. Patients who are hypoxemic and hypercapnic require assisted or controlled ventilation with a respirator; patients who are both hypoxemic and hypocapnic (usually patients in shock) may benefit from intubation and sedation with controlled ventilation via a volume-cycled respirator.

### The Patient on a Respirator (Ventilator)

Ventilators are used to do the work of breathing. Air is forced into the lung to give the patient adequate tidal volume (adequate sized breaths). Small bedside units have replaced the body or tank type respirator, the so-called "iron lung" which was widely used for the respiratory failure of acute poliomyelitis. The patient's respiration can be either assisted (patient cycled) or controlled (machine cycled). In assisted ventilation, the inspiration is initiated by the patient and is then boosted by the machine which has been preset as ordered by the physician. In many types of machines, after a set period of delay, the machine will trigger a breath if the patient's own effort fails to trigger the machine.

In controlled ventilation, the inspiration is initiated by the machine at a preset rate. The patient's spontaneous respiratory effort, if any, must be synchronized with the machine. As the machine is applied, the patient can be consulted regarding the rate and depth of respiration so that he gets the sense of maintaining some participation in the control of his own breathing. Fighting the respirator or becoming asynchronous with the respirator, on the part of the patient, is usually caused by inadequate alveolar ventilation, hypoxemia, or low cardiac output. Measures are then taken to overcome the patient's spontaneous breathing effort, such as a short period of manually controlled ventilation with an "Ambu" bag and 100 per cent oxygen. If this

is unsuccessful, drugs such as morphine or d-tubocurarine (curare) can be given in small intravenous doses by the physician to depress spontaneous respirations to the point where controlled ventilation can be initiated. Imagine how frightening this can be for the patient who is struggling to breathe on his own. He has to be convinced that the respiratory care team is concerned and competent to take over, temporarily, the work of breathing for him.

Ventilation is generally expressed as the number of liters of air breathed per minute, or minute ventilation. Minute ventilation is the product of the tidal volume, or the amount of air inhaled and exhaled, times the number of breaths per minute. When the physician orders ventilator therapy, he estimates the patient's tidal volume based on the norm that there is about 10 to 12 ml. of air exchanged per breath for each Kg. of body weight. Thus, a patient who weighs 154 lb., or 70 Kg. (2.2 Kg. = 1 lb.), and who breathes 15 times a minute would have a predicted minute ventilation of 10,500 ml. Since the upper respiratory tract conveys air, but does not take part in actual gas exchange, and since not all of the alveoli participate, there is a correction to be made for this so-called "dead space."

Physiologic dead space equals anatomic dead

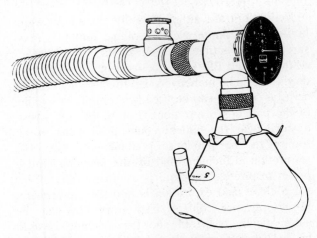

**Figure 60-3.** The Mark 12 Wright respirometer inserted into a semi-open breathing attachment to measure expiratory flow. When used in conjunction with a stopwatch, the respirometer (which shows the volume of gas passed through it) can be used to determine minute volumes. A catheter mount is supplied for use if the patient is intubated instead of using a face mask. (By kind permission of British Oxygen Co. Ltd., Pinnacles, Harlow, Essex, England)

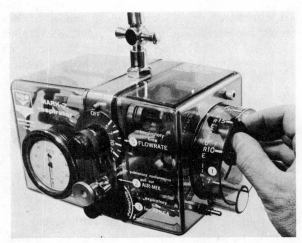

**Figure 60-4.** Mark 7 pressure cycled respirator. (Bird Corporation, Palm Springs, Calif.)

space plus alveolar dead space, or approximately 150 ml. per breath per pound for the average person. If he breathes 15 times a minute, then dead space minute volume is 2,250 ml. Therefore, true alveolar minute volume would be: 10,500 ml. minus 2,250 ml., equals 8,250 ml., or 8.25 liters. Minute volume and tidal volume can be easily measured in the patient on a ventilator by attaching a hand spirometer such as the Wright respirometer to the expiratory port of the respirator valve (see Fig. 60-3, p. 1071).

Ventilators are either pressure cycled (pressure limited) or volume cycled (volume limited). Pressure cycled ventilators, such as the Bird Mark 7 or the Bennett PR 1, can be used intermittently for deep breathing maneuvers or for the delivery of aerosols, or also can be used for continuous cycling of the patient's respirations. For respiratory assist, a valve near the patient connection opens in response to the patient's spontaneous effort. His respiration is then boosted by the machine until a preset inspiratory pressure is exceeded. The inflow valve closes and expiration is into the atmosphere. For respiratory control, inspiratory flow can be automatically triggered and the machine is used in conjunction with the cuffed tracheostomy or endotracheal tube. The physician determines inspiratory flow, sensitivity, rate, and expiratory pressure. Maximum pressure is about 40 to 45 cm. of water. Pressure-limited ventilators are small, are driven by compressed air or air-oxygen mixtures rather than electric power, are reasonable in price, but require frequent maintenance (Fig. 60-4).

If the patient on ventilatory assist is breathing too rapidly with small tidal volume, the machine will cycle too rapidly and the patient's condition will deteriorate. Controlled ventilation by the physician with 100 per cent oxygen and an anesthesia bag such as the "Ambu" until adequate alveolar ventilation is established has been found to be usually sufficient to synchronize the patient with the respirator.

In the volume-cycled or volume-limited respirator, a motor-driven piston pumps air or air-oxygen mixture. The Emerson postoperative ventilator (Fig. 60-5) and the Bennett MA-I volume-cycled respirator are examples. The rate of respiration and the volume of air per respiration or stroke (tidal volume) can be varied and are determined by the physician according to the patient's blood gases and predicted tidal volume needs. Volume-cycled machines are always used with a cuffed endotracheal tube if the condition is anticipated to be cleared in a short time, or the cuffed tracheostomy tube, for longer periods of treatment. They deliver the predetermined volume regardless of resistance of the lungs. They are more reliable and more expensive than pressure-cycled units. An example of efficient ventilation with such a machine would be the achievement of a tidal volume of 500 to 700 ml. with a respiratory rate of 12 to 14 breaths per minute, achieving a ventilation of 7 to 8 liters per minute.

Airway pressure depends on the amount of air delivered and the resistance of the lung to inflation. A safety or "pop-off" valve prevents excessive pressure. Increases or decreases in pressure can be signaled by an alarm built into or attached to the system. An elevation of pressure is an indication of obstruction usually due to retained secretions. A decrease in pressure is usually an indication of a lack of a closed, or airtight, system. The inflation of the cuff of the endotracheal or tracheostomy tube should be checked. Fall in pressure can also indicate a decrease in bronchoconstriction and mean progress for the patient. Supplemental oxygen and humidification can be provided with volume-cycled respirators. As with all types of mechanical equipment, precise knowledge of the principles of the instrument and the manufacturer's instructions is essential for all members of the health care team.

**Nursing Care.** Following are some important nursing considerations for the care of the patient on a respirator:

- One of the major problems leading to intubation and intensive respiratory care is retained secretions. Intubation buys time while the physician, nurses, and therapists direct their team efforts toward the basic problem. Secretions in the distal portions of the lungs cannot be cleared by a suctioning catheter. It should be appreciated also that positive pressure breathing does not adequately ventilate the entire lung parenchyma unless the patient is continuously repositioned every hour and secretions moved from the distal air passages to the mainstem bronchi and carina, where they can be cleared by suctioning or coughing. This is a nursing responsibility. Pulmonary physiotherapy techniques such as gentle vibration and percussion (clapping with cupped hands) over the lung fields from which secretions are to be removed need to be performed at frequent, regular intervals by the nurse or physiotherapist. Team efforts are also directed toward early mobilization of the patient by having him sit in a chair as soon as possible.
- Suctioning is done every hour or more frequently if necessary. Before the cuff is deflated, the upper airway is suctioned so that secretions do not gravitate downward. It is convenient to suction the patient at the fixed intervals when the cuff is routinely deflated to avoid necrosis of the tracheal mucosa. Color, consistency, and odor of secretions are noted. The cuff inflation should not exceed the quantity of air which is just sufficient to prevent the patient from talking or to prevent air escaping from the patient's mouth. For greater safety, 0.5 ml. of air can be removed after reaching the end-point.
- The patient must be in synchrony with the ventilator or else he is not getting the proper rate or volume. The physician is consulted if the patient is out of phase.
- Diffuse atelectasis can develop during constant-volume ventilation. In order to promote ventilation of dependent portions of the lungs, several techniques can be employed which simulate the normal sigh mechanism and produce periodic hyperinflation. The pressure of the pressure-cycled machine can be increased 10 to 20 cm. for several breaths every hour or several times an hour. Some volume-controlled machines, such as the Emerson postoperative ventilator, have a built-in sigh mechanism which is automatically activated every seven minutes or longer. Or, the patient's lungs can be inflated for several breaths manually with an anesthesia bag and 100 per cent oxygen.
- Gastric dilation and paralytic ileus are no uncommon problems of patients on respirator therapy. Gastrointestinal bleeding can also occur. Abdominal distention is reported promptly to the physician, who can initiate early use of gastric decompression. Vomiting with aspiration spells disaster for these patients. The patient's stools and gastric secretions should be checked for blood, and a fall in the hematocrit should be promptly reported.
- Positive-pressure breathing has an effect on systemic circulation since intrathoracic pressure which is raised to above atmospheric pressure decreases the gradient between the peripheral veins and the right atrium and decreases venous return to the heart. (This principle is utilized when IPPB is used to treat acute pulmonary edema.) To keep average intrathoracic pressure close to atmospheric and avoid fall in cardiac output for the patient not in pulmonary edema on controlled ventilation, the physician may order that inspiration comprise one-third of each respiration and expiration be twice as long as inspiration, or some other proportion in which the duration

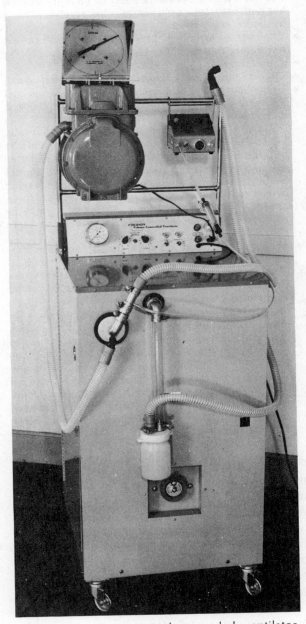

**Figure 60-5.** Emerson volume-cycled ventilator. (J. H. Emerson Co.)

of expiration exceeds that of inspiration. Settings on the machines are used to make this kind of adjustment. Any signs of decreased cardiac output are reported to the physician.

- Respiratory alkalosis from hyperventilation can occur in patients on respirators. The patient might complain of chest pain, numbness or tingling of the extremities, vertigo, or lightheadedness and muscle spasm, and may even develop tetany. This can sometimes be avoided in the susceptible patient if the respiratory rate is periodically decreased.
- Patients with tracheostomies may be on oral feedings, but patients with endotracheal tubes receive nothing by mouth.
- Vital signs including blood pressure, pulse, and respiratory rate should be checked hourly.
- Temperature is recorded every four hours.
- The patient on a ventilator should not be left alone.
- The patient's level of consciousness, color of lips and nailbeds, pupils, and muscle strengths are checked every hour.
- It must be remembered that the patient cannot talk, but can hear, and can usually write. A bell should be left with him at all times along with a "magic slate" or pad and pencil. The patient's dominant hand should be left free of intravenous needles, if possible, so that he can write more easily. Frightening aspects of the patient's condition should not be discussed where he may overhear the conversation and become more alarmed.
- Most respirator patients are conscious and alert during the major part of their illness. All are apprehensive; many are depressed, especially if they are victims of recurrent episodes of respiratory failure and between hospitalizations constantly have to fight the battle of breathlessness. Some patients may be bitter, having become acutely ill despite adhering closely to the home regimen prescribed for them. The person under age 65, not covered by Medicare, can incur tremendous debt from his intensive treatment. The patient becomes easily frustrated because of his inability to communicate verbally with physicians, nurses, inhalation therapists, and family. Explanations to the patient must continue, however. When the cuff is deflated, the patient can talk, using air flow from the respirator.

The patient knows that his life is dependent on the competence of people and the mechanics of machines. Accidental disconnection from the respirator, kinking of the tubes, or occlusion of them with a mucus plug can mean immediate asphyxiation. Once an accident occurs, fear of its recurrence can plague a patient and he will expend tremendous energy trying to guard his own life. A manual device such as an "Ambu" bag must be at the bedside of each patient in the event of mechanical breakdown of the ventilator or asynchrony creating an emergency. The patient must have the reassurance that he is under constant, competent supervision. When the patient breathes better, so does the staff!

**Weaning the Patient.** One of the considerations employed by the physician which indicates that the patient can be gradually removed from respirator support is that his vital capacity is at least 10 ml. per Kg. of body weight, or at least twice his normal tidal volume. Weaning should be initiated as soon as possible so that the patient's respiratory muscles can be restored to normal tone more quickly and also because the patient psychologically benefits from control of his own life processes and signs of improvement. Generally, the longer the patient has received artificial ventilation, the slower will be the weaning process. Also, whether or not the patient is successfully weaned from the respirator depends to a large extent on the quality of nursing care he received during the intensive treatment process. Weaning is best initiated early in the morning; the patient's responses are closely observed and the time intervals are increased during the day. Three to four minutes off the ventilator every half hour to start can test the patient's tolerance. Patients who were receiving volume-controlled assistance may be switched to a pressure-cycled respirator before weaning is attempted. The sensitivity can be gradually decreased on the pressure-cycled respirator so that more burden is put on the patient to initiate respiration himself.

While off the ventilator, the patient receives humidified oxygen. Some patients may require mild sedation to allay their anxiety. All patients require the constant presence of the nurse, who observes their tolerance, gives constant support to their own efforts, and is prepared to assist them back to respirator support if they are not up to the task of breathing on their own.

Even when weaning appears complete, the patient should be observed for several days by the specially prepared respiratory staff. This is especially true for the older, debilitated patient.

For after-crisis management of patients with chronic obstructive pulmonary disease, see Chapter 30, The Patient with Chronic Respiratory Disease.

## REFERENCES AND BIBLIOGRAPHY

Ayres, S., and Lagerson, J.: Pulmonary physiology at the bedside: Oxygen and carbon dioxide abnormalities, *Cardiovasc. Nurs.* 9:1, January-February 1973.

————, et al.: *Care of the Critically Ill,* ed. 2, New York, Appleton-Century-Crofts, 1974.

BROUGHTON, J.: Chest physical diagnosis for nurses and respiratory therapists, *Heart Lung* 1:200, March-April 1972.

CHERNIACK, R., et al.: *Respiration in Health and Disease,* ed. 2, Philadelphia, Saunders, 1972.

DIDIER, E.: Principles in the management of assisted ventilation, *Chest* 58:423 (Supplement No. 2), October 1970.

FINIGAN, M.: Ventilatory considerations in cardiac patients, *Nurs. Clin. N. Am.* 7:541, September 1972.

FUHS, M., et al.: Nursing in a respiratory intensive care unit, *Chest* (Supplement) 62:14S, August 1972.

HARGREAVES, A.: Emotional problems of patients with respiratory disease, *Nurs. Clin. N. Am.* 3:479, September 1968.

HUDSON, L. D.: The acute management of the chronic airway obstruction patient, *Heart Lung* 3:93, January-February 1974.

JACQUETTE, G.: To reduce hazards of tracheal suctioning, *Am. J. Nurs.* 71:2362, December 1971.

LAGERSON, J.: The cough—its effectiveness depends on you, *Resp. Care* 18:434, July-August 1973.

————: Nursing care of patients with chronic pulmonary insufficiency, *Nurs. Clin. N. Am.* 9:165, March 1974.

McCORMICK, K., and BIRNBAUM, M.: Acute ventilatory failure following thoracic trauma, *Nurs. Clin. N. Am.* 9:181, March 1974.

McCURDY, D.: Mixed metabolic and respiratory acid-base disturbances: Diagnosis and treatment, *Chest* (Supplement) 62:35S, August 1972.

National Tuberculosis and Respiratory Disease Association: *Cleaning and Sterilization of Inhalation Equipment,* New York, 1968.

NETT, L., and PETTY, T.: Acute respiratory failure, *Am. J. Nurs.* 67:1847, September 1967.

OAKES, A., et al.: Understanding blood gases, *Nurs. '73* 3:14, September 1973.

PETTY, T., and NETT, L.: After-crisis care in chronic airway obstruction, *Chest* (Supplement) 62:58S, August 1972.

RASTEGAR, A., and THIER, S.: Physiologic consequences and bodily adaptations to hyper- and hypocapnia, *Chest* (Supplement) 62:28S, August 1972.

SELECKY, P.: Tracheostomy: A review of present-day indications, complications, and care, *Heart Lung* 3:272, March-April 1974.

TINKER, J., and WEHNER, R.: The nurse and the ventilator, *Am. J. Nurs.* 74:1276, July 1974.

VOTTER, B. A.: Hand-operated emergency ventilation devices, *Heart Lung* 1:1277, March-April 1972.

WADE, J.: *Respiratory Nursing Care,* St. Louis, Mosby, 1973.

# The Patient with a
# Cardiac Arrhythmia

## CHAPTER 61

## NERVOUS CONTROL OF THE HEART

### Autonomic Nervous System

Although the heart has its own intrinsic control systems and can continue to operate without any outside nerve influences, there are times when efficacy of heart action can be greatly increased or decreased by regulatory impulses from the central nervous system. The nervous system is connected with the heart through two different sets of nerves, the parasympathetic nerves and the sympathetic nerves.

The vagus nerves which are part of the parasympathetic system, when stimulated, have the following four effects on the heart:

1. Decreased rate and rhythmicity of the S-A node
2. Decreased force of contraction of the cardiac muscle, particularly the atria
3. Decreased rate of conduction of impulses through the heart
4. Decreased blood flow through the coronary vessels

These can all be summarized by saying that parasympathetic stimulation decreases all activities of the heart. Usually the heart is stimulated by the parasympathetics during periods of rest; this allows the heart to rest at the same time the remainder of the body is resting and probably accounts for preservation of the resources of the heart.

Stimulation of the sympathetics has essentially the opposite effects on the heart:

1. Increased heart rate
2. Increased speed of impulse conduction through the heart
3. Increased vigor of cardiac contraction
4. Increased blood flow through the coronary arteries

These activities can be summarized by saying that sympathetic stimulation increases the activity of the heart as a pump, or increases the cardiac output. This effect is necessary when a person is subjected to stressful conditions such as exercise, disease, excessive heat, and other conditions that demand rapid flow through the circulatory system.

The postganglionic neurons of the sympathetic nervous system secrete epinephrine and norepinephrine, or adrenaline and noradrenaline. Therefore, these postganglionic neurons of the sympathetic system are said to be *adrenergic*.

It is thought that the effects of the sympathetic nervous system are mediated by receptors located throughout the body called adrenergic receptors. Adrenergic receptors are arbitrarily classified as alpha and beta on the basis of their characteristic responses. Adrenergic receptors in the *heart* are mainly of the *beta* category with stimulating effects on heart rate (positive chronotropic effect) and stimulating effects for muscular contraction or myocardial tone (positive inotropic effect).

Norepinephrine from sympathetic nerve endings and circulatory epinephrine from the adrenal glands stimulate beta adrenergic receptors in the heart. Certain agents can block this adrenergic or sympathetic action in the heart and are called, therefore, beta adrenergic blocking agents. (Only one, propranolol, is presently available for clinical use.) A beta adrenergic blocking agent would be expected, then, to have the opposite effect from a beta adrenergic stimulator, i.e., reduced heart rate (negative chronotropic effect) and reduced muscle contraction (negative inotropic effect). (See Chapter 59 for discussion of alpha and beta adrenergic stimulators and alpha adrenergic blockers.)

## The Valsalva Maneuver

This maneuver is accomplished with a forced expiration against a closed glottis. This can occur, for example, while straining to defecate or void, to lift oneself up in bed, or during gagging, vomiting, or severe coughing. During the Valsalva maneuver, intrathoracic pressure is increased and blood is trapped in the great veins preventing it from entering the chest and right atrium. The heart actually gets smaller in size and, after an initial decrease in heart rate due to vagal stimulation, the rate accelerates. When the breath is released, blood gushes into the heart and rapidly distends it. This "overshoot" results in tachycardia and increased blood pressure which stimulates pressor receptors in the carotid sinus and aorta. A reflex bradycardia then ensues which can prove fatal for the patient with a damaged heart. Although one might expect cardiac slowing during the maneuver due to powerful vagal reflexes, this is balanced by the "need" for a tachycardia in an attempt to compensate for the decreased venous return and decreased cardiac output and outweighs the influence of pulmonary vagal reflexes. Upon release, the pressure overshoot is associated with a bradycardia (Table 61-1).

## CARDIAC RHYTHMICITY AND ITS REGULATION

In order to pump blood, the heart must alternately relax and contract, allowing blood to enter its chambers during the relaxation phase and forcing it out during the contraction phase. The alternate contraction and relaxation is provided by an inherent rhythmicity of the cardiac muscle itself.

In the posterior wall of the right atrium immedi-

**Table 61-1. The Valsalva Maneuver Divided into Four Phases**

| | PHASE I (IMMEDIATELY AFTER INITIATION OF STRAINING—FIRST FEW BEATS [CONTROL]) | PHASE II (SHORTLY AFTER ONSET OF SUSTAINED STRAINING—THE PERIOD OF STRAIN) | PHASE III (IMMEDIATELY AFTER RELEASE) | PHASE IV (PERIOD OF OVERSHOOT) AND RESTITUTION TO CONTROL |
|---|---|---|---|---|
| Mean arterial blood pressure | Increased | Rapid decrease | No immediate change | Sharp increase |
| Stroke volume | No change | Rapid decrease (56%) | No immediate change | Sharp increase 6–15 beats after release |
| Pulse rate | Slight increase | Marked increase (tachycardia) | Increased | Marked decrease (bradycardia) |

ately beneath the point of entry of the superior vena cava is a small area known as the sino-atrial (S-A) node. This node has a rhythmic rate of contraction of muscle fibers at about 72 beats per minute. As one considers the muscle mass of the heart from atria to ventricles, one finds that the tissue retains its capacity to contract rhythmically, but the lower down the pacemaker site, the slower the inherent rate of the pacemaking tissue. An A-V node pacemaker functions at a rate of 40 to 60 times per minute, while a ventricular pacemaker functions around 20 to 40 times per minute. Because the sinus node has a faster inherent rate than the other portions of the heart, impulses originating in the S-A node spread into the atria and ventricles, stimulating these areas so rapidly that they cannot slow down to their natural rates of rhythm. As a result, in health the rhythm of the S-A node is called the pacemaker of the heart.

Cardiac muscle fibers are joined together in a kind of lattice-work formation. An electrical impulse arising in any single fiber eventually spreads over the membranes of all of the fibers. The normal muscle cell has more negative than positive ions inside the cell membrane and the electrical cardiac impulse is caused by sudden transfer of some of these ions through the membrane so that more positive than negative ions then appear on the inside. This process is called *depolarization*. Once depolarization has occurred, another normal cardiac impulse cannot be carried until the ions realign themselves to their original condition. This is called *repolarization*.

The metabolic systems of the cell can retransfer the ions through the membrane, but the time required for this is about 0.3 second. Therefore, a second impulse cannot be conducted during this period of time and the cell is said to be *refractory*.

Depolarization and repolarization produce an electrical field. Because of the ease with which body tissues conduct current, this electrical potential can be detected by electrodes placed on the external surface of the body and recorded by a machine known as the electrocardiograph.

Even though cardiac impulses can travel very well along cardiac muscle fibers, a special conduction route known as the *Purkinje* system exists in the ventricles to speed up the velocity of conduction. The Purkinje fibers transmit impulses about two to four times as rapidly as normal heart muscle. The purpose of the Purkinje system is to trans-

mit the cardiac impulses throughout the ventricles as rapidly as possible causing all portions to contract in proper sequence to exert a coordinated pumping effort.

Sequentially, the cardiac impulse originates in the S-A node and travels through the atria causing them to contract. A few hundredths of a second after leaving the S-A node the impulse reaches the A-V node where it is delayed a few hundredths of a second while the ventricles fill with blood. The Purkinje system fibers begin in the A-V node, extend through the bundle of His into the ventricular septum, where they divide into two major bundles, one spreading along the wall of the right ventricle and the other along the wall of the left ventricle. After the delay at the A-V node, the cardiac impulse spreads rapidly through the Purkinje system, thence to the ventricular musculature, causing both ventricles to contract in full force within the next few hundredths of a second.

The normal heart rhythm can be disturbed in a variety of ways. Some of these are the result of disease. Others are harmless adaptations in normal function. When arrhythmias occur in the absence of heart disease and are noted by the physician in the course of his examination, he may or may not mention them to the patient.

Each of us has had the sensation of a pounding heart, perhaps in a moment of fright when we are dodging an oncoming car. Most of the time we are not aware that our hearts are beating. Without our conscious awareness, the heart adjusts its work to the changing needs of the body. It can increase the amount of blood that it pumps in two ways: by beating more rapidly and by increasing the volume of blood pumped with each beat. Sudden fright often causes the heart to beat faster and more forcefully, and we become aware of our heartbeat.

These adjustments in heart action are beyond our conscious control. The stimulation of the sympathetic nervous system quickens the heart; the stimulation of the parasympathetic (vagus) system slows it. Both systems constantly affect the heart. In fright usually the stimulation of the sympathetic system causes a temporarily greater effect and, consequently, a faster and a fuller heartbeat.

In some very frightened or shocked people, however, vagal reflexes predominate and heart rate slows, cardiac output falls, and the person becomes weak or faint (vasovagal syncope). The patient should be assisted to a supine position to encourage cerebral blood flow until equilibrium is restored. Atropine sulfate may be ordered by the physician.

## CARDIAC ARRHYTHMIAS

In disease, the pacemaker of the heart can be too fast or too slow. The myocardial cells can become overly excitable or develop a shortened refractory period, or have a damaged Purkinje system or develop blocks in the conduction system. The cardiac arrhythmias that result can be major, that is, imminently life threatening, or they can be relatively minor. Because of their irregularity, all cardiac arrhythmias affect the rhythmic pumping action of the heart to some degree.

Many ambulatory patients receive treatment for cardiac arrhythmias and are able to live essentially normal lives. When their cardiac reserve, however, becomes overtaxed by coexisting illness, they become subject to more dangerous arrhythmias or more serious consequences of their underlying hemodynamic disturbance.

In recent years it has become evident that "sudden" cardiac arrest is really not so sudden, but is very often heralded by less dangerous warning arrhythmias. In the critically ill patient or the patient with heart disease, even "minor" arrhythmic changes can compromise cardiac function by causing a fall in cardiac output, thereby reducing coronary artery blood flow. Arrhythmias also increase myocardial oxygen need, lead to more dangerous arrhythmic complications, and make treatment of the patient's underlying disease more difficult and complex.

Many clinical states predispose to cardiac arrhythmias. Myocardial ischemia following infarction, disturbances in pH, inadequate ventilation, electrolyte imbalance, anxiety or pain—all can disturb heart rate, rhythm, or conduction.

In order to detect arrhythmic changes promptly so that treatment can be started or the underlying cause corrected, hospitalized cardiac patients or seriously ill patients receive continuous monitoring of their cardiac condition.

Because the nurse is available to the patient at all times, her technical role has expanded in recent years to encompass arrhythmia electrocardiography.

A cardiac monitor attached to a patient is useless unless accurate observations are made, interpreted correctly, and acted on appropriately. For example, the nurse may administer a p.r.n. medica-tion, notify the physician, or institute emergency measures required in the interim until the physician arrives.

The development of nursing skill in arrhythmia detection takes considerable study, supervised practice, and time. Only one lead of the ECG is generally necessary to accomplish nursing goals in arrhythmia analysis. The cardiologist reviews the entire 12-lead ECG and in addition to arrhythmia interpretation makes other cardiac diagnoses such as heart enlargement, electrolyte disturbance, ischemic tissue damage, necrosis, or intraventricular conduction delay on the basis of such data as the voltage, QRS interval, T wave changes, S-T segment changes, Q-T interval, and the presence of Q waves or U waves.

### Cardiac Monitor: Nursing Assessment Tool

The bedside cardiac monitor and a console at the nurses' station or a remote control monitoring system using radiotelemetry minimally provide for a continuous display on an oscilloscope of one lead of the patient's ECG. Additional channels may be available for monitoring other physiologic parameters. The efficiency of ECG monitoring depends to a great extent on electrode application. There are many models of cardiac monitors which vary according to the manufacturer, and many varieties of paste-on, superficial skin electrodes. As with all equipment, the manufacturer's manual should be studied and the recommendations utilized. Before electrode application, the chest area is shaved, if necessary, and the skin area cleansed with an antiseptic. Electrode sites are checked daily for inflammation.

The placement sites of electrodes are chosen so that the best cardiographic tracing appears on the oscilloscope (upright P waves and well-defined QRS).

A positive, negative, and ground electrode are required. For most patients, modifications of leads I or II are satisfactory, but the electrical axis of the patient's heart may make another lead necessary. For lead I, the negative electrode is placed beneath the right clavicle and the positive electrode beneath the left clavicle. For lead II, the negative electrode is beneath the right clavicle and the positive electrode on the left upper thigh (left leg). The ground electrode may be placed on the right side of the chest. Care should be taken that electrodes and nonallergenic adhesive tape are so

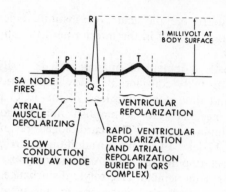

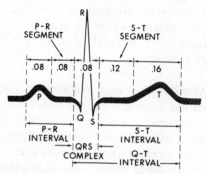

**Figure 61-1.** Basic electrocardiographic trace. (Hewlett-Packard Co., Medical Electronic Division, Palo Alto, Calif.)

placed that they do not interfere with the taking of the chest leads of the 12-lead ECG or the placement of paddles for defibrillation.

Marriott and Fogg (1970) recommend the $MCL_1$ hookup in which the positive electrode is placed in the $V_1$ position (fourth right interspace at the right sternal border), the negative electrode near the left shoulder (just under the outer fourth of the left clavicle), and the ground electrode near the right shoulder. This allows better distinction between left and right ventricular premature beats, bundle branch block and left ventricular ectopic beats, and right bundle branch block-type aberration. Placing electrodes in the $MCL_1$ position also leaves the chest clearer for physical examination and for placement of paddles for emergency cardioversion. However, many cardiac monitors, especially older models, are designed to count and respond to upright complexes, and since the electrocardiographic pattern from $MCL_1$ is essentially inverted, it may not be useful.

Generally, a high rate and low rate indicator is set on the cardiac monitor for each patient. Should the patient's pulse rate fall below or exceed these limits on a beat-to-beat basis, an audiovisual alarm system is activated. On some machines, a writeout may be concurrent with that appearing on the oscilloscope or may be written out from a solid state memory device employing mini-computers with a ten-second or longer delay. Hence, the cardiac rhythm immediately before the alarm situation can be identified. After the alarm, the nurse examines the cardiac tracing and observes the patient. Loosening of an electrode or excessive muscular activity can result in false alarms and an irregular monitor pattern. This fact should be explained to the patient so that he does not think that every alarm from his own monitoring system or those of other patients is due to an irregular heart rhythm.

If an arrhythmia is the source of the alarm, the nurse makes a decision regarding nursing intervention.

The alarm system should be ready for use at all times unless the nurse is directly with the patient doing something such as changing an electrode which would trigger the alarm. The cable that connects the electrodes to the cardiac monitor should be so secured that the patient has sufficient slack when he is moved or turns himself.

### Patient and Family Education

The patient and family need to know that a cardiac monitor is neither a dangerous nor a miraculous machine. It simply enables the patient's cardiac conduction to be displayed continuously. After an initial explanation, the nurse should attempt to get some feedback from the patient regarding its purpose, limitations, and so on. Needless apprehension can be built up if the patient fantasizes about this piece of machinery that blinks, beeps, and causes people to jump and take note when an alarm goes off. False alarms frighten patients. Every effort should be made to see that electrode placement and monitor connections are secure.

### Nursing Assessment and Intervention

Cardiac monitors are considered as aids to and not substitutes for nursing care and human contact with the patient. When going into the patient's room, the patient should be greeted and observed first; then his cardiac monitor pattern should be checked.

The patient with a disturbing arrhythmia needs the care of a staff who can recognize and assess early changes, who can intervene appropriately including obtaining medical help when indicated, who can accurately observe the patient's response to treatment, and who can appropriately manage their own anxiety, which is certain to increase in the presence of life-threatening arrhythmias. A skilled nurse recognizes that her own anxiety can compound the patient's if it is sensed by him. Staying with the patient between the necessary technical duties involved in treatment conveys to the patient that the nurse is not afraid of him or his arrhythmia, but is capable of carrying out necessary emergency treatment should the need arise. This kind of nursing behavior, however, takes a great deal of skill which the nurse needs support to develop. Opportunity for the nursing staff to learn about and discuss their own reactions and ways of helping themselves, and in turn, patients, under appropriate professional guidance, will ultimately improve the quality of care.

Though an arrhythmia can be diagnosed from an electrocardiogram rhythm strip, the effect of the arrhythmia on the patient's cardiac output is the crucial factor. A person with a normal heart who develops a sinus tachycardia (rate over 100) after running up a flight of stairs is showing a normal physiologic response. The patient with an acute myocardial infarction, however, who has a continued sinus tachycardia on bed rest, can add an intolerable workload to his already damaged heart. Observation of the cardiac monitor rhythm must be accompanied by observation of the patient. The advantage of continuous cardiac monitoring of the hospitalized patient is that changes in rhythm or rate can be detected early, reported to the physician, and treated promptly, before the clinical condition of the patient deteriorates.

Because of subjective feelings such as palpitations, "jolting" sensations in the chest, or a fluttering feeling, patients are often aware of their arrhythmias. Momentary dizziness or "stoppage of the heart" can be terrifying. These abnormal sensations increase anxiety. Studies have shown that anxiety and other emotional states, in turn, contribute to the onset, severity, persistence, and recur-

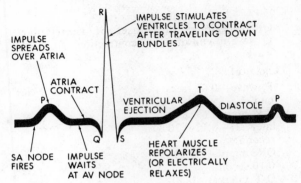

**Figure 61-2.** Electrical and mechanical events of basic ECG tracing. (Hewlett-Packard Co., Medical Electronic Division, Palo Alto, Calif.)

rence of cardiac arrhythmias (Wolf, 1969). When the patient is on a cardiac monitor and can observe the staff's anxiety over changes in his rhythm, he is apt to become more anxious.

## Basic Arrhythmia Electrocardiography*

Electrocardiographic display of a cardiac cycle (lead II) is shown in Figure 61-1 on page 1080. Figure 61-2 shows a correlation between electrical and mechanical events in a cardiac cycle.

| ELECTRICAL EVENTS | MECHANICAL EVENTS (follow electrical events) (Fig. 61-2) |
|---|---|
| P wave—Atrial depolarization | |
| INTERVALS | |
| P-R—Beginning of P wave to beginning of QRS complex | Atrial contraction |
| S-T—End of S wave to end of T wave | Period of maximal ventricular ejection |
| Q-T—Beginning of Q wave to end of T wave | Period from beginning to end of ventricular contraction |
| SEGMENTS | |
| P-R—End of P wave to beginning of Q wave | Delay of impulse at A-V node to allow atria to propel blood through valves into ventricles |
| S-T—End of S wave to beginning of T wave | Period of maximal ventricular ejection |

*The arrhythmia ECG tracings which follow are from the Magnetic Tape Recording Library of the Physiological Training Company, San Marino, Calif., reproduced on the Brush Instruments Recorder.

COMPLEX

QRS—Beginning of Q wave to end of S wave — Onset of ventricular contraction

DURATION

P wave—0.08 second

P-R interval (or P-Q interval)—0.12-0.20 second

QRS interval—0.07-0.10 second

Q-T interval—0.30-0.40 second

The electrocardiogram is recorded on calibrated paper. The vertical lines represent time, and each inch of ECG paper represents one second. Each inch is further subdivided into five segments by dark vertical lines. The space between each two dark lines is further subdivided by thin light lines into five smaller intervals, each representing 0.04 second.

The horizontal lines in the ECG are arranged so that ten small blocks (1 cm.) in the upright direction represent one millivolt.

One way to determine the rate of the heart from the electrocardiogram is to divide the number of seconds between two successive QRS complexes into 60 (60 seconds in one minute). For example, if there are 20 small blocks, or 0.8 second (20 × 0.04) between complexes, the heart rate would be 60 divided by 0.8, or 75 beats per minute.

A systematic approach to assessment of the patient with an arrhythmia includes knowing certain norms, gathering data and comparing this data with a set of facts characteristic of certain arrhythmias, then gathering data regarding the clinical state of the patient. For example, change in cardiac output can be reflected in blood pressure, pulse volume, skin color and degree of moisture, appearance and orientation of the patient, urinary output, chest pain, and dyspnea.

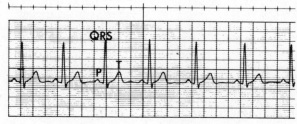

**Figure 61-3.** Normal sinus rhythm.

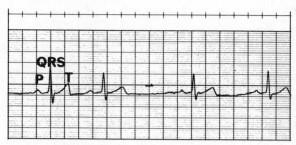

**Figure 61-4.** Sinus arrhythmia.

When the cardiac monitor pattern or rhythm strip is observed, the following steps are recommended:

- **Make an overall inspection of the strip. What are the gross abnormalities?**
- **Measure the atrial rate (P waves).**
- **Measure the ventricular rate (QRS complexes).**
- **Is the P-P interval the same as the R-R interval?**
- **Measure the P-R interval in several complexes.**
- **Measure the QRS width.**
- **Observe the configuration of the P wave and QRS.**
- **Observe the relationship of the P wave to the QRS. Does the P wave consistently precede the QRS? Does it follow the QRS? Are there more or less P waves than QRS's?**
- **Observe the S-T segment. Though the novice nurse does not routinely interpret the S-T segment, gross inspection of the strip can reveal changes in the S-T segment which can be referred to the physician for his interpretation. An example of this would be change in S-T segment occurring when the patient experiences chest pain or increases his activity.**
- **What does the dominant rhythm seem to be?**
- **What arrhythmias or irregularities are present?**
- **What is the clinical status of the patient?**
- **What kinds of therapy might the physician order?**
- **What would be the nursing intervention?**

**Normal sinus rhythm (NSR)** or regular sinus rhythm (RSR). The S-A node is the pacemaker and impulses are conducted normally through the conduction system (Fig. 61-3).

*Rate:* 60 to 100

*P waves:* Each has the same configuration and precedes the QRS.

*P-R interval:* 0.12 to 0.20 second

*QRS:* 0.07 to 0.10 second

*Significance:* Normal

*Treatment:* None

Atrial Arrhythmias

**Sinus Arrhythmia.** Strictly speaking this condition is not an "arrhythmia," but a normal variation. It is characterized by a slight change in rate usually occurring at regular intervals. The S-A node is the pacemaker and conduction through the ventricles is normal. To be classified as sinus arrhythmia, the longest and shortest R-R interval variation is 0.12 second or more (Fig. 61-4). It is common in young and old people and usually is related to respiration. On inspiration the heart rate speeds up due to stretching of the pleura which activates the Hering-Breuer reflex to cause vagal inhibition and an increase in rate. On expiration, there is vagal stimulation and cardiac slowing.

*Rate:* 60 to 100 but varies with inspiration and expiration
*Rhythm:* Irregular
*P waves:* Normal and precede each QRS
*P-R interval:* Normal
*QRS:* Normal
*Significance:* None
*Treatment:* None

**Sinus Bradycardia.** The pacemaker site is the S-A node but the rate is below 60 (Fig. 61-5). The rhythm is regular. The heart can be slow, normally in athletes and laborers who have normally enlarged hearts from regular strenuous exercise and greater than normal stroke volume. Emotional states, such as fear or shock, can result in increased vagal tone and slowing of the heart which can result in syncope. Bradycardia is sometimes seen in patients with increased intracranial pressure, hypothyroidism, or digitalis toxicity. Carotid sinus pressure, the Valsalva maneuver, and eyeball pressure result in vagal stimulation and slowing of the heart. Bradycardia can occur during anesthesia or following administration of morphine.

In acute myocardial infarction, sinus bradycardia is often an ominous sign of reflex vagal mechanisms. The slow rate may not be sufficient to maintain cardiac output in an already damaged heart. In addition, escape ectopic beats or rhythms such as idioventricular rhythm may take over as the primary pacemaker if their inherent rate is faster. This can increase ventricular irritability which is dangerous in myocardial infarction.

*Rate:* Below 60; a relative bradycardia may exist at a faster rate if it is insufficient to maintain cardiac output.
*Rhythm:* Regular
*P waves:* Normal and precede each QRS
*P-R interval:* Normal
*QRS:* Normal

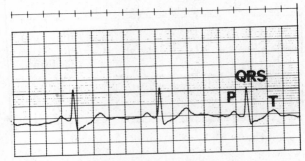

**Figure 61-5.** Sinus bradycardia.

*Significance:* Since cardiac output equals stroke volume times heart rate (c.o. = s.v. × h.r.), slow rate may not be sufficient for adequate cardiac output.
*Treatment:* Atropine sulfate 0.4 mg. IV may be ordered to override the vagal stimulus and increase sinus heart rate, thereby suppressing post-bradycardia idioventricular beats. Isoproterenol (Isuprel) may be ordered to increase the heart rate by stimulation of the S-A node. An artificial pacemaker may be inserted to keep the heart beating at a minimum rate to maintain cardiac output.

**Sinus Tachycardia.** Impulses are initiated by the S-A node and the rate is regular, but above 100 beats per minute (Fig. 61-6). Sinus tachycardia occurs in persons with normal hearts as a physiologic response to strenuous exercise or strong emotion. It can also occur with pain, fever, hyperthyroidism, hemorrhage, shock, or anemia. Cardiac output, coronary blood flow, and blood pressure can increase up to the rate of about 150 beats per minute. After that cardiac decompensation can occur. A decrease in vagal tone or an increase in sympathetic tone or both can result in sinus tachycardia. Tachycardia can be the initial evidence of heart failure.

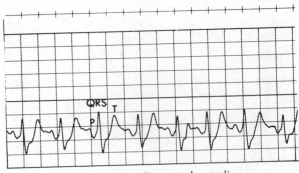

**Figure 61-6.** Sinus tachycardia.

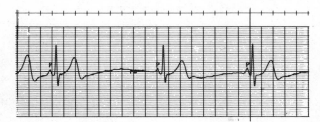

**Figure 61-7.** Sinus arrest (sinus pause).

*Rate:* 100 to 160
*Rhythm:* Regular
*P waves:* Normal, but may be obscured in T wave of previous cycle if rate is very fast
*P-R interval:* Normal
*QRS:* Normal
*Significance:* Can increase the work of the heart to the point of decompensation
*Treatment:* The underlying disease or the cause of the tachycardia must be treated. For example anxiety is alleviated, fever is reduced, oxygen is given for hypoxia, or digitalis may be ordered for congestive heart failure. The patient is kept to minimum activity until rate decreases to compensated level.

In persons with myocardial infarction or coronary artery disease, coronary insufficiency with chest pain can develop because coronary blood flow cannot keep up with the increased need of the myocardium imposed by the fast rate. With fast rates, diastole is shortened and the heart does not have sufficient time to fill. Congestive heart failure, chest pain or other symptoms of reduced cardiac output can occur.

**Sinus Arrest (Sinus Pause).** The S-A node fails to fire an impulse and there is a prolonged pause between two normal complexes (Fig. 61-7). Increased vagal tone, direct stimulation of the vagal center in the medulla, or reflex vagal stimulation such as occurs with gagging, ocular pressure, or carotid sinus pressure can result in sinus arrest. In

persons with normal hearts it is significant only if symptoms such as lightheadedness or faintness occur.

In persons with myocardial infarction or other heart disease, sinus arrest can indicate disease of the S-A node which encourages a lower foci to become the primary pacemaker. The condition can progress to complete atrial standstill. The physician is consulted before giving additional digitalis since sinus arrest can indicate digitalis toxicity.

*Rate:* Normal (basic rate)
*Rhythm:* Irregular
*P waves:* Normal when present
*P-R interval:* Normal
*QRS:* Normal
*Significance:* Can lead to more serious arrhythmias
*Treatment:* Withhold digitalis; atropine, isoproterenol (Isuprel) or a pacemaker

**Atrial Premature Beats (APB's).** An ectopic focus in the atria becomes more irritable than the S-A node and depolarizes the atria before the next normal P wave is due. The next sinus beat after the ectopic beat frequently occurs somewhat later than usual and the interval between the ectopic P wave and the next normal P wave is longer than the normal P-P interval. This is termed resetting of the S-A node, but the duration of the cycle preceding and the pause is less than two normal sinus cycles (not fully compensatory). The patient may complain of an "extra beat."

*Rate:* Within normal limits
*Rhythm:* Irregular
*P waves:* The premature beat has a different P wave configuration; if the rate is fast, the P wave may be obscured in the previous T wave.
*P-R interval:* Normal
*QRS:* Normal
*Significance:* Frequent APB's indicate atrial irritability; in the person with heart disease, they can be the forerunners of more serious atrial arrhythmias. In persons with normal hearts, they can result from nervous tension, ingestion of stimulants such as coffee, excessive use of tobacco, or infections.
*Treatment:* Depends on cause. In patients with heart disease, more than six APB's per minute are reported to the physician who may order an antiarrhythmic drug, such as procainamide, or sedation.

**Wandering Atrial Pacemaker (WAP).** The pacemaker site shifts within the S-A node, the atria, or close to the A-V node. This is a relatively innocuous rhythm but may be an early warning of a more serious atrial arrhythmia (Fig. 61-8). (A much

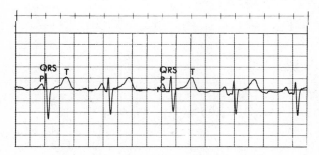

**Figure 61-8.** Wandering atrial pacemaker.

more serious kind of wandering pacemaker occurs when the pacemaker site "wanders" to different locations in atria, A-V node, or ventricles.)

*Rate:* Normal
*Rhythm:* May be slightly irregular
*P waves:* Vary in configuration indicating shifting pacemaker site
*P-R interval:* Varies in length; if pacemaker shifts close to A-V node, may be less than 0.10 second
*QRS:* Normal
*Significance:* May be early warning of more serious atrial arrhythmia
*Treatment:* None; observe for digitalis toxicity

**Paroxysmal Atrial Tachycardia (PAT).** An ectopic focus in the atria fires at a rate of 160 to 240 beats per minute (Fig. 61-9). The onset and cessation are usually abrupt, as the term paroxysmal indicates. The tachycardia can result in decreased cardiac output. Emotional stress, fatigue, toxic states, pregnancy, and thyrotoxicosis can precipitate attacks. In patients taking digitalis, PAT (especially with block) is considered highly suspicious of digitalis toxicity. PAT is also associated with rheumatic, arteriosclerotic, or hypertensive heart disease and acute myocardial infarction. Atrial tachycardia can be considered to be a burst of six or more APB's, equally spaced.

The ventricles generally respond to each atrial stimulus but occasionally, because of fatigue or ischemia of the A-V node or ventricles, some of the impulses from the atria can be blocked. The ventricles respond either regularly to every second, third, or fourth impulse (PAT with 2:1, 3:1, or 4:1 block) or they can respond in an irregular, random fashion. The patient may be anxious and agitated.

*Rate:* 160 to 240 (atrial); ventricular rate depends upon degree of A-V block.
*Rhythm:* Regular or varying with block
*P waves:* Usually have the same configuration preceding each QRS, but, due to fast rate, may be obscured. If P waves are not identifiable, rhythm may be termed *supraventricular tachycardia.*
*P-R interval:* May vary
*QRS:* Normal
*Significance:* Patients with normal hearts may tolerate rates around 180 with no evidence of circulatory insufficiency at rest. In diseased hearts, ventricular diastolic filling time is short and cardiac output falls. Angina pectoris due to diminished coronary blood flow, hypotension and shock, or acute congestive failure can develop.
*Treatment:* Digitalis is withheld. The physician is notified and may stimulate the vagus to slow the

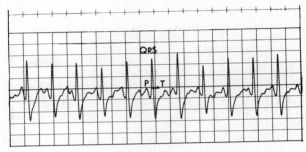

**Figure 61-9.** Atrial tachycardia.

heart by performing carotid sinus massage, having the patient gag or perform the Valsalva maneuver, or by giving edrophonium chloride (Tensilon). Other treatment includes use of a vasopressor such as metaraminol (Aramine) to elevate the blood pressure and stimulate the vagus reflexly followed once again by carotid sinus pressure or the Valsalva maneuver, sedation, digitalis, antiarrhythmics such as quinidine or procainamide, and withdrawal of irritants or intoxicants. In patients with myocardial infarction or other serious heart disease, electric cardioversion may be used if there are signs of congestive heart failure or shock.

**Atrial Flutter.** An ectopic focus in the atria discharges very rapidly, 240 to 360 times a minute (Fig. 61-10). The ventricle does not generally respond to each atrial stimulus. There may be a 2:1, 3:1, 4:1, or varying A-V block. This arrhythmia is associated with heart disease or digitalis intoxication. The clinical condition of the patient depends on the rate of ventricular response.

*Rate:* 240 to 360 (atrial). Ventricular rate varies according to degree of A-V block.
*Rhythm:* Regular if degree of A-V block is regular, irregular if block is varying
*P waves:* Have a regular "saw-tooth" appearance. These are called flutter waves.
*P-R interval:* May vary if A-V node becomes fatigued
*QRS:* Normal
*Significance:* A rapid ventricular response can lead to decreased cardiac output.

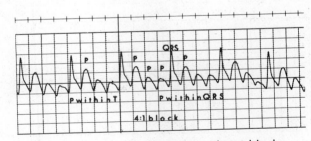

**Figure 61-10.** Atrial flutter with 4:1 block.

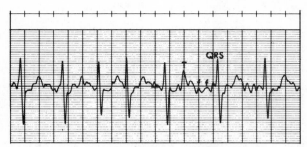

**Figure 61-11.** Atrial fibrillation.

*Treatment:* Digitalis is withheld if patient has been receiving this. Electric cardioversion is preferred by many physicians, especially if the patient's condition is deteriorating, because of the ease of treatment and the time factor involved in drug therapy. For slower treatment, digitalis is given to increase the block at the A-V node and thus prevent a rapid ventricular rate; then quinidine or procainamide may be given to convert the atrial arrhythmia.

**Atrial Fibrillation.** There is totally disorganized rapid atrial activity and the atria quiver rather than contract normally (Fig. 61-11). The ventricles respond to the atrial stimulus in an irregular fashion depending upon the sensitivity of the A-V node and the conduction system. Some of the ventricular beats are so weak that they are ineffective in opening the aortic valve and propelling blood, and a pulse deficit exists. An apical-radial pulse should be taken.

*Rate:* 350 to 800 (atrial). Ventricular rate varies but is irregular unless there is also a complete block at the A-V node in which case no atrial impulses are conducted and the lower pacemaker site produces a regular rhythm. In atrial fibrillation which is considered "controlled" either physiologically or by drugs, the ventricular rate is between 60 to 75 per minute. In uncontrolled atrial fibrillation, the ventricular rate is much faster.
*Rhythm:* Irregular

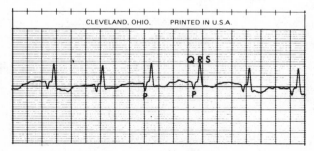

**Figure 61-12.** Junctional (A-V nodal) rhythm.

*P waves:* There are no P waves; there is an irregular rapid undulation of the baseline of the ECG; the atrial twichings are called f waves.
*P-R interval:* Since there are no P waves, the P-R interval is not measurable.
*QRS:* Normal
*Significance:* Loss of atrial contraction diminishes cardiac output by about 15 per cent. Irregular ventricular filling and rhythm diminish the pumping efficiency. Decrease in cardiac output can result in congestive heart failure.
*Treatment:* Digitalis may be given to slow the ventricular rate by its action on the A-V node; then, quinidine to convert the atria to normal rhythm. If the patient's condition is potentially deteriorating, electric cardioversion is used.

**Atrial Standstill.** When the S-A node fails to initiate an impulse (sinus arrest) or when the impulse from the S-A node is not conducted to the atria (sino-atrial block) for one or more cycles, the absence of atrial contraction is termed atrial standstill. Escape nodal or ventricular complexes initiated from a pacemaker site below the atria can continue in a regular manner.

*Rate:* Depends on pacemaker site
*Rhythm:* Regular
*P waves:* Absent
*P-R interval:* Absent
*QRS:* Normal in width if pacemaker site is in A-V node; 0.12 second or greater if pacemaker site is in ventricle
*Significance:* May be an early indication of ventricular standstill
*Treatment:* Digitalis and myocardial depressants are withheld. Artificial pacemaker may be indicated.

Junctional (A-V Nodal) Arrhythmias

**Premature Junctional (A-V Nodal) Beats (PNB's).** There is irritability in the area of the A-V node and an ectopic stimulus causes depolarization before the onset of the next impulse from the S-A node. There may or may not be a compensatory pause.

*Rate:* Normal
*Rhythm:* Irregular
*P waves:* Depend on pacemaker site of premature beat as in A-V nodal rhythm
*P-R interval:* Shortened
*QRS:* Normal
*Significance:* More than six PNB's per minute in patient with heart disease may indicate increasing myocardial irritability.
*Treatment:* Physician may order antiarrhythmic drug

**Junctional (A-V Nodal) Rhythm.** With this rhythm the predominant pacemaker of the heart is in the region of the A-V node. The intrinsic rate for the pacemaker here is 40 to 60 beats per minute (Fig. 61-12). The impulse spreads both downward to the ventricles and upward (retrograde) to the atria.

*Rate:* 40 to 60
*Rhythm:* Regular
*P waves:* Location and configuration of P waves depends on speed of conduction through junctional (A-V nodal) tissue. In lead II the normal upright wave may precede the QRS but may be inverted, may be obscured in the QRS, or may follow the QRS.
*P-R interval:* Shortened but length depends on site of pacemaker
*QRS:* Normal
*Significance:* The S-A node is depressed due to disease, excessive vagal activity, or drugs. The slow rate may be insufficient to maintain adequate cardiac output.
*Treatment:* Digitalis is withheld. Atropine sulfate may be given. An artificial pacemaker may be used.

**Junctional (A-V Nodal) Tachycardia.** Pacemaker site is in the region of the A-V node which is more irritable than the S-A node. Some would classify a rate above the upper limit of intrinsic rate (60 per minute) as a tachycardia. Other classifications are a rate of 140 to 160 per minute, or a rate above 100.

*Rate:* Rapid
*Rhythm:* Regular
*P waves:* As in A-V nodal rhythm
*P-R interval:* Shortened
*QRS:* Normal
*Significance:* See PAT
*Treatment:* Same as for PAT

**First Degree Heart Block.** Conduction of the sino-atrial impulse through the A-V node is delayed (Fig. 61-13). This may be caused by heart disease, edema around the A-V node, ischemia or direct damage, or digitalis. Antiarrhythmic drugs can overdepress the A-V node as can reflex vagal stimulation.

*Rate:* Normal
*Rhythm:* Normal
*P waves:* Normal
*P-R interval:* Prolonged beyond the upper normal limit of 0.20 second
*QRS:* Normal
*Significance:* May progress to higher degree of block
*Treatment:* Careful observation; digitalis or myocardial depressants may be withheld.

**Second Degree Heart Block.** Sino-atrial conduction is normal but one or more impulses are blocked, or kept from getting through the A-V

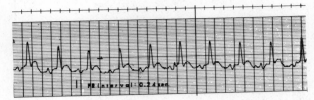

**Figure 61-13.** First degree heart block (baseline artifact).

node to depolarize the ventricle. The causes are the same as in first degree heart block. There are several varieties of second degree block.

WENCKEBACH TYPE (MOBITZ TYPE I). The P-R interval becomes progressively prolonged as the A-V node becomes more fatigued until one QRS complex is dropped. (One impulse is not conducted through to the ventricle.) The dropped beat allows time for recovery and the next P-R interval is usually normal. The P waves occur normally.

*Rate:* Atrial rate is normal. Ventricular rate is less than atrial rate due to occasional dropped beats.
*Rhythm:* Irregular, but the irregularity usually occurs in a regular pattern
*P waves:* Normal
*P-R interval:* Progressive prolongation until a QRS complex is dropped
*QRS:* Normal in configuration
*Significance:* Can progress to complete heart block and cardiac output can be compromised. The irregular ventricular response disturbs hemodynamics. The patient may feel a "thumping" in the chest or head since the ventricle has more time to fill after a dropped beat and thus ejects more blood. The patient may also have the feeling that his heart stops momentarily.
*Treatment:* Digitalis and myocardial depressants may be withheld. Atropine or isoproterenol or a temporary pacemaker may be ordered. Hypoxia is treated by adequate ventilation.

MOBITZ TYPE II. The P-R interval stays constant (though it may be prolonged) but some impulses are not conducted through to the ventricle

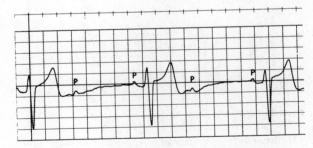

**Figure 61-14.** Second degree heart block (2:1).

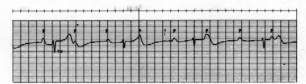

**Figure 61-15.** Complete heart block (third degree A-V block).

(Fig. 61-14). There can be an occasional dropped beat, or a pattern of response such as 2:1, 3:1, or 4:1 atrial-ventricular response.

*Rate:* Atrial rate usually normal. Ventricular rate varies usually in a pattern such as one-half or one-third the atrial rate (2:1, 3:1 A-V block).
*Rhythm:* Usually a regularly irregular pattern
*P waves:* Normal but not always followed by a QRS; there are two, three, or four P waves to each QRS.
*P-R interval:* Constant in conducted beats
*QRS:* Normal
*Significance:* Same as Wenckebach above
*Treatment:* Immediate pacemaker insertion if the patient has an acute myocardial infarction; otherwise same as Wenckebach above

**Complete Heart Block.** The atria and ventricles function without any relationship to each other; therefore P waves have no sequential relationship to QRS's though the rhythm of each is usually regular (Fig. 61-15). The S-A node functions normally; the main pacemaker in the heart is below the block in the A-V node. What might appear to be a P-R interval changes with each complex. However, there is really no P-R interval due to the complete interruption in conduction from atria to ventricles.

*Rate:* Atrial rate is normal; the ventricular rate is 20 to 40 beats per minute or faster.
*Rhythm:* Atrial and ventricular rhythms are regular.
*P waves:* Normal
*P-R interval:* None. Atria and ventricles beat independently.

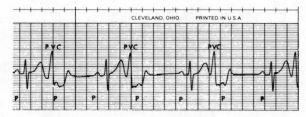

**Figure 61-16.** Ventricular premature beats (ventricular bigeminy).

*QRS:* Configuration is normal if pacemaker site is in A-V node below block, but widened if pacemaker site is in ventricle.
*Significance:* The slow ventricular rate is frequently ineffective in maintaining adequate cardiac output; angina, congestive failure, or Stokes-Adams seizures from cerebral hypoxia can occur; ventricular standstill or ventricular fibrillation may ensue.
*Treatment:* Digitalis is withheld; isoproterenol (Isuprel) may be ordered. Pacemaker is considered essential; adequate ventilation to correct hypoxia and treatment of other associated clinical conditions is needed.

### Ventricular Arrhythmias

**Ventricular Premature Beats (VPB's).** A VPB is a ventricular ectopic beat which occurs before depolarization of the ventricles by an atrial impulse is due (Fig. 61-16). Therefore it is not preceded by an atrial impulse and, since it is not dependent on an impulse from above, it is also called an idioventricular beat.

A VPB is followed usually by a long pause known as a "compensatory pause." This occurs because the normally occurring atrial impulse finds the ventricle refractory when it arrives, because it has not recovered from its depolarization by the VPB. The next normally occurring atrial impulse succeeds in depolarizing the ventricles. If the heart rate is very slow, the ventricles can repolarize after a VPB in sufficient time to receive the atrial stimulus precisely when it is due and there is an extra beat, but the basic rhythm is not interrupted. This is called an *interpolated* VPB.

*Rate:* Normal dominant rhythm
*Rhythm:* Irregular
*P waves:* Normal, but absent in idioventricular complexes
*P-R interval:* Normal if dominant rhythm is normal.
*QRS:* Bizarre in configuration; widened above 0.12 second in idioventricular complexes; T wave following VPB usually is opposite in direction to its QRS.
*Significance:* VPB's are very common; many people experience them at one time or another. They often cause a "flip-flop" sensation in the chest. Some people describe it as a "fluttering of the heart." The symptoms may be associated with pallor, nervousness, sweating, and faintness.

VPB's are usually harmless. Some people have them in response to anxiety and stress, and, as it so often happens, the symptoms then make the patient even more tense and fearful. Also, they may be associated with fatigue or excessive use of alcohol or tobacco.

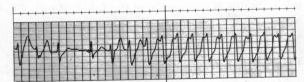

**Figure 61-17.** Ventricular tachycardia.

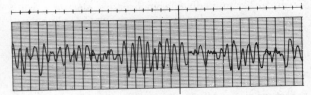

**Figure 61-18.** Ventricular fibrillation.

Although VPB's usually are unassociated with organic heart disease, the patient who is frequently troubled by them should consult his physician. A thorough examination is important in making certain that no organic heart disease exists and in assuring the patient that his heart is normal. Once the patient has received his physician's assurance that nothing is seriously wrong, he will find it easier to ignore the symptoms. This in itself often causes them to occur less frequently and to disappear more quickly.

In the presence of acute heart injury such as after cardiac surgery or in acute myocardial infarction, VPB's that occur in certain patterns are indicative of myocardial irritability and are precursors of lethal arrhythmias. These patterns or types are:

- More than six unifocal VPB's per minute. A run of ventricular bigeminy (a normal beat followed by a VPB) could meet this criteria also
- Runs, bursts, or salvos of VPB's, that is, two or more in a row
- Multifocal VPB's, that is, from more than one location in the ventricle
- A VPB whose R wave falls on the T wave of the preceding complex (Fig. 61-16)

*Treatment:* Digitalis may be withheld; myocardial depressant drugs such as lidocaine or procainamide are begun promptly if the patient has myocardial infarction, to prevent ventricular fibrillation.

**Ventricular Tachycardia.** This is a serious arrhythmia in which the pacemaker lies in an ectopic focus in one of the ventricles (Fig. 61-17). It is often associated with a severely damaged myocardium and if untreated can lead to ventricular fibrillation. Digitalis intoxication can also provoke it. Serious hemodynamic disturbances and vascular collapse can also occur. Coronary circulation is severely disturbed.

*Rate:* Atrial rate is normal. Ventricular rate usually is above the sinus rate, but any rate above the inherent ventricular rate of 40 can be considered tachycardic. Rate of 150 to 200 per minute is not uncommon.
*Rhythm:* Slightly irregular
*P waves:* Normal, but usually are not clearly seen
*P-R interval:* None; there is A-V dissociation

*QRS:* Wide, bizarre
*Significance:* Leads to ventricular fibrillation; cardiac output falls drastically; area of infarction can increase due to severe myocardial ischemia
*Treatment:* Synchronous or asynchronous electric cardioversion (countershock); myocardial depressant drug such as lidocaine. Careful diagnosis is essential. If ventricular tachycardia exists as an escape mechanism following A-V block, the use of myocardial depressants can produce ventricular asystole by suppressing the last remaining pacemaker site in the ventricle.

**Ventricular fibrillation** is rapid, ineffective twitching of the ventricles (Fig. 61-18). Since efficient contractions of the ventricles do not occur, there is a sudden drop in cardiac output, followed by death by cardiac arrest if the condition cannot be alleviated promptly. Ventricular fibrillation may result from myocardial ischemia which may occur in coronary artery disease, myocardial infarction, during the administration of general anesthesia, or from electric shock.

During an attack of ventricular fibrillation, the patient's pulse and blood pressure cannot be obtained, he loses consciousness, and he may have convulsions. Death follows unless the ventricles can be made to contract.

*Rate:* Neither atrial nor ventricular rates are measurable.
*Rhythm:* Totally chaotic
*P waves:* None
*P-R interval:* None
*QRS:* None; a series of irregular deflections occur on the ECG.
*Significance:* Almost always fatal unless aborted within three to four minutes; brain damage can occur earlier depending on patient's cerebral circulation.

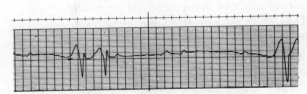

**Figure 61-19.** Ventricular asystole.

*Treatment:* Immediate asynchronous electric cardioversion (defibrillation) or external cardiopulmonary resuscitation if defibrillator is not immediately available

**Ventricular Asystole (Ventricular Standstill).**
There is no effective ventricular contraction and
therefore no cardiac output (Fig. 61-19).

*Rate:* None
*Rhythm:* None
*P waves:* May continue irregularly for short period of
time
*P-R interval:* None
*QRS:* None; usually a straight, isoelectric line appears
on the ECG.
*Significance:* Almost always fatal unless resuscitative
measures are instituted within four minutes
*Treatment:* Immediate precordial blow; cardiopulmo-
nary resuscitation.

### Additional Significant Arrhythmias

**A-V Dissociation.** This means that the atria
and ventricles beat independently of each other,
each under the stimulus of its own pacemaker.

Generally, if the atrial rate is faster than the
ventricular rate, some degree of A-V block is
present. Occasionally in incomplete A-V dissociation with block, an atrial impulse can get through
the A-V node and "capture" the ventricle when it
is refractory to its own pacemaker.

Another type of A-V dissociation occurs in fast
ventricular tachycardia when an irritable focus takes
over as the primary cardiac pacemaker. Since there
is no disease of the A-V node, atrial stimuli at a
slower rate are "interfered with" on their route to
the ventricle because the ventricle is in the refractory period from its own depolarization when atrial
stimuli arrive. This is called "interference dissociation."

In both cases, the approximate 15 per cent contribution of the atria to cardiac output is lost.

**Bundle Branch Block.** Recent studies have
shown the intraventricular conduction network to
be a "trifascicular" system consisting of the right
bundle branch (RBB) and anterior and posterior
divisions of the left bundle branch (LBB). Conduction blocks can occur at single or multiple points.
Thus there is a delay in the usual ventricular depolarization process since the normally fast conduction tissue of the Purkinje system cannot be
completely utilized. This is reflected in a widening
of the QRS (intraventricular conduction delay)
above 0.12 second. The site of the block is deter-

mined by the physician using the full 12-lead ECG
or by vectorcardiogram.

### TREATMENT OF CARDIAC ARRHYTHMIAS

Methods of treatment for cardiac arrhythmias
are aimed at:

1. Cardioversion (reversion) of the disturbed conduction to normal sinus rhythm, if possible
2. Where reversion to sinus rhythm is not possible, to
produce maximum physiologic improvement
3. Reduction of the number or severity of arrhythmic
episodes or prevention of acute life-threatening
attacks

Treatment for cardiac arrhythmias includes
mechanical, chemical (pharmacologic), and electrical modalities. Mechanical means include phy-
sician-administered carotid sinus pressure or directed patient performance of the Valsalva
maneuver, which slow the heart, or external cardiac compression.

### Drug Therapy

Drugs used in the treatment of cardiac arrhythmias include the following classifications:

DRUGS ACTING PRIMARILY ON TISSUES WITHIN
THE HEART
1. Myocardial depressants such as lidocaine
(Xylocaine), procainamide (Pronestyl) quinidine sulfate, propranolol (Inderal), dilantin
sodium, or bretylium tosylate
2. Drugs that increase cardiac rhythmicity and
contraction such as epinephrine or isoproterenol (Isuprel)
3. Drugs which depress conduction but increase
contractile force, such as digitalis preparations.
(Significantly, digitalis toxicity can cause every
arrhythmia it is used to treat!)
DRUGS ACTING ON THE AUTONOMIC NERVOUS
SYSTEM
1. Vagolytic or parasympathetic blocking agents
to increase heart rate, such as atropine sulfate
2. Vagal stimulants or parasympathomimetic
agents which slow the heart such as edrophonium (Tensilon) or neostigmine (Prostigmin)
3. Alpha and beta adrenergic stimulating drugs
such as epinephrine and isoproterenol (Isuprel)
4. Beta adrenergic blocking agents such as
propranolol

Quinidine and procainamide (Pronestyl) are two
drugs that are commonly employed to restore normal heart rhythm. Quinidine decreases the irritability and the contractility of the heart muscle. Also,
it lengthens the time necessary for the conduction

of impulses from the atria to the ventricles, and it lengthens the refractory period of heart muscle (the time between beats when the heart will not respond to another stimulus to contract). Although the mechanism of the action of quinidine in restoring normal heart rhythm is not completely understood, it is believed that these effects of quinidine on the heart are primarily responsible for its usefulness in restoring normal rhythm.

The dosage of quinidine is adjusted according to the patient's response. A usual oral dose would be 0.2 to 0.4 Gm. every four hours. Quinidine also may be given intramuscularly and rarely, intravenously. The effective dose may be a toxic one. The patient should be observed for faintness, fall in blood pressure, rapid weak pulse, nausea, vomiting, diarrhea, ringing in the ears, dizziness, headache, and visual disturbances. Some patients are allergic to quinidine. The patient might receive a small test dose before therapy is begun and be observed for any allergic reactions. Quinidine blood level can be determined in the laboratory.

Procainamide (Pronestyl) decreases the irritability of the heart muscle. It can be given intravenously and intramuscularly, as well as orally. The oral dose varies from 0.5 Gm to 1.0 Gm. every four hours. When a rapid effect is required, 100 to 200 mg. diluted in normal saline may be administered slowly intravenously by the physician while he monitors the patient's electrocardiographic response. Intravenous use may be followed by hypotension. Occasionally, depression of the white blood cells or a syndrome resembling lupus erythematosus results from repeated use of procainamide. When either drug is given intravenously, resuscitation equipment and drugs should be available.

The most frequently used drug for VPB's and ventricular tachycardia after acute myocardial infarction is lidocaine (Xylocaine), a local anesthetic which depresses ventricular irritability when given intravenously. (The exact mechanism of its electrophysiologic effect is not clear.) It is rapidly metabolized in the liver so that action dissipates within 10 to 20 minutes after intravenous injection. It is given by intravenous drip at a maintenance dose of 1 to 4 mg. per minute or by intravenous bolus dose of 1 mg. per Kg. of body weight (usually 50 to 100 mg). An hourly dose of more than 450 mg. is hazardous.

Lidocaine is contraindicated in the presence of A-V block, junctional (A-V nodal) and idioventricular rhythm since the last remaining spontaneous pacemaker can be abolished. Untoward reactions include apprehension, disorientation, euphoria, drowsiness, lightheadedness, numbness, sweating, and convulsions. Hypotension is possible.

When myocardial depressants are given, the ECG should be observed for junctional (A-V nodal) rhythm or intraventricular conduction delay. The P-R interval and QRS duration should be measured and any widening reported.

Whether or not the nurse gives intravenous medication depends on several factors. A major one is the nurse's level of preparation for assuming all the responsibilities involved, her assessment of her clinical competence as well as her limitations (which she must communicate to other members of the health care team), and the opportunity for the nurse to assess the patient's response to the IV drug. Another consideration is the institution's policies collaboratively arrived at by nurses, physicians, and hospital administrators. Influencing policy making are state nursing and medical practice acts, the definition of what constitutes an emergency, as well as opportunities for instruction, guidance, supervision, and continuing education for both nurses and physicians.

Propranolol (Inderal) blocks beta receptor sites in the myocardium from adrenergic (sympathetic) stimulation, thus producing a *decrease* in all of the following: heart rate (negative chronotropic effect), cardiac output, force of cardiac contraction (negative inotropic effect), and myocardial irritability. Since it is highly specific, the cardiac effects of calcium, digitalis, or the xanthines are not abolished when given simultaneously. It has effects on the conduction system similar to that of quinidine. It is used primarily in the treatment of atrial and ventricular tachyarrhythmias.

Propranolol may be given orally (10 to 30 mg. three or four times daily) or intravenously by a physician. The IV dose is 1 to 2 mg. diluted in 50 ml. of fluid infused slowly with constant ECG monitoring. The rate of infusion should not exceed 1 mg. per minute.

Side effects of propranolol can be bradycardia, heart block, sinus arrest, acute congestive heart failure, shock, or asystole. The patient may experience bronchoconstriction, and the drug is therefore potentially hazardous in patients with bronchial asthma or chronic obstructive lung disease. Minor

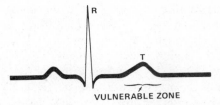

**Figure 61-20.** The vulnerable period of the cardiac cycle. (Hewlett-Packard Co., Medical Electronic Division, Palo Alto, Calif.)

side effects include nausea, diarrhea, mental depression, and fatigue.

## Electrical Therapy

Electrical cardioversion can be accomplished by the use of:

- Synchronized electrical cardioversion
- Unsynchronized electrical cardioversion (defibrillation)
- Artificial electrical pacing

**Synchronized electric cardioversion** is the delivery of a DC current by a machine which is programmed or synchronized so that electrical current is delivered to the heart usually just following the R wave of the QRS. It is necessary for the physician to avoid delivering the current during the so-called vulnerable period of the cardiac cycle, around the summit of the T wave (Fig. 61-20). The

current is delivered through paddles on the chest placed externally in such a way that the current traverses the heart (Fig. 61-21).

A shock delivered during the vulnerable period (the period of repolarization) could result in ventricular fibrillation.

Electric synchronous cardioversion is used to terminate rapid cardiac arrhythmias such as atrial flutter, atrial fibrillation, or ventricular tachycardia, all of which compromise cardiac output to some degree. The electric current completely depolarizes the entire myocardium at one time so that the fastest normal pacemaker can regain control of the pacing function. Electric cardioversion avoids the time element and potential side effects encountered in the use of drug therapy for cardioversion.

In elective electric cardioversion there is time for the physician to explain the procedure to the patient and obtain his consent. Because the patient is generally already anxious as a result of the tachycardia, explanation is limited to what the individual patient is able to comprehend. Where there is sufficient time, the physician may order an antiarrhythmic drug such as quinidine to be given orally several hours or a day prior to cardioversion so that a blood level of the drug will be achieved sufficient to maintain normal rhythm following cardioversion. Digitalis is sometimes withheld for a period prior to cardioversion because some believe that its presence in myocardial cells increases the incidence of ventricular irritability after cardioversion (Fig. 61-22).

The patient is attached to a cardiac monitor which has an attachment for, or an incorporated, cardioverter. An intravenous infusion is started. Generally the patient is given heavy sedation such as with intravenous diazepam (Valium), 2 to 5 mg., or light general anesthesia. Equipment and drugs used in cardiac arrest are immediately available. The cardioverter is activated and the physician selects the point of the cycle where the shock will be delivered. Gel is applied to the paddles, or a moist wet saline pad is placed under each paddle in such a position that there is no contact between paddles and the current will traverse the heart. The physician delivers the shock, usually in the range of 10 to 200 watt seconds. The patient's cardiac rhythm is observed on the monitor and his vital signs are taken. The nurse remains with the patient until he awakens.

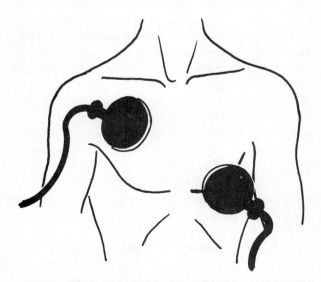

**Figure 61-21.** Position of paddles for synchronous cardioversion or defibrillation. (Hewlett-Packard Co., Medical Electronic Division, Palo Alto, Calif.)

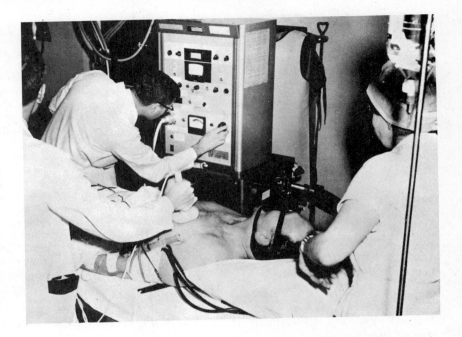

**Figure 61-22.** Electric cardioversion. The machine that the doctor is adjusting monitors heart rhythm; also, it can be used as here to apply an electric shock in an attempt to restore normal rhythm. The shock is applied through the electrode held on the patient's anterior chest by the physician and another electrode positioned against the posterior chest. The anesthetist is prepared to give the patient oxygen. (The Roosevelt Hospital, New York, N.Y.)

In order to avoid personnel injury from electric shock, the team must be alerted to stand away from the bed and to avoid touching any conducting source when the shock is delivered. To avoid fire hazard, the flow of oxygen is stopped while the shock is delivered.

**Defibrillation (Unsynchronized Electric Cardioversion).** The only treatment for ventricular fibrillation is immediate defibrillation. Without it, the patient will die. Since there is no QRS complex (no real ventricular depolarization), there is no need to avoid a vulnerable period. Cardiopulmonary resuscitation is given immediately before (while awaiting defibrillator) and after the shock and should never be ceased for longer than a period of five seconds since blood flow and blood pressure can drop to zero. Usually a defibrillating shock of 400 watt seconds is delivered.

Whether a nurse can defibrillate depends on her preparation and institutional policy, which is a collaborative decision of nurses, physicians, and administrators. Their decision is influenced by state nursing and medical practice acts. The nurse is responsible for seeing that her own performance is competent.

Ventricular tachycardia which is accompanied by hypotension and loss of consciousness is likewise an extreme emergency. The patient may be defibrillated under these circumstances rather than synchronously cardioverted.

## CARDIAC ARREST

Cardiac arrest is the sudden cessation of effective cardiac output. The electrical mechanism of cardiac arrest can be ventricular asystole or bradyarrhythmias, or ventricular tachyarrhythmias (ventricular tachycardia or ventricular fibrillation). An initially slow rhythm can induce myocardial hypoxia which can trigger ventricular fibrillation.

The severity of symptoms of cardiac arrest depends on the duration of the suspension of cardiac output. *Stokes-Adams syndrome* describes the loss of consciousness due to cerebral ischemia following ineffective ventricular contraction. The duration of loss of effective cardiac output and corresponding signs and symptoms are:

| | |
|---|---|
| 2 to 3 seconds: | palpitations |
| 3 to 5 seconds: | symptoms of cerebrovascular insufficiency with sensations of dizziness and distress |
| 5 to 10 seconds: | syncope with or without seizures (Stokes-Adams syndrome) |
| 30 to 90 seconds: | death usually occurs unless external stimulus reinitiates the circulation |

Some Stokes-Adams attacks are self-limited and the patient regains consciousness. In others, the full-blown clinical state of cardiac arrest develops. The treatment depends on the preceding arrhythmia. If ventricular fibrillation precedes unconscious-

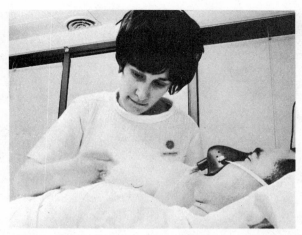

**Figure 61-23.** Nurse delivering a precordial blow to patient in cardiac arrest. (Photograph taken at Overlook Hospital, Summit, N.J., by Robert Goldstein for *Patient Care* magazine)

ness, defibrillation is the treatment. If heart block with a slow ventricular rate or ventricular asystole is the mechanism, cardiorespiratory action is maintained artificially until more definitive therapy such as the use of isoproterenol (Isuprel) or an artificial electronic pacemaker reinitiates effective circulation.

Care of the patient in cardiac arrest should encompass the following stages and maneuvers:

- **If the patient is on a cardiac monitor, respond to monitor alarm and check electrocardiographic pattern.**
- **In any situation, note the time. Go to the patient. Clear the A, airway. Note the B, breathing. Determine C, circulation by pulses and pupils. If the patient has neither a carotid pulse (or femoral) or respirations, and is disoriented or unconscious, deliver a sharp blow with the fist over the sternum (precordial blow) unless the patient has a chest injury. This has been shown to be sometimes effective in initiating cardiac action following ventricular asystole and ventricular fibrillation. The patient may be semiconscious, and needless to say an explanation will be required after the precordial blow! (Fig. 61-23.)**
- **Summon help.**
- **If necessary and possible, defibrillate immediately. In a hospital intensive care unit this should be within 30 seconds.**
- **Observe the following steps (ABCDE's):**
  1. **Airway should be established.**
  2. **Breathing, using the mouth-to-mouth method or assistive device if available. Give three to four maximal insufflations before initiating circulation so that oxygenated blood will be pumped.**
  3. **Circulation should be restored by closed chest cardiac compression. Check the pupils and carotid or femoral pulse.**
  4. **Definitive therapy is ordered by the physician, depending on the cause and length of the period of arrest. Sodium bicarbonate, usually 44.0 mEq. for every five to ten minutes in cardiac arrest is given to treat the metabolic acidosis which results from the accumulation of lactic acid as a by-product of anaerobic metabolism.**
  5. **Evaluation. Dilation of the pupils starts 45 seconds after cardiac arrest and is complete in one to two minutes. Since the pupil is the best index of brain oxygenation, pupillary response is the best indicator of the effectiveness of heart-lung resuscitation. Adequate oxygenation and good blood flow to the brain are present if the pupil constricts on exposure to flashlight.**

     **Pulses should be present during cardiac compression and the patient's color should improve if he is responding.**

The return of a relatively good ECG pattern is not an indication to stop resuscitation efforts. The patient can have sufficient circulation to produce a normal-looking ECG, but not enough cardiac output for functional circulation. Restoration of blood pressure and quality of the peripheral pulse are crucial indicators. The carotid pulse is the most reliable pulse and the last to disappear.

Some additional important points about cardiopulmonary resuscitation are:

**Airway.** A maximum backward tilt of the head is the easiest way to open an airway. Only an experienced person should attempt endotracheal intubation since cardiac massage cannot be halted for more than five seconds. Endotracheal intubation is not essential for an adequate airway. Secretions need to be wiped out or suctioned from the pharynx for an adequate airway. Establishment of an airway may be sufficient to permit spontaneous breathing to resume and restore circulation.

**Breathing.** One person extends the patient's neck, pulls the lower jaw upward and begins mouth-to-mouth resuscitation. The rescuer blows his breath into the patient's mouth, either directly, by tightly pressing his lips against the patient's mouth, or by means of a small tube.

Mouth-to-mouth breathing done effectively delivers about 18 per cent oxygen to the patient. A self-inflating bag, such as the Ambu bag, used with a face mask or endotracheal tube and oxygen, delivers about 50 per cent oxygen only if used correctly. Three to four maximal insufflations should be given before compression is started so that oxygenated blood will be circulated; then the pulse should be checked again. With two rescuers, one inflation should be interposed after each five compressions without any halting of compression (1:5 ratio or 12 breaths per minute). With one rescuer, two breaths are interposed after each fifteen compressions. The breather should see the chest rise and fall, feel the resistance of the lungs as they expand, and hear the noise of air escaping during exhalation.

Artificial breathing may cause distention of the stomach. This can lead to regurgitation, reduced lung volume, or the initiation of vagal reflexes.

A team member may exert moderate pressure between the umbilicus and the rib cage to expel the air. The patient's head should be lowered and turned to one side to avoid aspiration of gastric contents. Mouth-to-nose ventilation can be used if there is difficulty via the mouth-to-mouth route. Mechanical ventilators are also available when prolonged respiratory support is needed (see Chap. 60).

Artificial ventilation is not accompanied by cardiac compression if cardiac action is spontaneous.

**Cardiac Compression.** Rhythmic pressure applied over the lower half of the sternum results in compression of the heart and pulsatile arterial circulation. Correctly performed cardiac compression can result in a mean blood pressure of 40 to 50 mm. Hg in the carotid artery and a blood flow of up to 35 per cent of normal.

The patient is placed on his back on a firm surface, such as the floor, the pavement, a bed board, or even a large tray slipped under the patient's chest. (A soft mattress is depressed by pressure and would interfere with the massage.) As part of the emergency equipment, some hospitals keep a board that can be slipped between the patient and the bed. It makes a hard surface from the patient's waist to his shoulders (Fig. 61-24).

The rescuer kneels beside the patient, placing his hands at right angles on the lower sternum (Fig. 61-25). The hands, one on top of the other, are pressed vertically downward, pushing the sternum inward one and one-half to two inches, thus compressing the heart between the sternum and the spine and forcing the blood out of the heart. Only the heels of the hands are used. The fingers are kept up, out of contact with the patient's ribs.

Manual pressure is released, allowing the heart to fill with blood, and then pressure is reapplied.

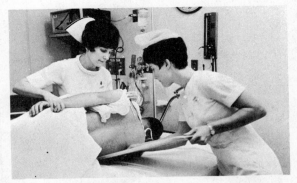

**Figure 61-24.** Nurses quickly place cardiac arrest board before initiating cardiac compression. (Photograph taken at Overlook Hospital, Summit, N.J., by Robert Goldstein for *Patient Care* magazine)

The cycle is repeated approximately 60 to 80 times per minute with breathing interposed.

Closed cardiac massage is not without its dangers. Hands that are misplaced too close to the diaphragm may rupture the liver. Hands that are misplaced to one side may break ribs. Considerable force is required to move the chest of an adult two inches.

When prolonged resuscitation or transportation of the patient is required, external cardiac com-

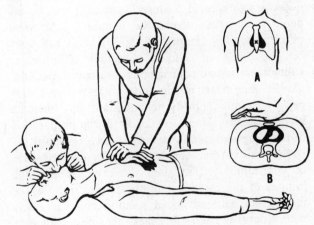

**Figure 61-25.** Technique of closed-chest cardiac massage. One rescuer gives mouth-to-mouth resuscitation. The other massages the heart by pressing downward on the patient's chest approximately 60 times a minute. (A) X indicates the area where pressure should be applied. (B) Manual pressure on the chest, compressing the heart and forcing blood out of it. (American Heart Association, Inc., New York, N.Y.; adapted from Kouwenhoven, W. B., et al.: Heart activation in cardiac arrest, *Modern Concepts of Cardiovascular Diseases* 30[2]:642)

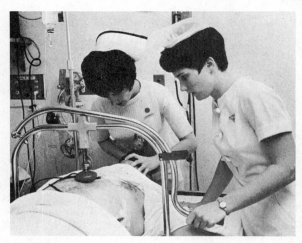

**Figure 61-26.** Nurse team initiates cardiopulmonary resuscitation following cardiac arrest.

pression machines are commercially available which are more consistent in the application of pressure than would be a number of different team members. The machine must be carefully and continually observed for correct placement and function (Fig. 61-26).

During the resuscitation effort the physician may give an intravenous or intracardiac injection of epinephrine and intravenous sodium bicarbonate as necessary to control acidosis. Lidocaine can be ordered to decrease ventricular irritability. Atropine or isoproterenol (Isuprel) to speed heart rate may be the drug of choice. Calcium chloride to strengthen cardiac contractions also may be administered once heart action starts. Vasopressors may be given intravenously to maintain an adequate blood pressure. The nurse assists in the preparation of the drug and monitors the patient's response.

External cardiac compression may be ineffective or contraindicated in such situations as crushing injuries of the chest or internal thoracic injuries, or in patients with advanced pulmonary emphysema with enlarged, fixed rib cages. The physician may elect to open the chest and do direct cardiac massage.

After successful cardiac resuscitation the patient needs to be observed closely. Vital signs are taken frequently; the patient's cardiac rhythm will be monitored. Oxygen will be given to reduce the onset of arrhythmias due to myocardial hypoxia. Oxygen administration is often monitored with ar-

terial blood gas studies. A nasogastric tube may be passed to prevent distention. Shock may have caused renal impairment.

Other complications for which the nurse should observe include flail chest, pneumothorax, hematoma of the liver, brain damage, fractured ribs or sternum, and fat embolism. After open heart massage there will be chest drainage tubes. The patient is observed for bleeding and infection. To minimize the chance of cerebral damage, some physicians order hypothermia for several days after cardiac arrest.

It is the nurse's responsibility to continue resuscitative efforts until medical help arrives, which is feasible in most institutions and areas of the United States. A sole rescuer, of course, would continue until exhausted. The decision to terminate resuscitation efforts is a medical one based on the patient's cerebral and cardiorespiratory response.

**Who Should Be Resuscitated?** Involved individuals from each agency should develop their own policies in response to this broad societal question. Generally speaking, cardiopulmonary resuscitation is a response to sudden, unexpected death. There is a generally agreed upon gap of time between so-called clinical death and actual physiologic death or irreversible cerebral change. The time period of three to four minutes, however, applies to persons with normal circulatory systems. Patients with previous cardiac or respiratory disease or cerebral arteriosclerosis have, of course, less "grace" period. Thus, there must always be a maximal sense of urgency in initiating ECPR and in continuing it because the longer ECPR is necessary, the less likely it is to succeed. ECPR is not indicated when it can be determined with a degree of certainty that cardiac arrest has persisted for more than five or six minutes, or somewhat longer in drowning. Nor is it indicated for patients with terminal cancer or end-stage irreversible disease of the liver, kidneys, heart, or brain. Old age, in itself, is not a contraindication to resuscitation.

Because the nurse is often the one who initiates resuscitation efforts, she should obtain more clear-cut guidelines for individual hospitalized patients through discussion with the patient's physician on admission. He, in turn, makes his judgment after evaluation of the patient's clinical condition and appropriate discussion with the patient and/or his family. These guidelines for the nurse should be written on the chart or other readily available source of information so that all nurses are aware of the situation. This avoids the regrettable situation of a nurse or intern instituting heroic efforts when they are not indicated, such as for the dying cancer patient. Discussion with the physician ahead of time is particularly important when patients are part of the general hospital division and not in an intensive care unit.

**Other Considerations.** Whether alone at night in a hospital ward in a previously undiscussed situation, on the street, or on the beach, the nurse needs to have guidelines for action in her own mind. In such areas of extended nursing activity she does in fact take the legal and moral responsibility for her own decisions and actions, or lack of action. Her performance expectations legally are those in keeping with her level of education and experience.

One of the challenging and difficult aspects of nursing where the risk of cardiac arrest is high is that many patients are not successfully resuscitated. Despite the best and most heroic efforts, patients do die. Recriminations, blame, and guilt feelings can occur when there are exaggerated expectations of one's own or a team's ability to save a life.

The nurse who elects to work in an area where mortality is high and emergency action is part of her role needs to reflect on the realities and risks involved. She needs to know her own human and professional assets and limitations, and work toward expertise within this framework. Rather than participate in emergency action solely because it is part of a job description, the realistic nurse knowingly takes the risks and can keep in perspective her own gradually improving skills as part of a team, the patient's chances for life, and what can be done for him. (See Chapter 58 for psychological considerations in the care of the cardiac arrest survivor, and Chapter 12 on care of the dying patient.)

Practice drills are essential so that a team is well prepared for such an emergency as cardiac arrest. After the stress of an emergency is over, an objective evaluation session with all team members present makes use of various events as opportunities for learning. Without this session, inefficiencies can be repeated.

## THE PATIENT WITH SYMPTOMATIC BRADYCARDIA

### Nursing Assessment and Intervention

Patients who are subject to Stokes-Adams seizures are often very apprehensive. They do not know when the next attack will occur and then they have only a few seconds to summon help before they become unconscious. It is not uncommon for patients to be admitted with acute physical injuries such as fractures or lacerations sustained during a Stokes-Adams seizure. Often attacks occur when the patient is away from his own community, and he may find himself admitted to an unfamiliar hospital under the care of personnel who are strangers to him. Stokes-Adams attacks may be associated with acute myocardial infarction; a patient with such an attack may be admitted to a cardiac monitoring unit. Since, however, the symptoms are cerebral, the patient may fear that he has a brain tumor or epilepsy or another neurologic condition.

A careful orientation of the patient to the hospital and community environment, close observation at all times, explanation of the cardiac monitor and other equipment and procedures, maintaining the patient's privacy and individual preferences, and offering to listen to the patient's fears are nursing measures which can alleviate anxiety.

A padded tongue depressor, gauze squares, and an oropharyngeal airway should be at the bedside, and side rails should be kept up. The patient's pulse is taken during a seizure or as soon as possible if he is not on a cardiac monitor. A marked decrease in pulse rate accompanied by signs and symptoms of cerebral ischemia is indicative of Stokes-Adams syndrome.

The staff is prepared for emergency measures. A sharp precordial blow is often sufficient to activate a pacemaker site somewhere in the conduction system or myocardium (see Fig. 61-23). If ventricular fibrillation is the mechanism, and the precordial blow is not effective, defibrillation is immediately essential. If the mechanism is sustained ventricular asystole, ECPR is initiated prior to definitive medical care.

Since attacks may be repetitious in acute ischemic conditions of the A-V node, the patient should not be left alone. He often gives clues to the onset by stating that he is getting "whoozy," feeling lightheaded, or going to faint. The reason for a precordial blow must be explained in terms that the individual patient can understand. He is often semiconscious and may think he is being abused! He can be assured that his heart is quite capable of beating, but the signals that help it to beat regularly are temporarily erratic.

The ambulatory patient who experiences symptoms and signs of transient cerebral ischemic attacks (TIA's) may be given a Holter monitor to wear as he goes about his usual daily routine (see Fig. 39-3). This device records the continuous ECG on tape which can be subjected to rapid review at a later time by the physician, who also reviews the log of activities kept by the patient. Cerebral symptoms may be due to low cardiac output resulting from cardiac arrhythmias.

While awaiting help after an attack, the patient is given oxygen and prevented from performing activities that cause vagal stimulation, thus slowing of the heart. This can happen if the patient strains to lift himself up from a recumbent position or to void or defecate. Also, it can occur in response to retching, severe coughing, drinking cold beverages, or during pharyngeal or tracheal suctioning.

Once the physician diagnoses Stokes-Adams syndrome or complete heart block he may elect to insert an artificial pacemaker. While awaiting the preparation of facilities, or if pacemaker facilities are not available, drug therapy is instituted. In an acute emergency, an external pacemaker is applied temporarily, but not activated unless essential.

## Drug Therapy

The drugs most frequently used are atropine sulfate, isoproterenol (Isuprel), and steroids. Atropine sulfate lessens the effect of the vagus nerve and therefore improves the rhythm of the S-A node and transmission of impulses over the Purkinje system. An emergency dose is 1 mg. (gr. $^1/_{60}$) intravenously. Because atropine increases intraocular pressure it is generally not given to patients with known glaucoma. Since patients in the older age group are glaucoma prone, the physician may order one drop of one per cent pilocarpine eyedrops in each eye every six hours if the patient requires frequent doses of atropine. Any blurring or change in vision should be promptly reported. The pupils are checked for dilation. Acute urinary retention can result from atropine administration. The voiding of patients receiving this drug must be closely monitored. Elderly males on bed rest, who may also have some prostatic hypertrophy, are particularly prone to this result of atropine. The patient will probably complain of dry mouth and thirst. Candy lozenges may relieve this.

Isoproterenol (Isuprel) is a very potent drug. In some facilities a physician must be present when it is given. Isuprel is useful for both its chronotropic (*rate* of contraction) and inotropic (*force* of contraction) effects. Isuprel enhances conduction by stimulating the S-A and A-V nodes, and it accelerates idioventricular pacemakers high in the bundle of His or bundle branches. In high doses or in sensitive patients, Isuprel can cause tachyarrhythmias and ventricular irritability. The drug is given diluted in an infusion and is titrated using a microdrip set to maintain the pulse rate ordered by the physician (usually 60 to 65 beats per minute). As the ventricular rate increases, the "piggy-backed" Isuprel infusion is slowed down or turned off and an unmedicated infusion turned on. The Isuprel is also ordered discontinued if dangerous forms of VPB's appear since these are precursors of ventricular fibrillation. Isuprel also increases stroke volume, cardiac output, and cardiac work, as well as heart rate.

Periods of sinus rhythm when Isuprel is turned off are not secure times for the staff because the change from sinus rhythm to complete heart block and low ventricular rate or asystole can occur quite abruptly.

When heart block is induced by inflammation and edema of or around the atrioventricular conduction system caused by a recent myocardial infarction or by myocarditis, corticosteroid therapy may be given.

## Pacemaker Therapy

An artificial cardiac pacemaker is used to stimulate the electrical activity of the heart and maintain the patient's ventricular rate at a minimum level for effective cardiac output. Formerly, an open-chest procedure was necessary to implant electrodes in the myocardium, so the use of a pacemaker was limited to "good risk" patients. Today, with the transvenous technique, a pacemaker can be inserted quickly in most patients under local anesthesia with minimal surgical risk and discomfort.

A pacemaker consists of electrodes connected

by wires (or leads) encased in a catheter to a pulse generator usually powered by batteries. The pulse generator can be implanted (permanent) or external (temporary) (Figs. 61-27 and 61-28).

**Indications.** The most frequent indication for permanent artificial pacing is to eliminate Stokes-Adams attacks associated with a variety of heart diseases, including coronary artery disease, rheumatic heart disease, and congenital malformations, or as a direct complication of cardiac surgery.

Since pacing increases heart rate, therefore cardiac output, it is also used to increase circulation in patients with slow heart rates with symptoms of right- or left-sided heart failure, angina, renal failure, or slow cerebration.

Formerly drugs such as ephedrine or isoproterenol (Isuprel) were used on a long-term basis to treat these conditions, but today pacing is considered to carry less risk than that associated with drug toxicity, changes in metabolic states of the patient, or the human failings associated with self-administration of drugs.

Temporary pacing is indicated in patients with acute myocardial infarction complicated by heart block, or other bradyarrhythmias, in digitalis toxicity with heart block, or in patients with slow heart rate and congestive failure who require digitalis. In most of these situations the pacemaker is removed when the normal sinus rhythm returns. In many patients the temporary pacemaker, though inserted, is not used but is left on "stand-by" as a precautionary measure should complications develop. Should the need arise, the prepared nurse activates the pacemaker. Today most temporary pacemakers are self-activating (the so-called "demand" pacemaker). Another indication for temporary pacing is to suppress rapid arrhythmias such as recurrent ventricular tachycardia which does not respond to drugs or electric cardioversion. The pacemaker is used to "overdrive" the ectopic focus and thus suppress it. Fast rates, such as around 150 beats per minute, may be needed, so the patient must be closely observed for his tolerance of the rapid rate.

Since there are many indications for pacing and several types of pacemakers, many still being researched, it is the responsibility of the nurse to know the objectives and precautions of the pacing treatment and the necessary observations of the patient; the nurse should study the product litera-

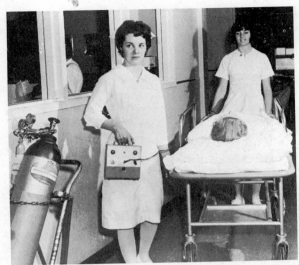

**Figure 61-27.** Transporting the patient with the temporary Electrodyne transistor pacemaker ready for use. (Electrodyne, division of Becton, Dickinson & Co.)

ture which describes the individual pacing unit. The physician determines the rate of the heartbeat and the amplitude of the pacing stimulus.

Some common terms used in the field of cardiac pacing are:

**External Pacing.** This is a form of temporary pacing used in dire emergencies in which a series of shocks of 50 to 150 volts is delivered to the heart through the chest wall via electrodes placed on the chest. It is painful if the patient is semiconscious, and it is often ineffective. It can be utilized in asystole or complete heart block, however, while awaiting a more adequate pacing technique or when transporting the patient via ambulance or from one hospital area to another. The battery life of an emergency pacemaker should be checked regularly by the engineering department so that it is effective when needed.

**Transvenous (Pervenous) or Endocardial Pacing.** An electrode catheter is passed through a peripheral vein such as the antecubital, external jugular, or subclavian vein into the right ventricle where it contacts the endocardial surface. The free end of the catheter is attached to an external pulse generating unit for temporary pacing. For permanent pacing, a subcutaneous pocket is prepared usually in the subclavicular area and the free end of the catheter is then passed through a tissue tunnel and connected

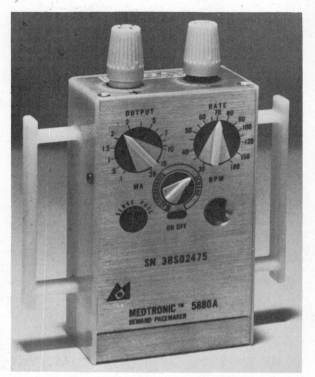

**Figure 61-28.** External demand pacemaker. (Medtronic, Inc.)

to the pulse generating unit which is implanted in the pocket.

**Epicardial Pacing.** At the time of cardiac surgery electrodes can be attached to the epicardium with fine sutures. For temporary pacing, the wires are brought out through the incision and attached to an external standby pulse generator. When cardiac rhythmicity is re-established the surgeon breaks the fine epicardial sutures with gentle traction and removes the electrodes. When permanent pacing cannot be accomplished transvenously, permanent epicardial electrodes can be implanted and the wires attached to an implanted pulse generator. The nursing care of the patient is complicated by the open-chest surgical approach.

**Fixed Rate (Asynchronous) Pacing.** The electrode catheter is placed in the right ventricle, thus ignoring the atrial contribution to cardiac output. The pulse generator is set by the physician to fire at a fixed rate of about 70 beats per minute and fires all the time regardless of what the patient's own conduction mechanism is capable of doing. At times, the patient's own mechanism can compete with that of the pacer, and this can be dangerous in

the patient with myocardial hypoxia, acidosis, drug toxicity, or other states in which the threshold for ventricular fibrillation is lowered. Should the pacer discharge its current into the vulnerable period of the cardiac cycle (around the summit of the T wave) ventricular tachycardia or fibrillation is a possible though infrequent result.

**Demand or Standby Pacing (R wave triggered).** Competition with the patient's spontaneous rhythm is avoided with this mode of pacing because of a special sensing circuit that recognizes a QRS complex. In one type of standby pacemaker (ventricular inhibited or ventricular suppressive) a pulse-blocking circuit prevents the pacer from issuing a pacing stimulus when the patient's spontaneous depolarization is detected. The temporary standby pacemaker functions in this manner as well as implanted units.

In another type of standby pacing (ventricular synchronous), the pacer issues a pulse when a spontaneous depolarization is sensed rather than withholding one. The pacer stimulus fires into the refractory period of the patient's own QRS and thus is ineffective as a stimulus. If the patient's ventricle fails to depolarize spontaneously after a set period of delay, the pacer-issued pulse depolarizes the ventricle and causes a ventricular contraction.

When standby pacemakers function they do so at a preset rate. Change in the set rate of implanted units can be accomplished in some cases (depending on the model) by use of a special needle, a magnet, or an external battery-powered programmer.

**Atrial Synchronous Pacing.** This mode is a more physiologic type of pacing. A catheter in the atrium detects the patient's own P wave, and it is relayed to an implanted unit where the impulse is delayed, similar to the normal delay at the A-V node; then it causes depolarization and contraction of the ventricle via another electrode catheter. Thus the rate can vary according to the patient's need up to a preset maximum, and the booster effect of atrial contraction is maintained. Should the atrial circuit fail, an automatic circuit initiates fixed-rate ventricular pacing. This type of pacemaker is used for younger, more active patients. If the atrial rate exceeds a preset limit of about 150, an automatic 2:1, 3:1, or 4:1 block will be induced. During the change in rate the patient might experience lightheadedness or a fainting feeling. A transthoracic or transvenous approach is used for implantation.

**Atrial Pacing.** When the A-V node and Purkinje system are intact and the problematic arrhythmia lies in the atria, a pacing electrode can be passed into the atria and attached to a pulse generator. In this way, the atrial boost to cardiac output is conserved. However, an atrial pacemaker is often unstable in its position.

**A-V Sequential Pacing.** The A-V sequential pacemaker has no output if cardiac function is normal. If no cardiac activity is sensed after a specific interval, it stimulates an atrial contraction. Its sensing circuit then allows time for the atrial-ventricular nodal delay, and if it does not sense ventricular activity it also stimulates a ventricular contraction.

**Unipolar or Bipolar Systems.** These terms refer to the type of electrical lead configuration. In a unipolar system, the stimulating electrode in the ventricle is the cathode, or negative electrode, and the anode can be a needle attached to the patient's skin in a temporary setup or the metal ground plate of a permanent implantable unit.

In a bipolar system, the two electrodes are incorporated in the end of the endocardial catheter which lies in the ventricle.

## The Surgical Period

When the physician decides that a pacemaker is to be inserted he explains this to the patient. A surgical consent is necessary. For most patients, the thought that their heart requires artificial electrical control is anxiety producing. They need time to talk about it and get used to the idea, but often there is very little time for this. The nurse should listen to the surgeon's explanation to the patient, and in her conversation with the patient review, clarify, and correct any misinterpretations that the patient or family might have in language that the patient can readily understand. For example, one patient who was a music teacher found the comparison of a fixed rate pacemaker with a metronome to be helpful. Some patients are relieved when they are told about the pacemaker since they no longer have to live with the uncertainty of recurring Stokes-Adams attacks.

A patient who is to have a transvenous pacemaker inserted may receive mild sedation.

If a portable image intensifier is available in a cardiac monitoring unit, transportation of the patient to another area is unnecessary. Electrodes for temporary external pacing are put in place if the patient must be moved. A portable pulse generator is taken along with the patient to the x-ray department in case of emergency; a pulse meter may be used en route. Image-intensifying fluoroscopic control is used to guide the pacing catheter into the ventricle. The patient care area must be equipped with a cardiac monitor, a defibrillator, and other equipment and drugs needed in the event of cardiac arrest. Ventricular fibrillation can be provoked mechanically by the catheter tip as it enters the ventricle.

For transvenous pacing, local anesthesia is used. The patient may find the procedure tedious and be uncomfortable from the supine position on a hard x-ray table. The patient hears what is going on though his eyes may be shielded. Strict surgical asepsis is essential. Contamination of the catheter or implantable pulse generator can result in infection and failure to pace properly.

The surgeon selects the correct pacing threshold and sets the voltage and rate. An amplitude of 6 mA. and rate of 70 is common.

Initially the pacing catheter floats in the ventricle but within a few days it becomes coated with a layer of fibrin, then endothelium, and eventually becomes embedded in the right ventricular trabeculae. Immediately after insertion, the electrocardiographic display might show complexes with varying electrical potentials because the tip of the catheter might not touch the ventricle with the same force at first. VPB's are more frequent during the early postimplant period, especially in patients who have received isoproterenol (Isuprel). The physician may order medication to suppress these. The patient may be returned for several days to an environment where cardiac monitoring, a defibrillator, and other emergency equipment and drugs are available.

## Postimplantation Care

Patients with newly inserted pacemakers are generally on an electrocardiographic monitor for an evaluation period after insertion. Each pacemaker has its own characteristic tracing. The electrical artifact or "blip" of the pacing stimulus should appear before the QRS of a ventricular pacer (Fig. 61-29).

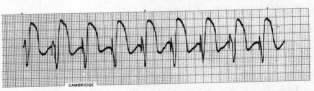

**Figure 61-29.** Paced ventricular rhythm. A pacemaker artifact precedes each widened QRS. (Sharp, L., and Rabin, B.: *Nursing in the Coronary Care Unit*, Philadelphia, Lippincott)

It is usually identified on the oscilloscope as a thin, straight stroke. Absence of the artifact may mean faulty monitoring equipment, or more seriously, failure to pace due to malposition of the catheter, dislodgment of the catheter, catheter breakage, or rise of the pacing threshold due to tissue reaction to the catheter or to infection. The location of the artifact is particularly important. If the paced rhythm competes with the patient's spontaneous rhythm, the artifact can fall in the vulnerable period of the cardiac cycle. Ventricular fibrillation is a possibility when electrical stimuli fall on or around the summit of the T wave. A competing beat can also fall in the vulnerable period of the previous beat.

Ventricular fibrillation in the event of competition is most apt to occur if the fibrillation threshold is reduced. Such conditions as drug toxicity or electrolyte imbalance can lower the fibrillation threshold. Most pacemakers today have a special shunting circuit which protects the pacemaker from damage during defibrillation, but if circumstances permit, the pacemaker should be disconnected, then reconnected immediately after the shock. Competition also results in an irregular ventricular rhythm which is disruptive of cardiac hemodynamics.

To assist in determining that each pacing stimulus results in effective ventricular contraction, the patient's pulse should be taken simultaneously with observation of the cardiac monitor.

The small pulse generator of a temporary pacing system should be placed so that it is immovable and there is no tension on the wires. The patient should not be able to manipulate the controls. Because of electrical hazards, wall outlets should never be used as electrical power sources for pacemakers. When the patient has a temporary pacemaker, a direct route exists from the external exit of the catheter (wire) to the heart. The exposed electrodes at the wire exit can be insulated at their junction with the pulse generator by placing the unit in a rubber glove. Only grounded electrical equipment should be used in the room and only one machine connected to a wall outlet should be used on the patient at one time. For example, when a 12-lead ECG is to be done, the single lead cardiac monitor should be disconnected immediately before the ECG machine is turned on.

Localized phlebitis and cellulitis can develop around the catheter exit site of a temporary pacemaker. The dressing should be checked for drainage and any patient discomfort reported to the physician. Dressings on an implantation incision should be checked for drainage and the wound inspected for complications. A catheter attached to Hemovac drainage may be inserted at the time of surgery for a few days to drain off fluid substances that can accumulate when tissues are disrupted.

If the patient develops singultus (hiccups), there can be current leakage across the diaphragm or perforation of the ventricle by the catheter. The physician should be consulted.

The extent of nursing care depends on the pre-pacemaker condition of the patient and whether the pacemaker is temporary or permanent. For example, if the patient developed heart block following acute myocardial infarction, he will continue to be on coronary precautions. After several days, the physician will observe the patient's cardiac response with the temporary pacemaker turned off; if the patient returns to sustained normal sinus rhythm, the temporary pacemaker will be removed after several evaluation periods. A permanent pacemaker may be necessary.

If a permanent pacemaker was implanted because of a gradually progressive bradycardia without acute infarction, the patient may be discharged after a few days' observation and teaching. If the patient had a thoracotomy for myocardial electrode implantation, his care will encompass chest drainage and other considerations of major surgery.

The physician should be consulted regarding the initiation of exercise of the shoulder on the side of the catheter insertion. Unless this is mobilized early, the elderly patient is apt to develop "frozen" shoulder.

Complications that occur with implanted pacemakers include inflammation as well as infection of the subcutaneous "pocket." Hemorrhage, pressure necrosis of the skin, or extrusion of the pulse generator can also occur.

Education Therapy for the Patient
with a Permanent Pacemaker

**Affective Considerations.** Initially the patient may not share the professional's view that the pacemaker is an awesome feat of modern technology. For the young person with heart block who wants to participate in all the activities of his age group, the pacemaker may indeed be viewed as a welcome relief from the unpredictability of Stokes-Adams attacks. However, most patients with permanent pacemakers are over age 60, and many have multiple health problems as well as difficulty in coping with the other developmental tasks of aging.

The person in his 40's who requires a permanent pacemaker following a myocardial infarction may initially perceive it as a constant reminder of the loss of highly valued bodily integrity, an unwelcome dependency, disruption in career goals, and temporary drastic change in family roles and responsibilities. For example, the long-distance truck driver may be bitter and angry over the loss of his job.

Listening to the patient's perception of his situation and encouraging the expression of feelings relieves tension and paves the way for more effective learning.

**Cognitive Aspects.** A family member or close associate should be included in the teaching program. The nurse, when possible, can teach groups of patients who then also have the opportunity to share their questions, thoughts, and feelings and derive support from each other.

The education program should contain information relative to the following points, but should be individualized according to such factors as patients' intellectual ability and motivation, as well as physiologic and emotional considerations.

- Basic anatomy and functioning of the heart and the electrophysiologic disturbance which necessitated the pacemaker.
- The type of pacemaker implanted, the way it functions, and its expected effect on the pulse.
- The activity prescription. The patient's prognosis and his activity depend on the underlying disease process, age, and degree of cardiac reserve. The pacemaker improves cardiac conduction, but cannot regenerate the diseased myocardium. Usually only those activities which might result in a direct blow to the pulse generator, such as karate, or which involves severe body twisting are restricted. Some patients may needlessly restrict activities such as sexual intercourse because of unfounded fears. The patient needs the opportunity to discuss activities with the nurse and physician and plan life realistically, using tolerance and enjoyment as guidelines.

Driving is prohibited during the period of wound healing but the physician may permit its resumption about a month postimplantation if the pacemaker is functioning well.

All pacemaker wearers should carry identification such as a Medic Alert emblem or a manufacturer's card on their person at all times with essential information such as type of pacemaker, date of implant, and paced rate.

Long-distance travel is not recommended around the time period that the battery is approaching the end of its predicted life expectancy. The pacemaker wearer who travels by airplane should have his pacemaker identification card available, as the pacemaker may activate an airport weapons detector device.

Return to work depends on overall cardiac function and is not limited by a pacemaker except in rare instances where there is dangerous exposure to electromagnetic fields. Despite the fact that in many cases patients are healthier, safer employees because they have a pacemaker, certain prejudices exist due to misinformation or fear of negative workman's compensation rulings, which keep such patients from resuming their former jobs or taking on new ones. The nurse can possibly overcome some of these prejudices through education of the public and employers.

- The importance of continuing health supervision. Some patients with congestive heart failure may continue to require diuretics and digitalis; those with symptoms of coronary insufficiency may require drug therapy. Because of distortion of the ECG by the pacemaker-produced configuration, clinical and enzyme changes are important in the diagnosis of acute myocardial infarction should this occur.
- Methods of pacemaker monitoring. The average life of a pacemaker unit is about two and one-half years, but this varies with the model. (The latest nuclear-powered pacemakers are predicted to last ten years.) Battery depletion is signaled by changing of the rate; battery exhaustion is the cause of 80 per cent of pacemaker failures. Other components can fail and result in decrease or increase in rate, including the very rapid rate of a "runaway" pacemaker, or absence of pacing. Symptoms of weakness or dizziness or reversion to other prepacemaker symptoms which indicate gradual or abrupt fall in cardiac output may be the patient's first clue. Immediate medical attention is essential.

Some physicians expect the patient or close associate to monitor the pulse, counting the rate for one full minute daily, relating the rate to the expected performance of the pacemaker, and reporting any changes. For example, a pulse rate which is faster than the set rate of a fixed-rate pacer can indicate component failure, while a slower rate can indicate battery depletion. A pulse rate below the set rate of a demand pacer may indicate lack of capture or faulty function of the unit.

Some physicians believe that routine pulse-taking is unproductive since significant rate change may be measured in milliseconds instrumentally before change can be detected in the patient's pulse. Some highly anxious patients may become more so if given the task of self-monitoring. In an attempt to detect early pacemaker failure and to change the pulse generator before the patient becomes symptomatic, regional clinics which ultilize instruments that measure the pacemaker spike intervals in milliseconds and waveform changes in the pacing artifact, as well as other parameters, have been established. Some patients are taught to use a data transmitter to send both pacemaker artifact and peripheral pulse (which deter-

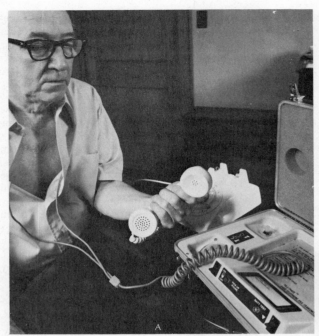
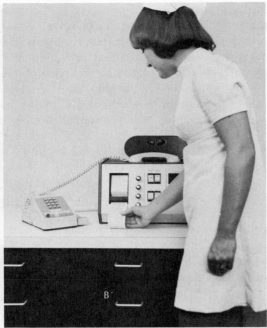

**Figure 61-30.** (A) The Teletrace<sup>(TM)</sup> Telephone ECG system for monitoring function of pacemaker in which battery depletion is signaled by rate change. (B) A receiver in the office converts the telephone transmitted signal from the patient into a digital display of pacemaker rate in pulses per minute, interval between pacemaker artifacts in milliseconds, and an ECG recording to verify ventricular capture. ECG information can also be used to monitor cardiac patients without pacemakers in conjunction with ECG recordings taken during office visits. (Medtronic, Inc.)

mines capture) over ordinary telephone lines to a pacemaker center where data is recorded and analyzed and reports sent to the patient's physician (Fig. 61-30). The transtelephonic technique provides a means of getting frequent data points to permit prediction of battery depletion. For some patients this system necessitates converting their demand pacer to a fixed rate mode by use of a magnet during the transmission. A telephone monitoring system is especially useful for invalids or others who experience difficulty in frequent travel to a regional clinic. One telephone monitoring system has reportedly reduced emergency hospital admissions from 35 per cent to 10 per cent (Stern).

Good pacemaker surveillance also reduces long-term costs by extending the pacemaker life to the last possible moment. Replacement costs including the pacemaker, surgeon's fee, and hospitalization are approximately $3,500. Medicare covers most of these costs but insurance coverage for younger patients varies among states.

• Electromagnetic interference (EMI). Though rare today because of the improvement in shielding around pulse generators, the circuitry of various types of pacemakers can respond to external electrical signals of sufficient magnitude. Depending on the type, the pacemaker may revert to a fixed rate, speed up excessively, slow down, fire irregularly, or fail to fire. The patient may have symptoms related to change in cardiac output such as dizziness or lightheadedness. Moving away from the source of interference generally permits the pacemaker to resume normal function. Radar installations, radio broadcast transmitters, and operating microwave ovens may cause difficulty, as may diathermy treatment or electrosurgical procedures involving cutting or cauterization. The patient should inform all his physicians, dentists, or other medical therapists that he is a pacemaker wearer. Earlier, gasoline engine ignition systems and small electrical devices held against the body such as electric shavers or hedge trimmers were noted to precipitate maulfunction in pacemakers. A patient's report of suspected malfunction should be respected and reported to the physician or clinic staff. A competent observer should accompany pacemaker wearers in areas of suspected difficulty until safety is established.

• The patient is instructed to inspect the implantation site at regular intervals and report swelling, discoloration, heat, pain, drainage, or change in contour. Direct pressure on the implantation site such as carrying a heavy object against it should be avoided.

With support from the nurse, physician, and family, the patient will be helped to become more secure and to understand that the pacemaker, rather than imposing limitations, maximizes the potential for cardiac rehabilitation. It often allows participation in social, occupational, and recreational activities which would be restricted in its absence.

## REFERENCES AND BIBLIOGRAPHY

### The Patient with a Cardiac Arrhythmia

AMSTERDAM, E. A., et al.: Use of bretylium tosylate in the management of cardiac arrhythmias, *Heart Lung* 1:269, March-April 1972.

ANDERSON, B.: Legal aspects of nursing care for cardiac patients, *Cardiovasc. Nurs.* 5:5, March-April 1969.

ANDREOLI, K., et al.: *Comprehensive Cardiac Care,* ed. 2, St. Louis, Mosby, 1971.

AZEVEDO, I., et al.: Reassessment of A-V junctional arrhythmias, *Heart Lung* 1:626, September-October 1972.

CASTELLANOS, A., and LEMBERG, L.: *Electrophysiology of Pacing and Cardioversion,* New York, Appleton-Century-Crofts, 1969.

DRUSS, R., and KORNFELD, D.: The survivors of cardiac arrest (a psychiatric study), *JAMA* 201:75, July 1967.

FISCH, C.: Electrophysiologic basis of clinical arrhythmias, *Heart Lung* 3:51, January-February 1974.

GANS, J. A.: Cardiac drugs today: Part 4. Antiarrhythmic drugs, *Nurs. '73* 3:29, August 1973.

GREEN, H.: Hazards of electronic equipment in critical care areas: A research approach, *Cardiovasc. Nurs.* 9:7, March-April 1973.

GROLLMAN, A.: How drugs work: The antiarrhythmics, *Consultant* 13:67, September 1973.

GUYTON, A.: *Textbook of Medical Physiology,* ed. 4, Philadelphia, Saunders, 1971.

JOHNSON, J.: Can you pass a test of life and death? *Emerg. Med.* 1:26, August 1969.

KLEIGER, R., and WOLFE, G.: Indications and contra-indications for cardioversion for arrhythmias, *Heart Lung* 2:552, July-August 1973.

LONG, M. L., et al.: Complications of central venous pressure monitoring: Cardiac arrhythmias and conduction disturbances, *Heart Lung* 2:416, May-June 1973.

MARRIOTT, H.: *Practical Electrocardiography,* ed. 5, Baltimore, Williams & Wilkins, 1972.

————, and FOGG, E.: Constant monitoring for cardiac dysrhythmias and blocks, *Mod. Conc. Cardiovasc. Dis.* 39:103, June 1970.

MELTZER, L., and DUNNING, A.: *Textbook of Coronary Care,* Philadelphia, Charles Press, 1972.

REGAN, W.: The new standing orders and their legal pitfalls, *RN* 31:38, April 1968.

RODMAN, M.: Drugs used in cardiovascular disease. Managing cardiac emergencies. Part 1, *RN* 36:71, March 1973.

ROSENBAUM, M.: The hemiblocks: Diagnostic criteria and clinical cardiology, *Mod. Conc. Cardiovasc. Dis.* 39:141, December 1970.

STUCKEY, J.: Atropine in bradycardia in the coronary-care unit and elsewhere, *Heart Lung* 2:666, September-October 1973.

UNGVARSKI, P., et al.: CPR-Current practice revisited. Basic life support. Advanced life support, *Am. J. Nurs.* 75:236, February 1975.

WINSOR, T.: The electrocardiogram in myocardial infarction, *Ciba Clin. Symp.* 20:107, October-November-December 1968.

WOLF, S.: Central autonomic influences on cardiac rate and rhythm, *Mod. Conc. Cardiovasc. Dis.* 38:29, June 1969.

### The Patient with an Artificial Pacemaker

BAIN, B.: Pacemakers and the patients who need them, *Am. J. Nurs.* 71:1582, August 1971.

BARSTOW, R.: Nursing care of patients with pacemakers, *Cardiovasc. Nurs.* 8:7, March-April 1972.

BELLING, D.: Nursing care of patients with mechanical cardiac pacemakers, *Nurs. Clin. N. Am.* 7:509, September 1972.

*Current Concepts of Cardiac Pacing and Cardioversion.* A Symposium, Philadelphia, Charles Press, 1971.

Defibrillation and external pacemakers, *Medtronic News* 2:3, 1971.

ESCHER, D.: Medical aspects of artificial pacing of the heart, *Cardiovasc. Nurs.* 8:1, January-February 1972.

FURMAN, S., and ESCHER, D.: *Principles and Techniques of Cardiac Pacing,* New York, Harper and Row, 1972.

GERMAIN, C. P.: The patient with a pacemaker, Chap. 7 in McIntyre, M. (ed.): *Heart Disease: New Dimensions of Nursing Care,* Garden Grove, Cal., Trainex Press, 1974.

————, and HANLEY, M. P., SR.: Metronome for a music teacher, *Am. J. Nurs.* 68:498, March 1968.

GREEN, W., and MOSS, A. J.: Psychological factors in the adjustment of patients with permanently implanted cardiac pacemakers, *Ann. Intern. Med.* 70:897, 1969.

KOS, B., and CULBERT, P.: Teaching patients about pacemakers, *Am. J. Nurs.* 71:523, March 1971.

MERKEL, R., and SOVIE, M.: Electrocution hazards with transvenous pacemaker electrodes, *Am. J. Nurs.* 68:2510, 1967.

Microwave oven effects on pacemakers, *Medtronic News* 2:4, 1970. (See also *JAMA* 212, No. 7, May 18, 1970.)

PARSONNET, V., et al.: Current views of indications, results, and complications of cardiac pacemakers, Chap. 41 in Russek, H., and Zohman, B. (eds.): *Cardiovascular Therapy: The Art and the Science,* Baltimore, Williams & Wilkens, 1971.

PENNOCK, R., et al.: Cardiac pacemaker function, *JAMA* 222:1379, 1972.

PRESTON, T. A., et al.: Management of stimulation and sensing problems in temporary cardiac pacing, *Heart Lung* 2:533, July-August 1973.

RAHMOELLER, G., and VEALE, J.: Pacing the heart electrically, *FDA Consumer* 18, November 1973.

SHILLING, E.: Pacemaker evaluation clinic, *Am. J. Nurs.* 73:1770, October 1973.

SPENCE, M., and LEMBERG, L.: Acute trifascicular block and congestive heart failure, *Heart Lung* 1:825, November-December 1972.

STERN, T.: Personal communication, Cardiac Data-corp, Inc.

WILLIAMS, C. D.: Exciting challenges in the future of pacemakers and clinics, *Heart Lung* 1:658, September-October 1972.

## Patient Education

*Living with Your Pacemaker,* New York, American Heart Association.

Patient information booklet on the pacemaker, Minneapolis, Minn., Medtronic, Inc.

# The Patient with Acute Myocardial Infarction

"Heart attack"—these two words often spell disaster for adults. Regardless of our level of sophistication in knowledge about the condition, as human beings we are all vulnerable to the threat of such a catastrophe or its actual occurrence.

A young man experiences severe chest pain and slumps over at his desk; an executive drops dead on the golf course; a father collapses in pain after an argument with a teen-aged son; an elderly female patient undergoing minor surgery has a hypotensive episode and awakens in a coronary care unit. All join the ranks of the 1.5 million people in the United States who yearly sustain acute myocardial infarction. Those who survive experience an acute disruption of their daily life activities. If they are fortunate to have an uneventful recovery, and make the adjustments to changed physical status, it is close to three months before normal activities can be resumed. Others are not so fortunate and may remain partially disabled with congestive heart failure, angina pectoris, or myocardial or emotional reserve below that necessary to resume their pre-infarction level of activity. All need the help and support of the health care team, families, employers, and friends to go on living as productively as possible. Some, who are able to use the time of prolonged rest in a constructive way philosophically, may be able to accept some losses and put new value on retained assets and thus continue to mature through the experience.

In myocardial infarction the interference with the blood supply to a portion of the muscle of the heart is so severe that necrosis of a part of the heart results. This may be precipitated by the occlusion of a coronary artery from capillary hemorrhage within an athero-sclerotic plaque or by the formation of a thrombus on one of the plaques. Myocardial infarction may occur without occlusion of an artery when there is a sudden reduction in the blood supply to the heart—for example, during shock or hemorrhage or during severe physical exertion—whenever, in fact, the need of the heart for blood is increased suddenly beyond that which the atherosclerotic arteries can deliver. Atherosclerosis is almost always the underlying cause of myocardial infarction. The narrowed, roughened vessels are very susceptible to obstruction.

## PATHOPHYSIOLOGY

The location of a myocardial infarction is most frequently in the left ventricle. The area of a myocardial infarction heals by scar tissue. The size of the scar determines the amount of cardiac reserve that is lost. Necrosis can extend through the thickness of the myocardial wall to the subendocardium (transmural infarction), involve part of the myocardium, or may just involve the subendocardial area which is furthest from the blood supply. Different terms are used to describe the area of the heart which is affected. For example, in most people the right coronary artery and its branches supply the posterior and inferior wall of the ventricle. Occlusion of this artery results in a so-called posterior wall or diaphragmatic infarction. Heart block is more common with this type of infarction because a branch of the right coronary vessel supplies the A-V node. The mortality rate associated with this is 40 per cent. Another branch supplies the S-A node.

The left coronary artery and its branches supply most of the anterior and apical portions of the left ventricle, the upper lateral left ventricular wall and left atrium, and the anterior portion of the interventricular septum. Infarctions from occlusion of these branches are termed anterior wall, or antero-septal. From 80 to 85 per cent of the coronary artery blood supply goes to the left coronary artery. If heart block results with occlusion of the left coronary artery system it generally means very extensive necrosis and 80 per cent mortality. The left anterior descending branch is termed the artery of sudden death.

Recurrent loss of myocardial cells (sequential small infarctions) with the formation of scar tissue eventually leads to congestive heart failure.

The stages of healing can be correlated with the period of restriction of cardiac workload. From the onset until about the third day, there is acute tissue degeneration and the infarct area is soft, mushy, and necrotic. It is dead tissue and therefore electrically inert. Dangerous arrhythmias are most apt to develop during this period, but they are thought to arise from the peri-infarction area which is ischemic and electrically unstable.

From the fourth to seventh days, softening of the infarcted area is greatest and there is danger of aneurysm formation. The weakened area in the ventricular wall may balloon out during systole. About the eighth to tenth day newly formed capillaries develop around the periphery of the infarct, but it is two to three weeks before there is a functionally significant collateral circulation.

Collagen begins to form about the twelfth day after the infarction. Rupture of the ventricle is likeliest during the first week. It is three to four weeks before the scar begins to grow firm and two to three months before a scar of maximum strength is formed.

## SYMPTOMS

The symptoms of myocardial infarction include sudden, severe pain in the chest, usually precordial or substernal, sometimes radiating to the shoulder and the arm, teeth, jaw, or throat, especially on the left side. The pain is more severe and of longer duration than that in angina pectoris, and it is not necessarily related to exertion. Patients sometimes describe it as "grinding" or "crushing" and so severe that every ounce of stamina is needed to endure it. Unlike that of angina pectoris, the pain of myocardial infarction is not relieved by rest or nitroglycerin. It may last several hours or as long as one or two days, and, finally, it becomes a soreness or an ache before it disappears entirely.

In some patients the pain is accompanied by symptoms of shock: pallor, sweating, faintness, a severe drop in blood pressure, and rapid, weak pulse brought about by sudden decrease in cardiac output.

It is not unusual for the patient to lose consciousness at the beginning of the attack and, as he regains consciousness, again to become aware of the excruciating pain in his chest. Sometimes the patient is more aware of feeling faint and weak than he is of chest pain. Nausea and vomiting may occur and lead the patient to believe that he is having an attack of acute indigestion.

The suddenness and severity of symptoms of acute

myocardial infarction have been described as being so stressful that primitive and virtually automatic responses to danger are aroused (Braceland, 1966). Fear and restlessness almost invariably occur, unless shock is so profound that the patient is unable to respond emotionally to the situation. Most patients are well aware of the seriousness of chest pain, and they are immediately apprehensive. Symptoms of left-sided heart failure—dyspnea, cyanosis, and cough—may appear if the pumping of the left ventricle is sufficiently impaired, and if congestion occurs in the lungs.

## FIRST AID

A nurse does not make a medical diagnosis; but understanding the possibility of myocardial infarction, knowing what to do, and, especially, what not to do, may save a patient's life. If the patient has had previous attacks of angina, he usually will have taken a nitroglycerin tablet and have stopped whatever he was doing. If these measures fail to relieve the pain within ten minutes, or if he has additional or atypical symptoms, he is kept at complete rest in the position most comfortable for him, and his physician called. If the physician cannot be reached immediately, as calmly as possible an ambulance should be summoned to take the patient to the nearest hospital emergency room. The nurse goes with the patient if possible. Cardiac arrest following acute myocardial infarction happens abruptly. The patient needs to be transferred as quickly as possible to a treatment facility where definitive measures such as defibrillation are available. Excessive emotion which results in the release of catecholamines into the blood (epinephrine and norepinephrine) can result in ventricular fibrillation. Because of this, the precautionary reasons for an ambulance ride and emergency room admission need to be explained to the patient in such a manner that he does not become more alarmed.

More than two-thirds of the 600,000 Americans who die each year of a myocardial infarction die before reaching a hospital. Sudden death is attributed in most cases to reversible ventricular fibrillation—excessive and uncoordinated electrical quivering of the ventricles arising from an irritable focus in ischemic tissue in the peri-infarction area. Cardiac output ceases and without adequate cerebral blood flow severe brain damage and death occur in three to four minutes. In many heart attack victims, at autopsy the heart muscle itself appears to be only minimally injured and the patient is said to have died from electrical failure rather than from pump or power failure. Sudden electrical deaths occur most often in younger men (and occasionally, women) who have not had the opportunity to develop collateral circulation. When their coronary artery occludes, myocardial hypoxia and other biochemical phenomena in the infarcted area lead to serious arrhythmias.

The majority of deaths from acute myocardial infarction occur in the first four hours after the onset of pain. Studies show that there is an average six- to ten-hour lapse in time between the onset of symptoms and admission to the hospital (A mobile CCU saves lives in New York City, *ICU* 3:12, 1969).

To prevent these out-of-hospital deaths, which often occur in young men with "hearts too good to die," a four-pronged approach becomes evident:

1. Prevention of coronary artery disease (see Chap. 36) and identification and treatment of those suspected to be coronary prone.
2. Education of the public to seek medical help promptly after the onset of characteristic symptoms. Preferably, this should be in a hospital with an emergency room and a coronary care unit where electrocardiographic monitoring and arrhythmia prophylaxis are continually available.
3. Bringing medical help to the stricken victim in the community in a fully equipped "mobile" coronary care unit or special ambulance, where, after stabilization of his condition, the victim can be transported under medical supervision to the hospital. A number of these mobile units are presently in operation while research is being carried out regarding their overall impact on the problem of sudden death.
4. Effective rehabilitation after an attack.

**Immediate Care.** Suggestions for the immediate care of any patient who experiences severe chest pains include:

- **The patient should be kept at complete rest. It is not helpful to get him undressed and into bed. Instead, he should rest in the position that is most comfortable for him. Any tight clothing, such as a collar and a belt, should be loosened so that it does not add to the patient's discomfort or interfere with his breathing. If he has dyspnea, he will be more comfortable with his head elevated. If he has symptoms of shock, he should be kept flat (provided that he experiences no respiratory distress). A blanket or coat can be used for warmth.**
- **A physician should be called immediately. Preferably, someone should remain with the patient. An immediate call for an ambulance may be indicated. The patient should not be permitted to get up and**

move about, even if he begins to feel better, until the physician has examined him. Above all, the patient should not undertake a trip home unattended.

• The pulse should be monitored at regular frequent intervals for rate, rhythm, and quality. If the patient has not suffered myocardial infarction, nothing will have been lost except a little time and effort. How much better is this kind of mistake than the feeling, "Oh, if I had only known how sick he was!"

• If the patient loses consciousness, go through the diagnostic ABC's of cardiac arrest (see Chap. 61), instituting cardiopulmonary resuscitative measures as indicated. (It is wise to have an oropharyngeal airway or resucitube in one's home or automobile for emergency use.) ECPR, properly performed, can pump sufficient blood to maintain the viability of the vital organs such as the brain, kidney, and heart until definitive medical therapy can be obtained. The longer the period of ECPR without definitive treatment, the poorer the patient's chances for survival.

## DIAGNOSTIC ASSESSMENT

The physician determines the diagnosis by history and physical examination and by certain special tests.

**A distinctive history** is a definite aid in diagnosis, but the medical history may be atypical. Diabetics frequently have atypical histories. Any additional data which the patient discloses in the nursing history should be shared with the physician. If the patient is anxious, which is often the case, he may not recall or may distort events leading up to his admission.

**Physical examination** includes nonauscultatory modes such as palpation with the fingers for heart size and vibrations (or thrills) as well as inspection of the chest. Auscultation of the heart and chest with the stethoscope can reveal heart murmurs, sounds of valve closure, changes in rhythm and rate, pericardial friction rub, and rales (moist, crackling sounds in the lungs). The presence of rales is an early finding in left ventricular failure and indicates pulmonary edema.

Auscultation of the heart and lungs at regular intervals should be performed by the prepared nurse so that treatment for heart failure can be instituted before the patient's condition deteriorates. Using the stethoscope the nurse can also detect rales and sudden heart murmurs which can indicate septal rupture or papillary muscle dysfunction. (See Chapters 29, 33, and 34 for physical assessment of the heart and lungs.)

**Electrocardiogram.** This is usually ordered promptly as soon as myocardial infarction is suspected, and it may be repeated several times (serial ECG's) in determining the diagnosis and in following the course of the illness.

**Laboratory Studies.** Necrosis of myocardial tissue results in the release of intracellular enzymes into the circulation. These enzymes are not specific for myocardial tissue alone, but are useful as a diagnostic aid in this as well as other conditions involving tissue damage. The CPK (creatine phosphokinase) and SGOT (serum glutamic oxalacetic transaminase) are especially used as indicators of the severity of tissue damage. Normal values vary according to laboratory methods.

The CPK begins to increase two to four hours after infarction, reaches its maximum in 24 to 36 hours, and returns to normal in three days. Intramuscular injections can also provoke a CPK elevation.

The SGOT begins to increase in 4 to 6 hours, reaches its maximum in 24 to 48 hours, and returns to normal in five days.

LDH (lactic dehydrogenase) may also be ordered. This enzyme begins to increase 8 to 10 hours after infarction, reaches its maximum in 48 to 72 hours, and returns to normal in 14 days. Shock, intramuscular injections, and congestive heart failure can also produce an elevated LDH.

Renewed damage to myocardial cells results in another increase in enzyme release (Coodley, 1967).

An elevated erythrocyte sedimentation rate and white blood cell count are less specific or valuable evidence of tissue necrosis in myocardial infarction.

**Temperature.** Fever is common after a day or so. Usually, it is low or moderate, and lasts four or five days. Fever is one of the body's responses to necrosis of tissue. The oral thermometer is most often used. Rectal temperature is most accurate, but is not used in some cardiac units because of the potential harm from vagal stimuli. The use of a well-lubricated rectal thermometer inserted gently with the patient in a comfortable, safe position should prevent harmful vagal stimulation which could result in cardiac slowing and the appearance of arrhythmias. Observing the cardiac monitor will indicate if another thermometer route should be used.

## THE CORONARY CARE UNIT

Some studies have shown that mortality of patients treated in specialized coronary care units has been reduced by at least one-third compared with traditional hospital care. Approximately 15 to 20 per cent of patients die compared with 30 to 35 per cent formerly. Today patients with chest pain or suspicious history of possible myocardial infarction are admitted to such a unit if one is available. For example, patients with cholecystitis, pericarditis, or pneumothorax may also be admitted with chest pain, and myocardial infarction has to be ruled out. Until all of the diagnostic data are available, patients are treated as if they have sustained an infarction. As many as 50 per cent of patients admitted to a well-managed CCU will not have a myocardial infarction.

The main purpose of the coronary care unit is to prevent death from complications following myocardial infarction, primarily arrhythmic or electrical deaths. Earlier emphasis was on the prompt institution of resuscitative measures. Today, however, the emphasis is on the prevention of the need for resuscitative measures by detecting early changes in the patient's condition. Thus all patients receive continuous close observation, including electrocardiographic monitoring for several days. The nursing staff receives specialized education in the early recognition of cardiac arrhythmias and other complications (Fig. 62-1). Prompt reporting of early warning signs enables the physician to institute treatment before complications become serious. Nursing care is directed toward the promotion of rest and healing, the prevention of complications, support of the patient through the experience, and the promotion of optimal rehabilitation.

The drama of the coronary care concept most often centers on heroic measures, "aggressive" treatment, and the numbers of lives saved. Just as dramatic and challenging to nursing, though in a different way, is the care of those patients who will not survive. One way to view the present statistics is that despite the current management of the patient in a well-operated CCU, one out of every five patients admitted and diagnosed as having a myocardial infarction will not live to be discharged from the hospital. Thus, coronary nursing embraces a wide range of intense human situations. The nurse who elects to work in the CCU views her role realistically when she realizes that a sizable aspect of it will be the care of patients and families facing the reality of death. If success is measured only by lives saved, then the death of a patient can be viewed as a failure. This view does not take into account human limitations. While giving the patient every advantage of knowledgeable and skilled care and

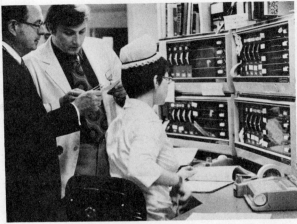

**Figure 62-1.** Nurse monitoring for cardiac arrhythmias enables prompt treatment to be instituted to prevent serious complications.

hope for his survival, one must come to grips with the fact that the best team efforts will not save all lives. The patient needs help to die with as much dignity as can be mustered out of the very gross realities of a resuscitation attempt in the event of sudden death; or sustained, listening, sensitive presence when his course is progressively downhill.

## ADMITTING THE PATIENT
### Nursing Assessment and Intervention

The same principles of nursing care apply whether the patient is admitted first to the emergency room and later transferred to the CCU or admitted directly to the CCU.

The appearance of the patient on admission can vary widely. He may neither look nor feel very ill, or he may be in deep cardiogenic shock. He may have received pain medication in his physician's office which gave relief, or he may be clutching his chest with muscle splinting of his shoulder and arm indicating severe pain. He may have a tachycardia—a normal response to abruptly leaving one's place of work in an ambulance with flashing lights and siren, or the tachycardia that means the early onset of heart failure. A bradycardia does not mean that the patient is not excited. Rather this can be an ominous sign of involvement of the S-A or A-V node or marked vagal tone. A slow rate can lead to myocardial hypoxia which fosters lethal cardiac arrhythmias. Vagal slowing of the heart can result from profound fear or drugs, such as morphine or digitalis. Slowing of the rate can mean the patient is in heart block if the A-V node is ischemic from the episode.

One patient may have a large area of muscle damaged; another, a relatively small area. The latter could, though, have more arrhythmic difficulty if the injury is in a critical site.

The common denominator of the group is that they all have had a close confrontation with death and are all prime candidates for cardiac arrest. All need a calm, confident, competent admitting nurse who can demonstrate by the way she greets the patient that he is in the best place for him to be under the circumstances. Frenzied activity and hurried or absent greeting or explanation only fosters the patient's feeling of disaster which can promote cardiac arrhythmias, including ventricular fibrillation. Time and speed are important, but they need to be tempered with an awareness of the patient's response to all that has happened and is happening about him so that more damage is not provoked. For example, it is understood that getting the patient on the cardiac monitor is important to assess his present condition and his response to drugs such as morphine or Demerol, and to detect lethal arrhythmias early. But ripping the alert patient's clothes apart and applying electrodes without warning or explanation can further activate the autonomic response to fright.

For each patient the admitting nurse has to determine priorities. Nursing intervention is based on an individual assessment. The life-saving activities always exert priority. Some other areas of nursing concern during the early admission period are:

- **Assisting the patient to bed and undressing him with minimal expenditure of effort. A roller placed next to the patient on the stretcher can be used so that the patient does not have to be lifted.**
- **Giving oxygen. Equipment ready for immediate use is at the bedside. Adequate oxygenation contributes to the relief of pain and the prevention of arrhythmias. Physicians differ in opinion regarding routine oxygen administration. Patients who are dyspneic, tachycardic, or cyanotic are given oxygen as an emergency measure. The danger is that some emergency patients, unknown to the local physician and nursing staff, may have chronic obstructive lung disease. Giving oxygen routinely at high concentration may result in respiratory arrest by depriving the patient of the hypoxic stimulus to respiration. Asking the patient or family promptly on admission if he has lung disease is necessary. Unit policies should offer guidelines for action. For example, oxygen may be**

given at a lowered concentration and the physician promptly notified. The patient's response is carefully observed. If he becomes pink, but increasingly drowsy without drugs, this is an emergency sign! (See Chap. 60.)
- **Placing chest electrodes for cardiac monitoring.**
- **Relieving pain. It is imperative to relieve pain, which is often severe, crushing, and the source of great fear. Arrhythmias and shock can follow severe pain. Also, arrhythmias and hypotension can follow the administration of a drug such as morphine given to relieve pain. Atropine is sometimes ordered to be given with morphine to prevent bradycardia and other vagal effects. A slow sinus rate with myocardial ischemia or hypoxia allows irritable sites in the ventricle to escape as potential primary pacemakers. The patient needs immediate treatment for escape or premature ventricular beats, but the treatment depends on the cause. Generally escape ventricular ectopic foci can be suppressed if the sinus pacemaker is kept above a minimal level. Premature ventricular beats (PVB's), on the other hand, are generally treated by a myocardial depressant such as lidocaine.**

The patient's response to the pain-relieving drug must be closely monitored. If he is not relieved in an hour the physician is called back. Often the pain is so severe that the narcotic does not completely relieve it, but makes it less intense and more bearable. Usually, the narcotic is given every three to four hours, as it is necessary, during the period when the pain is severe. Any depression of respiration, nausea, arrhythmias, and hypotension should be noted, particularly when morphine is given. The drug is given as often as it is required and permitted to control the pain. The period during which narcotics are needed usually lasts no more than one or two days; yet it is during this period that rest and the relief of apprehension are especially important.

Sometimes a patient is hesitant to accept narcotics for pain. If it is because he is allergic to certain drugs or has had an idiosyncratic reaction in the past, the physician should be notified so that another drug order can be obtained. On the other hand, the patient may fear addiction, or he may think that by accepting drugs frequently he is acknowledging how really sick he is. He may need help to cope with these thoughts and feelings but, in a state of severe pain, is hardly in a position to discuss them. The younger American male may be culturally habituated to thinking that complaining of pain is "sissy." In view of the blow to his virility that an acute infarction often engenders, he may try to prove (unconsciously) that he can grin and bear it.

There are times when words are not a substitute for action. If the patient is hesitant to accept medication for pain when it is objectively indicated, and he is not allergic, explain to the patient that you will give the drug as the physician ordered, but will discuss the situation with him when he obtains relief.

Oxygen should be given also since pain may be due to hypoxia and accumulation of metabolites in the infarcted area.

- **Intravenous infusion.** Because intravenous medications are commonly used to suppress arrhythmias and because cardiovascular collapse is an always-present threat, each myocardial infarction suspect has an intravenous route opened at admission and an infusion started to keep the vein opened. In an emergency, drugs can be quickly given and time is not wasted while a physician attempts to do a cut-down on a collapsed vein.

- **12-lead electrocardiogram.** This can be quickly taken by the nurse during the early admission period. Though the results do not markedly influence nursing care at this point (since all patients are treated with the same precautions) the record serves as a basis for later comparison and immediate arrhythmia treatment.

- **Observation of the patient** is an ongoing process initiated when the nurse first greets the patient. It is well to remember that observation is a two-way process—the patient also observes the nurse. How she looks and acts as she greets the patient gives him a message. Is she full of fear for him, and does this show in her eyes, her grim expression? Is she annoyed that he arrived at the change of shift and is her manner less than gentle when she undresses him or applies electrodes? Does she dart out of the room to the telephone when his ECG appears on the oscilloscope? How the nurse confronts the patient during this period can influence the entire course of his illness. He can get from her a message of hope, warm caring, competence, and concern or one that is cold, impersonal, pessimistic, scolding, or panicky. This capacity to sense feeling from another is called empathic observation.

Using one's sensory apparatus skillfully can quickly give much data:

1. **Eyes.** What does the patient look like? What is his color? Is he splinting his shoulder muscles from pain? Is he working hard to breathe (dyspneic)? Does he have a calm or apprehensive look in his eyes? Is he alert or somnolent? Are his neck veins distended? What does the oscilloscope show? What does the sphygmomanometer read?

2. **Ears.** What do you hear? Are the patient's respirations wheezing or stentorous? What are his baseline heart and lung sounds? These are used for immediate treatment or later comparison. What does the patient have to say? Is he in pain? If talking does not distress him further, he is asked what happened that brought him to the hospital. What questions does he have about the unit, the equipment, his condition?

3. **Touch.** Is the patient's skin cold and clammy? Warm and dry? Is there good skin turgor? What is the quality of his radial pulse? Full and bounding? Weak and thready? Is his abdomen or bladder distended?

4. **Smell.** What odors emanate from the patient? Does his breath smell like alcohol (the old home remedy for pain and other emergencies)? Is there the sweet fruity odor of diabetic acidosis? Is there the odor of perspiration? Of excreta?

Patients' needs for information and discussion vary widely. Today multimedia accounts of medical advances are readily available to the lay person, hence, patients generally are well informed. Even in the initial period after infarction, as pain subsides, some patients want answers to questions about risk factors, new equipment, and even cardiac arrest. A challenging aspect of nursing care is to answer questions accurately or, if the answer is not known by the nurse, to acknowledge this and suggest ways in which the patient can find the answers he is seeking. To give inaccurate information or to deny the patient's need for answers shows a lack of respect and can be destructive of the patient's confidence in the nursing staff.

Most patients can cope with their anxiety better if they are kept intellectually informed. Knowing why tests or treatments are done or obtaining information about their disease affords them some element of participation in and therefore control over life events. Other patients prefer to know very little and benefit from trusting their care without question to competent people who will make decisions for them.

How slowly or fast is the patient speaking? What is the pitch of his voice? What is the subject of his conversation? Is he talking about relatives who have died? Or relatives who have had heart attacks?

Does he have a language or other communication barrier? If the patient can't talk, who is the temporary voice for the patient? Did a relative or neighbor or employer bring him in to the hospital? What do they know about the incident or his past history?

Listening is an art. One patient may desperately need to express his fears immediately. Another may not have this need immediately, but it may appear later in the convalescent period. The nurse offers the opportunity for expression in such a way that the patient can feel free to take it or leave it in his own best interests.

Questions. In addition to the routine hospital admission procedures, some specific questions that should be asked the patient or family are:

What allergies does the patient have? Is he allergic to procaine (or Novocain)? The related drug lidocaine (Xylocaine) may be ordered for him if he has ventricular arrhythmias. An affirmative response should be discussed with the physician.

Does the patient have glaucoma? (Atropine sulfate, which increases intraocular pressure, is a frequently used drug in the coronary care unit.) Does he take eyedrops; a diuretic such as acetazolamide (Diamox) or chlorothiazide (Diuril)?

Is the patient a diabetic? The diabetic frequently has an atypical response to myocardial infarction. Does he take insulin or an oral hypoglycemic agent? When was the last dose taken? What has he eaten since?

Has the patient been taking anticoagulants, nitroglycerin, digitalis, or other cardiac drugs? When was the last dose taken? What other cardiac remedies are used? For example, one patient had a history of paroxysmal atrial tachycardia. To abort each attack the physician taught him to do a Valsalva maneuver to bring about vagal stimulation and slow the heart rate. In his present state of myocardial infarction, runs of ventricular tachycardia gave him the same sensation as PAT and he, from habit, dangerously reacted by doing the Valsalva maneuver.

What other drugs has the patient been taking that shouldn't be stopped? Examples are steroids and diphenylhydantoin (Dilantin) for epilepsy. Dilantin is also used as an antiarrhythmic drug.

Obtaining answers to these questions is a collaborative task of the physician and nurse. For example, the patient may arrive from the physician's office with some of this information written down. Or, the nurse may ask these questions if the patient is relatively unknown to the medical staff, or if the physician is not present, but has issued some emergency treatment orders. Medical and nursing staff then share pertinent information.

- Spiritual care. Generally all patients who are myocardial infarction suspects are listed as "critical." One role of the nurse is to expedite the availability of the patient's spiritual advisor. The suggestion of spiritual help from a clergyman of the patient's religion should be offered to the patient, or the family should be consulted regarding the patient's religious affiliation and usual practices if the patient is too ill to be questioned. The clergyman can be informed of the patient's emotional state prior to his visiting the patient, if this is significant. A study indicated that the suggestion of the reception of the Sacrament of the Sick by the priest to Catholic patients with myocardial infarction was more consoling than frightening (Cassem, 1969). The clergyman can also be supportive of the family during this time of crisis.
- Diet. Oral intake is restricted until specific orders are received. Because of the risk of cardiac arrest and aspiration, as well as the increased cardiac workload from digestion, intake for the critical period of the first three days is generally restricted to a clear to full liquid diet. Iced water or iced beverages are contraindicated because they are vagal stimulants. Coffee and tea contain stimulants which may increase heart rate and may also be restricted. Carbonated beverages are not served because they promote gaseous distention.

A low-calorie, low-cholesterol diet is now advocated in early convalescence as an educational exercise for future life style changes.

## OBJECTIVES OF CARE

Most of the time when the myocardial infarction patient arrives at the hospital, the heart damage has been done. The infarction can be extended, however, or other complications can develop. The objectives of care include the reduction of cardiac workload to prevent further damage and promote healing. This is accomplished through a program of optimal rest. Optimal rest includes helping the patient and family to accept and adjust to the experience. Successfully integrating it into his life experience is the foundation for effective rehabilitation.

### Rest and Activity

Optimal rest is a broad concept. Studies have shown that putting a patient to bed is not synonymous with putting him to rest. Prolonged bed rest favors the development of many complications which at worst can prove fatal, or at best prolong convalescence (Browse, 1965; Olson, 1967). Preventive measures, such as deep breathing and foot or leg exercises, aimed specifically at reducing the hazards of immobility, and a bowel hygiene program, are essential if the chief treatment of infarction—rest—is not to become a liability.

Unlike a broken leg which can be immobilized in plaster, the heart can never be immobilized. It works all the time, even when injured. It rests only during diastole. Therefore, the treatment of cardiac arrhythmias which adversely affect cardiac hemodynamics, or the use of a drug such as digitalis to enhance cardiac systole and the diastolic or resting period of the cardiac cycle, affords rest for the heart in the broad sense.

Levine and his colleagues (1966) who are proponents of the chair rest treatment of myocardial infarction advocate it on the physiologic basis that the heart works less in the sitting position than in the recumbent position. From the first day after infarction the patient is assisted (not lifted) to a chair placed next to the bed where he remains until fatigued. Time in the chair is gradually increased. Only cardiogenic shock, severe pain requiring narcotics which are apt to induce bradycardia, or blood pressure too low for adequate cerebral blood flow are contraindications. The patient is said to benefit from the reduced cardiac workload and reduction of anxiety associated with the hopelessness of long-term confinement to bed. Replication of the original study showed that "chair rest" as a treatment had no adverse effects on cardiovascular function. Hypotension, arrhythmias, vasovagal reactions, or other complications were not increased. Measures to prevent the complications of prolonged rest are necessary whether the patient is in a bed or a chair. The patient is permitted no more activity in the chair than he would be if confined to bed (Schmitt, et al., 1969).

The type of chair recommended is one with a straight backrest so that the buttocks do not sink down. The thighs should be parallel to the floor, or slanting downward. A slightly angled foot support may be used to allow comfortable extension of the legs.

Though the physician may order the chair or the bed or both, rest cannot be ordered. Nursing care assists the patient to find rest. The anxious, or fearful, or angry patient, or one under other strong emotion, may be pouring out catecholamines (epinephrine or norepinephrine) and subjecting his heart to the vigors of physical exercise though he may be sitting quietly in bed or in a chair. Appropriate precautions should be taken to protect patients who are allowed some activity. For example, to reduce electrical hazard only a battery-operated electric shaver should be used if the patient is attached to a cardiac monitor or some other device utilizing wall current.

The nurse finds out from the physician specifically what the patient may and may not do. This information is shared with every member of the nursing staff caring for the patient by appropriate notation on the nursing care plan so that one person does not let the patient feed himself at breakfast, while another, who arrives at lunch time, insists that he be fed. The patient often needs help to accept his plan of treatment. If he wonders why he is not treated the same way as the patient in the next bed or across the hall, he can be told that the conditions of no two patients are exactly alike, and that therefore the plan of treatment will differ.

Certain principles apply to a program of rest, regardless of the exact program that has been prescribed: The patient is not permitted to exert himself. Straining at stool is one common example. Knowing the patient's usual bowel routine and helping him to maintain it in the hospital if it does not violate any physiologic principles is one way to help the patient avoid constipation. The physician should be consulted regarding the use of stool softeners.

Studies have shown that the use of the bedside commode involves less energy expenditure than getting on and off and using the bedpan (Benton, et al., 1950). The risk of inadvertently performing the Valsalva maneuver is minimized. The patient still requires assistance in cleansing himself after defecation.

To avoid straining and bladder distention some physicians permit their male patients to stand at the side of the bed to void. A male orderly is an asset to assist them, especially elderly patients. Sometimes male patients suffer from urinary stream hesitancy if a female nurse is in the room. The patient should be given privacy, but assured that assistance is available when he is getting back to bed.

The Valsalva maneuver can also be accomplished when pushing oneself up in bed. Since it is sometimes physically impossible to move patients precisely when they wish to be moved, patients should be instructed to avoid the Valsalva maneuver by exhaling rather than holding the breath when moving in bed.

- Things are placed within easy reach—the glass of water, the radio, the call bell—so that the patient does not have to use effort to reach them.
- If the patient strenuously objects to certain activity restrictions, the nurse should consult the physician, who may permit more flexibility, or who may be more effectively persuasive than the nurse. Refusal to accept activity restrictions is sometimes a manifestation of denial. Since this is an unconscious defense against anxiety, reasoning with the patient often does not help. Attempting to force restrictions can only increase the patient's anxiety and cardiac workload. The physician may order sedation. The patient needs the nonjudgmental support of the nurse and family during this overwhelming adjustment period. Threatening or scolding increase his need for dangerous defense mechanisms. Supportive listening can reduce anxiety and the need for denial and gradually assist the patient to begin to acknowledge what has happened.
- The patient as well as the cardiac rhythm are observed during changes of activity. Physical and emotional strain (such as from an upsetting visitor) can be reflected in cardiac arrhythmias as well as increased pain, pulse rate, dyspnea. The nurse then uses her judgment in slowing down or eliminating the activity temporarily, then discussing it with the physician.
- Nursing care should be organized so that the patient is disturbed as little as possible. If medicines, TPR, and back care are needed at 4 P.M., they should be

done together, and the patient permitted to rest until supper time.

- If care is needed that may tire the patient, it is done slowly, with allowance for rest periods during care. Giving a bath and changing the bed may be fatiguing if they are undertaken all at once. In a well-staffed coronary unit, the bath can be given at any time of the day, according to the need and preference of the patient. Some patients who are not culturally accustomed to a daily bath may find this upsetting and consequently fatiguing. Attention to the essentials of skin hygiene to prevent complications such as skin breakdown from perspiration and pressure, along with mouth care, is sufficient during the critical period. Other patients may become upset if they do not have a daily bath. During illness the patient's cultural habits should be supported to the extent possible, even if they may be disagreeable to the nurse.
- There has been a gradual progression toward less stringent curtailment of activity following acute myocardial infarction (Harrison and Reeves, 1968). Today in many units patients without complications are permitted to start a program of conditioning exercises, self-care activities, and educational and craft activities in the coronary care unit (Phase I), gradually increasing energy expenditure levels during the remainder of hospitalization (Phase II) (Wenger, 1973).

The incidence of depression, venous thrombosis, and/or orthostatic hypotension has been reduced through the early mobilization of patients with diseases formerly treated by prolonged bed rest. The more scientific approach involves the prescription of various activities according to their energy expenditure level as well as the patient's response (see Chap. 39).

### Sedation

Sedatives or tranquilizers are sometimes ordered after narcotics are no longer necessary for pain. These drugs should facilitate the patient's rest and relaxation, but should not make him so somnolent that he no longer initiates deep breathing, leg exercises, or moving in bed. Older patients, especially, may have paradoxical reactions to sedative drugs and become hyperactive.

Prolonged deep sedation only postpones, but does not erase, the patient's need to deal with the realities of his situation. However, some believe that postponing discussion beyond the dangerous period of cardiac arrhythmias (the first three days) is beneficial, and therefore the patient is kept sedated and the nurse is advised to postpone encouraging discussion.

Others believe that since the patient's cardiac rhythm is being monitored, he can be given the opportunity to discuss what he wishes. The nurse's role is primarily that of a thoughtful, sensitive listener. If the nurse notes that arrhythmias or other signs of anxiety such as restlessness or hyperventilation appear as the patient talks about what is bothering him, then she can suggest temporarily stopping the discussion while the patient gets some rest and resuming the discussion at a later time. Sedation may be warranted as well as other rest-promoting nursing measures. The nurse who says she will come back later should do so. Relatively short periods should be allotted for conversation with the patient during the acute period so that he does not become fatigued. Frequent observation of the patient offers support and reassurance through the nurse's physical presence.

Sometimes signs of increasing anxiety are provoked by certain visitors, medical rounds (especially when a number of physicians physically examine the patient), or other persons or activities. Individual adjustments need to be made so that the patient's rest is insured. Other patients, especially elderly ones or those with language barriers, may be less anxious if visiting hours are more flexible and liberal.

### Observation

Observation and accurate reporting are essential. The location and the intensity of the chest pain, or whether there are any symptoms of dyspnea or cyanosis, should be carefully noted. Are physical or emotional activities associated with pain and/or arrhythmias? Absence of pain is not necessarily an indication that the patient is recovering. When the affected myocardial tissues die, the nerves in that portion of myocardium can no longer transmit impulses to the brain, and the pain ceases. Sometimes nurses are lulled into a false sense of security when the patient's pain abates or there is normal sinus rhythm. Vigilance cannot be relaxed; patients with myocardial infarction are disposed to sudden changes in their condition.

The patient's TPR and blood pressure are observed carefully. The temperature usually is taken every four hours. The rate and the quality of the pulse are noted. Blood pressure readings usually are ordered every two hours for the first several days. Intake and output are carefully noted for all patients for the first three days and longer if the patient has symptoms of congestive heart failure, or if shock has been severe.

(See Chaps. 34, 59, and 61 for specific observations regarding arrhythmias and their treatment, congestive heart failure, and cardiogenic shock.)

## Environment

Contrary to some presentations, a well-managed coronary care unit is not a noisy, hectic place with a continuous life-death drama. The principle of the unit is to prevent the drama of resuscitation efforts by close observation and early treatment of complications. There is an element of heightened awareness and periods of sustained tension because changes can occur suddenly. Since the primary principle of treatment for the patient with myocardial infarction is rest, ideally the hospital area where coronary patients are admitted should be separate from, but may be adjacent to, the surgical or medical intensive care area.

Though the patient may have a familiarity with the idea of a coronary care unit, coming upon it as he does abruptly and in the role of patient may make him more bewildered if he notices its difference compared with usual hospital wards. He may ask specific or general questions but due to his anxiety answers may have to be repeated on other occasions. He may initially distort what is in his environment. The greater the understanding the patient has of the purpose and function of the mechanical devices that surround him, the less fearful he is apt to be. Some questions need general answers. For example, if the patient asks "How long will I be here?" a general but frank response can be, "I don't know exactly. It depends on how things go for you and also on your doctor's recommendations. The laboratory tests take at least three days."

The more pleasant the overall environment of the CCU, the more orientation and diversionary devices that are in it such as calendars, clocks, artwork, and the opportunity for privacy, the greater the opportunity for the patient to maintain his orientation and emotional balance, as compared with a unit having a "fish-bowl" or "space-age" appearance.

## Emotional Support

The patient who suffers a myocardial infarction is beset by many fears. Among them are the fear of death and the fear of living with impending death. The patient must cope with these as well as threats to his physical integrity, change in body image and self-concept, sexual adequacy, loss of status at work, possible reduction of income or even loss of job, loss of prestige in social life, restriction of favorite activities, loss of ability to care for his or her family at least temporarily, and a potentially formidable barrier to the accomplishment of life goals. Many patients, because of early experiences, associate a heart attack with automatic and permanent invalidism. Though new therapies are available to aid recovery and assist in optimal rehabilitation, the patient's fears are not unfounded since heart attack is a major cause of mortality and morbidity.

All of the above threats to personal integrity—biological, psychological, and social—are so stressful that great anxiety is generated. Anxiety also arises from the appearance of symptoms which can signify sudden death to the patient—dyspnea, severe chest pain, or severe weakness. To cope with the anxiety, the patient unconsciously resorts to a level of defense mechanisms which he has matured beyond that needed when he is not under severe stress. The use of this level of defense is for most patients temporary; defenses such as denial, failure either to perceive what is happening or to respond emotionally to it; displacement of the sense of danger onto trivial issues such as food service; projection of the danger onto the family or even the staff; aggressive sexual behavior—all can be viewed as protective devices which can be removed when need for them is reduced.

Evidence of physical improvement, appropriate emotional support from staff and family, time, and the opportunity to express pentup emotions, thus making the experience less dreadful and easier to face, are factors which promote acceptance of the reality of the situation. The groundwork for rehabilitation depends upon acceptance, adjustment, and integration of the illness. Just when these initial defense mechanisms are let go by the patient depends on his preillness personality and the kind of care he receives. For some, this may occur in the coronary care unit; for others sometime later in the hospital stay, or after discharge. For successful rehabilitation, however, preferably sometime in the hospital experience the patient must face the realities of the event and take constructive steps to deal with them. Some patients may be able to accomplish this with little help from others; many are

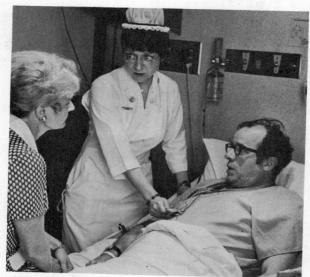

**Figure 62-2.** The myocardial infarction patient derives a sense of closeness from his wife's presence during a teaching session.

helped through nurse-led group sessions which may include spouses or other significant persons as well. All, however, need the help of a person who can listen to the expression of the thoughts and feelings about the fear of dying, family relationships, and changes in physical and job status. The nurse is in a unique position to help since she is with the patient so often, has an opportunity to build rapport through frequent contact with him, and is the only team member readily available to the patient when his usual resources are absent from the environment. The physician, clergyman, or friend can also function in a counseling role.

Prolonged use of inappropriate or harmful defense mechanisms gets in the way of other life goals such as work or home life. Therefore, the nurse needs to know what coping response the patient is employing, when to support it, and when and how, in collaboration with other members of the health care team, to intervene (Scalzi, 1973).

Patients with prolonged or inappropriate responses may require psychotherapy. Denial of the fact of illness or the feelings connected with it is initially a helpful response against overwhelming anxiety and should generally be supported during the emergency phase. Prolonged denial can lead the patient to perform restricted physical activities, thus threatening and restricting his life. Threats are not helpful. Listening to the patient's expression of feelings, conveying concern, allow-

ing more participation in decision making or reaching compromises regarding unprescribed activities are ways in which the nurse and physician can help the patient to cope. Denial is common during the preadmission phase and on the first and second hospital days.

The patient can be angry at the blow fate has struck him. He can express this in one way by showing exaggerated annoyance at things like cold food and the many interruptions, or by being critical of the staff. Or, he can turn his anger against himself and become markedly depressed. A certain amount of regression is natural and necessary and it can help the patient accept his forced initial role of dependence. But if prolonged, the desire to be taken care of can lead to needless chronic invalidism.

Some patients who are admitted to the CCU on an emergency basis want to sign themselves out of the hospital when they feel better physically. This usually occurs early in the hospital stay before the results of tests are returned and when the diagnosis of myocardial infarction is still uncertain. The physician should be notified immediately. Sometimes this is a manifestation of extreme denial; or it may be motivated by the pressure of reponsibilities to family or job. Threats of further damage if the diagnosis of myocardial infarction should be confirmed are often not helpful in inducing the patient to stay. The prepared nurse or other person with special counseling skills can help by finding out what the motivating factors are and seeking ways to offer immediate help, such as through referral to a social service agency. This may help the patient to reconsider. Often the physician speaks to the key people in the patient's life such as spouse, children, or clergyman to seek their assitance in persuading the patient to stay. When these measures fail some type of plan for care at home should be devised, such as through a community nursing agency. A refusal of treatment on the part of the patient may result in anger and frustration on the part of the physician.

Cassem and Hackett (1973) suggest that *depression* is usual following myocardial infarction, occurring around the third or fourth day in response to the realization that the heart has been damaged. Depression may be manifested by a look of sadness, expressions of hopelessness or futility, withdrawal, slowness in movement or speech, loss of appetite, or crying. The nurse can encourage the expression of feelings and relate to the patient that his feeling is usual for this phase of his illness and that crying or expressions of anger are acceptable. Diversionary materials such as radio, TV, or reading matter, or the addition or limitation of visitors may be helpful. Cassem and Hackett emphasize, however, that the most potent antidote to depression is return to physical activity, which should begin in a systematic way at least by the third day.

*Aggressive sexual behavior* by the male patient, either verbal or physical, such as deliberate exposure of the genitals or attempts to fondle the nurse, are viewed as attempts to counteract anxiety resulting from threats to sexual adequacy, loss of self-sufficiency and self-esteem, and decreased physical strength. Nursing intervention is based on an assessment of what the patient is seeking by his behavior. Discussing his behavior with him gives the nurse clues regarding ways that he can be helped to cope with his anxiety in a way more acceptable in our society. If the behavior makes the nurse uncomfortable or is unacceptable by her standards, she can with understanding and compassion honestly and simply tell the patient this. He may not be at all aware of the effects of his behavior. The patient's demonstration of his sexuality is a way of seeking reassurance of his manhood (sometimes unconsciously motivated) by evoking a response in the nurse; the nurse should also assess her own behavior and dress to see if it is provocative.

Ignoring the patient's behavior because of the nurse's discomfort can lead to staff isolation of the patient at a time when he is most in need of support, and may lead to an increase in the problematic behavior and more rejection—a vicious cycle.

Faced with many potential losses, small wonder that patients studied in a coronary care unit were found to experience many disturbing feelings—anxiety, anger, sorrow, depression, bitterness, clinginess, demandingness, and hopelessness (Sobel, 1969). This last feeling, intermittent hopelessness, was found to be the most difficult for the patient and for the nursing staff to deal with. An appropriate response by the staff to this feeling was derived from the simple truth that we do not know that a patient's situation is hopeless and that all of our medical knowledge and skills are employed to help him because there is some hope. The patient may persist in the feeling, but perhaps that is because there is a physiologic or other signal indicating his own demise. It was thought that the major

part of the struggle with hopelessness remained the patient's task to resolve. Helpful nursing action includes the capacity to confront the patient openly and humanly, to empathize with his situation, to think and feel about it and not turn away from him or rush to intervene in his painful human circumstance over which the nurse has little control. Being oneself with the patient involves honesty and frankness. Being able to say to a patient, "The other patient died," rather than "He was transferred," respects the patient's maturity and his capacity to employ defenses against facts which, temporarily, at least, are intolerable to him.

Recent reports indicate that survivors of cardiac arrest do not experience the chronic anxiety and emotional invalidism which was found among the initial studies done on survivors. There is a high degree of amnesia accompanying the experience. To avoid the need for fantasizing, Dobson, et al. (1971) advocate that the patient should be informed of his arrest at least by the next day. The patient can be told that his heart action was arrested and required assistance to resume its beat. The routine nature of the resuscitation should be stressed. The nurse can discuss with the patient his recollection of and feelings about the experience.

Inevitably some patients will die, many after a predictably downhill course. Assisting the patient to die with dignity is a formidable task in a coronary care unit where a resuscitation attempt is a general rule. Visitors and other patients become aware when such an attempt is in progress—from the increase in activity, numbers of personnel, and characteristic sounds. It is well for one staff member to be assigned to visit these people, explain what is happening, be responsive to their need to talk about the crisis, and stay with or find someone such as a clergyman to stay with them. Otherwise, a state of heightened anxiety pervades the environment with especially harmful physiologic and psychological consequences on other patients. The nurse can also use her judgment in permitting more flexible visiting routines for patients in extremely poor condition.

## TREATMENT OF COMPLICATIONS

**Arrhythmias. Disturbances of Heart Rate, Rhythm, and Conduction.** At least 80 per cent of myocardial infarction patients have some type of arrhythmia during the acute phase.

Over half of the deaths from myocardial infarction occur within 72 hours of admission to the hospital (Grace and Soscia, 1969). More than half of these deaths result from cardiac arrhythmias. Typically, the abnormal rhythm occurs suddenly within the first three days after the infarction, and it can be fatal within a few minutes. The arrhythmia can represent a transient abnormality in a heart that otherwise is capable of sustaining life and usual activity later. Consequently, prompt, effective treatment of arrhythmia assumes tremendous importance to the life of the patient. If he can be helped to survive the episode of ectopic rhythm, he may not die from myocardial infarction. (See Chapter 61 for nursing care and treatment of the patient with cardiac arrhythmias.)

**Venous Thrombosis.** This condition arises mostly in the veins of the lower extremities and pelvis. The exact cause is unknown. People who are ambulatory develop venous thrombosis also. Venous stasis, hypercoagulability of the blood, and external pressure against the veins, such as occurs in the side-lying position without a pillow between the legs, are thought to be involved. The use of elastic bandages, positioning pillows, foot and leg exercises on a regularly scheduled basis, and early return to physical activity are measures employed to prevent thrombus formation.

Some physicians treat all patients who have myocardial infarcts, regardless of the severity, with anticoagulants. Others reserve this treatment for patients whose heart damage has been severe, or for those who experience complications such as shock, congestive heart failure, or for the obese. Anticoagulants are given to decrease the likelihood of venous thrombosis and emboli and to prevent further increase in the size of a clot already formed.

Two types of anticoagulants may be given. Heparin prolongs the clotting time, thus decreasing the likelihood of clot formation; coumarin derivatives interfere with the utilization of vitamin K and prolong the prothrombin time, deterring the formation of clots. Often heparin and a coumarin derivative are administered simultaneously, since heparin takes effect promptly, whereas coumarin derivatives do not take effect for one or two days (Table 62-1).

When heparin is used the Lee-White test is done to determine the drug's effect on clotting time. Coagulation time is lengthened from the normal five to eight minutes to a therapeutic level of 30 to 60 minutes. If bleeding occurs, the antidote protamine sulfate is given. Blood transfusion may be necessary. Heparin can only be given parenterally. Because of heparin's predictable absorption and immediate action, as well as the pain incurred on subcutaneous injection, it is often given intravenously during the first few days of myocardial infarction. Hospital policy determines whether a physician or nurse actually injects the drug. A "heparin lock" permits dosages to be administered simply and painlessly at regular intervals. A pediatric scalp vein needle attached to polyethylene tubing is introduced percutaneously into a small arm vein and a 2-ml. syringe is attached to the catheter. The entire assembly is attached to the patient's arm. The catheter must remain filled with heparin between doses to prevent clotting.

Careful observation of prothrombin time is essential when coumarin derivatives are given. The nor-

**Table 62-1.  Commonly Used Anticoagulant Drugs**

| NONPROPRIETARY OR OFFICIAL NAME | TRADE NAME OR SYNONYM | INITIAL DOSE | MAINTENANCE DOSE | ONSET | PEAK EFFECT | DURATION |
|---|---|---|---|---|---|---|
| Bishydroxycoumarin U.S.P. | Dicumarol | 200–300 mg. | 25–200 mg.* | 24–72 hrs. | 36–48 hrs. | 5–6 days |
| Sodium Warfarin U.S.P. | Coumadin | 20–60 mg. | 2–10 mg.* | 24–36 hrs. | 36–72 hrs. | 4–5 days |
| Sodium Heparin Injection U.S.P. | | Bolus of 5,000 U.S.P. units IV | 10,000–30,000 units per liter by intravenous drip, 1 L. per 24 hrs., or with inlying needle, intermittent dose of 5,000–10,000 units every 4 to 6 hrs.; or 5,000–10,000 units into subcutaneous fatty tissues every 6-8 hrs.** | almost immediately | almost immediately | 4 hrs. |

*In accordance with prothrombin time determinations.
**In accordance with coagulation time.

mal prothrombin time is 14 to 18 seconds (Quick test). When coumarin derivatives are given, this is prolonged to approximately 24 to 30 seconds. If the prothrombin time is prolonged too much, there is danger of hemorrhage. The patient's prothrombin time is tested frequently throughout the period when anticoagulant therapy is given, and the dosage of the drug is adjusted accordingly. The usual procedure is for the physician to order one dose of the drug after checking the patient's prothrombin time. If the patient's prothrombin time is prolonged beyond 30 to 35 seconds, the anticoagulant usually is omitted on that day. Each order for an anticoagulant must be carefully obtained. One cannot assume that the drug ordered one day is to be repeated the next. Usually, only one dose at a time is ordered, such as "Coumadin 10 mg. today."

Considerable difference of opinion exists among physicians concerning the advisability of long-term anticoagulant therapy. If the patient is to continue anticoagulant treatment at home, it is often possible for the dosage to become so well regulated that tests of prothrombin time are needed only once a week, or at whatever interval ordered by the physician. It is essential for the patient to understand the importance of returning for tests of prothrombin time as long as he is taking the drug. The use of anticoagulants is dangerous unless it is carefully supervised by the physician or clinical nurse specialist. The patient is monitored for hematuria, ecchymoses (black and blue spots), bleeding gums, tarry stools, prolonged or excessive menstrual flow. If anticoagulant therapy is continued after the patient leaves the hospital, he is taught to watch for and to report promptly any unusual bleeding or tendency toward bruises. Large doses of aspirin may prolong the prothrombin time, and usual doses of ASA alter platelet function and thus may increase the danger of hemorrhage during anticoagulant therapy. The patient should be advised to consult his physician before taking aspirin or other over-the-counter drugs because of the danger of drug interactions. He should wear a Medic Alert emblem or carry a card stating the drug he is receiving and giving his physician's name and telephone number. The card informs an unknown physician that excessive bleeding may be a problem in emergency situations and enables him to contact the patient's physician.

Coumarin derivatives begin to act one to two days after administration. Their effect wears off slowly, too, persisting two to five days after the last dose. Prompt reporting of any bleeding tendency is especially important in the light of the duration of action after the drug has been discontinued. If bleeding occurs, the drug is discontinued temporarily. Vitamin $K_1$ (Mephyton) may be given orally or intravenously to control bleeding, or a transfusion may be necessary. For further information on anticoagulant drug therapy see Rodman, M. and Smith, D. W.: *Clinical Pharmacology in Nursing*, Philadelphia, Lippincott, 1974.

**Pulmonary Embolism.** Most pulmonary emboli arise from venous clots in the lower extremities and pelvis. Many do not cause pulmonary infarction. A lung scan and angiocardiogram would be necessary if embolectomy were contemplated. For the patient with myocardial infarction, however, this is extremely risky. Anticoagulation and vena caval ligation would probably be considered. (See Chapter 38 for further discussion of the problem of pulmonary embolism.)

**Arterial Emboli.** Anticoagulants are not thought to prevent arterial clot formation. A clot can form in the left ventricular cavity overlying the infarcted area (mural thrombus). Part of it can break off and enter the systemic arterial circulation and cause occlusion of peripheral arteries, resulting in a mottled, cold, pulseless extremity, or of arteries in the brain resulting in sudden stroke. Initial pulses in all extremities are important as a baseline. The nurse listens carefully to the patient's complaint of extremity pain and checks for differences in temperature of the extremities. Arteriotomy and embolectomy may be necessary. Any slight paralysis, slurring of speech, and drooping of a side of the face should be noted.

**Congestive Heart Failure.** See Chapters 34 and 59 for nursing care of the patient with congestive heart failure and pulmonary edema.

**Cardiogenic Shock.** This is a dreaded complication because of the high mortality rate. Seventy to 85 per cent of patients with this diagnosis die. The earlier shock is detected and treatment instituted the better are the patient's chances of survival.

Because some believe that this mortality cannot be reduced further by conventional therapy, and because the size of the infarction is not always related to the extreme degree of shock, research centers are developing and assessing mechanical circulatory

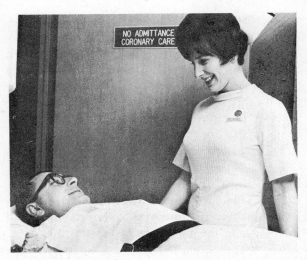

**Figure 62-3.** A well-cared-for patient is transferred from the coronary care unit. (Photograph taken at Overlook Hospital, Summit, N.J., by Robert Goldstein for *Patient Care* magazine)

assistance devices for the failing ventricle following myocardial infarction. For example, part of the circulation can be temporarily diverted from the heart through the use of an external pump oxygenator, or an invasive *counterpulsation* device such as the Kantrowitz balloon can be used. Recently a non-invasive relatively atraumatic mechanical circulatory assist device has become available (Medical Innovations, Inc.). An assist device is synchronized with cardiac events so that diastolic pressure in the aorta is increased, hence coronary artery blood flow is increased. Another effect is that systolic pressure, or the pressure against which the left ventricle contracts, is reduced, thus reducing myocardial oxygen consumption.

For nursing care of the patient in cardiogenic shock (pump failure), see Chapter 59.

**Other complications** which may be treated by emergency surgical intervention include papillary muscle dysfunction or rupture, and acute mitral insufficiency. Also ventricular aneurysm which decreases the pumping action of the heart, and causes angina or congestive failure may be surgically corrected as an emergency procedure or electively.

There can also be rupture of the interventricular septum characterized by a loud ejection systolic murmur. Dyspnea, rapid right heart failure, and shock result and the prognosis is poor though survival is possible with emergency surgery (see Chap. 63).

Cardiac rupture occurs when a soft necrotic area

gives way. Hemopericardium, cardiac tamponade, and sudden death ensue.

A relatively mild complication is the shoulder-hand syndrome or periarthritis of the shoulder which occurs during the convalescent period. It is characterized by pain, stiffness, and limitation of shoulder motion and sometimes swelling of the hand. The exact cause is unknown, but protective disuse of the shoulder during the acute period may be a contributory factor.

## PREPARATION FOR TRANSFER

Transfer from the coronary care unit generally means progress for the patient (Fig. 62-3). He has survived one critical period and can go to an area of the hospital where the close observation of the CCU is unavailable but also unnecessary. Like all "graduations," the step carries with it some anxiety. "Can I get along without my monitor? What happens if I need a nurse right away? What about my chest pain—I still have angina? Can they help me if I have a cardiac arrest?" are questions which the patient probably poses to himself.

Ideally, patients with a myocardial infarction should be transferred to a postcoronary division where specially prepared staff can help the patient through the transition period. Remote control monitoring or telemetry should be available in such an area. This is not always possible. The staff who receives the patient, however, must be aware that despite the fact that the patient may look and feel well and has survived his CCU stay, he is still critically ill and subject to all of the complications of acute myocardial infarction.

The patient should have the opportunity in the CCU to discuss his thoughts and feelings about the transfer. A length of time in the CCU without a cardiac monitor and IV (weaning period) gives the patient confidence that he can, in fact, survive without them. A realistic projection of the length of stay in the CCU and visits from the staff of the transfer unit help the patient to make the adjustment when the time comes. That there are adverse and serious cardiovascular effects in patients unprepared for the transfer has been documented (Klein, et al., 1968).

About 40 per cent of deaths due to AMI occur after discharge from the CCU. Some of these post-CCU deaths are sudden and unexpected while others occur in predictably terminal patients, with congestive heart failure or shock. Some deaths might be prevented by extended monitoring for cardiac arrhythmias. The convalescent unit must have a prepared staff and the necessary equipment for meeting cardiac emergencies.

If possible, nursing visits from the CCU staff should continue after transfer. When all units where coronary patients are cared for are physically adjacent, staff can circulate among units and thus have the opportunity to care for the patient during the various phases of hospitalization. The clinical specialist may be able to follow patients through various hospital areas and stimulate and coordinate continuity of nursing care.

## BEGINNING CONVALESCENCE

Of the approximately 80 per cent of patients who survive their first myocardial infarction, some will be troubled by angina or congestive heart failure. Most patients, however, will look and feel well after their transfer from the CCU. They continue to need nursing care, but care at this point involves more of the counseling, teaching, and socializing aspects of the nursing role, rather than technical or mother-surrogate components.

The convalescent period in the hospital focuses on gradually increasing the physical activity of the patient so that he can perform self-care activities by the time of discharge, and on patient education therapy. The teaching plan should include the nature of infarction and the process of repair; risk factor reduction such as cessation of smoking and dietary modification of fats or calories (see Chap. 39); physical activity rationale and type of exercise including sexual activity; control of associated diseases such as hypertension or diabetes; medication prescription, rationale, and monitoring for side effects; other cardiac treatment such as a pacemaker; patient monitoring of new or current cardiac symptoms and plans for obtaining medical care.

This is the period when the patient hopefully begins to come to grips with some of the changes in life that the infarction has precipitated. This can be a long-term process with much of the "rethinking" coming after discharge. For many, this time is one of profound philosophical dimension.

The nurse helps during this period by offering to be a listener as the patient attempts to work out his problems; by planning with the patient, family, or volunteer staff for appropriate diversion; and by teaching the patient and family or groups of patients and families.

An apprehensive family member can seem a burden to those on a staff who view their role solely in terms of working with the patient. But serious illness of one family member puts new burdens and responsibilities on others. For example, a wife who suddenly becomes breadwinner and sole active manager of the home and children, and a daily visitor as well, may begin to show signs of irritability and impatience with the patient or the staff.

Such reactions require understanding and help from both the physician and the nurse. When family members express dissatisfaction with the care given, it is difficult but important to consider possible reasons for their behavior and to help them feel more confident about the care that the patient is receiving.

A family member who might feel foolish or embarrassed to admit difficulty in coping with a situation may need to be encouraged to seek the care of a physician or nurse specialist. Family members who themselves receive support are in a better position to offer support to the patient.

If the patient needs nursing or homemaker assistance at home, or a stay in an intermediate care facility, referrals are instituted early in the convalescent period.

The nurse also contributes by assisting the patient to get answers to questions which may bother him, but which he may hesitate to ask. For example, it can be assumed that postcoronary patients will have questions about resumption of sex activity. Many are hesitant to ask questions about this. The nurse can detect clues that the patient may need help with this subject and can assist him and his spouse to formulate the questions and seek the physician's advice. When the limitations are reviewed and understood, the couple is in a better position to make their own decisions. A study of postcoronary males showed that conjugal sexual activity subjects the cardiovascular system to no more strain than many other activities of daily living. A conclusion of the study was that the postcoronary patient without cardiac decompensation can resume conjugal sexual activity when other physical activities are increased, usually about the ninth to twelfth weeks (Hellerstein, 1969). This of course, will vary with the individual patient, spouse, and the guidance of the physician. Points that the nurse might discuss with the patient are cited by Scalzi (1973).

Regardless of the specific diet order, the patient

whose activity is sharply restricted should not have gas-forming foods, such as baked beans, cauliflower, or cabbage. Many patients find that they are more comfortable if they eat four small meals daily rather than three large ones. Overeating may cause distention and flatulence or even an attack of angina. The patient should rest for half an hour after eating.

Most of the time the patient is eager to go home; often this is permitted in about three weeks, though there is a trend toward even earlier discharge. Sometimes, the patient returns home in an ambulance to minimize exertion during the trip. However, if the attack has been mild, he may be permitted to go home by car. Usually, he is instructed to gradually increase his activity by taking short walks or helping with light chores. Strenuous unprescribed physical exertion and emotional strain must be avoided. If all goes well, the patient may be permitted to return to work at the end of two to three months. The physician may advise working part-time, particularly at first.

There has been a trend in recent years toward a more scientific approach to the prescription of activity for patients after myocardial infarction and the enhancement of their physical fitness. Cardiac work evaluation centers, YMCA cardiac physical fitness programs, and each state's rehabilitation commission are examples of agencies which provide evaluation services.

(See Chapter 39 for rehabilitation of the cardiac patient.)

## PROGNOSIS

The term *cardiac neurosis* sometimes is used to describe patients who are so anxious about their heart function that they are unable to follow the physician's suggestions concerning increased activity. The following measures may help the patient to avoid this complication:

- **Avoid communicating apprehension concerning his condition to the patient. Sometimes the staff and the family spread apprehension and anxiety to the patient. Vigilance need not mean jumpiness.**
- **Allow the patient to discuss his reactions to the illness, if he wishes.**
- **Be concrete and specific in the instructions given the patient about the activities the physician recommends. For example, it is preferable to say, "Your doctor says you may walk to the end of the hall and back today. I'll walk with you," rather than "Your doctor says you can start taking a little more exercise**

**today." Knowing specifically how much and what sort of activity is considered safe for him, and that the nurse will be with him the first time he attempts it, can lessen the patient's anxiety.**

Although myocardial infarction is a serious event, constituting one of the major causes of death among older people, many patients not only survive the attack but also are able to return to work. Because the underlying condition of atherosclerosis is still present, the patient may have repeated attacks of myocardial infarction, or he may develop angina pectoris. Statistics concerning mortality apply to groups and not to specific individuals within the group. It is impossible to predict what the future holds for the individual patient. Some live comfortably and actively for many years afterward, such as former U.S. presidents Eisenhower and Johnson. Eight of the runners who completed a recent Boston marathon had recovered from a myocardial infarction.

Some patients may be helped by surgical techniques which improve the supply of blood to the heart muscle (see Chap. 63).

## REFERENCES AND BIBLIOGRAPHY

Andreoli, K., et al.: *Comprehensive Cardiac Care,* ed. 2, St. Louis, Mosby, 1971.

*Assessment of the Capability of External Pressure Circulatory Assist to Reduce the Morbidity and Mortality of Left Ventricular Failure Secondary to Acute Myocardial Infarction: A Clinical Study,* Revision 4, Waltham, Massachusetts, Medical Innovations, Inc., December 28, 1973.

Benton, J., et al.: Energy expended by patients on the bedpan and bedside commode, *JAMA* 114:1443, December 1950.

Boyek, J.: What heart patients want to know . . . and what to tell them, *Nurs. '72* 2:38, May 1972.

Braceland, F.: The coronary spectrum. Psychiatric aspects, *J. Rehab.* 32:53, March-April 1966.

Browse, N.: *The Physiology and Pathology of Bed Rest,* Springfield, Ill., Thomas, 1965.

Bunke, B.: Respiratory function after acute myocardial infarction: Implications for nursing, *Cardiovasc. Nurs.* 9:13, May-June 1973.

Cassem, N. H., et al.: How coronary patients respond to last rites, *Postgrad. Med.* 45:147, March 1969.

———, and Hackett, T.: Psychological rehabilitation of myocardial infarction patients in the acute phase, *Heart Lung* 2:382, May-June 1973.

Conrad, L.: The Valsalva maneuver: A clinical inquiry, *Am. J. Nurs.* 71:553, March 1971.

Coodley, E.: The new cardiac enzyme tests—how practical for diagnosing myocardial infarction? *Consultant* 7:13, September 1967.

CORDAY, E., and SWAN, H. J. C.: *Myocardial Infarction: New Perspectives in Diagnosis and Management,* Baltimore, Williams & Wilkins, 1973.

CORONA, D.: After the CCU, what? *RN* 36:42, June 1973.

DAVIS, M. Z.: Socioemotional components of coronary care, *Am. J. Nurs.* 72:704, April 1972.

DOBSON, M., et al.: Attitudes in long-term adjustment of patients surviving cardiac arrest, *British Med. J.* 3:207, 1971.

DUKE, M.: Bed rest in acute myocardial infarction: A study of physician practices, *Am. Heart J.* 82:486, 1971.

SISTER ELIZABETH, D. C.: A new dimension in the nursing care of coronary patients, *Hosp. Prog.* 68:104, 1968.

GERMAIN, C.: Nursing role variations in coronary care, *Hospitals* 43:147, September 1969.

————, and MINOGUE, W. F.: Precoronary care: Nursing considerations, *Cardiovasc. Nurs.* 8:1, May-June 1972.

GRACE, W., and SOSCIA, J.: Reducing mortality from acute myocardial infarction—current ideas, *Card. Dig.* 4:29, June 1969.

GRAHAM, L.: Patients' perceptions in the CCU, *Am. J. Nurs.* 69:1921, September 1969.

GOLDSTROM, D. K.: Cardiac rest: Bed or chair, *Am. J. Nurs.* 72:1812, October 1972.

HAFERHORN, V.: Assessing individual learning needs as a basis for patient teaching, *Nurs. Clin. N. Am.* 6:199, March 1971.

HARRISON, T., and REEVES, T.: *Principles and Problems of Ischemic Heart Disease,* Chicago, Year Book, 1968.

Headstart on a heart attack, *Emerg. Med.* 3:98, August 1971.

HELLERSTEIN, H.: Sexual activity and the post-coronary patient, *Med. Asp. Human Sexuality* 3:70, March 1969.

HOUSER, D. M.: Emergency cardiac care, *Nurs. Clin. N. Am.* 8:401, September 1973.

HURST, J., and LOGUE, R. B.: *The Heart,* ed. 2, New York, McGraw-Hill, 1970.

Inter-Society Commission for Heart Disease Resources: Resources for the optimal care of patients with acute myocardial infarction, *Circulation* 43, May 1971.

KLEIN, R.: "Heart attack" victims should discuss fears, *JAMA* 206:33, September 1968.

KLEIN, R., et al.: Transfer from a coronary care unit; some adverse responses, *Arch. Int. Med.* 122:104, August 1968.

LAVIN, M. A.: Bed exercises for acute cardiac patients, *Am. J. Nurs.* 73:1226, July 1973.

LEVINE, S.: Chair rest versus bed rest, *Hosp. Med.* 2:2, January 1966.

MELTZER, L., and DUNNING, A.: *Textbook of Coronary Care,* Philadelphia, Charles Press, 1972.

A mobile CCU saves lives in New York City, *ICU: A Review of the Literature on Intensive Care,* 3:12, 1969.

NARROW, B.: Rest is . . ., *Am. J. Nurs.* 67:1646, August 1967.

OLSON, E. (ed.): The hazards of immobility. A symposium, *Am. J. Nurs.* 67:780, April 1967.

PIEGAS, L. S., et al.: Use of the Swan-Ganz catheter in the diagnosis of ventricular septal defect after myocardial infarction, *Heart Lung* 2:539, July-August 1973.

PRANULIS, M.: Loss: A factor affecting the welfare of the coronary patient, *Nurs. Clin. N. Am.* 7:445, September 1972.

RACHLEY, C., and RUSSELL, R.: *Invasive Techniques For Hemodynamic Measurements,* New York, American Heart Association, 1973.

RODMAN, T., et al.: *The Physiologic and Pharmacologic Basis of Coronary Care Nursing,* St. Louis, Mosby, 1971.

ROSE, G.: Early mobilization and discharge after myocardial infarction, *Mod. Conc. Cardiovasc. Dis.* 41:59, December 1972.

ROYLE, J.: Coronary patients and their families receive incomplete care, *Canad. Nurse* 69:21, February 1973.

RUSSEK, H., and ZOHMAN, B. (eds.): *Coronary Heart Disease: A Medical-Surgical Symposium,* Philadelphia, Lippincott, 1971.

————: *Changing Concepts in Cardiovascular Disease,* Baltimore, Williams & Wilkins, 1972.

SCALZI, C.: Nursing management of behavioral responses following an acute myocardial infarction, *Heart Surg.* 2:62, January-February 1973.

SCHMITT, Y., et al.: Armchair treatment in the coronary care unit, *Nurs. Res.* 18:114, March-April 1969.

SHAPIRO, R.: Anticoagulant therapy, *Am. J. Nurs.* 74:439, March 1974.

SHARP, L., and RABIN, B.: *Nursing in the Coronary Care Unit,* Philadelphia, Lippincott, 1970.

SMITH, A. M., et al.: Serum enzymes in myocardial infarction, *Am. J. Nurs.* 73:277, February 1973.

SMITH, C. A.: Body image changes after myocardial infarction, *Nurs. Clin. N. Am.* 7:663, December 1972.

SOBEL, D.: Personalization on the coronary care unit, *Am. J. Nurs.* 69:1439, July 1969.

SOROFF, H., et al.: Physiologic support of heart action, *New Eng. J. Med.* 280:694, March 27, 1969.

SPENCE, M. I., et al.: Myocardial infarction, *Heart Lung* 1:543, July-August 1972.

TWERSKI, A.: Psychological considerations on the coronary care unit, *Cardiovasc. Nurs.* 7:65, March-April 1971.

TYZENHOUSE, P. S.: Myocardial infarction . . . its effect on the family, *Am. J. Nurs.* 73:1012, June 1973.

WENGER, N.: *Rehabilitation After Myocardial Infarction,* New York, American Heart Association, 1973.

WISHNIE, H., et al.: Psychological hazards of convalescence following myocardial infarction, *JAMA* 215:1292, February 22, 1971.

# The Patient Undergoing Heart Surgery

## CHAPTER 63

Few decisions require of the patient the degree of courage necessary to decide upon and to undergo open heart surgery. Though he may have been in failing health for some time, he is aware that the risk of death is real, and much higher than the risk incurred when undergoing most other types of surgery.

An individual can get along without a gallbladder or stomach, and though the adjustment may be difficult, he can make his way in this world with one eye, or one leg, or one kidney. Patients know, however, that they have but one heart, and trusting its repair to the hands of a surgeon and a team of strangers is a formidable threat when, to the patient, death can be one breath or one heartbeat away.

The idea of cutting into the heart is additionally stressful because society has associated the heart with many emotions. The red "heart" shaped valentine suggests joy and love while the expression "my heart in my throat" indicates fear. "I speak from the heart" describes the tendency to believe the heart is the seat of the emotions. "Getting to the heart of the matter" is an idiom which points up the belief that the heart is the critical part of the body.

Today, patients are more informed about medical practices than ever before. Television shows give information about hospital life through news and daytime serials, just as radio stations are constantly reporting current medical trends. The written media publish articles by both nonprofessional and professional persons. As cardiac surgery becomes more common, it is not unusual for prospective patients to have met others who have gone through the experience. Though some patients may misunderstand what they read or hear, or some information may be misleading, generally patients are in a better position today to make a more informed decision about having cardiac surgery. Thus they are apt to be less passive than formerly. They may raise more meaningful questions and have certain expectations regarding their care. Unless physicians, nurses, and other members of the cardiac surgical team are prepared to individualize their responses to patients, they may become quite threatened by sophisticated questioning. Few patients enter the hospital for heart surgery without preconceived ideas about the experience.

Several other factors contribute to the apprehension of the cardiac surgical patient. Because heart surgery is not performed in every hospital, many patients must go a considerable distance for the operation. Separation from familiar surroundings and absence of family members when they are needed most can cause intense loneliness when the patient realizes that the only people near him are relative strangers.

Uncertainties plague the patient. Can I trust these strangers? Do they behave as a team? Will my family be here? Will my operation be a success?

The patient who has decided to have surgery performed on his heart is taking a calculated risk for a longer and a more healthy life. Patients enter the hospital with varying degrees of emotional readiness to face the operation.

Age and developmental factors influence the patient's response. The patient with rheumatic heart disease who has grown up with activity limitations may perceive health as a terrifying unknown. The middle-aged, hard-driving executive with an active, dominant personality may desire a myocardial revascularization procedure so that he can resume a more vigorous life, but may dread the need to submit himself to the care and direction of others, particularly female nurses. Some patients may have unresolved conflicts about the wish to remain ill or the desire to get well. For some patients the psychic stress of heart surgery is so enormous that they cannot even acknowledge it. Such patients who deny the risk and seriousness of their surgery are frequently accusatory in the postoperative period, blaming pain or complication on the surgeon (Heller, 1974).

Team members involved in the care of the cardiac surgical patient work together to minimize stress and to help the patient to cope with the many biopsychosocial stressors which inevitably are part of the experience.

## THE EVOLUTION OF CARDIAC SURGICAL TECHNIQUES

**Extracardiac Surgery.** This technique was the first approach to cardiac surgery. As the terminology suggests, the corrective procedures were performed outside of the heart and its great vessels. Wiring of aneurysms, aspiration of pericardial fluid, and the suturing of traumatic wounds are examples of diseases amenable to surgical correction performed in this manner.

**Closed Intracardiac Surgery.** This technique evolved in the 1940s. The approach required the surgeon to perform cardiac repairs within a blood-filled beating heart, without his direct vision. The removal of foreign bodies, such as shrapnel or bullets, could be done in this manner. The surgeon could also enter the heart via the left atrial appendage and pass his finger across scarred, narrowed mitral valves. In this manner he opened the fused commissures of the valve, thus allowing for an increased blood flow across the orifice. The procedure was termed a transatrial digital mitral commissurotomy. Later, blunt instruments, such as a Gerbode or a Tubbs dilator, were designed to facilitate this technique.

**Open Intracardiac Surgery.** This approach developed in the mid 1950s. A major breakthrough was due to understanding the hemodynamics of cardiopulmonary bypass. This information allowed biomedical engineers and biological technicians, as well as many others, to collaborate their efforts and develop the artificial heart-lung machine.

With this device, the patient's blood that is normally returned to the heart is diverted to a machine that removes carbon dioxide, supplies oxygen, and then returns the blood to the aorta. This allows the surgeon to open the heart, stop the beating, and correct the pathology under direct vision while working in a bloodless field. Damaged cardiac valves can be critically inspected and reconstructed if necessary (valvuloplasty). Pathologic openings within the cardiac septums can also be corrected.

**Present Era of Replacement Surgery.** Today we are in an era of consideration and further development of a number of cardiovascular prostheses to repair many congenital and acquired defects. The

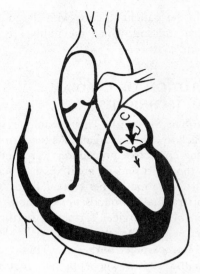

**Figure 63-1.** Mitral stenosis. The narrowed valve does not permit blood to flow freely from the left atrium to the left ventricle.

repair and/or replacement may be: complete or partial; artificial or tissue; temporary or permanent.

Presently researchers are studying the techniques for completely replacing the heart by using homotransplantation or by employing a totally mechanical device. Problems of immune rejection and ethical considerations have impeded homotransplantation while the inability to solve the problem of blood clot formation has prevented the use of a mechanical device for longer than a few days.

## CARDIAC SURGERY

Corrective surgery may be performed for

- Congenital heart lesions.* Approximately 1 per cent of adults beyond the second decade of life being con-

---

* Most of the congenital heart conditions amenable to surgery will not be discussed here, as they are corrected when it is possible during childhood. The most common congenital heart conditions that come to surgery are:

*Tetralogy of Fallot* consists of four defects: pulmonary stenosis, intraventricular septal defect, overriding of the aorta, and right ventricular hypertrophy.

*Patent ductus arteriosus* is a communication between the aorta and the pulmonary artery.

*Intra-atrial and intraventricular septal defects* are openings in the walls between the chambers of the heart.

*Pulmonary stenosis* obstructs the flow of blood from the right ventricle.

*Coarctation of the aorta,* a narrowing of the aorta, may be seen in young adults. It may cause hypertension of the upper extremities and the head, dizziness, retinal or cerebral hemorrhages. It is treated surgically by resection of the part of the aorta that contains the stricture and end-to-end anastomosis.

sidered for cardiac surgery are suffering from congenital pathology.

- Acquired heart lesions. Acquired heart disease refers to those pathological processes in the heart or great vessels that were not present at birth but have been incurred since that time and includes:

    **1.** Acquired valvular disease due to infectious processes
    **2.** Ischemic disease processes
    **3.** Traumatic injuries
    **4.** Tumors of the heart

### Acquired Valvular Diseases of the Heart

Acquired lesions of the valves are most frequently of rheumatic origin. The initial process occurs early in life, usually between 5 and 15 years of age. Because attacks may be relatively asymptomatic, only about half of those with acquired valvular disease have a definite history of rheumatic fever.

During the acute stages of rheumatic fever all sections of the heart may be involved. However, in approximately 15 or 20 years, after the acute disease process, permanent damage to the heart valves is recognized in about two-thirds of the individuals (Ellis, 1967).

The mitral valve is most commonly affected. Damage in females is three times more frequent than in males. The aortic valve is the next most commonly affected valve, but damage is three times more frequent in men. The tricuspid valve is less frequently involved and the pulmonic valve even less so. Disease may involve one, two, or three valves (Fig. 63-1).

During the active stages of rheumatic fever the normally delicate, pliable leaflets of the cardiac valves become inflamed. Microscopic examination may reveal deposits of fine translucent vegetation along the surface of the closure of the valves. Later in life, usually between 30 and 40 years of age, the once pliable leaflets may become nonflexible from scarring and become calcified and actually fuse together.

Other causes of acquired valvular diseases may be subacute or acute bacterial endocarditis which produces an inflammation of the lining of the heart including the lining of the valves. As a result, heart valves, particularly the mitral and aortic valves, can become scarred and function improperly.

Undiagnosed and/or untreated cases of syphilis can also affect the aortic valve. Trauma, such as from automobile accidents, can produce mitral or aortic insufficiency. Acute myocardial infarction may precipitate acute mitral insufficiency.

## Pathologic Valve Processes

A damaged heart valve may be stenotic, insufficient, or both. Aortic insufficiency is the most serious valvular disease.

**Stenotic Valves.** The valve can become so tightened and narrowed that its lumen is reduced to pencil-point size (stenosis of valve). The scarred valve opens upon cardiac contraction, but the reduced size of the lumen limits the amount of blood that can flow through it.

**Insufficient Valves.** As a result of the processes of scarring, fusion of the leaflets, and eventual calcification, the valves are no longer capable of closing properly and become "insufficient." Blood regurgitates backwards, through the incompetent valve.

## Surgical Repair of Valvular Heart Disease

Severely damaged aortic, mitral, or tricuspid valves can be dilated, reconstructed (valvuloplasty), or replaced by artificial valves or by tissue transplantation. Some patients require multiple replacements and as many as two or three damaged valves have been successfully replaced. The open heart surgical technique is almost always used. One reason for this is that the preoperative data indicating the degree of valve pliability may be in error and any attempt to correct the damage without replacement would be futile.

Mortality has been gradually decreasing. All patients do better if the valvular lesion is corrected before serious secondary involvement of the myocardium and lungs occurs.

## Cardiac Valve Replacement

**Ball Valves.** Currently in widest clinical use for the replacement of damaged valves is the Starr-Edwards ball valve (Fig. 63-2). Other variations of the design exist, but the primary hemodynamic principle is the same. The ball in the cage moves toward the top of the cage when the valve is open thus allowing blood to flow through the opening. The blood flows around the ball and enters the patient's circulatory system. During closure the ball falls back and sits firmly upon the rim, thus preventing the back flow of blood into the previous chamber.

**Flap Valves (Hinge, Disk, or Pivot Valves).** As a group these valves are usually more streamlined in design and less bulky than the ball valves. As a

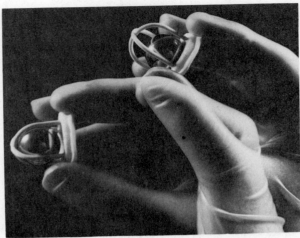

**Figure 63-2.** The Starr-Edwards ball valve is one of the most "popular" of artificial valves for the human heart. The double exposure photograph here shows the metal ball of this man-made valve in the closed (*left*) and open (*right*) positions. National Heart Institute surgeons have utilized the Starr-Edwards valve in many patients to replace natural mitral valves which have become damaged by rheumatic fever. Valves of similar design are also used to replace aortic and tricuspid valves in the human heart. The recently modified valve features a "cage" and sewing ring covered with porous synthetic fabric that, by allowing the ingrowth of living tissue, greatly minimizes the hazard of blood clot formation on these metal structures. The highly polished metal alloy (Stellite) ball is designed to reduce the size changes, fractures, and "sticking" seen occasionally in silicone rubber balls used over long periods of time. (National Institutes of Health)

result this type of valve occupies less space within the heart. In addition, the short cage requires less time for the traveling during the cardiac cycle; hence, complete closure and opening can be accomplished more readily.

While artificial valves differ in design and in the materials from which they are constructed they tend to share a number of common problems. Designs must be perfected in an effort to avoid the recipient's need for long-term anticoagulation therapy. A number of valves have a turbulent effect and cause destruction of blood cells. As valves are in use for prolonged periods of time, signs of wearing out, such as changes in the shape and size of the valves as well as strength and elasticity of the material from which they are constructed, are being noted.

**Tissue Transplantation.** Permanently damaged heart valves can also be removed and replaced by

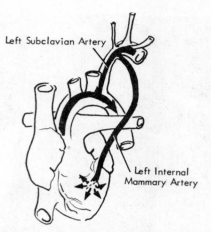

**Figure 63-3.** Vineberg revascularization procedure.

healthy tissue. This technique has been extensively employed in England and New Zealand and to a lesser degree in the United States.

Healthy valvular tissue (homografts) may be secured from animals, or from persons dying from other nonrelated causes. The tissue is obtained and processed under sterile conditions and can then be stored until the time a suitable recipient is found.

Tissue valves are more natural and some scientists believe they are superior to artificially constructed valves, when reviewed hemodynamically. Recipients do not need anticoagulation therapy as the valves are less likely to cause clotting complications. The possibility of rejection and the long-term followup of stability of valves are some of the questions being critically reviewed.

## Ischemic Heart Disease
### Myocardial Revascularization

Atherosclerotic heart disease is the leading type of heart disease in the United States. Hence, surgical techniques have been developed in an effort to increase the blood supply to the ischemic myocardium.

Although more than 2,000 revascularization operations are being performed yearly in the United States, this is a mere fraction of the total considered necessary to insure adequate care for the countless sufferers from coronary heart disease (Russek, 1971).

**Closed Technique (Indirect).** Until the late 1960s, a widely used technique to increase the supply of blood to the myocardium was the Vineberg procedure in which the internal mammary arteries are isolated then directly implanted, through a sur-

gically created tunnel, into the wall of the left ventricle (Fig. 63-3). The vast network of sinusoids in heart muscle provides open spaces through which the blood supply runs off into the ischemic portion. Revascularization, of course, is not immediate. The average convalescent period is about three months (Brogan, 1972). This procedure is not done very frequently at the present time because with most patients the results have only been temporary.

**Direct Open-Heart Approach.** The atherosclerotic deposits or clots obstructing the coronary arteries are frequently confined to a relatively short section of artery. Arterial transplants of blood vessel grafts have been employed to correct this. The surgical approach is directed toward bypassing the diseased area of the coronary artery by suturing a vein graft between the aorta and one or more coronary arteries beyond the site of obstruction.

Endarterectomy of the diseased vessel may also be employed either as the primary treatment or in conjunction with a vein graft. Carbon dioxide gas (gas endarterectomy) may be employed to separate the atheroma from the intima. The coronary artery is then surgically opened and the freed atheroma is removed in one piece.

While most patients undergoing direct coronary arterial surgery are operated upon electively, in recent years more attention has been given to attempts to reverse or prevent the effects of an acute myocardial infarction in a few highly selected patients. In these patients coronary arteriography and coronary bypass grafting using cardiopulmonary bypass are performed as emergency procedures.

## Septal Defects
### Atrial Septal Defect

An atrial septal defect is a hole in the cardiac septum that separates the right and the left atria. One low in the septum may reach the mitral and the tricuspid valves (Fig. 63-4).

Normally, the pressure within the heart is higher in the left atrium than in the right atrium; therefore, in a heart with an atrial septal defect blood flows from the left atrium through the hole to the right atrium. Because this blood already has been through the lungs, it is oxygenated. From the right atrium the blood goes to the right ventricle and back to the lungs. This inefficient functioning puts a strain on the right atrium, which enlarges in response to the extra load of blood. Over a period of time the right ventricle also enlarges and eventually so does the pulmonary artery. If the condition is not corrected, pulmonary vessel resistance may increase, and right-sided pulmonary hypertension occurs. The right ventricle becomes unable fully to empty itself of blood during each contraction because of the increased resistance in the pulmonary vessels. As a consequence, blood is backed up into the right atrium. When the pressure in this chamber grows higher than the pressure in the left atrium, there will be a reversal of the direction of leakage of blood. Now it will go from the right to the left through the defect in the wall. But the blood that goes from the right to the left has *not* been through the lungs; nevertheless it is sent on through the left atrium, the left ventricle and the aorta into the general circulation. Because the oxygen content of the blood being pumped from the left ventricle is lower than normal, the patient at this stage of the pathologic process can develop cyanosis.

Symptoms of right-sided failure include venous distention, ascites, and peripheral edema as blood backs up through the venous system network. Patients also may experience bouts of palpitation (usually due to atrial tachycardia), fatigue, and frequent respiratory infections. The condition may be complicated by mitral stenosis and a small aorta. Angiocardiography shows right ventricular hypertrophy. When the heart is catheterized, an increased oxygen content is found in the right atrium. If the catheter passes through the defect in the wall between the atria, the diagnosis is confirmed.

Patients who have a small defect may be symptom-free. If the defect is repaired by surgery before a right-to-left shunt develops, there is an excellent chance of complete closure of the defect, followed by a lessening of the secondary pathologic cardiac changes. Usually, surgery is of the open-heart type with use of the heart-lung machine and hypothermia. Unless severe pathologic changes have occurred before surgical repair is made, the mortality from this operation is low (1 to 3 per cent).

## Ventricular Septal Defect

A ventricular septal defect is a hole in the cardiac septum that separates the left and right ventricles. The opening may be in either the membranous or muscular portions of the ventricular septum. As described for an atrial septal defect, blood flow through a ventricular septal defect is from left to right in the early stages, and it is only late in the course of the illness that the blood flow may be reversed and

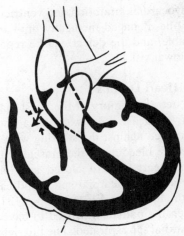

**Figure 63-4.** Atrial-septal defect. The abnormal hole in the wall between the right and the left atria at first allows a left-to-right leakage of blood. Later, there may be a right-to-left shunting of blood.

result in a right to left shunt. A congenital ventricular septal defect is uncommon in adults since the defect is usually repaired in childhood. The acquired ventricular septal defect, however, results from a myocardial infarction involving the ventricular septum. Often the symptoms present suddenly as severe right ventricular overload and failure. In these patients the defect may have to be repaired as an emergency using cardiopulmonary bypass. In other patients the physiologic abnormalities associated

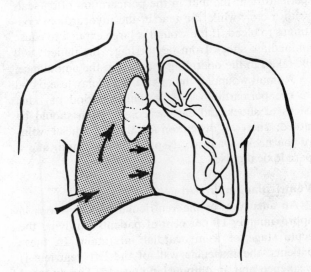

**Figure 63-5.** A chest wound that causes pneumothorax and collapse of the lung also can cause cardiac symptoms as the heart is forced out of its normal position.

with the myocardial infarction and ventricular septal defect may be managed medically until the patient is more stable, and the defect can be repaired electively at a lower risk.

### Traumatic Heart Lesions

A nonpenetrating injury of the chest may include bruising of the heart. For example, a patient who has been crushed against the steering wheel of a car may have some bleeding of the muscle of the heart. Because the heart is in a closed sac, blood will accumulate in the pericardial space and cause tamponade of the heart (see Fig. 63-5, p. 1131).

Most often the patient will need to have the fluid in the pericardial sac aspirated. The physician inserts a long needle into the pericardial sac (pericardiocentesis). During this procedure the patient is usually placed at approximately a 45-degree angle. One aspiration is sufficient in many patients. If the bleeding continues an open thoracotomy may be indicated to control the bleeding site. All patients with compressing chest injuries should have their apical pulse checked frequently. There may be inhibition of the vagus nerve, with a slowing pulse, and perhaps cardiac standstill. Cardiopulmonary resuscitation equipment must be available for instant use. The pain from a bruised heart may be masked by the pain from other chest injuries.

Direct trauma to the myocardium, such as a stab wound, also may cause leakage of blood into the pericardium; the tear in the pericardium often seals with a clot, while the tear in the myocardium continues to bleed. If the wound is large enough to cause immediate shock from hemorrhage, the patient will be taken to the operating room from the ambulance.

A small wound of the myocardium may lose blood to the pericardium over a longer period of time. Signs of shock and cardiac compression should be noted, such as distention of the superficial veins of the neck, cyanosis, dyspnea, hypotension, and a paradoxical pulse.

### Ventricular Aneurysm

An aneurysm of the ventricular wall develops in approximately 10 per cent of patients surviving the acute stage of a myocardial infarction. In these patients, the muscular wall of the left ventricle is weakened and an outpouching occurs. The diseased area dilates and produces a ballooning of the wall.

In some patients, the ventricular aneurysm may result in progressive congestive heart failure. Should this occur, surgical removal or exclusion of the aneurysm (by sutures) may significantly improve the patient. Often repair of the aneurysm is combined with direct coronary arterial surgery (bypass grafting).

### Tumors of the Heart

Primary tumors of the heart are rare. Benign lesions are three times more common among primary tumors than are malignancies.

The myxoma, a benign intracavitary tumor, comprises over half of all the reported cases of primary cardiac tumors. Its composition is such that it is often confused with a thrombus. The myxomas are noninvasive but portions can break off and serve as emboli.

Metastatic tumors, commonly from primary sites in breast, lung, or stomach can cause heart failure, arrhythmias, pericardial effusion, and the caval syndromes.

The clinical course usually depends upon the type of tumor and its location, that is, if it occupies space within the chambers of the heart or is contained within the muscle. Some smaller tumors have been noted only at autopsy. Over 90 per cent of the cases of left atrial myxomas were initially considered to be mitral valvular disease (Norman, 1967).

Surgery, using cardiopulmonary bypass, may be undertaken as cardiac failure may occur and the potential of embolization is often present. Benign tumors may stem from a pedicle and their removal is usually uncomplicated. Malignant tumors are more difficult to remove and the patient's prognosis is extremely poor.

## THE PREOPERATIVE PERIOD

The patient is usually hospitalized for one or two weeks prior to surgery for an extensive and exhausting medical evaluation. A thorough physical examination is imperative and a precise anatomic diagnosis of the cardiac lesion is desired.

The patient will be cared for by a large team of people, including surgeons, cardiologists, radiologists, nurses, dietitians, and technicians.

He will require a number of diagnostic tests that will take him into a variety of unfamiliar settings, such as cardiac and pulmonary diagnostic laboratories. He may also be moved from unit to unit within the hospital itself. He may be admitted to a medical unit for diagnostic workup until a definite diagnosis is made. If surgery is indicated he may be moved to a surgical unit until surgery and then to an intensive care unit until his critical postoperative period is over. This is usually within four or five days. The patient is then transferred back to a medical or surgical unit to recuperate for one to two weeks before discharge to the care of his private physician or local clinic.

One way to minimize the stress arising from the frequent relocation of the patient and the many diagnostic procedures is to afford the patient the opportunity to develop a trusting relationship through the assignment of a primary nurse who will be available to him through all phases of his experience, and who has advanced preparation as a cardiac surgical clinical nursing specialist.

### Nursing Assessment and Intervention

**Cognitive Factors.** The length of time for preoperative preparation and the amount of information the patient wants to know will vary. The nurse begins by trying to ascertain what the patient already knows. For example, Mr. A. has never seen a respirator. Ms. B. has used them at intervals during the past five years. Mr. A. needs different information than Ms. B. does. Hospital settings also have a patient-to-patient communication system. If the patient acquires information about the experiences accompanying cardiac surgery, it is wise to question him regarding his interpretation of it and correct any misinformation. The nurse should also ascertain that the patient's postoperative expectations are realistic. Often an anxious patient seeks reassurance by asking a number of persons the same question, and he is entitled to a similarly accurate response from each.

Whenever possible, family members should be included in the teaching program. They, too, are aware of the risks of surgery, and their anxieties may be somewhat diminished if they know what to expect when they visit the patient. (See p. 1135 for specific teaching points.)

**Affective Factors.** It is important to remember that two of the physiologic systems of the body that are involved in a major way, the circulatory and the respiratory, are the same systems directly affected by anxiety and stress-producing situations.

The nurse must be alert to the different ways anxiety is manifested and open the door to the expression of feelings. In submitting to cardiac surgery the patient is showing bravery in taking a calculated risk, and he can be assured that some degree of anxiety is an expected response. The patient who denies the significance of the experience ("It's no big deal") has his denial respected. However, his need for denial may be reduced and his opportunity to integrate the experience enhanced by supportive nursing measures, such as dealing with his specific fears and concerns, and keeping him informed as much as possible to minimize fears of the unknown.

**Sociocultural Considerations.** The patient's long illness and perhaps a previous hospitalization may have prevented his employment, and the high cost of past and present medical care, hospitalization, and surgery may leave him or his family drained physically, emotionally, and financially. If financial, home, job, or other problems exist help may be available through the social service department.

If the patient has come to the hospital from some distance, the clergyman of the patient's faith connected with the hospital's pastoral care department may substitute for the patient's usual clergyman. There will be time before surgery for them to establish a relationship. If the patient arrives from a foreign country and cannot communicate due to a language barrier, an interpreter must be found.

The nurse should recognize that there are cultural components in the response to stressful situations which will be reflected in the behavior of the patient and his family. Some patients are more expressive, and two patients from different cultures may be similarly expressive but for different reasons; for example, the one might be reacting to present reality factors, the other more to future concerns, such as the threat of invalidism or death.

### Nursing History

On admission, a nursing history is taken. The patient's perceptions and expectations related to his surgery and nursing care, how his illness has affected his usual living habits, and what he expects to have happen during his hospitalization are significant points to include. Questions about pain, dyspnea, elimination habits, locomotion, sensory losses and how he copes with these, and how he expects to get along after discharge give the patient opportunity to present problem areas in which nursing assistance may be required. The nursing care plan for each cardiac surgical patient has similarities, but each will differ according to the individual patient.

### Diagnostic Assessment

During the preoperative period, the patient undergoes many diagnostic procedures such as a cardiac catheterization and pulmonary function studies (see Chaps. 29 and 33).

When diagnostic procedures are completed the surgeon evaluates the data and discusses with the patient the findings and the recommended treatment. It is important for the nurse to know what the surgeon has explained to the patient. She can learn this either by being present at the explanation or by discussing with the surgeon later what he told the patient. Repeated experience has demonstrated that unanswered questions or varying explanations lead to the patient's increasing anxiety and lessened confidence in the staff.

### Physical Assessment

There are many obvious signs that are associated with the pathology of cardiac disease. A patient's posture may indicate difficulty in breathing. Facial expression may be tense if chest pain exists. Edema may be noted if fluid retention occurs. Distention of the neck veins may indicate increased venous pressure. Slurred speech, unsteady gait, and facial paralysis may all be clues to previous embolic pathology. Clubbing of fingers can suggest congenital pathology.

Vital signs, including rectal temperatures, are taken and recorded twice daily.

The nurse observes the patient when vital signs are taken. A weak, rapid, and/or irregular pulse may be felt and its effect on cardiac output reflected in the patient's color, level of alertness, degree of weakness, dyspnea or chest pain. Blood pressure can reveal hypertension or a reduced cardiac output. The rapid rate of respirations may indicate oxygen need or anxiety.

Physical examination of the heart and lungs by the nurse serves as a baseline for assessing early changes during the pre- and postoperative periods (see Chaps. 29 and 33).

### Infection Control

One advantage of the waiting period before surgery is to be more certain the patient is free from infection. Persons with cardiac disease and particularly those who have increased pulmonary pres-

sure are prone to lung congestion and frequent upper respiratory tract infections. Surgical candidates should be kept away from other patients with infectious diseases. Family or friends with respiratory infections should be encouraged to telephone or send cards rather than visit.

An antibiotic may be ordered preoperatively in an effort to prevent postoperative infections.

### Preparation of Surgical Site

Bacteria are found on all levels of the skin. A postsurgical wound infection could be fatal. It can spread to the sternum, mediastinum, and into the circulatory system. To prevent this, a scrub with an antibacterial preparation is ordered twice a day for ten minutes for several days prior to surgery. The patient is told why this is the only skin preparation to be used. Once he is taught the correct technique he may assume responsibility for the scrub if he is able to shower himself. The area to be covered includes front and back, from neck to knees. Special attention is paid to hairy areas, folds and ridges as the bacteria are more protected there. The hair is shampooed at least twice. Contraindications to the procedure may exist. The condition of the skin is noted and any irritations or allergies called to the physician's attention.

### Fluid and Electrolyte Balance

Patients undergoing cardiac surgery are usually on a reduced sodium diet preoperatively. The hospital prepared low sodium diet may not be very palatable to the patient. As he becomes more preoccupied with the thought of surgery he may not feel like eating. Careful attention is given to the patient's nutrition so that he receives the necessary carbohydrates, proteins, and fats. These play an essential part in the postoperative healing process.

There is a critical need for determining and maintaining fluid and electrolyte balance since most cardiac patients have some fluid retention preoperatively and receive diuretic therapy. Change in daily weight indicates the daily fluid loss or gain and on the day of surgery serves as a baseline for calculating the volume of fluid needed in the heart-lung machine during surgery. Some diuretics tend to deplete the serum potassium level. Although diuretics are usually discontinued prior to surgery the patient may require supplementary potassium. The physician may discontinue a digitalis preparation two days before surgery.

## Patient Education

One aim of preoperative teaching is to minimize the apprehension that can develop from fear of the unknown. Knowing what to expect helps the patient and his family to assist in the recovery process. The teaching-learning process is an opportunity for the patient to gain confidence in the staff and contributes to more open communication among patient, family, and staff.

The nurse in the teaching role must recognize that equipment, machines, and techniques—commonplace enough to the nurse—may be unfamiliar, and frightening to the patient. His anxiety level must be taken into consideration. The more some patients know, the better they are likely to cope. On the other hand, a suggestible patient with an already high anxiety level may become more anxious when detailed explanations are attempted and would benefit more from general explanations. For example, one patient wished to see the plastic valve that would replace her own mitral valve, but once she had seen it, her eyes widened with fear. Neither she nor the nurse had anticipated that the sight of the valve would be so upsetting. The patient stated she did not wish to see or to hear anything else about her surgery. She said she would handle whatever came as it came. However, the nurse returned later to discuss with the patient what was so frightening for her. Actually seeing the valve brought the surgery and all its risks into sharp focus. The opportunity to talk about her fears helped. There is a fine line between telling the patient enough to minimize fear and too much, so that fear is increased; and the line is different for each patient.

**Teaching Points.** Preoperatively the patient is taught the exercises that he will need to employ afterward. Of major importance is alternating dorsiflexion and hyperextension of the feet and alternating flexion of the knee and thigh to prevent venous stasis and promote the return of blood to the heart.

The patient also practices deep breathing and coughing maneuvers. Abdominal diaphragmatic breathing should be encouraged since it will help the patient expand his lungs more fully and exhale carbon dioxide more completely. He is advised to stop smoking in order to improve pulmonary function and prevent the vasospasm which is provoked by nicotine.

The patient usually requires a mechanical respirator (ventilator) postoperatively for assisted or controlled ventilation. Preoperative practice with it is indicated until the patient is familiar with how it works and how it feels.

As the day of surgery approaches the patient and family are acquainted with the following:

- **The purpose of the postsurgical unit, that is, to provide a central, well-equipped and well-staffed facility to provide around-the-clock care. The time and length of visiting hours—where they can wait, and how to obtain information regarding the patient's progress is explained. Some patients profit by a visit to the postsurgical unit to see the equipment and meet the nurse who will be caring for them.**
- **The immediate physical preparation that takes place before the patient enters the operating room—enema, shower, shave and skin preparation.**
- **The function of the cardiac monitor as well as each of the tubes that may be inserted just before surgery and removed several days afterward. There may be a cutdown, usually in the ankle or the arm (for hydration, drug administration and nutrition); a Foley catheter (for a more accurate measurement of urinary output); one or more chest tubes in the pleural space (for drainage and to help re-expand the lung); and perhaps a nasogastric tube (to prevent postoperative nausea).**
- **The fact that he will probably waken from anesthesia with an endotracheal tube and a mechanical respirator which will ease the workload of the heart by making breathing easier for him. A nasal oxygen catheter or mask may be used later.**
- **That he will not be given anything by mouth for a day or so but will resume a regular diet by the third or fourth postoperative day.**
- **The fact that pain will be intermittent and that analgesics will be given to relieve it.**
- **The usual situation is that most patients are placed on the serious list the evening prior to surgery and that opportunities are available for meeting religious needs.**
- **The fact that some but not all patients after the second to fifth day following open-heart surgery experience a period during which they lose track of time and their imaginations are quite active (see p. 1143, Postcardiotomy Delirium), that this is a temporary state and that should it occur the patient will be protected and cared for until the symptoms clear, usually within a few days.**
- **The fact that there will be dressings covering incisions on the chest and probably the groin.**

Attempts should be directed toward making general statements rather than specific statements about when tubes are removed, days spent in the intensive care unit and duration of postoperative hospital time. Any deviation from a specific prediction can be interpreted by the patient as a complication or failure of the surgical correction.

## OPERATING ROOM EXPERIENCE

The patient is usually very anxious upon leaving for the operating room as he may be only mildly sedated in an effort to limit depression of his vital centers. The primary nurse should accompany the patient and wait with him until the operating room nurse can take over and remain with the patient. The nursing care plan should accompany the patient to the operating room. Such information as a patient's hearing deficit and how it is best to communicate with him when he is without his hearing aid; or, orthopedic or other handicaps which warrant special consideration in positioning is included. A notation about the location of the family on the day of surgery, the patient's allergies and other pertinent data should also accompany him.

Previously acquired data is of great importance in planning his operating room nursing care. In many institutions, the operating room nurse sees the patient on the day before surgery and does some portion of the preoperative teaching.

When the patient arrives in the operating room he will be transferred to a surgical table in the "induction" or anesthesia room, which may be covered with a hypothermia mattress. An intracath is inserted or a cutdown may be done at this time. ECG monitor leads are fastened into place.

Following induction and intubation a venous pressure catheter may be inserted. The nurse assists in proper positioning of the patient. The unconscious patient requires good body alignment as well as freedom from acquiring pressure areas, abrasions and other injuries. A urethral catheter is inserted and the initial skin prep is begun before the patient is moved into the operating room.

The operating room team consists of surgeons, cardiologists, anesthesiologists, nurses, and pump technicians. The surgical approach is determined by the age of the patient, the pathology, the proposed surgery and the surgeon's preference. The incision may be extensive including the opening of the mediastinum and an extension of the incision to the right or left side of the lateral thoracic area. If the heart-lung machine is to be used an incision is made in the groin for insertion of the arterial line into the femoral artery. The duration of the procedure will vary but the patient is usually returned to the recovery unit three to four hours after arriving in the operating room.

### Aids to Heart Surgery

**Heart-Lung Machine, or Cardiopulmonary Bypass.** Open heart surgery is performed while the patient is being supported by the heart-lung machine.

A number of pumps and oxygenators are in use today. However, the principle underlying the use of the apparatus is to substitute temporarily for the patient's own heart and lungs during open heart surgery. The bypass can maintain circulation without damage to the organs of the body for a few hours (Fig. 63-6).

Just before surgery the machine is assembled. All parts that will come in contact with the blood priming solution are kept sterile. All connections are tightly secured to prevent the escape of the priming solution and to eliminate the entrance of air into the closed system. The apparatus is filled with a priming solution made up of electrolytes and fresh blood anticoagulated with heparin. The proportion of the varied solutions making up the priming solution as well as the rate of the flow of the perfusion will depend upon the weight of the patient as well as the type of apparatus being used.

**Oxygenator.** Three principal types of oxygenators are in use today. They include the bubble type, rotating disk, and the screen oxygenator. In the bubble type oxygenator, the bubble itself serves as the oxygenating surface. The gas bubbles must be small and multiple in order to come in contact with the large volume of unoxygenated blood. Problems with removing the bubbles from the oxygenated bloodstream have been documented. Hence, there is danger of producing microscopic gaseous emboli. The turbulence of the blood cells causes hemolysis, and there tends to be a denaturalization of the plasma protein. These problems limit the use of this apparatus. An advantage of this type of oxygenator is that it is disposable and requires a low priming volume and can be used without the addition of any blood. This is especially valuable for emergency surgery.

In the rotating disk oxygenator the venous blood is directed toward a series of small disks that expose the blood to a gaseous mixture of oxygen and carbon dioxide. Like the bubble oxygenator, it also produces some hemolysis by the agitation produced by the rotating disks but is said to cause less trauma.

The unit is simple to clean and sterilize and requires a minimal priming volume.

The screen oxygenator allows the venous blood, under the force of gravity, to filter down and through a series of stainless steel screens supported within a transparent chamber. The blood is exposed to an oxygen-rich gas mixture within the oxygenator and then returned to the patient's system. This oxygenator has no moving parts and there is little tendency toward foaming or trauma to the blood cell. It is used for prolonged surgery but does require more priming solution than either the bubble type or the rotating disk type oxygenator.

To put a patient on a conventional cardiopulmonary bypass machine, the chest is opened by either a median sternotomy or anterolateral incision. The pericardium is incised and the patient is heparinized. Catheters are inserted into the superior and inferior venae cavae. These catheters collect the venous blood by gravity. The blood (patient's and donor's) then passes through chambers in the machine, which in turn oxygenate it, remove carbon dioxide, warm or cool it to body temperature, filter out foam and bubbles, and pump it back into the body (arterial pump) through a catheter inserted into the left or right femoral artery in the groin. After the apparatus is working, and the heart is exposed, the heart's beating may be stopped temporarily, and the operation performed.

When the procedure has been completed, the venae cavae are unclamped, and the pumps are gradually slowed until the heart has resumed its function fully. The catheters are removed. Protamine sulfate is given to neutralize the anticoagulant effect of the heparin.

**Hypothermia and its Control.** An integral part of modern cardiopulmonary bypass technique is the ability rapidly to reduce and restore the patient's body temperature during the operation in an effort to take advantage of the benefits of lower perfusion rates. When surgery must be performed on a bloodless, still heart, cooling the body minimizes the danger that vital organs such as the brain and heart will be damaged by hypoxia. A lowering of body temperature means a lowering of metabolism, with less tissue need for oxygen. When the aorta has to be clamped during surgery, coronary circulation is interrupted. Cells that are cool will suffer less and have a greater chance for survival after the ex-

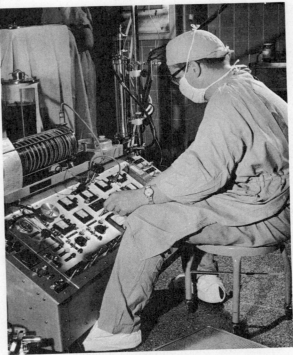

**Figure 63-6.** Heart-lung machine (blood pump-oxygenator). The machine takes over the job of pumping and oxygenating blood while surgeons operate inside the heart. This permits the surgeons a clear view of the inside of the stilled heart without its normal content of blood. Blood, just before it reaches the heart, is diverted into the heart-lung machine where gaseous wastes (carbon dioxide) are removed and it receives a fresh supply of oxygen. Blood is then pumped back into the body, entering through a main artery in the lower abdomen. (National Institutes of Health)

pected period of not receiving enough oxygen for their normal metabolic needs.

After the patient has been anesthetized, hypothermia may be induced by surface cooling employing rubber or plastic blankets containing tubing through which cold solutions are pumped. More commonly, however, cooling is accomplished after the patient is on cardiopulmonary bypass utilizing a heat exchanger. A heat exchanger is a tubular device placed in the pump circuit. It functions much like an automobile radiator in that blood passing through the heat exchanger is warmed or cooled by fluid circulated through adjacent (but separate) channels within the heat exchanger. The temperature of the blood and, therefore, the patient is controlled by varying the temperature of the "exchanging" fluid. This technique is known as core cooling in distinction to external or surface cooling.

When hypothermia is employed it is possible to cool the whole patient or only the patient's heart. Most often now the whole patient is cooled only to 25 to 30 degrees C utilizing the heart-lung machine and heat exchanger. When the surgeon desires to cool only the heart, the coronary arteries can be perfused by a separate circuit and heat exchanger or the heart may be cooled by ice cold saline placed in the pericardium about the heart. This latter technique is known as topical hypothermia. The decision to use systemic (whole body), regional or topical hypothermia depends upon the surgeon's preference, his experience, and the severity of cardiac lesion being repaired. Shivering should be prevented for it increases the metabolic activity of the brain cells by 100 per cent. It also raises the temperature and the need of tissues for oxygen. It uses up muscle and liver glycogen, leading to hypoglycemia. It also can cause hyperventilation and respiratory alkalosis.

An electric thermometer is placed in the patient's esophagus, and his temperature is watched constantly by the anesthesiologist. When the temperature is near the desired level, cooling is discontinued. There will be a downward drift of temperature even after the cooling device has been discontinued.

Rewarming is usually started when the intracardiac repair has advanced to the point when the surgeon can estimate the approximate time remaining for the completion of the repair and balance it with the anticipated rewarming time.

## POSTOPERATIVE NURSING CARE

Although it is often lifesaving, all cardiac surgery is a severe insult to the body. To make significant nursing assessments and diagnoses, and intervene appropriately, the nurse needs to understand the nature of the condition, how the abnormality affected the patient's cardiac function, how the surgery corrected it, and what his preoperative and operative experience was like.

### Preparing the Room

While the patient is undergoing surgery, the nurse checks to see that the postoperative unit is prepared to receive the patient. The equipment is checked to make sure that it is in working order. Consideration must be given to the elimination of electrical hazards. The equipment is placed about or near the patient's unit, so that it is available instantly if it is needed, but not in the way. If the unit is small, good planning is required to solve the space puzzle. Most hospitals in which a great deal of heart surgery is done have an open heart surgery recovery room permanently set up to receive postoperative heart patients.

### Transfer

The trip from the operating room to the recovery room or intensive care area should be well planned and go smoothly. If elevators are needed, arrangements should be made in advance as they should be awaiting the patient and the team.

The anesthesiologist, surgeons, and the operating room nurse usually accompany the patient to the recovery room. An endotracheal tube is in place and he receives oxygen from a small portable cylinder while being transported from the operating room. A portable suction apparatus also accompanies the patient.

The surgeon, operating room nurse, and the anesthesiologist provide information about the surgical procedure and the patient's response. Any problems during the operative course such as a prolonged pump time, bleeding problems or serious cardiac arrhythmias are cues to potential problem areas.

### Immediate Postoperative Care

As soon as he is lifted to the bed an intermittent positive pressure respirator is applied. Blood pressure, apical and radial pulses and respirations are taken. The leads for the cardiac monitor are applied so the nurse can notice immediately any change in cardiac rate or rhythm. The Foley catheter is attached to a closed urinary drainage system, and if a nasogastric tube is present, it is connected to the appropriate type of suction (single lumen tubes are to intermittent while double lumen tubes—most frequently used—are to continuous suction). The chest tubes are connected to underwater drainage. The nurse should also make a quick check of the intravenous and transfusion flow as the rate may have been accidentally changed while transferring the patient. It is also important to make certain that they are running well and not infiltrated.

If the patient is receiving a potent medication for the regulation of the heart rhythm or blood pressure, the line should be tagged and if possible it should be administered through an electronically metered machine to accurately regulate the rate of infusion. The venous pressure manometer is attached to the CVP catheter and positioned with the zero of the manometer at the level of the right atrium so the CVP pressure can be measured.

## Recovery from Anesthesia

If the patient has been on the heart-lung machine, the lightest possible anesthesia was given, and because hypothermia facilitates anesthesia, the patient usually is conscious when he comes to the recovery unit.

As soon as possible he should be told that the surgery is over. He may need to hear this several times. He may or may not be aware of the totality of the room, the people in it and the whole situation. He is aware of his discomfort and the one person with whom he attempts to speak. He cannot speak if the endotracheal tube is still in place. If he communicates that he is thirsty, he can be told that a drink now would not be indicated. Moistening his lips with a wet gauze might help.

## Responsibility to Family

Once the patient is in the recovery room, his family requires information and reassurance about his condition. The patient's surgeon has an important role in explaining what surgery was done, how the patient responded to it, and what the general outlook is at this time for the patient's recovery. The nurse, too, helps the members of the family understand and cope with the situation by such measures as reviewing with them what the surgeon has said, by listening to and supporting them, and by arranging for brief visits to the patient if this is indicated. The importance of the nurse learning what the surgeon explains to the family cannot be overemphasized as this forms the basis for the explanation which she gives.

No matter how well the preoperative education program is presented, the environment of the open-heart recovery room and the variety of equipment can prove very stressful to the patient and his visitors. Visitors, too, require support lest their looks of fear, sorrow and disbelief distress the postoperative patient.

## NURSING ASSESSMENT AND INTERVENTION

Most cardiac surgical patients are susceptible to a number of postoperative complications. Many have had long-standing pulmonary disease as well as enlarged hearts and myocardial reserve may be low. Patients may also have needed diuretics along with a restricted sodium intake and hence fluid and electrolyte balance may be disturbed.

Normal body processes undergo stress when subjected to hypothermia and perfusion. Acid-base and fluid balance, alveolar ventilation, and tissue oxygenation are examples of body processes subjected to disruption.

The concept of intensive care includes accurate, continuous, and comprehensive data collection regarding the patient's responses. Each physiologic system is observed and evaluated both separately and in relation to other body systems. The patient's psychological reaction is also considered because of the potent effect of emotions on the cardiovascular and respiratory response. Even minor deviations from the patient's baseline data suggest a potential critical situation.

## Activity

It is important to collaborate with the surgeon in helping the patient and family learn what activities can be safely assumed after discharge. Often families who have experienced a lifetime of caring both physically and emotionally for a patient will try to hold him back as they themselves cannot change their role from one which requires the patient to be dependent on them.

Age, the severity of illness preoperatively, the operative procedure, and the postoperative course are factors relevant to activity prescription. Most persons are capable of being up and about and doing a minimal amount of work upon discharge. They are encouraged to take rest periods as needed but are discouraged from thinking they will go home to bed rest.

Patients need help to realize that although they are up and about in the hospital, the hospital environment is such that it is not conducive to long periods of walking or visiting. It may be helpful to point out that the actual amount of time spent being up and about is perhaps only two or three hours a day, at most. Patients often get concerned when they get home and find they tire easily. They tend to equate the home with the hospital situation whereas the effects of deconditioning rather than the environment are the basis of their fatigue.

Because of the patient's lowered physical resistance crowds should be avoided since colds and upper respiratory infections can be easily acquired. Crowds also tend to tire the individual.

Driving is usually not permitted at this time due to the thoractomy incision that is still healing. Usually long trips are discouraged because the individual will need medical supervision for the first few weeks.

## Medical Followup

Cardiac surgical patients are given close medical followup for a brief period at the medical center after discharge.

If the patient is from a distant area, the need for medical followup, either by a physician or nurse specialist in an outpatient department or private office, is important and should be stressed to the patient. The visits are usually weekly for the first few weeks and usually become less frequent as time passes. Communication is made by the medical center physician to the physician who is to follow the patient. Information about the disease, surgical correction, and postoperative course is given, as well as the suggested medical regime after discharge.

Some patients are allowed to return to work six to twelve weeks postoperatively. Others have a more prolonged postoperative course. Most patients can, however, return to a more productive and satisfying way of life.

The patient can be expected to have ups and downs. Any person who has to curtail so many pleasures and so many of the normal experiences of life is bound to become discouraged, angry and resentful at times. It is important for the patient to keep in touch with his friends, even if it gives him a twinge of envy, to keep up with his interests and develop new ones, within his activity prescription. Instead of worrying about how much he cannot do, the patient can be encouraged to emphasize what he can do.

Self-centeredness is a natural consequence of a prolonged illness. As a result, the patient's relationships with others may suffer. As he recovers, he may require considerable time, patience, and perhaps some counseling to develop new attitudes and more mature relationships. This is an especially important area for the community health nurse or the nurse clinician in the outpatient department.

## The Circulatory System

In addition to apical and extremity pulse monitoring and auscultation of heart sounds, there are several other sources of data for the circulatory assessment.

**ECG Monitor.** The nurse must know the types of arrhythmias and understand their significance. Those such as ventricular premature beats (VPB's), ventricular tachycardia (VT), and various degrees of heart block are not uncommon, but they may be dangerous occurrences and should be reported to the surgeon immediately.

Patients with aortic valve prostheses frequently in their immediate postoperative period have an ECG picture that resembles an anterior to lateral wall infarction with a Q wave and S-T segment elevation in leads $V_3$ to $V_6$. After two to three days this abnormality usually disappears.

**Arterial Pressure Monitoring.** Cuff blood pressure measurement is taken frequently in the immediate postoperative period. Or, the patient may have his arterial blood pressure recorded directly and continuously on another channel of the monitoring device. A small polyethylene catheter may have been inserted in the patient's radial or femoral artery during surgery. The pressure in this artery is transmitted via the tip of the catheter through rigid plastic tubing to a pressure sensitive device such as a strain gauge or other type of transducer. The transducer converts the mechanical energy of pressure changes within the artery to electrical output. This is calibrated and equated to equivalent changes in millimeters of mercury which can be displayed on an oscilloscope or recorder. Small fluctuations in arterial blood pressure can be recorded and are obtainable at times when cuff blood pressures cannot be obtained. The arterial line also serves as a direct means by which blood for gas studies can be obtained.

The nurse is aided by the arterial monitoring device, but this also entails the responsibility for making certain that the recording is accurate. The nurse must calibrate the machine periodically.

Important points for nurses caring for patients with intra-arterial catheters are:

- **The nurse is responsible for maintaining a slow drip of heparinized saline into the arterial line at all times. A usual solution is normal saline with 2,000 units of heparin per liter.**
- **The line needs to be flushed after arterial blood samples are drawn if blood backs up into the arterial line, or if an inadequate pressure curve is noted on the screen. The use of "Intraflow," a commercially available continuous flush system, facilitates flushing the line without adjustment of the slow maintenance drip.**
- **All connections from patient to transducer and to syringe must be secure to prevent the introduction of air into the system or accidental separation which could result in exsanguination.**
- **All connections from patient to transducer must be kept free from contamination as infection can penetrate the catheter tract.**
- **The patient's position must be checked frequently to be sure the catheter is not kinked.**

Pulmonary artery pressure may also be monitored (see Chap. 59).

**Central Venous Pressure.** A central venous pressure reading is also done frequently. This line may also be used for drawing the venous blood samples that are necessary. The normal reading of the central venous pressure in or near the right atrium is estimated around 0 to 4 cm. of water. The numerical value is not as important as the occurrence of a change either increasing or decreasing. Because venous pressure is sensitive to an increased pressure in the respiratory system the patient should be off the ventilator at the time of the recording, or the fact that he is on the ventilator taken into account in interpreting the reading.

**Thermistor Probe.** Another indicator of the adequacy of the circulation is the tissue perfusion of the extremities. A thermister probe may be taped to the great toe, or the temperature, color, and character of the pulses in the feet can be used to estimate circulatory status.

**Artificial Pacemaker.** Some patients have pacemaker wires sewn on the epicardium and brought out through the chest wall. For most patients they are not connected continuously to a pacemaker unit but are connected when needed. Patients with a mitral valve prosthesis frequently have such standby pacers since edema around the sutures in the valve area is apt to develop several hours after surgery and can result in complete heart block. When not connected to the pacemaker unit, the wires need to be protected by being placed in a rubber glove and

taped to the chest so the patient will not inadvertently receive a microshock from contact with a metal surface or by a person that is touching the pacer wires at the same time they are in contact with a metal surface.

## Specific Circulatory Complications

**Emboli.** In mitral stenosis there is stasis of blood in the left atrium, and clots may have formed. Any clots observed during surgery are removed, but perhaps one escaped into the general circulation. There is no longer stasis of blood in the left atrium, and the free-flowing blood may push a clot along. Close observation should be made for symptoms of emboli in the legs, especially after a commissurotomy. Using the preoperative assessment data denoting the presence or absence of pulses in the lower extremities is important as the nurse evaluates the patient.

Embolization likewise is a danger after atrial fibrillation, which also allows blood to stay relatively still in the atrium, so that clots may form. After open heart surgery there is danger of air emboli affecting the brain. Neurologic symptoms, such as slurred speech, distortion of facial muscles or the tongue, and hemiparesis, may occur after air or a blood embolus to the brain. Dyspnea, cough, and expectoration of bloody sputum may indicate pulmonary embolism. An embolus to the spleen may cause sudden left flank pain, whereas an embolus to a kidney may result in hematuria and flank pain.

**Cardiac Tamponade.** Although the pericardium is left open to prevent the development of tamponade, blood clots sometimes prevent adequate drainage. One of the earliest indications is an increase in the central venous pressure. The alert nurse may then notice that the heart sounds appear muffled when listening to the chest. The paradoxical effect of respiration on the blood pressure can also be noted. The changing heights of systolic pressure on inspiration and expiration are easily detected if the arterial pressure transducer is connected to a readout machine. They can also be noted when taking a cuff pressure if the nurse slowly reduces the cuff pressure to find the level at which sounds are heard at the end of respiration and then continues to reduce the pressure until she finds the level at which the systolic sound is heard during inspiration as well as expiration. If respiration causes a difference greater than 10 mm. Hg it is considered to be a para-doxical effect and should be investigated as an indicator of tamponade. Other symptoms are lowered voltage on the ECG and a narrow pulse pressure.

### Respiratory Assessment

An endotracheal tube or tracheotomy with mechanical ventilation, assisted or controlled, is essential for the postoperative patient. A reduction in the patient's lung capacity may be due to the use of anesthetics or other drugs, a prolonged chronic disease process, pain or fear. The selection of the specific type of respirator to be used and the initial setting is the responsibility of the physician.

To evaluate the effectiveness of the breathing device and the patient's response the nurse can use a respirometer to be sure the patient is receiving an adequate tidal volume. Blood is drawn from the arterial line for blood gas analysis. In many units the nurse is responsible for drawing the blood, using the blood gas analyzer machine, and changing the respirations to maintain the blood gases at a prescribed level. The cyanosis of a patient's nail beds or lips may be a clue to inadequate ventilation, but in most patients cyanosis is not clinically evident until the $Po_2$ has dropped below 50 mm. Hg, so it is not a reliable indicator of early hypoxemia. Restlessness, flaring of the nares and a poorly moving chest cage are causes for concern. The prepared nurse can listen to the patient's lungs and note the presence of congestion or diminished breathing sounds. (See Chapters 29 and 60.) If the respiratory rate is increased the nurse must question if it is a result of an obstruction such as a mucus plug, improper positioning, splinting from incisional pain or circulatory insufficiency. The daily chest x-ray report is also valuable to the physician.

### Pain

If the patient complains of pain and the discomfort is not alleviated by positioning and other nursing measures, narcotics are given. The patient's vital signs and the cardiac monitor rhythm are checked before a drug is administered and periodically during the time of its effect. The dosage of narcotics given to patients who have had cardiac surgery is frequently less than average.

Since impaired circulation delays the action of pain medication given intramuscularly, medication in small amounts is given intravenously. While the patient is on the respirator, narcotics may be given to synchronize the patient with the respirator as well as for complaints of pain. After the patient is off the respirator, narcotics are given very sparingly because of the danger of respiratory depression.

### Assessment of Fluid-Electrolyte and Acid-Base Balance

The accurate monitoring of the patient's intake and output, including nasogastric drainage, along with his body weight, is most helpful in determining the type and amount of his fluid requirements. The type of intravenous solution that is ordered will depend upon the patient's need for nourishment as well as laboratory reports of serum electrolytes.

The rate of the infusion is adjusted according to the physician's order. He prescribes the total amount that will effect fluid replacement without overloading the cardiovascular system and the approximate hourly rate. This may need to be adjusted according to the patient's circulatory response. Hypovolemia must be avoided also as it may contribute to diminished tissue perfusion. Central venous pressure measurement is one guide to fluid replacement.

Urinary output via a Foley catheter is used to assess both circulatory and renal function. If tissue perfusion to the kidney is adequate to result in urine formation then it is assumed that perfusion of the other vital organs is adequate also. If the blood pressure and other measurements of circulatory function are normal but there is either scanty or no urine, renal shutdown may be present.

An hourly recording of urinary output is usually ordered. An hourly output of 30 ml. is adequate; output below this should be reported to the physician. Urinary output upon arrival in the intensive care unit is often elevated due to the osmotic diuretics used when the patient is on bypass. This situation corrects itself in a few hours. The patient may also have hemoglobinuria since lysis of blood cells can occur during prolonged cardiopulmonary bypass.

If the Foley catheter is irrigated to prevent clogging the amount of irrigating solution must be deducted from the total output. Specific gravity readings are taken hourly for information about the patient's hydration and how well his kidneys are concentrating the urine. Urine is usually tested for sugar, acetone, and pH as well.

If a nasogastric tube is in use, it must be kept open and the drainage recorded. Usually electrolyte solution is ordered to replace any gastric drainage. Most patients do not have nasogastric tubes initially, but need to be watched for signs of gastric distention which may exert pressure upon the diaphragm and move it upward, restricting respiratory movement.

## Chest Tube

The care of the chest tube is the same as for any patient who has had chest surgery (see Chap. 16). The nurse ascertains that chest tubes are not compressed, that there is no leak, and that the drainage flows through them. Unless the connecting tube lies lower than the wound, drainage will not take place. If drainage collects in the coils, the nurse changes the position of the tube so that the drainage flows into the collection bottle. Allowing drainage to remain stationary inside the tube may allow clotting and plugging of the tube. To prevent this the nurse should "milk" the tubes for their entire length at least once an hour. At this same interval the chest drainage is measured and level marked on the collection bottle. A running blood balance should be maintained at all times so the nurse can tell immediately whether the patient is ahead or behind on blood volume replacement. The surgeon usually orders chest drainage to be replaced volume for volume with fresh whole blood.

## Wound Care

As with other types of surgery, incisions are inspected regularly and dressings are changed using strict aseptic technique to prevent infection.

## Mobility

Mobility of patients is encouraged to prevent circulatory stasis and prevent the formation of thrombi. Active leg exercises are begun on the operative day when the patient's position is changed when possible. Anti-Embolism (Elastic) stockings are also used to prevent venous stasis.

The patient with a midline incision is turned to either side. After the patient has been lying on his back and turns toward his tubes, there often is a rush of bloody drainage as the accumulated fluid finds an escape. Each time the patient is assisted to turn, the chest drainage tubes must be checked to make sure the patient is not lying on them. Sometimes folded towels can be placed in such a way that they prevent the patient from lying on his drainage tubes.

Patients are often afraid to move as pain may accompany the turning as well as the fear of "coming apart." Skillful nursing care can help the patient tolerate the activity by carrying it out in the way which causes least pain and apprehension and which emphasizes the positive benefits of the procedure to the patient.

## Postcardiotomy Delirium

A high percentage of postoperative open-heart patients (approximately 25 per cent) develop a transient psychosis, usually after a lucid interval of two to five days. This state is characterized in some patients by perceptual illusions often related to the technology surrounding the patient such as the cardiac monitor or a respirator. Some patients experience proprioceptive distortions such as a floating sensation or thinking the bed is moving. Others develop confusion and disorientation especially at night and some have difficulty distinguishing between dreams and reality. Still others go on to experience hallucinations and paranoid elaborations which they may act upon. For example, a patient may believe he is a victim of a plot, pull out tubes or pacing wires or IV's and assault personnel. These symptoms generally clear up in a few days.

**Etiological Factors.** Heller (1974), describes the open heart recovery room as one of the most psychogenic environments ever created by the mind of man, noting also that all of the stresses of modern life produce hallucinations on a schizophrenic basis in only 1 per cent of the population. He describes many contributing factors:

- A patient who at some level is terrified about the possibility of sudden death, mutilation, and invalidism.
- Immobilization in bed by attachment to arterial and venous pressure lines, respirators, underwater chest drainage, gastric drainage, IV's, ECG monitor, and so on imprisons him. Not only is their bulk overwhelming, but strange noises come from them and personnel use peculiar language when referring to them. Activities such as irrigating tubes, turning dials, taking his blood, giving him blood, listening to

his heart, looking at the oscilloscope attached to him, tracheal suctioning, and a host of other activities are far removed from earlier illness experience.

- Possible anoxic or hypoxic episodes from preoperative insults to his brain, from cardiac failure or emboli or from low arterial blood pressure during surgery.
- The unphysiologic situation of cardiopulmonary bypass where the patient's blood is mixed with that of many others, oxygen bubbled through it, and passed through plastic tubing.
- Sensory deprivation due to placement in a room with no or few windows with lights on continuously.
- Periods of sensory overload such as during a crisis in his own recovery or one of his roommates.
- Sleep and dream deprivation due to frequent awakening for vital signs, coughing, positioning, suctioning.
- Castration anxiety associated with groin incisions.
- The personality type of the patient; those who find passivity difficult are most vulnerable.

**Prevention.** Research studies show that reduction in one or more of the factors will reduce the incidence of delirium. Incidence has been halved by a preoperative psychiatric research interview and follow-up visits postsurgery (Heller, 1974). The nurse can contribute to prevention by:

- **A preoperative explanation to the patient that there may be a period when he loses track of time and his imagination becomes very active, but that this is a common treatable, and transient, reaction.**
- **Encouraging the expression of thoughts and feelings before and after surgery.**
- **Early detection of delirium so that early treatment can be instituted. (Minor tranquilizers are used to reduce anxiety; a major tranquilizer such as chlorpromazine is used if agitation, illusions, delusions, or hallucinations occur.)**
- **Planning the patient's care to allow for the most physiologic sleep and dreaming; patients should be awakened for only urgent reasons.**
- **An attitude on the part of the nurse which conveys warmth and genuine concern, and a manner that conveys the firmness necessary to encourage progress.**
- **The promotion of as normal an environment as possible by such measures as frequent, patient-orienting statements regarding time, day, and weather; exposure to windows when possible; the use of wall clocks, calendars, transistor radios; and visitors within the patient's tolerance.**
- **Reduction of sensory overload by placement in private rooms or by drawing drapes when crises occur with other patients, but keeping the patient informed of what is happening and eliciting his feelings about the situation so he need not fantasize and increase his anxiety; dimming lights at night, toning down or tuning out auditory and visual stimuli from monitoring equipment.**

- **Including the patient in the plan of care.**
- **Encouraging return to physical activity such as chair sitting or ambulation as soon as medically permitted.**

## CARDIAC SURGICAL RESEARCH

In medical centers that have a strong teaching and research program, many parameters are monitored during the postoperative period. This type of monitoring provides valuable information on the complex pathophysiologic changes that some patients experience. Much of the surgery performed at such research centers is of greater complexity and on higher risk patients than the average heart surgery procedure. While uncomplicated heart surgery can be done with less than two hours pump time, complex procedures can require four hours or longer, with a resultant sharp increase in mortality. The complications that seem related to long pump time are low output syndrome, shock lung, and a bleeding diathesis which may be due to disseminated intravascular clotting (DIC) or the absence of essential clotting factors in the blood. For this high risk group continuous monitoring often includes measurement of cardiac output, left atrial or pulmonary artery pressure, and expired carbon dioxide tension. "In vivo" measuring devices may also be employed to get continuous measurements of $Po_2$, $Pco_2$, and pH rather than reliance on intermittent sampling procedures for blood gas determinations. Frequent measurement of blood lactic acid may also be made since this is more reliable than the pH for determining the severity of the acidosis accompanying shock. In critical patients measurements of the plasma colloid osmotic pressure (oncotic pressure) is indicated since comparison with the pulmonary artery pressure provides an index of the possibility of pulmonary edema. Studies that are being made seem to support the hypothesis that the administration of blood and plasma to maintain the colloid osmotic pressure between 21 to 25 torr will maintain an adequate circulating blood volume and increase the cardiac output as long as the pulmonary artery (or left atrial) pressure is not elevated. When pulmonary artery pressure is high, pulmonary edema is apt to occur, especially if the colloid osmotic pressure is low. These factors increase the need for the continuing development of the cardiac surgical nurse's knowledge and skills in the care of the critically ill patient.

## USUAL PROGRESSION OF INTENSIVE PATIENT CARE

As the patient's condition stabilizes the respirator is discontinued and the endotracheal tube is removed—usually in 24 to 48 hours. The patient may then be started on nasal oxygen and will be encouraged to use an intermittent positive pressure respirator for deep breathing and coughing. The Foley catheter, one intravenous line, the central venous pressure line and the arterial blood pressure line are all discontinued about a day later. The chest tubes may also be removed on the second or third postoperative day depending upon the amount of drainage that has been noted. If the patient has an artificial cardiac valve he is started on anticoagulants at this time. They are not started earlier because additional bleeding from the chest may occur. Digitalis preparations may be restarted. Antibiotics are continued intravenously for another four or five days and then if needed are given orally.

The patient's vital signs are taken every two hours at this stage and he begins progressively to ambulate. A restricted sodium liquid diet is ordered after the endotracheal tube is removed.

The patient who has had an endotracheal tube in place for a day or so will complain of a sore throat and excessive thirst for a few days after it is removed. If the patient is on restricted fluids he will need help, such as careful and consistent explanations, in remembering and abiding by this regime. Involving the patient in recording his intake and output gives him a chance to participate in his care, distribute his allotment with some personal choice and demonstrate understanding of the reasons for it.

As the patient's course continues to progress he begins to see signs of improvement (for example, ambulation) yet he is still feeling sick and remains in a potentially critical phase. While the need for constant observation and evaluation by the nurse is still important, she must attempt to prepare him for his return to a general medical or surgical unit within the next few days.

The nurse encourages the patient gradually to become more independent and lets him begin to regain confidence by doing things for himself. Gentle encouragement accompanied by support as he tries each new activity can help the patient to greater independence. The nurse guides his judgment and encourages him to make some decisions for himself. He can probably wash his face and hands and comb his hair by the second or third postoperative day. When some of his drainage tubes are removed he can be encouraged to put on his own pajamas, rather than wearing hospital gowns, as this will help him more toward viewing himself as convalescent.

## TRANSFERRING THE PATIENT

When it is time for the patient to be moved to another unit it is a nurse's responsibility to be certain that he knows when and where he will be moved, to accompany him in an effort to make the transfer as easy as possible, to introduce him to the new staff nurse, and to explain to the receiving nurse, in the presence of the patient, the patient's permitted activities. After leaving the room, the ICU nurse should review his written nursing care plan and pertinent hospital experiences and explain any recommendations she may have for his future care. The ECG is usually monitored for at least one more week.

The next two weeks are directed toward preparing the patient for discharge. Emphasis is on patient education and counseling.

Some patients become depressed and are confused or hostile, crying easily. They may say that they don't know why they are crying, but they just feel sorry for themselves. The patient may doubt that he will improve, or he may be afraid that he will. If he has been forced to limit his activities, he may now be unsure how to handle a new freedom. For example, a young adult who, because of his cardiac condition, is socially inexperienced in some respects such as dancing, may be self-conscious about initiating activities or skills which are well developed in his peers.

The expectation of what will happen after surgery can be important in the patient's postoperative adjustment. If he expected a complete cure and has had only partial relief of his symptoms, he may be resentful, and he may refuse to adhere to his low sodium diet or to the restrictions on his activities. The family may expect the postoperative patient to take the subway or the bus, whereas before they had been driving him. They may expect him to resume a full program of activities; he may or may not be able to do so.

These patient reactions are not unusual. The patient can be helped to identify what is troubling him and to express what he feels. His family may (or may not) be a comfort to him; they can be part of the counseling process also. If the depression is severe, the physician may order medication to help the patient through the period more comfortably. For some patients psychotherapy is beneficial.

During a crying episode one patient, who was usually a very independent businesswoman, was able to acknowledge that she just was lonely and could not wait for her family to come in, thus conveying her feelings of dependence and need for support. Other patients may request that a nurse stay and just listen and talk.

A common reaction in patients' behavior noted soon after the first four days postoperatively is questioning or hostile behavior. Patients who were able to discuss these feelings later said that they felt they were not making progress in their postoperative course because everything seemed the same. This feeling was compounded by members of the staff asking how they were doing. Apparently these patients were not capable of evaluating their progress, but wanted reassurance from others who had access to their hospital record and knew more about the details of their progress. Another reason for this depressed attitude is that patients tend to measure progress by new things occurring. In the first few days tubes are removed, ambulation begins, and fluids are taken. During the next week the patient's obvious criteria for measuring progress are limited. Listening to the patient's view of how he is doing may include his disappointment that he is not progressing faster than he is. Or, he may need the chance to say that he doesn't know how he is doing since nobody gives him any information about his progress. The nurse provides tangible and realistic reassurance by helping the patient to observe and evaluate signs of progress, such as increasing assumption of activities of daily living, and progressive ambulation.

## ACTIVITY PRESCRIPTION

Today the emphasis is on systematic prescription of activity for the cardiac patient in order to enhance his functional capacity. (See Chapter 39, Rehabilitation of Patients with Heart Disease.)

For the cardiac surgical patient careful assessment should be made of the patient's past activity and his attitude towards it. One person who was never sick before cardiac surgery led a very active life. While he was "taking it easy and convalescing" in the hospital the nurse found him chinning himself on the bathroom shower bar. When this was discussed the patient admitted he only did a few chin ups and that was reduced activity for him! In another instance, a patient who had a long history of very symptomatic cardiac illness had not done much for herself in some time. She did nothing for herself while in the hospital without prompting. She had to be helped to accept a new, more active role. Some patients who had problems sleeping flat in bed prior to surgery may still require a sitting position for sleep even after the symptoms are relieved. Even if a patient adjusts physiologically he may not be able to change his old habits immediately.

## Preparation for Discharge

Prior to discharge the nurse should review the patient's home situation. A patient may live alone and have no one to help him. Discharge to home may be unsuitable if a patient lives on an upper floor in a walkup building. Or, a patient may live in a crowded small apartment with a number of other persons including small children, where proper rest and limited activity would not be possible. On occasion a person may feel insecure and be afraid to go home and seeks some further assistance with convalescence in an extended care facility. Once there, the patient can slowly begin to get back to a more normal existence. Dressing in street clothes, going to a dining area for meals, and taking walks outside with some supervision gradually accustom the patient to activities of daily living.

If a patient needs domestic help at home, arrangements can be sought with the help of social service. If health supervision and some nursing care are to be given, a community nursing referral can be initiated several days prior to discharge so that there are no gaps in continuity of care.

## PATIENT EDUCATION

### Artificial Heart Valves

The nurse explains to the patient with an artificial heart valve that he may hear his valve clicking when he gets home. The hospital setting may be too noisy but the quiet atmosphere at home may allow the patient to hear the noise for the first time. This is especially true if the patient is thin and/or has a small chest cage. He should be assured that the clicking is normal and that an occasional skip of a heartbeat is common. The clicking sound may eventually disappear as new tissue grows around the valve edges. Sleeping on a foam rubber pillow may decrease the sound.

Permanent anticoagulation therapy is thought medically advisable in patients having prosthetic valves, as thrombus complications are a potential hazard. Prothrombin level should be between 20 and 30 per cent. The patient should know the action, dosage, tablet size, and plan of administration and monitoring of the drug and the signs of overdosage such as hematuria, hemoptysis, and large ecchymotic spots. Some patients are advised to keep a supply of vitamin $K_1$ on hand. He should also be alerted to the need for using nonsalicylate medications such as acetaminophen (Tylenol) and dextropropoxyphene (Darvon) for minor pain since salicylates potentiate the action of anticoagulants and not to take over-the-counter drugs without his physician's consent because of the danger of drug interactions. (See also Rodman, M. and Smith, D. W.: *Clinical Pharmacology in Nursing*, Philadelphia, Lippincott, 1974 for additional material on patient education.)

## ADDITIONAL DRUG THERAPY

A patient may go home on a digitalis preparation and perhaps a diuretic, potassium supplement, vitamin, and anticoagulant. He may have been on all or some of these prior to admission, but patient and family may require instruction concerning them. (See Chapter 34, The Patient with Congestive Heart Failure.)

Individualizing medication regimes is helpful in securing compliance. For example, a young patient took all her medications regularly except her diuretic which she often "forgot." On questioning further it was found that this medication was ordered "8 A.M. Mon.—Wed.—Fri." and this was the time she was going to college classes. The diuretic caused frequency and urgency which she could not tolerate. A smaller dose was prescribed to be taken b.i.d.

## DIET THERAPY

The patient may be discharged on a low sodium, low cholesterol diet. Helpful diet instructional ma-terials for the patient are available through local chapters of the American Heart Association. Dietitians should emphasize the need for a well-balanced nutritious diet as some patients are still slightly anemic at the time of discharge. (Not only can the bypass destroy red blood cells at the time of surgery, but the life span of the remaining ones is curtailed.)

## REFERENCES AND BIBLIOGRAPHY

ASPINALL, M. J.: *Nursing the Open-Heart Surgery Patient*, New York, McGraw-Hill, 1973.

BEAUMONT, E.: Hypo/hyperthermia equipment, Product Survey, *Nurs. '74* 4:35, April 1974.

BROGAN, M.: Nursing care of the patient experiencing cardiac surgery for coronary artery disease, *Nurs. Clin. N. Am.* 7:517, September 1972.

BROWN, G.: The post-operative heart patient, chap. 8, in McIntyre, M., ed.: *Heart Disease: New Dimensions of Nursing Care*, Garden Grove, Calif., Trainex Press, 1974.

CHOW, R.: Identifying professional nursing practice through research: Cardiosurgical patient care, *Int. J. Nurs. Stud.* 9:125, August 1972.

Defusing a coronary—with gas, *Life* 68:75, April 1970.

DeVILLIER, B.: Preoperative teaching of the cardiovascular patient, *Heart Lung* 2:522, July-August 1973.

ELLIS, H., JR.: *Surgery for Acquired Mitral Valve Disease*, Philadelphia, Saunders, 1967.

ELLIS, R.: Unusual sensory and thought disturbances after cardiac surgery, *Am. J. Nurs.* 72:2021, November 1972.

ELSBERRY, N. L.: Psychological responses to open heart surgery, *Nurs. Res.* 21:220, May-June 1972.

FINLAND, M.: Current problems in infective endocarditis: With special reference to cases acquired in hospital or after cardiac surgery, *Mod. Conc. Cardiovasc. Dis.* 41:53, November 1972.

FRANK, K. A., et al.: A survey of adjustment to cardiac surgery, *Arch. Intern. Med.* 130:735, 1972.

HELLER, S.: Sex after cardiac surgery, *Med. Asp. Human Sex. VIII:* 150, February 1974.

————: Psychological needs of the cardiac patient, Chapter 3, in McIntyre, M., ed.: *Heart Disease: New Dimensions of Nursing Care*, Garden Grove, Calif., Trainex Press, 1974.

HELLER, S., et al.: Psychiatric complications of open-heart surgery: A re-examination, *N. Eng. J. Med.* 283:1015, 1970.

HODGES, L. C.: Systems and nursing care of the cardiac surgical patient, *Nurs. Clin. N. Am.* 6:415, September 1971.

JOHNSON, D.: Cardiovascular care in the first person, *ANA Clinical Sessions* 1972, New York, Appleton-Century-Crofts, 1973:127.

JOLY, H., and WEIL, M.: Temperature of the great toe as an indication of the severity of shock, *Circulation* 35:131, 1969.

KOUCHOUHOS, N., and KIRKLIN, J.: Coronary bypass operations for ischemic heart disease, *Mod. Conc. Cardiovasc. Dis.* 41:10, October 1972.

LAYNE, O., et al.: Post-operative psychosis in cardiotomy; the role of organic and psychiatric factors, *N. Eng. J. Med.* 284:518, 1971.

LONG, M., et al.: Cardiopulmonary bypass, *Am. J. Nurs.* 74:860, May 1974.

MCFADDEN, E. H.: Sleep deprivation in patients having open-heart surgery, *Nurs. Res.* 20:249, May-June 1971.

MESERKO, V.: Pre-operative classes for cardiac patients, *Am. J. Nurs.* 73:665, April 1973.

MUNDTH, E. D., et al.: Myocardial revascularization during postinfarction shock, *Hosp. Pract.* 8:113, January 1973.

NORMAN, J., et al.: *Cardiac Surgery,* New York, Appleton-Century-Crofts, 1967.

Open-heart surgery. *RN* 34:OR-18, March 1971.

Optimal resources for cardiac surgery. ICHD Report. *Circulation* XLIV: Suppl. A-221, September 1971.

PARSONS, M.: The surgical intensive care nurse and cardiac surgery, *AORN* 18:124, July 1973.

REED, A. E.: Cardiopulmonary bypass, *AORN* 18:87, July 1973.

SCHECHTER, D., et al.: Post infarction complications—surgery may save your patient, *Consultant* 12:36, February 1972.

VERDERBER, A.: Cardiopulmonary bypass: Postoperative complications, *Am. J. Nurs.* 74:868, May 1974.

WALKER, B. B.: The postsurgery heart patient: Amount of uninterrupted time for sleep and rest during the first, second, and third postoperative days in a teaching hospital, *Nurs. Res.* 21:164, March-April 1972.

# The Patient in Renal Failure

Renal failure, acute or chronic, exists when a person's renal function is inadequate to maintain the normal volume and composition of his internal environment.

Advances in hemodialysis (the artificial kidney) and kidney transplantation within the past decade offer hope to many persons with serious kidney disease for a longer and more productive life. However, these measures have high economic and psychosocial costs. Hence it is a major goal of the nephrology team to help the person with serious kidney disease preserve the function of his own kidneys for as long as possible. Bernbeck (1973) notes that persons with only 10 to 25 per cent of remaining renal function can be maintained for years with only conservative therapy.

In fact, the vast majority of patients with chronic kidney disease receive "conservative" treatment: many are in the older age group. For these patients, the crux of therapy is medical and dietary prescription and nursing support of the patient and family through the many crises precipitated by the physical, emotional, and social changes the patient with progressive renal failure undergoes.

## ETIOLOGY

The problem resulting in uremia can be *prerenal,* within the kidney parenchyma itself (*renal*), or *postrenal.*

Conditions that markedly decrease the supply of blood to the kidneys, such as shock or thrombosis of the arteries supplying the kidneys, are in the prerenal category. If the ischemia is not immediately remedied, renal failure and uremia can result.

**1149**

The problem may be within the kidney itself as in acute renal tubular necrosis (lower nephron nephrosis) due for example to lethal doses of chemicals and drugs such as barbiturates, nephrotoxic antibiotics, bichloride of mercury, or carbon tetrachloride, or it may be due to transfusion with incompatible blood or severe ischemia. Chronic glomerulopathies such as those due to the streptococcus, systemic lupus erythematosus or diabetes mellitus, acute vascular or infectious disorders, and polycystic disease can result in progressive destruction of nephrons and progressively worsening renal insufficiency eventuating in end stage renal failure.

Postrenal problems such as obstruction of the lower urinary tract with ascending infection can cause damage to the kidney if not promptly treated.

## PREVENTION

Nurses, physicians, and the lay public have important roles in preventing kidney damage and in delaying the progression of renal insufficiency to the end stage of renal failure. Renal failure occurs more frequently when body fluid reserves are depleted. Nurses contribute to the prevention of prerenal insults and iatrogenic renal failure by planning with hospitalized patients a system of oral fluid intake, particularly for those patients who may be too old, too weak, disinterested, or otherwise unable to reach for the water pitcher on the bedside stand. Nursing orders are then entered on the patient's nursing care plan for the team to carry out.

Contrary to traditional hospital operation, a physician's order is not necessary for a patient's intake and output to be recorded. Rather all patients should be assessed for intake and output. Careful recording of intake and output for selected patients is frequently a judgment made by an alert nurse after her assessment of the patient. Physician consultation follows.

Withholding fluid and foods for long periods of time prior to general anesthesia can be dangerous, particularly in the elderly. The patient undergoing diagnostic tests who is given nothing by mouth before each procedure several days in a row (particularly when the preparation for x-rays such as the GI series requires several cleansing enemas) is a prime candidate for iatrogenic renal failure. The nurse must encourage fluids for as long as permitted preprocedure or preoperatively while taking the patient's cardiovascular status into consideration.

Intravenous fluids with central venous pressure monitoring may be ordered preoperatively by the physician to insure adequate blood flow to the kidney. The use of mannitol, the reduced form of the 6-carbon sugar mannose, is sometimes utilized to maintain urinary flow when renal ischemia is a potential hazard.

Lowered cardiac output due to such conditions as cardiac arrhythmias, anaphylactic shock, or accidental blood loss compromises renal blood flow. In addition to primary prevention of such states, careful nursing observation of the patient and prompt reporting of lowered blood pressure to the physician assists in initiating a course of action which minimizes the threat of kidney damage from prerenal causes.

Direct attack on kidney tissue may be prevented by the nurse in the teaching role who encourages patients with possible streptococcal infection to seek medical attention promptly to reduce the risk of glomerulonephritis. Assisting hypertensive patients to comply with their drug treatment program is another mode of prevention of kidney damage, since the kidney is a target organ for damage from hypertension. Alerting the public to the importance of keeping all drugs where they cannot be accidentally ingested is important, as some drugs are nephrotoxic.

Nurses and physicians, as well as ancillary personnel, must take utmost care to prevent the transfusion of incompatible blood. Massive hemolysis and kidney shutdown can result.

Preventive measures also include correct diagnosis and treatment of streptococcal infections, careful followup with renal function tests of patients taking prescribed drugs such as certain antibiotics which are nephrotoxic, and prompt relief of obstructions and treatment of infections of the urinary tract. Any patient with a disorder of the urinary tract can develop renal failure.

The earlier renal failure is recognized, the earlier the treatment can start, before there is severe damage to the electrolyte regulation of the body. Any decrease in a patient's urinary output below 500 ml. in a 24-hour period or 20 ml. per hour should be discussed with the physician. The nurse should remain alert for any symptoms that may indicate beginning uremia. When a patient who is usually cheerful and pleasant becomes irritable and complains of a headache, it may not be because he has had a disagreeable visit with his family or has experienced some other unpleasant episode. The reverse may be true; his interpersonal relations may suffer because his BUN is elevated.

## ACUTE RENAL FAILURE

Acute renal failure is a condition of recent onset and in many cases is completely reversible with prompt and adequate therapy. Some patients will die from the underlying condition such as shock due to severe burns while some will fail to regain renal function and will be in *chronic* renal failure.

Because acute renal failure usually occurs as a complication of an already serious medical or surgical condition signs and symptoms may be masked. Oliguria may be the only sign. After prerenal factors such as hypotension, volume depletion, or electrolyte imbalance are corrected and acute renal failure is confirmed, conservative medical management or dialytic therapy is decided upon by the physician.

## PATHOPHYSIOLOGY AND ASSESSMENT OF RELATED SYMPTOMS AND SIGNS

When kidney function is insufficient and such products as urea, other nonprotein nitrogens, creatinine, and uric acid accumulate in the blood, a state of azotemia is present. If unabated, the patient experiences the signs and symptoms of uremia.

Although uremia sometimes has a sudden onset with pronounced initial symptoms, it usually starts so slowly that it is not recognized immediately. The early symptoms may be no more than irritability, headaches, easy fatigability, vague gastrointestinal complaints, and malaise. The patient just does not feel right, and active life becomes increasingly difficult for him. The symptoms become more ominous as uremia advances and more and more products of metabolism—such as creatinine, uric acid, and sulfates are retained in the blood.

Skilled nursing observation of changes in the following areas can facilitate early detection of complications, increasing loss of function, or response to treatment.

### Urine

*Oliguria,* or decrease in normal urinary output may be present. However, the quantity of urine can be normal or even increased in volume when the kidneys are failing, but the specific gravity of the urine will be low since waste products appear in less than normal concentration. Total *anuria* is unusual in acute renal failure due to prerenal causes or intrarenal pathology. The daily urine volume in such instances is 75 to 300 ml. Total anuria is more indicative of obstruction of the urinary tract. Urinalysis may reveal elevated sodium, proteinuria, red blood cells and white blood cells.

### Circulatory System

Examination of the blood may show a gradual increase in the blood urea nitrogen (BUN) since the kidney's ability to excrete urea, the end product of protein metabolism, is impaired. The NPN test—nonprotein nitrogen—measures urea, creatinine, uric acid, and a few other less important protein end products and gives essentially the same information as the BUN. The BUN may become markedly elevated before any other symptoms are recognized. Mental clouding, confusion, and disorientation can accompany a rising BUN. Several factors influence BUN. Since BUN is the result of protein breakdown, a decrease in dietary protein intake could keep the BUN relatively low. On the other hand, the catabolic effects of infection, fever, GI bleeding, and steroids can cause an elevation of BUN.

Serum creatinine and urinary creatinine clearance as well as BUN are generally used to evaluate renal function. If, for example, a patient has a creatinine clearance of 12 ml. per min. he has essentially 12 per cent kidney function. Most patients are symptomatic (nausea, vomiting, diarrhea, insomnia) with a creatinine clearance of less than 10 ml. per min.

Patients with reduced glomerular filtration rate lose their ability to maintain sodium and fluid balance. So much sodium and water may be lost that the patient becomes dehydrated. Anorexia and vomiting intensify the losses. Muscular weakness and muscular cramps, more anorexia, and overall debility characterize hyponatremia (deficient blood sodium). More rarely, depending on the original pathology causing the uremia, the patient is edematous instead of dehydrated. Sodium and fluid retention can result in congestive heart failure. The nurse observes the patient for wheezing, dyspnea, and distended neck veins and auscultates for pulmonary rales, gallop rhythm, or pericardial friction rub.

In uremia, the blood level of calcium frequently is low because calcium is not reabsorbed in sufficient quantity from the glomerular filtrate. Early signs of calcium deficiency are numbness and tingling of the fingertips and toes, nose, and ears. This can pro-

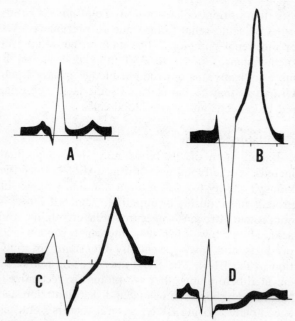

**Figure 64-1.** (A) Normal ECG. (B and C) Mild and severe hyperkalemia, characterized by lowered P waves and steepened T waves. (D) Hypokalemia with loss of T waves and a prominent U wave; difficult to distinguish from effects of cardiac drugs such as quinidine and digitalis. (Winsor, T.: Electrolyte abnormalities and the electrocardiogram, *JAMA* 203:109)

gress to symptoms of tetany, ranging from slight twitching to convulsions. Two tests for tetany are *Trousseau's* sign or *Chvostek's* sign. To elicit Trousseau's sign, the examiner grasps the patient's wrist sufficiently tightly to constrict the circulation for a few minutes. If the hand goes into a position of palmar flexion, a marked calcium deficit can be assumed. Chvostek's sign is present if twitching occurs when the face is lightly tapped just below the temple. Intravenous calcium chloride or calcium gluconate may be prescribed.

Also, with low serum calcium there may be hematemesis, or else blood in the stool. Because sodium bicarbonate may decrease serum calcium even further, twitching and muscle spasm may occur when this drug is given in treatment for acidosis.

When blood calcium and sodium are low, potassium levels may become abnormally high. Nausea, abdominal pain, diarrhea, and generalized weakness occur. Potassium retention is one of the most critical problems, since potassium intoxication causes cardiac arrhythmias, cardiac failure, and death if untreated. Frequent ECG's may be taken to observe the possible effects of increased potassium levels on the heart (Fig. 64-1). The nurse notes electrocardiographic changes and observes the patient for pulse irregularities and for signs of congestive heart failure.

Severe anemia is a common symptom of advancing renal failure. One theory explaining this is that seriously damaged kidneys are unable to produce adequate quantities of erythropoietin, which stimulates the bone marrow to produce red blood cells. Increased capillary fragility and prolonged bleeding time can result in purpura.

Hypertension commonly accompanies renal failure. Dimness or blurring of vision, and spots before the eyes may be the result of retinal hemorrhages caused by the hypertension. Adequate treatment of hypertension may improve renal function.

## Respiratory System

Dyspnea, pulmonary rales and other signs of congestive heart failure may become evident.

The normal kidney manufactures ammonia to react with the acid in urine, and also it excretes sulfate and phosphate acids. The diseased kidney fails to perform these functions, thus helping to create a severe metabolic acidosis. $CO_2$ combining power is markedly reduced. Nausea and vomiting, thirst and air hunger are symptoms of acidosis. The deep and rapid respirations (Kussmaul's breathing) are indicative of a respiratory attempt to compensate for the metabolic acidosis by blowing off $CO_2$.

## Nervous System

Though some patients remain mentally alert for a long period of time considering their electrolyte imbalance, mental processes are progressively slowed. There may be dizziness and irritability. Behavior can be totally unpredictable and even become psychotic. Cerebral edema can cause projectile vomiting, convulsions, and coma. Peripheral neuropathy, muscular weakness, twitching, cramping, neuritic pain, and headache may also occur.

## Gastrointestinal

Anorexia, nausea, and vomiting are often severe and lead to emaciation of the patient. Because uremia (urea) interferes with the normal clotting mechanisms of the blood, prolonged bleeding time results. Ulceration and bleeding of the gastrointestinal tract is a fairly common component of renal failure. The mucous membranes of the mouth often bleed and blood may be found is the feces. Hematemesis (vomiting of blood) is a frequent precursor of death in the patient with uremia. Relentless hiccoughing can also be present.

## Appearance and Skin

The patient with renal insufficiency is usually pale and he may have edema about the eyes and pitting edema of the ankles.

The patient may complain of torturing pruritus (itching of the skin) or "creepy crawling sensations." Since the skin also serves an excretory function, uremic frost, white crystals composed of waste products excreted by the skin instead of the kidneys, may become visible, especially in dark-skinned patients.

## Odor

Halitosis is generally marked and ulceration of the oral mucosa due to increased capillary fragility is common. The patient may have a generalized body odor suggestive of urine.

## PROGNOSIS AND TREATMENT

The prognosis in renal failure depends on the cause. If the primary cause can be removed or quickly remedied, such as in acute renal tubular necrosis (lower nephron nephrosis) or urinary tract obstruction, renal failure is reversible in about 80 per cent of such patients. In these cases the treatment objective is to keep the patient alive and free from complications during the two or three weeks required for regeneration of the damaged epithelium of the renal tubules. Adequate maintenance usually results in diuresis (a 24-hour urine volume of 1,000 ml. or more) during the second week. The patient is still seriously ill because kidney function gradually returns to normal over a period of several weeks.

Chronic renal diseases such as glomerular nephritis, nephrosis, pyelonephritis, polycystic kidneys and diabetic nephropathy progress to deterioration of the nephron involving either the glomeruli or the tubules or both (chronic renal failure) and ultimately, end stage renal disease. The onset of oliguria or anuria is ominous. Remissions can occur, however.

Treatment of acute renal failure can be nondialytic or by hemodialysis or peritoneal dialysis. Today hemodialysis is available in many centers and may be the treatment of choice but the patient's blood vessels might not be suitable for cannulation.

Peritoneal dialysis is readily available in every hospital, but may not be suitable for every patient for example, those with recent bowel surgery. The physician considers the patient's underlying condition and complications, and the available resources in the community.

## NONDIALYTIC MANAGEMENT; NURSING ASSESSMENT AND INTERVENTION

Many patients with acute renal failure develop it as a complication after some major medical or surgical problem. Thus they have their initial problem plus a serious setback to deal with. Patients with chronic renal insufficiency who become acutely symptomatic due, for example, to drug toxicity may fear that they are approaching end stage renal disease. The patient with uremia is often very ill and may even be comatose. For both patient (if conscious) and his significant others, fear of death is present. Added to this is the fear of losing control as the buildup of waste products in the blood affects the sensorium, causing the patient to become restless, confused, belligerent, disoriented, psychotic, or comatose. The nursing staff by their organization and manner can convey to the patient and his associates that they can be depended upon to keep the situation under control even though the patient may not be in control of himself.

Nursing care is often complex due to the underlying condition (i.e. burns, multiple trauma, diabetic arteriolar glomerulosclerosis). Skilled data gathering, communicating findings to the physician, collaborating with him and other team members in the treatment plan, and providing support to patient and family are important aspects of the nurse's role. Flexibility with visitors is a matter of nursing judgment. Some may be asked to participate in the patient's care. A person who has a calming, reassuring manner may sit quietly by the patient for long periods of time. This is especially true for older patients and those with cultural differences such as language, for whom the situation is particularly stressful. Guidelines to follow are that the visit does no harm and that patient and family can derive as much comfort as possible from the visit. When visitors remain in the waiting room, the nurse can offer support by going to them with reports about the condition of the patient. When the patient is irritable, the family can be helped to understand that his anger is not necessarily directed at them, but that it is rather the result of the accumulated chemicals in his blood stream.

Since infection, hyperkalemia, and fluid overload are the three main causes of death in patients with acute renal failure, the prevention of these complications is a major objective.

**Prevention of Infection.** Infectious processes increase protein catabolism and by increasing the workload of the kidneys hasten the onset or severity of uremia. Pulmonary complications are the most frequent cause of morbidity and mortality in acute renal failure (Muehrcke, 1969). Pulmonary secretions are more viscous and depression of the cough reflex and respiratory effort make it difficult for the patient to rid himself of secretions. Suctioning and positive pressure breathing are often necessary to prevent atelectasis in obtunded patients.

Frequent deep breathing, turning, effective coughing and pulmonary physical therapy are indicated. Strict aseptic technique must be used for catheterization and catheter care, wounds such as tracheostomy, and intravenous devices such as a central venous pressure monitoring line. Skin care and the prevention of decubitus ulcers is of utmost importance since the patient may be edematous or emaciated. Special, gentle mouth care is necessary to prevent stomatitis and parotitis.

To protect the patient, reverse isolation may be carried out. Implementation of the principles of medical asepsis is a nursing responsibility. The nurse exercises her professional judgment regarding placement of the patient, patient contact with staff and visitors, and instructs auxiliary personnel accordingly.

**Fluid Balance.** Fluid overload (hypervolemia) is monitored by recording intake and output, by measuring body weight daily using a bed scale or a bedside scale under constant conditions. Central venous pressure may also be monitored. The nurse should observe for periorbital, pedal or sacral edema and auscultate lungs and heart regularly for beginning signs of congestive heart failure. Water intoxication can be manifested by headache, lethargy, neuromuscular irritability, confusion, convulsions and coma. The physician determines how much fluid the patient can have based on exact measurements of intake and output via all routes, plus an estimation of insensible losses through the skin, lungs, burns or wounds. For most patients total intake for 24 hours is equal to the previous day's measured output plus approximately 500 ml. for usual insensible losses. Replacement solutions approximate the fluid losses from all sources in both amount and electrolyte composition. Hidden sources of intake which must be accounted for include ultrasonic nebulization.

In severe shutdown the patient may be limited to as little as 400 ml. intravenously (regulated to last 24 hours) and 100 ml. of oral fluid. Some days (depending on the output), tea, ginger ale or water are given with as much sugar or Coca-Cola syrup (to increase the caloric intake and for its protein-sparing effect) as the patient can tolerate. Sucking glucose ice chips made by freezing 20 to 50 per cent glucose in an ice tray can help with the problem of thirst while providing some calories. Ice chips can extend a small amount of fluid over 24 hours. To count intake accurately the nurse can measure in a graduate the same amount of ice which has been allowed to melt.

Unfortunately many fruit juices contain potassium and since the failing kidney cannot excrete excess potassium, most fruit juices are not permitted. Lemonade and cranberry juice may be permitted. Sucking on candy "sour balls" can increase the carbohydrate intake without adding potassium.

**Hyperkalemia.** When serum potassium is high cardiac arrest can occur. The uremic patient has constant cardiac monitoring for early detection of changes in the ECG indicative of high serum potassium (see Fig. 64-1).

The normal function of the kidney is the most efficient way to lower high serum potassium levels. When the kidney is not functioning normally, the use of drugs called *cation exchange resins,* given orally or by enemas, help to deplete the blood potassium. Such a resin is sodium polystyrene sulfate (Kayexalate-Winthrop). This is an inert, insoluble, synthetic substance which, when introduced into the gastrointestinal tract by mouth, gastric tube, or retention enema, exchanges sodium ions for potassium ions and thus decreases potassium intoxication. As a retention enema, 30 Gm. of the resin in 200 ml. of water may be ordered to be given over a 30 to 45 minute period and repeated if necessary in two to four hours. Kayexalate can be combined with the polyhydric alcohol, sorbitol, to facilitate its passage through the gastrointestinal tract. Since sodium ions are released in the intestine during electrolyte exchange, the patient's ability to handle the sodium must be carefully observed. In the digitalized patient, hypokalemia can result in digitalis intoxication with resultant cardiac arrhythmias. Daily serum potassium levels and electrocardiographic monitoring are essential.

In an emergency, hyperkalemia and the accompanying acidosis may be rapidly treated by giving sodium bicarbonate which drives K+ into the cells. One liter of 10 per cent glucose with or without regular insulin added can also be used to achieve an intracellular shift of potassium.

**Diet.** In severe failure, protein catabolism and the consequent demand on the kidneys for the excretion of protein end products is limited by restricting protein foods. To prevent endogenous protein breakdown in the patient seriously ill with renal disease, feedings should be spaced so that there are no long periods of fasting. If the patient awakens during the night, for instance, he should be given a high carbohydrate snack or drink.

**Activity.** In the acute stage metabolic demands are kept to a minimum by restricting activity to those measures necessary for preventing the hazards of bed rest. Chronic uremic patients in acute crises may have peripheral neuropathy and require considerable assistance from the nurse with passive, then active, assistive exercise to maintain function. Rapid progressive ambulation with the preservation of patient safety is the goal.

**Skin Care.** Pruritus can occur with or without "uremic frost." Uremic frost can be removed by bathing with a weak solution of vinegar (two tablespoons to a pint of water). An anesthetic ointment may be ordered to relieve the itching. Cleanliness helps, too; the patient may require two baths instead of one a day. Although the skin is not efficient for the disposal of such waste chemicals as uric acid, it is all that the body has available when the kidneys are not functioning, and a clean skin is always more efficient and more comfortable.

**Anemia.** Anemia, secondary to hematopoietic depression, is common. Usual hematinic drugs are of little value. Iron in the form of IV iron dextran in conjunction with androgen therapy has been used to increase and maintain the hematocrit at acceptable levels. The anemia contributes to the general weakness and lethargy of the chronic uremic patient. Blood transfusion with packed cells is given only if necessary to maintain the hematocrit above 25. Transfusion is avoided because of the risk of hepatitis, further suppression of the patient's own ability to build the hematocrit, and the danger of preformed antibodies interfering with the future chance of successful kidney transplantation, if this is an eventual goal. Frozen blood, though twice the cost of regular transfusion, reduces the risks.

**Recovery.** The period of oliguria may be brief or prolonged. If the patient with acute renal failure reaches the diuretic phase, nausea and vomiting subside and appetite returns. Urinary output can be quite large in volume because the patient loses surplus sodium and water previously present as edema. Hypovolemia and dehydration can occur. Decreased skin turgor, dry mucous membranes, hypotension, tachycardia and decreased body weight should be discussed promptly with the physician. Measurement of urine volume and composition and daily body weight are guides to fluid replacement and sodium intake.

Diet is usually low in protein and high in calories until renal function returns to normal.

If the kidneys do not recover and the patient is in a state of chronic renal failure, he will require an individually prescribed regime (see section on Chronic Renal Failure).

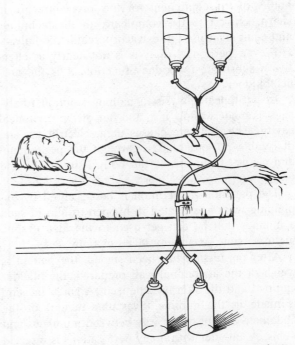

**Figure 64-2.** Peritoneal dialysis. After the solution flows into the patient it is allowed to remain in situ for the period of time ordered by the physician. During this time, dialysis takes place. Then the clamps on the lower bottles are opened and the solution is drained off.

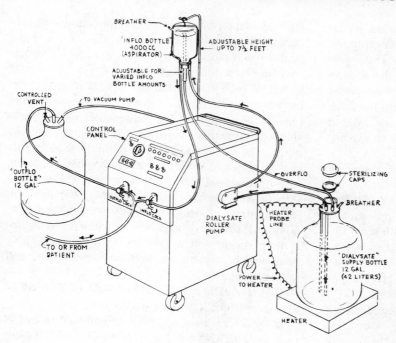

**Figure 64-3.** Automatic administration equipment for peritoneal dialysis. (Seattle Artificial Kidney Supply Company, Seattle, Wash.)

## Peritoneal Dialysis

The simplicity of peritoneal dialysis and the availability of the equipment for this procedure are in sharp contrast to the complexity of the technique and equipment used in extracorporeal hemodialysis. However, peritoneal dialysis is not nearly as effective a substitute for kidney function as is the artificial kidney.

In peritoneal dialysis, a bathing solution (dialysate) is made to flow into and out of the peritoneal cavity. The dialysate causes urea, electrolytes and dialyzable poisons to pass through the peritoneum and carries them out of the body (Figs. 64-2 and 64-3).

The patient's cooperation is best secured by explaining what is expected to happen to him in such a manner that he can get used to the idea despite his toxic state or anxiety level, or both.

After permission has been signed, the patient is weighed, the abdominal wall prepared, the bladder emptied and the skin anesthetized. A small incision is made in the midline (avascular region) of the abdomen, a third of the way between umbilicus and pubis. A catheter with many perforations is inserted by the physician so that the end lies free in the peritoneal cavity. The catheter is sutured in place and a dressing applied and sealed with adhesive tape. Blood pressure, pulse, and respirations are recorded.

Dialysate solutions are warmed to body temperature to prevent abdominal cramps and a drop in body temperature when the solution is instilled. Medication as ordered, such as potassium, heparin and antibiotics are added. The dialysate inflow tubing is attached to the catheter in the patient. The outflow tubing leading to a closed drainage system is clamped off.

Each peritoneal dialysis exchange consists of three periods: instillation, equilibration, and drainage. Each exchange should take about one hour.

**Instillation Period.** With the outflow tube clamped off, 2 liters of dialysate should run into the peritoneal cavity in 10 to 15 minutes. Gravity may be utilized by lowering the bed and raising the level of the bottles. If the drip is slow, the physician may need to reposition the catheter. When the bottles are empty, but the tubing is still filled with dialysate to prevent entrance of air, the inflow tube should be clamped. Instillation time, start and finish, the volume and type of dialysate, plus any medications added are recorded.

**Equilibration Period.** The solution is left in the abdomen the length of time ordered by the physician (usually 30 to 35 minutes).

**Drainage Period.** The outflow tube is unclamped and the dialysate allowed to drain into a receptacle, maintaining a closed sterile drainage system. Gravity drainage should occur rapidly in a steady, forceful stream. Drainage should take no longer than 10 to 15 minutes. If it does, the physician may need to irrigate the catheter to remove plugs, or he may need to reposition or replace the catheter. Turning the patient side to side or raising the head of the bed may promote drainage.

The time of the start and finish of the drainage period should be recorded. Note should be taken of the appearance of the fluid removed. It may be blood-tinged because of bleeding due to heparin, or cloudy from protein loss. The fluid removed should be carefully measured and the volume recorded. The difference between the volume instilled and the volume removed is recorded. The physician should be notified of excessive fluid retained or removed from the patient ($\pm 500$ ml.).

Commercially manufactured automatic cycling machines for peritoneal dialysis are available. The physician sets timing and volume devices and a pumping system delivers the dialysate to the patient from a large reservoir. Diffusion time and outflow are also automatically controlled. The patient's response is observed, particularly pain in the outflow cycle. Volume and timing are adjusted as necessary.

The number of exchanges performed in peritoneal dialysis varies and is ordered specifically by the physician. For example, peritoneal dialysis may be continued for 48 hours with 20 exchanges of 2 liters each 24-hour period. When dialysis is completed, the catheter is removed and a dry sterile dressing applied. A purse-string suture may be necessary. A bacteriologic culture may be obtained from the catheter tip as well as from the last dialysate drained. A postdialysis weight is obtained.

Several prostheses are available which provide ready access to the peritoneal cavity. These can be plugged when not in use. They are especially valuable for patients on chronic peritoneal dialysis. Daily care is minimal.

### Nursing Assessment and Intervention

Fluid and electrolyte shifts can occur rapidly during the dialysis. Accurate recording on a flow sheet facilitates ongoing assessment of the patient's status. Fluid volume status can be assessed by central venous pressure, and observation for congestive heart failure such as gallop rhythm and pulmonary rales. Hypovolemia is reflected in a fall in blood pressure and rapid pulse and is apt to occur when fluid removal is too rapid and when the dialysate has a high concentration of glucose.

Complications of peritoneal dialysis include hollow viscous perforation indicated by return of "urine" or liquid feces following catheter insertion. Intraperitoneal bleeding can occur. Fever, abdominal pain and tenderness, and cloudiness of the dialysate can be signs of peritonitis. Excessive absorption of glucose from the dialysate can result in hyperosmolar coma. Lethargy, confusion or other change in mental status is an indication for blood glucose measurement and notification of the physician.

Leakage around the catheter may require a purse-string suture. Pain in the left shoulder may be due to diaphragmatic irritation caused by the high concentration of glucose when present in the dialysate. Abdominal pain present at the end of the drainage period may be relieved by the next instillation or by procaine.

The procedure is tedious, and the patient may become bored and restless or anxious. It is not sufficient for the nurse to appear only when she has some task to do such as hanging bottles or measuring drainage. This conveys to the patient that the equipment is the major concern, not him, though he may recognize too that the technical aspects are important. Listening to the patient's reactions, being available to answer questions, providing physical comfort measures, or offering some tolerable diversion assists the patient through the procedure. A relative may sit quietly by; periodic sedation may be given throughout. The patient's position should be changed frequently and individual supportive nursing measures carried out. The patient undergoing peritoneal dialysis may eat and drink as permitted.

## HEMODIALYSIS

Extracorporeal (outside the body) hemodialysis via an artificial kidney is a process designed to bring blood into contact with a semipermeable membrane through which diffusion takes place. By "diffusion" is meant the spontaneous movement of solutes and solvent from areas of high concentration to areas of low concentration until a state of equilibrium is established.

With the improvements in design and availability of different types of artificial kidneys over the last decade as well as reliable techniques for quick and regular access to the circulation, hemodialysis is

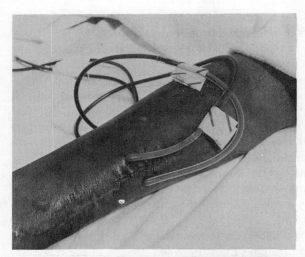

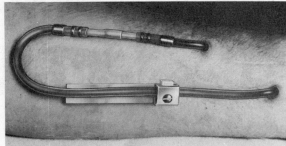

**Figure 64-4.** (*Top*) Recently performed external arteriovenous shunt of patient undergoing hemodialysis. (*Bottom*) External arteriovenous shunt between periods of use in hemodialysis. (Seattle Artificial Kidney Supply Company, Seattle, Wash.)

often the first choice of treatment for the hospitalized patient in acute renal failure. In addition, with the development of the internal arteriovenous shunt (Fig. 64-4), automatic monitoring devices on dialysis machines, and training programs, more than 10,000 patients with end stage renal disease are on long-term hemodialysis carried out two or three times weekly in limited care dialysis centers associated with hospitals, in mobile facilities, or in their own homes.

Nurses caring for patients receiving hemodialysis must have specialized preparation. The basic principles of treatment are the same for patients in acute and chronic failure. However, the hospitalized patient in acute failure is often critically ill and the complexity and instability of his underlying condition (burns, suicidal drug overdose, multiple trauma) differentiate his nursing needs from those of the patient on maintenance hemodialysis. The latter pa-

tient, after a training period, is often responsible for his own dialysis with the help of his selected assistant. However, such patients require the ongoing interest and support of the nephrology nurse and other members of the team due to the many complications of the disease and its treatment and the problems in adaptation to chronic illness characteristic of end stage renal disease. The psychiatric nursing clinical specialist can be an important resource in crisis management for individuals and groups (McClellan, 1972).

### Indications

Hemodialysis is utilized in acute renal failure for hypervolemia particularly with hypertension, for uncontrolled hyperkalemia, for symptomatic metabolic acidosis, for the relief of uremic symptoms (especially of the cardiovascular, gastrointestinal and nervous systems), for maintenance of the BUN less than 100 mg. per ml., and for dialyzable poisons. In some centers, prophylactic dialysis may be instituted before there is clinical deterioration of the patient in acute renal failure.

The indications are basically the same for the patient in chronic renal failure except that hyperkalemia is not generally a problem because of renal adaptive mechanisms and the absence of an acute catabolic state.

### The Artificial Kidney

Access to the patient's arteries and veins is necessary to attach him to the artificial kidney machine. Methods include a silastic-teflon external arteriovenous shunt, a surgically created internal arteriovenous fistula requiring needle "sticks" for each dialysis, autogenous vein grafts, or large vessel applique (the Thomas shunt). The patient's blood is removed from an artery, passed or pumped through the dialyzer and after a period of exposure to the dialysate the cleansed blood is returned to the body via a vein.

The basic types of artificial kidneys are the coil, the parallel flow (Kiil) and the hollow fiber (Figs. 64-5 and 64-6). Though more than 20 varieties have been manufactured certain principles apply to all.

The basic components are cellophane or Cuprophane which acts as the semipermeable membrane, and the solution (dialysate) in which it is immersed. Pores in the membrane similar in size to those of the glomerular capillaries permit water and metabolic end products and toxins to pass from the blood through the membrane into the dialysate but protein and red blood cells cannot. Any solute small enough to pass through the membrane will be removed if it does not have a matching concentration in the dialysate. Substances such as urea and creatinine, uric acid, ammonium, sulfate, phosphate and dangerously high levels of potassium can be removed. On the other hand, bacteria and viruses cannot cross from the dialysate into the blood. Blood samples taken pre- and postdialysis for substances such as urea, creatinine, sodium, potassium, chlorides, $CO_2$ and hematocrit are indicators of the efficiency of dialysis.

The dialysate consists of tap water to which has been added various chemicals to render the bath fluid similar to the composition of normal human plasma. Glucose or sorbitol or invert sugar is used to control osmolality. The composition of the dialysate is ordered by the physician according to the individual patient's need. For example, a potassium-free bath might be used for the hyperkalemic patient whereas a digitalized patient would require a bath higher in potassium to prevent hypokalemia and consequent digitalis toxicity. ECG monitoring and measurement of serum potassium are used to assess response. Calcium concentration of the dialysate must be kept high enough to prevent calcium loss from bones into the serum. In addition to osmosis, water is controlled by a process called ultrafiltration which allows for the correction of hypervolemia by increasing the outflow resistance of the blood and raising the blood circuit pressure above the dialysate pressure, thus forcing water out of the bloodstream. Different dialyzers have different ultrafiltration characteristics. The volume of blood in the dialyzer at any one time varies between 90 ml. to 250 ml. depending on the type of machine. The patient's blood volume deficit can be replaced with saline during dialysis to prevent hypotension and undesired weight loss. A pre- and postdialysis weight is taken. The dialysate is changed or recirculated intermittently to avoid the accumulation of toxins.

The length of time of a dialysis treatment varies according to type of machine and patient need. It may be from three to ten hours, two or three times a week. In acute renal failure, hemodialysis may be more frequent but it is started slowly and blood flow increased gradually to avoid rapid shifts of solute, water, or acid-base balance.

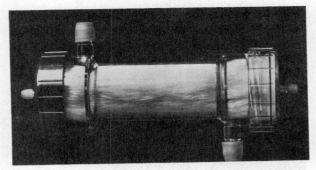

**Figure 64-5.** Cordis-Dow artificial kidney (C-DAK), a disposable capillary type dialyzer. (Cordis Corporation, Miami, Fla.)

During dialysis, heparin is administered by intermittent or continuous infusion (systemic heparinization) to prevent blood from clotting in the extracorporeal circuit of the dialyzer, or, to minimize the risk of systemic bleeding, regional heparinization may be used. This consists of infusing heparin into the blood as the blood passes from patient to dialyzer and protamine sulfate as the blood returns to the patient, to neutralize the heparin. Frequent clotting times are done. Artificial kidney clotting time is around 30 minutes while patient clotting time is as near normal as possible depending on the patient (6 to 17 minutes).

Well-developed observational, judgmental, and technical skills are necessary for the dialysis team to maintain the functional integrity of the dialysis system, to perform the dialysis procedure safely, and to know the potential problems and how to prevent or handle them such as separation of blood lines or coil ruptures.

Patient assessment factors include observation for

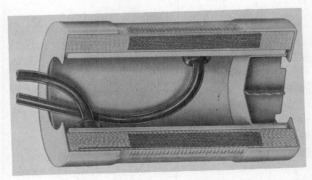

**Figure 64-6.** Coil dialyzer. (Extracorporeal Medical Specialities, Inc.)

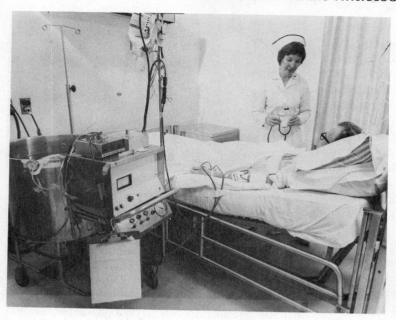

**Figure 64-7.** Nurse talks with hospitalized patient while observing his response to hemodialysis. (The New York Hospital, Cornell University Medical Center, New York, N.Y.)

bleeding, weight change, temperature, pulse, blood pressure, food and/or fluid intake, clotting time, and condition of the shunt. Leg blood pressures may need to be taken if both arms are needed to complete the blood circuit. The patient is observed for nausea, apprehension, dyspnea, restlessness, irritability, itching, flushing, pain, anxiety level, and level of consciousness (Fig. 64-7).

After dialysis, observation continues for bleeding (heparin rebound). The internal shunt is assessed by feeling for thrill or listening with a stethoscope for characteristic sound. Inspection of an external shunt should reveal a uniform red appearance to the column of blood. Other appearance may indicate clotting or potential clotting.

### Hepatitis

The staff of a dialysis unit is at particular risk for contracting infectious or serum hepatitis. Whereas patients with chronic renal failure usually have a subclinical response to infection with the virus of serum hepatitis, healthy hospital staff have clinical manifestations of the disease which are often severe. Serious outbreaks of hepatitis have occurred in dialysis units. Presently serological testing for the presence of Australia Antigen (AU-antigen; AuSH; hepatitis associated antigen-HAA; HB AG-hepatitis B antigen) in blood is the only screening method available for patients with suspected serum hepatitis. The antigen appears in the blood during the late incubation period, remains during the acute phase and disappears in the convalescent period. Hemodialysis patients can remain carriers for months or years.

Serum hepatitis is transmitted by contaminated blood through needle puncture, damaged skin, direct personal contact and possibly inhalation (Garibaldi, 1973). Accidental ingestion of the blood or feces of carriers is another possible mode of transmission which is why fingers, pencils, or other objects should not be put into the mouth.

Every dialysis unit should have a hepatitis prevention protocol. Personnel should wear gloves during "on and off" procedures to prevent contact with blood in tubing, membranes, syringes or needles. These should be disposed into plastic bag lined containers. Staff and patients should be regularly checked for the presence of Australia Antigen. It is recommended that any patient carrying the virus be isolated and prepared for home dialysis as soon as feasible. Staff carriers may be excluded from the unit until negative tests have been obtained.

Because of the risk of hepatitis, patients in chronic renal failure should not be given blood transfusions except when urgent. Transfusion should be with packed cells and the blood for transfusion should be negative for the presence of Australia Antigen. Patients should be instructed to carry out as much of the dialysis routine themselves and should use the same machine on each occasion.

Liver failure as a result of hepatitis is increasing as a cause of death in dialysis and transplant patients.

## CHRONIC RENAL FAILURE

Patients with chronic renal failure can be managed by conservative therapy, primarily diet and medications and treatment of uremic symptoms, until dialytic therapy becomes necessary. However, compliance with the treatment program may be an arduous task for the patient since dietary sodium, potassium, fluid and protein may be limited. Many drugs can be included such as diuretics, salt tablets, antihypertensives, exchange resins, and aluminum based antacids. A large part of the nurse's role is astute observation, patient education, and sustained support. Comprehending and remembering the rationale and components of his treatment regimen may be difficult for the patient due to the uremic state, so careful cognitive and affective assessment must be carried out.

Mental clouding with loss of interest and efficiency in work and subsequent loss of income as medical expenses mount, the shift of roles such as that of the male breadwinner and head of the household being necessarily assumed by the wife, or homemaking duties having to be assumed by a husband or children are examples of some of the sources of problems resulting from chronic renal failure. Diminished sexual desire and capability impose an added strain on a couple at a time when a satisfying sexual relationship would ordinarily offer a bulwark against the stress of life.

### Diet

Diets are prescribed in terms of total calories, total fluid intake, total protein, total sodium, and total potassium content. Low protein exchange diets are available (Muehrcke, et al., 1969).

Protein intake should be restricted to "high biologic value" proteins which contain only essential amino acids, thus promoting the metabolic utilization of urea which becomes available as a source of nonessential amino acid, reducing the BUN. The Giovanetti-Giordano diet is an 18 to 21 Gm. protein diet which can maintain the patient in positive nitrogen balance as long as all eight essential amino acids (which must be ingested every day) are supplied by egg protein and milk. The patient must ingest sufficient calories from carbohydrate and fat sources (2,000 to 3,000 calories per day) to prevent

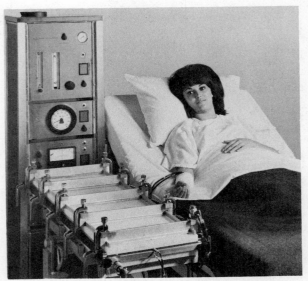

**Figure 64-8.** Bedside console and Kiil dialyzer. (Seattle Artificial Kidney Supply Company, Seattle, Wash.)

the use of body sources of protein such as muscle and liver to be broken down for fuel. This ingestion of calories is difficult because American calorie sources are also high in "low quality protein," for example, grain products and vegetables, and are not permitted on the Giovanetti diet. Sugars, jellies, jams, honey, and fat are high in calories and low in protein but are unappealing over a long period of time. A protein-free wheat starch flour is available for bread making but is not appealing to all.

Water deficiency (dehydration) and salt deficiency are causes of reduced renal function in chronic renal failure patients. Therefore, sodium is prescribed in maximum tolerable amounts to maintain extracellular fluid volume at normovolemic level. Fluids are prescribed as drugs are prescribed and are spread over the 24-hour day to prevent nocturnal dehydration. Since nocturia is often a problem taking fluids during the night is not difficult. Weight change, serum sodium concentration, urine volume, and maintenance of maximum glomerular filtration rate are guidelines for the prescription of fluid intake.

Hyperkalemia may be a problem in chronic renal failure if there is excessive potassium intake, intercurrent illness, or steroid administration in which the associated catabolic state liberates more potassium into the blood than the damaged kidneys can handle, or if there is exacerbation of the underlying renal disease. Dietary restriction of potassium may be necessary (see also p. 1154 for treatment of hyperkalemia).

In addition to the signs and symptoms described in the section on acute renal failure, patients with chronic renal failure can have the following common clinical manifestations.

### Clinical Manifestations

**Bone Lesions (Osteodystrophy).** Several processes lead to the development of bone disease. Patients with uremia tend to have inadequate absorption of dietary calcium and vitamin D resistance which also interferes with the absorption of calcium from the intestine. As glomerular filtration rate decreases, there is an increase in serum phosphate level (hyperphosphatemia) and a reciprocal decrease in serum calcium level. This stimulates overproduction of the hormone of the parathyroid glands which may enlarge. Parathyroid hormone acts to maintain normal serum calcium by causing calcium to be resorbed from bone. The resultant demineralization of bone (*renal osteomalacia*) contributes to pathologic fractures of the ribs from coughing, degeneration of hips, compression of vertebrae, fractures of other bones, and bone pain.

Calcium deposits can form in soft tissues (*metastatic calcification*), skin, blood vessels, the conjunctiva and cornea of the eye, in the viscera, and in the joints causing arthritis. *Osteitis fibrosa* is characterized by localized or generalized cystlike lesions in bones. Fractures occur easily and heal poorly.

The osteodystrophy of chronic renal failure is not relieved by hemodialysis, and every patient is a candidate for it. The treatment is aimed at reducing serum phosphorus to prevent reciprocal serum hypocalcemia with the consequent effects on bone demineralization and soft tissue calcification. Phosphate is lowered by reducing dietary intake of protein or by ingestion of an aluminum based antacid such as Amphogel or Basalgel (30 ml. four times a day). Aluminum binds phosphate in the intestine and prevents its absorption. The patient should understand that other types of antacids such as magnesium-based Mylanta or Maalox are not acceptable as substitutes. Large doses of vitamin D and calcium gluconate may be given but carry a high risk of serious complications. Subtotal parathyroidectomy may be performed to decrease production of the hormone. Monitoring of serum calcium, phosphorus, alkaline phosphatase, and a renal bone survey (x-rays of long bones, clavicles, digits, feet) must be done regularly to prevent undue bone destruction and metastatic calcification.

**Gastrointestinal Problems.** Anorexia, nausea and vomiting, and singultus (hiccoughs) are manifestations of the uremic state. The nausea and vomiting simulate the morning sickness of pregnancy. Fluids given throughout the night (nocturnal hydration) relieve the symptoms by preventing further decline in renal function and increase in renal failure. Chlorpromazine may give relief of symptoms. The low protein diet may lessen the symptoms. Hemodialysis produces marked symptomatic relief.

Ulcerations may occur anywhere in the gastrointestinal tract from the mouth to the anus. Pain, blood loss, and perforation can result.

Changes in composition and flow of saliva create an altered sense of taste. This, coupled with sometimes severe dietary restrictions, causes the patient to be disinterested in or rejecting of food with consequent cachexia.

**Cardiopulmonary Problems.** Fibrinous pericarditis can accompany uremia. A pericardial friction rub may be the only sign. However, severe substernal pain and pericardial tamponade can occur.

"Uremic pleuritis" also occurs. A pleural friction rub may be the only sign or pain can be present. The physician must distinguish this from pulmonary embolism. The "uremic lung," appearing on x-ray as a characteristic bilateral opacification with the appearance of "bat wings" is thought to be due to increased capillary permeability and transudation of fluid.

**Anemia.** A deficiency in erythropoietin, a hormone produced by the kidney which stimulates the bone marrow to produce red blood cells, is one cause of anemia in patients with chronic renal failure. Malabsorption of iron from the gastrointestinal tract, shortened life span of red blood cells and losses of small amounts of blood from the nose, gums, skin, or from sampling are contributing factors. Symptoms such as shortness of breath and angina pectoris are most likely to appear when the hematocrit is below 25 per cent. Normal hematocrit for men is 46 to 52 per cent and for women 40 to 45 per cent. This anemia is not improved by usual treatment or dialysis. Because of the risk of hepatitis, symptomatic anemia is treated by transfusion with packed red cells as infrequently as possible.

**Hypertension.** Hypertension is common, but there is difference of opinion regarding treatment of asymptomatic hypertension. Some believe that lowering elevated blood pressure induces decreased renal perfusion and further reduction of the glomerular filtration rate. Treatment may be reserved for target organ complications such as congestive heart failure or hypertensive encephalopathy. Hemodialysis may relieve hypertension by reducing extracellular fluid volume. In some patients only bilateral nephrectomy and maintenance hemodialysis is effective.

**Nervous System Manifestations.** Nervous system response in uremia has wide individual variation. While lethargy, somnolence, inability to concentrate, and confusion are common some patients might remain quite alert. High anxiety, agitation, frightening dreams, delusions, hallucinations, paranoid tendencies, or depression may occur in some while others may have a cheerful but inappropriate effect. Muscle twitching is common. Seizures can occur. The physician must distinguish the etiology of the convulsions. Hyponatremia, hypertensive encephalopathy, or tetany are also possible causes.

**Peripheral Neuropathy.** Deterioration of nerve function may occur gradually or relatively rapidly. Tingling and painful burning of the feet, restless legs, loss of sensation, reflexes, and muscle strength are the progressive symptoms and signs and paralysis can occur. Neuropathy can be relieved by dialysis though it may be intensified on the initiation of dialytic therapy.

**Acidosis.** Reduction of ammonia ($NH_3$) production, interference with buffer effect, and other mechanisms permit accumulation rather than excretion of hydrogen ions. Mildly symptomatic chronic renal failure patients with less than 15 mEq. of serum bicarbonate may be given an oral alkalinizing agent such as Shohl's solution. This contains 140 Gm. of citric acid and 98 Gm. of sodium citrate. If dissolved in water up to a volume of 1 liter, each ml. would contain 1 mEq. of sodium. A daily dose might be 25 to 75 ml. of the solution in three divided doses given in ginger ale or water. Severe acidosis is treated with intravenous sodium bicarbonate (Papper, March, 1971).

**Sexual Problems.** Many male patients in chronic renal failure have loss of libido and impotence as well. This additional strain on a couple's relationship may necessitate professional counseling to help preserve what strengths there are. Amenorrhea is often part of the uremic syndrome in women. With institution of dialysis and improved general health the above problems may be helped. Menstrual periods may be irregular or flow excessive. Heparinization during dialysis can aggravate this situation. The woman's gynecologist may need to be consulted.

### Patient Education

The success of the medical regime depends to a large extent on the patient's understanding of the disease and its treatment and his motivation to follow it. Bernbeck points out how the treatment program can be confusing to the patient. For example, dietary sodium intake may be restricted yet the patient may have to take sodium polystyrene sufonate (Kayexalate) to relieve hyperkalemia but which adds sodium. He may have to have sodium bicarbonate to control acidosis and then be given a potent diuretic such as furosemide to eliminate excess sodium. The patient needs to understand the concept of fluid restriction, and how to monitor his condition, such as observations for edema. Pills may be numerous and the patient may perceive medications such as Kayexalate and basic aluminum carbohydrate gel (Basalgel) as foul tasting.

These factors plus cost of medical care and drugs, monotony of diet, decreased physical strength, feelings of hopelessness and helplessness, fear of dying, and family conflicts strongly influence the patient's ability to comply with treatment. The nurse can help by listening to the patient's problems, clarifying misconceptions, and referring the patient to other sources of help such as the social worker and dietitian.

While successful conservative management is often very difficult, it does permit the patient to maintain a less altered life style than when maintenance hemodialysis is instituted.

A patient can get quite depressed when facing his dietary restriction, coupled with his lack of energy, his disinterest in what is going on around him, and his physical deterioration. If the patient is destined for a dialysis program in the future, the nurse can discuss some of his concerns with him. His diet will become liberalized, his nausea and vomiting will clear up, food will start to taste better, his itching will improve, as will his dry skin, his sensorium, and his sense of general well-being.

Some patients are not candidates for long-term hemodialysis. These patients and their families require sustained nursing support throughout the downward progression of the disease. (See Chapter 12 for care of the dying patient.)

## Maintenance Hemodialysis

In 1971 the National Dialysis Registry indicated that 3,700 patients were receiving maintenance hemodialysis and nearly 40 per cent of these were dialyzing at home. With the later passage of Public Law 92-603, Section 2991 (better known as HR-1) federal financing is provided for most patients with end-stage renal disease for whom dialytic intervention is indicated. With the resultant increase in the number and kind of dialysis units throughout the country, the former decision-making process regarding who were the more eligible candidates for the limited number of artificial kidneys need no longer apply. By July 1, 1974 over 14,000 persons were receiving maintenance hemo- or peritoneal dialysis.

The cost of dialysis in the home is reduced by about 60 per cent partly because of absence of professional staff. The patient is trained as his own dialysis technician. His assistant (usually the spouse but may be any close associate) enters the training program at a later time after the patient who is the primary person in home management has mastered certain parts of the program. A training progam can take several months. Many patients on home dialysis are awaiting kidney transplant.

Some homes are not physically suited to accommodate dialysis equipment. Initial costs in the home are about $10,500. A year's cost of supplies is about $3,000. Other homes are not suitable for socio-cultural reasons. Some patients prefer to dialyze in a center where they have some professional support as well as peer support. Age, emotional stability of the patient, other complicating diseases such as diabetes, and the ability of the home members to integrate dialysis into its way of life are other considerations.

Patients with chronic renal failure on a regular dialysis program can be expected to have a decrease in hypertension (thought to be due to a reduction of extracellular fluid volume or a better response to antihypertensive therapy), relief of uremic symptoms, return of appetite, improvement in libido and sexual functioning, and relief of peripheral neuropathy.

**Activity.** The patient should be encouraged to be as active as he can be. Many patients are able to return to work part-time or even full-time once a regular dialysis program has been initiated. However, most patients who are on pension or receive disability assistance cannot afford to financially give up such income for an insecure job situation that they simply physically may not be able to handle. A white-collar job that does not require much physical activity is certainly easier to perform than the job of a truck driver, farmer, or construction worker. As long as the patient performs some useful activity, it need not necessarily be the role of income provider to make a significant contribution to his self-worth and family integrity.

**Diet.** Even with maintenance hemodialysis diet is a principal and constant mode of therapy. However, protein is not as restricted. 40 Gm. to 70 Gm. protein diets may be prescribed. Sodium and potassium and fluid restriction may also be prescribed depending on the level of kidney function

**Psychosocial Aspects.** Studies have shown that the path of adaptation to maintenance hemodialysis is characterized by phases of denial, depression, and dependence. Reichsman and Levy (1972) found that patients experienced premaintenance dialysis depression followed by a "honeymoon" period after dialysis was initiated during which time patients felt better due to the relief of uremic symptoms. The end of the honeymoon period was usually precipitated by expectations of staff and family that the patient return to active and productive work. Disenchantment, discouragement, and unmet dependency needs were common, but most were able to achieve long term adaptation.

Patient and family need a great deal of support and should be viewed as an interacting system. Many complications accompany renal disease, and the impact that they can have on a family can be devastating. They can resent the demands placed on them and become angry at the patient even though they want him with them. They may withdraw from the patient if they view his disease as terminal. A strained family relationship may quite rapidly deteriorate when faced with the traumas and emotional drains imposed by near emergency situations during home dialysis, by life-threatening episodes of pericarditis, parathyroidectomy, hyperkalemia, air embolus, or unexplained seizures. Or a family may grow quite close as all members get involved in making their activities more enjoyable and challenging as they work out new menus, or find ways to vacation as a family and still dialyze on a regular basis.

Life with chronic illness and dependency on a machine for survival places a tremendous burden upon a patient and his significant others. Often the public may view the dialysis patient as "lucky" and expect the patient to feel this way. However the patient may feel angry, resentful at the loss of body integrity and forced change in life style and hate the machine and everything it represents.

Patients on maintenance dialysis can develop such problems as bone fractures, shunt and fistula complications, and increasing fatigue. They will always be chronically ill and have to face the threat of death. Periods of depression have resulted in overt suicide attempts in some patients or covert "giving up" by failing to follow diet or fluid restrictions. Unless the staff understands the unique needs and ways of responding of individuals and allows for and can accept the ventilation of feelings, staff can view patients as deliberately uncooperative, ungrateful, or unworthy of the time, effort, and money expended on their care. Patients, family, and staff may require crisis intervention or sustained psychotherapy to deal with the feelings and demands engendered by this extraordinary way of prolonging life. The cooperation of the team—nurses, physicians, technicians, dietitians, social workers, pharmacists, biochemists, biochemical engineers, and supply clerks is essential.

## RENAL TRANSPLANTATION

Some patients with end stage renal disease are candidates for kidney transplantation. Criteria may include creatinine clearance less than 5 ml. per minute, but the patient should not be critically ill, malnourished or infected. Age is also a factor. Most prospective recipients for renal transplantation are in maintenance dialysis programs. Some patients would rather remain on maintenance hemodialysis than risk the side effects of lifelong immunosuppressive therapy. Patients suffering from major disease symptoms not reversible with improved kidney function are not candidates for transplantation.

Well over 5,000 kidney transplantations have been performed throughout the world according to the ACS/NIH Organ Transplant Registry (Chicago, Illinois). World statistics of kidney transplantation in man indicate increasing success especially over the past decade. For example, from January 1967 to January 1969 percentage of graft survival at two years was 81 per cent, 73 per cent, and 40 per cent for sibling, parent, and cadaver transplants respectively. Some patients are alive and well eight to nine years after transplantation (Hamburger, 1972).

Several major problems are the subject of current research including methods of selection of cadaver donors, methods to prevent immunologic rejection of the transplanted kidney, and methods of monitoring the grafted patient to detect immunologic events in time to prevent damage.

### Immunologic Selection

Major methods of determining compatibility of donor and recipient are serologic determination of the leukocyte and/or platelet HL-A antigens and mixed culture of donor and recipient lymphocytes. All persons carry four HL-A antigens. Perfect compatibility exists when donor and recipient carry the same four HL-A antigens and have no detectable antigenic differences.

Kidney transplantation between identical twins carries no immunologic risk of rejection. Sibling donors are immunologically superior to parent donors.

### Donor Considerations

A proposed living related donor must be evaluated for the quality of immunologic compatibility; lack of hidden family pressure interfering with a free decision to be a donor; age; state of general health and studies of renal function and structure, including arteriography. The prospective donor must understand the future risks such as accidental damage to his remaining kidney. It may help him to know, for example, that the mortality risk to the healthy donor involved in having only one remaining kidney is much the same as that entailed by a United States male who drives a motor vehicle less than 8,000 miles per year (Merrill, 1965).

The surgical procedure (elective nephrectomy) will necessitate relief from full home and job responsibilities for a certain period of time with restriction against heavy lifting for about eight weeks postoperatively. Since many hospitalization insurance plans do not cover elective surgery, costs must be considered.

Generally, two hospitalizations are required: the first for evaluation for suitability as a donor and the second for the elective donor nephrectomy. In each instance, the donor enters the hospital as a well patient.

The nurse should recognize that the prospective donor may have ambivalent feelings as well as the normal anxiety associated with hospitalization. He may feel generous and noble; or on the other hand, resentful but obligated. Psychological evaluation is done in order to prevent a postsurgical hostile relationship with the recipient or significant others.

The evaluation period is one of anxious waiting and testing which can result in disappointment if the prospective donor does not meet the criteria.

Once approved and surgery is scheduled, pre- and postoperative nursing assessment and intervention for the patient with a nephrectomy is carried out. In addition to concern for his own needs, the donor is understandably concerned about the postsurgical response of the recipient.

### Cadaver Donor

Considerations in the selection of a cadaver donor in addition to immunologic compatibility include age, state of health before death (vascular or hypertensive disease is a contraindication), legal consent and clarity of the diagnosis of death, and length of time for which the kidney can be preserved.

### Recipient Considerations

When transplantation is proposed to the patient and family by the physician, they face a momentous decision. Careful initial explanation of the proposal, the surgical procedure, the expected outcomes and the risks for both donor and recipient must be followed by opportunities to question, to clarify, and to discuss the event with members of the nephrology team including the surgeons.

Transplantation should not be viewed as a cure but rather as a "trade-off" of one chronic illness for another. The recipient can be freed from dependency on a machine but faces lifelong immunosuppressive therapy with sometimes devastating side effects, especially if he is unaware that they can occur. The patient can be assured that in the event of failure of the transplant he can return to maintenance hemodialysis with the possibility of a second transplant. Since future dialyses are a possibility (temporary or maintenance), the patient is advised to preserve a functioning internal arteriovenous fistula such as by not permitting the vessels to be used for the withdrawal of blood specimens.

Visits with posttransplant patients can be arranged and can be a source of comfort to the prospective recipient and his significant others. The nurse encourages the patient and family to get as objective an account of the posttransplant risks and problems involved as possible. They should know that there is a possibility of early failure, that the patient with a renal transplant must be responsible for his lifelong immunosuppressive medication administration and that he is never without the fear of transplant rejection. The nurse's role is to help the patient and family understand the facts involved so that they can make a wise decision. It is not her role to attempt to make a decision for them either voluntarily or by entrapment. Once the decision is made, the nurse supports the patient in his decision as being right for him.

Bilateral nephrectomies may be performed eight weeks or so prior to transplantation particularly if hypertension is uncontrolled. Hemodialysis as well as dietary and other measures to keep the patient in optimal condition for surgery are continued. Cystograms are performed to assess the bladder and ureters for structural abnormalities.

A patient awaiting a cadaver transplant has a period of additional stress after his decision has been made. There may be considerable delay between the decision time and the availability of a suitable kidney.

### Preoperative Care

The nursing assessment and intervention is that for the patient undergoing major renal, urinary tract, and blood vessel surgery. In addition, immunosuppressive drug therapy is initiated. Blood transfusions are given only if urgent and are specially prepared to reduce the number of lymphocytes. The recipient is placed on the seriously ill list and is helped to obtain pastoral counseling if he wishes it. The patient and family should know that isolation precautions during the critical postoperative period preclude usual visiting periods.

The patient who has been in a hemodialysis program is usually accustomed to being self-responsible and very well informed of his status such as his usual blood chemistry values. The transplant team is new to him and may have a different viewpoint about the extent of patient information and education. This can result in a major source of stress for the recipient who often needs as much information as possible to remain in control of his situation. Thus it is essential that nursing intervention be based on an individual cognitive, affective, and psychomotor assessment.

### Postoperative Considerations

Usual nursing assessment and intervention for the patient with kidney, urinary tract, and major blood vessel surgery is indicated.

Immunosuppressive therapy required in renal transplantation lowers the white blood cell count, lymphocytes in particular. Thus, the patient's resistance to infection is lowered. To minimize exposure to infection the postoperative transplant patient remains in a single room and the environment is kept as clean as possible. Meticulous care must be taken when handling all urinary drainage systems. Aseptic technique is essential for catheter care, intravenous monitoring lines and fluids, irrigations, and dressing changes. Only personnel essential to patient care are permitted to enter the room; they do a surgical scrub and wear a sterile gown and mask. The patient remains in this setting for four to five days after the transplantation and he may become lonely, bored and irritable. The nurse who makes herself available to this patient at times other than when she has technical functions to perform conveys the message that she is interested in him for himself. Encouraging the patient to air his thoughts and feelings about his present situation and future plans assists him to assess his life realistically and to examine alternatives. Frequent communication carried by the nurse from family to patient, and vice versa, can minimize the chances of cumulative tension.

Assessment factors include weight, temperature, pulse, respiration, blood pressure, intake and output from all sources, serum electrolytes, and hematocrit. Urinary drainage is tested for protein, sugar, pH, specific gravity, electrolytes, and creatinine clearance. Intravenous fluid replacement is guided by amount of urinary output and electrolyte studies.

Immediate satisfactory function of the grafted kidney (living donor or cadaver) after the circulation is restored is the usual situation. There is an early high volume output due to osmolar diuresis which diminishes to normal volume in 48 to 72 hours. Fluid volume maintenance and electrolyte balance are crucial considerations. In cases where the transplanted kidney does not function adequately, hemodialysis may be performed. This decreased function may result from acute renal failure due for example to mechanical obstruction, thrombosis, or rejection. The usual symptoms of rejection are decreased urinary output, fever, swelling and tenderness of the transplant site, proteinuria, lymphocytes in the urine, elevated serum creatinine, sudden weight gain (edema), and hypertension. Acute renal failure may be reversible and the patient is maintained on hemodialysis, until with adjustment in immunosuppressive therapy, the transplanted kidney functions adequately. Rejection, if severe, may necessitate removal of the transplanted kidney and management with maintenance dialysis.

## Immunosuppression

Immunosuppression after renal transplantation is accomplished most often by medications such as azathioprine (Imuran), corticosteroids such as prednisone, or antilymphocyte globulin. Surgical cannulation of the thoracic duct and drainage of lymph to deplete the lymphocyte count may be initiated preoperatively.

Azathioprine (Imuran) is often the immunosuppressive agent of first choice whereas prednisone may be used primarily during rejection crises. Azathioprine therapy may predispose the patient to virus infections (herpes simplex, herpes zoster, and viral hepatitis), bone marrow aplasia and certain malignant diseases. Steroids on a long-term basis are one of the most serious hazards of kidney transplantation. They encourage microbial and viral infections and relatively large doses result in a Cushingoid appearance, buffalo hump, abdominal striae and protuberance. These changes in body image may be extremely upsetting to the patient. Other side effects of steroid therapy include peptic ulcer, gastrointestinal hemorrhage, and diabetes mellitus. Bone disorders, especially bilateral aseptic necrosis of the femoral head, may result in crippling.

Antilymphocyte sera produce pain and an inflammatory reaction at the injection site within two to six hours and which fades in a few hours. Fever also occurs. Thrombocytopenia and thrombocytosis are possible.

## Long-Term Care

Immediate return of blood pressure to normal in previously hypertensive patients is common, along with improvement in the state of the retina with improved visual acuity. In the first few months after successful transplantation there is dramatic improvement in the general condition of the patient. Red cell count returns to normal, peripheral neuropathy resolves, cardiovascular complications improve and there is a slow correction of disturbances of calcium and phosphorus metabolism. Menstruation returns when uremia was accompanied by amenorrhea. Restoration to full health ranges from weeks to six or ten months after transplantation (Hamburger, et al., 1972).

While rejection crises can occur at any time, death is usually due to extrarenal complications of immunosuppressive therapy such as infections, hepatitis, and malignant tumors.

The patient requires lifelong medical supervision for monitoring of function and histology of the transplanted kidney and complications of immunologic therapy. He is told the side effects of immunosuppressive therapy and what and when to report to the physician. He may be required to test his urine for protein daily. He also makes a daily record of his temperature, weight, and urine output. Any change in these observations is reported to the physician immediately. Avoidance of infection and prompt reporting of early signs are stressed in the patient education program.

In spite of these responsibilities the successful transplant patient is advised to resume normal life. A full program of work and recreation, including sports, is advocated. Transplant patients are aware of the possibility of rejection and this brings with it fear and uncertainty. They may need subsequent hospitalizations for drug dosage adjustment. All need sustained support from the nephrology team. In one large institution the average renal transplant patient was 28 years old and married. Having spent a sizable portion of their lives chronically ill, renal transplantation offers patients with end-stage renal disease cautious optimism for a more normal life.

## Resources for Patients with Kidney Disease

The Ruth Gottscho Foundation, 916 Ridgewood Road, Millburn, N.J. 07041 provides anatomical gift donor cards and literature such as *Dialysis Centers for Traveling Kidney Patients.*

National Association of Patients on Hemodialysis and Transplantation (NAPHT), 505 Northern Boulevard, Great Neck, New York 11021.

National Kidney Foundation, 116 E. 27th St., New York, N.Y. 10016. (Contact local affiliate.)

## REFERENCES AND BIBLIOGRAPHY

BELL, P., and CALMAN, K.: *Surgical Aspects of Haemodialysis,* Edinburgh, Churchill Livingstone, 1974.

BERNBECK, L.: Conservative care of patients with renal failure, Chap. 5 in Schlotter, L. (ed.): *Nursing and the Nephrology Patient,* Flushing, N.Y., Medical Examination Publ. Co., 1973.

CRAVEN, R. F., and SHARP, B. H.: The effects of illness on family functions, *Nurs. Forum* 11:186, 1972.

CUMMINGS, J.: Hemodialysis—The pressures and how patients respond, *Am. J. Nurs.* 70:70, January 1970.

Death of an angel. Nursing grand rounds. *Nurs. '73* 3:52, June 1973.

DENOUR, A. K.: Psychotherapy with patients on chronic haemodialysis, *Brit. J. Psychiat.* 116:207, February 1970.

DENOUR, A. K., and CZACZKES, J. W.: Resistance to home dialysis, *Psychiat. Med.* 1:207, July 1971.

DUNEA, G.: Peritoneal dialysis and hemodialysis, *Med. Clin. N. Am.* 55:155, January 1971.

FEELEY, E.: Mr. Stevens . . . was he really seeking death? *Nurs. '74* 4:62, January 1974.

FRENCH, R.: *The Nurse's Guide to Diagnostic Procedures,* ed. 3, New York, McGraw-Hill, 1971.

FRIEDMAN, E. A.: Psychological adjustment to maintenance hemodialysis, 1, *N.Y. J. Med.* 70:629, March 1, 1970.

————: Psychological adjustment to maintenance hemodialysis, 11, *N.Y. J. Med.* 70:767, March 15, 1970.

FOY, AUDREY: Dreams of patients and staff, *Am. J. Nurs.* 70:80, January 1970.

GARIBALDI, R. A., et al.: Hemodialysis-associated hepatitis, *JAMA* 225:384, July 23, 1973.

GLASSMAN, B. M., et al.: Personality correlates of survival in a long-term hemodialysis program, *Arch. Gen. Psychiat.* 22:566, June 1970.

GOLDSTEIN, A. M., et al.: Suicide in chronic hemodialysis patients from an external locus of control framework, *Am. J. Psychiat.* 127:1204, March 1971.

GUTCH, C., and STONER, M.: *Review of Hemodialysis for Nurses and Dialysis Personnel,* St. Louis, Mosby, 1971.

HALL, R. C. W.: Psychiatric complications of chronic renal hemodialysis and renal transplantation, *The New Physician* 20:255, April 1971.

HALPER, I. S.: Psychiatric observations in a chronic hemodialysis program, *Med. Clin. N. Am.* 55:177, January 1971.

HAMBURGER, J., et al.: *Renal Transplantation: Theory and Practice,* Baltimore, Williams & Wilkins, 1972.

HAMPERS, C., et al.: *Long-Term Hemodialysis,* ed. 2, New York, Grune and Stratton, 1973.

HARRINGTON, J., and BRENER, E.: *Patient Care in Renal Failure,* Philadelphia, Saunders, 1973.

HASSETT, M.: Teaching hemodialysis to the family unit, *Nurs. Clin. N. Am.* 7:349, June 1972.

Hemodialysis—some facts and figures, *Am. J. Nurs.* 70:73, January 1970.

*Hemodialysis Manual.* U.S. Department of HEW Publ. No. (HSM) 72-7002.

KROAH, J.: An exploratory study of the strategies that renal nurses use in response to the emotional reactions and behaviors of hemodialysis patients, *Image* 5:16, No. 2, 1972.

Kossoris, P.: Family therapy: An adjunct to hemo-dialysis and transplantation, *Am. J. Nurs.* 70:1730, August 1970.

Lennon, E.: The surgical dialysis patient, *Nurs. Clin. N. Am.* 4:443, September 1969.

Martin, A.: Renal transplantation: Surgical technique and complications, *Am. J. Nurs.* 68:1240, June 1968.

Martin, M.: Home dialysis, *J. Rehab.* 38:18, May-June 1972.

McClellan, M. S.: Crisis groups in special care areas, *Nurs. Clin. N. Am.* 7:363, June 1972.

Merrill, J.: *The Treatment of Renal Failure,* ed. 2, New York, Grune and Stratton, 1965.

Muehrcke, R., et al.: *Acute Renal Failure,* St. Louis, Mosby, 1969.

O'Neill, M.: Guidelines for teaching home dialysis, *Nurs. Clin. N. Am.* 6:641, December 1971.

————: Home dialysis: A most encompassing nurs-ing situation, *ANA Clin. Sess.* 1972, New York, Appleton-Century-Crofts, 1973:141.

Papper, S.: Renal failure, *Med. Clin. N. Am.* 55:335, March 1971.

————: *Clinical Nephrology,* Boston, Little, Brown, 1971.

Preston, B.: Trailer dialysis: A new concept in a self-care facility, Ch. 13 in Schlotter, L. (ed.): *Nursing and the Nephrology Patient,* Flushing, N. Y., Medi-cal Examination Publ. Co., 1973.

Rappaport, F.: *A Second Look at Life: Transplanta-tion and Dialysis Patients: Their Own Stories,* New York, Grune and Stratton, 1973.

Read, M.: External arteriovenous shunts, *Am. J. Nurs.* 72:8, January 1972.

Reichsman, F., and Levy, R.: Problems in adaptation to maintenance hemodialysis, *Arch. Intern. Med.* 130:859, December 1972.

Rodriquez, D.: Moral issues in hemodialysis and renal transplantation, *Nurs. Forum* 10:201, 1971.

Schlotter, L. (ed.): *Nursing and the Nephrology Pa-tient: A Symposium on Current Trends and Issues,* Flushing, N. Y., Medical Examination Publ. Co., 1973.

Simmons, R.: Family tension in the search for a kidney donor, *JAMA* 215:909, February 8, 1971.

Thorwald, J.: *The Patients. The Kidney Patients,* Zurich, Droemer Knaur Verlay Schoeller & Co., 1971.

Wang, F.: Conservative management of chronic renal failure, *Med. Clin. N. Am.* 55:137, January 1971.

When the patient's kidneys shut down, *Nurs. Update* 4:1, March 1973.

Winsor, T.: Electrolyte abnormalities and the electro-cardiogram, *JAMA* 203:109, 1968.

# The Burned Patient

Suddenly a well person sustains serious burns, and is confronted with problems resulting from pain, mutilation, fear of death, disfigurement, separation, immobilization, helplessness, and possible abandonment. Together with his own injuries and problems he may be grieving over the death of others involved in the accident such as spouse or children or coworkers. He may experience guilt over the cause of the accident to others and anger that this catastrophe should have happened to him. If he lives he has a long battle with prevention of infection, continuing pain from dressing changes; scarring; changes in body image, finances, social relationships, even motivation to continue living; and reconstructive surgery.

The nurse who elects to care for burned patients is in a difficult position. Recognizing and sympathizing with the patient and all his problems, she is the one who also inflicts pain by necessary procedures when she probably views her role more in terms of providing comfort. However, she can earn the satisfaction of helping the patient to recover by the intensive care she gives, with other members of the burn team, over the weeks and months of the patient's illness.

National Safety Council statistics indicate that 6,700 persons died in fires and of burn injuries in 1970, and 250,000 suffered disabling injuries. About 90 per cent of burns occur at home or in the home neighborhood. Space heaters (usually gas), matches, outdoor fires, and gas hot-water heaters are responsible for more than half the burn injuries. Combustible clothing, gasoline, barbecue starters, paint thinners, cigarette lighter fluid, cigarettes, and bedding that has been set on fire are also responsible for burn injuries.

Thermal burns are caused by such factors as the heat of flame, scalding water or food, and steam. Poison gases, electricity, strong acids (such as nitric and sulfuric), and strong alkalies (such as lye and caustic soda) can cause chemical changes in tissue that are similar to the changes caused by thermal burns.

## TYPES OF BURNS

A *first-degree burn* is characterized by erythema. It does not blister. There may be a small amount of edema in and under the burn. Only the corium layer of the epidermis is involved. There is no necrosis of skin, and systemic derangement is minimal. It peels in three to six days.

A *second-degree burn* is characterized by a blister that contains water and electrolytes in ratios similar to those in plasma. The fluid comes from local vessels (lymphatics and capillaries) and cells. It is carried away by the lymphatics, but not so rapidly as it accumulates. The interstitial spaces soon are flooded. Most or all of the epithelial layers are involved, but the deepest layers of skin are not burned, and therefore re-epithelization can occur. A second-degree burn heals without scarring in 10 to 14 days (Fig. 65-1).

A *third-degree burn* destroys the entire dermis down to the subcutaneous fat. Massive edema is present, collected deep in the wounded tissue, but there is no blister. There is necrosis of tissue. This is the kind of burn that causes scarring.

In a *fourth-degree burn* not only is the full thickness of skin destroyed, but also tissue underneath the skin. This may include subcutaneous tissue, fascia, muscle, tendon, and bone.

The diagnosis of the depth of a burn often is difficult. There may be a combination of all degrees of burn. Both locally and systemically, the deeper the burn, the greater the damage.

The second measure of damage is the extent of the area: the larger the burn area, the greater is the damage to the body. Severe sunburn (first-degree) over 85 per cent of the body will cause a much greater disturbance of fluid and electrolyte regulation than a third-degree burn on the tip of a forefinger. Since physicians base their prescriptions for fluid replacement therapy both on the degree and the extent of the body surface injured, the diagnosis includes both these factors. The "Rule of Nines"

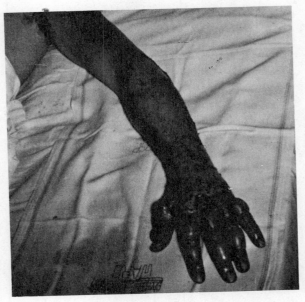

**Figure 65-1.** Second-degree burn of hand and arm. The picture was taken eight hours postburn. The appearance of the blebs is typical. This wound was treated by exposure to the air and healed without complication. The arm is kept on sterile towels.

(Fig. 65-2) is one method of estimating how much of the patient's skin surface is involved.

Burns caused by *electricity* are characteristically deep, involving not only the skin, but also blood vessels, muscles, tendons, and bones. Pain may be only slight when the cutaneous nerves are destroyed, but the later functional disturbance may be devastating. The area of necrosis frequently is deeper than it appears at first. The burn is caused by the transformation of the energy of the electric current into heat as it passes through body tissue. At first the skin is white; then it becomes black. Muscles contract, sometimes violently enough to fracture bones. The electrical shock may cause ventricular fibrillation so that a primary first aid need may be cardiopulmonary resuscitation while the victim is rushed to a facility for defibrillation. In extensive electrical burns later rehabilitation may require bone grafts and repair of hernias caused by weakened muscle tissue as well as plastic surgery to relieve contractures.

## PROGNOSIS

Burns over 40 per cent of the skin are likely to be fatal. Prognosis depends on the depth of the burn,

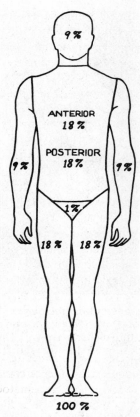

ANTERIOR 18 %

POSTERIOR 18 %

9 %

9 %      9 %

1 %

18 %    18 %

100 %

**Figure 65-2.** The "Rule of Nines," a simplified method for estimating the per cent of the body surface covered by burns. According to this method, the entire head is 9 per cent of the body surface area; each entire arm is 9 per cent; each entire leg is 18 per cent; the genital region is 1 per cent; the front torso is 18 per cent; and the back torso is 18 per cent. Doctors often sketch the area burned on a diagram such as this to facilitate the calculation of the per cent of the body burned.

as well as the extent of the area. Few patients with more than 70 per cent burns live.

A severe burn disrupts the functioning of the body to such an extent that a patient who already has some organic malfunction or other injuries is in grave danger of losing his life, even with considerably less than a 40 per cent burn. A kidney disorder, a chronic lung infection, or hypertension becomes a very serious matter. The very young and the very old have a greater mortality rate than other age groups.

In recent years such large strides have been made in the treatment of burn shock and wound infection that patients are saved today who would have died several years ago. This is especially true of patients

who are not very young or very old, and who have no pre-existing disease. However, those patients saved from dying in shock may later succumb to other complications, such as pulmonary failure, septicemia, and renal failure. The prevention of infection and other complications has always been an important nursing consideration in the care of the burned patient.

In general the seriousness of any given burn injury can be assessed and the injury categorized as minor, moderate, or critical. Minor burns are second-degree burns of less than 15 per cent of the total body surface area and third-degree burns of less than 2 per cent of the body surface area. Minor burns can usually be managed on an outpatient basis and rarely require hospitalization. Moderately severe burns are those second-degree burns of 15 to 30 per cent of the body surface area and third-degree burns of less than 10 per cent of the body surface area except those involving the hands, face, and feet. Burns of this magnitude can usually be managed satisfactorily in community hospitals and ordinarily do not require hospitalization in a specialized burn unit. Critical burns are those second-degree burns of over 30 per cent of the body surface area, third-degree burns of the face, hands, and feet or involving more than 10 per cent of the body surface area, as well as burns complicated by respiratory tract injury, major soft tissue injury, and fractures. Additionally, electrical burns are usually placed in this category due to the specialized problems which must be dealt with. Critical burn patients require highly specialized nursing and physician care and should be hospitalized on a special burn unit or in a regional specialized burn center. In such units, clinical nurse specialists assume a high level of responsibility for the complex care of severely burned patients. They also supervise others with special preparation such as the burn care technician (BCT).

Nursing assessment and intervention for the various phases of recovery from burns require unique considerations. Each phase is discussed separately below.

## EMERGENT PERIOD

### First Aid

If the clothes are flaming, the first thing to do is to put out the fire. A blanket, a coat, or a loose rug can be used. Outdoors, if there is nothing to smother the flames, the person is slowly rolled on the ground.

Using sand or dirt to cover him should be avoided; this can lead to infection.

If the burn is due to a chemical, it should be diluted by flushing the area with copious quantities of clean, cool water as quickly as possible. The longer the chemical is on the skin, the more it burns. Ideally, the water should be sterile, but chances are sterile water will not be available.

General principles of first aid apply. An airway must be established and bleeding related to associated injuries controlled before wound care is initiated.

Any clothing that does not adhere to the skin should be removed. Rings, bracelets, and wristwatches are taken off before edema forms and causes constriction. If the patient has to be transported, the burned area should be covered with the cleanest dressing obtainable, or the patient can be wrapped in a clean sheet. No two body surfaces should be wrapped together: fingers are bandaged separately, and a pad is placed between the arms and the trunk. No oil, ointment, or any other medication should be put on the burns, since it would have to be removed after the patient enters the hospital, adding to the trauma that the skin already has received. If the face has been burned, the eyes should be rinsed in large amounts of clean, cool water, and a drop of mineral or liquid petrolatum oil should be instilled in each to protect the cornea from specks of dust and dirt.

If there will be a delay before the patient is seen by a physician (as might happen in a large-scale disaster, such as an explosion aboard ship or in an enemy attack), and if the patient is conscious and not nauseous or vomiting, sips of a mixture of one teaspoon of table salt and half a teaspoon of soda bicarbonate (or baking soda) mixed in a quart of water can be given. The salt provides some of the sodium lost to the body as it is poured into the edematous tissues, and the baking soda is a base to help to correct the acidosis of burns. A record of intake and output should be kept.

## Shock Phase

Soon after the body suffers a burn, the burned area is flooded with fluid containing electrolytes and protein. Edema results from increased capillary permeability, increased osmotic pressure, and vasodilation. Protein molecules, which usually are too large to pass through the capillary walls, in this instance move freely from the bloodstream into the

injured skin through damaged capillary walls, pulling even more water with them. Some areas swell more than others. For instance, the hands and the face become more edematous than the middle of the back. The amount of fluid lost to the body as a result of the burn is large. Some of this fluid is held in the wound and thus is unavailable to the rest of the body, and some leaves the body entirely, seeping through the wound and when the blisters break. Water vapor, an additional source of fluid loss, passes from the body into the air through the burn eschar 75 times faster than through normal skin. Water vapor in large amounts can pass constantly through eschars that look dry.

Potassium ions are transferred from the damaged tissue to the bloodstream. Sodium and protein leave the body in the exudate from the wounds. The result is that the body is flooded with potassium, and it is lacking in sodium. Red blood cells are trapped and held in the wounds.

The water that goes from the bloodstream into the wounds causes a fall in the volume of blood in the normal paths and avenues of the circulatory system. The blood thickens as a consequence. This hemoconcentration makes the hematocrit* rise from its normal figure (about 45), since there is less and less fluid to dilute the solid components of the blood. Blood pressure drops, and the kidneys may receive insufficient blood to process urine. Less blood is available to maintain circulation. The heart beats faster and harder to push the sludge along. The result of this process is shock.

These fluid shifts proceed rapidly for the first eight hours after the accident, and they continue for about two days. Then the process slowly tapers off. The amount of fluid and electrolytes lost is related to the extent and the depth of the burn, and the resulting shock may be fatal. Timing is vital. Replacement therapy with fluids and electrolytes needs to be started soon after the burn, because the fluid shifts rapidly. Starting replacement therapy before irreversible shock has set in may make the difference between life and death.

Not all those who have been burned go into shock; it depends on the extent and the degree of the burn, the age and the general physical condition of the

---

*A *hematocrit* is a test to determine the relative amount of solids and fluids in blood—in other words, the concentration of blood. The name is used also for the apparatus employed in making the test.

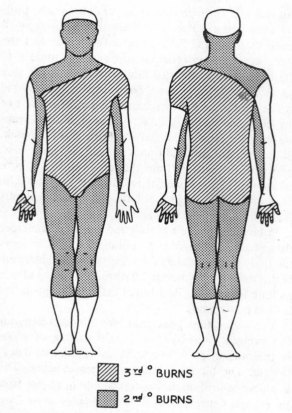

3 ʳᵈ ° BURNS

2 ⁿᵈ ° BURNS

**Figure 65-3.** Diagram used to calculate the per cent of burns: second-degree, 48½ per cent; third-degree, 31 per cent; total, 79½ per cent.

patient. An 80-year-old woman with hypertension may go into shock with a 10 per cent burn, which might not put a younger, healthier person into shock.

### Assessment and Intervention

Everything said about the severely burned patient in this chapter can apply also, with modification, to the patient with a milder or less extensive burn. A patient with a 1 per cent burn is not likely to go into shock, but the basic pathology remains the same. Infection, contractures, and emotional disturbances can occur with a ½ per cent burn as with a 32 per cent burn.

A great deal needs to be done within the first hour of a severely burned patient's admission. Because the patient needs such complex and intensive attention, it is usual for a team of physicians, nurses, and various therapists and technicians to care for him during the emergency period. Several treatments may be performed simultaneously, and time is important. One physician may perform the tracheostomy, another computes the patient's fluid and electrolyte requirements, and a third cares for the wounds. Ideally, the team includes several nurses, but in practice only one nurse may be available. She has a double role: to assist the physicians and to render direct care to the patient. She also has a role in comforting the family and helping them to understand what care is being given and in what ways they can help. For example, some family members may donate blood.

Tetanus prophylaxis should be ordered at the time of admission for all patients.

**Preparation.** Any hospital unit to which burned patients are admitted needs to have the equipment necessary for the emergency assembled and in readiness for immediate use. There is no time to hunt through the cabinet for sterile gloves or to run to central supply for a cutdown set. Sterile goods should be periodically checked to make sure that they are not outdated. Some hospitals keep the necessary equipment on a burn cart that can be rolled to a patient's room.

Because the room is crowded with equipment and busy with the activity of many people, having equipment that is needed right at hand and ready for instant use helps to prevent confusion. Preplanning helps the emergency team to function smoothly.

While emergency treatment is being carried out, a bed can be prepared for the patient as follows: a plastic sheet is placed next to the mattress and a sterile bottom sheet is covered by three sterile draw sheets (one at the top, one at the middle, and one at the bottom of the bed), or disposable sheets can be used. This arrangement of draw sheets allows wet linen to be changed with minimal handling of the patient. Sterile sheets are pinned in place on the side rails. A bed cradle is kept in readiness to place over the patient.

Since the introduction of topical antibacterial agents in skin care of burns, some hospitals use regularly cleaned linen instead of sterile sheets and gowns with no apparent risk to the patient. Isolation technique may be used by staff and visitors, who wear a clean gown or scrub dress and mask to protect the patient from organisms which they carry.

Some hospitals have burn units, including the ventilation system, isolated from the rest of the hospital so that exposure to microorganisms is minimized.

**Fluid Therapy.** If there is no cardiorespiratory distress, the severely burned patient's most urgent need is the replacement of the fluid lost, so that an adequate blood volume is maintained, and irreversible shock is avoided. To determine the amount and the type of fluid to give, the physician estimates the extent of the burn and its severity. He usually draws a diagram of the burn area (such as that in Fig. 65-3), and he may use the "Rule of Nines" as a basis of his calculations. Several burn and fluid replacement formulas are available. One such formula is the Brooke formula:

FIRST 24-HOUR PERIOD:

Colloids (blood plasma or dextran), 0.5 ml. × weight in kilograms × per cent of body burn.
Electrolyte (such as lactated Ringer's solution), 1.5 ml. × weight in kilograms × per cent of body burn.
Dextrose in water, 2,000 ml.

Rigid adherence to a formula is impossible. Adjustments are determined by the physician according to urinary output and central venous pressure.

It is recommended that one half of the total fluid volume calculated according to the above formula should be administered within the first eight hours after injury and the remaining half should be administered during the remaining sixteen hours of the first 24-hour period. This is necessary because the rate of fluid loss is greatest immediately after injury and progressively declines over the first 48 to 72 hours after injury.

SECOND 24 HOURS:

Colloid: ½ to ⅔ of the first 24-hour requirement.
Electrolye: ½ to ⅔ of the first 24-hour requirement.
Dextrose in water, 2,000 ml.

Another burn fluid replacement formula which has become increasingly popular of late is the Parkland fluid regimen. Since it has been demonstrated that very little colloid can be retained within the vascular system during the first 24 hours after injury, many physicians have reasoned that colloid should not be administered during this period of time. Instead, the fluid losses are replaced solely by the administration of an electrolyte solution, and colloid is given only after the first 24 hours. The Parkland regimen dictates that during the first 24 hours postburn, lactated Ringer's solution should be given in the amount of 4 ml. per kilogram of body weight per per cent of body surface burn. This regimen has been highly successful in the fluid resuscitation of patients during the shock phase after burn injury. However, when a patient is resuscitated according to this formula, the amount of edema that develops appears to be significantly greater than when the Brooke formula is utilized.

In the emergency room a cutdown may be done or an intracath is inserted and intravenous fluid started. Blood is sent to the laboratory for typing and crossmatching, hematocrit, serum protein, complete blood count (CBC), blood urea nitrogen (BUN), sodium, chloride, potassium, and sugar. Arterial blood gas studies may be done.

A Foley catheter is inserted and the volume of urine is measured every hour. The urine is inspected for any visible abnormalities such as blood or purulence and is tested for specific gravity, pH, sugar, acetone, and protein on a regular basis during this critical period.

The amount of urine excreted is an indication as to whether the patient's fluid requirements are being met. Urine should be produced in at least the rate of 30 to 50 ml. an hour. When there is less than 20 ml. an hour the physician may speed up the infusions or increase colloid. If the amount is over 50 ml. an hour, the rate of fluid intake is reduced. When the urine flow is less than 10 ml. an hour, or over 80 ml. an hour, the patient is in danger. Too little urine means either renal shutdown or hypovolemia which leads to shock; too much urine may mean an overload of fluids and congestive heart failure. Either situation is serious and demands immediate medical attention. It is the nurse's responsibility to monitor fluid therapy by measuring the amount of intake and output every hour and recording it on the flow sheet and by noting the patient's blood pressure and pulse at least every hour. Central venous pressure measurement may also be used to guide fluid administration. A rising CVP (above 15 cm.) heralds pulmonary edema. These parameters and hematocrit reports are discussed with the physician and a plan for titrating fluid therapy is developed for each patient. (See also Chapter 59 for care of the patient in shock.)

Restlessness in a patient who has been quiet may be an indication that fluid replacement has not kept pace with fluid loss, and it should be reported immediately to the physician. Not all patients in burn shock are unconscious. A patient may be extremely thirsty, and this thirst can be relieved by replacement of the lost fluids. In the hospital the nurse awaits the physician's orders before she gives any patient anything to drink. No cracked ice, milk, fruit juice, or anything else is given. Unlimited tap water, if it is tolerated, would lead to water intoxication. If the patient is given anything to drink, an electrolyte solution probably will be ordered in preference to plain water. Even though the patient finds the salty solution highly palatable, the nurse should be careful to give him only sips at first, and she should not give any more than 200 ml. an hour unless the physician orders a different amount. Citrus fruit juices (and other potassium-containing fluids) are not given to the patient during the first few days postburn, unless specifically ordered. Many burned patients develop gastric distention, which leads to vomiting. Vomiting is to be avoided, because of the danger of aspiration, and because more valuable fluids and electrolytes are lost.

The large amount of fluid that the patient loses through his skin causes hypermetabolism, due to heat loss as water is evaporated from the burned areas. If the patient loses 5,000 ml. of water a day this way, he needs 2,880 calories just to maintain his body temperature—calories that he cannot ingest. This is above and beyond his need to maintain body weight.

**Pain Therapy.** To relieve the pain of the burns, the physician may give morphine intravenously. It is not given subcutaneously or intramuscularly to a patient in shock; the sluggish circulation would hinder its absorption. However, because morphine is a respiratory depressant, it may not be used at all, especially in a patient with burns of the head and the neck. Instead, intravenous barbiturates may be used for sedation. When medication for pain is ordered, the nurse should prepare it promptly. Subsequently, p.r.n. orders for medication to relieve pain should be given only when the patient is actually in pain (not, for example, for restlessness), since depressants are dangerous.

Intramuscular antibiotics usually are given. Cortisone is not generally used because it masks symptoms of infection.

**Pulmonary Therapy.** The nurse makes continuous, careful observations for respiratory difficulty, especially in patients with burns of the face and the neck. Patients who breathe in fumes of the fire will have respiratory tract damage, even in the absence of burns of the face.

Respiratory rate change (under 8 or over 20 per minute), dyspnea, hoarseness, stridor (harsh, high-pitched sound), cyanosis, coughing, darkened or blood-tinged sputum, restlessness, anxiety, chest pain, and hypo- or hypertension are indicators of possible pulmonary complications and should be discussed promptly with the physician. The prepared nurse can gather further data through auscultation of the chest for rales and rhonchi, quality of breath sounds, areas of absence of aeration, etc.

Arterial blood gases are measured in the burned patient with possible pulmonary complications to determine his oxygenation status and acid-base balance. Oxygen may be ordered or the patient may require assisted or controlled mechanical respiration (Fig. 65-4).

Whenever the patient is burned indoors there is danger of respiratory tract damage from inhaling smoke. Respiratory failure is a major cause of death in the first 48 hours. Labored respiration is the most frequent, and coughing is the second most frequent, symptom of respiratory tract damage in the burned patient.

The prognosis of the cyanotic patient usually is grave. Cyanosis may be difficult to see because the usual sites of observation for it may be burned. If the hands and face are burned, perhaps color may be observed in a toenail.

Blood-tinged or smoke-stained sputum is an ominous sign. Those patients who have respiratory tract damage and survive later almost always develop respiratory tract infection. Purulent sputum is coughed up three to four days postburn. The congestion, obstruction (usually in the smaller bronchi), and edema lead to atelectasis and pulmonary edema, which may threaten the patient's life. Every new respiratory symptom should be discussed immediately with the physician.

A constant inhalation of warm or cold nebulized air or oxygen keeps tracheal secretions liquefied and easier to cough up.

---

**Figure 65-4.** (A) This severely burned patient with respiratory tract damage requires mechanical ventilatory support. (B) Escharotomy has been performed to facilitate breathing and circulation. Linear incision through dead tissue releases the thick, hard constricting eschar, allowing for expansion. (C) Initial cleansing is necessary to remove debris so that accurate evaluation of wounds and infection control measures can take place. (D and E) To prepare healthy granulation tissue for grafting, daily debridement is carried out in a hydrotherapy tub (D), or when the patient's dressings are changed (E). (Reprinted with permission from *Nursing the Burned Patient*, Feller, Archambeault, 1974, National Institute for Burn Medicine, Ann Arbor, Mich.)

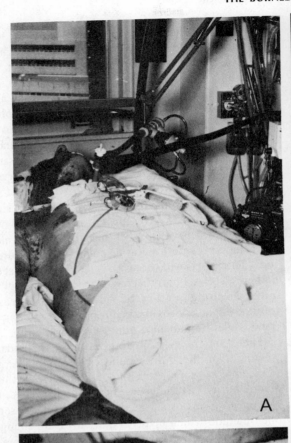

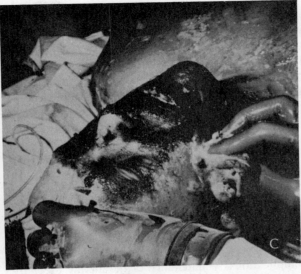

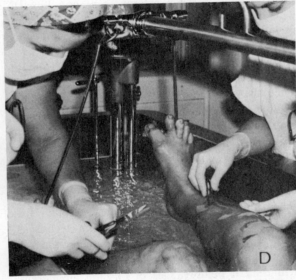

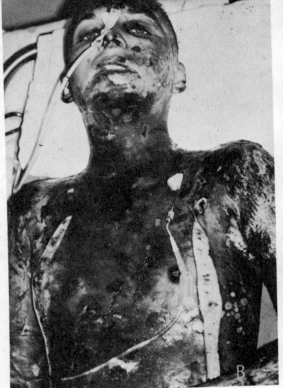

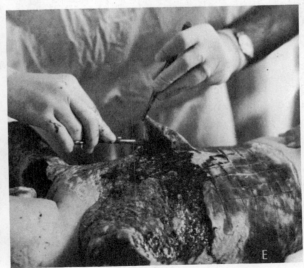

A regular schedule of deep breathing and coughing is carried out to minimize respiratory complications. Change of position is helpful but may be limited due to the burn wounds. If possible, the patient with potential respiratory complications is placed in semi- or high-Fowler's position and is turned side-to-side.

The patient with carbon monoxide intoxication appears confused. His color is often pink even though he is hypoxic. The cherry red of carbon monoxide poisoning can hide the purple-blue of cyanosis; and unless oxygen therapy is given the patient may suffer brain damage.

Patients with a history of having been burned in an enclosed space or who have severe burns of the face and neck can be predicted to have pulmonary complications. Maintenance of the airway by endotracheal tube or tracheostomy, aminophylline to dilate bronchi, and immediate steroids to decrease the inflammatory process may be ordered (Feller and Archambeault, 1973).

A way of breathing which is different from the normal route increases the burned patient's sense of helplessness. He requires adequate explanation, a planned communication system, and the reassurance derived from a nurse's competence and supportive presence.

The care of a tracheostomy in a burned patient is somewhat different from that of a patient whose respiratory passages have not been burned. As the tracheostomy wound easily becomes infected, suctioning should be done using aseptic technique, with sterile glove and fresh sterile catheter for each suctioning. Suctioning must be very gentle to avoid starting small hemorrhages or causing an increase in edema that would lead to further obstruction. Unlike the suctioning of patients whose respiratory passages have not been burned, the suction should be turned off whenever the catheter is moved. After suctioning, the nurse helps the patient in deep breathing, which is important to reinflate any alveoli that have been caused to collapse, leading to atelectasis.

Pulmonary edema may be caused by burns of the respiratory tract or also may be an indication of an overload of fluid, or too much absorption of fluid from an ultrasonic nebulizer.

Sometimes eschar around the chest and neck constricts respirations, and the surgeon may perform an escharotomy (a relaxing incision through the thickened, dead eschar, see Fig. 65-4). (See Chapter 28 for care of the patient with a tracheostomy and Chapter 60 for care of the patient with ventilatory insufficiency and failure.)

**Wound Therapy.** Treatment of the burned areas varies according to the conditions and the physician's preferences. Whatever method is employed, the object of the skin care is to keep the wound as clean and as free from microorganisms as possible.

On admission, the burn wounds are gently cleansed of dirt and debris, usually with gauze and a surgical detergent followed by a saline rinse. Loose sloughing skin or blisters are removed with forceps and scissors. Intact blisters are left alone since they provide a natural, painless, sterile dressing. The unburned areas of the body must be bathed also. A hydrotherapy tub is very useful for initial cleansing (see Fig. 65-4); shaving the areas of the body that approximate the burn wound can be done while the patient is submerged in the tub.

There are, in general, four primary methods of treatment of the burn wound. These include: (1) immediate or early excision of all areas of third-degree burns, (2) the use of occlusive dressings, (3) the open or exposure method, and (4) the semi-open method which involves daily dressing changes.

In recent years, several highly effective topical antibacterial agents have been introduced, which have revolutionized concepts of treatment of the burn wound and have resulted in a definite decrease in the mortality rate of serious burns. The mainstays of burn wound therapy presently include frequent debridement, cleansing of the burn wound, and the use of one of the several currently available topical antibacterial agents, with or without dressings.

Primary or early excision of third-degree burns is presently utilized primarily in the treatment of third-degree burns of very limited extent (less than 10 per cent of the total body surface area) and in the treatment of electrical burns.

The exposure method of treatment, the semi-open technique, and the occlusive dressings technique (closed technique) currently are utilized in the majority of patients with major burns, in combination with the use of one of the topical antibacterial agents. Included among these effective topical germicidal agents are mafenide acetate (Sulfamylon), 0.5 per cent silver nitrate solution, gentamicin sulfate ointment (Garamycin ointment), and silver sulfadiazine (Silvadene).

**Initial Care.** Care of the burn wound is initiated after all immediate, life-saving treatment has been instituted.

After thorough cleansing of the burn wound, one of the topical germicidal agents is usually selected and applied.

Mafenide (Sulfamylon) is a cream-base sulfa drug that has proved highly effective in preventing burn wound infection. After cleansing of the burn wound as described above, the cream is applied to all burned surfaces in a fairly thick layer; the gloved hand or a spatula is used. Thereafter, the patient's wounds are cleansed daily, preferably by immersion in a Hubbard tank. After thorough cleansing and washing in the Hubbard tank, the cream is reapplied. If the patient is ambulatory, cleansing may be performed in a shower. If a Hubbard tank is not available, cleansing may also be performed in a bathtub.

Complications resulting from the use of mafenide include skin rash resulting from sensitization to the drug, mild pain (usually of short duration) at the site of application of the drug, and metabolic acidosis. Mafenide is a carbonic anhydrase inhibitor and results in a diminished ability of the body to produce bicarbonate and consequently a metabolic acidosis. (See Chapter 60 for care of the patient with metabolic acidosis.)

Silver nitrate solution, 0.5 per cent, has also proved to be a highly effective topical antibacterial agent. After initial cleansing of the burn wound, occlusive dressings of fine-mesh gauze without a filler are applied and the dressings are kept constantly saturated with the silver nitrate solution. Dressings are then changed at specified intervals, from every 12 hours to three to five days. Disadvantages of the use of the 0.5 per cent silver nitrate solution include staining, hyponatremia, and hypokalemia.

A third effective topical antibacterial agent is gentamicin ointment or cream. The gentamicin ointment is usually used in the impregnated-gauze form. The gauze impregnated with the ointment is applied to the burn wound after cleansing as described above, and an occlusive dressing is applied over the gauze.

Silver sulfadiazine is one of the newest topical antibacterial agents and is a combination of the silver ion and the sulfa drug, sulfadiazine. Early trials have revealed this to be an effective topical chemotherapeutic agent somewhat similar to mafe-

nide. The principal advantage appears to be a decreased incidence of the complications frequently associated with the use of mafenide.

**Dressing Changes.** Regardless of the topical agent used for the semi-open technique, burn wounds are generally cleansed at least once every 24 hours.

Burned patients experience pain from dressing changes. This pain can be intensified by anticipatory anxiety and by grief, anger, or other emotions caused by viewing the burned areas.

Analgesics, to be helpful, should be given 20 to 30 minutes prior to the procedure so that they will start to take effect. The anxiety component of the pain experience can be reduced (and thus the pain sensation) by the patient's increasing confidence in the technical competence of the dressing team and their encouragement of his expressions of his thoughts and feelings about his situation. Some of these expressions might not be pleasing to the team, but for the most part they are valid expressions of the outrage which is a usual response to such an experience.

**Debridement.** Debridement, the removal of eschar (the leathery covering or scab consisting of dead tissue and exudate), is an important part of wound care (see Fig. 65-4). It is necessary in order to prepare a clean surface of granulation tissue which will accept skin grafts to close the burn wound. A natural mechanical debridement occurs with the removal of fine-mesh gauze from the wound since a thin layer of liquefying eschar is removed at the same time. In enzymatic debridement, commercially prepared concentrated enzymes can be applied to a wound to dissolve the eschar.

Sharp debridement, using forceps and scissors, is performed daily at the time of the dressing change. The eschar, which is dead tissue and therefore has no nerve endings or bleeding vessels, is loosened and cut at least one-fourth of an inch away from the body. Should bleeding occur from accidental tearing of the granulation tissue, it is controlled by pressure, a local clotting agent, or ligation of the bleeding vessel if necessary.

Debridement is performed at the time of each dressing change or wound cleansing until wound healing has occurred or a suitable granulating bed has developed. Skin grafting to obtain permanent wound closure is begun as early as possible by the surgeon (see Chap. 57).

**Closed Technique.** Many layers of coarse gauze

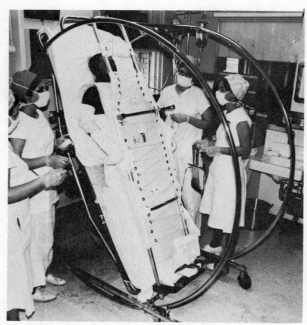

**Figure 65-5.** The CircOlectric bed provides access to a patient's extensive burn wounds, facilitates position change, and prevents sustained pressure on burned areas. (Reprinted with permission from the text "Nursing the Burned Patient," Feller, Archambeault, 1974, National Institute for Burn Medicine, 200 North Ingalls Street, Ann Arbor, Michigan.)

dressings are used to cover the burn, and these may be left intact for two to ten days.

Because bandaging immobilizes the part, good alignment and proper splinting are necessary to help to prevent deformities. The hands should be bandaged in the position of function with the injured hand grasping a roll of gauze; the wrist should be straight. The leg should not be in outward rotation; nor should the foot be pronated. No two skin surfaces should be touching. Medicated gauze is placed between the fingers, the folds of the genitalia, the arm and the trunk, and the ear and the scalp. Uniform pressure is important; tight uneven constriction, especially around the limb, may interfere with circulation.

The physician may leave an unburned finger or toe out of the bandage so that the color can be checked as a test for the adequacy of circulation. This exposed part should be observed for color and touch to test its warmth at least every four hours. Drainage is to be expected. When the bandage becomes wet from exudate the physician should change it. A wet bandage forms an easy avenue of access for microorganisms to invade the burned tissue. Sterile waterproof material should be used to protect dressings around the perineum from contamination when the patient urinates or defecates, and the perineal area is cleansed promptly afterwards.

**Open Technique.** Exposure treatment is used for less extensive burns and for areas which are hard to dress, such as the perineum. Because the burn wounds are constantly open to contamination, the patient may be on isolation precautions. Because there are no dressings to absorb exudates, bed linen or sterile towels must be frequently changed.

In some hospitals the burned patient is put to bed inside a germ-free plastic tent (Kress, et al., 1968). Everything that enters the enclosed environment is first sterilized when possible. If only a limb is burned, that part may be encased in a plastic tent to prevent contamination.

Patients treated by the exposure method find every draft painful, and therefore a draft should be avoided. The patient is especially likely to feel cold because, due to the injury of these tissues, the superficial vascular bed cannot contract to retain body heat and because no covering is placed on him. The regulation of room temperature is therefore especially important. The room temperature should be adjusted to the patient's temperature. If the patient becomes cold, his discomfort is increased; if too warm, further vasodilation occurs with additional loss of fluids by perspiration. If an electric thermometer is available, rectal temperature readings can be taken frequently without disturbing the patient. In the absence of an electric thermometer, his temperature has to be taken very carefully at frequent intervals. When direct care is not being given to the patient, a sterile blanket stretched across the top of the side rails and securely pinned there may help to keep him warm, or the blanket can be pinned over a cradle which contains an electric light for warmth (Artz and Moncrief, 1969). Another method for providing warmth to the burned patient is by the use of ordinary portable home hair dryers. The warm air produced by the dryer can be directed on the patient.

Although immobilization of the skin is important, the patient must breathe deeply at frequent intervals as a precaution against hypostatic pneumonia. Also his position must be changed at intervals. If he is burned front and back, the air must be able to reach both sides. The patient may be

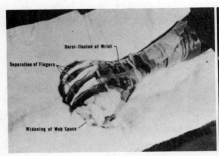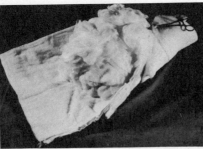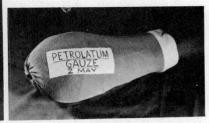

**Figure 65-6.** Placing a dressing on a burned hand. (*Left*) A single layer of gauze, lightly filmed with petrolatum or petroleum, is applied. The skin surfaces are separated, and the hand is placed in a position of function. (*Center*) It is covered with fluffed gauze. (*Right*) A stockinette, adhesive tape anchor and dated label complete the dressing. (Artz, C. P., and Moncrief, E.: *The Treatment of Burns,* ed. 2, Philadelphia, Saunders)

placed in a Stryker frame or CircOlectric bed to facilitate turning (Fig. 65-5). If he is not on a special bed, he may prefer to move unaided, because touching him causes pain. Flotation therapy, or the use of a nylon fish net stretched and secured tightly to a Bradford frame are other methods which allow air circulation and prevent pressure maceration of circumferential burns of the trunk or thigh (Noonan, et al., 1968; Crews, 1967). In any circumstance, care must be taken not to jar the bed, to hurry the patient, or to be rough in any way. The less he is touched, the better. When he is turned, hands should be placed only on the unburned skin even though sterile rubber gloves are worn. Portions of the patient that are not burned should be exercised regularly to maintain muscle tone. Sheets should be changed when they are wet, but any skin that is stuck to the sheet by dried exudate should not be pulled away. The area is wet with a continuous flow of warm sterile saline using a bulb syringe, and the skin and the sheet are separated very slowly and gently.

Burns of the face inhibit normal moistening of the lips, and the patient's dehydration contributes to crust formation of the mouth. Oral hygiene is given as frequently as is necessary to keep the patient's mouth clean, moist, and comfortable. Hydrogen peroxide and water, half and half, is good for removing crust inside the mouth and may be followed by glycerine flavored with lemon juice applied on an applicator stick.

## Other Considerations in the Emergent Period

A Levin tube may be passed to help to prevent the gastric distention, nausea, and vomiting so commonly associated with a severe burn.

To prevent Curling's ulcer, a frequent complication of severe burn, antacid therapy (one ounce antacid every two hours) via nasogastric tube initially may be started on admission and continued until autografting is completed (Feller and Archambeault, 1973).

Patients whose eyes are closed with edema may fear that they are blind. The physician may forcibly open an eye to demonstrate to the patient that he will be able to see as soon as the edema subsides. When the face is burned, the physician may order irrigations of the eyes with sterile saline, or he may order moist sterile saline pads. Blindness, even though temporary, is severely frightening to the patient.

Whenever possible, the patient should be given relief from the turmoil of all the activity during the first busy hours of emergency treatment. Once all the equipment is set up, treatment should be consolidated, so that the patient has some periods of rest. For example, his temperature can be taken during the same interval in which he is assisted to cough, offered fluids, and turned.

The burned patient has had no time to prepare himself for entry into the hospital or for the emotional shock of the experience. With a severe burn he knows that at best there will be pain, at least temporary disfigurement, and a long hospitalization; at worst, there may be crippling disfigurement or death. The patient needs relief from fear. During the emergency period time must be spent to give him encouragement. He cannot be promised that he will not die or be disfigured, but he can be assured that he is getting the best care that is available, that everything will be done for his comfort, that today's therapy helps many burned patients to recover completely, and that the burn team is personally taking an interest in his welfare and the nursing staff will be immediately available.

In the care of a patient with severe burns, many people make demands on the nurse, and she must know what needs to be done first, and what duties can be delegated to others. The situation calls for a nurse who moves quickly without adding confusion, who can function as a member of a team, and who can translate compassion for the patient into effective action and soothing words. This level of expertise can be arrived at after a good deal of study, supervised clinical experience, and familiarity with the equipment and specialized procedures. The nurse, too, sometimes needs support to cope with all the demands upon her in the emergency care of the burned patient.

## ACUTE PERIOD

The acute period starts with the end of the emergent period. It is termed "acute" because of the many complications that can occur. If the burn is a partial-thickness injury, this period lasts 10 to 20 days until healing takes place spontaneously. If the burns were full thickness, the acute period lasts until the wounds are covered with autografts; severe complications are possible until full-thickness burn wounds are reduced to less than 2 per cent of the body surface (Feller and Archambeault, 1973).

**Pathology.** For about two days after the burn, edema accumulates and fluid seeps out through the wounds. Sometime between the second and the fourth day (or sometimes much longer) the fluid that has gone to the burned tissues and has not left the body moves to the bloodstream. This is the period of diuresis, in which urinary output suddenly changes from a trickle to a flood. (One patient put out 11,000 ml. on the third day.) For this reason the physician restricts intake, especially intravenously. The patient looks thinner, and actually he is losing weight. Daily weights are taken when possible to keep careful track of the loss. A bed scale may be used, or the patient may be able to stand up momentarily to be weighed. The great outpouring of fluid into the bloodstream swells the volume of circulating fluid, and it may tax the heart with resultant pulmonary edema. The patient is observed carefully for any respiratory distress and especially for the sound of moist rales.

This is the period when the patient's body is changing from its emergency response to the burn injury to repairing the damage. There is spontaneous nitrogen balance (which will aid in rebuilding proteins), and local re-epithelization has started. The patient is beginning to recover.

### Nursing Assessment and Intervention

**Fluids and Nutrition.** Intravenous therapy may be discontinued at the period of diuresis, assuming that there are no gastrointestinal disturbances. It is not uncommon for patients with severe burns to suffer not only from vomiting and gastric distention but also from paralytic ileus. Oral fluids are tolerated better by some patients if the fluids are given by a slow nasogastric drip rather than by mouth. Unless specifically ordered otherwise, any type of oral feeding is started very slowly—not more than 500 ml. the first day. If the patient tolerates this well, the intake is slowly increased up to 2,500 ml. or the amount that is ordered. The patient is observed for distention, vomiting, and diarrhea. Early oral fluids may be an electrolyte solution or a salty broth; later they may be changed gradually to a protein drink. Patients rarely can tolerate solid foods until the beginning of the second week. Accurate records of intake are continued. Once diuresis is well established the hourly recording of urinary output probably will be replaced by measurement and recording q. 8 h. Daily specimens for specific gravity, sugar, and protein still may be required. As long as the patient has an indwelling catheter in place, irrigation every four or six hours may be ordered.

**Medications.** Burned patients develop severe deficiencies of vitamin C. This vitamin and others may be given intravenously or by mouth. If the patient still is in pain and has no respiratory problems, morphine may be ordered. Meperidine (Demerol) may be used. Prophylactic antibiotics usually are continued. Because the patient may not have many accessible sites for injection, the needle must be injected carefully; tearing the skin must be avoided. More than 3 ml. should not be given in any one place.

**Preventing Complications.** The patient still needs turning at one- to two-hour intervals, deep breathing and coughing (which may be a painful problem in burns of the thorax), exercise of the unburned portions of his body, and rest of the burned areas in a position to prevent contractures.

If the hands are bandaged, they may be suspended on IV poles, or the limbs may be splinted (in the position of function) for immobilization. If they are, they have their position shifted by the nurse. Because the patient is in bed for a long period, good body alignment is important, whether the patient is bandaged or exposed (Fig. 65-7). Contractures due to poor positioning are easily acquired because the patient finds comfort in the nonfunctional position. The patient needs the nurse to help him keep long-term goals in mind and prevent additional complications. Sandbags can be used against unburned portions of the legs to keep them from outward rotation. A footboard should be kept in place unless the soles of the feet are burned. The hand should not be permitted to droop over the edge of a pillow; it should be positioned in slight dorsiflexion.

Elevation and immobilization are still two important aspects of positioning the patient during this and the earlier phase of treatment. However, to prevent bedsores and pneumonia, immobilization has to be tempered by very gentle repositioning of the patient. If the burn wound is exposed, the nurse should be aware as she turns the patient that a crack in the skin is an invitation for bacterial invasion. Change of position is important, regardless of the type of skin treatment: exposed, bandaged, splinted. The physical therapist is a vital part of the team. He should be consulted for problems in positioning.

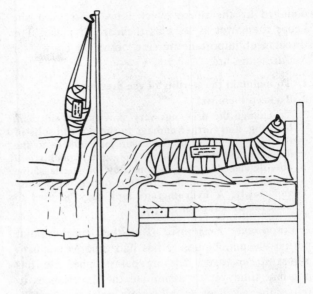

**Figure 65-7.** Elevation of a bandaged burned hand by suspension on an IV pole. The leg is elevated on pillows. Elevation helps to reduce edema. Both the arm and the leg are kept in good body alignment.

**Skin Care.** The patient must be prevented from picking at the eschar. If the patient is irrational or otherwise cannot resist the temptation, his hands may have to be wrapped during the periods when he is alone. A single layer of fine-mesh gauze may cover the wound to avoid picking.

If wet dressings are ordered, they usually are

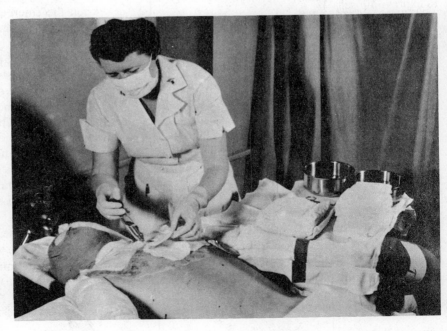

**Figure 65-8.** The nurse is wetting the dressing over a grafted burn to loosen the gauze so that she can remove it without pulling off the graft. She is using an Asepto syringe, and the sterile solution is warmed to body temperature. This patient is on a Stryker frame. For this sterile procedure she wears gloves and a mask. (Artz, C. P., and Moncrief, E.: *The Treatment of Burns*, ed. 2, Philadelphia, Saunders)

changed by the nurse every four hours, and she keeps them wet as long as they are in place. The three most important nursing points in caring for wet dressings are:

1. **To maintain the sterility of the dressings**
2. **To keep them wet**
3. **To change the dressings very slowly to avoid pain, bleeding, and further damage to the skin. In spite of the moisture some of the tissue may adhere to the dressing, and pulling the dressing away quickly will also detach skin. A generous flow of sterile saline should be used and the dressings pulled very gently and slowly. A hydrotherapy tank may be used to soak the dressings off.**

**Emotional Response.** By the turning-point period the patient barely has had time to begin to adjust to an overwhelming catastrophe. He has not had time yet to assimilate the experience, to relive the accident in his mind, and to come to grips with his feelings about it. Although he probably is no longer in constant pain, he still is uncomfortable. He is separated from loved ones, he may still feel the emotional pain of the accident, and perhaps he has not yet thought through all the implications of a long and costly hospitalization. He is probably still too ill to talk much about how he feels.

The nurse helps the patient to become aware of his progress, and implies that he is on the way to recovery. When the patient starts to talk about what happened, then the nurse can encourage him to express himself.

Family members may be shocked at the rapid changes in the patient's appearance. The burn itself may be seen as ugly and disfiguring, and the change from marked edema to leanness in a few days is startling. It is necessary to know what the physician has said to the family about such subjects as scarring.

Before members of the family enter the patient's room, it is helpful to tell them that although his face will seem swollen, this swelling will not last. Also they can be cautioned that if they reflect shock at his appearance, which is temporary, the patient's fears concerning disfigurement will be confirmed in spite of what they may say to the contrary. The family also needs the chance to express their fears to the nurse, who should be available to them before they enter the room and again when they leave. If they are willing they can be taught to assist the patient with his feeding, deep breathing, or dressings if these will be continued at home.

Any questions that can be answered need answering. The patient may be worrying about something needlessly—for example, scarring or blindness, or returning to his usual life style. The patient needs the opportunity to express his concerns. Some questions can be answered immediately, some may be referred to the appropriate therapist, and the unknowns can be shared with a good listener.

Diversion may help the patient to keep from prolonged brooding. What can the patient do that he likes to do during the long period of healing? Television, reading, radio? He should be asked about his special interests. The occupational therapist may be able to arrange a program. A patient who is flat on his back may be able to watch television or the hall through a prism lens or by a strategically placed mirror. Initially, with mirrors, the patient may become frightened by his appearance. The patient's bed can be placed where he cannot easily see himself in the mirror until the edema phase is over, and until he has had a chance to see his chest or his arms start to heal. The patient's concept of his appearance can be a vital factor in restoring relations with his family and his friends. "How do I look?" and "Will people be repelled by my appearance?" may worry the patient.

## RECOVERY

When the emergency is over, the body must repair itself. The energy that was required to meet the emergency was greatly in excess of normal. Because large areas of fat deposits have been used and the caloric intake over the first five days or so has been low, patients often are emaciated. As much as 20 pounds may be lost, even if the loss of edema is not considered. The debilitation is dangerous, because it reduces the patient's resistance to infection, it delays the healing of the skin, and it impedes the growth of new granulation tissue and the progress of new skin grafts. Accordingly, the nurse does everything possible to improve the patient's nutrition.

The drying of the skin wounds becomes evident early in this phase, starting about the fifth or the sixth day and continuing until the dead skin sloughs away, about two to three weeks after the burn occurred.

**Nutrition.** Nutrition may make the difference between an uncomplicated recovery and progressive emaciation. The patient's physiologic need for food usually is greater than his appetite. He still is sick, and he feels weak and not equal to eating the high caloric, high protein diet that he needs.

Gradually, his diet is increased to 3,000 to 6,000 calories and 2 to 3 Gm. of protein per kilogram of body weight per day. Vitamins are given; vitamin C may be ordered up to 1,000 mg. a day. This large intake is essential, but it is a problem for the patient and the nurse alike. Protein-enriched drinks help to fulfill the protein requirement without excess bulk, and they should be served in any way that the patient can ingest them (warm, iced, at bedtime, etc.). The patient on such a large intake needs to be observed carefully for distention, diarrhea, and vomiting. If these signs of gastric distress occur, the intake may have to be reduced, slowing the patient's nutritional recovery. Oral hygiene is essential to promote appetite.

When a patient has burns of over 50 per cent of total body area, intravenous hyperalimentation therapy may be instituted around the third week as an additional source of amino acids, calories, vitamins, and minerals until grafting is completed or the patient's oral intake is adequate for his needs. (See Chapter 40 for a discussion of hyperalimentation therapy.)

Solid foods are begun cautiously about the second week (or sooner, if possible), and they are increased rapidly if the patient tolerates them. The patient needs foods that he likes. Conferences between patient, family, dietitian, and nurse will help the patient to feel that he is contributing to his recovery by participating in his treatment. Also, it will serve to emphasize to the patient the importance of nutrition and the necessity of eating what is offered. The nurse can point out to the patient that every mouthful he swallows is another building brick for a patch of skin. His usual eating habits should be adhered to as much as possible.

Except in extensive third-degree burns, long-term debilitation usually results from neglect and indifferent nursing care. Inspired and ingenious nursing care is the challenge. During this period patients usually are weighed twice a week. The patient can be encouraged to keep a record of his progress as well as of his intake and output.

**Skin Care.** EXPOSURE. By about the third week, or longer with local antibacterial treatment, the crusts of second-degree burns spontaneously separate, leaving pink, thin, new skin. Now immobilization of the burned parts is replaced by exercise and physiotherapy to recondition muscles and to encourage circulation and healing. In third-degree burns the crust cracks, and it is at this time that grafting may be done.

BANDAGES. Dressings may be changed about once a week. Frequently, these changes are so painful that anesthesia is needed. Dressings on third-degree burns may be changed daily until the skin is grafted.

GRAFTING. (See Chapter 57 for a discussion of plastic surgery.) In third-degree burns an early grafting procedure may be done to cover large denuded areas. After the recovery period, grafts may be used to improve appearance or function when scar tissues limit motion.

Grafts may be permanent or temporary. When they are used initially to cover the burned areas, they are not expected to stay on the patient, but they are used to protect the denuded areas. Frequently skin must be donated to the patient from another person or animal because the patient with extensive burns does not have sufficient unburned skin left to cover the burned areas.

Grafts obtained from another human being either living or cadaver are called homografts (allografts). Grafts obtained from a different species are termed heterografts (xenografts). The most commonly used animal for obtaining heterografts is the pig. Pigskin heterografts (porcine skin dressings) are currently available from several commercial sources and are thus much more convenient to obtain and use than are homografts. Homografts or heterografts are applied to deep second-degree burns and freshly debrided third-degree burns. Homografts and heterografts act as temporary physiologic dressings. They are used to alleviate pain, lessen fluid loss, and hasten the reduction of infection in the burned area. They are replaced after no longer than five days by other homografts or heterografts until the site is ready for autografting. Split-thickness grafts may be done as early as two days after the burn. Corrective grafting may take the form of split-thickness, full-thickness or pinch grafts. The skin for such grafts is taken from the patient's own body (autografts). They are permanent and usually they should take about two weeks to heal. In contrast, homografts and heterografts, being foreign tissue to the patient, will eventually be rejected by the patient. The patient should expect pain for a day or two. Full-thickness skin loss requires complete skin replacement. Grafting may be done every 10 to 12 days until coverage is complete. Recently devised instruments and techniques are now available to slit and expand autografts so that an area two or more times the area of the donor site can be covered. Hospitalization is long and the procedures are multiple. The maintenance of the patient's nutrition and his morale is important. Diversional therapy is a help.

**Complications.** This is a phase all too frequently plagued by complications. The trouble may have had its origin in an earlier period, finally to manifest itself in the recovery period. For example, burned areas may be contaminated during the excitement of the shock period, and the symptoms of infection may become evident a few days later, after the organisms have had time to multiply and to thrive. The prevention of complications in the severely burned patient is one of the greatest challenges that nursing has to offer. Although patients usually receive ample attention while they are in shock, it is harder to continue to give them the concentrated care that they need over a period of months.

INFECTION. Dead tissue, warmed by body temperature and bathed in the fluid exudate from the wound, provides a favorable environment for the growth of microorganisms. There are two sources of infection of the burned skin: bacteria beneath the burned tissue and contamination of the wounds from the outside. The body's great barrier to bacteria—the skin—has been broken, and the patient's resistance has been lowered by poor nutrition and exhaustion.

Wound infection and septicemia are responsible for a large number of the deaths of burned patients who survive the shock period. The predominant infecting organisms are *Pseudomonas aeruginosa* (*Bacillus pyocyaneus*) and hemolytic *Staphylococcus aureus*. Besides the overall lowered resistance of the burned patient, edema and thrombosis in the traumatized subcutaneous tissue obstruct bacterial-fighting mechanisms. Second-degree burns rarely become infected, but there always is some infection in third-degree burns. Tetanus and, equally

dangerous, gas-gangrene infection may occur, although they are rare.

An increase in temperature may be the first indication of infection, and it should be brought to the physician's attention. Temperature characteristically mounts rapidly, rarely below 102 degrees F. The pulse is rapid and yet regular. The odor or the appearance of the burn (if it is exposed) may change. The odor of the burned area should be noted at least once a day. The odor of infection is different from that of burn exudate. On the other hand, a dry-appearing crust may harbor copious amounts of pus beneath its surface. By close and frequent contact with the patient, the nurse is in an excellent position to be the first observer of infection, and she should remain alert to its possible existence.

Treatment may include continuous saline soaks and such antibiotics as colistimethate (Coly-Mycin) for *Pseudomonas* and sodium methicillin (Staphcillin) for *Staphylococcus*. The physician may order dressing changes every four hours with removal of the dead tissue loosened by the soaks. When large areas of the body are kept wet in an otherwise exposed patient, it is difficult to prevent chilling and the introduction of additional contamination. The saline should be warmed to normal body temperature before it is applied to the dressings.

Septicemia may result in oliguria, hypotension, tachypnea, paralytic ileus, disorientation (related to the degree of the fever), and cardiac failure. The patient may need oxygen, nasogastric suction, and blood; and intravenous fluid therapy may have to be resumed or increased.

Aspirin and sponging of the unburned areas may be ordered for the fever. It is not easy to sponge a burned patient. Only those portions of his body that are covered by unbroken skin should be sponged. If there is a high fever, the patient may be placed on a hypothermic blanket.

KIDNEY FAILURE. Some studies report that this complication of burns is second only to infection as a cause of death of those patients who survive the shock phase (Crews, 1967). Among other pathologic changes, the decreased circulating blood volume leads to lowered renal blood flow and glomerular filtration rate. The increased viscosity of the blood may fill the kidney capillaries and cause stasis there, which also leads to decreased glomerular filtration. Oliguria or anuria are usual symptoms, but occasionally there is diuresis. If this complication is going to occur, it usually does so by the tenth to the twelfth day postburn. (See Chapter 64 for care of the patient in renal failure.)

CYSTITIS. Any patient with an indwelling catheter may develop a bladder infection.

CURLING'S ULCER. For unknown reasons, burned patients sometimes develop a gastrointestinal ulcer. It may be gastric, duodenal, single, or multiple. Ulcers are more common in patients with extensive burns, but may be seen in any burned patient. The symptom most suggestive of an ulcer that has not perforated a blood vessel is onset of, or increase in, anorexia, associated with abdominal distention due to gastric dilation. As the patient recovers physiologic balance from the widespread disturbances caused by the burn, his appetite should slowly improve. If there is reversal of this trend, it should be reported to the physician. Gross or occult blood in the stool might be noted, or it may be apparent in the nasogastric tube drainage or vomitus. Some patients have no symptoms until there is sudden gastrointestinal hemorrhage. Emergency surgery is necessary to stop the bleeding. The peak incidence of onset of a Curling's ulcer is at the end of the first week postburn (Moncrief, et al., 1964). As noted above, prophylactic antacids are sometimes ordered from the time of admission.

GASTROINTESTINAL DISTURBANCES. Dilatation of the stomach may occur, characterized by regurgitation of fluid, discomfort, anorexia, and nausea. The patient may be dyspneic, because the bloated stomach is pressing on the diaphragm, interfering with respiration. Also, fecal impaction may follow paralytic ileus.

ANEMIA. A number of factors contribute to the burned patient's anemia. Heat causes red blood cell destruction or makes them abnormally fragile which shortens their life. Red blood cells are trapped in dilated capillaries. Infection depresses the function of hematopoietic tissue. Blood is lost from granulating wounds at dressing changes. The treatment is blood transfusions and a high-protein and iron-rich diet, with iron supplements.

CONTRACTURES. Due to the pull of tightening scar tissue, patients with third-degree burns may develop contractures that are both disfiguring and crippling. For example, a healed third-degree burn of the right side of the neck can twist and hold the head in a permanently fixed position. To mini-

mize contractures, parts with third-degree burns sometimes can be held in extension during the period of immobilization with splints, sandbags, or casts. As soon as healing has advanced sufficiently so that movement will not crack the eschar, a program of physical therapy is started—perhaps whirlpool baths, and underwater and then dry exercises, both passive and active. If contractures develop nonetheless, plastic surgery is indicated.

THROMBOPHLEBITIS. This may occur in the vein in which the indwelling catheter is inserted. Pain and streaks of redness on that limb are signs.

DECUBITUS ULCERS. Conditions are ripe for this complication. The patient has lost much body protein. He is immobilized for a time; therefore some areas of his body are compressed between the hard bed and an even harder bone. Frequent turning and good skin care to unburned areas help to prevent decubitus ulcers.

RESPIRATORY PROBLEMS. Pneumonia also can follow immobilization and debilitation. A patient with burns of the chest finds it painful to cough up secretions, but he must be encouraged to do so. Atelectasis may be caused by the aspiration of gastric contents following tube feedings or vomiting, as well as by mucus plugs retained in the respiratory passages.

ADRENOCORTICAL INSUFFICIENCY, STRESS-DIABETES, HEPATIC CRISIS. These are other conditions that can occur when severe burns overtax the patient's adaptability.

## REHABILITATION

This phase of treatment begins when the burned area is less than 20 per cent of the total body surface. The patient is encouraged to participate progressively in self-care activities. The burn care team is cognizant of rehabilitation goals from the time of the patient's admission. However, preparing him for discharge for a productive place in society and for functional and cosmetic reconstruction are specific goals of this period. Their accomplishment, however, may take five years or longer.

During this time the patient and family may need the assistance of the community health nurse, psychiatric nursing specialist, plastic surgeon, social worker, occupational and physical therapist, and State Division of Vocational Rehabilitation, among others.

A person burned over 50 per cent of his body requires initial specialized hospital care for about four months. Greater emphasis on the prevention of fires and other types of causes of thermal injuries is a responsibility of all team members to reduce the toll of human tragedies from burns.

## REFERENCES AND BIBLIOGRAPHY

ARTZ, C.: The burned patient: Newer concepts of medical and nursing management, Chap. 14 in Kintzel, K. (ed.): *Advanced Concepts in Clinical Nursing,* Philadelphia, Lippincott, 1971.

———, and MONCRIEF, J.: *The Treatment of Burns,* ed. 2, Philadelphia, Saunders, 1969.

BARTLETT, R., and ALLYN, P.: Pulmonary management of the burned patient, *Heart Lung* 2:714, September-October 1973.

BAXTER, C., et al.: Fluid and electrolyte therapy of burn shock, *Heart Lung* 2:707, September-October 1973.

BENNETT, J. P.: Skin grafting and the treatment of burns, *Nurs. Times* 66:1584, December 10, 1970.

BOWDEN, M.: Helping the burn patient return home, *AORN* 13:69, January 1971.

———, and FULLER, I.: Family reaction to a severe burn, *Am. J. Nurs.* 73:317, February 1973.

Burn care. *Nurs. '72* 2:32, July 1972.

The burned patient. A symposium in critical care. *Heart Lung* 2:686, September-October 1973.

CHUTZ, SR. A., D. C.: *The Development of a Nursing Categorization of Burn Patients and a Burn Patient Nursing Care Index,* The League Exchange No. 88, New York National League for Nursing, 1969.

CREWS, E.: *A Practical Manual for the Treatment of Burns,* ed. 2, Springfield, Ill., Thomas, 1967.

DAVIDSON, S. P.: Nursing management of emotional reactions of severely burned patients during the acute phase, *Heart Lung* 2:370, May-June 1973.

———, and NOYES, R.: Psychiatric consultation on a burn unit, *Am. J. Nurs.* 73:1715, October 1973.

FELLER, I., and ARCHAMBEAULT, C.: *Nursing the Burned Patient,* Michigan, Institute for Burn Medicine, 1973.

———, et al.: The team approach to total rehabilitation of the severely burned patient, *Heart Lung* 2:701, September-October 1973.

HARTFORD, C. E.: The early treatment of burns, *Nurs. Clin. N. Am.* 8:447, September 1973.

HUNT, J., et al.: Burn-wound management, *Heart Lung* 2:690, September-October 1973.

JACOBY, F.: *Nursing Care of the Patient with Burns,* St. Louis, Mosby, 1972.

KRESS, B. R., et al.: Isolated in a life-island, *Canad. Nurse* 64:48, May 1968.

MINCKLEY, M.: Expert nursing care for burned patients, *Am. J. Nurs.* 70:1888, September 1970.

MONCRIEF, J. A., et al.: Curling's ulcer, *J. Trauma* 4:481, 1964.

NOONAN, J., et al.: Two burned patients in flotation therapy, *Am. J. Nurs.* 68:316, February 1968.

POTTER, B.: Even the air is isolated in this burn unit, *Mod. Hosp.* 110:95, March 1968.

RODMAN, M.: What's new in drugs. Burn treatment (silver sulfadiazine), *RN* 37:80, June 1974.

SCHLICHTMANN, K.: Adaptive mechanisms in a selected group of burned patients, *ANA Clinical Sessions 1968,* New York, Appleton-Century-Crofts, 1969.

SCHNEIDER, J., et al.: Burn patient care. The psychiatrist's role, *AORN* 14:58, August 1971.

SHAW, B.: Current therapy for burns, *RN* 34:33, March 1971.

SHUCK, J.: The use of homografts in burn therapy, *Surg. Clin. N. Am.* 50:1325, June 1970.

SILVERSTEIN, P.: The development of porcine cutaneous xenograft as a biologic dressing, *Hosp. Care* 4:4, March 1973.

STINSON, V.: Porcine skin dressings for burns (pictorial), *Am. J. Nurs.* 74:111, January 1974.

WILLIAMS, B. P.: The burned patient's need for teaching, *Nurs. Clin. N. Am.* 6:615, December 1971.

WILLIS, B., et al.: Positioning and splinting the burned patient, *Heart Lung* 2:696, September-October 1973.

WOOD-SMITH, D., and POROWSKI, P. (eds.): *Nursing Care of the Plastic Surgery Patient,* St. Louis, Mosby, 1967.

# Index